# PERIANESTHESIA NURSING

## NURSING

### A Critical Care Approach

# PERIANESTHESIA NURSING

## A Critical Care Approach

### Cecil B. Drain
PhD, RN, CRNA, FAAN, FASAHP

Professor & Dean, School of Allied Health Professions
Virginia Commonwealth University
Medical College of Virginia Campus
Richmond, Virginia

### Jan Odom-Forren
RN, BSN, MS, CPAN, FAAN

Perianesthesia/Perioperative Consultant
Co-editor, Journal of PeriAnesthesia Nursing
Louisville, Kentucky

FIFTH EDITION

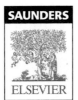

# SAUNDERS
ELSEVIER

11830 Westline Industrial Drive
St. Louis, Missouri 63146

PERIANESTHESIA NURSING: A CRITICAL CARE APPROACH

ISBN: 978-1-4160-3474-2

---

### Notice

Perianesthesia nursing is an ever-changing field. Standard safety precautions must be followed, but as new research and clinical experience broaden our knowledge, changes in treatment and drug therapy may become necessary or appropriate. Readers are advised to check the most current product information provided by the manufacturer of each drug to be administered to verify the recommended dose, the method and duration of administration, and contraindications. It is the responsibility of the licensed prescriber, relying on experience and knowledge of the patient, to determine dosages and the best treatment for each individual patient. Neither the publisher nor the author assumes any liability for any injury and/or damage to persons or property arising from this publication.

The Publisher

---

Library of Congress Control Number: 2007938354
Previous editions copyrighted 2003, 1994, 1987, 1979
ISBN-13: 978-1-4160-3474-2

*Editor:* Tamara Myers
*Developmental Editor:* Charlene R.M. Ketchum
*Editorial Assistant:* Kelly Brinkman
*Publishing Services Manager:* Jeff Patterson
*Project Manager:* Jeanne Genz
*Designer:* Elaine Rickles

## Working together to grow libraries in developing countries

www.elsevier.com | www.bookaid.org | www.sabre.org

**ELSEVIER**  **BOOK AID** International  **Sabre Foundation**

Printed in Canada

Last digit is the print number:  9  8  7  6  5  4  3  2  1

As I complete this edition of the "Blue Book," I realize that it has been my distinct honor and pleasure to be the author of this book since 1979. The "Blue Book" did so much. It was the first book totally dedicated to the art and science of Recovery Room Nursing and had a major impact on the development of the national organization, the American Society of PeriAnesthesia Nurses (ASPAN), in 1980. It served *as the* professional text to facilitate the development of Postanesthesia Care Unit (PACU) Nursing as a specialty of nursing.

Most rewarding to me are the many lives touched through this book. So many of you have shared with me how much you liked the book and, even more importantly, how the book helped to serve as the text of choice in preparing to take the ASPAN certification examination to be a Certified PeriAnesthesia Nurse (CPAN).

It is interesting how technology has made such a difference in the preparation of the manuscript for this book. For the first edition, all of the chapters were written by hand on legal paper in a small hospital room while taking call or at home in the late hours of the night. The time it took to prepare a manuscript by hand was amazing; I missed many meals, social events, and sporting events. But with new technology, that time factor has lessened, allowing more time for research and making each new edition better than the previous.

The intent of this book from its inception was to present the appropriate components of perianesthesia nursing; to present the anatomy, physiology, pathophysiology, and pharmacology of the various processes; and to supply the appropriate nursing care concepts to ensure a favorable outcome for the patient in all the aspects of the surgical stay: preoperative, intraoperative, and postoperative.

This specialty has always been evolving, and the book has always tried to symbolize the many positive changes. Because I always felt that the care of the PACU patient was nursing practice in the critical care arena, the subtitle "A Critical Care Approach" was added to the second edition of the book. In doing so, the book reflected the strong movement of having a critical care of the patient component. This specialty evolution was symbolized during the writing of the fourth edition, when we moved to perianesthesia nursing as the specialty, as opposed to postanesthesia. Now, in the fifth edition, we continue to support the concept of *PeriAnesthesia Nursing: A Critical Care Approach.* This edition symbolizes the focus now on a critical care nursing approach throughout the entire preoperative, intraoperative, and postoperative hospitalization process.

It was a very difficult task to find the right coauthor for this book. I felt a strong responsibility to find someone who understood the philosophy of the book, who is considered to be an extremely respected leader in the ASPAN community, who is ethically strong, and who will carry on the traditions of the book. I found all of these qualities in Ms. Jan Odom-Forren, whom I have known for years. She is a great leader, a great writer, and a most trusted friend. I really was able to put her career into perspective when I wrote her letter of support for the American Academy of Nursing, of which she is now a Fellow.

It became quite obvious that the person of choice was staring me right in the face. Ms. Odom-Forren is the best person that I could ever select because she possesses all the qualities that I was seeking. I am confident that Ms. Odom-Forren will carry on the excellent traditions of the book and in fact make it even better in the future editions.

I cannot thank Mr. Bob Wright enough; he is a great man who provided me with needed education on all aspects of writing such a textbook. Mr. Wright, as I understand it, even stayed an extra few months on the job just to finish the first edition of the "Blue Book" before he retired. He was and always will be held in very high esteem by myself and the many authors he served over the years. After Bob Wright retired from Saunders, the nursing editor was Ms. Judith Paseczky, a very professional person who certainly helped me to make the second edition a wonderful experience. Next came Mr. Dan Ruth, a great friend, who really helped to heighten the excellence of the book. His copyeditor, Ms. Susan L. Bielitsky, was the best, and

I appreciate her continued support. As the book moved to Elsevier for the fourth edition, Mr. Michael Ledbetter was so very helpful in making the transition and providing the necessary upgrades to the book. The preparation of this edition has been special. My Elsevier team, Tamara Myers, Charlene Ketchum, and Kelly Brinkman, made the preparation of this edition a very positive experience as they have been so wonderful and supportive. They brought Ms. Odom-Forren and me together for a week in St. Louis where we all, working together, were able to orchestrate this great fifth edition. During that week, I had the opportunity to work with Ms. Odom-Forren and to provide her with the necessary history and philosophy of the book, which will ensure the book's continued success and excellence.

I must also thank Dr. Sue Christoph and the many contributing authors who certainly helped to make the "Blue Book" and the second edition a reality. I especially want to acknowledge Ms. Marie Dutton, who wrote the neurosurgical anatomy and physiology and the care of the neurosurgical patient chapters in the "Blue Book." Her chapters, to this day, are considered to be classic, and I appreciate her being part of the book.

It has been the greatest of honors to serve the perianesthesia nursing community by providing a textbook that has endured the test of time. It has been my honor and privilege to be *your* author for the last 30 years. In parting, it seems appropriate to dedicate this special edition to my wife of 43 years, Cindy; my children, Tim, Steve, and Katie; and my grandchildren; Dr. Jan Odom-Forren, may she have many happy days because of this book; and lastly, each of you, the perianesthesia nurses. I hope that this book will help you "to be all you can be" as a professional nurse, specializing in the most exciting specialty of them all: the art and science of PeriAnesthesia Nursing.

**Cecil B. Drain**

*To the staff in the PACU at Humana Hospital Audubon (now Norton Audubon Hospital), Louisville, KY, who first taught me what perianesthesia nursing was all about*

*To the PACU staff at Forrest General Hospital in Hattiesburg, MS, who took me further on my journey in this specialty and supported all my endeavors*

*To my new work colleagues in Phase II Recovery, Baptist Hospital East, Louisville, KY, whose clinical expertise is an inspiration*

*To my family who support me and make writing possible: Gary, Kelsey, and Brittny Forren; Andrew and Patrick Odom*

*To my mother, Ada Pittman, and my father, Johnny Pittman (1928-1994)*

*To my mentor, colleague, and friend, Cecil Drain, who offered me the opportunity of a lifetime to coauthor his esteemed and well-known perianesthesia book*

**Jan Odom-Forren**

**Kay Ball, RN, BSN, MSA, CNOR, FAAN**
Perioperative Consultant/Educator
K & D Medical, Inc
Lewis Center, Ohio
*Chapter 26: Transition from the Operating Room to the PACU*

**Chuck Biddle, PhD, CRNA**
Professor of Nurse Anesthesia
Virginia Commonwealth University
Richmond, Virginia
*Chapter 9: Research*

**Michael J. Boss, MD**
Resident in Anesthesiology
Virginia Commonwealth University
Department of Anesthesiology
Richmond, Virginia
*Chapter 31: Pain Management in the PACU*

**Joni M. Brady, RN, MSN, CAPA**
*Breathline* Editor
American Society of PeriAnesthesia Nurses
Stuttgart, Germany
*Chapter 39: Care of the Thyroid and Parathyroid Surgical Patient & Chapter 44: Care of the Plastic Surgical Patient*

**Nancy Burden, RN, MS, CPAN, CAPA**
Director of Ambulatory Surgery
BayCare Health System
New Port Richey, Florida
*Chapter 46: Care of the Ambulatory Surgical Patient*

**Joseph F. Burkard, DNSc, CRNA**
United States Navy
San Diego, California
*Chapter 51: Care of the Pregnant Patient*

**Matthew D. Byrne, RN, MS, CPAN**
Adjunct Instructor
College of St Benedict/St John's University
St Joseph, Minnesota
*Chapter 39: Care of the Thyroid and Parathyroid Surgical Patient & Chapter 44: Care of the Plastic Surgical Patient*

**Thomas Corey Davis, CRNA, MSNA**
Assistant Professor, Director of Clinical Education
Department of Nurse Anesthesia
Virginia Commonwealth University
Richmond, Virginia
*Chapter 24: Local Anesthetics & Chapter 25: Regional Anesthetics*

**Philip H. Ewing, MD**
Pediatric Emergency Medicine Fellow
Children's Medical Center of Dallas
University of Texas Southwestern Medical Center
Dallas, Texas
*Chapter 31: Pain Management in the PACU*

**Michael D. Fallacaro, DNS, CRNA**
Professor and Chairman, Department of Nurse Anesthesia
Virginia Commonwealth University
Richmond, Virginia
*Chapter 4: Patient Safety in the PACU*

**Ken Faulkner, MDiv, MA**
Assistant Professor, Program in Patient Counseling
Virginia Commonwealth University
Richmond, Virginia
*Chapter 8: Ethics of Health Care in the PACU*

**Mary Bryant Ford, MSNA, CRNA**
Staff Nurse Anesthetist
Virginia Commonwealth University Health System
Richmond, Virginia
*Chapter 45: Care of the Thermally Injured Patient*

**Marie Fiascone Gerardo, MS, RN-C, ANP, CCRN**
Neurology Nurse Practitioner
Neurological Associates, Inc
Richmond, Virginia
*Chapter 6: Managed Care and Its Impact on the PACU*

**William Hartland, Jr, PhD, CRNA**
Associate Professor, Director of Education
Department of Nurse Anesthesia
Virginia Commonwealth University
Richmond, Virginia
*Chapter 57: Cardiopulmonary Resuscitation in the
   PACU*

**Melody S. Heffline, MSN, RN, APRN,BC, ACNP**
Acute Care Nurse Practitioner
Southern Surgical Group
West Columbia, South Carolina
*Chapter 36: Care of the Vascular Surgical Patient*

**Vallire D. Hooper, MSN, RN, CPAN, FAAN**
PeriAnesthesia Consultant, Assistant Professor
School of Nursing, Medical College of Georgia
Augusta, Georgia
*Chapter 47: Care of the Laser/Laproscopic
   Surgical Patient & Chapter 53: Care of the
   Patient with Thermal Imbalance*

**Donna Landriscina, RN, MSNA, CRNA**
Assistant Professor and Assistant Director of
   Education
Department of Nurse Anesthesia
Virginia Commonwealth University
Richmond, Virginia
*Chapter 46: Care of the Pediatric Patient*

**Stephen P. Long, MD**
Medical Director, Commonwealth Pain Specialists
Clinical Associate Professor
Department of Anesthesiology
Virginia Commonwealth University
Richmond, Virginia
*Chapter 31: Pain Management in the PACU*

**Mary Beth Flynn Makic, PhD, RN, CNS, CCNS, CCRN**
Clinical Nurse Specialist and Educator
University of Colorado Hospital
Denver, Colorado
*Chapter 55: Care of the Intensive Care Unit
   Patient in the PACU*

**Myrna Eileen Mamaril, MS, RN, CPAN, CAPA**
Nurse Manager, Perianethesia Services
University of Colorado Hospital
Denver, Colorado
*Chapter 54: Care of the Shock Trauma Patient &
   Chapter 55: Care of the Intensive Care Unit
   Patient in the PACU*

**Colleen Medley, BSN, RN, CPAN**
Division Officer of PACU
Naval Medical Center San Diego
San Diego, California
*Chapter 56: Bioterrorism and Its Impact on the PACU*

**Carole Muto, RN, BSN, CPAN**
Staff Nurse
Stereotactic Radiosurgery Department
Thomas Jefferson University Hospital
Jefferson Hospital for Neuroscience
Philadelphia, Pennsylvania
*Chapter 33: Care of the Ophthalmic Surgical Patient*

**Denise O'Brien, MSN, APRN,BC, CPAN, CAPA, FAAN**
Clinical Nurse Specialist, Department of
   Operating Rooms/PACU
University of Michigan Health Systems
Ann Arbor, Michigan
*Chapter 1: Space Planning and Basic Equipment
   Systems, Chapter 28: Patient Education and
   Care of the Perianesthesia Patient, Chapter 29:
   Postanesthesia Care Complications &
   Chapter 40: Care of the Gastrointestinal,
   Abdominal, and Anorectal Surgical Patient*

**Donna M. DeFazio Quinn, BSN, MBA, RN, CPAN, CAPA**
Director
Orthopaedic Surgery Center
Concord, New Hampshire
*Chapter 2: Perianesthesia Nursing as a Specialty
   & Chapter 3: Management and Policies*

**Audrey R. Roberson, MSN, RN, CPAN**
Nurse Clinician, Perioperative Surgical Services
Virginia Commonwealth University Health
   System
Richmond, Virginia
*Chapter 8: Ethics of Health Care in the PACU*

**Nancy M. Saufl, MS, RN, CPAN, CAPA**
Preadmission Testing Coordinator
Florida Hospital Memorial System
Ormond Beach, Florida
*Chapter 37: Care of the Orthopedic Patient &
   Chapter 43: Care of the Breast Surgical Patient*

**Lois Schick, MBA, MNA, RN, CPAN, CAPA**
Per Diem Staff Nurse
Exempla Lutheran Medical Center
Littleton Adentist Hospital
Lakewood, Colorado
*Chapter 27: Assessment and Monitoring of the
   Perianesthesia Patient*

**Patricia C. Seifert, RN, MSN, CNOR, CRNFA, FAAN**
Education Coordinator, Cardiovascular
   Operating Room
Inova Heart and Vascular Institute
Falls Church, Virginia
*Chapter 35: Care of the Cardiac Surgical
   Patient*

**Beverly A. Smith, BSN, RN, CPAN, CAPA**
Nurse Manager, UH PACU
University of Michigan Health System
Ann Arbor, Michigan
*Chapter 1: Space Planning and Basic Equipment
Systems*

**Lisa Sturm, MPH, CIC**
Supervisor
Surgical Infection Control and Epidemiology
University of Michigan Health System
Ann Arbor, Michigan
*Chapter 5: Infection Control in the PACU*

**Alexander Tartaglia, DMin, BCC**
Associate Professor and Chair,
Program in Patient Counseling
Associate Dean, School of Allied Health
Professions
Virginia Commonwealth University
Richmond, Virginia
*Chapter 8: Ethics of Health Care in the
PACU*

**Candace Taylor, BSN, RN, CPAN**
PACU Supervisor, Patient Safety Officer
Cedar Oaks Surgery Center
Warrensburg, Missouri
*Chapter 41: Care of the Genitourinary Surgical
Patient*

**Kimberly F. Taylor, PhD**
Assistant Professor
Department of Gerontology
Virginia Commonwealth University
Richmond, Virginia
*Chapter 50: Care of the Geriatric Patient*

**E. Ayn Welleford, PhD**
Chair and Associate Professor
Department of Gerontology
Virginia Commonwealth University
Richmond, Virginia
*Chapter 50: Care of the Geriatric Patient*

**Kenneth R. White, PhD, RN, FACHE**
Charles P. Cardwell, Jr, Professor of Health
Administration and Professor of Nursing
Department of Health Administration
Virginia Commonwealth University
Richmond, Virginia
*Chapter 6: Managed Care and Its Impact on the
PACU*

**Wendy K. Winer, RN, BSN, CNOR**
Endoscopic Surgery Specialist, RNFA
Center for Women's Care & Reproductive
Surgery
Atlanta, Georgia
*Chapter 42: Care of the Obstetric and
Gynecologic Surgical Patient*

**Suzanne M. Wright, MSNA, CRNA**
Assistant Professor
Director, Center for Research in Human
Simulation
Department of Nurse Anesthesia
Virginia Commonwealth University
Richmond, Virginia
*Chapter 4: Crisis Resource Management in the
PACU & Chapter 30: Assessment and
Management of the Airway*

The authors also acknowledge the following
consultants and contributors to previous
editions:

**Marie H. Dutton, RN, MS[†]**
Ellicott City, Maryland
*Chapter 10: The Nervous System & Chapter 38:
Care of the Neurosurgical Patient*

**Karen N. Swisher, MS, JD**
Associate Professor
Department of Health Administration
Virginia Commonwealth University
Richmond, Virginia
*Chapter 7: Legal Issues in the PACU*

**John J. Nagelhout, PhD, CRNA, FAAN**
Program Director, School of Anesthesia
Kaiser Permanente
Pasadena, California
*Chapter 19: Basic Principles of Pharmacology &
Chapter 20: Inhalational Agents*

[†]Deceased.

**Kay Ball, RN, BSN, MSA, CNOR, FAAN**
Perioperative Consultant/Educator
K & D Medical, Inc
Lewis Center, Ohio

**Jan Belden, MSN, APRN, BC**
Nurse Practitioner, Pain Management
Advanced Nursing Practice
Loma Linda University Medical Center
Loma Linda, California

**Marcia Bixby, RN, MS, CS, CCRN**
Beth Israel Deaconess Medical Center
Boston, Massachusetts

**Imad F. Btaiche, PharmD, BCNSP**
Clinical Associate Professor
Department of Clinical Sciences
University of Michigan
Ann Arbor, Michigan

**Nancy Burden, RN, MS, CPAN, CAPA**
Director of Ambulatory Surgery
BayCare Health System
New Port Richey, Florida

**Deborah Caswell, RN, MSN, NP-C**
Assistant Director, Nurse Practitioner
Gonda (Goldschmied) Vascular Center
University of California,
    Los Angeles Center for Health Sciences
Los Angeles, California

**Paul S. Dalby, MBA, RRT-NPS, RPFT**
Department Director,
    Respiratory Care Services
Virginia Commonwealth University
    Medical Center
Richmond, Virginia

**Nancy Eksterowicz, MSN, RN**
Pain Services Advanced Practice Nurse
University of Virginia Health System
Patient Care Services
Charlottesville, Virginia

**Marjorie A. Geisz-Everson, MS**
Instructor
LSUHSC Nurse Anesthesia Program
New Orleans, Louisiana

**Julie Goelmbiewski, PharmD**
Clinical Associate Professor
Departments of Pharmacy Practice &
    Anesthesiology
University of Illinois Medical Center at
    Chicago
Chicago, Illinois

**Judy Graham-Garcia, MN, CRNA, FNP, ACNP**
Staff Nurse Anesthetist
Anaesthesia Associates of Massachusetts
Boston, Massachusetts

**Vallire D. Hooper, MSN, RN, CPAN, FAAN**
PeriAnesthesia Consultant,
    Assistant Professor
School of Nursing,
    Medical College of Georgia
Augusta, Georgia

**Kathy Kendrick, RN, BSN, CPAN**
Nurse Educator, Day Surgery and PACU
Children's Healthcare of Atlanta at Egleston
Atlanta, Georgia

**Lemont Kier, BS, PhD**
Professor of Medical Chemistry and
    Nurse Anesthesiology
Virginia Commonwealth University
Richmond, Virginia

**Melissa Koehle, RN, BN, MEd**
Organizational Learning Consultant
Interior Health Authority
Registered Nurse, PACU
Kelowna General Hospital
Kelowna, British Columbia, Canada

**Shelly J. Lane, PhD, OTR/L, FAOTA**
Professor and Chair, Occupational Therapy
Assistant Dean of Research
Virginia Commonwealth University
Richmond, Virginia

**Debra Pecka Malina, CRNA, MA, MBA, APN**
Independent Contractor and Coordinator of
　Clinical Education
University of Tennessee Health Science
　Center Nurse Anesthesia Option
Memphis, Tennessee

**Kathleen J. Menard, RN, BSN, CPAN, CAPA**
Clinical Nurse III
PACU/Interventional Radiology–Memorial
　Campus
UMass Memorial Medical Center
Worcester, Massachusetts

**Teresa Nadder, PhD, CLS (NCA), MT (ASCP)**
Chairman and Associate Professor
Department of Clinical Laboratory Sciences
Virginia Commonwealth University
Richmond, Virginia

**Denise O'Brien, MSN, APRN, BC, CPAN, CAPA,
　FAAN**
Clinical Nurse Specialist, Department
　of Operating Rooms/PACU
University of Michigan Health Systems
Ann Arbor, Michigan

**Judith H. Poole, PhD, RNC**
Nurse Manager
Birthing Care/Special Maternity Care
Presbyterian Hospital
Charlotte, North Carolina

**Donna M. DeFazio Quinn, BSN, MBA, RN, CPAN,
　CAPA**
Director
Orthopaedic Surgery Center
Concord, New Hampshire

**Patricia Radovich, MSN, CNS, FCCM**
Clinical Nurse Specialist,
　Hepatology/Liver Transplantation
Loma Linda University Medical Center
Loma Linda, California

**Jacqueline Ross, MSN, RN, CPAN**
Perianesthesia Consultant, Risk Management
　Analyst
OHIC
Chagrin Falls, Ohio

**Debbie Crowe Sandlin, RN, CPAN**
Nurse Manager Peri-Operative Surgical Services
Southern Hills Medical Center
Nashville, Tennessee

**Nancy M. Saufl, MS, RN, CPAN, CAPA**
Preadmission Testing Coordinator

Florida Hospital Memorial System
Ormond Beach, Florida

**Lois Schick, MBA, MN, RN, CPAN, CAPA**
Per Diem Staff Nurse
Exempla Lutheran Medical Center
Littleton Adventist Hospital
Lakewood, Colorado

**Mavis N. Schorn, RN, MS, CNM**
Assistant Professor
Director, Nurse–Midwifery Program
Vanderbilt University School of Nursing
Nashville, Tennessee

**Elizabeth Monti Seibert, MSN, CRNA, PhD**
Associate Professor
Department of Nurse Anesthesia
Virginia Commonwealth University
Richmond, Virginia

**Susan S. Shelander, RN-CPAN**
Director of Recruitment/Retention
Memorial Hermann Healthcare System
Houston, Texas

**Sharon Summers, PhD, RN, ARNP**
Retired
Overland Park, Kansas

**Karen Swenson, PhD, RN, AOCN**
Oncology Research Manager
Park Nicollet Institute
St. Louis Park, Minnesota

**Alexander Tartaglia, DMin, BCC**
Associate Professor and Chair,
　Program in Patient Counseling
Associate Dean, School of Allied Health
　Professions
Virginia Commonwealth University
Richmond, Virginia

**Keiko L. Torgersen, BSN, MSM, RNC**
Commander, 60th Medical Operations Squadron
60th Medical Group
Vacaville, California

**Cathy Trame, RN, MS, CNS, BC**
Clinical Nurse Specialist for Pain Services
Miami Valley Hospital
Dayton, Ohio

**Victor A. Yanchick, BS, MS, PhD**
Dean
School of Pharmacology
Virginia Commonwealth University
Richmond, Virginia

The fifth edition of this book represents a significant milestone for all of us in Perianesthesia Nursing. First published in 1979, *The Recovery Room*, or as it was often referred to, the "Blue Book," has evolved into the standard textbook for perianesthesia nurses. We are so honored that this fifth edition continues the tradition of excellence, providing the practicing perianesthesia nurse with the most comprehensive knowledge base for this nursing specialty available under one cover. The title of this fifth edition, *Perianesthesia Nursing: A Critical Care Approach*, reflects the evolving professionalism of this advanced nursing practice specialty. In 1983, under the aegis of the American Society of Post Anesthesia Nurses (ASPAN), the term *postanesthesia care unit (PACU)* was chosen to designate the postoperative work area and the term *postanesthesia nurse* was chosen to indicate the nurse specializing in that area of patient care. Now, in accordance with the advance practice concepts, the term *perianesthesia nurse* is accepted as defining the nursing practice to include the entire nursing care of the patient that is to undergo a surgical procedure.

All the chapters in this fifth edition have been restructured to help the reader understand and retain the information presented. Each chapter now contains a opening paragraph that serves to introduce the reader to the topic to be discussed. After the introduction, a complete section on the definitions of terms particular to the chapter topic is presented, and then the chapter topic is presented in detail. The final portion of the chapter now contains a summary of the material presented and an extensive listing of the references that the reader can use should further reading about the topic be desired.

This book is organized into five major sections. Section I, "The Postanesthesia Care Unit," focuses on the postanesthesia facilities and equipment, the specialty of perianesthesia nursing, and management and policy issues. The chapter on crisis resource management in the PACU looks at the newest techniques in the care of the patient with use of technology such

as anesthesia simulators and provides the most up-to-date concepts in regard to patient safety. Because of the tremendous concern about infection control, a new chapter has been developed to provide the perianesthesia nurse with the most current information on epidemiology and infection control. The health care system continues to change, and particularly, in the PACU, so a chapter is devoted to managed care and its impact on the PACU. Another focus area that is having a major impact on perianesthesia nursing is legal issues associated with the nursing practice in the PACU. The legal issues chapter was revised to ensure that the perianesthesia nurse has the most current information so that nursing practice is legally sound. Another area of interest for perianesthesia nurses is in regard to the ethics in health care. Hence, the chapter on ethics of health care and specifically of perianesthesia nursing has been completely updated to reflect the most current information on many of the ethical issues facing the perianesthesia nurse in the practice setting. Another new chapter that has been added to the fifth edition is on research. This chapter should serve as an introduction to the research process along with many suggestions on focus areas of research that can be conducted during the perianesthesia experience. The chapter also introduces the reader to evidenced-based practice.

Section II deals with the physiologic considerations in the PACU. All of the chapters have been updated to reflect the current concepts in anatomy and physiology, including the most recent information available concerning the care and treatment of patients with acquired immunodeficiency syndrome. Because of numerous requests by readers, the chapter on fluids and electrolytes has been updated significantly to reflect the new and most current laboratory nomenclature.

Section III, "Concepts in Anesthetic Agents," presents the reader with up-to-date pharmacologic considerations of postanesthesia care. The first chapter presents a complete overview of pharmacology, including uptake and distribution, pharmacokinetic and pharmacodynamic principles, drug-drug interactions in the

PACU, and the influence of herbal medications on postanesthesia emergence of the patient. Also, this chapter contains an extensive table on most of the drugs used in perianesthesia care. Because of advances in research and applications of intravenous anesthetic agents, this content has been divided into two separate chapters that cover opioid and nonopioid intravenous anesthetic agents. Also, the regional anesthesia chapter, which was presented in a single chapter in the previous edition, has been divided into a chapter focusing on local anesthestics and another chapter discussing the use of regional anesthesia.

Section IV addresses the nursing care in the PACU for various surgical specialties. Many of the chapters in this section have been completely revised by guest authors. Chapter 26 looks at the transition of the patient from the operating room to the PACU. Chapter 27, "Assessment and Monitoring of the Perianesthesia Patient," includes an all-new section on monitoring equipment and data interpretation. This update is especially important because of the many technologic advances in the PACU that have occurred in the last 5 years. The next chapter presents not only the overall care of the perianesthesia patient but now also includes a complete discussion on the area of patient education. A new chapter was developed to better address the postanesthesia complications. As opposed to having a discussion of these complications throughout the book, this new chapter should serve the reader well by conveniently addressing the complications in depth in one area. Chapter 30 explores the art and science of airway management, with special attention to intubation and extubation of the trachea. This addition was in response to frequent requests by users of the previous edition for more information with a greater focus on the newest technology of airway management. Also updated in this text is Chapter 31, "Pain Management in the PACU," which includes discussions on related physiology and pharmacology.

Section V, "Special Considerations," has been revised and condensed in this edition. Chapter 45, "Care of the Patient with Thermal Imbalance," has a complete update and discussion of the care of patients with hyperthermia and hypothermia; with the almost daily advances in surgical technology in the use of laser and laparoscopic surgery, a complete update is presented to reflect the use of this new technology and its implications to perianesthesia nursing care. Chapter 54 addresses the needs and care of the shock trauma patient, a topic currently receiving an exceptional amount of attention in professional meetings and literature. In response to many requests by perianesthesia nurses, a chapter has been added on the "Care of the Intensive Care Patient in the PACU." This chapter serves as a conduit in the description of critical care nursing practice in the PACU. Because of the times we live in and the impact of perianesthesia nursing, the chapter focusing on bioterrorism and its impact on the PACU has been updated to reflect the most current thinking in regard to this public health concern.

The success of any multiauthored book is in large part dependent on the expertise and commitment of the contributors. The contributors to this book were invited because they are acknowledged authorities in their fields. With their help, it is hoped that this book will continue to inform and guide students, teachers, and clinicians in the critical care specialty of perianesthesia nursing. As in previous editions, we welcome all evaluations and suggestions for improvement.

Cecil B. Drain
Jan Odom-Forren

# Contents

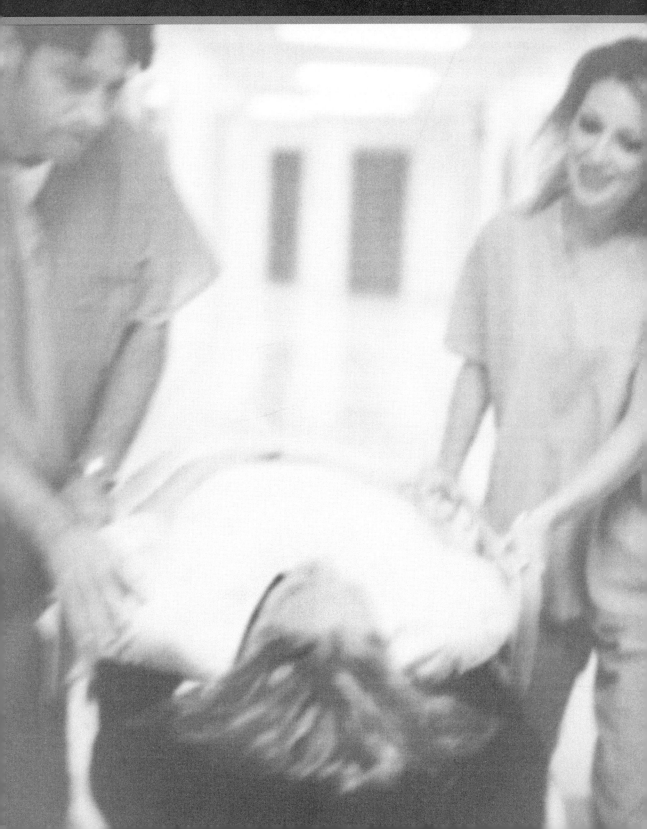

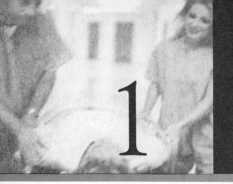

# SPACE PLANNING AND BASIC EQUIPMENT SYSTEMS

*Denise O'Brien, MSN, APRN,BC, CPAN, CAPA, FAAN*
*Beverly Smith, BSN, RN, CPAN, CAPA*

From the birth of the recovery room in the 1940s to the postanesthesia care unit (PACU) of the 21st century, the look and function of this room (or unit) have been in a constant state of evolution. Throughout the last six decades, surgical procedures have become more extensive and complicated and thus require more specially prepared nursing staff and equipment for care of the patients.

The first recovery rooms were established for centralization of patients and personnel. The PACUs of today have evolved from general care to an intensive care specialty that provides a range of nursing care, from neonatal to geriatric and from outpatient or same-day surgery to inpatient surgery. The PACU now must be flexible to serve all perianesthesia phases and patient acuities. The design of the space is critical to the ability of the staff to care safely and efficiently for a range of patients.

## SPACE

Many factors are considered in the design of a PACU. Before the architect or design firm is consulted, the users of the space (i.e., perianesthesia nurses, anesthesia providers, and clerical staff) should come together to answer the following questions regarding the function of the space:
- Is this new construction or is the current space to be remodeled?
- How will the space be used?
- Will a separate preoperative holding area be created or will preoperative functions be carried out in this space?
- Is this space a PACU Phase I and/or PACU Phase II?
- What patient population will be served (i.e., outpatient, same-day admission, and/or inpatient)?
- What patient age groups will be served (i.e., neonatal, pediatric, adult only, or combined age groups)?

Current and future programs in the Department of Surgery and the institutional demographics are also important considerations. The following questions should be answered:
- How many operating rooms or suites will this area serve?
- How many operations will be done per day?
- How many different surgical services will be served?
- What types of procedures will be done?
- Will some patients need prolonged monitoring or observation?
- What type of anesthesia practices will impact this area (i.e., regional anesthesia program, acute or chronic pain service)?
- What is the average patient acuity (i.e., American Society of Anesthesiologists [ASA] physical status classification)?
- Will nonsurgical or procedural patients that need anesthesia undergo recovery in this same space?

### Define the Use

Flexibility is an important consideration. One of the first factors for consideration is how the space will be used. Will the bays be used strictly for postoperative care, or will the unit need the flexibility of preoperative use? Many institutions have a separate area dedicated to preadmission testing or screening. This area is best located near the surgical clinics and testing areas (i.e., blood draw station and radiology and cardiology [electrocardiography] departments). However, consideration should be given to how the preoperative holding area will be designed and used. Because of the cost of construction and the limited hours of use, most administrators are reluctant to build space that has only a single function and that does not lend itself to change as the users or programs evolve. Therefore, all disciplines that use or expect to use the area need to engage in the discussion related to space usage so that future needs can be anticipated. The department of anesthesia will have input regarding preoperative needs (e.g., a preadmission testing or screening area and day-of-surgery preoperative procedures).

Perianesthesia nurses have knowledge of the entire process from preadmission testing to discharge the day of surgery. The staff in the department of surgery need to have input regarding types of operations, new surgical techniques, and the need for prolonged observation before discharge. Clerical services personnel should have input related to the flow of patients and record and paperwork systems. Input from environmental services personnel is related to needs of janitorial space and house cleaning supplies and equipment. Central supply personnel should be consulted regarding the space needed for storage of disposable supplies and linen for ready availability on the unit. Patient equipment personnel should give input regarding space needed to deliver and store reusable equipment, including stretchers, beds, wheelchairs, infusion pumps, patient-controlled analgesia (PCA)/ epidural pumps, implantable cardioverter defibrillators (ICDs).

Adequate time for consultation with all of the potential users and ancillary personnel who will use or provide services in the space is wise. One needs only a brief talk with staff who has been forced to "make do" with poorly designed space to understand the importance of this first step in the design process.

## Determine the Location

The same factors that influence the building of a housing development or retail shops in one place versus another can be applied to this discussion of perianesthesia space needs. A new construction design typically offers greater probability of optimization of design than remodeling does. Nevertheless, all of the factors should be considered to ensure that the end result best serves the unit's needs. Whether the result is a free-standing ambulatory surgery center or an inpatient hospital setting, the first consideration should be ease of access for the patients and family. Parking should be easily accessible and plentiful, and the entrance should be located adjacent to the parking garage or lot. The patient reception and waiting area should be near the entrance to decrease the patient anxiety and frustration that results from a search for the area.

The second consideration should be egress. A logical patient flow—with adjacent areas that naturally follow the patients' transit through the unit—should be established for maximization of staff efficiency and decreased steps between areas. The waiting area should be adjacent to the preoperative holding area. PACU

Phase I and PACU Phase II should be adjacent but with separate entrances from the operating rooms (ORs) for safety and efficiency. In an inpatient setting, a separate elevator is ideal for patients of the OR to be transported to general care and intensive care units (ICUs). This separate elevator is a matter of safety for patients going to an ICU and maximizes staff efficiency for patients going to general care. With remodeling, great care should be taken to determine that the design shows consideration of these factors and incorporation whenever possible.

## Components of the Space

Several key components must be incorporated into the design of the space. The first element that needs determination is the number of patient bays necessary. Before this number can be calculated, consideration must be given to several key factors that influence that number.

- How are the bays to be used? Will they be used for preoperative care only, PACU only, PACU Phase II only? Or will they be used interchangeably for all phases of care?
- Are they also to be used for preoperative care, or is a separate space available for that function?
- How many ORs does the preoperative area and PACU service, and how many cases are done per day?
- Does the PACU service other procedure areas of the hospital (i.e., cardiac catheterization/ electrophysiology laboratory, electroconvulsive therapy treatments, medical procedures [endoscopy, bronchoscopy], radiology and angiography, anesthesia pain service [chronic and acute])? If so, how many cases per day and at what time of day?
- Are the patients adults, children, or both?
- What is the scheduling method used by the department of surgery? How many different surgical services are served?
- What is the hospital bed capacity and usual census?
- Do patients wait long periods for inpatient beds?
- Is the PACU used for ICU, telemetry, or general care overflow? If so, how often and for how many patients at one time?
- Does the department of anesthesia have a regional anesthesia program? Do they need space for these services?
- What is the average patient acuity (i.e., ASA physical status classification)?
- What is the average length of stay for different patient types (i.e. outpatient, inpatient, same-day admission)?

For an inpatient hospital PACU that services a combined patient population of inpatients and same-day admission patients, a ratio of 1.5 to 2 PACU bays per OR is necessary to safely care for the patients and not back up the OR. For an ambulatory surgery center with a limited number of surgical services and types of procedures, 2.5 to 3 PACU Phase I and PACU Phase II (combined) bays are necessary. The shorter surgical procedures necessitate an increased number of PACU slots because the recovery time may be two to three times the length of the procedure. If pediatric cases are done in either setting, the number of bays may need to be increased because this patient population necessitates 1:1 nursing care for a longer time than does a solely adult population.

Cases of antibiotic-resistant organisms and tuberculosis infections have been on the rise over the past several years. As a result, the need for negative pressure isolation or body substance isolation should be considered in the design. Geographic location and patient population demographics should be reviewed to determine the number of isolation rooms needed. Every PACU should have at least one negative pressure room. However, if the institution services a more susceptible population, more rooms may be necessary. Consultation with the institution's infectious diseases department is advisable to ensure that the design meets institutional policy and is prepared to serve the patient population.

Another consideration in the design of patient bays is size and means of separation. Most states have building codes that define the minimum square footage of each bay (e.g., State of Michigan Health Care Facilities code is 80 square feet). However, consideration should be given to how the bays are to be used. If they are strictly for patients of PACU Phase I, the minimum required square footage may be adequate. If they are for anesthesia preoperative procedures or anesthesia pain procedures that necessitate equipment such as fluoroscopy or bronchoscopy, the size may need to be increased (to as much as 150 square feet). Also, if the bays are to be used alternatively as PACU Phase I or PACU Phase II and then as observation for 23-hour admissions, they may need to be large enough to accommodate a patient bed, table, or lounge chair. Building some of the bays larger to accommodate these future needs may also be wise, but one should keep in mind that the size of the bays affects the configuration of the space.

Patient privacy needs to be considered in determination of the means of separation between patient bays. Typically, PACU bays are open spaces defined only by a curtain that can be pulled for privacy. The open floor plan maximizes patient safety and staff efficiency in the higher acuity PACU Phase I setting. With preoperative and PACU Phase II care, patient acuity is typically lower and continual observation of patients is usually not necessary. Patients are more alert and families are generally present, so the need for privacy is increased. Half walls may be considered in these spaces. A half wall (i.e., floor-to-ceiling wall one third to half the depth of the bay) gives more privacy to the patient and family from the sights and sounds of the adjacent bays. However, this configuration still allows the clinicians to observe patients and be readily available for acute needs.

The bays should be carefully arranged for maximized staffing efficiency within the constraints of the American Society of PeriAnesthesia Nurses (ASPAN) staffing resource guidelines. The PACU Phase I staffing recommendation is a maximum of two patients per registered nurse (RN), less for an unstable condition or a pediatric patient. For PACU Phase II staffing, the recommendation is a maximum of three patients to one RN, less for a patient with an unstable condition who needs transfer or a pediatric patient without family or staff support. Grouping of slots in multiples of two or three allows the most efficient, safe staffing. Careful consideration should be given as to how the space will be used (i.e., as preoperative care, PACU Phase I or PACU Phase II, or interchangeably).

The ASPAN standards do not define staffing ratios for preoperative cases. Ideal safe staffing ratios are determined by individual institutions on the basis of the particular patient population, the number of ORs, the OR turnover time, and the number of preoperative procedures done with anesthesia. The amount of nursing time necessary to prepare for surgery depends on the patient's age, the amount of preparation done in the surgery clinic, and the patient's knowledge base and anxiety level. Patients who are well prepared when they arrive for surgery need less preoperative nursing time. The number of ORs, the average length of procedures, and turnover time affect how many patients are in the preoperative area at one time and how much time they wait before going into the OR. In a small ambulatory surgery center, one or more rooms may be used for quick procedures that necessitate little equipment or cleaning to ready the OR for the next patient. In this case, two patients for that same OR may need to be in the preoperative area at the same time. Another factor that affects preoperative staffing is the number and type of anesthesia preoperative procedures. Again, in a small ambulatory surgery center, most procedures may be done with a general anesthetic or sedation; thus, the preparation time is shorter. Conversely, a teaching institution may have a patient population with significant comorbid conditions that necessitate monitoring lines (i.e., pulmonary artery catheters, arterial lines, central lines, etc.). Also, many institutions have a pain service that offers patients epidural catheters or extremity blocks for postoperative pain management. These patients occupy the preoperative holding area bay for a longer period and may need nursing assistance for sedation or monitoring during and after the procedure until they go into the OR. In these situations, a ratio of three to five patients to one RN is safe and efficient. However, staffing should be flexible to decrease the number of patients per RN as the patient acuity rises or the need for nursing care and monitoring increases.

For space that is flexible for any need, preoperative or postoperative care, all of the headwalls should be designed uniformly to allow flexibility day to day or in the future as institutional needs change. During new construction, when the walls are open, the addition of piped-in medical gases and vacuum for suction at each bay is simple and cost effective. For the care of critically ill patients in PACU Phase I, each bay should have a minimum of two oxygen outlets, one air outlet, and three vacuum outlets for suction. In a free-standing ambulatory surgery center that never serves a critically ill inpatient population it may be more prudent to decrease the number of oxygen and vacuum outlets. However, consideration should be given to the possibility of a patient with a surgical or anesthesia complication that necessitates more intensive care. The other elements of the headwall design include electrical outlets and data and telephone jacks. Again, whether the unit is new construction or renovation, a plan for maximum care and future needs is wise. Each bay should have adequate electrical outlets to service a variety of pieces of equipment, including a patient bed, a forced air warming/cooling device, multiple infusion pumps, a ventilator, a physiologic monitor, a computer, a compression device, and a patient-controlled analgesia machine. Telephone and data jacks should be installed to service the current standard of practice and future needs. Today, most physiologic monitors are computers that need a data jack. Technology development will bring online data entry to the bedside. Planning for adequate data jacks to support this future need is wise and necessary.

Another important component of the design of the patient care bay is lighting. Adequate light needs to be available for admission assessment and emergency situations. Large overhead lights provide the best source of light to meet this safety need. Consideration should be given to the patient in stable condition for whom bright lighting is not a safety concern. Wall-mounted lights, overhead canned lights on a dimmer, or low-watt lighting provide the appropriate ambience for the patient and still allow the nurse to provide safe care.

Another important component of the patient bay is storage. Some emergency equipment must be stored at each bay for ready availability to the practitioners. However, careful planning should occur to avoid clutter that would hamper the nurses' ability to quickly access equipment. Many different systems are available to service this need. Before any system is purchased, the items to be stored and the space needed must be assessed. Another point for consideration is what constitutes "emergent" equipment and what is at the bedside for convenience. Figure 1-1 shows one example of a storage system with a rail attached to the wall and a series of baskets that clamp onto the rail. The baskets are available in different shapes and sizes and can be moved along the rail to suit the user. A storage cart complements this system; it contains items that need to be readily available for efficiency but are not needed emergently.

The ability to care for patients in the PACU safely and efficiently is dependent on the layout of the room. Beyond the confines of the patient bay and its components, immediate access to supplies, equipment, and service areas is essential. Box 1-1 contains a list of the space and service areas needed for the function of the preoperative holding area and PACU. Many of the supplies, pieces of equipment, and service areas overlap, which should be considered in the design. If service areas are strategically placed, they can service two units and thus increase staff efficiency while decreasing the cost of building and maintenance.

The amount of duplication can be decreased with determination of the components that may be shared. These spaces should be placed between two units or in close proximity to one another. This thoughtful careful planning allows for safe efficient care and minimization of duplication and cost.

Staff needs are an important consideration in the design. Staff lounge and toilets adjacent to the unit are essential. They allow staff the opportunity to take breaks consistent with the workflow. Because of the dynamic nature of the preoperative holding area and PACU,

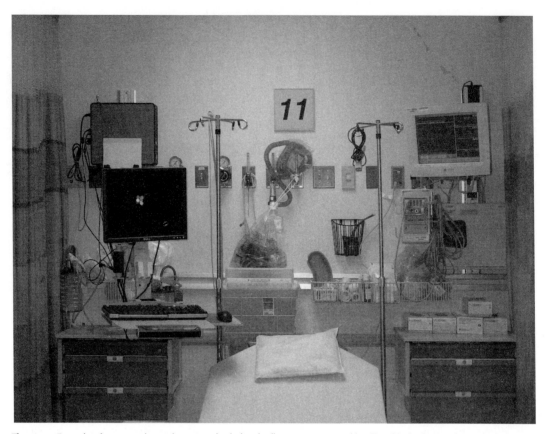

**Fig. 1-1**   Example of preoperative and postanesthesia headwall storage system with adjustable baskets and storage drawers.

scheduling of breaks consistent with staff members' requests is sometimes difficult. Facilities that are immediately adjacent to the unit allow flexibility of scheduling and ensure the availability of staff in the event of an emergency.

Ergonomics and efficiency are important elements in the design of the space and the equipment. For patient safety, the nurse must be able to visualize the patient from every point in the room. Essential equipment should be in the room so the nurse can constantly monitor the patient while obtaining and using the equipment. A bedside table and chair should be available for every staff member for sitting at the patient's bedside and documenting during observation. Tables, chairs, and computer monitors and keyboards should be adjustable to fit multiple users. With an aging workforce, the lack of adequate adjustable furnishings could lead to increased injury and exacerbate the growing nursing shortage.

Another component of the space is the reception and waiting area, which varies depending on the location (i.e., inpatient hospital-based versus free-standing ambulatory surgery center).

In either location, several items need to be incorporated. If possible, preoperative patients and their families should wait in a separate location than the families of patients in the OR or PACU. Preoperative patient anxiety may increase when a physician is seen with another family or a family is visibly upset. Also, the sight and smell of food and drink are inconsiderate to a patient who has been fasting. Conversely, families of patients in the OR or PACU want to stay in close proximity to their loved ones and need to be readily available to clinical staff; therefore, they need to be able to eat and drink in the waiting area. Also, the waiting areas should accommodate a variety of needs so that waiting patients and families can be entertained or distracted or work, if necessary. Some considerations are: an area dedicated to Internet access with computer work stations and data connections for laptops, a television area, a quiet area for reading, a children's play area with toys, and furniture appropriate to the patient population served. Consultation rooms should be available for private consultation between physicians and patients and families.

## Box 1-1 Support Areas and Equipment*

**PREOPERATIVE HOLDING AREA**
- Clean storage
- Dirty utility
- Patient toilet
- Equipment storage (e.g., stretchers, beds, wheelchairs, infusion pumps, transducer set-ups)
- Procedure carts
- Blanket warmer
- Emergency cart
- Medication dispensing unit (e.g., Pyxis, Omnicell)
- Point-of-care testing (blood gas laboratory)
- Medical records storage
- Radiograph view box
- Bulletin board for patient education material

**PACU PHASE I**
- Clean storage
- Dirty utility
- Medication dispensing unit (e.g., Pyxis, Omnicell)
- Blanket warmer
- Emergency cart
- Equipment storage (e.g., stretchers, beds, wheelchairs, infusion pumps, warmers, PCA/epidurals, ICDs)
- Point-of-care testing (blood gas laboratory)
- Radiographic view box

- Patient toilet
- Patient nourishment
- Medical records
- Procedure carts
- Patient education bulletin board
- Nursing station
- Physician dictation
- Staff toilet
- Staff lounge
- Staff locker room

**PACU PHASE II**
- Clean storage
- Dirty utility
- Medication dispensing unit (e.g., Pyxis, Omnicell)
- Patient toilet
- Emergency cart
- Equipment storage (stretchers, beds, wheelchairs, etc.)
- Blanket warmer
- Patient nourishment
- Patient education bulletin board
- Nursing station
- Physician dictation
- Staff toilet
- Staff lounge
- Staff locker room

*This list is not meant to be all-inclusive. It should serve as a guide to help determine the needs of the institution.

## Standard Equipment

The type and amount of equipment needed for the safe care of preoperative and postanesthesia patients vary to some extent on the basis of environment and patient population. However, some basic items are essential in any setting.

Types of equipment can be divided into three categories: emergent, readily available, and necessary. Emergency cases in the PACU typically start as a result of airway compromise, so the availability of supplies (e.g., resuscitation bag, oral/nasal airways, suction catheters, and lubricant) at the bedside is prudent. Intubation equipment should be readily available as part of the emergency cart or as a separate container or bag of anesthesia supplies. Box 1-2 provides a list of suggested items to be stocked in an anesthesia PACU emergency bag. In addition, ASPAN's Standards for PeriAnesthesia Nursing Practice 2006-2008 Resource 6 provides a list of suggested emergency medications and equipment for a preoperative holding area, PACU Phase I, and PACU Phase II.

Malignant hyperthermia (MH) is a rare but potentially fatal complication of general anesthesia. An MH box or cart or the equivalent supplies in the PACU Phase I is essential. The Malignant Hyperthermia Association of the United States has a recommended list of supplies for MH emergency cases (Box 1-3). (See also Chapter 53.)

Institutions where intensive care patients recover in the PACU should have available a "travel box" of medications and supplies for use in transportation. Table 1-1 lists the types of medications and supplies that may be included in this box.

Readily available bedside supplies may vary between institutions depending on the types of patients and volume. However, some essential supplies should be at every patient bedside. In addition to the aforementioned airway supplies, several means of oxygen delivery (see Chapter 28), a variety of suction catheters and tubing, gloves, emesis basins, and tissues should be immediately available at the bedside.

---

**Box 1-2   Contents of Anesthesia PACU Emergency Bag**

**PACU EMERGENCY BAG**
*Main Compartment*
- Endotracheal (ET) tubes with stylet and syringe (6.0, 7.0, and 8.0)
- Extra ET tube (5.0, 5.5, 6.0, 6.5, 7.0, 7.5, 8.0)
- Light wand with ET tube
- Bougie
- Laryngoscope with blades (MAC 3 and 4, Miller 2 and 4)
- Face mask, clear (2)
- Pediatric ET tubes (2.5, 3.0, 3.5, and 4.0)
- Succinylcholine
- Sodium pentothal

*Front Compartment*
- Guedel airway (red, green, and yellow)
- Disposable airway
- Yankauer
- Breathing circuit
- Nasopharyngeal airway (6.5, 7.5, and 8.5)

*Side Pocket*
- Syringes
- Alcohol swabs

*Back Pocket Emergency Kit*
- Cricothyrotomy
- Nasal cannula
- Laryngeal mask airway (LMA) 3, 4, 5
- 60-mL syringes (2)

---

Bedside supplies should be limited to only essential items to ensure they are stocked and easily retrievable by all personnel.

Other supplies that need to be readily available can be stored in a variety of ways. If the clean storage room is in close proximity to all patient bays and has a user-friendly system, equipment may be left there and retrieved at the time it is needed. If the room design does not allow for quick retrieval of supplies from the clean storage room, consideration should be given to a storage system located in the immediate proximity of patient bays. This system could be a cart that would be moved from bay to bay or built-in cupboards that would service several bays. The staff's involvement in the choice of a storage system is essential so that their needs are met.

Institutions that have 24-hour equipment delivery service do not need to store such items as intravenous (IV) pumps, pneumatic compression devices, forced air warming devices, and IV poles for transport. However, if these items are not readily available, they should be stored on the unit.

Pain management is an essential part of the patient care delivered in the PACU. If the institution uses IV patient-controlled analgesia pumps and epidural pumps for patient-controlled analgesia, a supply of these pieces of equipment should be kept in the PACU for ready availability. The PACU is an ICU and should therefore have a ventilator available at all times; individual institutional policy governs which department is responsible for the set up and maintenance of any ventilators.

---

**Box 1-3   Malignant Hyperthermia Cart or Kit Supplies**

An MH cart or kit that contains the following drugs, equipment, supplies, and forms should be immediately accessible to operating rooms and the PACU.

**DRUGS**
1. Dantrolene sodium IV, 36 vials (each diluted with 60-mL sterile water)
2. Sterile water for injection USP (without a bacteriostatic agent) to reconstitute dantrolene, 1000 mL (2)
3. Sodium bicarbonate (8.4%), 50 mL (5)
4. Furosemide, 40 mg/amp (4 ampules)
5. D50, 50-mL vials (2)
6. Calcium chloride (10%; 2)
7. Regular insulin, 100 units/mL (1; refrigerated)
8. Lidocaine HCl (2%), 1 box (2 g) or 20-mL vials (5)

**GENERAL EQUIPMENT**
1. Syringes (60 mL; 5) to dilute dantrolene
2. Mini spike IV additive pins (2) and MultiAd fluid transfer sets (2; to reconstitute dantrolene)

**Box 1-3    Malignant Hyperthermia Cart or Kit Supplies—cont'd**

3. Angiocatheters: 20-gauge, 2-inch; 22-gauge, 1-inch; 24-gauge, 3/4-inch (4 each; for IV access and arterial line)
4. Nasogastric (NG) tubes: sizes appropriate for the patient population
5. Blood pump
6. Irrigation tray with piston syringe (1) for NG irrigation
7. Toomy irrigation syringes (60 mL; 2) for NG irrigation
8. Large clear plastic bags for ice
9. Bucket for ice
10. Disposable cold packs (4)

**MONITORING EQUIPMENT**
1. Esophageal temperature probes
2. Central venous pressure (CVP) kits (sizes appropriate to the patient population)
3. Transducer kit

**DRIP SUPPLIES**
1. D5W, 250 mL (1)
2. Microdrip IV set (1)

**NURSING SUPPLIES**
1. Large sterile Steri-Drape (for rapid drape of wound)
2. Three-way irrigating Foley catheters: sizes appropriate for the patient population
3. Urine meter (1)
4. Toomy irrigation syringe (60 mL; 2)
5. Rectal tubes: sizes (Malecot drain) 14F, 16F, 32F, 34F
6. Large clear plastic bags for ice (4)
7. Small plastic bags for ice (4)
8. Tray for ice

**LABORATORY TESTING SUPPLIES**
1. Syringes (3 mL) or arterial blood gas (ABG) kits (6)
2. Blood specimen tubes (each test should have 2 pediatric and 2 large tubes): A for creatine kinase (CK), myoglobin, sequential multiple analysis (SMA), 19 (lactate dehydrogenase [LDH], electrolytes, thyroid studies); B for prothrombin time/partial thromboplastin time (PT/PTT), fibrinogen, fibrin split products; C for complete blood cell count (CBC), platelets; D for blood gas syringe (lactic acid level)
3. Urine cup (2): myoglobin level
4. Urine dipstick: hemoglobin

**FORMS**
1. Laboratory request forms: ABG form (6); hematology form (2); chemistry form (2); coagulation form (2); urinalysis form (2); physician order form (2)
2. Adverse Metabolic Reaction to Anesthesia (AMRA) report form (obtained from Malignant Hyperthermia Association of United States)
3. Consult form

## Table 1-1   Travel Box Contents

| Contents | Quota | Contents | Quota |
|---|---|---|---|
| **COMMON MEDICATIONS** | | **COMMON SUPPLIES** | |
| Atropine 0.1 mg/mL, 10-mL syringe | 1 | 0.9% NaCl, 20-mL vial | 2 |
| Atropine 0.4 mg/mL, 1-mL vial | 1 | 1-inch wide tape | 1 |
| Calcium chloride 10%, 10-mL vial | 1 | Alcohol preparation | 10 |
| Dextrose 50%, 50-mL vial | 1 | Angiocatheter, size 18, 20, 22, 24 | 1 of each size |
| Diphenhydramine 50 mg/mL, 1-mL vial | 1 | Blood drawing butterfly needle | 3 |
| Dopamine 400 mg/mL, 5-mL vial | 2 | Gauze, sterile 4 × 4 | 5 |
| Epinephrine 1:10,000, 10-mL syringe | 2 | Hemostat | 1 |
| Flumazenil 1 mg/10 mL, 10-mL vial | 1 | Needle, 21 g | 4 |
| Furosemide 100 mg 10-mL vial | 1 | Needle, 18 g | 4 |
| IV bags, 250-mL D5W | 1 | Oral airway | 1 |
| Labetalol 5 mg/mL, 20-mL vial | 1 | Suction catheter pediatric | 2 |
| Lidocaine 2%, 5-mL syringe | 1 | Suction catheter adult 14F | 2 |
| Mannitol 25%, 50-mL vial and filter needle | 4 | Syringe, 1 mL | 4 |
| NaHCO$_3$ pediatric bristoject 4.2%, 10 mL | 2 | Syringe, 3-mL w needle | 4 |
| NaHCO$_3$ adult bristoject 8.4%, 50 mL | 1 | Syringe, 10 mL | 4 |
| Naloxone HCl 0.4 mg/mL, 1 mL | 1 | Syringe, 20 mL | 4 |
| Nitroglycerin SL 0.4 mg, #25 tabs | 1 | Syringe pump tubing | 1 |
| Phenytoin 100 mg, syringe 2 mL | 10 | Tourniquet | 1 |
| Prochlorperazine 10 mg/2 mL, 2-mL vial | 1 | Venoset, universal | 1 |
| 0.9% NaCl, 50-mL IV bag | 1 | Total Parenteral Nutrition (TPN) filter | 1 |
| | | Yankauer suction catheter | 1 |

## SUMMARY

Many changes in the care of postanesthesia patients have occurred in the last 60 years, and continued change is inevitable. Thoughtful planning and interdisciplinary communication are essential for the space and equipment to continue to meet the patient care needs in perianesthesia care areas.

## BIBLIOGRAPHY

American Society of PeriAnesthesia Nurses: *Standards of perianesthesia nursing practice 2006-2008*, Cherry Hill, NJ, 2006.

Feeley TW, Macario A: The postanesthesia care unit. In Miller RD: *Miller's anesthesia*, ed 6, Philadelphia, 2005, Saunders.

Israel JS, DeKornfeld TJ: *Recovery room care*, ed 2, Chicago, 1987, Year Book Medical Publishers.

Malignant Hyperthermia Association of the United States: available at http://www.mhaus.org.

American Society of PeriAnesthesia Nurses: *Historical information*, available at www.aspan.org/historical.htm.

Michigan State Government: Department of Consumer & Industry Services: *Minimum design standards for health care facilities in Michigan*, available at www.cis.state.mi.us/bhs/hfes/pdfs/standard.pdf.

# 2

## PERIANESTHESIA NURSING AS A SPECIALTY

*Donna M. DeFazio Quinn, BSN, MBA, RN, CPAN, CAPA*

Recognition of perianesthesia nursing as a critical care specialty has been well established. This past decade has been witness to a number of significant factors that have influenced the practice of perianesthesia nursing. Among these factors are the emphasis on cost containment in health care, declining reimbursement for medical services, the aging and increased acuity level of the population, advances in technology, advances in pharmaceutical therapy, and fasttracking of patients through the postanesthesia care unit (PACU).

Perianesthesia nursing is practiced in a variety of settings, both inpatient and outpatient and within the hospital setting and in free-standing practice settings (Box 2-1). The perianesthesia environment is delineated by the following phases: preanesthesia phase, postanesthesia Phase I, postanesthesia Phase II, and Extended Observation (formerly known as Phase III)[1] that assist the patient with transition through the surgical event.

The continued emphasis on cost containment has stimulated the regionalization of health care and the development of tertiary care centers in major cities, and primary care has increasingly moved to ambulatory settings. As a consequence, perianesthesia nursing is practiced in a variety of settings, from the physician's office to recovery care centers to highly specialized PACUs in dedicated medical centers, such as eye institutes and surgical hospitals. At the same time, in an effort at cost containment, hospitals have increased the use of the PACU for special procedures, such as electroconvulsive therapy (ECT), elective cardioversion, and endoscopic examination. In addition, the PACU is used for services such as pain clinics, preoperative holding areas (for both inpatient and outpatient services), and overflow units when intensive care unit or inpatient beds are full. Although some of these changes seem to create less than optimal conditions for patient care, the creative collaboration of all health care practitioners is imperative to meet the challenges of the rapidly changing health care environment. PACUs have the unique opportunity to be innovative and creative in implementation of methods to meet these changes.

The increasingly competitive business environment for health care and technologic advances has significantly increased the use of ambulatory surgical settings. The emergence of surgical hospitals has added to the equation. These multispecialty facilities provide both inpatient and outpatient surgical services. By functioning much the same as an ambulatory surgery center (ASC), the surgical hospital operates in a cost-effective mode. The focus is on quick turnovers and a user-friendly atmosphere—hallmarks that make the ASC successful.

The acuity of inpatient cases has also greatly increased. In addition, the increasing age of the population in the United States means many surgical patients have a number of concomitant chronic problems, such as chronic obstructive lung disease, diabetes mellitus, and chronic heart conditions. The provision of quality care in the PACU necessitates a strong knowledgeable leader with excellent skills and a highly skilled nursing staff. In addition to the promotion and support of the nursing staff, attention must be paid to the organizational and operational structure of the unit.

Fasttracking has become a popular concept in the PACU. Fasttracking involves admission of patients from the operating room directly to PACU Phase II and a bypass of PACU Phase I.[1] Policies and procedures on fasttracking should be developed collaboratively with the involvement of nursing and anesthesia personnel. Policies should address patient selection, criteria for direct admission to PACU Phase II, patient monitoring, and discharge criteria. Nurses in the PACU Phase II unit must be competent to handle any unexpected outcome that may or may not be a direct result of fasttracking.

In an effort to define the role of the perianesthesia nurse, the American Society of PeriAnesthesia Nurses (ASPAN) has published a formal Scope of Practice document (Box 2-2) that

## Box 2-1    Perianesthesia Practice Settings

- Hospital (Inpatient and Outpatient Units)
  - PACU
  - Ambulatory Surgery Unit
  - Endoscopy Unit
  - Radiology Unit
  - Obstetric Unit
  - Cardiology Unit
  - Oncology Unit
  - Pain Management Unit
  - Special Care Unit
- Surgical Hospital
- Free-standing Ambulatory Surgery Unit
- Recovery Care Center
- Office-based Setting
  - Physician (Medical/Surgical)
  - Dental
  - Plastic Surgery

addresses the core, dimensions, boundaries, and intersections of perianesthesia nursing practice.[1]

The perianesthesia environment can be both challenging and rewarding for nurses who choose to work in this specialty area. Nurses who enjoy a fast pace and unexpected emergencies, balanced with critical independent decision-making skills, thrive in the PACU.

## ORGANIZATIONAL STRUCTURE

One person should be ultimately responsible for the management of the PACU. Typically, this person is the nurse manager, director, supervisor, clinical leader, or head nurse. For the purpose of clarity, this person will be referred to as the nurse manager. The nurse manager is responsible for the administrative control of the PACU and may report directly to the surgical or the anesthesia service, depending on the institution's organizational structure.

## Box 2-2    Scope of Practice: Perianesthesia Nursing

The American Society of PeriAnesthesia Nurses (ASPAN), the professional organization for the specialty of perianesthesia nursing, is responsible for the definition and establishment of the scope of perianesthesia nursing. In doing so, ASPAN recognizes the role of the American Nurses Association (ANA) in defining the scope of practice for the nursing profession as a whole.

ASPAN supports the ANA Social Policy Statement 2003.[1] This statement charges specialty nursing organizations with definition of their individual scope of practice and identification of the characteristics within their unique specialty areas.

Evolving professional and societal demands have necessitated a statement that clarifies the scope of perianesthesia nursing practice. Given rapid changes in health care delivery, trends, and technologies, the task of definition of this scope is complex. This document allows for flexibility in response to emerging issues and technologies in health care delivery and the practice of perianesthesia nursing.

The Scope of Perianesthesia Nursing Practice involves the assessment for, diagnosis of, intervention for, and evaluation of physical or psychosocial problems or risks for problems that may result from the administration of sedation/analgesia or anesthetic agents and techniques. The practice is systematic in nature and includes the nursing process, decision making, analytic and scientific thinking, and inquiry. The unique knowledge base regarding sedation/analgesia and anesthetic agents and techniques, the physiologic and psychologic responses to them, and the vulnerability of the patient subjected to them is coupled with all the principles of age-specific medical-surgical and critical care nursing.

ASPAN has the responsibility to promote cultural sensitivity within the specialty in nursing practice, education, research, and leadership. ASPAN strives to promote an environment in which the perianesthesia nurse can deliver quality care among a diverse population within a multidisciplinary health care team.

This scope of practice includes, but is not limited to:
- Preanesthesia Level of Care
- Preadmission
- Day of Surgery/Procedure
- Postanesthesia Levels of Care
- Phase I
- Phase II
- Extended Observation

The delivery of care includes, but is not limited to, the following environments:
- Hospitals
- Ambulatory Surgery Units or Centers

## Box 2-2   Scope of Practice: Perianesthesia Nursing—cont'd

- Procedure Areas (i.e., Cardiology, ECT, Gastrointestinal (GI)/Endoscopy, Interventional and Diagnostic Radiology, Oncology, Pain Management, etc.)
- Labor and Delivery
- Office-based Settings

This specialty of perianesthesia nursing encompasses the care of the patient and family or significant other along the perianesthesia continuum of care: Preanesthesia, Postanesthesia Phase I, Phase II, and Extended Observation. Characteristics unique to perianesthesia practice are discussed in the next section.

### PREANESTHESIA PHASE
#### Preadmission
The nursing roles in this phase focus on preparation of the patient, family, or significant other physically, psychologically, socioculturally, and spiritually for the experience. Interviewing and assessment techniques are used for identification of potential or actual problems that may result. Education and interventions are initiated for optimization of positive outcomes.

#### Day of Surgery/Procedure
The nursing roles in this phase focus on validation of existing information and completion of preparation of the patient, family, or significant other physically and emotionally for the experience.

#### Postanesthesia Phase I
The nursing roles in this phase focus on provision of postanesthesia nursing care to the patient in the immediate postanesthesia period, for transition to Phase II, the inpatient setting, or an intensive care setting for continued care. Basic life-sustaining needs are of the highest priority. Constant vigilance is necessary during this phase.

#### Postanesthesia Phase II
The nursing roles in this phase focus on preparation of the patient, family, or significant other for care in the home, Extended Observation, or an extended care environment.

#### Extended Observation (formerly known as Phase III)
The nursing roles in this phase focus on the provision of ongoing care for those patients who need extended observation or intervention after discharge from Phase I or Phase II.

Perianesthesia nursing roles include those of patient care, research, administration, management, education, consultation, and advocacy. The specialty practice of perianesthesia nursing is defined through the implementation of specific role functions that are delineated in documents including ASPAN's Perianesthesia Nursing Core Curriculum: Preoperative, Phase I and Phase II PACU Nursing and the Standards of Perianesthesia Nursing Practice.[1] The scope of perianesthesia nursing practice is also regulated by policies and procedures dictated by the hospital or facility, state and federal regulatory agencies, and national accreditation bodies.

Professional behaviors inherent in perianesthesia practice are the acquisition and application of a specialized body of knowledge and skills, accountability and responsibility, communication, autonomy, and collaborative relationships with others. Certification in perianesthesia nursing (Certified Post Anesthesia Nurse [CPAN] and Certified Ambulatory Perianesthesia nurse [CAPA]) is recognized by ASPAN as it validates the defined body of knowledge for perianesthesia nursing practice. Resources to support this defined body of knowledge and nursing practice include ASPAN's Perianesthesia Nursing Core Curriculum: Preoperative, Phase I and Phase II PACU Nursing, Standards of Perianesthesia Nursing Practice, and Competency Based Orientation and Credentialing Program.[1,2]

ASPAN interacts with other professional groups to advance the delivery of quality care. These include but may not be limited to:
- American Association of Colleges of Nursing (AACN)
- American Association of Critical Care Nurses (AACCN)
- American Association of Nurse Anesthetists (AANA)
- American Board of Perianesthesia Nursing Certification (ABPANC)
- American Nurses Association (ANA)

*Continued*

## Box 2-2   Scope of Practice: Perianesthesia Nursing—cont'd

- American Radiological Nurses Association (ARNA)
- American Society of Anesthesiologists (ASA)
- American Society of Pain Management Nurses (ASPMN)
- American Society of Plastic Surgical Nurses (ASPSN)
- Anesthesia Patient Safety Foundation (APSF)
- Association of Women's Health, Obstetric and Neonatal Nurses (AWHONN)
- Association of periOperative Registered Nurses (AORN)
- British Anaesthetic & Recovery Nurses Association (BARNA)
- Federated Ambulatory Surgery Association (FASA)
- National Association of Perianesthesia Nurses of Canada (NAPANC)
- National League for Nursing (NLN)
- National Student Nurses Association (NSNA)
- Nursing Organizations Alliance (NOA)
- Society for Ambulatory Anesthesia (SAMBA)
- Society of Gastroenterology Nurses and Associates (SGNA)
- Society of Office Based Anesthesia (SOBA)

The Perianesthesia Nursing Scope of Practice document defines the specialty practice of perianesthesia nursing. The intent of this document is conceptualization of practice and provision of education to practitioners, educators, researchers, and administrators and information to other health professions, legislators, and the public about perianesthesia nursing's participation in and contribution to health care.

From The American Society of PeriAnesthesia Nurses (ASPAN): *2006-2008 Standards of Perianesthesia Nursing Practice: Scope of Practice Perianesthesia Nursing,* Cherry Hill, NJ, 2006, ASPAN.

The chief of anesthesiology should be the medical director of the PACU. In large institutions, if the chief of anesthesiology cannot fill this role because of other duties, the chief may appoint a designee to this position. The medical director works closely with the nurse manager to develop policies and procedures and to assist with continuing education activities for the nursing staff. The director may also be involved in the development and implementation of continuous quality improvement activities in the unit. Maintenance of a good working relationship between the perianesthesia nurse manager and the medical director of the unit is essential so that areas of concern can be addressed in a collaborative productive fashion.

## STAFFING

### Nurse Manager

As a general rule, each institution identifies the qualifications needed for the nurse manager. The nurse manager should have, at minimum, a baccalaureate degree in nursing and, preferably, a master's degree in nursing or another health-related field, with an emphasis on administration and business. A minimum of 5 years of experience in acute care nursing, with at least 2 of those years in the PACU, is desirable. In addition, the nurse manager should also have previous management experience.

The nurse manager of the PACU should have a strong medical-surgical and perianesthesia background, preferably with critical care experience. The nurse manager should also obtain certification as either a Certified Postanesthesia Nurse (CPAN) or a Certified Ambulatory Perianesthesia nurse (CAPA).[2] Active involvement in ASPAN ensures that the unit is informed about the latest professional developments.[3]

The nurse manager of the PACU is responsible for planning, organizing, implementing, and evaluating the activities of both the nursing staff and the patient care functions. In addition, the manager is responsible for staff scheduling, assignments, performance evaluation, counseling, hiring and firing, educational program coordination (including the development and implementation of a unit-specific orientation program), and the unit budget formulation and monitoring. The nurse manager is also responsible for developing and implementing both standards of care and the unit's quality improvement program and for evaluating and monitoring the effectiveness of the quality improvement program.

The perianesthesia nurse manager needs skills in time management, decision making, organization, financial management, communication, interpersonal relations, and conflict resolution. In addition, the manager should have the ability to negotiate and collaborate with other departments and health care team members.

The nurse manager should also project a positive nursing image.

## Clinical Nurse Specialist

The clinical nurse specialist (CNS) in the PACU can be identified by a number of different titles, including, but not limited to: advanced practice nurse (APN), nurse practitioner, clinical leader, resource nurse, and nurse consultant. For the purpose of this discussion, the nurse in this role is referred to as the CNS.

The CNS usually is a master's prepared nurse. Although currently no graduate perianesthesia nursing curriculum exists, the nurse in this role should posses advanced clinical expertise in perianesthesia nursing.[1] The CNS should be certified in postanesthesia nursing (CPAN) or ambulatory perianesthesia nursing (CAPA). Each institution develops role requirements for the role of the CNS. Examples of activities that may involve the CNS are included in Box 2-3.

Qualifications of the CNS include, but are not limited to, the following: strong leadership skills, clinical expertise in the perianesthesia setting, excellent communication skills, the ability to share knowledge, the ability to work in a collaborative manner with all members of the health care team, the capability to incorporate nursing research into practice, and the ability to multitask.

The CNS works closely with the nurse manager to achieve the mission and goals of the PACU. In addition, the CNS is involved in ensuring the clinical competencies of each perianesthesia nurse as required by The Joint Commission (TJC).

The CNS role should include involvement in quality improvement activities of the PACU.

The CNS can play an important part in the development of an effective monitoring and evaluation program. This nurse is instrumental in implementing corrective action to correct deficiencies and improve patient outcome. Research activities should be ongoing in the PACU. Research can serve to strengthen the identity of perianesthesia nursing as a specialty. The CNS can be invaluable in assisting staff members to develop and implement a research project.

The CNS is also the resource person for clinical problem solving and dissemination of information of an advanced nature. In addition, the CNS can ensure that standards of practice are implemented consistently throughout the organization. As a liaison, the CNS can work closely with units outside the PACU that are involved in patient recovery. These areas include labor and delivery, endoscopy, or special procedure units. The CNS can also be instrumental in collaborating with free-standing ASCs if the hospital is so affiliated.

The role of the CNS is an important one. Through skill and expertise, the CNS can offer support and encouragement to staff members, thereby promoting satisfaction and teamwork in the PACU. These factors ultimately lead to continued individual and professional growth among team members.

## Staff Nurses

Selection of quality nursing personnel for the PACU is of the utmost importance. The nurse manager, in conjunction with the CNS, should establish qualifications for PACU nursing personnel. These qualifications along with required expectations should be written and used in all employment proceedings. This practice tends to preclude, or at least minimize, subsequent problems such as job dissatisfaction, unsatisfactory work performance, and staff turnover and also helps ensure a smoothly functioning PACU.

The following qualifications should be considered in establishment of selection criteria. The nurse who considers employment in the PACU should have an interest in perianesthesia nursing. The nurse must have a solid foundation of the nursing care needed to provide preanesthesia and postanesthesia care to patients[1] and should be committed to providing high-quality individualized patient care. The candidate should also possess exceptional communications skills to communicate in a positive manner with all members of the health care team. The nurse should have the ability to form good working relationships with all members of the health care team and be a positive team player. The perianesthesia nurse should be capable of making intelligent

---

### Box 2-3 Examples of Clinical Nurse Specialist Activities

- Education of PACU clinical staff (RNs, LPNs, UAPs)
- Education of hospital and facility staff who receive patients from the PACU
- Development and implementation of new programs and services
- Development and implementation of patient and family education programs
- Quality improvement activities
- Liaison between management and staff nurses
- Liaison between departments (anesthesia, operating room, surgical units, critical care units)
- Evaluation of clinical staff outside the PACU (e.g., surgical units, critical care units)

independent decisions and initiating appropriate action as necessary and should be willing to accept the responsibility that accompanies working in a critical care unit. The ability to be flexible is of the utmost importance for nurses working in the PACU. In addition, the nurse should also have excellent patient teaching skills. Additional qualities to consider include the ability to coordinate care being rendered by a variety of health care team members and the ability to function effectively in a crisis situation.

The nurse who seeks employment in the PACU should also express an interest in and have the ability to learn the scientific principles and theory underlying patient care and the technologic aspects of perianesthesia nursing. The person should be in good health, dependable, and motivated and should express an intention to stay at least 1 year in the PACU after completing the unit orientation. The orientation and training of a perianesthesia nurse requires significant time, energy, and money. Temporary assignment to the PACU is not worthwhile, except as a student learning experience.

The "cross training" of nurses to the PACU may be a feasible solution in hospitals or facilities where staffing is a concern. The nurse who is cross trained to the PACU should fulfill the required competencies of competent support staff as outlined in Resource 7 of ASPAN's *2006-2008 Standards of Perianesthesia Nursing Practice.*[1]

The PACU nurse should have a baccalaureate degree in nursing[1] and at least 1 year of general medical-surgical nursing. Critical care experience is suggested. The perianesthesia nurse must also be able to adapt to changes in the health care setting. Continuous restructuring and reengineering of hospital practices has led to turmoil in some institutions. Nurses must be able to accept and adapt to the constant changing environment of the future.

Certification by one of the professional nursing associations (Table 2-1) shows commitment to professional excellence and should be considered positively in the selection of perianesthesia nurses. Ideally, candidates for PACU positions who have attained a CPAN or CAPA credential should be given preference in hiring. Commitments to other professional nursing organizations should also help the candidate to be considered for a PACU position.

Certification in basic cardiac life support (BCLS) and advanced cardiac life support (ACLS) is required of all nurses who work in the PACU. For units with a high volume of pediatric patients, certification in pediatric advanced life support (PALS) is also

| Table 2-1 | Certification by Professional Nursing Associations |
|---|---|
| **Professional Association** | **Credential** |
| American Nurses Association | Medical-surgical certification |
| American Association of Critical Care Nurses | CCRN |
| American Society of PeriAnesthesia Nurses | CPAN or CAPA |
| Association of peri-Operative Registered Nurses | CNOR |
| Emergency Nurses Association | CEN |

recommended. Application of BCLS in the PACU or ambulatory surgical unit helps sustain a patient's condition in crisis until ACLS techniques can be instituted. ACLS includes training in dysrhythmia recognition, intravenous infusion, blood gas interpretation, defibrillation, intubation, and emergency drug administration. If the perianesthesia nurse responds quickly and efficiently during crisis situations, the patient's chance of survival increases.

Assignment of nursing personnel to the PACU should be permanent, and staff members should not be routinely rotated to other units. Staffing in the PACU is dependent on volume, patient acuity, patient flow processes, and the physical layout of the unit.[1] Two registered nurses, one of whom is competent in perianesthesia nursing, should be in attendance at all times when a patient is receiving care.[1] Refer to ASPAN's *2006-2008 Standards of Perianesthesia Nursing Practice*, Resource 3, Patient Classification/Recommended Staffing Guidelines, for detailed information concerning staffing requirements for Phase I, Phase II, and Extended Observation.[1]

As previously noted, the PACU should also have a registered nurse who functions in the position of clinical nurse specialist (CNS). The CNS's role encompasses many spectra, including education, direct patient care, quality improvement, research, and consultation. The CNS works closely with all members of the PACU team to assess and provide ongoing support and continuing education to meet the individual staff member needs.

The role of education includes providing or arranging for continuing education of all PACU nursing staff. Support for continuing education activities increases satisfaction within the work environment, promotes stability of staff, and, in turn, decreases turnover in the PACU. Perianesthesia nurses take pride in their competence to deliver safe patient care. Opportunities to broaden and expand the perianesthesia nurse's knowledge base should be fostered. Direct patient care is provided by working individually with staff members to ensure the necessary training, support, and guidance that eventually enables the nurse to function efficiently and competently. This process allows for consistent teaching and evaluation on an individual level.

The ultimate goal of the PACU is delivery of quality patient care. To accomplish this goal, continuous professional nursing judgment is necessary; therefore only professional registered nurses ideally should be assigned patient care.

### Ancillary Personnel

Minimal numbers of ancillary personnel should be assigned to the unit to support the registered nurses. Licensed practical or vocational nurses (LPNs or LVNs) assigned to the PACU are restricted in their roles. A registered nurse must be the primary nursing care provider in the PACU, thereby limiting the role of the practical nurse in the PACU setting to one that does not allow functioning to fullest capacity. Orderlies and nurses' aides could be assigned to the unit to perform technical tasks that are helpful to the nurse. These tasks include restocking supplies; assisting with transfer of patients; and running errands to the laboratory, central supply, or other locations.

The PACU may employ unlicensed assistive personnel (UAP). When working with UAPs, the registered nurse (RN) is responsible for knowing the policies and procedures as set forth by the individual institution. UAPs can be a valuable asset to the PACU, but the RN should remain cognizant of the fact that nursing care cannot be delegated to UAPs. UAPs can assist the nurse by performing nonnursing related tasks. Ultimately, the RN is responsible and accountable for the safe delivery of nursing care. Refer to ASPAN's position statement on Registered Nurse Utilization of UAPs[1] for additional information.

A skilled secretary-clerk is a definite asset to the PACU. A person adept at handling and redirecting the numerous phone calls to the PACU and proficient in clerical duties makes the job of the perianesthesia nurse much easier. The proficient secretary can assist the unit by acting as the liaison to family members. Frequent updates on the status of the patient helps reassure family members that the surgery is progressing as planned. The secretary-clerk

should possess excellent communication skills because this is the person who communicates to a wide spectrum of individuals—from patient and family members to physicians and other health care workers.

Because the patient's first contact is usually with this position, the secretary-clerk must possess exceptional customer service skills. An individual who gives the impression that the patient is the most important contact of the day is certainly the individual wanted on the front line.

### Staffing Patterns

Ideally, staffing patterns are developed based on the acuity of the patients who receive care in the PACU. Managers need to assess the acuity of the patients scheduled and staff accordingly. Historic data can also be used to predict staffing needs. Unfortunately, the operating room schedule and the PACU environment do not follow a predictable path. Unforeseen emergencies infiltrate daily operations, causing even the best-made plans to go awry. Contingency staffing plans in place to deal with such fluctuations is thus the best practice. For example, a contingency plan could include the addition of "on-call" or "per diem" staff members or "cross-trained" nurses from other departments.

The staffing pattern developed for the PACU must include consideration for the length of patient stay, the type of surgical procedures performed, the type of anesthesia administered, and the patient population served. In addition, the skill level of the staff must be considered. According to ASPAN's 2006-2008 *Standards of Perianesthesia Nursing Practice*, two licensed nurses, one of whom is a registered nurse competent in PACU nursing, should be present whenever a patient is recovering in a PACU Phase I or II.[1] Institutions that are unable to meet this ASPAN standard must have a policy that outlines the manner in which services are provided in the PACU and delineate how direct access to emergency assistance is accomplished. Other creative means to meet this standard include patient recovery in an area where additional staff are present, such as the intensive care unit, or the assignment of the operating room staff nurse to remain available during the recovery process.

## BASIC STAFF ORIENTATION PROGRAM

The orientation program for the PACU should be designed to specifically meet the needs of the nurse who works in the PACU. The program should include formal lectures and discussions and informal demonstrations and supervised practice. The orientation program should be structured to include objectives, content, and resources and also include the method used to evaluate the orientee's progress. The orientee should be provided with materials that clearly delineate the structure of the orientation program. The expectations the orientee faces should be absolutely clear to everyone.

Each nurse who undergoes orientation to the PACU should have an individually assigned preceptor. The preceptor works closely with the orientee to ensure individual needs are met and deficiencies are promptly addressed. In addition, anesthesia provider, surgeons, the CNS, and other nurses in the PACU should be involved in the orientation program. Fostering of seasoned nurses to prepare and present short lectures or skill demonstrations not only recognizes the nurse for individual expertise but also displays the manager's confidence in the individual's ability to provide quality patient care. Lectures and presentations should be geared toward the specific needs of the orientee.

Experienced staff members should support and encourage new staff members. Nurses who are made to feel a part of a team are certainly more likely to stay, whereas nurses who are unhappy leave. Orientation of a new staff nurse is costly and time-consuming; therefore, implementation of all possible measures to limit staff turnover is essential. Working to create a stable cohesive staff helps with staff morale. This process begins at orientation.

Objectives should be clearly stated, and methods for evaluation of the achievement of the objectives should be clearly outlined. A notebook of the objectives, resources, evaluation forms, pertinent PACU policies and procedures, and other valuable resources should be given to each orientee. The notebook should be carefully reviewed with each orientee. A clear understanding of objectives and expectations in the beginning avoids problems in the long term.

Traditionally, nursing orientation programs used methods that focused on the new nurse acquiring the knowledge necessary to perform the job but lacked direct application to apply that knowledge. Competency-based orientation focuses on acquiring the knowledge necessary to perform the job and additionally encompasses applying that knowledge to real-life situations. Competency-based orientation is effective because it allows an expert clinician to transfer knowledge and skills to the novice learner. The learner now becomes responsible for the progress and the preceptor facilitates and guides the learner.

## Content of the Orientation Program

The content of the PACU orientation program should include the topics presented in Box 2-4. Additional material, as appropriate to the practice setting, should also be included.

The length of the orientation program should be tailored to meet the individual needs and previous experience of the orientees. Consideration should be given to the expectations placed on the orientees. Will they be expected to perform in a "call" situation at the conclusion of the orientation period, or will an experienced perianesthesia nurse be working with them for an indefinite period? The orientation period should be at least 3 months for nurses without previous PACU experience. During this time, the orientee should work full time. An experienced perianesthesia nurse should complete a 6-week orientation program before placement in the position of functioning without special supervision.

During the orientation period, careful and constant communication must be maintained between the nurse manager, the orientee, and the preceptor. Evaluation by the nurse manager and preceptor should be ongoing, and the orientee should receive a formal written evaluation at the end of the orientation. The orientee should clearly understand the expectations as set forth by the perianesthesia nurse manager, and the orientee and preceptor should discuss progress daily. If issues arise, the manager may need to step in and clearly review progress and expectations with the orientee. In some cases, for various reasons, an orientee may clearly not fit into the perianesthesia environment. In these circumstances, the best solution is to assist the orientee in gaining the required prerequisite skills rather than allowing the orientee to flounder in an environment in which success is not possible.

## DEVELOPMENT OF EXPERTISE

Expertise in nursing involves the overlapping of the following three basic components of nursing: knowledge, skill, and experience. Mastering any one or two of these components never equates with expertise. The expert nurse uses a complex linkage of knowledge, experience, skill, clue identification, gut feelings, logic, and intuition in problem-solving or the nursing process. As the nurse gains knowledge and experience through formal and informal programs, nursing intuition begins to develop. Intuition may be thought of as identification of a deviation from the expected or the feeling that "something just doesn't seem right." Over time, with experience and practice, the nurse becomes proficient. The accumulation

## Box 2-4   Suggested Topics for a PACU Orientation Program

**REVIEW OF THE ANATOMY AND PHYSIOLOGY OF THE CARDIORESPIRATORY SYSTEM**
- Pathophysiologic processes of the cardiorespiratory system
- Factors that alter circulatory or respiratory function after surgery and anesthesia
- Position
- Type of incision
- Medication
- Blood loss and replacement; intake and output
- Anesthetic agent used
- Type of operative procedure
- Monitoring techniques
- Hemodynamic monitoring
- Pulse oximetry
- Cardiac dysrhythmias
- Identification and treatment
- ACLS or PALS certification
- Airway maintenance, equipment, and techniques, pharmacologic and nonpharmacologic
  - Evaluation of treatment
  - Techniques for maintenance of a patent airway
  - Administration of oxygen
  - Use of suction equipment
- Ventilatory support, equipment, and procedures
  - Ambu bag
  - Airway insertion
- Cardiorespiratory arrest and its management
  - Use of monitor-defibrillator
  - Emergency medications
- Pain management
  - Assessment of patient's pain level in all age groups
  - Use of pain scales
  - Documentation of pain level
  - Treatment methods, including patient education
- Treatment of hypotension or hypertension
- Interpretation of laboratory values
- Identification and treatment of malignant hyperthermia

**REVIEW OF OTHER PHYSIOLOGIC CONSIDERATIONS IN THE PACU**
- Neurologic system
- Musculoskeletal system
- Genitourinary system
  - Fluid and electrolyte balance
  - Fluid and electrolyte imbalance
- Gastrointestinal system
- Integumentary system
  - Identification of risk factors
  - Preventive measures

- Pediatric-adolescent physiology
  - Age-specific competencies
  - Patient education strategies
- Geriatric physiology
  - Age-specific competencies
  - Patient education strategies
- Physiology of pregnancy

**ANESTHESIA**
- Administration and properties of selected agents (include all agents routinely used in the institution)
  - Intravenous agents
  - Muscle relaxants
  - Conduction anesthesia
  - Reversal agents
- Intravenous conscious sedation (IVCS)
  - Policies and procedures
  - Medications used
- Nursing implications

**CARE OF THE PATIENT IN THE PACU**
- Preoperative preparation
  - Physical assessment
  - Implementation of comfort measures
  - Nursing interventions to decrease anxiety
- Consent (surgical and anesthesia)
- Intravenous insertion
- Correct site policy (facility specific)
- Postoperative care
  - Physical assessment of the patient after surgery
  - General PACU care
    - Psychologic considerations
    - Anxiety
    - Coping responses
- The stir-up regimen
- Intravenous therapy and blood transfusion
- Infection control
  - Universal precautions
  - Occupational Safety and Health Administration regulations
- General comfort and safety measures
- Specific care needed after surgical procedures
  - Ear, nose, and throat surgery
  - Ocular surgery
  - Cardiothoracic surgery
  - Neurosurgery
  - Orthopedic surgery
  - Genitourinary surgery
  - Gastrointestinal surgery
  - Gynecologic and obstetric surgery
  - Plastic surgery
  - Vascular surgery

*Continued*

---

**Box 2-4   Suggested Topics for a PACU Orientation Program—cont'd**

**CARE OF THE PATIENT IN THE PACU—cont'd**
- Special considerations for the pediatric-adolescent patient
- Special procedures, such as ECT and pain blocks
- Postoperative medications
  - Pain control medications (intravenous, intramuscular, oral, epidural, patient-controlled analgesia, and pain pumps)
  - Age-dependent assessment measures
  - Numeric, visual analog, or faces scale
  - Antiemetics
  - Others (antihypertensives, antiarrhythmics)
- Patient and family teaching
  - Preprocedure
  - Postprocedure
- Thermoregulation
  - Hypothermia
  - Hyperthermia (malignant hyperthermia)
- Department specifics
  - Layout
  - Policies and procedures
  - Preparation of patient units
- Documentation
  - Policies and procedures
  - Electronic charting
- Orientation program
  - Goals and expectations
  - Performance evaluation
  - Competency assessment

---

of knowledge, along with the chance to practice the skills acquired, leads to competence.

Once the nurse finishes the formal PACU orientation program, the nurse should work continuously on improving background theory and skills. This improvement may be accomplished with active participation in on-the-job training, nursing inservice programs presented on the unit, outside reading, membership in ASPAN and other state and local professional nursing organizations, and attendance at both in-house and outside-sponsored seminars and educational offerings. Constant review of basic knowledge and procedures is essential. Keeping abreast of new scientific information and innovations is necessary to ensure quality care.

Once the orientee has worked in the perianesthesia environment for at least a year and believes that sufficient knowledge and experience have been gained, certification as a CPAN or CAPA should be considered. Certification is one method of promoting to consumers and peers that the quality of services they receive is enhanced because the nurses caring for them attained either a CPAN or CAPA credential.

Inclusion of funds in budgeting to send nurses to important educational and information-sharing meetings for the unit is essential. An investment made to stimulate the professional development of the nursing staff is directly reflected in the level of nursing care provided to the patient.

## COMPETENCY ASSESSMENT

Once the orientation period has ended, the assurance that staff members remain competent is essential. Integration of a competency checklist with the annual performance evaluation is one method to ensure competency. Assessment of competency on an annual basis provides a number of benefits. Staff members are forced to review procedures and equipment that may not be routinely used.

Assessment of competency can be divided into two aspects. The first aspect of staff competence assessment relates to policies and procedures and could include facility standards and national standards as set forth by organizations such as ASPAN. Some competencies that managers may want to address include, but are not limited to, the following:
- Unit-specific administrative policies and procedures
- Patient confidentiality and patient rights
- Fire safety and patient safety issues, including The Joint Commission's National Patient Safety Goals[4]
- Environment of care issues
- Infection control practices
- Thermoregulation, including hypothermia[1] and hyperthermia
- Variance/occurrence reporting
- Compliance policies
- Medications commonly administered in the practice setting, including intravenous conscious sedation, anesthetic agents, antiemetics, and analgesics
- Age-specific competencies (pediatric, adolescent, adult, geriatric)

A complete list of Recommended Competencies for the Perianesthesia Nurse can be found in ASPAN's 2006-2008 *Standards of Perianesthesia Nursing Practice*.[1]

The second aspect of assessment of staff competence relates to equipment. Evaluation of staff members is essential to ensure their skills and knowledge in the operation of and caring for equipment used in the practice setting is proficient. Specific equipment competencies include, but are not limited to, the following:

- Monitors, including electrocardiography (EKG), pulse oximetry, and noninvasive blood pressure
- Defibrillator (defibrillation, cardioversion, external pacing)
- Warming devices
- Infusion pumps
- Ventilators

Managers should develop processes to assess the previously named activities. For assessment of equipment competence, employees must be able to appropriately demonstrate proper use of the specific piece of equipment. For assessment of competence of policies and procedures, unit-specific tests can be developed.

In an effort to streamline processes, assessment of competence of the new orientee and of senior staff members should follow the same path. Competency assessment methods differ. The new orientee may be required to demonstrate the step-by-step process of defibrillation and to verbalize the rationale for each step. In contrast, the seasoned nurse may be required to just demonstrate the process.

Incorporation of competency assessments into monthly staff meetings may also be helpful. One method is the assignment of a staff member to present a short inservice on a specific piece of equipment or a specific policy to the staff. Competence can then be assessed with a follow-up posttest or return demonstration from the staff. Documentation can either be a checklist that outlines the step-by-step return demonstration or the posttest that is filed in employee personnel files to document competence in the specific skill.

Quality management and improvement activities may uncover a specific deficiency. In this instance, development of a program to educate staff on the proper skills needed is important. After completion of the education, the nurse manager can follow up with a competency assessment of the problem-prone activity.

Perianesthesia nursing is unique in that the nurse has only a small amount of time to assess the patient, identify a plan of care, implement the plan, and then evaluate the effectiveness of the plan before care is turned over to someone else, be it another nursing professional, a family member, or simply the patient. The skill and expertise needed to provide quality care in the fast-paced environment takes time to obtain. Nurses who are motivated to learn, like a fast-paced environment, and work well in teams enjoy the challenges of the PACU work environment.

## THE PACU WORK ENVIRONMENT

The PACU work environment is a complex one. Patient care activities can range from simple recovery after local anesthesia to complicated assessment and planning for the patient in critical condition. In addition, the PACU is generally set up as an open unit with limited division between patients. Inherent in the system is the need for nurses to work together as a cohesive team.

Unification of the PACU team is challenging to say the least. Factors that can influence the ability of the team to work together include the generation gap, the aging workforce, and each individual team member's ability to deal with stress and burnout.

## THE GENERATION GAP

Discovery of individuals from two, three, or even four different generations in the work force today is unsurprising. A good manager understands that reaching each generation may require a different approach. Learning how to approach the diverse workforce is key to a successful and cohesive unit. Gerke[5] describes the diversity of the four different generations in Table 2-2. Imagine the chaos that can erupt when individuals from four different generations are placed in an environment where they must work together.

The traditional, mature, veteran, GI, or silent generation, as it has been called, is the older generation. These individuals grew up in a time when the world was at war. They lived through the Depression and experienced hard times. They are usually hard working, dedicated, and loyal in their values. They possess a wealth of knowledge. The traditional generation of workers commonly respect authority and believe that rewards need to be earned. In the work force, they prefer to be managed in a hierarchical fashion. They respect titles and rank and believe that sacrifice and hard work are rewarded.[5]

The Baby Boomers are a competitive lot. Known as boomers or the sandwich generation, this group grew up in a time of educational and economic growth. As a result, they sought to find a solution to any problem they encountered. The fast-paced environment to which they are accustomed led to many inventions that accommodate their lifestyle. They often place a high value on materialism and are not opposed to working long hours to get what they want.

**Table 2-2   Generational Diversity**

| | Mature (1922-1943) | Baby Boomers (1943-1960) | Generation X (1960-1980) | Nexters (1980-2000) |
|---|---|---|---|---|
| How many? | 52 million | 73.2 million | 70.1 million | 69.7 million |
| Popular names used for generations | Traditionalist<br>GIs<br>Mature<br>WWII generation<br>Silent generation<br>Seniors | Baby Boomers<br>Sandwich generation | Xers<br>Twenty-somethings<br>Latchkey kids | Millenials<br>Generation Y<br>Generation 2001<br>Nintendo generation<br>Generation Net<br>Internet generation<br>Dotcom generation<br>Generation "why" |
| Defining events | Great Depression<br>WWII<br>Korean War<br>Radio<br>Rise of labor unions<br>Family<br>Patriotism | Prosperity<br>Civil rights movement<br>Women's liberation<br>Vietnam<br>Television<br>Space race<br>Assassination of John F.<br>  Kennedy and Martin Luther<br>  King, Jr<br>Cold War<br>Suburbia<br>Birth control pill<br>Cuban missile crisis | *Watergate, Nixon resigns*<br>Single-parent homes<br>AIDS<br>Computers<br>Challenger disaster<br>Fall of Berlin Wall<br>Persian Gulf War<br>Exxon Valdez oil spill | New millennium<br>Computers<br>School violence<br>Columbine High School<br>Oklahoma City bombing<br>"It takes a village"<br>Girl's movement<br>Multiculturalism<br>2000 Political race<br>Stock market decline<br>September 11, 2001<br>War in Iraq |
| Core values | Hard work<br>Dedication<br>Loyalty<br>Detail-oriented<br>Conformity<br>Law and order<br>Respect for<br>  authority | Optimism<br>Team orientation<br>Personal gratification<br>Health and wellness<br>Personal growth<br>Youth<br>Work<br>Involvement | Diversity<br>Thinking globally<br>Balance<br>Technoliteracy<br>Fun<br>Informality<br>Self reliance<br>Pragmatism | Optimism<br>Civic duty<br>Confidence<br>Achievement<br>Sociability<br>Morality<br>Street smarts<br>Diversity |

| | | | | |
|---|---|---|---|---|
| | Delayed reward<br>Duty<br>Adherence to rules<br>Honor<br>Status quo<br>Focus on family, country, others | Struggle with change<br>Seeking to find internal meaning<br>Struggle with self awareness<br>Materialistic | Embrace change<br>Free time<br>Embrace self awareness<br>Ecologic awareness<br>Materialism not a driving factor | Change masters<br>Faster, faster |
| Education | Institutions<br>Majority grade school or high school graduates | Institutions<br>Majority high school graduates, increase in college graduates<br>Time to graduate, 4.5 years<br>SAT scores in 1965, 969<br>Major: English literature, psychology, and sociology | Institutions blended with virtual media<br>Majority college graduates<br>Time to graduate from college, 5.8 years<br>SAT scores in 1990, 900<br>Major: business and computer science | Multimedia in institutions, computer-based learning<br>Lifelong learning |
| Work | Hierarchy<br>Seniority rules<br>Male breadwinner<br>Lifetime career or profession<br>Low risk takers<br>Diversity threatening<br>Externally motivated<br>Labor unions<br>Majority full-time workers<br>Honest day of work for honest day of pay<br>Grateful for a job<br>Large teams<br>Retirement age, 62 to 64 years | Shared leadership often just lip service<br>Value long-term employee<br>Increase of women in management and full-time workers<br>Second career after age 50 years<br>Struggle with diversity<br>Want wealth today<br>Tested on the job<br>Job defines them<br>50-hour to 60-hour weeks<br>Many have two jobs<br>Benefit packages<br>Struggle with pleasing the boss and pleasing self<br>Commune-size teams<br>Pension plans<br>Retirement age, 65 to 67 years | Responsive competitive teams<br>Virtual teams<br>Brutally honest<br>Equal male and female workers and managers<br>Working at home, virtually<br>Decrease in unemployment<br>Work is just a job<br>Do not want to work more than 40 hours a week<br>Want flexible hours<br>Multitasking<br>Parallel processing<br>Technology wizards<br>Retirement age, 67 to 70 years<br>Increase in volunteers<br>Multiple careers in a lifetime | Civic-minded teams<br>Increase technologic conferencing<br>50% work from home<br>Low unemployment<br>8 careers in a lifetime<br>Resilient<br>Teamwork ethic<br>Can-do attitude<br>Technologically savvy<br>Expect to work 50 hours<br>Confidence in the establishment<br>High productivity<br>Collective consensus driven<br>Demand pay equity<br>Will reestablish the middle class<br>Will change the spirit from for-profit to not-for profit sector<br>Retirement after 70 years of age |

*Continued*

**Table 2-2  Generational Diversity—cont'd**

| | Mature (1922-1943) | Baby Boomers (1943-1960) | Generation X (1960-1980) | Nexters (1980-2000) |
|---|---|---|---|---|
| View of authority | Distance between boss and worker | Untrustworthy<br>Not credible unless they are boss<br>Love/hate | Disdain authority<br>Refuse to pay dues<br>Demand competent managers<br>Unimpressed | Trust in centralized authority<br>Will downgrade CEO and executive salaries<br>Polite |
| Rewards and recognition | Valued, to be earned | Valued, deserved | Valued, demand | Inclusively valued |
| Preferred leadership | Hierarchy | Consensus | Competence | Pulling together |
| Work ethic | Dedicated | Driven | Balanced | Determined |

Adapted from Gerke ML: Understanding and leading the quad matrix: four generations in the workplace: the traditional generation, boomers, gen-x, nexters, *Semin Nurse Manag* 9(3):173–181, 2001.

The Baby Boomers often do not trust those in power. Instead, they choose to have a love-hate relationship with the boss and sometimes would like it even better if they were the boss.

Individuals of generation X, also known as Xers, twenty-somethings, baby busters, or post-boomers, were the latchkey kids who grew up fending for themselves. This group adapts easily to change. Members of generation X cause chaos in the workplace because, in addition to showing their feelings upfront, they often want flexible hours and do not want to work more than 40 hours a week. They are also the group that is most likely to have no problem doing 10 things at once. They embrace the technologic advances presented to them. What they achieve in technologic know-how, they may lack in people skills. They work hard, and they want to see that hard work pay off immediately. Xers want to advance their career now. If that means they need to change jobs to advance, they do, and they do not waste time thinking twice about it. As children, this generation watched their parents work long hours in search of success. This generation seeks employment opportunities where they can find a balance between work and home life. Generation Xers do not feel loyalty to one employer and seek different opportunities in search of money and job satisfaction. Because of this, they are often looked on as disloyal and uncommitted, when in fact they are loyal to their profession but unwilling to sacrifice their personal life for success.[5]

The nexters, generation Y, generation next, millennial generation, and net generation, as they are known, often are the most educated group of individuals. They have been bombarded with learning since they were born. They are not afraid of technology and in fact have never known life without it. They communicate via the Internet, cell phones, text messaging, and e-mail.[5] This group of individuals seeks out educational opportunities because they consider learning a lifetime endeavor.

So what happens when staff members from two, three, or even four of these generations are required to work together as a team? The different values that each brings to the group are sure to cause conflict, yet when each group is nurtured appropriately, the end result of a cohesive team is not unrealistic. Creative ways to meld the group are sure to be each manager's challenge. Bridging the generation gap requires creative thinking on the manager's part.

The traditional group has a wealth of knowledge and experience to bring to the group. Uncovering ways that allow the veterans to share their expertise is key. Their knowledge can be channeled into inservice educational programs, preceptorships, and development of staff competencies. The traditional group operates in the "old-fashioned" mode. Common courtesies of "please" and "thank you" are important to remember in communications with this group. A written note of appreciation to the traditional member of the team goes a long way.

The Baby Boomers should also be valued for their knowledge and experience. Sometimes, unlike the traditionals, they live in a competitive environment. The Baby Boomers serve well as preceptors and educators. They also tend to like recognition for their accomplishments in a more public way. Achievements such as certifications should be published in the organization's newsletter. Baby Boomers like to be in the spotlight and receive recognition for their accomplishments.

Generation Xers may have lived their early years with only one parent. They are in search of parental figures, and the traditional and Baby Boomers can fit well into this role. This group of individuals likes to control their own destinies. Managers do well if they just present the task to be accomplished and let the individual establish the means to accomplish the end goal. The generation Xers typically do not do well with politics in the work place. They also want to work in a positive happy environment.

The nexters thrive on new learning opportunities. Traditional nursing focused on one area of expertise, whether medical, surgical, or intensive care nursing. This group wants to learn it all. The nurse manager can establish opportunities for this group to expand their knowledge base by allowing them to attend conferences and seminars. They can also be invaluable in assisting nurses of the older generations with computers and other technologic equipment.

Creation of a work environment where all employees work together in harmony takes a great deal of work on the manager's part. Managers need to embrace this concept and use strategies to build a work place in which all team members work in unity. Recognition and appreciation of the differences that each generation brings to the workplace can assist in decreasing tension and building a harmonious work environment.[6] The key is finding ways in which members from all the groups can work together and accept each other for what they are without trying to change each other's beliefs. Young nurses need to be aware that voicing their opinions may be looked on as disrespectful from older nurses. On the other hand, the older nurses need to realize that when given the chance, younger nurses may have something valuable to contribute to the work environment.[5]

When nurses from the different generations work together, an opportunity exists to explore new and different ways to do things. The challenge is getting nurses to acknowledge and appreciate each other's differences.[5] Realistically, no work place is always free of strife, but it certainly can be a place where conflict and low morale surface only on rare occasions.

## AGING NURSING POPULATION

Unsurprisingly, the average age of a nurse is approximately 45 years.[6] New career opportunities are steering prospective nurses toward what are seen as more appealing career paths. Seasoned nurses need to reexamine their views of their own profession and begin encouraging others to enter the field. After all, who will take care of this aging population if no new recruits join the field?

As the average age of a nurse increases, managers need to begin to find ways to accommodate staff members so they do not leave the profession. Many seasoned nurses feel they have "paid their dues" and do not want to work the "off shifts" or be "on-call" any longer. Physically, they are getting tired.

Creative managers develop mechanisms to keep this group in the work force. We can no longer afford to let their experience and expertise be tossed aside. Flexible staffing schedules for these individuals can be considered. Job sharing and split shifts are other possibilities. If the individual tires easily because the environment is too fast paced, another valued position in the department can be considered. Can the nurse perform the required quality monitoring activities that no one ever seems to have time to do? What about precepting that new nurse? Or developing required competency assessment of staff? Granted, enough of these positions may not be found for all the staff members, but creativity in addressing this issue certainly impacts retention.

Although the method may not be popular among younger nurses, another creative way to promote retention of older nurses is elimination of the "on-call" requirement. Policies can be established to delineate the number of years of service to the unit and the minimum age the nurse must be to be excused of taking call. This policy could be a win-win situation in a unit where younger nurses are motivated to take additional call for monetary reasons whereas the older nurse is more established in life. Creativity should not be overlooked when establishing policies. Perhaps instead of the total elimination of call for the older nurses, a reduced call policy is implemented. In this scenario, for example, in a unit where call is required one night a week, the senior nurse may only be required to take call one night every other week. An astute manager works with the nursing staff to brainstorm ideas and implement policies that not only meet the needs of the unit but at the same time assist in retention of senior nurses.

The perianesthesia arena has been fortunate in that many nurses want to transfer into this specialty. Many critical care nurses in need of a change frequently transfer into the specialty, with the expection that the perianesthesia unit is slow paced, which could not be farther from the truth. The PACU is not the place to transfer as one winds down one's career. In fact, many nurses, regardless of age, find the pace to be harried. Prioritization and good organizational skills are essential to avoid an overwhelmed feeling. The current administrative strategy of use of the PACU as a "dumping ground" when no beds are available in the hospital's emergency department, critical care unit, or surgical unit is also an issue that impacts staff morale. When morale is low, staff retention becomes even more difficult.

Managers need to seek out those factors that keep the older work force employed. Is it shorter hours or a more flexible schedule? Better lighting so that they can see? More ergonomically correct furniture? Better health care benefits? Whatever those factors are, methods to meet these needs should be investigated and implemented if at all possible.

The continued employment of the aging work force is key to the future of this specialty. Sharing the knowledge, experience, expertise, and wisdom that one has garnered over the years is crucial to the future of perianesthesia nursing.

## STRESS AND BURNOUT IN THE PERIANESTHESIA NURSE

Stress is a word that is often too familiar to the perianesthesia nurse. Stress occurs when forces from the outside world affect the individual.[7] Stress is the body's response to any demand, whether the demand is caused by or results in a pleasant or an unpleasant condition.

Stress can be either positive or negative (i.e., good or bad). The body responds to good or bad stress in essentially the same physiologic manner. The difference between the two responses is the body's ability to relax after the stress is encountered. Left untreated, stress can act as a negative force that, in turn, can lead to physical ailments. Many adaptive methods are available to assist people who are dealing with stress. The real challenge, however, is successful employment of these adaptive measures.

Development of the ability to deal with daily stressors is essential, but before daily stress can be dealt with, one must first be able to recognize it. Stress can manifest itself differently in each person. Recognition of one's own individual response to stress is essential. Learning to recognize the individual message the body sends is a first step. Do you feel tightness in your chest? Heart palpitations? A nervous feeling in your gut? Something click in your head? Recognition of stress early is of benefit in the long term because early detection makes stress easier to manage.

### Stress in the Perianesthesia Setting

Behavioral symptoms of stress are exhibited in a number of ways (Box 2-5). When several people in the PACU exhibit symptoms of burnout, the unit is faced with problems such as low morale, interpersonal conflict, decreased productivity, and lack of teamwork.

Too often, individual coping methods for dealing with stress can have the reverse effect. Use of drugs, pain medications, or alcohol or smoking or eating can worsen the stress and make the individual more reactive to further stress.[8]

In the perianesthesia setting, burnout may result from the lack of positive feedback received from patients who do not remember the nurse who took care of them. In the inpatient setting, the perianesthesia nurse rarely has the opportunity to see the positive results of care unless postoperative visits are a part of the PACU routine. Positive reinforcement by peers and the manager aids in building self esteem for the perianesthesia nurse. Perianesthesia nurses must learn to take care of themselves as well as they care for their patients. We as caregivers must be able to care for ourselves first if we are to remain productive.

Perianesthesia nurses are susceptible to burnout and experience many of the same frustrations as other nurses. In the past, the incidence rate of burnout in the PACU was low. The reasons for this low rate have not been fully explained, but the regular hours and the social support gleaned from the close relationships developed with the entire surgical team seem to assist in the prevention of burnout. Presently, nurses in the perianesthesia setting are under increasing stress. Perianesthesia nurses are mandated to work long hours and extra shifts, many times to care for patients in the PACU who cannot be transferred to a hospital bed. The PACU is becoming a holding unit when no beds are available or nursing staff is insufficient to care for the patient on the nursing units. These same nurses are "called in" to staff the PACU for an entire shift and then are needed to work their designated shifts. Therefore, the nurses' feelings of being overworked and underappreciated are understandable. In these situations, the feelings of abuse do not take long to surface as stress, burnout, and resentment.

Managers need to be tuned in to how the staff is feeling. When stress is a factor, how does one deal with it at work, at home, and in everyday life? The nurse manager plays an important role in dealing with a staff that is overworked, understaffed, and stressed for any number of reasons. The manager must be able to offer support and guidance to nursing staff members so that they are better able to deal with the numerous stressful situations they face every day.

The manager should reassure staff members that their concerns are legitimate (when they are). Listening to staff concerns with an active ear can also assist staff nurses to deal with their own frustrations. Sometimes, just the ability to vent concerns helps the situation. Managers should offer possible solutions to problems.

In some instances, rewarding the staff for their efforts can assist in increasing morale. Rewards do not necessarily have to be monetary. Examples of simple yet effective rewards include:

- Handwritten notes from the manager that acknowledge the staff member's hard work
- Small gifts such as a fragrant hand lotion or lip moisturizer
- Provision of coverage so the nurse can attend a child's or grandchild's school play
- Approval for the nurse to attend an outside conference or workshop
- Supply of the ingredients for ice cream sundaes for the unit

Rewards do not necessarily need to come from the manager. In a cohesive team, any team member may surprise colleagues with something special. Accepting each other's differences yet working cohesively is the key.

| Box 2-5    **Behavioral Symptoms of Stress** |
| --- |

Temper outbursts
Restlessness
Impatience
Forgetfulness
Boredom
Mood swings
Difficulty with concentration

| Box 2-6    Causes of Stress in the PACU |
|---|
| Understaffing<br>Critical patients<br>Changes in policies<br>Working overtime<br>Lack of sleep<br>Additional responsibilities |

As stated previously, stress in the PACU can be caused by a number of factors (Box 2-6). Understaffing, critical patients, changes in policies, working overtime, lack of sleep, and additional responsibilities all contribute to stress. How does the perianesthesia nurse deal with the continuous evolution of change in the workplace? The perianesthesia nurse must first recognize the existence of the problem. Once this has been accomplished, the nurse can take three possible directions: (1) eliminate the stress; (2) resist or minimize the stress; or (3) accept the stress.

Elimination of the stress sometimes seems like the best way to go and eliminates the need to face the problem. However, total elimination of the stress factor is not always possible. In circumstances in which the stress can be totally removed, the nurse may face undesirable consequences as a result of the elimination. For example, if working with a certain physician causes a great deal of stress, switching assignments with another nurse may be possible. The two nurses may be able to come to an agreement that one cares for all of Dr X's patients if the other cares for all of Dr Y's. Each nurse individually must weigh the consequences of always caring for Dr X's patients. On the other hand, if the consequence is of no concern to the nurse, then elimination of the stressor through this option is the way to achieve the ultimate goal of avoidance of Dr Y. One must also consider that in reality the day may come when the nurse will have to care for Dr Y's patients, which is especially true in a setting in which nurses are called in for emergencies.

The second approach is to minimize the stress element. Is reduction of the stress factor possible so that its effect becomes minimal? Does acceptance of the responsibility to preceptor yet another staff nurse push a senior nurse over the edge? The nurse may already be in the process of orienting two new staff members. As much as the nurse may enjoy this process, the nurse may have to decline. The level of energy needed to be a preceptor is high. In this instance, refusal of the assignment is possibly the alternative to choose. With choices that ultimately affect well being, guilt should not be the deciding factor. Nurses tend to feel guilty when they make unpopular decisions. Overcoming the feeling of guilt is essential if true acceptance of the decision is expected.

Another part of stress reduction is to set priorities. The ability to look at one's current responsibilities and honestly assess what is important to accomplish at a particular time is a necessary step in stress reduction. Whenever possible, one should avoid procrastinating about tasks that are disliked but must be completed. Sometimes, getting the "dislikes" out of the way first allows for thorough enjoyment of the work that remains. For the older generations of nurses, changing from a paper documentation system to an electronic form may be a huge stressor. Offers of support and encouragement, and ample time for learning the new electronic system, are crucial. At the same time, pairing the veteran nurse with a nexter who has the patience and ability to teach can prove to be a valuable experience for both. The veteran nurse gains experience and the nexter feels a contribution to knowledge and expertise.

The third approach to dealing with stress is acceptance. Some stress factors cannot be alleviated and must be accepted. These include realities such as divorce, death, or resignation of a favorite peer or manager. Although these events are difficult to manage, accepting them and moving ahead is one way to handle the stress. With management of the stressors that cannot be eliminated, the nurse is able to achieve the goal of final acceptance.

Perianesthesia nurses must take time out to reward themselves and set aside time for their personal needs. Too often nurses are absorbed in everyday activities and are quick to give helpful advice to others yet neglect to follow their own advice. For example, nurses should set aside 30 minutes three times a week for exercise. Nurses do not need to be world-class athletes, but a brisk 30-minute walk three times a week is certainly in order. Nurses should also take time to work on their favorite hobby or craft or engage in another enjoyable activity, such as sports, cross stitching, or sewing. They should set aside some time to read that bestseller they have been saving. Relaxation is an important element necessary to successfully reduce stress. Time should be taken to enjoy free time. Every spare moment should not be filled with work. The best way to relax may be to just do nothing.

Activities such as bicycling, hiking, and swimming are also ways to reduce stress.

When the body is physically fit, it is better able to handle stress. Nurses should also eat well and get plenty of rest. Nutrition plays an important part in maintenance of a healthy lifestyle; avoidance of sugar, salt, caffeine, and alcohol is important. Eating well is essential for health maintenance, which, in turn, assists the body in dealing with stress. Rest is vital for the rejuvenation of body cells.

Managing stress is important for the perianesthesia nurse. Once the nurse has identified the stressors in life, they require conscious responses. Eliminating, minimizing, and accepting the different stressors allow the opportunity to experience a more productive and enjoyable life.

## SUMMARY

What makes perianesthesia nurses so special? The answer is the ability to blend expert clinical knowledge that is based on experience, education, and collegial sharing with caring practices that come from within and from being a nurse. This special ability to provide the highest level of quality care with the minimal amount of resources gives perianesthesia nurses pride.

The specialty of perianesthesia nursing is a little more than two decades in age. Perianesthesia nurses have expanded their roles to include all phases of postanesthesia care, from preadmission to discharge. Perianesthesia nurses work in a myriad of settings that include high-level trauma hospitals, ambulatory surgery centers, preadmission holding units, physician offices, and dental offices. The future will bring even more challenges for this specialty as we continue to face reforms in healthcare delivery. The perianesthesia nurse must be flexible enough to handle competently and efficiently whatever situations arise to allow the specialty of postanesthesia nursing to survive. The "specialness" of perianesthesia nursing will continue to develop and flourish as each individual nurse strives to gain that special expertise prevalent in PACUs across the country.

## REFERENCES

1. American Society of PeriAnesthesia Nurses: *2006–2008 Standards of perianesthesia, nursing practice*, Cherry Hill, NJ, 2006.
2. American Board of Perianesthesia Nursing Certification, available at www.cpancapa.org.
3. American Society of PeriAnesthesia Nurses, available at www.aspan.org.
4. The Joint Commission (TJC), available at www.jointcommission.org/patientsafety/nationalpatientsafetygoals/npsg_intro.htm, accessed January 17, 2007.
5. Gerke ML: Understanding and leading the quad matrix: four generations in the workplace: the traditional generation, boomers, gen-X, nexters, *Semin Nurs Manag* 9(3):173-181, 2001.
6. Weston MJ: Integrating generational perspectives in nursing, *OJIN Online J Issues Nursing* 11(2), 2006, available at www.nursingworld.org/ojin/topic30/tpc30_1.htm, accessed January 12, 2007.
7. *Stress*, available at www.medicinenet.com/stress/htm, accessed January 29, 2007.
8. McHaney DF, Varner J: Accommodating the needs of the registered nurse workforce, *Ala Nurse* 33(3):24-25, 2006.

## BIBLIOGRAPHY

American Society of PeriAnesthesia Nurses: *Competency-based orientation credentialing program manual, 2002 edition*, Cherry Hill, NJ, 2002, The Society.

Aps C: Postoperative critical care: overnight intensive recovery, *Br J Anaesth* 89(2):344, 2002.

Bahlman DT, Johnson FC: Using technology to improve and support communication and workflow processes, *AORN J* 82(1):65-73, 2005.

Bethune G, Sherrod D, Youngblood L: 101 tips to retain a happy, healthy staff, *Nurs Management* 36(4):24-29, 2005.

Boychuk Duchscher JE, Cowin L: Multigenerational nurses in the workplace, *J Nurse Admin* 34(11):493-501, 2004.

Carayon P, Gurses AP: A human factors engineering conceptual framework of nursing workload and patient safety in intensive care units, *Intensive Crit Care Nurs* 21(5):284-301, 2005.

Cioffi C: Nurses' experiences of caring for culturally diverse patients in an acute care setting, *Contemp Nurse* 20(1):78-86, 2005.

Clausing SL, Kurtz DL, Prendeville J, et al: Generational diversity: the Nexters, *AORN J* 78(3):373-379, 2003.

Cohen JD: The aging nursing workforce: how to retain experienced nurses, *J Healthcare Management* 51(4):233-245, 2006.

Cutilli CC: Do your patients understand? Providing culturally congruent patient education, *Orthop Nurs* 25(3):218-224, 2006.

Deleskey K: Factors affecting nurses' decisions to join and maintain membership in professional associations, *J Perianesth Nurs* 18(1):8-17, 2003.

Dexter F, Epstein RH, Penning DH: Statistical analysis of postanesthesia care unit staffing at a surgical suite with frequent delays in admission from the operating room: a case study, *Anesth Anal* 92(4):947-949, 2001.

Dexter F, Wachtel RE, Epstein RH: Impact of average patient acuity on staffing of the Phase I PACU, *J Perianesth Nurs* 21(5):303-310, 2006.

Ellison DJ: A guideline for incorporating holistic nursing interventions into perianesthesia practice, *J Perianesth Nurs* 20(1):19-22, 2005.

Fields M, Zwisler S: Guiding across the generations: rediscovering nursing's promise, *Semin Nurse Management* 9(3):154-156, 2001.

Force MV: The relationship between effective nurse managers and nursing retention, *J Nurs Admin* 35(7-8):336-341, 2005.

Galanti GA: Applying cultural competence to perianesthesia nursing, *J Perianesth Nurs* 21(2):97-102, 2006.

Glover DE, Newkirk LE, Cole LM, et al: Perioperative clinical nurse specialist role delineation: a systematic review, *AORN J* 84(6):1017-1030, 2006.

Harrington L: Program development: role of the clinical nurse specialist in implementing a fast-track postanesthesia care unit, *AACN Clin Issues* 16(1):78-88, 2005.

Hart SM: Generational diversity: impact on recruitment and retention of registered nurses, *J Nurs Adm* 36(1):10-12, 2006.

Hayhurst A, Saylor C, Stuenkel D: Work environmental factors and retention of nurses, *J Nurs Care Qual* 20(3):283-288, 2005.

Hu J, Herrick C, Hodgin KA: Managing the multigenerational nursing team, *Health Care Manag (Frederick)* 23(4):334-340, 2004.

Humphreys S: Patient autonomy: legal and ethical issues in the postanesthetic care unit, *Br J Perioper Nurs* 15(1):35-43, 2005.

Iacono MV: Perianesthesia nurse management perspective: evidence-based practice, *J Perianesth Nurs* 21(3):195-199, 2006.

Janiszewzki GH: The nursing shortage in the United States of America: an integrative review of the literature, *J Adv Nurs* 43:335-343, 2003.

Johnson SA, Romanello ML: Generational diversity: teaching and learning approaches, *Nurse Educ* 30(5):212-216, 2005.

Jones ML: Role development and effective practice in specialist and advanced practice roles in acute hospital settings: systematic review and metasynthesis, *J Adv Nurs* 49(2):191-209, 2005.

Kanaskie ML: Mentoring: a staff retention tool, *Crit Care Nurse Q* 29(3):248-252, 2006.

Kane-Urrabazzo C: Management's role in shaping organizational culture, *J Nurs Manag* 14(3):188-194, 2006.

Kassulke S: Becoming a Magnet hospital: the role of the perianesthesia nurse, *J Perianesth Nurs* 19(2):71-77, 2004.

Kerridge RK: Perioperative patient management, *Best Pract Res Clin Obstet Gynaecol* 20(1):23-40, 2006.

Kiekkas P, Poulopoulou M, Papahatzi A, et al: Workload of postanaesthesia care unit nurses and intensive care overflow, *Br J Nurs* 14(8):434-438, 2005.

Kupperschmidt BR: Addressing multigenerational conflict: mutual respect and carefronting as strategy, *OJIN Online J Issues Nursing* 11(2), 2006, available at www.nursingworld.org/ojin/topic30/tpc30_3.htm, accessed January 7, 2007.

Lavoie-Tremblay M, O'Brien-Pallas L, Viens C, et al: Towards an integrated appraoach for the management of aging nurses, *J Nurs Manag* 14(3):207-212, 2006.

Leners DW, Wilson VW, Connor P, et al: Mentorship: increasing retention probabilities, *J Nurs Manag* 14(8):652-654, 2006.

Lynn MR, Redman RW: Faces of the nursing shortage: influences on staff nurses' intention to leave their positions or nursing, *J Nurs Admin* 35(5):264-270, 2005.

Mamaril ME: Standards of postanesthesia nursing practice: advocating patient safety, *J Perianesth Nurs* 18(3):168-172, 2003.

Marcon E, Dexter F: Impact of surgical sequencing on post anesthesia care unit staffing, *Health Care Manag Sci* 9(1):87-98, 2006.

Marcon E, Kharraja S, Smolski N, et al: Determining the number of beds in the postanesthesia care unit: a computer simulation flow approach, *Anesthesia Analgesia* 93:1415-1423, 2003.

Meyer MA, Sokal SM, Sandberg W, et al: Incoming! A web tracking application for PACU and postsurgical patients, *J Surg Res* 132(2):153-158, 2006.

Miller ET: Bridging the generation gap, *Rehabil Nurs* 32(1):2-3, 2007.

O'Brien-Pallas L, Duffield C, Alksnis C: Who will be there to nurse? Retention of nurses nearing retirement, *J Nurs Admin* 34:298-302, 2004.

Palese A, Pantali G, Saiani L: The management of a multigenerational nursing team with differing qualifications: a qualitative study, *Health Care Manag (Frederick)* 25(2):173-183, 2006.

Pasero C, Belden J: Evidence-based perianesthesia care: accelerated postoperative recovery programs, *J Perianesth Nurs* 21(3):168-176, 2006.

Sadler JJ: Who wants to be a nurse: motivation of the new generation, *J Prof Nurs* 19(3):173-175, 2003.

Santos SR, Carroll CA, Cox KS, et al: Baby boomer nurses bearing the burden of care: a four-site study of stress, strain, and coping for inpatient registered nurses, *J Nurs Adm* 33:243-250, 2003.

Schuster M, Standl T: Cost drivers in anesthesia: manpower, technique and other factors, *Curr Opin Anaesthesiol* 19(2):177-184, 2006.

Sherman RO: Leading a multigenerational nursing workforce: issues, challenges and strategies, *Online J Issues Nurs* 11(2):3, 2006, available at www.nursingworld.org/ojin/topic30/tpc30_2.htm, accessed January 7, 2007.

Shermont H, Krepcio D: The impact of culture change on nurse retention, *J Nurs Adm* 36(9):407-415, 2006.

Sievers B, Wolf S: Achieving clinical nurse specialist competencies and outcomes through interdisciplinary education, *Clin Nurse Spec* 20(2):75-80, 2006.

Skillman SM, Palazzo L, Keepnews D, et al: Characteristics of registered nurses in rural versus urban areas: implications for strategies to alleviate nursing shortages in the United States, *J Rural Health* 22(2):151-157, 2006.

Sokal SM, Craft DL, Chang Y, et al: Maximizing operating room and recovery room capacity in an era of constrained resources, *Arch Surg* 14(4):389-393, 2006.

Song D, Chung F, Ronayne M, et al: Fast-tracking (bypassing the PACU) does not reduce nursing workload after ambulatory surgery, *Br J Anaesth* 93(6):768-774, 2004.

Weissman C: The enhanced postoperative care system, *J Clin Anesth* 17(4):314-322, 2005.

White PF, Rawal S, Nguyen J, et al: PACU fast-tracking: an alternative to "bypassing" the PACU for facilitating the recovery process after ambulatory surgery, *J Perianesth Nurs* 18(4):247-253, 2003.

Windle PE: Moving beyond the barriers for evidence-based practice implementation, *J Perianesth Nurs* 21(3):208-211, 2006.

THE POSTANESTHESIA CARE UNIT

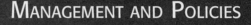

# 3

# MANAGEMENT AND POLICIES

*Donna M. DeFazio Quinn, BSN, MBA, RN, CPAN, CAPA*

All management procedures and policies of the postanesthesia care unit (PACU) should be established through joint efforts of the PACU staff, the nurse manager, and the medical director of the unit. These procedures and policies should be written and readily available to all staff working in the PACU and all physicians using the area for care of patients.

Policies are guidelines that give direction and have been approved by the administration of the institution. Procedures specify how a policy is to be implemented and are either managerial in scope or specific to clinical nursing methods. The PACU policies and procedures should be reviewed periodically so that appropriate changes can be made when necessary. Policies and procedures must always reflect the actual practice of the unit.

Changes in the clinical situation of the facility and advances in science and technology make revision of policies and procedures a continuous challenge. Some suggested areas that often require a written policy for the PACU are noted in Box 3-1. Policies and procedures must be tailored to meet the individual unit's needs.

## PURPOSE OF THE PACU

The PACU is designed and staffed for intensive observation and care of patients after a procedure for which an anesthetic agent has been necessary. Criteria for admission to the PACU should be clearly outlined, and exceptions to the policy should be specifically delineated.

The effects on staffing and the use of PACU beds for a multitude of services have created a special concern—the use of the PACU for performance of special procedures or for observation of patients who have undergone special procedures, such as cardiac catheterization, arteriography or other specialized radiologic tests, and electroshock therapy. A recent development is use of the PACU for patients of the intensive care unit (ICU) or telemetry or emergency departments when no beds are available in those units in the hospital. A shortage of

hospital beds has also turned the PACU into a holding area for surgical patients. Specific policies and procedures should address any special procedures performed in the unit and nursing care of these nonsurgical patients.

## STAFF

The nursing staff should consist of registered professional nurses who provide direct patient care (see Chapter 2). Each unit also should have a clinical nurse specialist for orientation and educational needs and for expertise in direct care of the patients. The clinical nurse specialist also functions in research and consultative roles. Licensed vocational or practical nurses may be employed in the area to assist the professional nurse, but they must be supervised by a registered nurse at all times. Some units use licensed vocational or practical nurses as members of their transport teams. Unlicensed assistive personnel must be under the direct supervision of a registered nurse.

Student nurses should not be used to staff the PACU. Students are assigned to the PACU primarily for observation. Any patient care delivered by student nurses should be accomplished only under the direct supervision of a permanent staff nurse. No private duty or "float" nurses should be used to staff the PACU unless they have been specially oriented and possess current PACU competencies.

### Retaining Nursing Staff in the PACU
Abundant information now alerts us to the existing nursing shortage—one that will only worsen over time. This shortage is multifaceted. One factor is the imminent retirement of baby boomer nurses. At the same time, fewer nurses are graduating and demand for nurses is growing. Simultaneously, many colleges and universities have seen the recent number of nursing applicants increase, only to be turned away because of the lack of qualified nursing educators.

Nursing as a whole has begun to address the shrinking number of its practitioners. One issue

## Box 3-1  Suggested Policies and Procedures for the PACU

- Purpose and structure of the unit
  - Facility and unit philosophy and objectives
  - Scope of service (patient population)
  - Mission, vision, and values statements
- Administrative
  - Administrative organizational chart
  - Chain of command
  - Governing body
  - Job descriptions
  - Staffing patterns
  - Hours of operation
  - Standards of care
- Medical staff
  - Physician privileges
  - Physician credentialing procedure
  - Medical advisory committee
- Patient rights
  - Rights and responsibility statement
  - Ethical treatment
  - Patient grievance process
  - Advance directives
  - Health Insurance Portability and Accountability Act (HIPAA) privacy notice
- Admission
  - Criteria
  - Population served
  - Preoperative assessment
- Discharge
  - Criteria and scoring system
  - Patient instructions
  - Responsible adult escort
- Anesthesia requirements
  - Anesthesia consent
  - Monitoring of patients who receive anesthesia
  - Fast-tracking guidelines
- Consents
  - Informed consent
  - Minors
  - Power of attorney
  - Sterilization
  - Administration of blood products
  - "Do Not Resuscitate" (DNR) orders
  - Experimental treatment
  - Procurement of forensic evidence
  - Electroconvulsive therapy
  - Cardioversion
  - Hepatitis B immunization
  - Release of medical information
- Emergency procedures
  - Emergency eye wash station
  - CPR, basic cardiac life support (BCLS), and advanced cardiac life support (ACLS) standards
- Malignant hyperthermia crisis
- Cardiac arrest
- Equipment
  - Operative
  - Emergency
  - Preventative maintenance program
  - Repairs
  - Medical device reporting
  - Biomedical engineering requests
- Facilities management
  - Emergency generator protocol
  - Maintenance of fire warning system
  - Preventative maintenance program
  - Occupational Safety and Health Administration (OSHA) regulations
- Environment of care plans
  - Safety management
  - Utilities management
  - Life safety management
  - Medical equipment management
  - Employee safety
  - Security management
  - Hazardous materials management
  - Emergency preparedness
- Infection control
  - Universal precautions
  - Personal protective equipment
  - Disposal of contaminated needles and sharps
  - Transmission-based precautions
  - Hepatitis B vaccine
  - Handwashing
  - Housekeeping procedures
  - OR attire
  - Traffic patterns
  - Visitors
  - Restricted areas
- Information systems
  - Description and use of systems
  - Confidentiality and security agreements
  - System backup and retention policy
  - System access and password policy
- Employee health
  - Annual requirements
  - Tuberculosis (TB) testing requirements
  - Sick leave
  - Worker's compensation
- Patient care
  - PACU standards of care
  - National, state, and facility standards of care
  - Nurse:patient ratios
  - Preoperative testing requirements
  - Moderate sedation and analgesia guidelines
  - Postoperative monitoring procedures
  - Patient education requirements

| **Box 3-1    Suggested Policies and Procedures for the PACU—cont'd** |
|---|

- Physician orders
  - Standing preoperative orders
  - Standing anesthesia orders
  - Standing orders for specialty services (i.e., ophthalmology; total joint, etc.)
- Quality management and performance improvement
  - Overview of quality management and performance improvement program
  - Goals of quality management and performance improvement program
  - Description of indicators and benchmarks
- Patient records
  - Consents
  - Confidentiality and HIPAA requirements
  - Electronic documentation
  - Order of medical record
  - Medical record retention
  - Release of information
- Safety
  - Fire safety
  - Electrical safety
  - Hazardous material training

- Emergency preparedness training
- Glutaraldehyde exposure monitoring
- Waste gas monitoring
- Exposure control plan
- Postexposure follow-up
- Bomb threat
- Violence in the workplace
- Body mechanics
- Radiation safety
- Control of radioactive materials
- Staff member rules and responsibilities
  - Orientation
  - Confidentiality
  - Security
  - Competency requirements
  - Performance appraisals
  - Required education and certification
  - Conflict of interest statement
- Supplies
  - Procurement and ordering
  - Sterilization
  - Storage
  - Annual inventory

Adapted from Quinn DMD, Shick L: *PeriAnesthesia core curriculum: preoperative, Phase I and Phase II PACU nursing,* Philadelphia, 2004, Saunders.

is the professional image of nursing. Some believe that cost-cutting activities in health care that resulted in layoffs a few years ago discouraged some young people from entering a profession with an uncertain future. Other articles have mentioned verbal abuse from physicians, low salary ceilings, inflexible working hours, and mandatory overtime as deciding factors. Also considered are the expanded options of female college students. Female students of today can pursue more options than baby boomers had available. These options have pulled some of the young people to other professions.

Recruitment into nursing and into specific hospitals is a widely discussed topic. Once nurses are recruited into the perianesthesia setting, retention of these experienced staff members becomes a major challenge. Some research has defined that the nurse manager leadership behaviors had the most influence on retention of hospital staff nurses (Box 3-2).

Retention of qualified nurses is fast becoming a priority for nursing administration. In exit interviews, nurses cite an unhealthy work environment as the reason they leave the workplace. Issues continue in the treatment of nurses towards each other. Some reasons often given for nurses who leave the workplace include lack of support,

mentoring, and clear direction.[1] Nurses are not exempt from conflict in the workplace. As trite as it may seem, females are generally expected to work harmoniously together in a "sister-like" fashion. This belief could not be farther from the truth. When issues of conflict arise, some individuals may find confronting the situation to establish resolution to be difficult. As a result, an ongoing underlying current of tension may exist on the unit. Box 3-3 identifies some strategies that the nurse manager may use to build a supportive workplace.

Other factors linked to job satisfaction and retention have been flexible work schedules, appropriate pay scales, and shared governance. Flexible schedules and a shared governance philosophy are created and controlled by the manager. Managers need to reassess age-old beliefs that nurses must work set shifts. The 7:00 AM to 3:30 PM shift is a thing of the past. A creative manager works with the nursing staff to accommodate individual work schedules. The mother who needs to put her children on the school bus before work may prefer to work 8:00 AM to 4:30 PM instead of the traditional 7:00 AM to 3:30 PM. For mothers or fathers who work the evening shift, a 5:00 PM to 1:00 AM shift may be a better fit to accommodate childcare issues. Implementation of a 10-hour shift

---

**Box 3-2  Retention Practices for Nurse Managers**

- Peer interviews
  - Use appropriately educated staff to collaborate in interview process
- Use of preceptors for new hires
  - Provide support for new hire and positive reinforcement for preceptor
- High-risk retention monitoring
  - Develop specific plans of action to retain those nurses at high risk for transfer
- Supplies and resources available to do the job
  - Find out from staff any barriers to doing their jobs (e.g., supplies) and then take action
- Individual career plan with each employee
  - Each employee should have an individualized career development plan
- Regular feedback
  - Guarantee formal feedback to staff at least twice a year
- Open communication in unit
  - Make open communication a priority; staff with staff and manager with staff
- Unit as a team
  - Make outside activities available for the unit; rely on staff input into unit goals

Modified from *The advisory board company: becoming a chief retention officer*, Washington, DC, 2001, The Advisory Board Company: Nursing Executive Center.

---

or a split shift assists in covering the gaps. Creative staffing solutions are key to staff retention and employee satisfaction.

Creation of an environment conducive to staff growth and development is the manager's responsibility. A survey conducted by the American Academy of Nursing in 1982 identified variables in nursing that attracted and retained quality nurses. These variables include nursing autonomy and personal and job satisfaction, and nursing practice that resulted in excellence.[2] As a result of this survey, the Magnet Recognition Program was established for recognition of health care organizations that provide nursing excellence.[3] Facilities that strive for recognition as a Magnet facility have identified that the nurses employed at the facility provide quality patient care. Nurses who believe they have the support and resources needed to provide quality patient care are more apt to be satisfied in the workplace.

Nurse managers need to be cognizant of the workplace environment. When strife is evident in the unit, the issues need to be identified and dealt with immediately to avoid a deluge of conflict, which can soon translate to discord among the staff.

## SHARED GOVERNANCE

Many units use a participative type of management. A well-documented fact is that nurses want to be treated as professionals and desire autonomy and participation. A concept used by many hospitals to meet these needs is shared governance. In this form of management, the PACU nurse assumes more authority and responsibility and shares management skills and duties with peers. The overall structure is that of self management, with the staff involved in the decision-making processes that affect nursing practice and management.

---

**Box 3-3  Management Strategies to Build a Supportive Workplace**

- Forge honest and open relationships
- Set realistic expectations
- Demonstrate how to deal effectively with colleagues who disagree or disapprove
- Recognize when being "nice" prevents discussion and resolution of issues
- Acknowledge conflicts and find solutions
- Recognize that some competitive tensions will always exist and talk them through
- Openly discuss how dealing with the issues can lead to optimism, movement, and growth
- Lead with respect for each person and empathy for the inevitable workplace tensions that will arise

From Vestal K: Conflict and competition in the workplace, *Nurse Leader* 4(6):6-7, 2006.

Committees that address the needs of the unit, the employees, and the patients are established. Usually, a nursing practice committee is in charge of any decisions about policies and procedures or practice issues; a quality management committee is in charge of quality management and performance improvement activities for the unit; and an educational committee is responsible for meeting the educational needs of the unit. Other unit-specific committees that have been used are equipment supply, budget and finance, communications, and statistics.

The nurse manager becomes a facilitator and a resource person for the staff. Most nurse managers retain responsibilities such as employee evaluations, interviews, and liaison with administration or physicians. The challenge for the nurse manager within this system of management is to maintain a vision and to impart that vision to the staff. In addition, the nurse manager must learn how to relinquish control and to support the decisions of the staff.

## SELF-SCHEDULING

One option for scheduling of staff is a system that is completely coordinated by the staff nurses that also recognizes professional nurses as capable of making crucial decisions about their practices. The schedule is developed and implemented by nurses and other staff in the unit. The nurses are given preestablished requirements that must be filled. They can be as creative and flexible as they want in developing the staffing schedule. Advantages include decreased amount of time spent by the nurse manager on scheduling, increased team building by the staff, increased job satisfaction and autonomy of the staff, and decreased staff turnover.

## PATIENT CLASSIFICATION

Most PACUs have some type of patient classification system (PCS). The most accurate PCSs are those that base the patient classification on length of stay in the PACU and intensity of the care needed. The PCS can be used to justify staffing and charges for the PACU stay. For example, a patient with a classification of 1 has a lower charge than a patient with a classification of 3.

Development of a PCS for the PACU is difficult at best. Many variables must be considered; for example, the length of stay of each patient varies and the acuity of one patient can change within a short period. Moreover, patient populations can range from pediatric to geriatric and can include minor to extensive surgical procedures.

The advantages of a PCS include a more accurate assessment of the nursing time and energy needed for each patient, which, in turn, allows a manager to estimate staffing requirements on the basis of the next day's schedule. Other advantages may include knowledge of the peak workload each day and patient charges that reflect not only the length of stay but also patient acuity and the intensity of nursing care needed. PACU nurses also feel that the type of workload in the PACU is acknowledged and that management is responsive to the staffing needs.

## VISITORS

Visiting may be allowed if staffing and the physical structure of the unit permit. Traditionally, family visitation in the PACU has not been allowed. The restrictions have been because of the lack of privacy, the acuity of the patients, and the fast turnover that is common to the PACU. However, the value of visitation in the PACU is a point of discussion among perianesthesia nurses. The catalyst behind the change has been, in part, the extended PACU stays many patients now need. For example, some patients may have a prolonged stay in the PACU while they wait for critical care, telemetry, or a surgical bed on the nursing unit. As the incidence rate of morning admissions increases, the incidence rate of extended PACU stays also increases because of lack of postoperative bed availability. In some hospitals, the PACU is used to help with emergency department overflow.

The nursing care in the PACU historically has concentrated on the patient. However, family members also need nursing interventions. Because of this need, many PACUs are adapting critical care unit visiting policies, which may include a 5-minute visit each hour or a 20-minute visit every 4 hours. Other criteria may include a limit of two family members at one time and visitation changes if warranted by the unit needs or patient condition. Privacy of other patients in the PACU must also be a priority.

Other situations in which visitation may be permitted include the following:
- Death of the patient may be imminent.
- The patient must return to surgery.
- The patient is a child whose physical and emotional well being may depend on the calming effect of the parent's presence.
- The patient's well being depends on the presence of a significant other. Patients in this

category include persons with mental disabilities, mental illnesses, or profound sensory deficits.

- The patient needs a translator because of language differences.

As facilities renovate or build new surgical suites, patient privacy must be taken into consideration. The design of the perianesthesia area should accommodate patients who need an extended PACU stay. Amenities should allow for patient comfort and privacy, including the ability for family members to visit.

## PATIENT RECORDS

Every patient admitted to the PACU should have a postanesthesia record. Whether traditional paper documentation or electronic format is used, the record should be an accurate account of the patient's perianesthesia stay. Anecdotal notes should detail admission observations. The assessment, planning, and implementation phases of the nursing process should be documented as should an evaluation of the patient's response to the care provided. A discharge summary should also be included.

The current trend in many institutions is toward a fully electronic medical record. The computerized record for the surgical patient may begin in the preoperative phase and follow the patient to the PACU. Advantages of a computerized medical record include immediate access by other health care practitioners involved in the patient's care and a time saver for nurses because data entry is often accomplished with drop-down menus much like a checklist. Disadvantages may include the cost of installation and education and the time necessary to orient the staff to the system.

## DISCHARGE OF THE PATIENT FROM THE PACU

Written criteria for discharge of the patient from the PACU must be available and should include when: (1) the patient regained consciousness and was oriented to time and place (provided the patient was oriented to time and place before surgery); (2) the airway was clear and the danger of vomiting and aspiration passed; and (3) circulatory and respiratory vital signs were stabilized. The criteria for discharge of a patient from the PACU vary by the unit or the location of transfer from the PACU, by the anesthetic technique, and by the physiologic status. Ultimately, the physician is in charge of the patient's discharge from the PACU. Predetermined criteria can be applied if the

criteria have been approved by the physician staff.

Use of a numeric scoring system for assessment of the patient's recovery from anesthesia is common. Many institutions have incorporated the postanesthesia recovery score as criteria for discharge. Box 3-4 shows an example of two discharge scoring systems. The Aldrete Scoring System was introduced by Aldrete and Kroulik in 1970 and was modified later by Dr. Aldrete to reflect oxygen saturation instead of color. The Post Anesthetic Discharge Scoring System (PADSS) is used for assessment of readiness of the patient to be discharged home or to an Extended Observation area. The policy of the unit determines the appropriate score for discharge from the PACU. The patient must have a preestablished score to be discharged from the PACU. Scores lower than the preestablished level necessitate evaluation by the anesthesia provider or surgeon and possible disposition to a special care or critical care unit.

Clinical assessment must also be used in determination of a patient's readiness for discharge from the PACU. This scoring system does not include detailed observations such as urinary output, bleeding or other drainage, changing requirements for hemodynamic support, temperature trends, or patient's pain management needs. All of these criteria should be considered in determination of readiness for discharge.

Because patient conditions vary with surgical procedure, anesthesia used, use of analgesics, and patient response, no specific time requirements for the PACU stay can be stated. Professional judgment is needed to determine when the patient is ready for discharge from the PACU. A complete accurate report is required from the PACU nurse to the nurse who will be responsible for the care of the patient. Hand-off communication has been identified as an area in which patient safety can be compromised if not performed accurately.

When ambulatory surgical patients are discharged to home, other criteria should be assessed. These criteria may include the following: control of pain acceptable to the patient, control of nausea, ambulation in a manner consistent with the procedure and previous ability, and a responsible adult present to accompany the patient home.

Some PACUs require the patient to void or tolerate oral fluids before discharge to home. Home care instructions should be written and taught to the patient and responsible adult, both of whom should verbalize an understanding of the instructions. Emergency and routine

## Box 3-4   Discharge Scoring Systems

### THE ALDRETE SCORING SYSTEM

**Respiration**
- Ability to take deep breath and cough = 2
- Dyspnea/shallow breathing = 1
- Apnea = 0

**$O_2$ Saturation**
- Maintenance of > 92% on room air = 2
- $O_2$ inhalation needed to maintain $O_2$ saturation > 90% = 1
- $O_2$ saturation < 90% even with supplemental oxygen = 0

**Consciousness**
- Fully awake = 2
- Arousable on calling = 1
- Not responding = 0

**Circulation**
- Blood pressure (BP) ± 20 mm Hg preoperative value = 2
- BP ± 20 to 50 mm Hg preoperative value = 1
- BP ± 50 mm Hg preoperative value = 0

**Activity**
- Ability to move 4 extremities = 2
- Ability to move 3 extremities = 1
- Ability to move 0 extremities = 0

### THE POST ANESTHETIC DISCHARGE SCORING SYSTEM (PADSS)

**Vital signs**
- BP and pulse within 20% preoperative value = 2
- BP and pulse with 20% to 40% preoperative value = 1
- BP and pulse within > 40% preoperative value = 0

**Activity**
- Steady gait, no dizziness, or preoperative level met = 2
- Assistance needed = 1
- Inability to ambulate = 0

**Nausea and Vomiting**
- Minimal or treated with oral medication = 2
- Moderate or treated with parenteral medication = 1
- Severe or continues despite treatment = 0

**Pain**
- Controlled with oral analgesics and acceptable to patient:
- Yes = 2
- No = 1

**Surgical Bleeding**
- Minimal or no dressing changes = 2
- Moderate or up to two dressing changes needed = 1
- Severe or more than three dressing changes needed = 0

From Ead H: From Aldrete to PADSS: reviewing discharge criteria after ambulatory surgery, *J Perianesthesia Nurs* 21(4):259-267, 2006.

phone numbers should be included with the instructions.

Patients should receive a follow-up visit by the anesthesia provider and be released as appropriate. In instances in which the nursing staff of the PACU is appropriately educated, a policy that defines discharge criteria and allows the nurse to discharge the patient may be in effect. Discharge criteria should be developed to meet appropriate standards but should be individualized to each PACU.

## FASTTRACKING

*Fasttracking* refers to the bypass of PACU Phase I and admission of the patient directly from the operating room (OR) to Phase II PACU. A Phase I bypass for the patient with general or regional anesthesia should only be practiced in the ambulatory setting. The patient needs to meet all Phase I discharge criteria in the OR before admission to Phase II PACU.

Contributing factors to the practice of fasttracking are technologic advancements in surgery, shorter-acting anesthetic agents, and improved pain management. Patients awaken faster and have fewer side effects and complications.

One advantage of bypassed care in PACU Phase I is a decrease in the expensive costs of a critical care area for patients who do not need those services. The total length of stay in the facility is also decreased for the ambulatory surgery patient. Patients have reported higher

## Box 3-5   Collaborative Plan for Fasttracking

- Establish multidisciplinary workgroup, including anesthesia, Perianesthesia Phase I and II nurses, surgeons, perioperative nurses
- Define criteria for appropriate patient selection
- Develop a program to address preoperative education of patient and family
- Define appropriate selection and management of anesthetic agents
- Develop assessment criteria for evaluation of patient readiness for bypass of Phase I at the end of the surgical procedure
- Determine discharge criteria
- Develop a mechanism to monitor and report patient outcomes

Modified from American Society of PeriAnesthesia Nurses: *A position statement on fast tracking*, Cherry Hill, NJ, 2006, ASPAN.

satisfaction rates with the opportunity for earlier discharge.

Facilities need to avoid implementation of a program of fasttracking without identified criteria. Inappropriate bypass of Phase I PACU results in patients admitted to Phase II in severe pain, with respiratory distress, or with emotional anxiety. The American Society of PeriAnesthesia Nurses (ASPAN) has developed a position on fasttracking because this practice has not been well defined (Box 3-5).

## STANDARDS OF CARE

Standards of postanesthesia nursing practice have been published and are available from ASPAN. These standards have been devised to stand alone or be used in conjunction with other health care standards. They provide a basic framework for nurses who practice in all phases of postanesthesia care. A copy of these standards may be obtained from the ASPAN National Office, 10 Melrose Avenue, Suite 110, Cherry Hill, NJ 08003-3696, or ordered via the ASPAN website at www.aspan.org.

All preanesthesia, postanesthesia, and ambulatory surgical nurses should be familiar with these standards of practice, and a copy of the standards should be available on each unit. The PACU may develop its own standards specific to the hospital that use the ASPAN standards as a reference or may adopt the ASPAN standards for use. If the PACU adopts the ASPAN standards, they must be adopted in their entirety or a policy must be added to note any exceptions. Any written standards must be attainable reflections of the actual practice.

Nurses must possess a minimum standard of knowledge and ability. Standards are objective and are the same for patients and staff members, which means that an inexperienced nurse in the PACU is held to the same standard as an experienced nurse. Standards are commonly used today in legal proceedings to measure the care a patient received. The ASPAN standards have already been used in court proceedings, and many medical malpractice attorneys have a copy of the ASPAN Standards of Perianesthesia Nursing Practice in their libraries.

## QUALITY MANAGEMENT/PERFORMANCE IMPROVEMENT

Each PACU should have a planned quality management and performance improvement program. Performance improvement programs differ from the quality management programs of the past in that the emphasis on inspection has changed to an emphasis on continuous improvement. Performance improvement is based on overall improvement of the system and includes the consumer in that process. A consumer is any person who uses output at any point in the system. Examples include the patient who receives care in the PACU or the PACU nurse who receives supplies from a central materials supply location.

The Joint Commission has established standards that focus on the role of the nursing staff in quality improvement. Every nurse is responsible for quality management and performance improvement. The result is an effective program that has a positive impact on the process and outcome of care. Patient care problems can be prevented, or basic operating procedures or systems can be changed and improved.

One of the aspects of a quality management and performance improvement program is interdisciplinary participation in these activities. The common focus is on quality patient care and service and how they can be improved. Departmental boundaries fade with a common focus on the patient. In the past, each department had its own plan developed with occasional interdepartmental and interdisciplinary participation. Today, the focus of quality management and performance improvement activities must be practiced with no boundaries between departments and disciplines. The focus is on improved patient care and a seamless continuum.

Monitoring and evaluation are still parts of the quality management process. Expansions include the role of leadership in quality improvement; the scope of assessment from strictly clinical to other systems and processes that affect patients; and the focus on the processes, and not performances, of individual staff members and how they can be improved.

Examples of performance improvement activities might include reduction in the time the pharmacy takes to respond to PACU needs, improvement in the system to decrease the length of time patients remain in the PACU waiting for beds, a change in staffing patterns in the PACU or ambulatory care areas to meet patient care needs, or a patient education program written for all outpatients discharged with a venous access device to ensure that all patients receive the same quality education.

## SUMMARY

This chapter has focused on the management of a PACU and an ambulatory care setting involved in postanesthesia care. Important policies and management techniques were discussed along with aspects of nursing satisfaction and retention and quality improvement.

## REFERENCES

1. Vestal K: Conflict and competition in the workplace, *Nurse Leader* 4(6):6-7, 2006.
2. Lewis C, Matthews J: Magnet program designates exceptional nursing services, *AJN* 98(12):51-52, 1998.
3. ANCC Magnet recognition program: available at http://nursingworld.org/ancc/magnet/index.html, accessed February 2007.

## BIBLIOGRAPHY

American Society of PeriAnesthesia Nurses: *Competency-based orientation credentialing program manual 2002 edition*, Cherry Hill, NJ, 2002, The Society.

American Society of PeriAnesthesia Nurses: *2006-2008 Standards of perianesthesia nursing practice*, Cherry Hill, NJ, 2006, The Society.

Andrews DR, Dziegielewski SF: The nurse manager: job satisfaction, the nursing shortage and retention, *J Nurs Manag* 13(4):286-295, 2005.

Andrews J, Manthorpe J, Watson R: Employment transitions for older nurses: a qualitative study, *J Adv Nurs* 51(3):298-306, 2005.

Arruda EH: Better retention through nursing theory, *J Nurs Manag* 36(4):16-18, 2005.

Bahlman DT, Johnson FC: Using technology to improve and support communication and workflow processes, *AORN J* 82(1):65-73, 2005.

Bethune G, Sherrod D, Youngblood L: 101 tips to retain a happy, healthy staff, *Nurs Manage* 36(4):24-29, 2005.

Bond LM, Flickinger D, Aytes L, et al: Effects of preoperative teaching of the use of a pain scale with patients in the PACU, *J Perianesth Nurs* 20(5):333-340, 2005.

Blythe J, Baumann A, Zeytinoglu I, et al: Full-time or part-time work in nursing: preferences, tradeoffs and choices, *Healthcare Q* 8(3):69-77, 2005.

Buchanan M: Playing for keeps: improvement in nurse recruitment must be matched by retention, *Nurs Stand* 19(27):27, 2005.

Burden N: Regulatory compliance in the ambulatory surgery setting: a process improvement approach, *J Perianesth Nurse* 18(3):173-181, 2003.

Caramanica L, Roy J: Evidence-based practice: creating the environment for practice excellence, *Nurse Leader* 4(6):38-41, 2006.

Chan CS, Molassiotis A: The effects of an educational programme on the anxiety and satisfaction level of parents having parent present induction and visitation in a postanaesthesia care unit, *Paediatric Anaesthesia* 12(2):131-139, 2002.

Cohen JD: The aging nursing workforce: how to retain experienced nurses, *J Healthcare Management* 51(4):233-245, 2006.

Cutilli CC: Do your patients understand? Providing culturally congruent patient education, *Orthop Nurs* 25(3):218-224, 2006.

Deleskey K: Factors affecting nurses' decisions to join and maintain membership in professional associations, *J Perianesth Nurs* 18(1):8-17, 2003.

Dexter F, Epstein RH, Penning DH: Statistical analysis of postanesthesia care unit staffing at a surgical suite with frequent delays in admission from the operating room: a case study, *Anesth Anal* 92(4):947-949, 2001.

Dexter F, Wachtel RE, Epstein RH: Impact of average patient acuity on staffing of the phase I PACU, *J Perianesth Nurs* 21(5):303-310, 2006.

Drenkard KN: Sustaning Magnet: keeping the forces alive, *Nurs Adm Q* 29(3):214-222, 2005.

Duncan PG, Shandro J, Bachand R, et al: A pilot study of recovery room bypass ("fast-track protocol") in a community hospital, *Can J Anaesth* 48(7):630-636, 2001.

Ead H: From Aldrete to PADSS: reviewing discharge criteria after ambulatory surgery, *J Perianesth Nurs* 21(4):259-267, 2006.

Ellison DJ: A guideline for incorporating holistic nursing interventions into perianesthesia practice, *J Perianesth Nurs* 20(1):19-22, 2005.

Ervin NE: Does patient satisfaction contribute to nursing care quality? *J Nurs Adm* 36(3):126-130, 2006.

Fitzgerald M, Milberger P, Tomlinson PS, et al: Clinical nurse specialist participation on a collaborative research project: barriers and benefits, *Clin Nurse Spec* 17(1):44-49, 2003.

Force MV: The relationship between effective nurse managers and nursing retention, *J Nurs Adm* 35(7-8):336-341, 2005.

Fredman B, Sheffer O, Zohar E, et al: Fast-track eligibility of geriatric patient undergoing short urologic surgery procedures, *Anesth Anal* 94(3):560-564, 2002.

Frith K, Montgomery M: Perceptions, knowledge, and commitment of clinical staff to shared governance, *Nurse Adm Q* 30(3):273-284, 2006.

Galanti GA: Applying cultural competence to perianesthesia nursing, *J Perianesth Nurs* 21(2):97-102, 2006.

Gerke ML: Understanding and leading the quad matrix: four generations in the workplace: the traditional generation, boomers, gen-X, nexters, *Semin Nurs Manag* 9(3):173-181, 2001.

Gibbs VC: Patient safety practices in the operating room: correct-site surgery and nothing left behind, *Surg Clin North Am* 85(6):1307-1319, 2005.

Glover DE, Newkirk LE, Cole LM, et al: Perioperative clinical nurse specialist role delineation: a systematic review, *AORN J* 84(6):1017-1030, 2006.

Gmah L: Hand offs: a link to improving patient safety, *AORN J* 83(1):227-230, 2006.

Harrington L: Program development: role of the clinical nurse specialist in implementing a fast-track postanesthesia care unit, *AACN Clin Issues* 16(1):78-88, 2005.

Hart SM: Generational diversity: impact on recruitment and retention of registered nurses, *J Nurs Adm* 36(1):10-12, 2006.

Hayhurst A, Saylor C, Stuenkel D: Work environmental factors and retention of nurses, *J Nurs Care Qual* 20(3):283-288, 2005.

Hu J, Herrick C, Hodgin KA: Managing the multigenerational nursing team, *Health Care Manag (Frederick)* 23(4):334-340, 2004.

Humphreys S: Patient autonomy: legal and ethical issues in the postanesthetic care unit, *Br J Perioper Nurs* 15(1):35-43, 2005.

Iacono MV: Perianesthesia nurse management perspective: evidence-based practice, *J Perianesth Nurs* 21(3):195-199, 2006.

Janiszewzki GH: The nursing shortage in the United States of America: an integrative review of the literature, *J Adv Nurs* 43(4):335-343, 2003.

Jevtovic-Todorovic V: Standards of care for ambulatory surgery: are we up to speed, *Minerva Anesthesiol* 72(1-2):13-20, 2006.

Johnson K, Hallsey D, Meredith RL, et al: A nurse-driven system for improving patient quality outcomes, *J Nurs Care Quality* 21(2):168-175, 2006.

Johnson SA, Romanello ML: Generational diversity: teaching and learning approaches, *Nurse Educ* 30(5):212-216, 2005.

Jones ML: Role development and effective practice in specialist and advanced practice roles in acute hospital settings: systematic review and metasynthesis, *J Adv Nurs* 49(2):191-209, 2005.

Kain ZN, Mayes LC, Caldwell-Andrews AA, et al: Preoperative anxiety, postoperative pain, and behavioral recovery in young children undergoing surgery, *Pediatrics* 118(2):651-658, 2006.

Kanaskie ML: Mentoring: a staff retention tool, *Crit Care Nurse Q* 29(3):248-252, 2006.

Kane-Urrabazzo C: Management's role in shaping organizational cutlture, *J Nurs Manage* 14(3):188-194, 2006.

Kassulke S: Becoming a Magnet hospital: the role of the perianesthesia nurse, *J Perianesth Nurs* 19(2):71-77, 2004.

Kerridge RK: Perioperative patient management, *Best Pract Res Clin Obstet Gynaecol* 20(1):23-40, 2006.

Kiekkas P, Poulopoulou M, Papahatzi A, et al: Workload of postanaesthesia care unit nurses and intensive care overflow, *Br J Nurs* 14(8):434-438, 2005.

Kleiman S: Discovering cultural aspects of nurse-patient relationships, *J Cult Divers* 13(2):83-86, 2006.

Kyrkjebo JM: Teaching quality improvement in the classroom and clinic: getting it wrong and getting it right, *J Nurs Educ* 45(3):109-116, 2006.

Lavoie-Tremblay M, O'Brien-Pallas L, Viens C, et al: Towards an integrated approach for the management of aging nurses, *J Nurs Manag* 14(3):207-212, 2006.

Leary C, Allen SJ: Navigating the path of leadership: 12 qualities of an effective charge nurse, *Nurse Leader* 4(6):22-23, 2006.

Leners DW, Wilson VW, Connor P, et al: Mentorship: increasing retention probabilities, *J Nurs Manag* 14(8):652-654, 2006.

Lynn MR, Redman RW: Faces of the nursing shortage: influences on staff nurses' intention to leave their positions or nursing, *J Nurs Admin* 35(5):264-270, 2005.

Mamaril ME: Standards of postanesthesia nursing practice: advocating patient safety, *J Perianesth Nurs* 18(3):168-172, 2003.

Mamaril ME, Ross JM, Krenzischek D, et al: The ASPAN's EBP conceptual model: framework for perianesthesia practice and research, *J Perianesth Nurs* 21(3):157-167, 2006.

Marcon E, Dexter F: Impact of surgical sequencing on post anesthesia care unit staffing, *Health Care Manag Sci* 9(1):87-98, 2006.

Marcon E, Kharraja S, Smolski N, et al: Determining the number of beds in the postanesthesia care unit: a computer simulation flow approach, *Anesth Analgesia* 93:1415-1423, 2003.

McHaney DF, Varner J: Accommodating the needs of the registered nurse workforce, *Ala Nurse* 33(3):24-25, 2006.

Meyer MA, Sokal SM, Sandberg W, et al: Incoming! A web tracking application for PACU and post-surgical patients, *J Surg Res* 132(2):153-158, 2006.

Newhouse R: ASPAN and the organizational EBP vision: synergistic opportunities for perianesthesia nurses, *J Perianesth Nurs* 21(3):190-194, 2006.

Ninger L: Planning a family visit program for PACU, *OR Manager* 19(12):20-22, 2003.

O'Brien-Pallas L, Duffield C, Alksnis C: Who will be there to nurse? Retention of nurses nearing retirement, *J Nurs Admin* 34(6):298-302, 2004.

Pasero C, Belden J: Evidence-based perianesthesia care: accelerated postoperative recovery programs, *J Perianesth Nurs* 21(3):168-176, 2006.

Robinson P: Master the steps to performance improvement: plan, do, study, act to enhance your facility's patient care initiatives, *Nurs Manag* 35(5):45-48, 2004.

Rogers LM: Meeting the Center for Medicare & Medicaid Services requirements for quality assessment and performance improvement: a model for hospitals, *J Nurs Care Quality* 21(4):325-330, 2006.

Runy LA: Nurse retention: an executive's guide to keeping one of your hospital's most valuable resources, *Hosp Health Netw* 80(1):53-62, 2006.

Sadler JJ: Who wants to be a nurse: motivation of the new generation, *J Prof Nurs* 19(3):173-175, 2003.

Santos SR, Carroll CA, Cox KS, et al: Baby boomer nurses bearing the burden of care: a four-site study of stress, strain, and coping for inpatient registered nurses, *J Nurs Adm* 33(4):243-250, 2003.

Scott L, Caress AL: Shared governance and shared leadership: meeting the challenges of implementation, *J Nurs Manag* 13(1):4-12, 2005.

Sherman RO: Leading a multigenerational nursing workforce: issues, challenges and strategies, *Online J Issues Nurs* 11(2):3, 2006, available at www.nursingworld.org/ojin/topic30/tpc30_2.htm, accessed January 7, 2007.

Shermont H, Krepcio D: The impact of culture change on nurse retention, *J Nurs Adm* 36(9):407-415, 2006.

Sievers B, Wolf S: Achieving clinical nurse specialist competencies and outcomes through interdisciplinary education, *Clin Nurse Spec* 20(2):75-80, 2006.

Skillman SM, Palazzo L, Keepnews D, et al: Characteristics of registered nurses in rural versus urban areas: implications for strategies to alleviate nursing shortages in the United States, *J Rural Health* 22(2):151-157, 2006.

Sokal SM, Craft DL, Chang Y, et al: Maximizing operating room and recovery room capacity in an era of constrained resources, *Arch Surg* 14(4):389-393, 2006.

Song D, Chung F, Ronayne M, et al: Fast-tracking (bypassing the PACU) does not reduce nursing workload after ambulatory surgery, *Br J Anaesth* 93(6):768-774, 2004.

Smykowski L, Rodriguez W: The post anesthesia care unit experience: a family-centered approach, *J Nurs Care Quality* 18(1):5-15, 2003.

Vestal K: Conflict and competition in the workplace, *Nurse Leader* 4(6):6-7, 2006.

Weissman C: The enhanced postoperative care system, *J Clin Anesth* 17(4):314-322, 2005.

Weston, MJ: Integrating generational perspectives in nursing, *OJIN Online J Issues Nursing* 11(2), 2006, available at www.nursingworld.org/ojin/topic30/tpc30_1.htm, accessed January 12, 2007.

White PF, Rawal S, Nguyen J, et al: PACU fast-tracking: an alternative to "bypassing" the PACU for facilitating the recovery process after ambulatory surgery, *J Perianesth Nurs* 18(4):247-253, 2003.

Wilson M: Giving postanesthesia care in the critical care unit, *Dimens Crit Care Nurs* 19(2):38-43, 2000.

Windle PE: Moving beyond the barriers for evidence-based practice implementation, *J Perianesth Nurs* 21(3):208-211, 2006.

Zuzelo P, McGoldick TB, Seminara P, et al: Shared governance and EBP: a logical partnership, *Nurse Manag* 37(6):45-50, 2006.

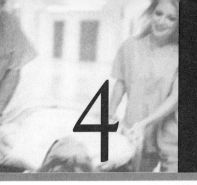

# 4 CRISIS RESOURCE MANAGEMENT IN THE PACU

*Michael D. Fallacaro, DNS, CRNA*
*Suzanne M. Wright, MSNA, CRNA*

Emergency and urgent situations that necessitate immediate intervention are not uncommon in postanesthesia care units (PACUs), but procedures do not always go smoothly as physicians and nurses care for the patient. The evolutionary nature of health care requires responsiveness to change on the part of academic programs that prepare professionals for roles in the health care field. Both changing delivery system methods and innovative technology currently impact the educational needs of health care providers. Technologic advances have altered the skills necessary for increasingly complex equipment and postoperative procedures. The heightened acuity of surgical patients also impacts on postanesthesia nursing practice. Certain pathophysiologic conditions can lead to critical incidents in the perioperative period. The rarity of such conditions or events challenges traditional methods of educational preparation. Furthermore, although critical events rarely occur, when they do, they can be life threatening, which is especially relevant for nurses who practice with limited support or resources. Urban and suburban areas have more resources available and more anesthesia providers available. However, the increasing acuity of patients, new procedures and equipment, and the increased emphasis on ambulatory or *same-day* surgery are changing anesthesia delivery and postanesthesia care. Although routine anesthesia practice involves a set of basic skills for routine anesthesia administration, complex skills are needed for an effective response to rare critical anesthesia events that often occur after anesthesia. Most recently, didactic instruction supported with hands-on patient care has been the method used by educators to prepare providers in management of events. Technologic advancements in human simulation may now offer the potential to support or enhance current methods, with experiential learning offered in rare and critical episodes. Thus, an innovative form of training may change the way patients receive care in the future. Crisis Resource Management (CRM) training uses human factors, expertise, and patient simulators to better prepare medical teams to function effectively in their dynamic work environments.

Since World War II, aviation has used flight simulators as a safe yet realistic training environment for pilots. Investigations into airline crashes have shown that pilot technical skills were not usually the cause of accidents.[1] Teamwork and crew communication were often the cause of the incident. Airline crew team training was initiated in the 1980s when the fact that cockpit and cabin crews and the ground personnel and air traffic controllers needed to learn to work cohesively to prevent disasters became apparent. Although the practice has never been empirically validated, simulation training has become the mainstay of aviation training. Pilots train extensively in all emergency procedures in the simulator to become proficient in crisis management before the situation could occur on an actual flight.

Similar training in medicine is now possible with the introduction of full-sized human patient simulators in the early 1990s. Dr. David Gaba and colleagues at Stanford University in Palo Alto, California, adapted the principles of CRM training to the medical domain.[2] They found that the principles were as applicable in anesthesiology as they were in aviation. Both fields were dynamic, necessitated rapid decision making, and required that teams of individuals work together effectively to prevent loss of life. Since then, critical care medicine, emergency medicine, and trauma teams have also begun using simulation and CRM training. Although the initial emphasis was on the training of physicians, the technique is now used to train nurse anesthetists, nurse practitioners, critical care nurses, paramedics, and other allied health personnel. Simulation has also been incorporated into many curricula for health care providers and continues to expand its role in education and training for improved patient care.

## HUMAN FACTORS TRAINING AND THE SYSTEMS APPROACH TO MEDICAL ERROR

Have you ever locked your keys in the car with the motor running or put the car in reverse prematurely? These "slips," although seemingly significant at the time, can pale in importance in comparison with a nurse who accidentally administers the wrong medication to a patient or who forgets to deliver the proper concentration of oxygen. Yet, in principle, the fundamental human nature of these errors of omission is the same. Nothing is more concerning to a patient than the possibility that the outcome of treatment may be determined by a mistake the health care provider might make by virtue of being less than perfect.

CRM training addresses the medical management of critical events with a strong emphasis on the human factors aspects. Its primary focus is on improvement of human performance in complex work environments for the promotion of better decision making, teamwork, and outcomes for the patient. This emphasis recently has become an area of intense interest in medicine. The Institute of Medicine's report on human error attracted media and public attention. Cooper et al[3] noted that more than 80% of incidents in anesthesia were preventable. Similar error rates have been found in other industries, such as aviation and nuclear power.[4]

Human error is an inevitable part of complex and rapidly changing work domains, such as aviation, anesthesiology, and critical care medicine. Human error in any discipline can lead to critical incidents with catastrophic outcomes. Major incidents, such as the crash of the Concorde jet in 2000, gain media interest and prompt public attention and action primarily because of the drama and scope of the event in terms of lives altered or lost. Unfortunately, until recently, human error–related accidents in health care tended to be less visible to the public, primarily because these events usually impact one patient at a time.

Human factors theorists have identified particular circumstances and error types and can help train individuals to recognize the signs of errant problem solving. Although human error can never be eradicated, it can certainly be better managed.[5] Aviation has tended toward the teaching of "error management" techniques rather than an aim for human perfection. Numerous organizations that focus primarily on patient safety measures and funding of research in this area have evolved. One such organization, the Anesthesia Patient Safety Foundation (APSF), has funded many studies[6] in recent

years for the facilitation of human factors research and training in the field of anesthesiology. Moreover, the recently organized National Patient Safety Foundation (NPSF) has broadened the study to all medical specialties. Both groups believe that further study and improved training can improve patient outcomes and safety.

Reason[7] operationalized error into the following three terms: slips, lapses, and mistakes. A *slip* is defined as an error of execution. It is observable and can simply involve the human action of picking up the wrong syringe or turning the wrong knob on an oxygen flowmeter. A *lapse* is not observable and involves the inability of a person to correctly recall something from memory, such as the mixture of a lidocaine drip. Finally, a *mistake* is an error in planning instead of execution. Here a nurse may have planned to place a suction catheter down an endotracheal tube for extubation of the patient with application of full suction. Although the execution was technically correct, the lungs were left devoid of oxygen in the process, which was a mistake in planning.

A common misconception is that errors only happen to lazy incompetent individuals who lack vigilance. On the contrary, errors can happen to any individual despite vigilance and motivation. When errors occur, we need to avoid placing blame on the individual; rather, we should strive toward a more enlightened view—to understand the breakdown in the system and the resulting harm to a patient. Two compelling themes surface from human factors research: (1) humans are prone to err; and (2) most errors are not the result of personal inadequacy or carelessness but instead are the product of defects in the design of health care environmental systems in which that work occurs. An illustrative case follows.

Sarah, an experienced PACU nurse, was well into her double shift by the time the patient arrived in the unit at 2 AM. A 36-year-old woman involved in a motor vehicle accident had just undergone an exploratory laparotomy and splenectomy for intraabdominal bleeding. Thirty minutes after the patient's arrival, an alarm sounded. Sarah noted that the patient's heart rate was 36 bpm and dropping. Following unit protocol, Sarah quickly reached into the medication cart for atropine and intravenously administered a 0.4-mg dose. Almost instantly, the patient's blood pressure soared to 300 mm systolic on the arterial line monitor and the patient went into cardiac arrest. Despite full resuscitative efforts, the patient did not respond.

Later, as Sarah was cleaning up the bedside stand of all the medications used in the code, she found an empty phenylephrine vial that had not been used during the resuscitation. That she had inadvertently given the patient a 10-mg bolus of phenylephrine instead of the intended atropine then became obvious to Sarah.

A follow-up root cause investigation discovered that the pharmacy had recently stocked phenylephrine next to atropine in the medication drawer. Both the drugs were manufactured by the same company and came in the exact same size vials, with the same color snap-off caps. The label for atropine was a light red color, and the phenylephrine label was pink. Instead of the blame being placed on the nurse, the suggestion was made to the pharmacy that the vials immediately be tagged with a black colored "A" atop the atropine and that the two drugs be physically separated from one another in the medication cart. The manufacturer was also notified and encouraged to change the labeling system.

Although initially one might question how a nurse could not read the label and give a wrong medication, in retrospect, one might easily see how an experienced nurse could slip while emergently reaching for a medication in a familiar vial. This slip is analogous to a once all-too-common error among anesthetists that concerned gas flow meters. At one time, anesthesia gas delivery systems had two similar gas control knobs: one to deliver oxygen and one to deliver nitrous oxide. Slips occurred when anesthetists inadvertently turned up the nitrous oxide when they had intended to turn up the oxygen, which resulted in a hypoxic gas mixture being delivered to the patient. A human factors approach was taken to remedy this problem. The oxygen knob was redesigned with deep indentations, whereas the nitrous oxide knob remained smooth. The anesthetist then was able to tell by touch alone that the correct knob was in hand. The anesthesia machine was also given a built-in fail-safe mechanism that did not allow the delivery of a hypoxic mixture regardless of how high the nitrous flow was set. This approach to the problem effectively prevented any further patient from receiving a hypoxic mixture. Accidents and accident reporting were viewed in these examples as opportunities to design more robust systems to prevent the same type of injury from ever occurring again.

Historically, an adverse outcome results in blame toward the caregivers at the patient end, akin to the "pilot error" verdict after an airline disaster. Yet careful study of the larger system in which the incident occurs usually yields many factors that contributed to the event.[8] Lack of training, improper equipment maintenance, poor staffing, or an illegible order transcribed incorrectly can individually or jointly contribute

to a critical event. In other words, a cascade of events, not just a single event, often results in the adverse outcome. CRM training advocates this systems approach to adverse outcome investigations. It seeks answers from a broader perspective of the entire system to find the contributing factors. A look at policies and administrative decisions that either supported or derailed a critical incident is a radical departure from the traditional "frame and blame" punitive approach used in medicine. This approach should not be interpreted as lessening the responsibility of the person who made an error but as gaining a better understanding of why the error occurred; only then can the system be adjusted to better prevent reoccurrence. CRM training strives to make practitioners aware of systemic factors and how to work effectively within the context of a large system that may not always support their efforts. The goal is for trainees to learn from the mistakes of others through an open exchange of information. In this way, students can come to understand the cascade of events that leads to mistakes and can avoid similar errors. Largely, anesthesia providers who err are no different than other professionals who do their best in challenging environments. In the past, when a mistake was made, a good practitioner who may have helped so many was then blamed and shamed. A career ended and a life was shattered, which created an additional victim to join the patient who was harmed by the human flaw of being less than perfect.

Today when mistakes happen, we look not only at the care provider but also at the entire system. Anesthetists are at the "sharp end"; they interface directly with the patient. Many "blunt end" factors, such as equipment manufacturers, hospital administrations, and other institutional effects, significantly contribute to placing and equipping anesthetists at that sharp end. When error occurs, however, we tend to focus blame solely on the sharp end person and ignore the contributions of those blunt end phenomena. This approach must change.

## CRISIS MANAGEMENT PRINCIPLES

The acronym "ERR WATCH" (Box 4-1) was developed by Dr. Joanne Fletcher[9] to help the practitioner recall the eight essential elements of crisis management. ERR WATCH also serves as a reminder that the goal of crisis management is the reduction of the element of human error in any given situation. The human factor in performance is one of prime importance. Limitations exist in a health care provider's ability to quickly and accurately process rapidly changing

---

**Box 4-1  Err Watch Principles**

- Know Your **Environment**
  - Know equipment function, troubleshooting, and plans for failure
  - Be aware of staffing levels throughout shift
- Use Your **Resources**
  - Be aware of personal limitations
  - Use texts and references as resources
  - Plan ahead for probable problems
- Frequent **Reevaluation**
  - Evaluate treatments for untoward effects or effectiveness
  - Gather information from all available sources
  - Maintain situation awareness
- Manage Your **Workload**
  - Prioritize patient needs
  - Preload and offload tasks
  - Delegate tasks to others
- **Attention Allocation**
  - Limited resource
  - Avoid fixation errors
- **Teamwork**
  - Communicate changes and new information
  - Use shared mental models
- **Communication**
  - Use closed loop communication
  - Avoid blame and criticism of others
  - Focus on patient needs
- Call for **Help**
  - Global check before report
  - Give a clear concise report to incoming staff
  - Assign duties as needed

---

information during a crisis. Once these limitations are understood, many opportunities can be found to improve performance.

The role of PACU nurses is unique in health care delivery. Nurses not only must be familiar with a wide variety of pathologies and surgical treatments, but they also must be trained and prepared to provide care for a multitude of patient populations, including neonates, small children, adults, and the elderly, all within a single shift. In addition, PACU nurses interact with staff and physicians from many disciplines and must be able to function with an often unpredictable workload. The following sections discuss these crisis management principles in detail from the perspective of a PACU nurse.

## Environment

The perioperative period is a potentially tumultuous time for surgical patients. Therefore, the typical postanesthesia care unit represents a complex and dynamic work environment for

nurses. The acuity of postsurgical patients, dependency on technology and complex equipment, and inadequate staffing levels contribute to the uncertainty of the environment.

The inherent risk associated with the surgical experience follows patients to the postanesthesia care unit. Each patient brings an underlying medical pathology that may not be recognized until the recovery period. Such pathology can include obstructive sleep apnea, coronary artery disease, and electrolyte imbalances. PACU nurses must be cognizant of the ill effects of such conditions and be prepared to act on them if necessary.

A multitude of sophisticated monitors and equipment are involved in the care of patients after surgery. Nurses often rely heavily on technical specialists for maintenance and proper functioning of this equipment. Although nurses work with routine equipment on a daily basis, they may need additional training to deal with troubleshooting and the possibility of catastrophic failure of life-sustaining equipment, such as ventilators, dialysis machines, and intraaortic balloon pumps. Seconds can be critical if the patient is disconnected from any of these life-supporting devices. The nurse's focus remains on the patient while the specialist concentrates on the equipment. However, a crossover of skills is necessary. Therefore, opportunities for education regarding critical equipment in the environment should be offered to PACU nurses to facilitate an exchange of information and to develop contingency plans for major equipment failures should they occur. Familiarity with such emergency plans is essential and can save lives.

Unit staffing has a major influence on the PACU nurse's role as a care provider. Open unit layouts are advantageous because nurses are expected to simultaneously monitor and assess multiple patients. Maintenance of an overall awareness of staffing levels throughout a shift enables the nurse to make appropriate assignments and exert some control over the environment. Staffing that appears adequate at one point can quickly become inadequate, unsafe, and inept as staff are called to transport and admit patients, take breaks, or attend meetings. As staffing becomes insufficient, so does the opportunity for assistance should it be needed in an emergency.

## Resources

Resources are assets that are available to the PACU nurse. The appropriate use of resources allows for safe and effective care for patients after surgery. Often, resources are overlooked in an emergency. A primary resource available to the nurse is one's individual self. A nurse's knowledge and skills are indispensable in caring for patients in the recovery room. However, recognition of personal limitations is also a necessary component of delivery of safe care. An honest self appraisal may reveal multiple factors that influence performance and vigilance.[10] Lack of sleep, boredom, concerns over personal matters, illness, and the influence of medications can adversely impact performance. Because nurses are human, they are not entirely immune to these influences. Knowledge of these factors and communication of them to coworkers can go a long way to overcome their deleterious effects. A request for a lighter assignment may ultimately be safer than an attempt to overcome fatigue after an all night session with a sick child. The expectation that every nurse can perform optimally every day is unrealistic.

Critical care texts, drug formularies, and pharmacology manuals provide essential references for many drugs and dosages that are not used routinely. Institutional protocols and procedure guidelines should be kept on the unit for reference as needed. A review of reference manuals is prudent with care of a patient whose condition is atypical. Given the volumes of knowledge related to nursing care, one cannot stay current in all areas without use of these resources. Advanced Cardiac Life Support (ACLS) algorithm cards, for example, are invaluable in the event of cardiac arrest when recall of the detailed protocols is difficult. Many practitioners carry a personal notebook of medications, precalculated dosages, and protocols for quick access if necessary.

Planning ahead for rare but life-threatening emergencies is propitious. For example, while caring for a patient at risk for myocardial ischemia, the PACU nurse should consider a judicious review of cardiac drugs used to treat ischemia. Should the problem actually occur, the nurse will be more effective and better prepared to intervene.

## Reevaluation

The critical aspects of an emergency often cause nurses to lose sight of the proverbial big picture. Thus, the purpose of reevaluation is twofold: first, to evaluate the effectiveness of treatment, and then, to provide more comprehensive insight to the problem. For example, a nurse may become involved in initiating a cardiac arrest response yet forget to turn the oxygen to 100% on the ventilator. A scan of all monitors and machines to see whether anything else is changing has value. With every intervention, a continuous

risk-benefit analysis must be carried out. Reevaluation helps draw the focus outward to see whether parameters that were overlooked initially have changed. With baseline data, a better understanding of the trends in these parameters can be realized. The ability to stand back and absorb the situation in its entirety is referred to as "situational awareness" in human factors literature.[11] Situational awareness allows one to grasp the impact of significant changes and to plan instead of merely react to the situation. With continuous reevaluation of the patient, the PACU nurse can report more effectively to incoming help. The PACU nurse is able to detail what has been done and to prioritize subsequent interventions, which helps new team members contribute positively and effectively.

## Workload

A typical day in any critical care unit is filled with multiple tasks. Most nurses quickly learn to distribute their workload throughout the shift and to prioritize patient care needs as conditions change. Experienced nurses frequently use tactics known as preloading and offloading to balance the demands of patient care. *Preloading* is defined as early preparation for an upcoming procedure. *Offloading* is the opposite. An example of offloading is catching up on the narrative chart after care has been rendered. These two tactics can dramatically decrease the workload during busy periods.

An unexpected emergency dramatically and precipitously increases workload. Additional help is essential in completion of the multitude of tasks required during this critical time. As new staff members arrive, they should be assigned a specific task that is appropriate to their training and experience. The charge nurse can page attending physicians and other support personnel and reassign patient care responsibilities to ensure coverage. Registered nurses can administer medications, change ventilator settings, and assist in procedures, and aides can run laboratory work, obtain blood from the blood bank, or obtain equipment.

## Attention Allocation

Attention is a limited resource. One can accurately follow only two to three rapidly changing variables at any one time. Direct patient care activities further reduce the number of variables one can manage simultaneously. The uncertain nature of a crisis presents a great opportunity for error, which makes comprehension and analysis of the situation difficult for one individual. Someone must be available to make observations, commit to decisions, and continuously evaluate the patient's condition. These duties are the responsibility of the team leader in a code situation but may fall to the primary nurse unless more expert help arrives.

Fixation and pauses in thinking are common for health care providers involved in a critical incident. *Fixation errors* occur in dynamic situations and are often difficult events from which to recover. For example, a nurse may recognize a decrease in oxygen saturation and elevated peak airway pressures and, with that information, treat the patient for bronchospasm. At the same time, the nurse may fail to note the accompanying hypotension, flushing, and rash that signal an allergic reaction. This failure is an example of a "this and only this" fixation error in which one has a reasonable diagnosis in mind and manipulates any additional changes to fit that diagnosis. A second common pitfall is an "anything but this" fixation error, in which treatment is delayed while one seeks additional information in the face of a crisis. The nurse essentially identifies the problem but continues to look for a more manageable diagnosis. The third type of fixation error is an "everything's okay" error, in which the health care professional denies a problem in evolution. All health care providers are vulnerable to these errors during an emergency. These errors are the result of an overtaxed brain that precludes effective work given the immense workload.

### Teamwork

Nurses in the PACU routinely use teamwork to care for critically ill patients. Flexible assignments, assistance with turning patients, or preparation of medications are just a few ways nurses work together to accomplish their goals.

During a critical event, however, teamwork needs to change dramatically. Additional staff with variable expertise join the team. Physicians arrive and begin to order treatments, drugs, and tests. The original PACU team of nurses now becomes multidisciplinary and takes on a new character. New physician residents may be reluctant to take on a leadership role or several may attempt to be the leader simultaneously. Orders may be shouted into the air, directed at no particular individual. A previously orderly environment may rapidly become chaotic and disorganized.

Multidisciplinary team training at major institutions has shown excellent results in crisis management. Physicians are trained in leadership skills, and the other team members are taught to be productive and effective team members. Team members are encouraged to give their input to the leader, to inform leaders of significant changes, to report the administration of drugs and treatments, and to critique problem solving. Information from any source may provide the answer in an ambiguous situation. Recognition that every member of the team has the potential to make valuable contributions is important. The team supports the leader in maintaining good situational awareness and in making the best possible decisions. Ideally, the leader should be willing to consider input from all team members, communicate diagnosis and plans for treatment, and keep team members informed of progress. By doing so, the team leader keeps the entire team focused on the immediate needs of the patient and further encourages their active role in optimizing the patient's condition.

### Communication

Great leadership and teamwork cannot occur without the ability to communicate effectively. The military uses "closed loop" communication to ensure that orders are received and understood properly. People must be addressed by name to attract their attention. Once the message is stated clearly, one should look for verbal confirmation that the message was received correctly. "Give some Bicarb" is better stated as "Suzanne, give 1 amp of Bicarb IV now." Suzanne, in turn, should state "I am giving 1 amp of Bicarb IV now." As Suzanne completes the task, she should inform the leader that it has been done, which verifies that she has successfully completed the task and that she is now free to participate in other additional tasks.

High noise levels accompany an emergency situation as many people try to talk at the same time. Speaking in a calm quiet voice does more to attract attention than another shout in the melee. Again, preceding the statement with the person's name helps gain attention. Repeating the name may be necessary to divert the person from other activities.

Conflict is common in emotionally charged situations. The media have published several accounts of hostile interactions between health care providers that actually led to violence. To avoid escalation of existing hostility, speak in impersonal terms and avoid making judgments and placing blame on others.

### Call for Help

Nurses are used to working in teams. They rarely have trouble calling for additional help as needed for physical tasks, such as getting the code cart, starting additional intravenous (IV) lines, or hanging blood. Value is found in a second person's opinion in management of a critical situation. Many people believe that they lose credibility with colleagues if they call for assistance in this type of situation. Merit exists in the adage "it's what's right for the patient, not who is right." A call for a second opinion from someone with more expertise is a wise move, not a weak one.

Before help arrives, a global scan of the patient, the equipment, and the monitors is a good practice. This requisite knowledge provides a set of baseline data with which to compare as the treatment progresses and allows the nurse to provide a full report to incoming assistants. When help arrives, incoming staff should receive a brief succinct report on what has happened and any treatment that has begun. Information in the report need not include insignificant details but should convey the information necessary to explicate the situation at hand.

The ERR WATCH principles make good sense. Most PACU nurses can use them daily in their practice and have them available when an emergency situation occurs. These principles are universal and can be used to effectively improve performance and positively influence the care given to the postsurgical patient in the recovery room.

## SIMULATION IN CRM TRAINING

*Simulation* is the implementation of artificial representations of complex real-world processes with a sufficient level of fidelity to achieve particular goals.[12] Simulation imitates real phenomena and processes to capture key characteristics and behaviors of real life events. It is an innovative instructional approach that enhances learning and promotes a sense of empowerment on the part of learners by involving them in the decisions that influence their learning. Through simulation, trainees are challenged in novel ways and take more responsibility in their learning. A critical feature of simulation as a learning tool is that learners have the ability to interact with their surroundings experimentally.[12] With use of high-fidelity simulated environments, educators and trainers can create models of crisis and chaos where the risk to a real patient is absent.

CRM training for PACU personnel incorporates human patient simulators in high-fidelity critical care environments to simulate rare but life-threatening recovery room crises, including inability to ventilate, anaphylactic shock, and cardiac arrest, to name a few. Human patient simulators, sometimes referred to as mannequins, are full-body representations of patients that demonstrate physiologic parameters, such as blood pressure, heart rate, airway pressure, oxygen saturation, and central venous and pulmonary pressures. Different models of human patient simulators offer varying degrees of realism, including bleeding, urination, sweating, drooling, pupil constriction and dilation, seizures, chest movement, and peripheral pulses. Standard monitoring equipment is used to display physiologically appropriate measurements of all invasive and noninvasive values. Simulators also have the ability to breathe spontaneously with measurable exhaled carbon dioxide. Furthermore, trainees can assess heart, breath, and bowel sounds. The addition of various props can transform the patient into a full-term parturient, an elderly gentleman, or even a young athlete. Placed within a realistic setting, the human patient simulator becomes lifelike as it converses with trainees via an instructor-speaker microphone.

Human patient simulators come with an accompanying laptop computer and software and are operated by a controller, usually a member of the training team. The controller can 'steer' the human patient simulator to respond to trainee interventions, such as drug and fluid administration, cardiac defibrillation, intubation, and oxygenation. Human patient simulators are highly effective in contributing to the realism necessary to achieve educational objectives.

CRM emphasizes the integration of crisis management principles, including decision making, task management, leadership, communication, situational awareness, and teamwork, in the training of recovery room nurses and team members to manage critical events and crisis situations. Identification and mastering of ideal case management behaviors, including preparation, anticipation, and vigilance, are also a significant goal of CRM training. In addition, factors such as production pressure, problem evolution, and abstract reasoning and their influence on the provider to act efficiently are considered and explored.[13]

CRM training is an experiential teaching approach that brings the daunting characteristics of a perioperative crisis to life and ultimately intends to improve efficiency, effectiveness, and safety in the delivery of care to surgical patients. Most CRM training courses have a similar structure that incorporates assigned readings that describe basic principles, a course introduction that details the overall concept, an orientation to the simulated critical care environment, and video-taped critical incident scenarios of which the learner is an active participant carrying out the duties of a recovery room team member under the extreme conditions of a postanesthesia emergency. During a simulated scenario, one learner out of the group is randomly selected to be in the "hot seat" as the team leader while the other members of the group participate in various roles as team members. During a CRM training course, the trainee is able to not only actively apply crisis resource management principles during a crisis but also observe other learners applying these same principles while fulfilling other team member roles.

A video-playback detailed debriefing session, usually facilitated by course faculty, immediately follows the scenario in an adjacent classroom. *Debriefing* is a discussion among students, guided by faculty, that encourages reflective thought and self review.[14] Debriefing is regarded as an integral part of CRM and occurs in a positive, supportive, nonjudgmental, and non-evaluative environment that allows all participants an opportunity to share their experience, offer comments, and discuss concerns.[14] The primary goal of debriefing is the discussion of the CRM principles as they relate to the outcome. The discussion is focused on essential crisis management principles such as communication, teamwork, and decision making. Trainees are often surprised at their performances as they view the videotape and are able to scrutinize their interaction with other team members. Most importantly, the group examines CRM strategies that may be used to prevent future errors in similar situations. Most participants complete the course feeling better prepared to navigate the complexity inherent in critical events characteristic of the PACU.

### Variety of Teaching Goals

Simulation centers provide a safe place for the training of health care providers. Mistakes made during sessions do not harm actual patients. Procedures can be done repeatedly until the trainee gains a desired level of confidence and proficiency. New employees can learn the unit's routines or how to admit and care for various types of patients. PACU personnel can work with the actual unit equipment to better understand its operation. Existing staff can use the simulator to practice rarely performed procedures, learn new skills, or orient to new equipment. A review of ACLS protocols is just one example of the potential use of simulation. Personnel can gain experience in the diagnosis and management of rare life-threatening medical crises rarely witnessed in any other setting. Several institutions have developed morbidity and mortality conferences with simulation to recreate real cases. Through simulation, many topics can be taught either individually or as part of a more comprehensive critical care course.

For effective management, most critical incidents require the collaboration of multiple team members, including physicians and nurses. Simulation provides an opportunity for training health care teams to work collectively and maximize their potential. Studies in aviation and medicine have found that lack of teamwork skills—not the requisite technical knowledge—resulted in most disasters. Until the introduction of full-scale human patient simulators, the training of teams was never formalized. Now, actual teams of nurses, respiratory therapists, physicians, and other health care providers can interact realistically and learn to communicate and function together as a cohesive unit. This type of training has been performed at various sites and has been found to be effective at improving team performance.[15,16]

## SUMMARY

Technical knowledge and skills alone are not adequate for functioning in the complex environment of critical care. Patients today are sicker than ever before. With this increased acuity also comes an increasing number of critical events that need prompt and accurate management. Each problem has many possible outcomes that depend largely on the actions or inactions of caregivers. Every patient deserves to have well-trained and knowledgeable care providers that can manage not only the usual events associated with recovery but also the unexpected ones. CRM training and simulation offer a new approach to help PACU nurses meet these challenges successfully. Like the patients for whom they care, health care professionals are human, and humans are imperfect, which is something that cannot be changed. But through advanced simulation training in preventable mishaps, coupled with an enlightened systems approach to looking at error, one can best prepare and enable providers to avoid mistakes before they occur.

## REFERENCES

1.   Helmreich RL, Foushee HC: Why crew resource management? Empirical and theoretical bases of human factors training in aviation. In Wiener EL, Kanki BG, Helmreich RL, editors: *Cockpit resource management*, San Diego, 1993, Academic Press.

THE POSTANESTHESIA CARE UNIT

2. Howard SK, Gaba DM, Fish KJ, et al: Anesthesia crisis resource management training: teaching anesthesiologists to handle critical incidents, *Aviat Space Environ Med* 63(9):763-770, 1992.

3. Cooper JB, Newbower RS, Long CD, et al: Preventable anesthesia mishaps: a study of human factors, *Anesthesiology* 49:399-406, 1978.

4. Cook RI, Woods DD: Human error in medicine. In Bogner MS, editor: *Operating at the sharp end: the complexity of human error*, Hillsdale, NJ, 1994, Lawrence Erlbaum Associates.

5. Helmreich RL: On error management: lessons from aviation, *Br Med J* 320:781-785, 2000.

6. *Topics of previous APSF grants*, available at http://www.gasnet.org/societies/apsf/foundation/topics/topics.html. Accessed October 3, 2001.

7. Reason J: *Human error*, New York, 1990, Cambridge University Press.

8. Gaba DM, Fish KJ, Howard SK: *Crisis management in anesthesiology*, New York, 1994, Churchill Livingstone.

9. Fletcher JL: AANA journal course: update for nurse anesthetists; ERR WATCH: anesthesia crisis resource management from the nurse anesthetist's perspective, *AANA J* 66(6):595-602, 1998.

10. Howard SK, Smith BE, Gaba DM, et al: Performance of well-rested vs. highly-fatigued residents: a simulator study, *Anesthesiology* 87:A981, 1997.

11. Gaba DM, Howard SK, Small SD: Situation awareness in anesthesiology, *Human Factors* 37(1):20-31, 1995.

12. Doyle DJ: (2006). *Simulation in medical education: focus on anesthesiology*, available at www.med-ed-online.org/f0000053.htm. Accessed November 5, 2006.

13. Gaba DM, Howard SK, Fish KJ, et al: Simulation-based training in anesthesia crisis resource management (ACRM): a decade of experience, *Simulation Gaming* 32(2):175-193, 2001.

14. Savoldelli GL, Naik VN, Park J, et al: Value of debriefing during simulated crisis management, *Anesthesiology* 105(2):279-285, 2006.

15. Lippert A, Ostergaard HT, White J, et al: The knowledge and performance of the cardiopulmonary resuscitation team, *Anesthesiology* 90:A-1212, 2000.

16. Sexton B, Marsch S, Helmreich R, et al: Participant evaluation of team oriented medical simulation, available at http://www.Psy.utexas.edu/psy/Helmreich/evaltoms.htm. Accessed October 3, 2001.

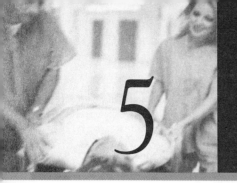

# 5

# INFECTION CONTROL IN THE PACU

*Lisa Sturm, MPH, CIC*

The increasing prevalence rate of multidrug resistant organisms combined with the increasing complexity of care and the volume of patients seen in a busy perianesthesia unit underscores the importance of having a developed infection control program in place.

Patients with a wide range of infectious diseases, some communicable, are commonly cared for in the preoperative and postoperative settings. The goal of infection control is prevention of the transmission of pathogenic microorganisms between patients, staff, and visitors. A multitude of variables needs to be managed for this prevention, ranging from environment, to equipment, to health care worker (HCW) behaviors and practices.

The following policies and procedures that are based on published guidelines and recommendations can help minimize the infectious risks present in a perianesthesia unit. Education, compliance, monitoring, and quality improvement are essential to the success of the infection control efforts.

## DEFINITIONS

**Adverse Events:** Untoward, undesirable, and usually unanticipated events, such as death of a patient, an employee, or a visitor in a health care organization. Incidents such as patient falls or improper administration of medications are also considered adverse events even if there is no permanent effect on the patient.

**Airborne Transmission:** (Microorganisms that are) carried or transported by the air.

**Antibiotic Resistance:** The selective pressure of antimicrobial therapy has resulted in the evolution of bacteria that are resistant to certain antibiotics. The resistance patterns of the microbes are constantly changing. These patterns are affected by patterns of antibiotic use, the prevalence of specific microorganisms, the mechanisms of resistance in these organisms, resistance transfer from one organism to another, and the patient population. The risk of infection or colonization with antibiotic-resistant

microorganisms is higher among sicker and debilitated patients and in settings of high antimicrobial use and invasive technology (e.g., intensive care unit [ICU]). Infections from antibiotic-resistant organisms are difficult to treat and are often associated with high morbidity rates. These microbes can be spread from patient to patient through transient hand carriage and environmental contamination.

**Antimicrobial Prophylaxis:** Antibiotics that are given before the surgical incision for prevention of a surgical wound infection.

**Artificial Nails:** Nails with products affixed to them, such as gel, tips, jewelry, overlays, and wraps.

**Attributable Mortality Rate:** The death rate (expression of the number of deaths in a population during a specified time frame) that can be linked to a particular cause or source.

**Barrier Precautions:** The use of garb (e.g., masks, hair coverings, gowns, gloves) for protection to either the health care worker or the patient.

**Bloodborne:** Microorganisms that are carried or transmitted via the blood or fluids that contain blood.

**Bloodborne Pathogens:** Pathogenic microorganisms that are present in human blood and can cause disease in humans. These pathogens include, but are not limited to, hepatitis B virus (HBV) and human immunodeficiency virus (HIV).

**Catheter-Related Bloodstream Infections (CRBSI):** Bacteremia or fungemia in a patient with an intravascular central venous catheter.

**Central Venous Catheter:** A vascular access device that terminates at or close to the heart or one of the great vessels. An umbilical artery or vein catheter is considered a central line.

**Chlorhexidine Gluconate (CHG):** An antibacterial that is effective against a wide variety of gram-negative and gram-positive organisms and used as a topical antiinfective for the skin and mucous membranes.

***Clostridium difficile:*** A bacterium that causes diarrhea and more serious intestinal conditions such as colitis. It is found in the normal gastro-intestinal (GI) flora in about 3% of healthy adults and in 10% to 30% or more of hospitalized patients. Antibiotic use, even a short course given for prophylaxis or treatment of infections, often changes the normal GI flora, which can lead to *C. difficile* overgrowth and toxin production. *C. difficile* accounts for 15% to 25% of all antibiotic-associated diarrhea. *C. difficile* colitis occurs in all ages but is most frequent in middle-aged and elderly adults or patients with debilitated conditions. *C. difficile* is shed in feces and is spread primarily via the hands of health care personnel who have touched a contaminated surface or item and via direct contact with a contaminated item. Hand hygiene performed with soap and water and thorough disinfection of the environment reduce the risk of spreading *C. difficile*.

**Colonization:** Microorganisms that have become established in a habitat in a host but do not cause disease (infection) in this habitat.

**Contact (direct or indirect):** (Microorganisms that are) spread from contaminated hands or objects.

**Contact Dermatitis:** Inflammation of the skin that results from direct exposure to an irritant.

**Contaminated Sharps:** Any contaminated object that can penetrate the skin, including, but not limited to, needles, scalpels, broken glass, broken capillary tubes, and exposed ends of dental wires.

**Cross Transmission:** Horizontal transmission of an organism in the health care setting; patient to patient.

**Disinfection:** To render free from infection, especially with destruction of harmful microorganisms.

**Droplet Transmission:** (Microorganisms that are) carried on airborne droplets of saliva or sputum.

**Epidemiology:** A branch of medical science that deals with the incidence, distribution, and control of disease in a population.

**Exposure Control Plan:** A formal document as defined by the Occupational Safety and Health Administration (OSHA) Regulations (Standards, 29 CFR) Bloodborne Pathogens 1910.1030; to exist in any institution with occupational exposure. The document is designed to outline the steps necessary to eliminate or minimize employee exposure.

**Extended Spectrum Beta-Lactamases (ESBL):** Beta-lactamase is a type of enzyme responsible for bacterial resistance to beta-lactam antibiotics. Among these are penicillins, cephalosporins, carbapenems, and others. In the mid 1980s, new types of beta-lactamase were produced by

*Klebsiella* and *Escherichia coli* that could hydrolyze the extended spectrum cephalosporins. These are collectively termed the extended spectrum beta-lactamases (ESBLs).

**Fecal-Oral:** Microorganisms that are spread through contaminated feces and are ingested.

**Health Care-Associated Infections (HAI):** Acquired or occurring in the health care setting.

**Health Care Worker Flora:** The microorganisms (as bacteria or fungi) that live in or on the body of personnel that work in a health care institution.

**Hypothermia:** Subnormal temperature of the body, defined as temperature less than 36°C.

**Immunocompromised:** Impairment or weakening of the immune system.

**Medical Waste/Regulated Waste:** Liquid or semiliquid blood or other potentially infectious materials; contaminated items that release blood or other potentially infectious materials in a liquid or semiliquid state if compressed; items that are caked with dried blood or other potentially infectious materials and are capable of releasing these materials during handling; contaminated sharps; and pathologic and microbiologic wastes that contain blood or other potentially infectious materials.

**Microbial Colony Counts:** Enumeration via direct count of viable isolated bacterial or fungal cells or spores capable of growth on solid culture media. Each colony (i.e., microbial colony-forming unit) represents the progeny of a single cell in the original inoculum. The method is used routinely by environmental microbiologists for quantification of organisms in air, food, and water; by clinicians for measurement of patient microbial load; and in antimicrobial drug testing.

**Moist Body Substances:** All body fluids, including blood, body cavity fluids, breast milk, urine, feces, wound or other skin drainage, respiratory and oral secretions, mucous membranes.

**Mucous Membranes:** Mucous membranes line cavities or canals of the body that open to the outside, including the eyes, ears, mouth, nose, and genitals.

**Multidrug Resistant Organisms (MDRO):** Microorganisms, predominantly bacteria, that are resistant to one or more classes of antimicrobial agents. Although the names of certain MDROs describe resistance to only one agent (e.g., methicillin-resistant *Staphylococcus aureus* [MRSA], vancomycin-resistant *Enterococcus* [VRE]), these pathogens are frequently resistant to most available antimicrobial agents. These highly resistant organisms deserve special attention in health care facilities. In addition to MRSA and VRE, certain gram-negative bacteria, including those that produce extended spectrum beta-lactamases (ESBLs) and others that are resistant to multiple classes of antimicrobial agents, are of particular concern.

**N95 Respirator:** An air-purifying filtering-facepiece respirator that is more than 95% efficient at removal of 0.3-μm particles and is not resistant to oil.

**Negative-Pressure Isolation Rooms:** The difference in air pressure between two areas. A room that is under negative pressure has a lower pressure than adjacent areas, which keeps air from flowing out of the room and into adjacent rooms or areas.

**Normothermia:** Normal body temperature (i.e., 36° C to 38° C).

**Nosocomial Infections:** Term used historically to denote infections that are acquired or occur in a hospital.

**One-Handed "Scoop" Technique:** A method of capping a needle if deemed necessary to do so. The needle cap is set on a stable surface and not touched. The needled device then is placed inside the cap with one hand. The cap then is secured into place with the other hand.

**Parenteral Exposure:** Piercing of mucous membranes or the skin barrier through such events as needlesticks, human bites, cuts, and abrasions.

**Pathogenic Microorganisms:** An organism of microscopic or ultramicroscopic size that is capable of causing disease.

**Personal Protective Equipment (PPE):** Specialized clothing or equipment worn by an employee for protection against a hazard. General work clothes (e.g., uniforms, pants, shirts or blouses) not intended to function as protection against a hazard are not considered to be personal protective equipment.

**Seroconversion Risk:** The likelihood of conversion from negative virus status to positive virus status.

**Susceptible:** Little resistance to a specific infectious disease.

**Transient Contamination:** A microorganism that exists temporarily on the hands of a health care worker and is not part of the normal flora of the skin.

**Vancomycin-Resistant Enterococcus (VRE):** A strain of *Enterococcus* bacteria that normally lives in the intestines and sometimes the urinary tract of all people. VRE has learned to resist or survive most antibiotics, including a strong antibiotic called vancomycin. VRE is acquired via direct contact (touching) with objects or surfaces that are contaminated with VRE. VRE is not spread through the air. People at risk for VRE are those who have chronic illnesses, have undergone recent surgery, have weakened immune systems, or have recently taken certain antibiotics.

**Vector:** Microorganisms that are spread through insects.

## MANAGING THE ENVIRONMENT AND EQUIPMENT

### Environment

A safe and clean environment is essential for a reduction in the risk of transmission of microorganisms. Most equipment that comes into contact with patients in a perianesthesia unit is considered to have a low risk of infection transmission, most notably if the equipment is noninvasive and only comes into contact with intact skin. Examples of these items are electrodes, stethoscopes, blood pressure cuffs, the outside surfaces of equipment (e.g., ventilators, intravenous pumps), and larger surfaces (e.g., tables, wheelchairs, bedside stands, floors, and walls). Depending on the item and the nature of the contamination, simple surface cleaning is all that is necessary to ensure safety between patient use. Many hospital-grade disinfectants are combined with a cleaning component so that both cleaning and disinfection can be achieved in one step. Disinfection wipes are an appropriate option as well because of their active ingredient. If visible blood or body fluid is present, then an Environmental Protection Agency (EPA)–approved hospital grade disinfectant (e.g., a quaternary ammonium compound, 70% isopropyl, properly diluted bleach, or phenolic) is required per the OSHA Bloodborne Pathogen Standard.[1]

### Laundry

The risk of actual disease transmission from soiled linen is negligible, although laundry may harbor large numbers of pathogenic microorganisms. Simple hygienic practices for the processing and storage of linen are recommended for a reduction in the likelihood of transmission of infectious diseases.

Soiled linen should be handled as little as possible and with minimal agitation for prevention of gross microbial contamination of the air and of persons who handle the linen. All soiled linen should be bagged or placed in containers in the care unit. It should never be sorted or rinsed in the location of use. Linen heavily contaminated with blood or other body fluids should be bagged and transported in a manner that prevents leakage.

Commercial laundry facilities often use water temperatures of at least 160° F and 50 to 150 ppm of chlorine bleach for removal of significant quantities of microorganisms from grossly contaminated linen. Commercial dry cleaning of fabrics soiled with blood also renders these items free of the risk of pathogen transmission. Lastly, clean linen should be handled, transported, and stored by methods that ensure its cleanliness.

## Furnishings

All furnishings in a perianesthesia environment should be evaluated before purchase and assessed for the ability to resist staining and tearing. Absorbent upholstery should be avoided if the likelihood of contamination is present. Torn mattress pads and seating should be repaired or replaced promptly for prevention of contamination.

## Sinks

The number and accessibility of sinks in the perianesthesia care unit is important for increased compliance with hand washing. The Guidelines for Design and Construction of Hospital and Health Care Facilities, published and updated periodically by the American Institute of Architects (AIA), should be referenced for current sink allotment recommendations. The guidelines are conceived as minimal construction requirements for hospitals, and the document includes engineering systems, infection control, and safety and architectural guidelines for design and construction. The Joint Commission (TJC) states that the AIA guidelines should be used during new construction. The current AIA guidelines recommend at least one hand washing station with hands-free or wrist blade–operable controls for every four beds in a postanesthetic care unit (PACU).[2]

## Bays and Isolation Rooms

Appropriate space allotment and other design features for patient bays and rooms during new construction and renovation can be obtained from the AIA guidelines reference. Additional local and state stipulations may apply. Provisions should be available for the isolation of infectious patients, but an airborne (respiratory) infection isolation room is not required in a preoperative or postanesthetic care unit. However, each individual setting needs to conduct an infection control risk assessment for the need for an isolation room based on the epidemiology of airborne diseases (e.g., frequency of tuberculosis in the community, medically or surgically treated in the institution).

## Traffic Flow

The movement of staff, patients, visitors, and equipment in the preoperative and PACU setting is an important consideration in the design or renovation of space. Areas in which invasive procedures (e.g., central line insertions) take place should be away from main traffic areas and entrances and exits to reduce the likelihood of contamination.

# GENERAL INFECTION CONTROL PRACTICES

## Handwashing

The benefits of hand hygiene in a hospital setting were first recognized by Ignaz Semmelweis in 1847 after the death of his friend from an infection that he contracted after his finger was accidentally punctured with a knife during a postmortem examination. The friend's autopsy showed a pathologic situation similar to that of the women who were dying from puerperal fever in one of the obstetric clinics. Semmelweis immediately proposed a connection between cadaveric contamination and puerperal fever and made a detailed study of the mortality statistics of the obstetric clinic attended to by physicians who also performed autopsies with the statistics of the midwives' clinics. The midwives did not participate in autopsies. He concluded that he and the students carried the infecting particles on their hands from the autopsy room to the patients they examined in the clinic setting. Semmelweis concluded that some unknown "cadaveric material" caused childbed fever. He instituted a policy requiring use of a solution of chlorinated lime for washing hands between autopsy work and the examination of patients and the mortality rate dropped from its then-current level of 12.24% to 2.38%, comparable with the midwives' clinics' rates.[3]

To this day, hand hygiene remains of paramount importance for prevention of the spread of disease-causing germs in the perianesthesia setting. Hands should be washed with soap and water for at least 20 seconds with a hospital-approved liquid or foam soap (bar soap should be avoided). If hands are not visibly soiled, an alcohol-based hand rub can be used. Alcohol-based hand rubs significantly reduce the number of microorganisms on skin, are fast acting, and cause less skin irritation.[4] They should not be used if the hands are visibly contaminated with blood, body fluids, or soiling. Hand hygiene should be minimally performed before and after patient care, after handling of soiled equipment or linen, after removal of gloves, after use of the restroom, before and after eating, or whenever hands are soiled. Health care personnel should avoid wearing artificial nails and keep natural nails less than one quarter of an inch long if they care for patients at high risk of acquiring infections (e.g., patients in intensive care units or in transplant units).

Adherence of hand hygiene has been studied in observational studies of HCWs. Compliance rates to follow recommended hand hygiene procedures have been poor, with mean baseline rates of 5% to 81% (overall average, 40%). Perceived barriers to adherence with hand hygiene include skin irritation, inaccessible hand-hygiene supplies, interference with HCW-patient relationships, priority of care (i.e., the patient's needs are given priority over hand hygiene), wearing of gloves, forgetfulness, lack of knowledge of hand hygiene policy, insufficient time for hand hygiene, high workload and understaffing, and the lack of scientific information or education indicating a definitive impact of improved hand hygiene on health care–associated infection rates.[5-11]

Frequent and repeated use of hand hygiene products, particularly soaps and other detergents, is a primary cause of chronic irritant contact dermatitis among HCWs.[12] For minimization of this condition, health care workers should use hospital-approved hand lotion frequently and regularly on their hands. Small personal-use containers or multiuse pumps that are smaller than 16 oz (and not refilled) should be used. Lotions that contain petroleum or other oil emollients may affect the integrity of latex gloves; therefore, compatibility between the lotion and its possible effects on gloves should be considered at the time of product selection.[1] Lastly, certain moisturizing products and surfactants have been shown to interfere with the residual activity of CHG, a skin antiseptic in liquid soap. Compatibility between a lotion and its possible effects on the efficacy of certain antiseptic soaps should be considered at the time of product selection.

### Personal Protective Equipment (PPE)

The most common PPE used by health care workers is gloves. The Centers for Disease Control has recommended that HCWs wear gloves to: (1) reduce the risk of personnel acquiring infections from patients; (2) prevent health care worker flora from being transmitted to patients; and (3) reduce transient contamination of the hands of personnel by flora that can be transmitted from one patient to another.[13] OSHA mandates that gloves be worn during all patient care activities that may involve exposure to blood or body fluids that may be contaminated with blood.[1] They should also be worn for direct contact with mucous membranes, nonintact skin, open wounds, or items potentially contaminated with moist body substances. Gloves should also be worn in vascular access procedures. The effectiveness of

gloves in prevention of contamination of HCWs' hands has been confirmed in several clinical studies. Two of these studies, which involved personnel caring for patients with C. difficile or VRE, revealed that wearing gloves prevented hand contamination among most personnel who had direct contact with patients.[14-16] Wearing of gloves also prevented personnel from acquiring VRE on their hands when touching contaminated environmental surfaces.[16] Prevention of heavy contamination of the hands is considered important because hand washing or hand antisepsis may not remove all potential pathogens when hands are heavily contaminated.[17,18]

Additional forms of PPE include fluid-resistant gowns, aprons, or other protective clothing. These should be worn to protect clothing and all areas of exposed skin when contact with moist body substances is reasonably anticipated. Gowns shall be used once and discarded after use. Face protection, such as masks and protective eyewear (goggles or glasses with side shields), should be worn to prevent contact of blood or other moist body substances with the mucous membranes of the nose and mouth, which may occur when moist body substances are splashed, sprayed, or splattered. Face shields may be worn in place of protective eyewear and masks.

### Standard Precautions

Standard Precautions synthesize the major features of Universal Precautions (Blood and Body Fluid Precaution, designed to reduce the risk of transmission of bloodborne pathogens) and body substance isolation (BSI; designed to reduce the risk of transmission of pathogens from moist body substances) and apply to all patients who receive care in hospitals, regardless of diagnosis or presumed infection status. Standard Precautions apply to: (1) blood; (2) all body fluids, secretions, and excretions, except sweat, regardless of whether or not they contain visible blood; (3) nonintact skin; and (4) mucous membranes. Standard Precautions are designed to reduce the risk of transmission of microorganisms from both recognized and unrecognized sources of infection in hospitals.[19]

In addition to the aforementioned use of hand hygiene and PPE, Standard Precautions also encompass the management of patient care equipment. They stipulate that used patient care equipment that is soiled with blood, body fluids, secretions, and excretions should be managed in a manner that prevents skin and mucous membrane exposures, contamination of clothing, and transfer of microorganisms to other patients and environments. Reusable equipment should be cleaned and reprocessed appropriately before use for the care of another patient, and single-use items (or items labeled disposable) should not be reprocessed and reused and should be discarded properly.

Standard Precautions also encompass the practices of environmental control (e.g., that the hospital has adequate procedures for the routine care, cleaning, and disinfection of environmental surfaces, beds, bedrails, bedside equipment, and other frequently touched surfaces) and ensure that these procedures are followed. Lastly, Standard Precautions reiterate the importance of the Occupational Health and Bloodborne Pathogens Rule and proper patient placement for prevention of transmission of disease, both of which are discussed in later sections of this chapter.

## MANAGEMENT OF THE INFECTED OR CONTAGIOUS PATIENT

The "chain of infection" is a concept that shows the essential requirements for the perpetuation of a disease-causing microorganism (Fig. 5-1). All infectious diseases are caused by a microorganism (e.g. bacteria, virus, mold or fungi, or parasite). For survival, each microorganism sustains itself in a source. The source may be a living host, such as a human or animal, or a nonliving source, such as biohazardous waste, laboratory specimen, etc. To cause disease, the microorganism must have a portal of exit from the source (e.g., respiratory tract, spill) and a method of spread. The six main methods of spread for infectious diseases include airborne, droplet, contact (direct or indirect), bloodborne, vector, and fecal-oral. With its unique method of spread, an organism must find a way to enter its

next host. The entry point may be the same as the exit from the source of the infection (such as respiratory route to respiratory route or blood to blood), or it may be different (such as fecal exit to oral entry). The last component to the chain of infection is the susceptible person. A person may be more susceptible because of underlying illness, such as immunocompromise from chemotherapy or AIDS, or because of the risks of an open incision or invasive procedure. Likewise, a person may be less susceptible to the infection as a result of history of vaccination or natural immunity from past exposure or disease.

### Communicable Diseases of Concern

Every institution should have a method of identification of patients who pose a public health risk to others, and each perianesthesia unit needs to be aware of the process used for this identification. Certain communicable diseases should be clearly documented in the patient's medical record, and the patient should be appropriately placed into precautions or isolation per institutional policy to minimize the infectious risks to others. Infectious diseases that warrant immediate attention include, but are not limited to, bacterial meningitis (or meningitis of unknown infectious etiology), measles (rubeola), mumps, rubella, chickenpox, tuberculosis, and severe acute respiratory syndrome (SARS). Each individual state in the United States publishes it own Reportable Disease listing that stipulates reporting requirements. Typically, diseases are reported to the local public health department by the physician or the infection control department. Communication is essential between the patient, health care provider, reporting department in the institution, and public health department to ensure that the chain of infection is broken.

### Antibiotic-resistant Organisms

In addition to the communicable diseases that pose an infectious risk to others, antibiotic-resistant organisms pose a significant threat to others if not properly controlled and managed. Aside from the cross-transmission risks, these organisms also cause an increase in lengths of stay, costs, and mortality rates.[20-25] The most common organisms include MRSA and VRE. Certain strains of *Staphylococcus aureus* also have intermediate susceptibility or are resistant to vancomycin (i.e., vancomycin-intermediate *S. aureus* [VISA], vancomycin-resistant *S. aureus* [VRSA]). In addition to the gram-positive organisms are certain gram-negative bacteria, including those that produce ESBLs and others that are resistant to multiple

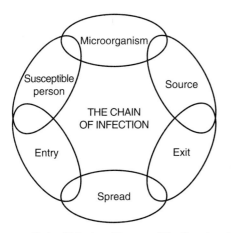

**Fig. 5-1** Chain of infection. (*Courtesy of The Department of Infection Control & Epidemiology at the University of Michigan Hospitals & Health Centers, Ann Arbor, Mich.*)

classes of antibiotics. Examples of resistant gram-negative bacteria include *E. coli*, *Klebsiella pneumoniae*, *Acinetobacter baumannii*, and organisms such as *Stenotrophomonas maltophilia*.

Because of the differences in the pathogens, the diseases they cause, their routes of transmission, the patients they infect, and the intensity of patient care activities, each institution needs to have tailored infection control strategies. The perianesthesia personnel should be familiar with the epidemiology of the institution's antibiotic-resistant organisms. This information can typically be obtained from the microbiology department or infection control department.

Patients who are vulnerable to colonization and infection include those with severe disease, especially those with compromised host defenses from underlying medical conditions; recent surgery; or indwelling medical devices (e.g., urinary catheters or endotracheal tubes). Hospitalized patients, especially patients in the ICU, tend to have more risk factors than nonhospitalized patients do and have the highest infection rates. Increasing numbers of infections with MDROs also have been reported in non-ICU areas of hospitals.[26]

Ample epidemiologic evidence suggests that MDROs are carried from one person to another via the hands of health care workers. Hands are easily contaminated during the process of care giving or from contact with environmental surfaces in close proximity to the patient. The latter is especially important when patients have diarrhea and the reservoir of the MDRO is the gastrointestinal tract. Studies of poor compliance to hand hygiene policies and glove use indicate a greater likelihood that HCWs will transmit MDROs to other patients. Thus, strategies to increase and monitor adherence to policies are important components of MDRO control programs.[21]

An institutional control program for MDRO includes administrative support, judicious use of antimicrobials, surveillance (routine and enhanced), Standard and contact precautions, environmental measures, education, and decolonization.

## Isolation and Precautions

The Centers for Disease Control (CDC) Hospital Infection Control Practices Advisory Committee (HICPAC) has a published guideline that outlines recommendations for isolation precautions in hospitals. Two tiers of HICPAC isolation precautions exist. The first is referred to as Standard Precautions, and the second is precautions designed only for the care of specified patients. These additional Transmission-based precautions are for patients known or suspected to be infected by epidemiologically important pathogens spread via airborne or droplet transmission or via contact with dry skin or contaminated surfaces.

## Standard Precautions

Standard Precautions apply to all patients who receive care in hospitals, regardless of diagnosis or presumed infection status. Standard precautions apply to: (1) blood; (2) all body fluids, secretions, and excretions *except* sweat, regardless of whether or not they contain visible blood; (3) nonintact skin; and (4) mucous membranes. Standard Precautions are designed to reduce the risk of transmission of microorganisms from both recognized and unrecognized sources of infection in hospitals. Handwashing is a critical component of Standard Precautions.

## Transmission-based Precautions

Transmission-based precautions are designed for patients who need additional precautions above and beyond Standard Precautions to interrupt transmission of the infectious organism. The three types of transmission-based precautions are airborne precautions, droplet precautions, and contact precautions. These precautions may be combined for diseases that have multiple routes of transmission. When used either singularly or in combination, they are to be used *in addition* to standard precautions.

Airborne precautions are designed to reduce the risk of airborne transmission of infectious agents. Airborne transmission occurs with dissemination of either airborne droplet nuclei (5 µm or smaller in size of evaporated droplets that may remain suspended in the air for long periods of time) or dust particles that contain the infectious agent. Microorganisms carried in this manner can be dispersed widely by air currents and may become inhaled by or deposited on a susceptible host within the same room or over a longer distance from the source patient, depending on environmental factors; therefore, negative-pressure isolation rooms are necessary for placement of these patients. If such a room is not available, the patient should be given a mask to wear and should be segregated away from other patients. Prompt transfer of such patients to negative-pressure isolation rooms should be undertaken to minimize the risk of transmission. During transport, the patient should be masked. Personnel who transport the patient should not be masked. Examples of diseases that require airborne precautions include pulmonary tuberculosis, chickenpox, and disseminated zoster (shingles). Personnel who care for patients in airborne precautions must wear respiratory protection (N95 respirator) when entering the room of a patient with known or suspected infectious pulmonary tuberculosis.[22,23] Susceptible persons should not enter the room of patients known or suspected to have measles (rubeola) or varicella (chickenpox) if other immune caregivers are available. If susceptible persons must enter the room of a patient known or suspected to have measles (rubeola) or varicella, they should wear respiratory protection (N95 respirator).[23] Persons who are immune to measles or varicella need not wear respiratory protection.

Droplet precautions are designed to reduce the risk of droplet transmission of infectious agents. Droplet transmission involves contact of the conjunctivae or the mucous membranes of the nose or mouth of a susceptible person with large-particle droplets (larger than 5 micrometers in size) that contain microorganisms generated from an infected person. Droplets are generated from the source person primarily during coughing, sneezing, or talking and during the performance of certain procedures such as suctioning and bronchoscopy. Transmission via large-particle droplets necessitates close contact because droplets do not remain suspended in the air and generally travel only short distances, usually 3 feet or less, through the air. Because droplets do not remain suspended in the air, a negative-pressure room is not needed to prevent droplet transmission. Health care workers should wear gowns, gloves, masks, and eye protection when within 3 feet of an infected patient. Because the environment can play a role in harboring contamination, prompt clean up of visible contamination should be performed. In addition, multiple-patient care items (e.g., blood pressure cuffs, stethoscopes) should be disinfected before use on another patient. Hands can become contaminated through holes in gloves or during removal of PPE and therefore should be promptly washed after patient care and removal of PPE. During patient transportation, patient dispersal of droplets is minimized with masking of the patient.

Contact precautions are designed to reduce the risk of transmission of infectious organisms with direct or indirect contact. Direct-contact transmission involves skin-to-skin contact and physical transfer of microorganisms to a susceptible person from an infected or colonized person, such as occurs when personnel turn patients, empty drainage bags, or perform other patient care activities that require physical contact. Indirect-contact transmission involves contact of a susceptible person with a contaminated intermediate object, usually inanimate, in the patient's environment. Examples of diseases that require Contact precautions include VRE, MRSA, *C. difficile*, lice, and scabies. Health care workers should wear disposable gowns and gloves when providing direct care to patients in contact precautions. As in droplet precautions, a clean environment is critical to minimize transmission of disease and should be promptly and thoroughly disinfected if contaminated and on patient discharge from the area. Hand-washing is of paramount importance in interruption of the spread of infections from patients in contact precautions and should be practiced diligently. Patients in contact precaution can be safely transported in a wheelchair or stretcher without any special requirements. However, a clean barrier (e.g., sheet, gown) should be placed between them and the transport vehicle, which should be disinfected before use on another patient. Health care workers should avoid wearing dirty gowns and gloves during transport to avoid contamination of public spaces.

A synopsis of the types of precautions and the patients who need the precautions is listed in Table 5-1. Although prospective identification of all patients who need these enhanced precautions is not possible, certain clinical syndromes and conditions carry a sufficiently high risk to warrant the empiric addition of enhanced precautions while a more definitive diagnosis is pursued. A listing of such conditions and the recommended precautions beyond Standard Precautions is beyond the scope of this chapter but can be referred to in the CDC HICPAC Isolation Guidelines.

Patients who are immunocompromised vary in their susceptibility to healthcare-associated infections, depending on the severity and duration of immuposuppression. They generally are at increased risk for bacterial, fungal, parasitic, and viral infections from both endogenous (own flora) and exogenous (external) sources. The use of standard precautions for all patients and transmission-based precautions for specified patients, as recommended in this guideline, should reduce the acquisition by these patients of institutionally acquired bacteria from other patients and environments.

### Prevention of Health Care–Associated Infections

Currently, between 5% and 10% of patients admitted to acute care hospitals acquire one or more infections, and the risks have steadily increased during recent decades. These adverse events affect approximately 2 million patients

*Text continued on page 66*

**Table 5-1    Type and Duration of Precautions Needed for Selected Infections and Conditions**

| Infection/Condition | PRECAUTIONS Type* | Duration† |
|---|---|---|
| Abscess | | |
|   Draining, major[1] | C | DI |
|   Draining, minor or limited[2] | S | |
| Acquired immunodeficiency syndrome[3] | S | |
| Adenovirus infection, in infants and young children | D,C | DI |
| Anthrax | | |
|   Cutaneous | S | |
|   Pulmonary | S | |
| Aspergillosis | S | |
| Bronchiolitis (see respiratory infections in infants and young children) | | |
| Candidiasis, all forms, including mucocutaneous | S | |
| Cellulitis, uncontrolled drainage | C | DI |
| Chickenpox (varicella; see F[4] for varicella exposure) | A,C | F[4] |
| *Chlamydia trachomatis* | | |
|   Conjunctivitis | S | |
|   Genital | S | |
|   Respiratory | S | |
| Closed-cavity infection | | |
|   Draining, limited or minor | S | |
|   Not draining | S | |
| *Clostridium* | | |
|   *C. botulinum* | S | |
|   *C. difficile* | C | DI |
|   *C. perfringens* | | |
|     Food poisoning | S | |
|     Gas gangrene | S | |
| Congenital rubella | C | F[5] |
| Conjunctivitis | | |
|   Acute bacterial | S | |
|   *Chlamydia* | S | |
|   Gonococcal | S | |
|   Acute viral (acute hemorrhagic) | C | DI |
| Creutzfeldt-Jakob disease | S[6] | |
| Cytomegalovirus infection, neonatal or immunosuppressed | S | |
| Decubitus ulcer, infected | | |
|   Major[1] | C | DI |
|   Minor or limited[2] | S | |
| Diarrhea, acute infective etiology suspected (see gastroenteritis) | | |
| Diphtheria | | |
|   Cutaneous C CN[7] | | |
|   Pharyngeal D CN | | |
| Endometritis | S | |
| Enterobiasis (pinworm disease, oxyuriasis) | S | |
| Enterocolitis, *C. difficile* | C | DI |
| Epiglottitis, from *Haemophilus influenzae* | D | U (24 h) |
| Epstein-Barr virus infection, including infectious mononucleosis | S | |
| Erythema infectiosum (also see Parvovirus B19) | S | |
| *Escherichia coli* gastroenteritis (see gastroenteritis) | | |

**Table 5-1  Type and Duration of Precautions Needed for Selected Infections and Conditions—cont'd**

| Infection/Condition | Type* | Duration† |
|---|---|---|
| Food poisoning | | |
| Botulism | S | |
| *Clostridium perfringens* or *welchii* | S | |
| Staphylococcal | S | |
| Furunculosis-staphylococcal | | |
| Infants and young children | C | DI |
| Gangrene (gas gangrene) | S | |
| Gastroenteritis | | |
| *Campylobacter* species | S[9] | |
| Cholera | S[9] | |
| *C. difficile* | C | DI |
| *Cryptosporidium species* | S[9] | |
| *E. coli* | | |
| Enterohemorrhagic O157:H7 | S[9] | |
| Diapered or incontinent | C | DI |
| Other species | S[9] | |
| *Giardia lamblia* | S[9] | |
| Rotavirus | S[9] | |
| Diapered or incontinent | C | DI |
| *Salmonella* species (including *S. typhi*) | S[9] | |
| *Shigella* species | S[9] | |
| Diapered or incontinent | C | DI |
| *Vibrio parahaemolyticus* | S[9] | |
| Viral (if not covered elsewhere) | S[9] | |
| *Yersinia enterocolitica* | S[9] | |
| German measles (see rubella) | | |
| Giardiasis (see gastroenteritis) | | |
| Gonococcal ophthalmia neonatorum (gonorrheal ophthalmia, acute conjunctivitis of newborn) | S | |
| Gonorrhea | S | |
| Granuloma inguinale (donovanosis, granuloma venereum) | S | |
| Guillain-Barré syndrome | S | |
| Hand, foot, and mouth disease (see enteroviral infection) | | |
| *Hantavirus* pulmonary syndrome | S | |
| *Helicobacter pylori* | S | |
| Hemorrhagic fevers (for example, Lassa and Ebola) | C[8] | DI |
| Hepatitis, viral | | |
| Type A | S | |
| Patients who are diapered or incontinent | C | F[8] |
| Type B–HbsAg-positive | S | |
| Type C and other unspecified non-A, non-B | S | |
| Type E | S | |
| Herpangina (see enteroviral infection) | | |
| Herpes simplex (*Herpesvirus hominis*) | | |
| Encephalitis | S | |
| Neonatal[11] (see F[11] for neonatal exposure) | C | DI |
| Mucocutaneous, disseminated or primary, severe | C | DI |
| Mucocutaneous, recurrent (skin, oral, genital) | S | |
| Herpes zoster (varicella-zoster) | | |
| Localized in patient with immunocompromise, or disseminated | A, C | D[12] |

*Continued*

## Table 5-1  Type and Duration of Precautions Needed for Selected Infections and Conditions—cont'd

| | PRECAUTIONS | |
|---|---|---|
| Infection/Condition | Type* | Duration† |
| Localized in healthy patient | S[12] | |
| Histoplasmosis | S | |
| HIV (see human immunodeficiency virus) | S | |
| Hookworm disease (ancylostomiasis, uncinariasis) | S | |
| Human immunodeficiency virus (HIV) infection[3] | S | |
| Impetigo | C | U (24 h) |
| Infectious mononucleosis | S | |
| Influenza | D[13] | DI |
| Kawasaki syndrome | S | |
| Lassa fever | C[8] | DI |
| Legionnaires' disease | S | |
| Lice (pediculosis) | C | U (24 h) |
| Listeriosis | S | |
| Lyme disease | S | |
| Malaria | S | |
| Measles (rubeola), all presentations | A | DI |
| Meningitis | | |
| Aseptic (nonbacterial or viral meningitis; also see enteroviral infections) | S | |
| Bacterial, gram-negative enteric, in neonates | S | |
| Fungal | S | |
| *Haemophilus influenzae*, known or suspected | D | U (24 h) |
| *Neisseria meningitidis* (meningococcal) known or suspected | D | U (24 h) |
| Pneumococcal | S | |
| Tuberculosis[14] | S | |
| Other diagnosed bacterial | S | |
| Meningococcal pneumonia | D | U (24 h) |
| Meningococcemia (meningococcal sepsis) | D | U (24 h) |
| Mucormycosis | S | |
| Multidrug-resistant organisms, infection or colonization[15] | | |
| Gastrointestinal | C | CN |
| Respiratory | C | CN |
| Pneumococcal | S | |
| Skin, wound, or burn | C | CN |
| Mumps (infectious parotitis) | D | F[16] |
| Mycobacteria, nontuberculosis (atypical) | | |
| Pulmonary | S | |
| Wound | S | |
| Norwalk agent gastroenteritis (see viral gastroenteritis) | | |
| Parainfluenza virus infection, respiratory in infants and young children | C | DI |
| Parvovirus B19 | D | F[17] |
| Pediculosis (lice) | C | U (24 h) |
| Pertussis (whooping cough) | D | F[18] |
| Pinworm infection | S | |
| Plague | | |
| Bubonic | S | |
| Pneumonic | D | U (72 h) |
| Pleurodynia (see enteroviral infection) | | |
| Pneumonia | | |
| Adenovirus | D,C | DI |
| Bacterial not listed elsewhere (including gram-negative bacterial) | S | |

| Table 5-1 | Type and Duration of Precautions Needed for Selected Infections and Conditions—cont'd | | |
|---|---|---|---|
| | | Precautions | |
| Infection/Condition | | Type* | Duration† |
| *Burkholderia cepacia* in patients with cystic fibrosis (CF), including respiratory tract colonization | | S[19] | |
| *Chlamydia* | | S | |
| Fungal | | S | |
| *Haemophilus influenzae* | | | |
| Adults | | S | |
| Infants and children (any age) | | D | U (24 h) |
| *Legionella* | | S | |
| Meningococcal | | D | U (24 h) |
| Multidrug-resistant bacterial (see multidrug-resistant organisms) | | | |
| *Mycoplasma* (primary atypical pneumonia) | | D | DI |
| Pneumococcal | | S | |
| Multidrug-resistant (see multidrug-resistant organisms) | | | |
| *Pneumocystis carinii* | | S[20] | |
| *Pseudomonas cepacia* (see *Burkholderia cepacia*) | | S[19] | |
| *Staphylococcus aureus* | | S | |
| *Streptococcus*, group A | | | |
| Adults | | S | |
| Infants and young children | | D | U (24h) |
| Viral | | | |
| Adults | | S | |
| Infants and young children (see respiratory infectious disease, acute) | | | |
| Poliomyelitis | | S | |
| Psittacosis (ornithosis) | | S | |
| Q fever | | S | |
| Rabies | | S | |
| Rat-bite fever (*Streptobacillus moniliformis* disease, *Spirillum minus* disease) | | S | |
| Relapsing fever | | S | |
| Resistant bacterial infection or colonization (see multidrug-resistant organisms) | | | |
| Respiratory infectious disease, acute (if not covered elsewhere) | | | |
| Adults | | S | |
| Infants and young children | | C | DI |
| Respiratory syncytial virus infection, in infants and young children, and adults with immunocompromise | | C | DI |
| Reye's syndrome | | S | |
| Rheumatic fever | | S | |
| Rickettsial fevers, tickborne (Rocky Mountain spotted fever, tickborne typhus fever) | | S | |
| Rickettsialpox (vesicular rickettsiosis) | | S | |
| Ringworm (dermatophytosis, dermatomycosis, tinea) | | S | |
| Ritter's disease (staphylococcal scalded skin syndrome) | | S | |
| Rocky Mountain spotted fever | | S | |
| Roseola infantum (exanthem subitum) | | S | |
| Rotavirus infection (see gastroenteritis) | | | |
| Rubella (German measles; also see congenital rubella) | | D | F[21] |
| Salmonellosis (see gastroenteritis) | | | |
| Scabies | | C | U (24 h) |

*Continued*

**Table 5-1    Type and Duration of Precautions Needed for Selected Infections and Conditions—cont'd**

| Infection/Condition | Type* | Duration† |
|---|---|---|
| | **PRECAUTIONS** | |
| Scalded skin syndrome, staphylococcal (Ritter's disease) | S | |
| Schistosomiasis (bilharziasis) | S | |
| Shigellosis (see gastroenteritis) | | |
| Sporotrichosis | S | |
| *Spirillum minus* disease (rat-bite fever) | S | |
| Staphylococcal disease (*S. aureus*) | | |
|   Skin, wound, or burn | | |
|     Major[1] | C | DI |
|     Minor or limited[2] | S | |
|   Enterocolitis | S[j] | |
|   Multidrug-resistant (see multidrug-resistant organisms) | | |
|   Pneumonia | S | |
|   Scalded skin syndrome | S | |
|   Toxic shock syndrome | S | |
| *Streptobacillus moniliformis* disease (rat-bite fever) | S | |
| Streptococcal disease (group A streptococcus) | | |
|   Skin, wound, or burn | | |
|     Major[1] | C | U (24 h) |
|     Minor or limited[2] | S | |
|   Endometritis (puerperal sepsis) | S | |
|   Pharyngitis in infants and young children | D | U (24 h) |
|   Pneumonia in infants and young children | D | U (24 h) |
|   Scarlet fever in infants and young children | D | U (24 h) |
| Streptococcal disease (group B streptococcus), neonatal | S | |
| Streptococcal disease (not group A or B) unless covered elsewhere | S | |
|   Multidrug-resistant (see multidrug-resistant organisms) | | |
| Syphilis | S | |
| Tapeworm disease | S | |
| Tetanus | S | |
| Tinea (fungus infection dermatophytosis, dermatomycosis, ringworm) | S | |
| Toxic shock syndrome (staphylococcal disease) | S | |
| Tuberculosis | | |
|   Extrapulmonary, draining lesion (including scrofula) | S | |
|   Extrapulmonary, meningitis[14] | S | |
|   Pulmonary, confirmed or suspected or laryngeal disease | A | F[22] |
|   Skin-test positive with no evidence of current pulmonary disease | S | |
| Urinary tract infection (including pyelonephritis), with or without urinary catheter | S | |
| Varicella (chickenpox) | A,C | F[4] |
| Viral diseases | | |
|   Respiratory (if not covered elsewhere) | | |
|     Adults | S | |
|     Infants and young children (see respiratory infectious disease, acute) | | |
| Whooping cough (pertussis) | D | F[19] |
| Wound infections | | |
|   Major[1] | C | DI |
|   Minor or limited[2] | S | |
| Zoster (varicella-zoster) | | |

## Table 5-1 Type and Duration of Precautions Needed for Selected Infections and Conditions—cont'd

| | PRECAUTIONS | |
| --- | --- | --- |
| Infection/Condition | Type[*] | Duration[†] |
| Localized in patient with immunocompromise, disseminated | A,C | DI[12] |
| Localized in healthy patient | S[12] | |

Modified from Garner JS, Hospital Infection Control Practices Advisory Committee: Appendix A: type and duration of precautions needed for selected infections and conditions in guideline for isolation precautions in hospitals, *Infect Control Hosp Epidemiol* 17:53-80, 1996; *Am J Infect Control* 24:24-52, 1996.

[*]Type of precautions: A, Airborne; C, Contact; D, Droplet; S, Standard. When A, C, and D are specified, also use S.

[†]Duration of precautions: *CN*, Until off antibiotics and culture-negative; *DI*, duration of illness (with wound lesions, DI means until they stop draining); *U*, until time specified in hours (h) after initiation of effective therapy; *F*, see footnote.

[1]No dressing or dressing does not contain drainage adequately.

[2]Dressing covers and contains drainage adequately.

[3]Also see syndromes or conditions listed in Table 5-2.

[4]Maintain precautions until all lesions are crusted. The average incubation period for varicella is 10 to 16 days, with a range of 10 to 21 days. After exposure, use varicella zoster immune globulin (VZIG) when appropriate and discharge susceptible patients if possible. Place exposed susceptible patients on Airborne Precautions beginning 10 days after exposure and continuing until 21 days after last exposure (up to 28 days if VZIG has been given). Susceptible persons should not enter the room of patients on precautions if other immune caregivers are available.

[5]Place infant on precautions during any admission until 1 year of age, unless nasopharyngeal and urine cultures are negative for virus after age 3 months.

[6]Additional special precautions are necessary for handling and decontamination of blood, body fluids and tissues, and contaminated items from patients with confirmed or suspected disease. See latest College of American Pathologists (Northfield, Ill) guidelines or other references.

[7]Until two cultures taken at least 24 hours apart have negative results.

[8]Call state health department and CDC for specific advice about management of a suspected case. During the 1995 Ebola outbreak in Zaire, interim recommendations were published (1997). Pending a comprehensive review of the epidemiologic data from the outbreak and evaluation of the interim recommendations, the 1988 guidelines for management of patients with suspected viral hemorrhagic infections (2016) will be reviewed and updated if indicated.

[9]Use Contact Precautions for diapered or incontinent children less than 6 years of age for duration of illness.

[10]Maintain precautions in infants and children less than 3 years of age for duration of hospitalization; in children 3 to 14 years of age, until 2 weeks after onset of symptoms; and in others, until 1 week after onset of symptoms.

[11]For infants delivered vaginally or via C-section and if mother has active infection and membranes have been ruptured for more than 4 to 6 hours.

[12]Persons susceptible to varicella are also at risk for development of varicella when exposed to patients with herpes zoster lesions; therefore, susceptibles should not enter the room if other immune caregivers are available.

[13]The Guideline for Prevention of Nosocomial Pneumonia (1995, 1996) recommends surveillance, vaccination, antiviral agents, and use of private rooms with negative air pressure as much as feasible for patients for whom influenza is suspected or diagnosed. Many hospitals encounter logistic difficulties and physical plant limitations with admission of multiple patients with suspected influenza during community outbreaks. If sufficient private rooms are unavailable, consider cohorting patients or, at the very least, avoid room sharing with patients at high risk. See Guideline for Prevention of Nosocomial Pneumonia (1995, 1996) for additional prevention and control strategies.

[14]Patient should be examined for evidence of current (active) pulmonary tuberculosis. If evidence exists, additional precautions are necessary (see tuberculosis).

[15]Resistant bacteria judged by the infection control program, based on current state, regional, or national recommendations, to be of special clinical and epidemiologic significance.

[16]For 9 days after onset of swelling.

[17]Maintain precautions for duration of hospitalization when chronic disease occurs in a patient with immunodeficiency. For patients with transient aplastic crisis or red-cell crisis, maintain precautions for 7 days.

[18]Maintain precautions until 5 days after patient is placed on effective therapy.

[19]Avoid cohorting or placement in the same room with a patient with CF who is not infected or colonized with *B cepacia*. Persons with CF who visit or provide care and are not infected or colonized with *B cepacia* may elect to wear a mask when within 3 ft of a colonized or infected patient.

[20]Avoid placement in the same room with a patient with immunocompromise.

[21]Until 7 days after onset of rash.

[22]Discontinue precautions *only* when patient with tuberculosis (TB) is on effective therapy, is improving clinically, and has three consecutive negative sputum smears collected on different days or when TB is ruled out. Also see CDC Guidelines for Preventing the Transmission of Tuberculosis in Health-Care Facilities (PDF; 23).

each year in the United States, result in some 90,000 deaths, and add an estimated $4.5 to $5.7 billion per year to the costs of patient care.[24] These infections are referred to as nosocomial infections or as, the more recent terminology, health care–associated infections (HAI).

Most HAIs (in descending order of frequency) are caused from urinary tract infections (UTIs), surgical site infections (SSIs), bloodstream infections (BSIs), and pneumonia. The perianesthesia nurse can play a major role in prevention of all of these infections in the surgical population by adhering to time-honored practices such as asepsis and recommended standards of care supported by the literature (often times referred to as evidence-based care). Published guidelines are available from the CDC on prevention of surgical site infections, intravascular catheter infections, and pneumonia. Refer to the bibliography for complete references.

One area of surgical patient quality improvement where perianesthesia nurses can play a significantly active role is the Surgical Care Improvement Project (SCIP), originated by The Centers for Medicare & Medicaid Services (CMS). This project is a national quality partnership of organizations focused on improvement of surgical care with significant reduction in surgical complications. The SCIP goal is reduction of the incidence rate of surgical complications nationally by 25% by the year 2010. Partners in SCIP believe that a meaningful reduction in surgical complications depends on surgeons, anesthesia providers, nurses, pharmacists, infection control professionals, and hospital executives working together to intensify their commitment to making surgical care improvement a priority.[25] SCIP has identified seven processes or outcome measures related to infection prevention. They are listed in Table 5-2.

The CDC estimates that approximately 500,000 SSIs occur annually in the United States.[26] Patients who have SSIs are up to 60% more likely to spend time in an intensive care unit, are five times more likely to be readmitted to the hospital, and have twice the mortality rate compared with patients without an SSI.[27] A targeted process within the SCIP initiative to reduce SSIs is with the appropriate antimicrobial prophylaxis administration process because, despite evidence of effectiveness of antimicrobials to prevent SSIs, previous studies have shown inappropriate timing, selection, and excess duration of administration of antimicrobial prophylaxis. The SCIP measures are: (1) the proportion of patients who have parenteral antimicrobial prophylaxis initiated within 1 hour before the surgical incision; (2) the proportion of patients who are provided a prophylactic antimicrobial agent that is consistent with currently published guidelines; and (3) the proportion of patients whose prophylactic antimicrobial therapy is discontinued within 24 hours after the end of surgery.[28]

Two additional process measures gaining momentum in the surgical population because of the SCIP initiative are glucose control and normothermia. Currently, the measures are limited to specific patient populations undergoing surgery, consistent with evidence-based medicine. SCIP CMS infection indicator 4 addresses patients for cardiac surgery and the postoperative serum glucose. This recommendation was in part the result of studies such as Latham et al,[29] who concluded that diabetes (odd ratio [OR], 2.76; $P < .001$) and postoperative hyperglycemia (OR, 2.02; $P = .007$) were independently associated with development of SSIs. SCIP CMS infection indicator 7 addresses normothermia in the colorectal surgery population. Kurz, Sessler, and Lenhart reported SSIs in 18 of 96 patients undergoing colorectal surgery who were

---

**Table 5-2   SCIP Process Measures for Prevention of Infection**

SCIP INF 1: Prophylactic antibiotic received within 1 h before surgical incision.

SCIP INF 2: Prophylactic antibiotic selection for surgical patients.

SCIP INF 3: Prophylactic antibiotics discontinued within 24 h after surgery end time (48 h for patients for cardiac surgery).

SCIP INF 4: Patients for cardiac surgery with controlled 6 AM postoperative serum glucose.

SCIP INF 5: Postoperative wound infection diagnosed during index hospitalization (OUTCOME).

SCIP INF 6: Surgery patients with appropriate hair removal.

SCIP INF 7: Patients for colorectal surgery with immediate postoperative normothermia.

---

*INF*, Infections.

Modified from MedQIC: *Surgical Care Improvement Project*, available at http://www.medqic.org/dcs/ContentServer?cid= 1137346750659&pagename=Medqic%2FContent%2FParentShellTemplate&parentName=TopicCat&c=MQParents, accessed March 1, 2007.

hypothermic (19%) but in only 6 of 104 patients who were normothermic (6%; P = .009).[30]

Another SCIP process targeted towards SSI reduction is the issue of appropriate hair removal at the surgical site. The CDC Surgical Site Infection Prevention Guidelines state that preoperative shaving of the surgical site the night before an operation is associated with a significantly higher SSI risk than either the use of depilatory agents or no hair removal.[31-36] Shaving immediately before the operation compared with shaving within 24 hours before surgery was associated with decreased SSI rates (3.1% versus 7.1%); if shaving was performed more than 24 hours before the operation, the SSI rate exceeded 20%.[33] In addition to when the hair is removed, how it is removed is important as well. In one study, SSI rates were 5.6% in patients who had hair removed with razor shave compared with a 0.6% rate among those who had hair removed with depilatory or who had no hair removed.[33] The increased SSI risk associated with shaving has been attributed to microscopic cuts in the skin that later serve as foci for bacterial multiplication. On the basis of the data, the SCIP recommendation is avoidance of shaving surgical sites or, use of clippers only if hair removal is necessary immediately before surgery.

The role of the perianesthesia nurse relative to the SCIP initiative varies because of institutional differences in ordering and administration of surgical prophylaxis, glucose control, maintenance of normothermia, and surgical site hair removal. Nonetheless, active collaboration with the initiative is essential for optimal outcomes.

Another recommendation from the CDC SSI Prevention Guidelines relates to a patient's skin hygiene before surgery. A preoperative antiseptic shower or bath decreases skin microbial colony counts. In a study of more than 700 patients who received two preoperative antiseptic showers, chlorhexidine reduced bacterial colony counts nine fold (2.83 to 0.3), compared with other products.[37] Although other studies corroborate these findings,[38,39] a Cochrane Review found no added benefit of CHG over other antimicrobial soaps.[40] CHG-containing products need several applications to attain maximal antimicrobial benefit, so repeated antiseptic showers are usually indicated.[39] Although preoperative showers reduce the skin's microbial colony counts, they have not definitively been shown to reduce SSI rates.[41] However, from a basic hygiene perspective, a patient's skin should be as clean as possible before surgery. Products are now on the market that allow for quick and easy skin cleansing in the perioperative setting. They are CHG based and waterless.

Intravascular devices are regularly inserted into patients in the perianesthesia setting. Care must be taken during insertion and line management to prevent bloodstream infections. The incidence rate of catheter-related bloodstream infections (CRBSI) varies considerably by type of catheter, frequency of catheter manipulation, and patient-related factors (e.g., underlying disease and acuity of illness). Peripheral venous catheters are the devices most frequently used for vascular access. Although the incidence rate of local or bloodstream infections (BSIs) associated with peripheral venous catheters is usually low, serious infectious complications produce considerable annual morbidity rates because of the frequency with which such catheters are used. However, most serious catheter-related infections are associated with central venous catheters (CVCs). A total of 250,000 cases of CVC-associated BSIs has been estimated to occur annually.[42] In this case, attributable mortality rate is an estimated 12% to 25% for each infection, and the marginal cost to the health care system is $25,000 per episode.[42]

In the perianesthesia setting, the biggest impact on prevention of CVC-associated BSIs is control of the insertion process and adherence to aseptic technique. Best practice recommendations for skin preparation include use of an appropriate antiseptic before catheter insertion and during dressing changes. A 2% chlorahexidine-based preparation is preferred, but tincture of iodine, an iodophor, or 70% alcohol can also be used.[43-46]

The level of barrier precautions needed to prevent infection during insertion of CVCs is more stringent then what is required for peripheral venous or arterial catheters. Maximal sterile barrier precautions (e.g., cap, mask, sterile gown, sterile gloves, and large sterile drape) during the insertion of CVCs substantially reduces the incidence rate of CRBSI compared with standard precautions (e.g., sterile gloves and small drapes).[47,48] To further reduce the likelihood of contamination of the line, injection ports should be cleaned with 70% alcohol or an iodophor before the system is accessed and all stopcocks should be capped when not in use.[49-51]

## OCCUPATIONAL HEALTH

The perianesthesia nurse is at risk of occupational exposure to bloodborne pathogens, such as HIV, HBV, and the hepatitis C virus (HCV). Seroconversion risk after exposure to HIV is 0.3%, to HBV is 15% to 30% (if unvaccinated), and to HCV is 3% to 10%. Exposure to blood from a patient can occur from parenteral exposure to contaminated sharps (e.g., needlestick injury) or splashes to mucous membranes with blood or body fluids. If a nurse is stuck with a needle or other sharp or gets blood or other potentially infectious materials in the eyes, nose, or mouth or on broken skin, the exposed area should be immediately flooded with water and any wound cleaned with soap and water or a skin disinfectant if available. The incident should be immediately reported to the employer, and the nurse should seek medical attention.

The Occupational Safety and Health Administration Bloodborne Pathogen (OSHA BBP) Standard outlines the appropriate measures an institution must have in place to control for employee exposures. Each institution is required to have an exposure control plan to be in compliance with the OSHA BBP Standard, which outlines the policies, procedures, and training requirements of the HCWs. Each perianesthesia setting should evaluate its practices and ensure that it has the appropriate safety devices, personal protective equipment, and training to minimize risks to the employees who work there.

Recommendations for minimization of exposures include taking care to prevent injuries: with use of needles, scalpels, and other sharp instruments or devices; with handling of sharp instruments after procedures; with cleaning of used instruments; and with disposal of used needles. Used needles should never be recapped or otherwise manipulated with both hands, or any other technique that involves directing the point of a needle toward any part of the body used; rather, either a one-handed scoop technique or a mechanical device designed for holding the needle sheath should be used. Used needles from disposable syringes should not be removed by hand and should not be bent, broken, or otherwise manipulated by hand. Used disposable syringes and needles, scalpel blades, and other sharp items should be disposed in appropriate puncture-resistant containers that are located as close as practical to the area in which the items were used, and reusable syringes and needles should be placed in a puncture-resistant container for transport to the reprocessing area.

For minimization of exposure to mucous membranes, all procedures that involve blood or other potentially infectious materials shall be performed in such a manner as to minimize splashing, spraying, spattering, and generation of droplets of these substances. PPE should be provided at no cost to employees and should be readily accessible.

Eating, drinking, smoking, applying cosmetics or lip balm, and handling contact lenses are prohibited in work areas with a reasonable likelihood of occupational exposure. Food and drink shall not be kept in refrigerators, freezers, shelves, or cabinets or on countertops or bench tops where blood or other potentially infectious materials are present.

Medical waste must be managed properly and in compliance with the OSHA BBP Standard. Regulated waste should be placed in containers that are closable; constructed to contain all contents and prevent leakage of fluids during handling, storage, transport, or shipping; labeled or color-coded per the Standard; and closed before removal to prevent spillage or protrusion of contents during handling, storage, transport, or shipping.

The employer should make the HBV vaccination series available to all employees who have occupational exposure and should provide postexposure evaluation and follow-up to all employees who have had an exposure incident.

Perianesthesia nurses should protect themselves against infection from HBV with vaccination with the HBV vaccine, unless contraindicated for medical reasons. With proper administration, the vaccine is about 90% (80% to 95%) effective in prevention of infection in susceptible vaccinees. Immunity produced by this vaccination possibly will decrease with time and boosters will have to be given to ensure protection.[52] Per OSHA Standards, this vaccine must be made available at no cost to the employee and must be accompanied by the necessary training requirements.

Training and training records are an important component in the OSHA BBP Standard. Training records shall include the following information: the dates of the training sessions, the contents or a summary of the training sessions, the names and qualifications of persons who conduct the training, and the names and job titles of all persons who attend the training sessions. Training records shall be maintained for 3 years from the date on which the training occurred.

Twenty-four states, Puerto Rico, and the Virgin Islands have OSHA-approved State Plans and have adopted their own standards and enforcement policies. For the most part, these States adopt standards that are identical to Federal OSHA. However, some States have adopted different standards applicable to this topic or may have different enforcement policies.

In 2001, the OSHA BBP Standard was revised to reflect the stipulations of the Needlestick Safety and Prevention Act passed by the U.S. Congress in 2000. This Act requires the use of engineering and work practice controls to eliminate or minimize employee exposure to bloodborne pathogens. It requires that the institution perform an annual consideration and implementation of appropriate commercially available and effective safer medical devices designed to eliminate or minimize occupational exposure. It also requires solicitation of input from nonmanagerial employees responsible for direct patient care, who are potentially exposed to injuries from contaminated sharps, in the identification, evaluation, and selection of effective engineering and work practice controls and the documentation of the solicitation in the exposure control plan.

In addition to the HBV vaccine, additional vaccines are recommended to ensure that personnel are immune to vaccine-preventable diseases. Optimal use of vaccines can prevent transmission of vaccine-preventable diseases and eliminate unnecessary work restriction. Prevention of illness through comprehensive personnel immunization programs is far more cost effective than case management and outbreak control. Mandatory immunization programs, which include both newly hired and currently employed persons, are more effective than voluntary programs in ensuring that susceptible persons are vaccinated.[53] National guidelines for immunization of and postexposure prophylaxis for health care personnel are provided by the U.S. Public Health Service's Advisory Committee on Immunization Practices.[54]

## SUMMARY

Provision of care in a perianesthesia unit is not without infectious risks for patients and the health care worker in the environment. Adherence to published guidelines and institutional policies for minimization of infectious risks is paramount for optimal patient and employee outcomes. Simple tasks such as hand washing can significantly reduce the incidence rate of health care–associated infections and reduce the transmission of disease. Additional measures to ensure a safe and clean environment and equipment further lower the risks. Lastly, the perianesthesia nursing team can play a significant role in the quality improvement process of the surgical patient and can greatly impact outcomes that benefit the patient and the institution.

## REFERENCES

1. Occupational Safety and Health Administration: 29CFR Part 1910:1030: Occupational exposure to bloodborne pathogens: final rule, federal register, OSHA, Washington, DC, 1991.
2. AIA Facilities Guidelines Institute: *Guidelines for design and construction of healthcare facilities,* ed 2006, Washington, DC, 2006, AIA.
3. Wikipedia, the free encyclopedia: *Ignaz Semmelweis,* available at http://en.wikipedia.org/w/index.php?title=Ignaz_Semmelweis&oldid=91899744, accessed December 10, 2006.
4. Centers for Disease Control and Prevention: Guideline for hand hygiene in health-care settings, *MMWR* 51(RR-16), 2002.
5. Pittet D, Mourouga P, Perneger TV: Members of the Infection Control Program: Compliance with handwashing in a teaching hospital, *Ann Intern Med* 130:26-130, 1999.
6. Larson E, Killien M: Factors influencing handwashing behavior of patient care personnel, *Am J Infect Control* 10:93-99, 1982.
7. Conly JM, Hill S, Ross J, et al: Handwashing practices in an intensive care unit: the effects of an educational program and its relationship to infection rates, *Am J Infect Control* 17:330-339, 1989.
8. Dubbert PM, Dolce J, Richter W, et al: Increasing ICU staff handwashing: effects of education and group feedback, *Infect Control Hosp Epid* 11:191-193, 1990.
9. Larson E, Kretzer EK: Compliance with handwashing and barrier precautions, *J Hosp Infect* 30(suppl):88-106, 1995.
10. Sproat LJ, Inglis TJJ: A multicentre survey of hand hygiene practice in intensive care units, *J Hosp Infect* 26:137-148, 1994.
11. Kretzer EK, Larson EL: Behavioral interventions to improve infection control practices, *Am J Infect Control* 26:245-253, 1998.
12. Tupker RA: Detergents and cleansers. In van der Valk PGM, Maibach HI, editors: *The irritant contact dermatitis syndrome,* New York, 1996, CRC Press.
13. Garner JS, Simmons BP: Guideline for isolation precautions in hospitals, *Infect Control* 4(suppl 4):245-325, 1983.
14. McFarland LV, Mulligan ME, Kwok RYY, et al: Nosocomial acquisition of *Clostridium difficile* infection, *N Engl J Med* 320:204-210, 1989.
15. Pittet D, Dharan S, Touveneau S, et al: Bacterial contamination of the hands of hospital staff during routine patient care, *Arch Intern Med* 159:821-826, 1999.
16. Tenorio AR, Badri SM, Sahgal NB, et al: Effectiveness of gloves in the prevention of hand carriage of vancomycin-resistant *Enterococcus* species by health care workers after patient care, *Clin Infect Dis* 32:826-829, 2001.
17. Ehrenkranz NJ, Alfonso BC: Failure of bland soap handwash to prevent hand transfer of

patient bacteria to urethral catheters, *Infect Control Hosp Epidemiol* 12:654-662, 1991.

18. Kjrlen H: Andersen BM: Handwashing and disinfection of heavily contaminated hands—effective or ineffective? *J Hosp Infect* 21:61-71, 1992.

19. Garner JS, Hospital Infection Control Practices Advisory Committee: Guideline for isolation precautions in hospitals, *Infect Control Hosp Epidemiol* 17:53-80, 1996; *Am J Infect Control* 24:24–52, 1996.

20. http://Seigel, JD, Rhinehart E, Jackson M, Chiarello L, and the Healthcare Infection Control Practices Advisory Committee: Management of multidrug resistant organisms in healthcare settings 2006. Available at http://www.cdc.gov/ncidod/dhqp/pdf/ar/mdro Guideline2006.pdf. Accessed May 21, 2007.

21. Institute for Healthcare Improvement: *Reducing hospital acquired infections*, available at http://www.ihi.org/IHI/Programs/Innovation Communities/IMPACTICReducingHospital-AcquiredInfections.htm, accessed March 2007.

22. Centers for Disease Control and Prevention: Guidelines for preventing the transmission of tuberculosis in health-care facilities, *MMWR* 43(RR-13):1-132, 1994; *Federal Register* 59(208):54242-54303, 1994.

23. Department of Health and Human Services, Department of Labor: Respiratory protective devices: final rules and notice, *Federal Register* 60(110):30336-30402, 1995.

24. Burke JP: Infection control—a problem for patient safety, *N Engl J Med* 348:651-656, 2003.

25. MedQIC: *Surgical care improvement project*, available at http://www.medqic.org/dcs/ContentServer?cid=1137346750659&pagename=Medqic%2FContent%2FParentShellTemplate&parentName=TopicCat&c=MQ Parents, accessed March 1, 2007.

26. Wong ES: Surgical site infection. In Mayhall DG, editor: *Hospital epidemiology and infection control*, ed 2, Philadelphia, 1999, Lippincott.

27. Kirkland KB, Briggs JP, Trivette SL, et al: The impact of surgical site infections in the 1990s—attributable mortality, excess length of hospitalization, and extra costs, *Infect Control Hosp Epidemiol* 20:725-730, 1999.

28. Bratzler DW, Houck PM: Antimicrobial prophylaxis for surgery: an advisory statement from the National Surgical Infection Prevention Project, *Clin Infect Dis* 38:1706-1715, 2004.

29. Latham R, Lancaster AD, Covington JF, et al: The association of diabetes and glucose control with surgical-site infections among cardiothoracic surgery patients, *Infect Control Hosp Epidemiol* 22(10):604-606, 2001.

30. Kurz A, Sessler DI, Lenhardt R: Perioperative normothermia to reduce the incidence of surgical-wound infection and shorten hospitalization, *N Engl J Med* 334:1209-1215, 1996.

31. Cruse PJ, Foord R: The epidemiology of wound infection: a 10-year prospective study of 62,939 wounds, *Surg Clin North Am* 60(1): 27-40, 1980.

32. Mishriki SF, Law DJ, Jeffery PJ: Factors affecting the incidence of postoperative wound infection, *J Hosp Infect* 16:223-230, 1990.

33. Seropian R, Reynolds BM: Wound infections after preoperative depilatory versus razor preparation, *Am J Surg* 121:251-254, 1971.

34. Hamilton HW, Hamilton KR, Lone FJ: Preoperative hair removal, *Can J Surg* 20: 269-271, 1977.

35. Olson MM, MacCallum J, McQuarrie DG: Preoperative hair removal with clippers does not increase infection rate in clean surgical wounds, *Surg Gynecol Obstet* 162: 181-182, 1986.

36. Mehta G, Prakash B, Karmoker S: Computer assisted analysis of wound infection in neurosurgery, *J Hosp Infect* 11:244-252, 1988.

37. Garibaldi RA: Prevention of intraoperative wound contamination with chlorhexidine shower and scrub, *J Hosp Infect* 11(Suppl B): 5-9, 1988.

38. Paulson DS: Efficacy evaluation of a 4% chlorhexidine gluconate as a full-body shower wash, *Am J Infect Control* 21(4):205-209, 1993.

39. Hayek LJ, Emerson JM, Gardner AM: A placebo-controlled trial of the effect of two preoperative baths or showers with chlorhexidine detergent on postoperative baths or showers with chlorhexidine detergent on postoperative wound infection rates, *J Hosp Infect* 10:165-172, 1987.

40. Webster J, Osborne S: Preoperative bathing or showering with skin antiseptics to prevent surgical site infection, *Cochrane Database of Systematic Reviews* 2(CD004985), 2006.

41. Rotter ML, Larsen SO, Cooke EM, et al: A comparison of the effects of preoperative whole-body bathing with detergent alone and with detergent containing chlorhexidine gluconate on the frequency of wound infections after clean surgery, The European Working Party on Control of Hospital Infections, *J Hosp Infect* 11:310-320, 1998.

42. Kluger DM, Maki DG: *The relative risk of intravascular device related bloodstream infections in adults [abstract]*, Proceeding of the Abstracts of the 39th Interscience Conference on Antimicrobial Agents and Chemotherapy, American Society for Microbiology, 1999, San Francisco.

43. Maki DG, Ringer M, Alvarado CJ: Prospective randomised trial of povidone-iodine, alcohol, and chlorhexidine for prevention of infection associated with central venous and arterial catheters, *Lancet* 338:339-343, 1991.

44. Garland JS, Buck RK, Maloney P, et al: Comparison of 10% povidone-iodine and 0.5% chlorhexidine gluconate for the prevention of peripheral intravenous catheter colonization in neonates: a prospective trial, *Pediatr Infect Dis J* 14:510-516, 1995.

45. Little JR, Murray PR, Traynor PS, et al: A randomized trial of povidone-iodine compared with iodine tincture for venipuncture site disinfection: effects on rates of blood culture contamination, *Am J Med* 107:119-125, 1999.

46. Mimoz O, Pieroni L, Lawrence C, et al: Prospective, randomized trial of two antiseptic solutions for prevention of central venous or arterial catheter colonization and infection in intensive care unit patients, *Crit Care Med* 24:1818-1823, 1996.

47. Mermel LA, McCormick RD, Springman SR, et al: The pathogenesis and epidemiology of catheter-related infection with pulmonary artery Swan-Ganz catheters: a prospective study utilizing molecular subtyping, *Am J Med* 91(suppl):S197-S205, 1991.

48. Raad II, Hohn DC, Gilbreath BJ, et al: Prevention of central venous catheter-related infections by using maximal sterile barrier precautions during insertion, *Infect Control Hosp Epidemiol* 15:231-238, 1994.

49. Luebke MA, Arduino MJ, Duda DL, et al: Comparison of the microbial barrier properties of a needleless and a conventional needle-based intravenous access system, *Am J Infect Control* 26:437-441, 1998.

50. Salzman MB, Isenberg HD, Rubin LG: Use of disinfectants to reduce microbial contamination of hubs of vascular catheters, *J Clin Microbiol* 31:475-479, 1993.

51. Plott RT, Wagner RF Jr, Tyring SK: Iatrogenic contamination of multidose vials in simulated use: a reassessment of current patient injection technique, *Arch Dermatol* 126:1441-1444, 1990.

52. Occupational Safety and Health Administration: *CPL 2-2OSHA instruction: subject: hepatitis B risks in the health care system,* 1983, Office of Occupational Medicine, Washington DC.

53. Bolyard EA, Tablan OC, Williams WW: The Hospital Infection Control Practices Advisory Committee: Guideline for infection control in health care personnel, *Am J Infect Control* 26(3):289-354, 1998.

54. Advisory Committee on Immunization Practices (AICP): Immunization of health-care workers: recommendations of the Advisory Committee on Immunization Practices (ACIP) and the Hospital Infection Control Practices Advisory Committee (HICPAC), *MMWR* 46(RR-18):1-42, 1997.

## BIBLIOGRAPHY

Allen A, Badgwell JM: The post anesthesia care unit: unique contribution, unique risk, *J Perianesth Nurs* 11(4):248-258, 1996.

Benson L, et al: The effects of surfactant systems and moisturizing products on the residual activity of a chlorhexidine gluconate handwash using a pigskin substrate, *Infect Control Hospital Epidemiol* 11(2):67-70, 1990.

Block S: *Disinfection, sterilization and preservation,* ed 5, Philadelphia, 2001, Lippincott.

Bratzler DW, Houck PM, Surgical Infection Prevention Guideline Writers Workgroup: Antimicrobial prophylaxis for surgery: an advisory statement from the National Surgical Infection Prevention Project, *Am J Surg* 189(4):395-404, 2005.

Chin J: The use of hepatitis B virus vaccine, *N Engl J Med* 307:678-679, 1982.

Guidelines for preventing infections associated with the insertion and maintenance of short-term indwelling urethral catheters in acute care, *J Hosp Infect* 47(Suppl):S39–S46, 2001.

Guidelines for preventing the transmission of *Mycobacterium tuberculosis* in health-care settings, *MMWR* 54(RR17);1-141, 2005.

Guidelines for the prevention of intravascular catheter-related infections, *MMWR* 51(RR-10): 1-2, 2002.

*Needlestick Safety and Prevention Act: public law 106-430, 106th Congress,* available at http://frwebgate.access.gpo.gov/cgi-bin/getdoc.cgi?dbname=106_cong_public_laws&docid=f:publ430.106. Accessed May 21, 2007.

Kerr CM, Savage GT: Managing exposure to tuberculosis in the PACU: CDC guidelines and cost analysis, *J Perianesth Nurs* 11(3):143-146, 1996.

Mangram AJ, Horan TC, Pearson ML, et al: Guidelines for the prevention of surgical site infections, 1999, Hospital Infection Control Practices Advisory Committee, *Infect Control Hosp Epidemiol* 20(4):250-278, 1999.

Recommendations for Preventing the Spread of Vancomycin Resistance Recommendations of the Hospital Infection Control Practices Advisory Committee, *MMWR* 44(RR12):1–13, 1995.

Sullivan EE: The use of contact and airborne precautions in the perianesthesia setting, *J Perianesth Nurs* 17(3):190-192, 2002.

Sullivan EE: Off with her nails, *J Perianesth Nurs* 18(6):417-418, 2003.

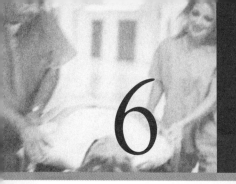

# 6

# MANAGED CARE AND ITS IMPACT ON THE PACU

Kenneth R. White, PhD, RN, FACHE
Marie Fiascone Gerardo, MS, RN-C, ANP, CCRN

## MANAGED CARE AND PERIANESTHESIA NURSING

The health care delivery system in the United States is a multifaceted multipurpose organization that historically has emphasized care for acutely ill persons and relies on medical science and technology to solve health care problems. Therefore, a health care system more accurately described as an "illness care" system has evolved. Today's health care system is influenced by health promotion and illness prevention strategies and gradually is shifting to wellness care and improvement of the health status of communities.

The health care financing system mirrors the health care delivery system in complexity and reflects its priorities. The financing of health care has also focused on acute care and critical conditions rather than the prevention of chronic degenerative diseases and wellness. The health care financing structure includes both government (public) and private components and is increasingly challenged to meet the needs of a growing elderly population and access to health care for all those in need.

Health care is increasing in cost and complexity because of the advancement of technology and improved methods of diagnosis and treatment. The U.S. Center for Medicare and Medicaid Services (CMS) reports that national health care expenditures were $1.8 trillion in 2004, a 6-year trend of growth below 8%.[1] Private spending for health care continued to grow more rapidly in 2003 than did public spending. Private spending grew by 8.6%, whereas public spending grew 7.8%. But this trend reversed in 2004, with private spending growing 7.6% and public spending growing 8.2%. The CMS estimates that national health expenditures are projected to reach 17.4% of the gross domestic product (GDP) by 2011[2] after declining from 13.4% in 1993 to 13% in 1999.[1] However, access, affordability, and availability of the continuum of health care services for those who need it remain critical issues that face health care providers and consumers.

Today, as a consequence of fundamental changes in the social and economic environment of health care, recognition that economic judgment is essential at all levels of decision making is widespread. Economic analysis is needed not only at the level of national health policymaking and the institutional level but also at the individual level as providers make decisions about the best way to use their time and resources for the best clinical outcomes for patients, which means that health care professionals must examine the services to ensure that decisions are worth the costs. Economic pressures demand this level of analysis to improve efficiencies while controlling costs and delivering quality services.

In addition to the federal government's role in regulating health services, a market system is controlling use, consumption, and availability of health services. In a market system, the market, rather than some other entity such as a national or state government, determines the distribution of resources. One market force, managed care, refers to an organized system of care delivery that coordinates a broad range of patient services and monitors care to ensure that it is appropriate and provided in the most efficient and cost-effective way.[3] Managed care plans are health insurance products designed as a lower cost alternative to fee-for-service health care services. A fee-for-service (FFS) system asks providers, mainly physicians and hospitals, how much they spent and reimburses them for costs. Alternatively, managed care plans selectively contract with hospitals and physicians for a prospective determination of how much will be reimbursed for health care services for the plan's enrollees. Thus, through a stricter review of service use, various managed care plans (i.e., health maintenance organizations, preferred provider organizations, and others) provide alternative forms of less expensive health care.

The burgeoning enrollments in managed care plans significantly changed the health care economy. Debates continue about the overall effects of managed care and whether health care costs have been "managed." One certainty is that the role of nurses has expanded to include a focus on managing the economic impact of care. Nurses more than ever are at the forefront of identifying less expensive ways to deliver quality health care services while integrating health promotion strategies. This chapter provides a broad overview of the ways that the health care delivery system is financed, including the aspects and trends of managed care, and the roles for nurses in economic decision making for the cost of care in the perianesthesia unit.

## Health Care Delivery Structure

The health care delivery system is a complex web of public and private services and programs developed to provide care at the federal, state, and local levels.

***Role of the Federal Government.*** Federal health care activities are implemented by the Department of Health and Human Services (DHHS). This department oversees two divisions: the Public Health Service Division and the Human Services Division (Fig. 6-1). Within each division are several agencies, some of which have a direct influence on health care delivery.

In the Public Health Service Division, the National Institutes of Health (NIH), the Food and Drug Administration (FDA), and the Centers for Disease Control and Prevention (CDC) are the primary federal agencies that conduct research and establish policy aimed at the protection of the health and safety of the U.S. population.

In the Human Services Operating Division, the CMS plays a principal role in operating the multibillion dollar federal health insurance programs, Medicare and Medicaid, which provide health coverage to about one in every four Americans.[4] Medicare provides health insurance for 42.4 million elderly (over age 65 years) and disabled Americans. Medicaid, a joint federal-state program, provides health coverage for 52 million enrolled low-income persons, including 26.3 million children.[1]

Another federal agency that contributes to the health care system is the Veterans Health Administration. This agency provides health care services to eligible veterans of military services in the Armed Forces.

***Role of State and Local Governments.*** Although state programs vary greatly, state health departments are responsible for the oversight of a particular state's health needs. State and local health departments have the responsibility for evaluation and regulation of health care practices and coadministration of the Medicaid program with the federal government. These agencies work closely in developing approaches and solutions to community health problems.

***Role of Private Entities.*** Private health care organizations consist of: (1) providers: hospitals, long-term care facilities, hospices, home health agencies, ambulatory care centers, and others; and (2) payers: insurance companies, employers, and individuals. Health care provider organizations are concerned about the health status of the communities served; thus, they have a vested interest in keeping people healthy and providing health care services that are needed.

Insurance companies provide health care coverage for those who pay monthly premiums. Employers pay most of these premiums, although

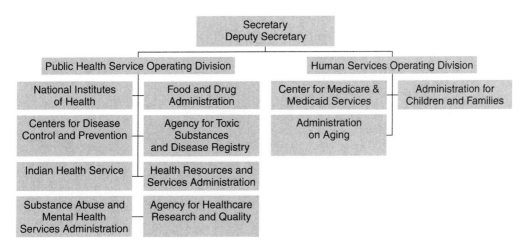

**Fig. 6-1** Operating divisions of U.S. Department of Health and Human Services.

patients themselves pay copayments and must meet deductible amounts before the insurance coverage begins to pay for services.

## Who Pays for Health Care?

Health care is one of the most expensive necessities of life. Consequently, many approaches to financing the health care system, both public and private, exist. Financing health care may be categorized as the source of payment—direct personal payment, private insurance payment, or government health plan payment.

*Direct Personal Payment.* Direct personal payment pays for health care costs that are not covered by insurance plans and are paid out of pocket by consumers. In 2004, average health care consumers spent 17.1% of their budgets in direct out-of-pocket expenditures for health care, as opposed to 13.8% on food and tobacco and 14.9% on housing.[5] This amount represents a major shift in spending patterns. Although consumers are paying more out of pocket, employers continue to pay most of the costs of health care, thus reflecting the increasing availability of private and government insurance plans.

*Private Insurance Payment.* Most health care consumers are covered by private insurance plans, many of which are paid all or in part by employers. In 2005, private insurance covered an estimated 72% of U.S. citizens.[6] In addition to the 14% covered by public insurance, 18% of U.S. citizens at some point in any given year were left without health insurance and access to health care. The proportion of noncitizens without health insurance coverage jumps to 32.3%.[6]

The large and growing numbers of uninsured have been attributed to changes in the private insurance market, reductions in employer-sponsored health policies, and limited availability of dependent coverage (Figs. 6-2 and 6-3).

*Government Health Insurance.* The two major health-related social insurance programs in the United States, Medicare and Medicaid, were enacted in 1965.

Medicare was designed to provide health care to individuals 65 years of age and older, the group with the greatest health care needs and fewest resources. Medicare is organized into three sections.

Part A of Medicare pays more than $100 billion to hospital and home health agencies. The Part A program is financed primarily through a mandatory payroll deduction (FICA tax). The FICA tax is 1.45% of earnings (paid by each employee and also by the employer) or 2.9% for self-employed persons.

Through Part B of Medicare, nearly $50 billion is paid to the facility operators and physicians in the outpatient setting. The Part B is financed: (1) through premium payments ($72.80 per month in 2005), which are usually deducted from the monthly Social Security benefit checks of those who are enrolled in Part B; and (2) through contributions from general revenue of the U.S. Treasury. Beneficiary premiums are currently set to cover 25% of the average expenditures for aged beneficiaries.

When managed care plans receive premium payments from Medicare, they are obligated to

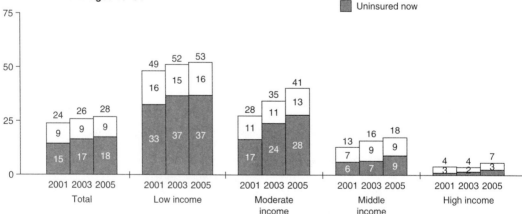

**Fig. 6-2**  Uninsured rates among adults based on income.
*From The Commonwealth Fund Biennial Health Insurance Surveys (2001, 2003, and 2005).*

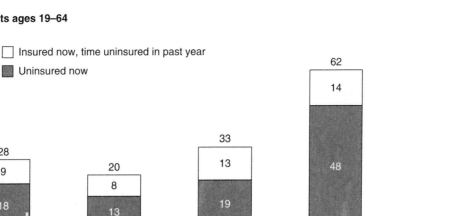

**Percent of adults ages 19–64**

**Fig. 6-3** Uninsured rates are highest among Hispanics and African Americans. *From the Commonwealth Fund Biennial Health Insurance Survey (2005).*

pay for covered services for each enrolled beneficiary. This arrangement is known as Part C of Medicare.

In 2005, a new supplement to Medicare was introduced for prescription drug coverage and is known as Medicare Part D. As of mid 2006, 38 million Medicare beneficiaries were enrolled in this program, nearly 91% of all enrollees. The average premium cost for Part D is $265 per year, in addition to a 25% copayment for many medications.[7]

Medicaid is a financial aid program designed to provide medical assistance to low-income persons who are aged, disabled, blind, or members of families with dependent children. Jointly, the program is sponsored by the federal and state governments. Although the federal government provides broad guidelines for operation of Medicaid, states have wide latitude in determination of eligibility and benefit criteria.

### Changing Patterns of Financing Care

As the foregoing discussion emphasized, the health care system in the United States does not meet the needs of all its citizens and non-citizens, despite constantly increasing expenditures. Growth in spending persists; the number of uninsured continues to rise; and efforts to control rising costs have not given the desired outcome of stabilization of the health care expenditures as a percentage of the gross domestic product. Although many attempts have been made to reform the U.S. health care system, the most recent activity comes from the market system of purchasers and consumers. Control of expenditures through a managed care strategy

has slowed but not arrested the dramatic rate of cost escalation.

***Managed Care Strategy.*** The impetus for managed care has arisen from the purchasers of health care, the government and employers, who are increasingly frustrated by escalating health care costs. Managed care works by shifting the financial risk of health care from the insurer (government or private insurance plans) to the individual providers (physicians, nurse practitioners, and others) and institutional providers (hospitals, nursing homes, home health agencies, and others). Providers are paid set preestablished fees in a capitated or heavily discounted FFS arrangement. Capitation is a set dollar payment per patient per unit of time (usually per month) that is paid to cover a specified set of services and administrative costs without regard to the actual number of services provided. Discounting FFS pays for services rendered is another way of preestablishing fees. With either system, providers are held accountable for providing all health services necessary to the members or beneficiaries of the managed care plan for this set level of payment.

The advantage of managed care is primarily reduction of costs with patients ensured to receive a standard level of quality health care services. However, criticisms of managed care are that the cost concerns may outweigh the quality concerns and that some patients may be restricted in their use of needed services merely to save money. Also, evidence is somewhat equivocal about the overall cost savings under managed care.[5] However, a preponderance of the evidence suggests that managed care is effective in controlling costs and excessive use of services without compromising quality.[7] For these reasons, managed care seems likely to remain an important aspect of the U.S. health care system for years to come.

**Role of Case Managers.** One way to reduce the fragmentation of health care delivery and to coordinate services so that patients are moved from more expensive to less expensive sites of care is the use of case managers. Case managers assess a patient's overall needs for different health services, delineate comprehensive patient outcomes, identify and procure the most cost-effective means of meeting those outcomes, and evaluate the effectiveness of the provided services. Case managers oversee the complete continuum of care from preadmission through rehabilitation. Case managers also coordinate services through the continuum of care for patients with chronic conditions. Although nurses commonly fill this role, many different models of case management exist.

**Implications for Perianesthesia Nurses.** The spread of managed care has impacted the way that health care is delivered, not only for the nursing profession and health care provider organizations but also for the individual nurse at the bedside. Implications for nursing include facilitating access to care to those without health insurance, increasing collaboration with other health care providers for more prevention and education about health promotion and disease prevention, and increasing productivity and efficiency in providing direct and indirect patient care. For individual nurses, understanding the economics of health delivery and the advent of managed care is the first step in delivering cost-effective care without compromising—rather, perhaps, improving—quality.

## Cost of Care in the Postanesthesia Care Unit (PACU)

Historically, surgical services were the most financially profitable area in the hospital. The advent of managed care and managed costs dramatically reduced the revenue generated by these areas. Most surgical cases are now reimbursed at a fixed rate regardless of the costs incurred by the facility. This shift in reimbursement strategy has caused hospitals and ambulatory surgery centers to look for ways to minimize their costs to maximize their revenues. Drugs, equipment (both reusable and disposable), prosthetics, linen use, and the numerous other incidental components have been examined to determine cost-effective procedures.

Charges do not necessarily reflect the cost incurred by the hospital to provide services to a patient because charges often reflect the market forces of supply and demand and do not necessarily maintain a constant relationship with costs.[8] Charges may also be deliberately higher to cover costs for other departments that have no reimbursement, such as medical records and risk management.

The actual cost of provision of services is much more difficult to calculate because of the wide array of items used to provide a service. Therefore, most facilities use a charge structure that they believe reflects the cost of a service or procedure to patients. Total cost can be determined by adding together the cost of each component expended to complete a particular surgical case or procedure. The total cost is then compared with the charge for the surgery or the negotiated payer reimbursement; the difference determines the level of profit or loss for that procedure or surgery.[9] Costs are subdivided into fixed and variable categories.

**Fixed Costs.** Fixed costs are one-time costs, such as capital expenditures. Examples of this type of cost include monitors, stretchers, intravenous (IV) pumps, and the bricks and mortar of the facility itself. Fixed costs do not change in proportion to the number of procedures or surgeries performed.[8]

**Variable Costs.** Variable costs vary with the volume of patients who receive care. These costs are linked directly to the number of surgical cases.[8] Dressings, medications, laundry, oxygen and ventilator tubing, electrocardiographic (EKG) electrodes, and the salaries of most staff members are variable costs. Labor (staff) costs are further subdivided into direct and indirect costs.

Direct labor costs represent the amount paid to employees for the length of time spent in performance of patient care. Direct labor costs for a PACU are calculated by multiplying the average hourly wage rate of each job class by the number of hours provided in each class and adding the results together.[9] These costs are variable because the number of patients cared for directly impacts the cost.

Indirect labor costs are made up of the salaries of those not involved in the provision of direct patient care. The nurse manager, unit secretaries, and any other staff who do not provide direct patient care are in this category. This category also contains any portion of staff salaries that are derived from attendance at meetings, inservice education, or other nonpatient care activities.

## How Nursing Contributes to Management of the Cost of Care

In the perianesthesia setting, labor represents the highest percentage of costs.[9] In an often quoted study, labor is 98% of the cost of care in a PACU.[10] As revenues declined after the implementation of managed care, most facilities developed strategies that included reduction or elimination of paid time for meetings and education to reduce labor costs. In addition, facilities shifted away from hiring full-time employees, who carry higher benefit costs, to more part-time and hourly employees who have fewer, if any, benefit costs. Cost containment always is an important strategy to ensure the financial viability of health care facilities. Nurses play important roles in identifying areas and process improvement opportunities that result in cost savings for an organization while providing efficient and effective quality patient care.

**Quality Versus Cost.** When nurses talk about cost and quality, many seem to put the concepts on opposite ends of a spectrum, as if the two were mutually exclusive, which may be the result of a knowledge deficit regarding the financial aspects of patient care. Nursing as a profession typically attracts individuals who value the capacity that the human touch has for promoting healing and a sense of well being, which is not a quantifiable value. In addition, the concept of quality lacks a shared definition. *Quality* means different things to different people and organizations; however, the cost of providing care seems less important than ensuring that patients have a positive experience of the health care system. Typically, once nurses develop an understanding of how money flows through an organization, they become some of the best advocates for cost-reduction strategies. The individuals at the bedside usually know where money is wasted and how the system can be improved to benefit all parties involved. All they need is to be involved in the decision-making process.

**Patient Education.** The perianesthesia nurse can begin setting the tone of the patient experience during preoperative teaching. A discussion of what the patient anticipates can help to guide care in the PACU. This exchange provides the opportunity for the nurse to explain the postoperative course and for the patient to share expectations and concerns. Ambulatory surgery patients assume that the procedure and recovery will consume most of the operative day.[11] A discovery of what is meaningful to the patient can help set expectations that are easily met by the PACU staff. This type of exchange and follow through in care costs little and can provide the patient and family with a better PACU experience.

Nurses who work in the ambulatory surgery setting have the additional challenge of providing extensive discharge teaching. Preprinted instructions are a necessity because patients only remember about 10% to 15% of what they are told. Perianesthesia nurses must be involved in the creation of these materials and should serve on the patient education committee in their facility. In addition, nurses in this area are in a unique position to track the quality of care via the incidence rate of infections. Typically, ambulatory care centers call patients 24 hours after discharge for determination of how the patient is progressing and for assessment for any concerns.

Some facilities have instituted a 72-hour call back to identify postoperative infections that may be related to quality issues at the hospital. These infections are typically underreported because most patients return to their primary care providers or surgeons for follow-up and no tracking mechanism is in place to quantify this issue.

**Use of Clinical Guidelines.** The American Society of PeriAnesthesia Nurses (ASPAN) is responsible for defining the practice of perianesthesia nursing.[12] ASPAN's mission is to advance nursing practice through education, research, and standards. Perianesthesia nurses should familiarize themselves with the mission and standards of this organization. Pain and comfort, staffing, hypothermia, postoperative nausea and vomiting (PONV), postoperative discharge nausea and vomiting (PDNV), and intensive care unit (ICU) overflow guidelines are available on the web site and should be used by PACUs. These are some of the major issues that face perianesthesia nurses today and are some of the costliest issues. Appropriate use of these guidelines can aid in provision of optimal patient care with control of costs.

### Evidence-based Strategies

Evidence-based medicine refers to the way in which treatment options are chosen. Many traditional strategies for patient care are not supported by research. A simple example is the alcohol sponge bath that nurses in the past performed when a patient had a fever. We now know that this bath is actually detrimental in most cases because it promotes shivering, increases oxygen consumption, and increases carbon dioxide production, which can be harmful to the patient. The practice made sense at the time, but research proved otherwise.

In the perianesthesia setting, a variety of research has been done on the prevention and management of nausea, returning a patient's condition to normothermia, and pain management. These studies provide necessary guidance to assist nurses in making care decisions regarding the patients entrusted to them.

A principal PACU nursing intervention is the assistance of a patient's return to a normothermic state. Shivering increases oxygen demands and can cause airway obstruction and increased somnolence in postoperative patients. In 1999, Mahoney and Odom[13] published a metaanalysis of 20 studies (N = 1575) that provided evidence that patients had a significantly higher risk for adverse outcomes when their temperatures fell just a few degrees below normal during surgery. Patients who had temperatures in the 34°C to 36°C range had higher hospital costs, between $2500 and $7000, more because of adverse events. The study's analysis also revealed that the most effective heating device was the forced warm air unit. This information is very important and can also be used by PACU nurses.

Pain management is equally important to restoring normothermia. Unfortunately, health care providers consistently use too little pain medication. This practice is becoming a growing concern for the consumer as studies typically prove this to be true. Perianesthesia nurses are in a unique position to initiate appropriate pain management and set the tone of the patient's experience. Nurses are educated to combine strategies to maximize pain relief. These other strategies cost little but can be very effective and even reduce the need for pharmaceutical management. Chapter 31 is devoted to the pharmacology of pain management.

In 1999, Medina[14] investigated the relationship between the sound level in a PACU and the use of analgesics. The study revealed that more analgesics were dispensed after periods of medium and high sound levels than were given in periods after low sound levels. This research supported findings from previous studies that sound influences the perception of pain and the use of analgesics.

Sound can easily be controlled in the PACU setting. Health care providers often become immune to the noise level in the care environment. Studies have shown that minor modifications have the ability to improve the patient experience and decrease the cost of the PACU stay by reducing the need for medication.

**Outcomes Research.** The first outcomes researcher in nursing was Florence Nightingale. She used data to link mortality rates with patients' diagnoses and treatments. She also developed the first uniform hospital discharge data set.[15] Outcomes research is a rapidly growing field with enormous potential to provide critical information to the health care and pharmaceutical industries. The overall aim of outcomes research is to improve health care

and achieve optimal benefit from the available resources with the assessment of the outcomes of different medical treatments. The emphasis in this area of research is on the benefits to the patient. Economic, health, and clinical concerns combine for examination of the influence of the treatment on the patient's quality of life, the functional status of the patient, and patient satisfaction with treatment.[15]

**Cost-benefit Analysis.** Cost-benefit analysis is an economic principle used for evaluation of outcomes. This approach promotes the efficient use of scarce resources with the methodology with which projects are evaluated and alternatives are compared.[5] The value of the project is determined in dollar amounts, and the consequences are measured in dollars.[16] The cost of pharmaceuticals and the patient's length of stay have become the primary focus of cost reduction efforts by many health care facilities. The overarching goal is the appropriate use of medications based on their efficiency and effectiveness to decrease the length of stay or to decrease the unnecessary use of diagnostic tests and a prolonged hospital stay that results from ineffective or inefficient treatment.[15]

A study still frequently cited in the literature is a cost-benefit analysis regarding PACU issues conducted in 1995 by Dexter and Tinker.[10] They developed computer simulations to determine whether the cost of PACU care could be reduced. They examined three hypotheses. First, they looked at the influence of shorter acting anesthetics. Second, they examined the hypothetic elimination of nausea and vomiting. Finally, they adjusted operating room scheduling practices to determine whether that could reduce PACU costs. They found that the use of drugs with "faster recovery" only decreased PACU costs if operating rooms were scheduled to run later each day (not a popular concept with surgeons). Because all patients do not leave at the same time, the idea that a decrease in the length of time in the PACU decreases the cost is unlikely. If nausea and vomiting could be eliminated in the percentage of patients who typically experience this phenomenon, the total time to discharge would have decreased by 4.8%. The largest impact on PACU costs was the distribution of admissions. Currently, as the day progresses, admissions increase. If the bulk of the admissions could occur in the earliest hours, personnel could leave sooner in the day and therefore, labor costs would be reduced. This is not a likely scenario, given the other hospital systems and personnel involved in surgical services. This study also determined that supplies and medications account for only 2% of PACU charges, whereas personnel costs account for almost all the costs in the PACU.

The latest trend in postanesthesia care is referred to as fasttracking, which is the process in which patients are moved rapidly through the phases of recovery from anesthesia and are discharged home faster. Advancements in surgery techniques and anesthetic agents have been the major contributors to this trend in the ambulatory surgery setting.[17] The ASPAN recognized two distinct models of fasttracking in the perianesthesia setting. The first is PACU Phase I bypass where the most intensive monitoring takes place directly after the patient leaves the surgical suite. Phase I is generally referred to as the first hour after surgery. Estimates are that a hospital can save between $50,000 and $158,000 annually in salaries and supplies by allowing patients who meet selective criteria to bypass Phase I and proceed directly to the Phase II setting.[17] The second model is referred to as rapid PACU progression (RPP). In this model, the patient progresses rapidly through the Phase I PACU in as little as 15 to 20 minutes after admission, which also results in a reduced length of stay in the PACU because of aggressive nursing care based on the individual biopsychosocial and emotional needs of the patient.[17] Time savings do not translate into cost savings unless the fasttracking process leads to savings in personnel costs or enhanced productivity.[18]

A 2004 analysis by Song et al[18] examined nursing workload in PACUs that fasttracked patients. They found that the accelerated recovery process was not associated with any increased patient discomfort or postoperative side effects. Their study also determined that a reduction in the time to discharge or a bypass of the PACU phase I reduced nursing workload significantly. The postoperative personnel costs are typically fixed costs in the traditional hospital setting. Therefore, a realization of cost savings in the PACU by fasttracking patients is difficult.

A study by Sandberg and others[19] examined fasttracking for patients for laparoscopic cholecystectomy. The study was conducted at Massachusetts General Hospital and examined the efficiency and efficacy of moving patients rapidly through the PACU process. The authors concluded that they could free up at least one surgical bed per six surgeons if they adopted a direct PACU discharge pathway, which would result in fewer delays for the surgical service while maintaining quality patient care. They planned to disseminate this process throughout the rest of the surgical department.

***Cost-effectiveness Analysis.*** Placement of a monetary value on life and health in addition to a value for other intangible costs and benefits is difficult. Cost-effectiveness analysis is offered as a more practical approach to decision making than cost-benefit analysis.[5] In this type of analysis, one assumes that the objective is desirable, although the benefits cannot be measured in monetary terms. The cost is still determined in dollar amounts, but the consequences are measured in nondollar amount, such as life years gained or disability prevented.[16]

Anesthetic drugs can vary widely in cost. Newer more expensive drugs are used for induction of anesthesia with the promise that they provide more rapid awakening and less nausea and vomiting. Since the development and marketing of 5-HT3 antagonists, the successful management of postoperative nausea and vomiting has become more expensive.[15] The choice for the newer drug is made based on the hope that it will allow patients to be discharged sooner. In reality, little evidence suggests that earlier discharge is possible or that it decreases costs. Why do facilities switch to the more expensive drug? Typically they do so because they believe it will provide a better experience for the patient, something which is much more difficult to assign a dollar amount. The evaluation of the cost effectiveness of an antiemetic must include the risk from any given anesthetic, the procedure performed, the patient-risk profile, and the value that the patient places on avoiding nausea.

A cost is associated with postoperative nausea and vomiting (PONV). In a 2006 study by Habib et al,[20] the researchers looked at the use of antiemetics both for the prophylaxis and the treatment of PONV and for the assessment of the resource utilization and duration of the PACU stay. They looked at adult patients who had inpatient surgery with general anesthesia between January 2004 and February 2005 at Duke Medical Center. A total of 3641 patients were included in the analysis, and 2689 (79%) had received prophylactic antiemetics. The incidence rate of vomiting was significantly less in patients who had been given PONV prophylaxis (3% versus 16%). Vomiting results in a higher PACU cost ($138 dollars per patient) than nausea ($85 dollars per patient). This is an area where nursing can intervene with complementary techniques to minimize these side effects. Music therapy, aromatherapy, and accupoint stimulation are areas currently being studied to see how they can be incorporated into PACU care.[21]

**Short-term Outcomes.** In the PACU, short-term outcomes are those outcomes that are desirable for a patient to experience in the first 12 hours after surgery. Perianesthesia nurses can conduct cost-effectiveness research regarding nursing interventions that reduce the need for pain medication, reduce the incidence rate of nausea and vomiting, and promote a faster return to normothermia. The ability to positively alter these experiences for patients results in improved short-term outcomes.

The impact of preoperative education can also be assessed as a short-term outcome. Identification of reductions in patient anxiety, the ability to perform certain postoperative maneuvers (such as incentive spirometry) correctly, and recalling home care instructions can help to evaluate the effectiveness of teaching.

**Long-term Outcomes.** For the purposes of perianesthesia nursing, long-term outcomes can be defined as those that occur within 12 to 72 hours. These may include correctly following postoperative instructions for activity and pain management, the identification of wound problems by the patient, and the appropriate use of follow-up services. Nursing research can be directed to determine the effectiveness of discharge teaching methodologies and strategies for PACU nurses.

## SUMMARY

Our pluralistic health care system is designed to combine public and private health care delivery services and financing. Management of the economic issues related to patient care is necessary to control the costs of health care. Nurses are perfectly situated to assist with strategies that cut costs while simultaneously improving quality and health status of individuals.

Perianesthesia nurses should be part of education committees and policy and standards committees and should have a place on product committees. Perianesthesia nursing can make significant contributions to understanding the surgical experience of the patient. Many opportunities exist for research to determine the best practices of the art and science of nursing in this field.

## REFERENCES

1. Centers for Medicare & Medicaid Services: *Highlights: national health expenditures*, 2004, available at http://www.cms.hhs.gov/National HealthExpendData/02_NationalHealthAccounts Historical.asp#TopOfPage, accessed October 2, 2006.

2. Heffler S, et al: *Health spending projections for 2002-2012*, available at http://content.healthaffairs.org/cgi/content/full/hlthaff.w3.54v1/DC1, accessed November 1, 2006.

3. Griffith JR, White KR: *The well-managed healthcare organization*, ed 6, Chicago, 2007, Health Administration Press.

4. Department of Health and Human Services: *HHS agencies*, available at www.hhs.gov/agencies/, accessed October 22, 2001.

5. Folland S, Goodman A, Stano M: Cost-benefit analysis and other tools of economic evaluation. In *The economics of health and healthcare*, ed 5, Upper Saddle River, NJ, 2007, Prentice Hall.

6. 2005 Biennial Health Insurance Survey: The Commonwealth Fund, available at http://www.cmwf.org/surveys/surveys_show.htm?doc_id=367929, accessed November 1, 2006.

7. Centers for Medicare & Medicaid Services: (2006). Medicare prescription drug coverage, available at http://www.medicare.gov/pdphome.asp, accessed November 1, 2006.

8. Macario A, Glenn D, Dexter F: What can the post anesthesia care unit manager do to decrease costs in the post anesthesia care unit? *J Perianesth Nurs* 14(5):284-293, 1999.

9. Kahl K, Preston B: Identifying the cost of patient care in the postanesthesia care setting, *J Post Anesth Nurs* 3(3):198-202, 1998.

10. Dexter F, Tinker J: Analysis of strategies to decrease postanesthesia care unit costs, *Anesthesiol* 82(1):94-101, 1995.

11. Phillips B: Patients' assessment of ambulatory anesthesia and surgery, *J Clin Anesth* 4:355-358, 1992.

12. ASPAN: *ASPAN mission statement*, available at http://www.aspan.org/Foundation.htm, accessed December 15, 2006.

13. Mahoney CB, Odom J: Maintaining intraoperative normothermia: a meta-analysis of outcomes with costs, *AANA J* 67:155-164, 1999.

14. Medina M: *The relationship between sound levels in the postanesthesia care unit and use of analgesics*, unpublished master's thesis, 1999, Uniformed Services University of Health Sciences.

15. Windle P: Outcomes research: a paradigm shift for nursing research, *J Perianesth Nurs* 20: 351-353, 2005.

16. Aday L, et al: Efficiency: concepts and methods. In Aday LA, Begley CE, Lairson DR: *Evaluating the healthcare system*, ed 3, Chicago, 2004, Health Administration Press.

17. Mamaril M: Fast-tracking the postanesthesia patient: the pros and cons, *J Perianesth Nurs* 15(2):89-93, 2000.

18. Song D, Chung F, Ronayne M, et al: Fast-tracking (bypassing the PACU) does not reduce

nursing workload after ambulatory surgery, *Br J Anesthesia* 93(6):768-774, 2004.

19. Sandberg W, Canty T, Sokal S, et al: Financial and operational impact of a direct-from-PACU discharge pathway for laparoscopic cholecystectomy patients, *Surgery* 140(3):372-378, 2006.

20. Habib AS, Chen YT, Taguchi A, et al: Postoperative nausea and vomiting following inpatient surgeries in a teaching hospital: a retrospective database analysis, *Curr Med Res Opin* 22(6):1093-1099, 2006.

21. Mamaril M, Windle P, Burkard J: Prevention and management of postoperative nausea and vomiting: a look at complementary techniques, *J Perianesth Nurs* 12(6):404-410, 2006.

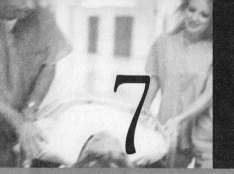

# 7

# LEGAL ISSUES IN THE PACU

Cecil B. Drain, PhD, RN, CRNA, FAAN, FASAHP

The perianesthesia nurse, as a licensed professional nurse, is subject to a set of standards that must be followed for continuance to practice nursing; the standards are such as a reasonable and prudent nurse would follow in the state of practice. If the action of a perianesthesia nurse is not reasonable for a perianesthesia nurse and the action causes injury to the patient, a malpractice lawsuit may be the outcome.

Because the legal field has a host of new terminology, the first section of this chapter includes definitions with examples and boxes. Next, the chapter presents specific case law to show how some cases transpired. Because most of the litigation in the perianesthesia period falls into the operating room phase, all the cases cited are from this area. However, the perianesthesia nurse is hoped to have a better understanding of the litigation process with a review of these cases.

The legal component of nursing practice is often viewed as unpredictable and frightening and as out to harm the perianesthesia practitioner. If the perianesthesia nurse becomes involved in a legal action, a presumption of only negative effects usually occurs, in addition to a feeling of terror. After reading this chapter, the perianesthesia nurse hopefully will find the law to be a helpful tool to ensure safe practices. The intended outcome of this chapter is the facilitation of the perianesthesia nurse as a legally educated nurse, able to protect oneself when dealing with legal issues.

## DEFINITIONS

**Advance Directive:** A written document, sometimes called a living will, recognized by state law that provides directions for care of a person in the event that person is unable to make decisions on treatment choices.

**Advocacy:** Acting in behalf of the patient in an effort to protect that person's rights to make his or her own decisions.

**Confidentiality:** A special relationship that exists between the patient and the perianesthesia nurse in which the information discussed is not shared with a third party who is not directly involved in the patient's care. Disclosure of confidential information exposes the perianesthesia nurse to liability for invasion of the patient's privacy and breech of confidentiality malpractice claims.

**Consent:** A voluntary act on the part of the patient to grant someone a type of care.

**Damages:** Viewed as the sum of money a court or jury awards as compensation for a tort action. Damages can be broken down into *general damages*, which are given for intangible wrongs, such as pain and suffering, disfigurement, interference with ordinary enjoyment of life, and loss of consortium (marital services), that are inherent in the injury itself; *special damages*, which are the patient's out-of-pocket expenses, such as medical care, lost wages, and rehabilitation costs; and *punitive damages*, which are the damages sought as punishment for those whose conduct goes beyond normal malpractice.

**Defamation:** Refers to damage caused to someone's reputation. If the damaging information is written, the defamation is called *libel*; if it is spoken, it is called *slander*.

**Defendant:** A person who is accused of wrongdoing; in a malpractice claim, the defendant can be a perianesthesia nurse.

**Defensive Charting:** Extensive documentation that is accurate and factual in the medical record (see Box 7-1).

**Deposition:** Out-of-court oral testimony given under oath before a court reporter. The deposition can involve expert witnesses, fact witnesses, defendants, or plaintiffs and can be used to impeach (find inconsistencies or untruths) testimony in trials.

**Ethics:** The distinction between right and wrong based on knowledge, not just opinions.

**Expert Witness:** A person with specific knowledge, skills, and experience regarding a specific area, such as perianesthesia nursing, who testifies to the ultimate issue, such as: What was the duty or was the duty violated? Did the violation cause injury? What could the defendant have done to prevent the injury? Did malpractice occur?

## Box 7-1 Guidelines for Defensive Charting

- All entries should be accurate and factual.
- Make corrections appropriately and according to agency or hospital policies. DO NOT EVER obliterate or destroy any information that is or has been in the chart.
- If information exists that should have been charted and was not, the perianesthesia nurse should make a "late entry," noting the time the charting actually occurred and the specific time the charting reflects.
- All identified patient problems, nursing actions taken, and patient responses should be noted. Do not describe a patient problem without including the nursing actions taken and the patient response.
- Documentation of why you did not do something that you would routinely do is often as important as documentation of why you did do something. An example of this situation is a patient who refuses ambulation; the notation would be, "patient refused to ambulate because of..."
- Be as objective as possible in charting.
- Each page of the chart should contain the current date and time.
- Each page of the chart should include the full name and professional designation of every person who makes an entry on that page.
- Follow through with who saw the patient and what measures were initiated, especially in such instances as when the physician visited and calls that were made to the physician for a problem, and record the physician's response, the nursing actions, and the patient's response.
- Make sure your notes are LEGIBLE and CLEARLY reflect the information to be documented to assure that the information makes sense and is accurately portrayed.
- Pertinent notes from other providers should also be reviewed to ensure that the medical record shows a coordination of health care team efforts and thoughts.

Adapted from Zerwekh J, Claborn J: *Nursing today: transitions and trends*, ed 5, St Louis, 2006, Mosby.

**Health Insurance Portability and Accountability Act (HIPAA):** This law was enacted to ensure privacy rights and describes how personal health information (PHI) may be used and how a patient can obtain access to the information.

**Impaired Nurse:** A nurse who is unable to function effectively because of some type of substance abuse, such as alcohol, prescription drugs, and illegal drugs.

**Informed Consent:** The patient's approval (or that of the patient's legal representative) to a specific care service; informed consent is a legal document. Informed consent can be waived for urgent medical or surgical intervention as long this exception is so stated in an institutional policy. Types of consents are admission agreement, blood transfusion consent, surgical consent, research consent, and special consent, such as for the use of restraints, client photographs, organ donation, or autopsy.

**Intentional Tort:** Consequences of actions that can be reasonably foreseen, violate duty, or cause injury; in this case, an expert witness is not necessary to bring a case. The actions are closely related to criminal acts in that they involve intent to do wrong. Types of intentional torts include assault and battery, false imprisonment, and defamation.

**Interrogatory:** The process of discovery of the facts regarding a case through a set of written questions exchanged through the attorneys that represent the parties involved in the case.

**Jurisdiction:** The court's authority to accept or decide cases, which can be based on location or subject matter of the case.

**Law:** Perianesthesia nurses are governed by civil and criminal law when they are in the role as providers of services, employees of institutions, and private citizens. The types of laws are presented in Box 7-2.

**Liability:** Proof of liability is described in Box 7-3.

**Malpractice:** Determined if the perianesthesia nurse owed a duty to the client and did not carry out that duty and the client was injured because the nurse failed to perform the duty. The elements of negligence are applied to determination of malpractice, and usually an expert witness is used to establish standard of care and prove the violation resulted in injury.

**Minors:** A patient who is under the legal age (usually 18 years) as defined by state statute and may not give legal consent; consent must be obtained by a parent or the legal guardian.

**Negligence:** Failure to provide care that a reasonable person ordinarily would provide in a similar circumstance. The elements that must

---

### Box 7-2    Types of Laws

**CONTRACT LAW**

A law that is concerned with enforcement of an agreement among private individuals.

**CIVIL LAW**

A type of law that is concerned with relationships among persons and the protection of a person's rights. Violation of this type of law may cause harm to an individual or property, but no grave threat to society exists.

**CRIMINAL LAW**

A type of law that is concerned with relationships between individuals and governments and with acts that threaten society and its order; a crime is an offense against society that violates a law and is defined as a misdemeanor (less serious in nature) or a felony (serious in nature).

**TORT LAW**

A tort is a civil wrong, other than a breach in contract, in which the law allows an injured person to seek damages from a person who caused the injury.

---

be established to prove negligence are: (1) an established relationship. (2) the duty established by profession; and (3) a violation of that duty that results in injury.

**Nurse Practice Act:** A series of statutes that have been enacted by every state legislature to regulate the practice of nursing. In essence, the statutes define the scope of nursing practice and distinguish between nursing practice and medical practice; every professional nurse must review and understand the provisions of the Nurse Practice Act in the state or province in which the nurse works.

**Patient's Bill of Rights:** A document of client rights that reflects acknowledgement of the client's right to participate in one's own health care, with an emphasis on client autonomy and several laws and standards that pertain to the client's rights. A description of the patient's rights during hospitalization is in Box 7-4.

**Plaintiff:** The person who files the lawsuit and seeks damages for a perceived wrongdoing; usually the patient or the patient's family.

### Box 7-3    Elements Needed to Prove Liability

- *Duty:* At the time of injury, a duty existed between the plaintiff and the defendant.
- *Breach of Duty:* The defendant breached duty of care to the plaintiff.
- *Proximate Cause:* The breach of duty was the legal cause of injury to the plaintiff.
- *Damage or Injury:* The plaintiff experienced injury or damages or both and can be compensated by law.

**Post hoc, ergo propter hoc:** "After this, therefore because of this"; the theory of the injury has been bypassed as the injury occurred, and that by itself indicates a failure to do what was reasonable and prudent.

**Res ipsa loquitur:** "The thing speaks for itself." This can be invoked in a medical malpractice case if the case meets the following four criteria or tests: (1) the injury is considered to occur only during failure to exercise ordinary care, skill, or diligence; (2) the injurious actions are under the exclusive control of the practitioner; (3) the patient makes no contribution to the injury; and (4) the reasons for the injury are more attributable to the nurse than to the patient. Allows *post hoc* reasoning.

**Standard of Care:** Standards based on various types of evidence as to what is reasonable and prudent behavior for a perianesthesia nurse (health care professional). These standards are usually outlined by the state or province Nurse Practice Acts.

**Statute:** Documented rules for living in a state (state law) or the United States (federal law) that are passed by state legislatures and by Congress.

**Tort:** A civil wrong (not criminal), other than a breach in contract, in which the law allows an injured person to seek damages from the person who caused the injury.

## MEDICAL MALPRACTICE IN PERSPECTIVE

A 61-year-old woman enters the hospital for "routine" elective surgery on a deviated septum in the nose. Neither the attending surgeon nor the attending anesthesiologist are present when the patient undergoes extubation by the nurse

---

**Box 7-4    Patient Rights When Hospitalized**

- Right to considerate and respectful care.
- Right to be informed about illness, possible treatments, and likely outcome and to discuss this information with the physician.
- Right to know the names and roles of the persons who are involved in care.
- Right to consent to or refuse a treatment.
- Right to have an advance directive.
- Right to privacy.
- Right to expect that medical records are confidential.
- Right to review the medical record and to have information explained.
- Right to expect that the hospital will provide necessary health services.
- Right to know whether the hospital has relationships with outside parties that may influence treatment or care.
- Right to consent or refuse to take part in research.
- Right to be told of realistic care alternatives when hospital care is no longer appropriate.
- Right to know about hospital rules that affect treatment and about changes and payment methods.

From Christensen B, Kockrow E: *Foundations of nursing*, ed 4, St Louis, 2003, Mosby.

---

anesthetist. The extubation does not go well, and the patient's final diagnosis is a persistent vegetative state. During the medical malpractice trial, the jury learns that both the surgeon and the anesthesiologist were in other operating rooms during the extubation and that each thought that the other was with this particular patient. In addition, the jury hears testimony that the anesthesiologist did not evaluate the patient between the operating room and the postanesthesia care unit (PACU) unit. The jury is not pleased with the sequence of events and awards the plaintiff $9.6 million in compensatory damages and an additional $3.5 million in punitive damages.[1]

Medical malpractice cases, such as this case, with large jury verdicts are often widely publicized in the media. The cases are used to illustrate medical malpractice that can be neatly categorized into risk management issues to be discussed by hospital attorneys during grand rounds. During this process, the so-called blame game becomes all too easy to play. Is this case a case of inappropriate medical supervision, or are other issues, such as the lack of informed consent, involved? Regardless of the cause and effect, jury verdicts this large are sure to get the attention of both the public and health care providers, and in doing so, the blame game is further perpetuated. Perhaps hospital employees are fired or physicians lose their hospital privileges. Medical malpractice insurance premiums may rise dramatically, and some practitioners may be unable to retain professional malpractice coverage. Hospital administrators tell everyone to "try harder" to avoid similar mistakes; otherwise,

medical practice in the operating room often continues just about the same as before the tragic incident.[2,3] The important learning lessons from this—and from other medical mistakes—often go undetected and unlearned because we have too narrowly focused medical mistakes as the result of individual error. As Dr. Lucian Leape aptly notes:

> Ironically, that unique nature of medical injury, or more precisely, our reaction to it, has been the major barrier to reducing medical errors and injury. Shame, guilt, and fear prevent many physicians from discussing their mistakes, being honest with patients, and being able to look beyond their individual errors to correct underlying systems failures. They can only try harder. For many lawyers, a sense of just cause, in some cases moral outrage, similarly blinds them to alternatives to tort litigation. Both are misplaced. And both have been manifestly unsuccessful in preventing medical injuries. We have created a monster.[4]

Analysis of medical malpractice issues therefore requires an understanding of the complex relationship between law and medicine and the role that both professions can play in development of health care policy in the United States. Medical malpractice has been an issue of intense public debate since the 1970s, with periodic allegations that America is in a "malpractice crisis." Usually, this perception of a malpractice "crisis" comes from many physicians dismayed at what they perceive to be excessively large jury verdicts against them and at a growing number of legal claims against the medical profession, larger premium payments for professional malpractice insurance, the decreasing availability of malpractice insurance at any cost, and clinical practice changes physicians sometimes believe they must make to avoid litigation.[5,6] Physicians argued that they had to practice defensive medicine, including unnecessary tests and treatments, not to benefit their patients but to avoid potential liability.[7] This practice, in turn, created a significant increase in the cost of medicine to the consumer, often in the government's Medicaid and Medicare programs. Consequently, in 1970, the Secretary of Health, Education, and Welfare established a major Commission on Medical Malpractice to investigate the entire system. The results of this study, published in 1972, were not what many physicians expected to hear from the federal government:

> The Commission found that there were a large number of doctor-caused injuries for which claims were never made; that 75 percent of jury verdicts were for the defendant; that malpractice insurance was available, albeit at rising premiums; that most hospitals had experienced little litigation; that defensive medicine was widely believed to exist but impossible to measure, because of difficulties in identifying services provided solely or primarily to avoid legal liability; and that state licensing agencies had little authority, staff, or inclination to discipline incompetent or "impaired" physicians.[8]

With the desired results not achieved from this 1972 commission study, a number of medical organizations throughout the United States began a concerted effort to lobby state legislatures to create various statutory "tort reform" remedies in an effort to alleviate the societal costs of this perceived malpractice crisis. Almost every state has passed some sort of medical malpractice tort reform legislation to date, although these state statutes vary considerably and no particular pattern exists.

Examples of state tort reform remedies include limits imposed on the monetary amount received for pain and suffering or a limit in the total amount recovered in a medical malpractice action. Many states also require submission of a malpractice case to a medical screening board before a patient can bring a legal action to court, and other states require submission of a medical malpractice case to arbitration and restriction of attorney contingent fee systems.[9,10] The most contentious tort reform issue to date has been placement of a statutory "cap" on total medical malpractices damages. Some state courts have held that these statutes are reasonable and constitutional under the circumstances to protect health care providers and health care services within a state, but other courts have held such statutes to be unconstitutional because they arbitrarily favor health care providers at the expense of other professionals and lay persons within a particular state.[11]

In practice, however, such tort reform has done little to alleviate the concerns of physicians and patients regarding the cost and quality of medicine.[12] Some evidence suggests that certain tort reform legislation, such as that which directly limits physician liability through caps on medical malpractice damage awards, the limitation or abolition of punitive damages, and the abolition of mandatory prejudgment interest, may reduce hospital expenditures somewhat, at least in certain populations.[13] However, if these tort reform remedies have done little to reduce the frequency and severity of malpractice cases, what else might work?

Traditionally, the medical malpractice liability system serves two principal roles: (1) compensation is provided for patients injured as the result of negligence on the part of players in the health care system; and (2) an incentive is provided for physicians and other health care providers to practice better quality medicine. Until recently, little empiric research had been published to show the prevalence rate of negligence within the health care system. This lack of research changed dramatically, beginning in the early 1990s, with the publication of a series of research results commonly called the Harvard Medical Practice Study. This study was a population-based study of injuries that resulted from medical care during hospitalizations in New York. A review of thousands of medical records indicated that nearly 4% of patients had an injury that caused the hospital stay to be prolonged or that resulted in measurable disability. Indeed, 14% of those patients identified as having had a medical injury died as a result of the injury.[14] In a follow up on the initial review of medical records, the authors identified patients who had filed claims against physicians and hospitals and discovered that only a fraction of those patients who were injured as the result of medical negligence filed claims and that compensation awarded was based primarily on the severity of injury rather than a finding of negligence. The authors concluded that:

> the civil justice system only infrequently compensates injured patients and rarely identifies and holds healthcare providers accountable

for substandard medical care. Although malpractice litigation may fulfill its social objectives crudely, support for its preservation persists in part because of the perception that other methods of ensuring a high quality of care and redressing patients' grievances have proved to be inadequate.[15]

At about the same time the Harvard study was conducted, the federal government was in the process of passing the Health Care Quality Improvement Act of 1986. One critical underlying assumption of this new law is that medical malpractice, not merely medical malpractice litigation, is increasing and that professional review can remedy this problem. Major portions of this act were designed to give immunity to physicians and others who participate in peer review processes, but the act also requires the reporting of medical malpractice payouts to the Secretary of Health and Human Services for inclusion into a national databank and also to state boards of medical examiners. The databank was created in large part to prevent unethical or incompetent health care practitioners from moving from state to state without any disclosure or discovery of previous negligence or incompetent performance.[16,17] To date, little research has been published on the efficacy of this databank, and little is known about the impact of this databank on physician practice or quality of health care to date.

## Sources for Identification of Malpractice in the PACU

Despite this medical-legal conundrum, much can be learned in the area of risk management from individual malpractice claims. National malpractice carriers, such as the St. Paul Fire and Marine Insurance Company, are able to give more detailed and "countrywide" data that involve medical malpractice claims, and a closed claims study by the American Society of Anesthesiologists (ASA), with a reported database of more than 4000 cases that represent 35 insurance companies, has substantially helped medical professionals understand and analyze the legal consequences of adverse outcomes.[18] These closed claim data, however, do not contain the "near misses" or the bad outcomes without damages. The American Association of Nurse Anesthetists further examined adverse outcomes of anesthesia care provided by nurse anesthetists with use of the St. Paul databank.[19] A data bank created in the American Society of PeriAnesthesia Nurses (ASPAN) is anticipated in the near future.

A *claim* is a demand for financial compensation for an injury that results from medical care. On rare occasions, hospitals or providers may pay for these claims out of pocket. Most claims are reported to the commercial malpractice insurance carrier who then investigates the claim, determines liability issues, and either settles the case out of court, denies liability altogether, or goes to trial. A few claims are dropped by the claimant before trial or are handled via arbitration or mediation. Trained reviewers who use the professional Practice Manual for the Certified Registered Nurse Anesthetist (CRNA) along with available medical records and other information collected by the insurance carrier for investigative purposes are used to determine whether appropriate medical care was given and whether anyone on the treatment team could have prevented the adverse event.

The nurse anesthesia study found that "lack of vigilance contributed to 79% of damaging events and adverse outcomes and that in 62% of the incidents, the CRNA could have taken action to prevent harm to the patient. Vigilance was defined as state or quality of being watchful to detect any occurrences that might harm a patient during an anesthetic."[20] Most of the results of this study were predictable. For example, many of the claims involved inadequate preinduction of anesthesia activities, and almost half of all claims were deemed to have been preventable by the CRNA. The study concluded with the note that patients with ASA I and II are at risk for damaging events and adverse outcomes and that just over half the claims provided inappropriate care, which indicates that the filing of a legal claim by the plaintiff or patient does not necessarily imply that substandard or inappropriate anesthesia care was provided.

In a review of the limited legal cases that involve the PACU, most of the litigation occurs between the operating room and the PACU. Most of the cases involve the standard of care for physicians, anesthesia personnel, and operating room nurses as they accompany the patient to the PACU. And most of the involvement of the perianesthesia nurse in these cases continues to be the written documentation on the patient on arrival to the PACU. Hence, Chapter 26 in this book discusses the transfer of the patient from the operating room (OR) to the PACU. Only a few legal cases deal with litigation regarding the PACU stay of the patient. These cases involve the management of the patient's airway. Airway management, from a legal point of view, appears to be the major legal issue in the PACU. Therefore,

Chapter 30 on airway management was developed not only to provide knowledge about this important aspect of care in the emergence phase of anesthesia but also to aid in prevention of litigation that focuses on this area of care.

As mentioned previously, the National Practitioner Databank (NPDB) is a central source of information regarding malpractice payments for physicians, nurses, nurse anesthetists, and dentists. The databank became operational on September 1, 1990, and, as of 1998, had more than 195,000 reports of malpractice payments, adverse licensure, clinical privileging, professional society membership, Drug Enforcement Agency (DEA) actions, and Medicare/Medicaid exclusions actions concerning licensed professionals. Approximately 30,000 reports are added each year.[21] Nurse anesthetists are identified separately from other nursing specialties in the databank. Analysis of information in the databank is limited by the codes that the submitter must use. Anesthesia-related malpractice codes include assessment, monitoring, equipment testing, wrong agent or equipment, intubation, equipment use, improper technique or induction, positioning, consent issues, and "other." The most frequently reported malpractice reason code for both physicians and nurse anesthetists was "anesthesia not otherwise coded," followed by "failure to monitor."[22]

Understanding where and how medical mistakes happen is just half the picture. In hospitals, patients sometimes have iatrogenic adverse outcomes induced through the effects of treatment by a physician, nosocomial infections, or other accidents. But is a bad outcome necessarily medical malpractice? Translation of a medical mishap or mistake into medical malpractice takes a deeper understanding of how American laws define and prove medical malpractice.

### Medical Malpractice Issues in the Perianesthesia Period: A Traditional Overview

Because of the quantification of legal cases that involve nurse anesthetists, many of those cases will be cited. We hope to never be able to gather a significant number of medical malpractice cases that directly involve PACU care. However, when and if these cases are published, they will be featured in this chapter in the future. The discussion of standards and locality has major significance to perianesthesia nursing.

Many state laws that govern legal claims for medical malpractice specify that the actions or inactions of nurses and doctors may be the basis for a medical malpractice lawsuit.[23,24] The legal formula used in most medical malpractice cases is that a physician, or other health care practitioner, must have and use the knowledge, skill, and care ordinarily possessed and used by members of the profession in good standing and that a doctor or nurse is liable if he or she does not have them.[25,26] American states are split on whether the standard of care for a health care practitioner should be judged by practitioners in the "same or similar locality" or according to a "national standard" of medical care. A national standard is normally used in cases of medical specialists.[27,28] For example, a Louisiana court, in a medical malpractice case that involved a specialist nurse, stated the following:

> A nurse who practices [his or] her profession in a particular specialty owes to [his or] her patients the duty of possessing the degree of knowledge or skill ordinarily possessed by members of [his or] her profession actively practicing in such a specialty under similar circumstances. It is the nurse's duty to exercise the degree of skill ordinarily employed, under similar circumstances, by members of the nursing profession in good standing who practice their profession in the same specialty and to use reasonable care and diligence, along with his/her best judgment, in the application of his/her skill in the case.[29]

In the decision of whether a nurse was negligent and legally liable for malpractice, the court therefore needs to compare the particular nurse's professional behavior with that of a reasonably prudent nurse under the same or similar circumstances. Thus, in a case that involves injury or death from a highly technical bad outcome that involved anesthesia, the court's first question might be the following:

> whether the nurse was a nurse anesthetist or a general registered nurse specially tasked to work with anesthesia. A nurse anesthetist would probably be held to a higher standard [of care]. Nurse anesthetists are organized into a professional association (the American Association of Nurse Anesthetists) that has issued protocols for patient treatment. A nurse anesthetist would be expected to satisfy those standards, whereas a general registered nurse might not.... A court may agree that these specialist associations help define the appropriate standard of care for nurses regularly practicing within that specialty. ...[In this scenario] the standard [of care] is implicitly national in application.[30]

After an evaluation of previous court decisions, the perianesthesia nurse can be said to be held to a higher standard of care. Perianesthesia nurses have their own organization

(American Society of PeriAnesthesia Nurses), their own journal (Journal of PeriAnesthesia Nursing), and their own certifying examination for that specialty of nursing, Certified Post-anesthesia Nurse (CPAN). Hence, one may say that a perianesthesia nurse with CPAN certification is held to a higher standard than a nurse who has not specialized in that particular functional area of the profession of nursing.

Legal liability for nurse malpractice generally falls on the responsible nurse or the nurse's employer (e.g., the hospital) and perhaps on the supervising physician as well under the legal doctrine of *respondent superior*. American tort law generally assigns shared responsibility for the nurse's malpractice to the employer, the supervising physician, or both under the doctrine of joint and several liability; thus, both the nurse and the *respondent superior* codefendants are liable for the full judgment against them, which gives the plaintiff-patient the option of suing the nurse (and the liability insurance carrier), the nurse's codefendant employer, and any other codefendants (and the liability insurance carriers). However, a nurse who has committed malpractice is still primarily liable for damages to the patient-plaintiff:

The mere fact that the plaintiff may focus collection efforts against a wealthier [or so-called "deep pockets"] codefendant, such as the nurse's employer, does not eliminate the nurse's liability (or the possibility that the nurse's employer will take some adverse job action, such as discipline or termination, or that the state licensing board will suspend or revoke the nurse's license). A nurse must be satisfied that he or she has [adequate] malpractice insurance, provided by either the self or the employer. In selecting the amount of coverage, the nurse should be aware of any caps or limits on damages that exist under state law.[31]

So with this traditional approach to medical malpractice actions, the blame game continues, for doctors, nurses, and other health care providers.

## A New Approach to Medical Malpractice
The continuing focus on blaming health care providers—and attorneys—for the current medical malpractice crisis has left little inclination for developing a more systematic analysis of medical malpractice. Sources of this perceived medical malpractice crisis certainly involve more than incompetent physicians or hungry attorneys ready to litigate at a moment's notice. First, a

significant contribution to an increase in medical error is the simple fact that more people are receiving more complicated medical treatment than ever before, largely in part because of new Medicare and Medicaid programs that began in the 1960s. Second, the increasing complexity of medical technology and drug advancements has created more injuries, which many times are considered a presumed risk of modern medicine. Third, an aggressive marketing of medical products and services directly to patient consumers often has created unrealistic patient expectations regarding favorable outcomes of medical treatment.[32] Finally, the role of insurance for both health care providers (in the form of liability insurance) and patients (in the form of health insurance) inadvertently insulates and cloaks the real financial risks involved in providing and receiving medical care.

Virtually all physicians carry some form of medical malpractice insurance, and because this insurance is loss rated and not experience rated and because it usually provides no deductible, physicians often bear little knowledge or accountability of the costs of malpractice injuries. Most patients in the United States, on the other hand, have insurance that covers most costs of medical treatment, which leaves little incentive for patients to inquire about the costs and risks of medical treatment or otherwise shop around for the most quality-oriented health care providers.[33,34]

Although empiric research has contributed greatly to our understanding of medical malpractice, consideration should also be given to the outstanding qualitative research conducted today. This research seeks information through questionnaires and opinions of what people believe to be reasonable behavioral conduct. Subjective in nature, such opinions often lead to hypotheses, which are eventually tested with quantitative methodologies. Few studies have questioned patient or plaintiff motives for suing health care providers because of the difficulty of conducting such research and the limitations involved in the results. These studies, however, are useful in showing a serious breakdown in physician/patient communication, in individual perceptions on medical outcomes, and the stark reality that sometimes medicine does not have all the answers when bad things happen to good people. Clearly, more research is needed to better understand the complex interdependent nature of the doctor/patient relationship.[35,36]

One study published almost 10 years ago developed a questionnaire given to several hundred families in Florida who had filed malpractice claims that alleged that physicians and other health care practitioners who provided medical care during the perinatal period and immediate postpartum period deviated from community and national medical standards and caused death or permanent injury to infants. The responses of the families were fascinating. Families were asked open-ended questions that led to multiple responses for each question. When asked, "What was wrong with the care you or your child received?" these families alleged that physicians failed to recognize fetal distress (53%), manage fetal distress appropriately (57%), perform a cesarean section (33%), or be available when needed (29%). In response to why the families filed the medical malpractice lawsuits, many stated they did so on the advice of a family member or a close friend. Some filed a lawsuit because they needed money to pay for long-term care of the infant, and many filed when they realized that the physician had failed to be completely honest and open with them about what had happened. Several others filed because they believed that the courtroom was the only forum in which they could find out what had really happened with the physicians who provided care. A good number responded that they filed legal action as a way to deter subsequent medical malpractice by the physician or to seek revenge.

A central theme throughout this study was an apparent lack of communication and trust between the physician and the family. Respondents stated they believed their physicians would not talk with them, answer questions, or listen to them and that their physicians had misled them or that no one involved in providing medical care during the perinatal period ever told them that their infants might have permanent medical problems.[37]

A review of current legal and medical literature revealed no end to the blame game. After all, tort liability depends on an identifiable victim and an identifiable wrongdoer, both connected by causation. Medicine, too, in its morbidity and mortality (M&M) conferences, grand rounds, physician credentialing, and the federal databank, depends on identification of individual physicians, nurses, and other health care providers that cause individual medical mistakes. This system all changed, however, with the publication of the 1999 report by the Institute of Medicine, *To Err is Human: Building a Safer Health System.*[38]

## A Systematic Approach for Analysis of Medical Mistakes

Health care providers and the general public are familiar with the well-publicized statistics in the 1999 Institute of Medicine's report that medical errors kill between 44,000 and 98,000 people a year in American hospitals. If these statistics are true, medical mistakes today are the fifth leading cause of death in the United States. If true, this number is equivalent to the rate of three fully loaded jumbo jets crashing every other day. More importantly, if true, our prized American health care system, which is often cited as the finest in the world, may in reality constitute a public health menace of epidemic proportions.[39] Although the debate continues regarding exactly how many patients are actually harmed through medical error, those who work in the health care industry find such statistics alarming but not unexpected. After all, the previously mentioned 1984 Harvard Study clearly showed that the number of medical malpractice cases in the courts was just the tip of the iceberg in sampling the true number of negligent incidents. The central message of this report, that errors are caused by faulty systems and not by faulty people, is nothing new or surprising to those in the medical field. Indeed, the whole focus of a management perspective to the delivery of health care has been written and researched for decades and is well established in the curriculum of any graduate hospital administration program.[40]

The major recommendations of this report were considered a number of years ago by anesthesiologists—long before "systems analysis" or "continuous quality improvement" became popular buzzwords—when consistent monitoring of patients for anesthesia was established as a new standard of care.[41-44] Anesthesiologists had found that their own skyrocketing medical malpractice insurance was too expensive. To correct this imbalance, they took a number of steps to reduce their own liability with a systems approach to anesthetic-related accidents.[45,46]

A systems approach to identification and prevention of medical errors gets away from the blame game, which tends to emphasize individual fault, and focuses instead on the underlying causes of medical error as part of a comprehensive process for managing patients and their medical care. Certainly, a nurse who gives a wrong medication to a patient is at fault because he or she did not read the label properly, but a closer examination of the process of giving medication to patients reveals that many medications have similar names, similar labels, and similar packaging formats and sometimes are stocked together, making the final medical error easier to commit. Rather than an emphasis and focus on the individual nursing error, a systems approach analyzes the entire process of ordering, stocking, delivering, and administering medications to patients. Rational redesign and evaluation of this systematic process must depend on sound empiric data of how, when, and where these medical mistakes occur. "Data collection must [then] be followed by careful epidemiological analysis and the dissemination of both anecdotal and statistical insights into prevention."[47]

If data collection on medical errors is critical for a systems approach to prevention of future medical errors, it is also controversial. For one thing, a traditional malpractice litigation system largely depends on discovery of such reports to help substantiate medical error and assess legal blame. Although laws designed to protect various medical documents and records from lawyer discovery and use in court exist, these laws have many loopholes and are often disregarded during actual litigation.[48] Moreover, many physicians do not believe that reporting medical errors contributes to the quality of medical care, and hospital administrators appear to agree with this questionable philosophy because the departments of risk management and quality improvement in many hospitals are substantively different enterprises.[49]

Reporting of medical mistakes, whether voluntary or mandatory, requires a working definition of what a medical mistake encompasses. Reportable mistakes should include errors that resulted in no harm to the patient. For example, assume a physician writes a prescription for a 1% solution of a drug, but the pharmacist misreads the physician's handwriting and prepares a 10% solution instead. A nurse who is about to administer this medication notices this unusually high concentration and brings her concern to the attention of the prescribing physician, who corrects the dosage. This error, which does not injure the patient, is still an example of the kind of information that is essential for the development of a sound systems approach to prevent medication errors. Thus, "if physicians, nurses, pharmacists, and administrators are to succeed in reducing errors in hospital care, they will need to fundamentally change the way they think about errors and why they occur."[50] As Palmer restates this systems approach to patient safety:

> Reaching the goal of patient safety requires a paradigm shift in the way we think about prevention of accidents in law. Rather than continue to debate about liability as instrumental or as an obstacle to increased safety in health care, we need to acknowledge that the single goal of preventing patient injuries requires a new and dynamic way of

conceptualizing law so that knowledge about safety will continue to grow. In this new view, medical liability—the imposition of civil liability for damages on healthcare professionals and organizations—is acknowledged to be an imperfect system for enhancing patient safety. The goal is not to perfect or eliminate medical liability under the banner of efficiency or rationality. Rather, the goal of a new conceptualization of the role of law is to assess the capacity of the legal system to adopt new ways of viewing safety.[51]

A systems approach to patient safety therefore requires administrators, academics, and licensed professionals to look beyond individual mistakes and to analyze more closely the underlying goals of a health care system. Despite the efforts of many talented proponents and dedicated professionals in their attempts to restructure the health care system, improvement of patient safety has not been a major goal. Mergers, acquisitions, and affiliations have been commonplace within the health plan, hospital, and physician sectors. Yet all this organizational turmoil has resulted in little change in the way health care is delivered to patients and with little evidence of improvement in either quality or cost in the United States. The discrepancy between what Americans should receive in health care and what they actually receive is so great that the Committee on Quality of Health Care in America published *Crossing the Quality Chasm: A New Health System for the 21st Century*, which stresses that a redesign of the American health care system should include underlying goals focused on medical care that is safe, effective, patient centered, timely, efficient, and equitable.[52] Although some medical errors are the result of poorly designed systems, some errors are the result of variances in physician practices. From this perspective, more focus should be placed on medical outcomes and clinical guidelines as a way of establishing the standard of care in medicine.

## Individual Liability and the Standard of Care

In the past, nurses and physicians attended continuing medical education lectures, sometimes presented by attorneys who elaborated on the elements of medical malpractice negligence cases. These attorneys normally analyzed and discussed selected appellate court cases that were published in various trade journals.[53] Sometimes, the attorneys went into great detail about a particularly interesting medical malpractice case, similar to the case mentioned at the beginning of this chapter, and then concluded that medical providers needed to try harder to avoid being sued.

As previously stated, health care providers have a duty to act in accordance with the specific norms or standards established by the profession, which are commonly called the standard of care. Whether the perianesthesia nurse has performed at full potential and in complete good faith may not matter. Instead, the perianesthesia nurse must have conformed to the standard of a prudent perianesthesia nurse under similar circumstances. Unfortunately, no clear definition of a standard of care for a particular patient during particular circumstances exists. The standards for evaluation of the delivery of professional nursing services are not normally established by either judge or jury. Instead, the nursing profession itself sets the standards of practice and the courts enforce these standards in tort suits. This practice requires that both plaintiff and defense attorneys present evidence of the standard of care by use of expert medical witnesses, almost always other perianesthesia nurses who practice nursing under similar circumstances as the defendant nurse. No clear definitions of the standard of care for a particular situation exist. Medical and nursing expert witnesses rely heavily on their own personal experiences from practice; they may use medical treatises or journals as evidence; they may cite from nursing and medical reference books; and because substantial regional variations exist in the use of many procedures, experts may rely more on anecdotal experiences with little regard for differences in outcome. Some experts comment that the system is not very good because determination of which medical expert is more believable to the jury generally boils down to a "battle of the experts." Often attorneys on both sides attempt to impeach the qualifications of the expert witness on the other side, questioning qualifications or perhaps attempting to prove that the expert medical witness is unqualified because he or she is not familiar with the practice of medicine in a particular locality or a particular area of expertise. Box 7-5 presents ways that a perianesthesia nurse can protect against litigation. Box 7-6 provides suggestions for the perianesthesia nurse called on to give a deposition or make a mandated court appearance.

The development and proliferation of clinical practice guidelines is one of the transforming forces in current medical practice and has aided both plaintiff and defense attorneys in developing a more objective case on behalf of their clients. In this area, clinical practice

guidelines can be very useful.[54] As one author states:

> The consistent use of well-developed and medically appropriate practice guidelines has two potentially compelling benefits. First, scientifically reliable guidelines can improve medical practice by reducing the incidence of misdiagnoses and inappropriate treatment decisions.... Second, if major inroads are made into the process of creating and disseminating guidelines, their use may improve the process of malpractice litigation when the

---

**Box 7-5    How to Protect Against Litigation**

- Adhere to accepted standard of care
- Assure that major aspects of care are met: responsibility, technical competence, and nursing judgment
- Appropriate documentation (see Box 7-1)
  - Document what you see and do
  - Do not judge in documentation
  - Do not alter the records
- Avoid medication errors
  - Violation of the classic five "rights" of medication administration
    - Right drug
    - Right patient
    - Right amount
    - Right route
    - Right time
  - Claims based on medication errors are augmented when the perianesthesia nurse:
    - Fails to record the medication administration properly
    - Fails to recognize side effects or contraindications
    - Fails to know patient's allergies
- Recognize and respond to complications
- Ensure that all equipment functions properly
- Adequately assess, monitor, and obtain assistance
- Ensure adequate communication with all members of the health care team
- Report ALL incidents or occurrences
- Properly supervise nursing staff, students, or technicians
- Protect a patient's privacy
- Assure that informed consent has been given by the patient
- Follow up on ordered tests
- Record phone calls or e-mails
- Cooperate in defense of case because of tendency of denial

| **Box 7-6** **Suggested Behaviors for the Perianesthesia Nurse Giving a Deposition** |
| --- |

- Look and act like a professional, indicating that you must be prepared.
- Be clear, accurate, and concise; do not guess.
- Never give opinions unless asked for them; try to stick to the facts.
- Speak slowly and in a well-modulated tone of voice.
- Do NOT allow yourself to be rattled by the opposing attorney.
- If you do not remember a question or do not understand it, ask for it to be repeated or clarified. Do not get caught in the trap of allowing the attorney to use long multipart questions in an effort to confuse you.
- If you have made a statement and later realize it is not correct, do not be afraid to say so, rather than skirt issues or contradict yourself.
- Do not allow yourself to be goaded into an angry or emotional response; remember you can always ask for a break during a deposition to collect yourself and your thoughts.
- Avoid the use of "always" and "never" and vague comments like "maybe," "I think," or "possibly."
- Do not answer more than is asked for by the question.

practice of medicine goes awry or when insurance coverage is denied. Clinical practice guidelines are being used by both plaintiff and defense attorneys as evidence of the standard of care in medicine. For this very reason, it may be more useful for practitioners, including nurse anesthetists, to review and implement guidelines rather than to review and analyze published malpractice cases on the same subject![55]

Several definitions of *clinical practice guidelines* exist, and the term itself has various synonyms, including clinical pathways, critical pathways, clinical paradigms, practice parameters, treatment protocols, and evidence-based medicine standards. Regardless of the name, the definition includes "systematically developed statements to assist practitioners and patient decisions about appropriate health care for specific clinical conditions."[56] Most guidelines attempt to improve physician decision making by detailing appropriate indications for specific medical interventions.[57]

As in other areas of patient safety and quality of care, anesthesiologists have been leaders in embracing viable and realistic practice guidelines by developing practice parameters in pacemaker practice. The ASA has reviewed claims data from malpractice insurance carriers with the goal of ascertaining whether common patterns were seen with certain injuries. The ASA discovered that a high percentage of accidents could have been avoided with use of equipment designed to measure the amount of oxygen in a patient's blood during administration of anesthesia. The challenges of developing such a practice parameter that could be considered the standard of care were described 12 years ago in the Journal of the American Medical Association (JAMA).[58]

Since the publication of this JAMA article, extensive research has been underway at federal, state, and private sector levels to develop viable practice guidelines and to disseminate such information on the Internet. Managed care organizations have embraced practice guidelines in the belief that their use will help control medical costs. A number of health care providers, feeling financial pressure to use such practice guidelines, have rebelled against their use believing that they will lead to a "cookbook" practice of medicine. Although this claim is partly valid, more compelling reasons for health care providers to embrace practice guidelines exist. American medicine is subject to too much variation in practice, according to some commentators, and physicians and nurses are now inundated with increased research on practice guidelines. Keeping up with all the medical advances made and published worldwide is simply impossible. Between 1966 and 1995, for example, the number of clinical research articles based on randomized clinical trials jumped from about 100 to 10,000 annually.[59,60]

Accordingly, the advantages of use of evidenced-based guidelines in medical practice are gaining more widespread approval among health care providers. The Institute of Medicine declared that professional societies can contribute to improvement in patient safety through the promulgation and promotion of practice guidelines and that such guidelines can be written through a more interdisciplinary approach to medical care. Practice guidelines are among the most widely used methods of modification of physician behavior and improvement of patient safety. Moreover, practice guidelines were cited in the most recent report on patient safety practices as evidence that guidelines are effective in positively influencing the medical process and outcome of care. Most significantly, medical practice guidelines are increasingly cited in court litigation and are used as evidence of a medical standard of care.[61] They can also be raised as an affirmative defense by physicians and nurses in medical malpractice suits to show compliance with accepted medical practice. Several states have legislated the use of such medical practice guidelines and provide tort immunity for health care practitioners in exchange for following such guidelines. Finally, because these medical practice guidelines are widely published on the Internet, failure to access such information is likely to become an important piece of evidence in a malpractice suit because the failure is evidence that a physician or nurse has failed to stay current in his or her field of practice. With more focus on practice guidelines based on medical outcomes, health care practitioners, more importantly than ever, must understand the sources of medical malpractice to develop practice guidelines aimed at these patient safety areas.

## RISK MANAGEMENT SUGGESTIONS

Health care providers remain deeply committed to the care and safety of their patients. However, focus on the blame game—singling out individuals for punishment and retribution and reliance on the court system for compensation to injured patients—have done little to increase patient care overall in American hospitals. The complex nature of the health care industry simply does not lend itself to this process of blaming individuals and allowing the courts to compensate injured patients. Instead, medical professionals should embrace and encourage a systematic approach to defining quality of patient care and improving patient safety. To this end, the blame game will hopefully give way to developing a root cause analysis of medical mistakes and a systematic approach for making patient safety a priority in hospitals. This is not to say that individual accountability or liability will disappear altogether—it will not. However, a systematic approach to individual liability will result in more focus on detailed credentialing processes, better assessment of professionals within certain job constraints, better licensing techniques, and better continuing educational programs, all geared to keep professionals competent and qualified for the particular tasks that they must do. With this new way of ascertaining how medical mistakes are made and how they can be avoided, health care attorneys can provide their clients valuable risk management. Some of the more important tips include the following:

- Report and investigate all near misses. We can all learn from our mistakes, and mistakes that do not cause harm are just as important to understand and investigate as those that do cause harm.
- Be sure that your hospital has a system to report and investigate all medical mistakes by encouraging and rewarding those who report personal mistakes rather than punishing them. Develop a systematic process to question potential medical errors before they happen. Time and again, members of a health care team see problems coming but are afraid to question the authority of the person who is about to make a mistake.
- Nurses are sometimes afraid to question physician's orders, yet their internal doubt can often save a patient's life. Develop a policy on questioning authority and use it. Every medical team member has the responsibility for patient outcome. You cannot hide behind the physician's cloak of authority any longer.
- Empower and actively involve your patients in the determination of their own standard of medical care. In an age of patient autonomy and informed consent, patient involvement is taking on new meaning. Informed consent is no longer a signature on a piece of paper but a process of communication. The more patients know what to expect from their own treatment protocol, the better they are able to help you do your job and improve their own safety during your care.
- Embrace medical protocols and electronic checklists into your practice. Human errors that involve equipment misuse remain a big concern for patients for anesthesia. Studies indicate that indexed electronic checklists are superior to either memorized or nonindexed paper checklists in reducing errors of omission. Airline pilots never fly without them, and neither should you.
- Embrace the use of clinical guidelines in your practice. Just as checklists and protocols can avoid many human mistakes made as the result of doing a repetitious task, clinical guidelines can avoid human mistakes made as the result of judgmental error. Guidelines are just that—guidelines—and are not a definitive standard of care. However, clinical guidelines help you "armor plate" the medical record and justify in the record when you find it necessary to deviate from the guidelines. Untoward risks are part of medical care, but justifying what decision you make when you make it really helps in defending your medical actions later.

**Box 7-7    Ways to Reduce Errors in Hospitals**

- Reduce mental errors by reducing stress and fatigue.
- Expand knowledge and develop programs to minimize inevitable errors by simplifying steps and systems.
- Avoid reliance on memory; simplify tasks and standardize procedures.
- Reduce drug errors of all types by systematizing and using dedicated staff for use of drug delivery systems.
- Standardize equipment, such as same location in each unit, and identify equipment that is prone to cause errors.
- Training and education: use of simulators and performance certification.
- Use a process of care approach, whereby decision making is standardized, and development of error reduction program.
- Improve structure of department by having leadership direction that is multidisciplinary with outcome measures and reporting along with use of external benchmarks.
- Be responsive to change and resource allocation.

- Know what your malpractice insurance covers, excludes, and provides for you. Even with all the previously listed recommendations, medical mistakes happen and involvement in a legal claim is often the first time medical professionals learn what insurance they do or do not have. As an employee, you may be covered under a hospital "house" policy. Read that policy and know your coverage. If your job description changes dramatically, be sure to get written clarification of your coverage from your insurance carrier. All health care professionals should make appointments with their insurance agents to review their medical malpractice policies provision by provision. You may be surprised at the exclusions within your policy. Sexual misconduct with a patient is obviously excluded, but often, intentional acts are excluded as well. Know what this means; ask for examples; and know your coverage dollar amount limitation and your tail policy, if any.

A focus on patient safety rather than a sole focus on medical malpractice must involve the coordinated efforts of several sectors of our society. First, the legal community must support and implement appropriate tort reform to protect medical incident reports from legal discovery, especially those that involve near miss medical incidents. If this reform is not feasible, legal discovery should be limited in medical malpractice cases to encourage physicians and other health care providers to freely report and investigate all medical mistakes and near mistakes as they happen. Second, medical licensing boards and accreditation agencies must monitor more closely the quality of those licensed to practice in the various medical specialties. The granting of licenses by medical licensing boards to physicians and other health care providers with a failure to follow up with required continuing medical education as part of the license renewal process is no longer acceptable. Third, real leadership is needed on the part of hospital administrators, physicians, and nurse administrators to incorporate patient safety and the reduction of medical errors as a specific goal, which requires a real change in the way hospitals hire, monitor, and manage their human resources. Fourth, patients must take responsibility for their own medical care and treatment.

Most importantly, physicians and nurses need to accept the notion that error is an inevitable accompaniment of the human condition and that medical error must be accepted as evidence of a systems flaw, not a character flaw. Until this change happens, that substantial progress in reduction of medical errors is unlikely. However, as Box 7-7 suggests, some methods exist to reduce errors in hospitals and specifically the PACU.

## SUMMARY

The intent of this chapter is to introduce the perianesthesia nurse to the legal components of being a licensed professional nurse. Hopefully, the extensive definition section aids in developing an understating of the legal system and how it impacts perianesthesia care. Cases were cited in an effort to show how the legal system functions; and finally, with the use of tables and boxes, ideas were presented to help the perianesthesia nurse understand the importance of defensive charting, patient rights, methods to protect the perianesthesia nurse from litigation, and some ideas on the appropriate actions for giving a deposition. The perianesthesia nurse is hoped to gain a good understanding of the legal process and become more confident when faced with the law. Certainly, continuing education, critical thinking, and use of good common sense help in dealing with the legal issues that touch every perianesthesia nurse everyday. Also, nurses should be involved with such activities as patient safety through simulation and quality and risk management processes in the institution. Another important element to the legal component to perianesthesia practice is to get involved and visit the hearings conducted by the state board of nursing and the state legislature. With involvement in these legal processes and functions, perianesthesia nurses become more aware of how to protect themselves legally in their practice setting; more importantly, with a better understanding of the legal process, the perianesthesia nurse can influence the direction of many health care issues locally, statewide, and nationally.

## REFERENCES

1. Watkins versus Cleveland Clinic Found, 719 N.E.2d 1052 (Ohio 1998).
2. O'Connell J: *The blame game: injuries, insurance, and injustice*, Lexington, MA, 1987, Lexington Books.
3. Reason J: Human error: models and management, *Br Med J* 320–328, 2000.
4. Leape LL: Foreword: preventing medical accidents: is "systems analysis" the answer? *Am J Law Med* 27:27-37, 2001.
5. Law SA, Polan S: *Pain and profit: the politics of malpractice*, ed 1, New York, 1978, Harper & Row.
6. Robinson GO: The medical malpractice crisis of the 1970s: a retrospective, *Law Contemp Problems* 49:5-25, 1986.
7. Kessler D, McClellan M: Do doctors practice defensive medicine? *Q J Econ* 353-362, 1996.
8. Rosenblatt RE, Law SA, Rosenbaum S: *Law and the American health care system*, Westbury, NY, 1997, Foundation Press.
9. Sanders J: Off to the races: the 1980s tort crisis and the law reform process, *Houston Law Review* 27:207-227, 1990.
10. Viscusi WK, Born P: Medical malpractice in the wake of liability reform, *J Legal Studies* 24:463, 1995.
11. Smith DR: Battling a tort frontier: constitutional attacks on medical malpractice laws, *Oklahoma Law Review* 38:195-206, 1995.
12. US Congress Office of Technology Assessment: *Impact of legal reforms on medical malpractice cases*, Washington, 1993, U.S. Government Printing Office.
13. Kessler DP, McClellan MB: Do doctors practice defensive medicine? *Q J Econ* 111(2):353-359, 1996.
14. Harvard Medical Practice Study: *Patients, doctors, and lawyers: medical injury, malpractice litigation, and patient compensation in New York*, 1990.
15. Localio AJ, Lawthers AG, Brennan TA: Relation between malpractice claims and adverse events due to negligence, *N Engl J Med* 325:245-251, 1991.
16. 42 U.S.C.A. section 1101 et seq.; 54 Fed. Reg. 42, 722.
17. Mullan F: The national practitioner databank: report from the first year, *JAMA* 268(1): 73-80, 1992.
18. Caplan R: *Adverse outcomes in anesthesia practice, 1995 annual refresher course lectures*, Park Ridge, IL, 1995, The American Society of Anesthesiologists.
19. Jordan LM, Oshel RE: Nurse anesthetist malpractice and the national practitioner databank, *AANA J* 66(6):292-303, 1998.
20. Jordan LM, et al: Data-driven practice improvement: the AANA foundation closed malpractice claims study, *AANA J* 69(4):304-311, 2001.
21. National Practitioner Data Bank: available at *www.npdb.com*, accessed February 16, 2007.
22. Jordan LM, et al: Data-driven practice improvement: the AANA foundation closed malpractice claims study, *AANA J* 69(4):301-311, 2001.
23. Andrews M: *Nurse's legal handbook*, ed 3, Spring House, PA, 1996, Springhouse Corp.
24. Gic J: Nursing and the law. In *Legal medicine*, ed 7, St Louis, 2007, Mosby.
25. William P, Keeton P: *The law of torts*, ed 5, St Paul, MN, 1984, West Publishing Co.
26. Pegalis S, Wachsman H: *American law of medical malpractice*, ed 2, Deerfield, IL, 1992, Clark Boardman Callaghan.
27. Annotation, 18 A.L.R. 4th 603, 1982.
28. Prosser WL, Keeton P: *Prosser & Keeton on torts*, ed 5, St. Paul, MN, 1984, West Publishing Co.
29. King versus Department of Health and Hospitals, 728 So. 2d 1027, 1030 (La. Ct. App.) writ denied 741 So. 2d 656 (La. 1999).
30. Gic JA: Nursing and the law. In *Legal medicine*, ed 7, St Louis, 2007, Mosby.
31. Gic JA: Nursing and the law. In *Legal medicine*, ed 7, St Louis, 2007, Mosby.
32. Michael S: Do we really know anything about the behavior of the tort litigation system—and why not? *U Penn Law Review* 140:1147-1158, 1992.
33. Danzon PM: *Medical malpractice: theory evidence and public policy*, Cambridge, MA, 1985, Harvard University Press.
34. Kessler DP, McClellan MB: The effects of malpractice and liability reforms on physicians' perceptions of medical care, *Law Contemp Problems* 60:81-92, 1997.
35. Merz JF: On a decision-making paradigm of medical informed consent, *J Legal Med* 14 (231):242, 1993.

36. May ML, Stengel DB: Who sues their doctors? How patients handle medical grievances, *Law Soc Rev* 24:105-119, 1992.

37. Hickson GB, Clayton EW, Githens P, et al: Factors that prompted families to file medical malpractice claims following perinatal injuries, *JAMA* 267:10,1359-1363, 1992.

38. Kohn LT, Corrigan JM, Donaldson MS, editors: *To err is human: building a safer health system*, Washington, 2000, Academy Press.

39. Hayward RA, Hofer TP: Estimating hospital deaths due to medical errors: preventability is in the eye of the reviewer, *JAMA* 286(4): 415-420, 2001.

40. Department of Health Administration, Virginia Commonwealth University: available at *http://www.had.vcu.edu*. Accessed February 20, 2007.

41. Eichhorn JH, et al: Standards for patient monitoring during anesthesia at Harvard Medical School, *JAMA* 256:1017-1026, 1986.

42. Tinker JH, et al: Role of monitoring devices in prevention of anesthetic mishaps: a closed claim analysis, *Anesthesiology* 71:541-555, 1989.

43. Cote CJ: A single blind study of combined pulse oximetry and capnography in children, *Anesthesiology* 74:980-992, 1991.

44. Cooper JP, Gaba DM: A strategy for preventing anesthesia accidents, *Int Anesthesiol Clin* 27:122-130, 1989.

45. Anesthesia Patient Safety Foundation: available at *www.gasnet.org/societies/apsf*, Accessed February 15, 2007.

46. Gellhorn W: Medical malpractice litigation (U.S.): medical mishap compensation (N.Z.), *Cornell L Rev* 73:170-176, 1988.

47. Studdert DM, Brennan TA: No-fault compensation for medical injuries: the prospect for error prevention, *JAMA* 286(2):266-274, 2001.

48. Scheutzow SO, Gillis SL: Confidentiality and privilege of peer review information: more imagined than real, *J Law Health* 7:140-148, 1992.

49. Brennan TA, Berwick DM: *New rules: regulations, markets, and the quality of American health care*, San Francisco, 1996, Jossey-Bass.

50. Lucian L, et al: Promoting patient safety by preventing medical error, *JAMA* 280(16):422-434, 1998.

51. Palmer LI: Patient safety, risk reduction, and the law, *Houston L Rev* 36:86-94, 1999.

52. Institute of Medicine: *Crossing the quality chasm: a new health system for the 21st century*, Washington, 2001, National Academy Press.

53. Blumenreich G: The importance of following procedures in anesthesia, *AANA J* 68(2) 240-251, 2000.

54. National Guidelines Clearinghouse: available at *www.guideline.gov/index.asp*, accessed February 15, 2007.

55. Finder JM: The future of practice guidelines: should they constitute conclusive evidence of the standard of care? *Health Matrix* 10:67-76, 2000.

56. Field MJ, Lohr KN, editors: *Clinical practice guidelines: directions for a new program*, Washington, 1990, National Academy Press.

57. Sheetz ML: Toward controlled clinical care through clinical practice guidelines: the legal liability for developers and issuers of clinical pathways, *Brooklyn L Rev* 63:1341-1366, 1997.

58. Hirshfeld EB: Should practice parameters be the standard of care in malpractice litigation? *JAMA* 266:20, 2886-2894, 1991.

59. Furrow BR: Broadcasting clinical guidelines on the Internet: will physicians tune in? *Am J Law Med* 25:403-409, 1998.

60. Chassin MR: Is health care ready for six sigma quality? *Milbank Q* 76:565-574, 1998.

61. Agency for HealthCare Research and Quality, Pub. No. 01-E057: Making health care safer: a critical analysis of patient safety practices, Rockville, MD, 2001, available at www.ahrq.gov/clinic/ptsafety. Accessed February 22, 2007.

## BIBLIOGRAPHY

Brent N.: *Nurses and the law: a guide to principles and applications*, ed 2, Philadelphia, 2001, Saunders.

Christensen B, Kockrow E: *Foundations of nursing*, ed 4, St Louis, 2003, Mosby.

Education on litigation, *Audio Digest Anesthesiology* 48(10):1-4, 2006.

King versus Department of Health and Hospitals, 728 So. 2d 1027, 1030 (La. Ct. App.) writ denied 741 So. 2d 656 (La. 1999).

Legal and ethical issues, part 1, *Audio Digest Anesthesiology* 46(8):1-4, 2004.

Legal and ethical issues, part 2, *Audio Digest Anesthesiology* 46(9):1-4, 2004.

Malpractice lawsuits: a attorney's perspective, *Audio Digest Anesthesiology* 46(18):1-4, 2004.

Medicolegal issues, *Audio Digest Anesthesiology* 47(24):1-4, 2005.

Pegalis S, Wachsman H: *American law of medical malpractice*, ed 2, Deerfield, IL, 1992, Clark Boardman Callaghan.

Silvestri L: *Saunders comprehensive review for NCLEX-RN® examination*, ed 3, Philadelphia, 2005, Saunders.

Staunton P, Chiarella M: Nursing and the law, ed 5, New York, 2003, Churchill Livingstone.

The law and you, *Audio Digest Anesthesiology* 44(17): 1-4, 2002.

William P, Keeton P: *The law of torts*, ed 5, St. Paul, MN, 1984, West Publishing Co.

Alexander Tartaglia, MDiv, BCC
Ken Faulkner, MDiv, MA
Audrey R. Roberson, MS, RN, CPAN

Concern for ethical practice in the care of patients has a long tradition. Beginning with the ancients Hammurabi and Hippocrates, clinicians have identified the need to develop superior technical skills and an understanding of the application of those skills with use of sound moral judgment. This chapter assists the perianesthesia nurse in development of a framework for understanding ethical obligations to patients, surrogates, and colleagues. Beginning with a definition of ethics, the chapter offers an historic review of landmark cases that contribute to the development of bioethics as a distinct discipline. It describes and outlines the common principles used in the analysis and resolution of ethical concerns.

The chapter proceeds to examine ethical concerns most commonly encountered by perianesthesia professionals, including patient safety, privacy, and informed consent, with particular attention to "do not resuscitate" orders in the perioperative context. It offers practical guidance to assist clinicians in seeking strategies toward the resolution of ethical dilemmas.

## UNDERSTANDING ETHICS

Understanding the nature of ethical reflection requires the establishment of a common language and definition of terms. Foundational questions about the nature of ethics and morality precede movement to particular ethical issues within the moral context of the clinical setting. What do we mean when we use the terms ethics and morality? What is the nature of a moral dilemma? What is the goal of ethical reflection? How can we know which rules, principles, standards, or guidelines are best for determination of appropriate ethical behavior in the resolution of everyday dilemmas?

The terms ethics and morality, while obviously related, are distinct. Ethics is derived from the Greek root ethos, meaning character.[1]

Morality or morals is derived from the Latin word mores or moralis, meaning customs, character, or habit.[1] The ancient terms do have a shared meaning. Today, persons engaged in the formal discipline of ethical reflection have a more distinct understanding. Beauchamp and Childress understand ethics as a "generic term for various ways of understanding and examining the moral life" and morality as "norms about right or wrong human conduct that are so widely shared that they form a stable (although usually incomplete) social consensus."[2] Morality informs persons in society as to what behavior or conduct may be considered good or right. Questions of morality include: What is the right thing to do in this circumstance? How ought I act in this situation?

Ethics is the formal analysis, study, and reflection on how individuals answer basic questions of moral behavior. As a discipline, ethics is most often associated with the fields of philosophy and theology. As a method of reflection, it asks certain types of questions, such as: How do I determine what is good or bad? How do I justify my actions, and what reasons, rules, principles, standards, or guidelines should direct my decisions? Understood as a formal discipline engaged in the systematic assessment of the morals that exist in the lives of individuals and society, ethics has a two-fold task. One task is descriptive in nature, which means ethics may simply describe in an orderly fashion those values or norms of good or bad behavior that are a part of the social context. The other task is normative, which means that ethics seeks to clarify, justify, and correct those values and norms as they apply in certain circumstances.

The goal of ethical reflection, particularly in health care, has the practical function of assisting individuals or groups in the resolution of moral dilemmas. A dilemma occurs when one is faced with a choice between two or more equally desirable but mutually exclusive options.

A moral dilemma is present when a moral obligation exists on both sides of the choice to perform or refrain from performing an action and ethical reasons can be found to support either of the alternatives. [3] The essence of a moral dilemma is *conflict*. That is, a moral dilemma occurs when an individual or society experiences a conflict between competing values, duties, and obligations in a given situation.

A classic example of a moral dilemma in health care that continues to evade resolution in American society is the permissibility of abortion. Those who support reproductive or abortion rights argue on the basis of a woman's right to decide what happens to her own body and her freedom of choice to determine whether or not to give birth. Supporters of abortion rights give greater weight to the moral status of the mother, as an independent and autonomous agent, than to the developing fetus. Those who oppose abortion argue that the fetus is also a living human with its own independent moral status and, as a human life, deserves equal protection and the same right to a full life as the mother. The conflict is not so much between the mother and the fetus but rather the values and obligations that are owed to each party. Some value the autonomy of the mother more than the fetus. Others value the independent moral status of the developing fetus over the mother's. In this situation, one cannot equally honor both sets of values or obligations; thus, the moral dilemma. A dilemma exists because a reasonable individual can appreciate the need to respect the rights of a woman to make decisions concerning her own body and by association her own destiny and, at the same time, can respect the value of the unborn human life that has the same potential to develop into an equally autonomous individual. As a result, we remain conflicted about which obligation should prevail. This simplified version of the abortion debate illustrates the conflict of competing values that are inherent in any moral dilemma.

## THE EMERGENCE OF BIOETHICS

Ethical reflection can apply to any arena of life, but in the last few decades, a new term has come to signify ethical reflection in the health care field: *bioethics*, or more precisely, *biomedical ethics*. Bioethics is the application of ethical study and reflection to the life sciences. More recently, the term *clinical ethics* has been used to define ethical reflection in the clinical context of the actual care of patients. Many of the ethical concerns that confront professionals in the perianesthesia context are, by nature, clinical ethics issues.

The emergence of bioethics as a field within health care responds to a series of emerging problems in the second half of the 20th century. This period represents a time in American history of social foment related to developing individual and civil rights concerns, to the recognition that society has become increasingly pluralistic, and to the rapid development of technologic advances in medicine. Each of these concurrent historic forces led to novel moral challenges and the need for new ways to address the transformative dilemmas. For many years, medical ethics remained under the purview of physicians who almost exclusively governed decision making for patients, with any discussion or reflection on difficult moral problems encountered in the delivery of care or in medical research kept private. After 1950, a number of noteworthy medical and legal cases emerged in the context of a rapidly changing society, which led to challenges to "paternalism" and gave rise to bioethics as a new interdisciplinary discipline. David Rothman describes this historic development as one in which physicians slowly became "strangers at the bedside" as other professions more frequently weighed in on the deliberations of medical decision making and other recurring ethical dilemmas. "In the post-World War II period, a social process that had been under way for some time reached its culmination: the doctor turned into a stranger, and the hospital became a strange institution. Doctors became a group apart from their patients and from society as well, encapsulated in a very isolated and isolating universe."[4] Isolation occurred in part because the old paternalistic ways of governing health care by physicians began to break down in the face of increasing social challenges. Physicians could no longer maintain sole discretion in addressing problems and shaping policy. Individuals from the fields of philosophy, religion, law, journalism, and social sciences began to pay attention to the rumblings of problems in health care and began to organize to address their concerns. A more informed citizenry began to demand a more active voice in decision making and oversight in the delivery of medical care.

## PARADIGMATIC CASES

In addition to the larger social movements, the history of the development of bioethics has been fueled by noteworthy medical and legal cases. These cases are significant for leading to profound changes in the way similar medical cases would forever be viewed. These cases reshaped health policy, law, and reformed ethical practices in the way other patients in similar circumstances would be treated. They led to a different way of perceiving and valuing the moral obligations owed to patients by physicians, researchers, and other health care professionals.

## Research with Human Subjects

Among the most sweeping reform in the second half of the 20th century was in the arena of medical research with human subjects. For much of medicine's history, the improvement of care for patients has been through the trial and error method of experimentation. Few therapies, when initially applied, had any guarantee of success, and some were fraught with the risk of further injury or debilitation to the patient. Early medical researchers were practicing physicians whose small-scale experiments were conducted solely for therapeutic benefit. The goal of experimentation was undertaken not as much to benefit future patients as to heal the very individual under the immediate care of the practicing physician.[5] Most research was, at least in its intent, benevolent and humanistic with the Hippocratic ideal of "doing no harm" providing the guiding norm of the experimenter's conduct. Nonetheless, two key events revealed how flagrantly this norm can be ignored when the focus shifts to utilitarian goals other than the safety and welfare of humans.

Nazi Germany will forever be remembered for the terrible war crimes committed against the human race. Millions of victims lost their lives not only to the actual military conflict of World War II but also to the mass exterminations of innocent members of "undesirable" ethnic groups and other minorities. The techniques for these exterminations were perfected by Nazi physicians whose gruesome acts were later publicly revealed in the Nuremberg war criminal trials and documented by American observer Dr. Leo Alexander.[6] The trials revealed how physicians and administrators conspired to engage in medical experiments, such as forced sterilizations, poisonings, the infliction of simulated combat injuries, and exposure to infections and extreme weather conditions, and ultimately, the refinement of euthanasia techniques on those deemed mentally or physically "defective." There were approximately 275,000 victims over a 10-year span of time. After these staggering revelations, an international tribunal of judges developed what is now known as the Nuremberg Code, a statement of 10 principles that govern the ethical conduct of medical experimentation with human subjects. At the heart of the code stands the requirement that the "voluntary consent of the human subject is absolutely essential" and that freedom from coercion, force, duress, or deception be a condition of participation in any form of experimentation. Expanding the moral framework for the conduct of medical research in the Nuremberg Code, the World Medical Association adopted the Helsinki Declaration in 1964.

Unfortunately, the efforts of Nuremberg and Helsinki did not end the problems with human research. Even within the United States, these important principles did not filter into the consciousness or conduct of physician experimenters, which became all too apparent in the infamous research project now known as the Tuskegee Syphilis Study. From 1932 to 1972, the United States Public Health Service (USPHS), later known as the Centers for Disease Control (CDC), engaged in a research study that involved 400 African-American men in Macon County, Alabama. During the course of 40 years, what began as a small time-limited project to improve the treatment of syphilis among poor minorities expanded into a full-blown plan marked by deception and discrimination that yielded no new information about the disease and offered no bona fide treatment for subjects.[7] When the study first began in the early 1930s, the treatment for syphilis consisted of a difficult regimen of arsenic and mercury vaccinations. Although the treatment offered some control, this method proved to be no definitive cure for the illness. The study was initiated with hopes of understanding the disease and finding the definitive cure but evolved merely into an observation of how the disease progressed through its various stages, culminating, in many cases, with death.

Participants in the study were led to believe that they were being provided real treatment for what the physician researchers called "bad blood," a euphemistic term for any kind of blood-related condition. Treatment amounted essentially to various placebos combined with painful nontherapeutic spinal taps. Subjects were induced to participate in the study through the offer of free treatment, meals, and transportation. Free burial insurance was promised on the condition that the research subjects permit an autopsy on their deaths for documentation of the effects of the end stages of the disease. Even after World War II, when the curative antibiotic of penicillin became widely available, subjects of the study were prohibited from receiving penicillin so that researchers might continue to track the disease's impact on the unsuspecting subjects' bodies. The deception and coercion continued until the young USPHS (CDC) investigator Peter Buxtun learned of the project from a colleague. Frustrated in his attempts to end the study by working within the USPHS, Buxtun turned to the press, and reporter Jean Heller broke the story in July 1972.[8]

The public and political outcry that followed the revelation of the study culminated in its immediate suspension and Congressional passage of the Federal Research Act of 1974, which created two significant entities.[9] First, the act established what is now known as the Office for Human Research Protections (OHRP), which mandates that all institutions that receive federal funding for research with human subjects maintain Institutional Review Boards (IRBs) with oversight for the safety and ethical treatment of research subjects. Second, the act established the National Commission for the Protection of Human Subjects of Biomedical and Behavioral Research. The Commission, composed of physicians, researchers, attorneys, theologians, and philosophers, was assigned to craft guidelines that would serve as a moral foundation for future human research regulation.[5] By 1979, the Commission had arrived at a policy statement known as the Belmont Report.[10] The report highlighted three basic ethical principles that guide all medical research involving humans in the United States. The principle of *respect for persons* requires that participation in research be based on the voluntary informed consent of the subject of the study. The principle of *beneficence* calls for a comprehensive risk/benefit assessment that weighs the potential harm against the potential benefit to the current subjects or future patients. The principle of *justice* requires that research subjects be chosen equitably (unlike Tuskegee) and that a fundamental fairness in both benefits gained and risks incurred be shared by research participants. Justice also requires that the more vulnerable of society, such as children, prisoners, pregnant women, and the mentally challenged, be given added protection in research.

Reforms and regulations that emerged from Tuskegee and the Belmont Report now ensure that essential elements be present in every medical or behavioral research study that involves persons. These elements are voluntary participation, informed consent, comprehension by the subject of the nature and purpose of the study, full disclosure of risks and benefits, disclosure of alternatives to participation in research (as in the case of treatment associated with clinical trials), and the option to withdraw from the study without penalty.

## End-of-life Cases

Controversial patient care cases that involve end-of-life decision making hold a prominent place in the development of the bioethics movement. Three cases are particularly noteworthy; all involved young women, each of whom was severely incapacitated and unable to participate in the decisions to forgo life-sustaining therapy. One of the first landmark cases is that of Karen Ann Quinlan.[11] Karen was a 21-year-old woman in New Jersey who, in 1975, suffered a severe anoxic brain injury after an accidental overdose of alcohol and drugs. Karen never regained consciousness and remained dependent on a ventilator for breathing and a feeding tube for nutrition and hydration. Eventually, she was given the diagnosis of being in a persistent vegetative state (PVS), a neurologic condition characterized by a "complete unawareness of the self and the environment, accompanied by sleep-wake cycles with either complete or partial preservation of the hypothalamic and brainstem autonomic functions."[12] Patients with PVS display "eyes open" unconsciousness and may have gross involuntary movements yet do not respond to external stimuli or engage in any purposeful activity. After some months, Karen's parents came to the realization that their daughter would likely never regain consciousness or the ability to have any meaningful interaction with others. Following what they believed would be her own wishes, they asked physicians to remove the ventilator and allow Karen to die a natural death. Karen's physicians adamantly opposed this idea, believing this to be an act of euthanasia, or worse, murder. Karen's parents then petitioned the courts for help, and her case eventually came before the New Jersey Supreme Court. The Supreme Court ruled in favor of Karen's parents on the basis that Karen had a fundamental right to privacy and the right not to have treatment continued against her will. The Court wrote that "the State's interest (to preserve life) weakens and the individual's right to privacy grows as the degree of bodily invasion increases and the prognosis grows dim. Ultimately there comes a point at which the individual's rights overcome the State's interest."[11] Physicians slowly weaned Karen from the ventilator while continuing her tube feedings and hydration (Karen's parents never asked for the removal of the tube). Remarkably, Karen lived another 10 years before she died in a nursing home in 1986.

A second landmark case is that of Nancy Cruzan, a case sometimes referred to as the first "right to die" case to go before the United States Supreme Court.[13] In 1983, Nancy was a 24-year-old woman who lost control of her vehicle on an icy road late one night in Missouri. She was found lying face down in a ditch after being ejected from her overturned car; Nancy had stopped breathing and had no detectable heartbeat for a brief period of time. Rescue personnel intervened to restore her respiratory and cardiac function. Like Karen Ann Quinlan, Nancy had had an anoxic brain injury that led to the eventual diagnosis of a PVS. Nancy was eventually transferred from an acute care setting to a rehabilitation facility where, despite years of effort, no improvements were seen in her condition. Unlike Karen Ann, Nancy was not dependent on a ventilator but was similarly sustained with a gastrostomy tube for feeding and hydration. Fours years after her injury, Nancy's parents asked physicians to remove the feeding tube with the understanding that Nancy would die. They contended that Nancy had remarked about never wanting to be artificially sustained if she could not be "at least halfway normal."[13] Physicians resisted, and Nancy's parents turned to the courts for help. The Supreme Court of Missouri ruled against them with the argument that sufficient evidence of Nancy's true wishes did not exist to justify the withdrawal of life support, particularly in light of the consequence of death. Denial of the Cruzans' wishes on Nancy's behalf led to an appeal to the U.S. Supreme Court and set the stage for one of the most famous medical legal cases ever in the nation's history.

The U.S. Supreme Court received the case in December 1989 and issued a ruling in June the next year. In somewhat of a "split decision," the Court, on Constitutional grounds, affirmed both certain rights and requirements for all parties in determination of a course of action in cases like Cruzan's. First, the Court acknowledged an individual's right to refuse treatment, even such treatment as life-sustaining tube feeding and hydration. Yet the Court went on to say that the state of Missouri could require "clear and convincing evidence" that such refusal was made while that person was still competent. On these grounds, the Cruzan case was remanded to Missouri for further adjudication. The emergence of new evidence that indicated that Nancy would not have wanted life-sustaining treatment in her current condition led to a Missouri lower court permitting the withdrawal of the feeding tube. Nancy died in December 1990.

The Cruzan case, and the memory of the Quinlan case before it, propelled the creation of federal legislation designed for individuals to state their desire to refuse life-sustaining treatment under the conditions set forth by the Supreme Court, even if rendered incompetent and unable to communicate. The Patient Self-Determination Act of 1990 established on a national level the legitimacy of previously written advance directives as valid legal expressions of an individual's desire for nontreatment in end of life circumstances.[14] These advance directives, often referred to as living wills (and in many states including durable power of attorney for health care decisions), in theory meet the "clear and convincing" evidence standard required by the Supreme Court. Currently, all 50 states recognize and honor some form of written advance directives. However, problems persist in these difficult cases in both the interpretation of generalized written statements and the infrequency of use among the public.[15,16] As the next case shows, the absence of clear communication and understanding among family members over end-of-life wishes in medical care sometimes yields disastrous consequences.

The case of Terri Schiavo is the most recent of the series of tragic end-of-life cases to be pushed onto the national stage.[17,18] Terri was a 26-year-old woman in 1990 when she had a cardiac arrest most likely as a result of an electrolyte imbalance from an ongoing eating disorder. Like Quinlan and Cruzan before her, she had a severe anoxic injury that rendered her, for 15 years, a total care patient in a PVS, dependent on a percutaneous endoscopic gastrostomy (PEG) tube for nutrition and hydration. Early on in her care, Terri's husband, Michael, and her parents, Bob and Mary Schindler, were united in efforts to keep Terri alive and restore her to some level of conscious functioning. Within a few years, Michael came to the conclusion that Terri would not make any recovery and sought to remove the feeding tube to allow Terri to die. The Schindlers, deeply religious, vehemently opposed this request. They believed that removal of the tube was an act of murder and that continued aggressive effort could restore Terri to wakefulness. The Schindlers also questioned the diagnosis of PVS; they believed that Terri both recognized and communicated with them in her own limited way.

Fundamental disagreement between Michael and the Schindlers over Terri's fate led to a bitter and international public dispute waged in the courts for more than a decade. The Schindlers petitioned to have Michael removed as Terri's guardian and garnered the support of the Florida state legislature and Governor Jeb Bush, who signed a one-time stay (known as Terri's law) forbidding the removal of the feeding tube pending further legal appeal.

On three separate instances, the U.S. Supreme Court refused to hear the case, each time affirming the appropriateness of lower court findings in favor of Michael Schiavo. In the end, Michael's position as Terri's guardian was upheld and the courts allowed the removal of the PEG tube. Terri died on March 31, 2005, with her husband at her side. After her death, Michael permitted, at the request of the Schindlers, a neuropathologic autopsy that revealed severe atrophy of the brain. The official cause of death by the medical examiner was listed as "complications from anoxic encephalopathy."[19]

The cases of Quinlan, Cruzan, and Schiavo reveal the ongoing struggle that clinicians and families face in making decisions on behalf of patients with incapacitated conditions. The legacy of these cases highlights the continuing difficulties in withdrawing or withholding treatment in the care of patients with life-threatening conditions and little or no hope of recovery. A lack of public consensus has limited the development of social and institutional policy to guide clinicians. Even the closest of kin can sometimes be unclear about what their loved ones would desire in critical cases.[20]

## GUIDING PRINCIPLES

With insight gained from history with research with human subjects and from the difficult end-of-life cases, the bioethics movement developed new ways of valuing and examining ethical dilemmas in patient care. A consensus has emerged on a set of guiding principles to assist health care professionals in the wide variety of clinical situations they may encounter. Tom Beauchamp and James Childress advance the clearest interpretation of these principles emerging over time from the common morality of society and the particular context of the clinical environment. These principles are *respect for autonomy, nonmaleficence, beneficence,* and *justice.*[2]

*Respect for autonomy* refers to the norm of respect for the decision-making capacities of autonomous individuals. Defined as self rule or self governance, autonomy means that competent adults have the fundamental right to determine what happens to their bodies and to make choices in treatment options that are consistent with their own beliefs and values.[2] Autonomy is grounded in respect for persons and the inherent dignity and worth of each individual and is reflected in the Code of Ethics of the American Nurses Association.[21] In the clinical setting, the autonomy of the patient is often challenged by the vulnerabilities created by

severe illness and by the lack of understanding of the complexities of the modern health care institution, such as the medical language and jargon used by professionals. The obligation of clinical caregivers is to uphold autonomy by engaging in an ongoing process of informed consent, maintaining privacy and confidentiality, and enhancing, to the greatest degree possible, the mental and emotional capacity of the patient for participating in decision making. In the American context, autonomy is often thought of as the first and most important of the four principles.

*Nonmaleficence* refers to the obligation of clinicians to prevent harm to patients under their care or to minimize risks of harm to the fullest extent possible. This norm is often linked to the medical framework of the Hippocratic admonition, *Primum non nocere,* translated to mean "Above all, do no harm."[2] The potential for harm to patients in health care can be understood in both broad and narrow terms. Nursing in particular frames this in the ethical obligation to advocate for processes that minimize harm and maximize comfort and support for patients.[22] Minimally, nonmaleficence refers to the effort made by clinicians to limit physical pain, disability, or even death as a consequence of the treatment process itself. More broadly, it refers to the duty to alleviate the emotional and spiritual suffering of the patient undergoing the traumatic experience of institutionalization, separation from loved ones, and the inability to make a living among other challenges.

*Beneficence* is the principle that speaks to the duty of promoting the ultimate welfare of the patient above all other concerns. In common usage, beneficence speaks to acts of mercy, kindness, and charity.[2] In this sense, beneficence and nonmaleficence may be thought of as two sides of the same coin. Nonmaleficence emphasizes not harming the patient in the effort to do good. Beneficence supports doing good for the patient. Once again, the obligation to serve as a patient advocate in a manner that promotes health, well being, and especially safety is a component of sound ethical practice for the nursing professional. In health care, beneficence speaks to the humanitarian values that should undergird decision making and treatments offered to vulnerable persons. That the word hospital is associated with the term hospitality is no accident. Beneficence affirms that patients should be treated as valued guests in what can often be a foreboding institutional environment. It also suggests that although clinicians often are tempted by interests that conflict with the patient's welfare, they should seek to set aside those interests or minimize their impact as much as possible, in an effort to maintain professional integrity.

The last and perhaps most elusive principle promoted is the principle of *justice*. The elusiveness of justice is the result, in part, of the wide variety of ways it is defined and understood in society. Within the context of health care, justice is best understood as the obligation of clinicians to distribute *fairly* the medical benefits, risks, and costs associated with the provision of health care.[2] In this sense, persons in similar circumstances are treated similarly. The challenges to the fairness principle are immeasurable in the modern American health care system. Global challenges are most visible in the debates concerning universal health insurance, equity of access, and financing the health care industry. Clinical challenges to justice are more evident in the struggle to evenly allocate scarce resources, such as organs for transplant and blood products, and access to care, services, and beds in emergency and critical care areas. Justice for the practicing nurse might be understood again in terms of advocacy, this time in the promotion of equality in the provision of quality care through the use of appropriate standards of practice for all patients.[22]

## PERIANESTHESIA ETHICS

Nursing professionals face a complex maze of ethical issues within the perioperative context. The intensity of a fast-paced environment with limited room for error demands not only clinical competence but critical thinking, quick judgment, and clear communication. Vigilance regarding professional functioning and ethical practice is essential for the achievement of positive clinical outcomes within a morally sound arena. Although many issues exist, the ethical issues faced by perianesthesia nurses can be captured within three general categories: (1) informed consent; (2) privacy and confidentiality; and (3) patient safety.

### Informed Consent

*Informed consent* is the process of communication between a patient and physician that results in the authorization or understanding for a specific medical intervention.[23] Informed consent is rooted in respect for persons, patient autonomy, and self determination and formalizes a component of the covenant between the patient and the physician. It is built on the principles of trust and truth telling regarding the use of a particular intervention or treatment to achieve a desired medical outcome.

Despite the clarity of definition for the informed consent process, multiple questions or potential ethical conflicts can arise for nursing staff within the perioperative period. A simple question such as "What were they going to do again?" asked by an anxious patient in the preoperative holding area can set off a series of internal alarms in the mind of a nurse. Does the patient need reassurance or more information? Is it a momentary failure of memory or a lack of adequate understanding of the procedure that prompted the question? Who secured the consent of the patient? How was the request approach conducted? How does the nurse understand the professional and ethical obligations in the face of a seemingly unsure patient and the pressure of a tight operating room schedule?

The nurse might begin by seeking verification of a signed written consent form. But although the presence of the form might satisfy the "technical" act of granting consent, it may or may not fulfill the ethical obligation. Informed consent is more than a means of securing a signature. Rather, it is a process of open two-way communication that implies full disclosure and provides detailed information on the nature of a specific procedure. A comprehensive informed consent process not only reviews the diagnosis and purpose of the intervention but also outlines its potential risks and benefits. It includes alternative treatment options, if any, and the risks and benefits of forgoing the treatment procedure. Informed consent assumes that the threshold elements of patient capacity and voluntary nature are met.[24]

Questions may also arise regarding the duration and scope of a signed informed consent. The nurse in the previous scenario may have noticed that the signed consent was properly secured but completed in the surgeon's office nearly 90 days ago. Should the consent still be valid for the patient who is now unsure about the nature of the procedure? What if, once inside the operating room, the surgeon determines that a change or expansion to the original procedure is indicated? Is the consent still valid? How much latitude is afforded the surgeon? What is the nurse's obligation to confirm that the patient understood the potential surgical outcomes?

Informed consent requires that the process be completed by a clinician able to provide the intervention and in a manner that allows time and space for patients to ask questions, seek clarification, and discuss potential options for care. The content of these discussions should be documented and communicated to members of the interdisciplinary team. An adequate informed consent process is further challenged by potential language barriers, such as complex medical terminology, cultural diversity, and functional limitations among populations with cognitive impairments.[25,26] All of these issues underscore the significance of effective communication in the patient-physician relationship and among members of the interdisciplinary team.

What then is the ethical responsibility of the nurse in the holding area who is faced with the patient's question of uncertainty and the surgical team's schedule? To what extent is the nurse's ethical obligation to serve as a patient advocate in support of an informed decision? How might the nurse's obligation be impacted for the patient who adds the statement, "At least my surgeon promised to be there for the entire operation," when the nurse knows of that particular surgeon's tendency toward intermittent presence while residents perform most operations? What if the nurse understood from a colleague that the patient's original consent was provided under pressure to comply? Specific questions such as these identify just a few of the immediate moral dilemmas that have implications for clinical practice and patient outcomes.

*Resuscitation in the Perioperative Context.* A special circumstance of informed consent in the perioperative context is the issue of resuscitation for patients with preexisting "do not resuscitate" (DNR) orders. Cardiopulmonary resuscitation (CPR) is the only medical procedure routinely performed in a hospital without the expressed consent of a patient. Routine management of the patient who is under the influence of anesthesia shares some of the same interventions and characteristics of resuscitation. As such, the practice of routine suspension of DNR orders for patients during anesthesia care in the operating room was commonly accepted through the 1980s.

By the mid 1990s, a growing dissatisfaction existed with this practice. The evolution of increased respect for patient autonomy evolved from changes in medical practice and the Patient Self-Determination Act of 1990. Complicating matters was an apparent lack of consistency within organizational policies regarding physician obligation to inform patients with existing DNR orders that they would be resuscitated during the perioperative period. Respect for patient autonomy and concern for adequate informed consent procedures challenged old practices and forced the issue onto the agendas of key professional organizations. Emerging from these conversations was support for the practice of required reconsideration. A comprehensive conversation regarding a patient's DNR status during the administration of anesthesia is recommended between the physician and the patient or surrogate, with the result documented and communicated among health care team members. Required reconsideration has since become the predominant recommended approach supported by the American Society of PeriAnesthesia Nurses, the American College of Surgeons, the American Society of Anesthesiologists, the Association of Operating Room Nurses, and the American Association of Nurse Anesthetists.[27-31]

Despite the majority movement toward required reconsideration, a lack of consensus remains on the application of this practice among anesthesiologists, nurse anesthetists, and other perianesthesia nurses. Variation among hospital policies that guide the use of CPR for patients with preexisting DNR orders who undergo surgical intervention and anesthesia reflects this diversity of opinion. Presently, three distinct approaches to addressing this issue dominate the landscape. These approaches include: routine or automatic suspension of DNR orders for a defined time period, required reconsideration of the DNR status with a means approach, and required reconsideration of the DNR status with a goals-oriented approach.

A decreasing but still not uncommon practice is the automatic suspension of DNR orders for this category of patients. Complications related to maintenance of a DNR order are well documented in the literature. These complications include: (1) many of the elements of routine care for a patient undergoing general anesthesia are considered resuscitation; (2) failure to exercise resuscitative efforts for this category of patients without certainty of the cause of an arrest is inconsistent with the principles of beneficence and nonmaleficence; (3) failure to suspend DNR orders places the surgeon in an unintended ethical dilemma between patient preferences and surgical outcomes that may be used to evaluate physician practice; and (4) the very ethos of the operating room is to sustain life and reluctance is found for practices that might otherwise introduce an avoidable death to that context.

The argument for supporting unrestrained resuscitation is one of clarity for both clinicians and patients or surrogates, but other arguments may also support this position.[32] This position reduces the burden on the provider to differentiate whether the underlying cause of a cardiopulmonary arrest is related to the routine effect of anesthesia rather than the result of the patient's underlying disease process. A resuscitative effort that leads to an unintended outcome for the patient, such as extended ventilator dependency period, can be reversed with later removal of mechanical support in compliance with the patient's previously expressed wishes. Unrestrained resuscitation also simplifies the content of conversation between the provider and the patient or surrogate and becomes a matter of informing the patient or surrogate of hospital policy, thus eliminating discussion about which interventions would and would not be performed during the perioperative period. Another interpretation is that the practice relieves the patient or surrogate of the burden of a complicated decision in the face of a series of "what if" scenarios that may or may not emerge during surgery.

The minimal ethical obligation in the case of automatic suspension of DNR orders is an intentional and comprehensive conversation between the physician (surgeon or anesthesiologist) and the patient or surrogate before sedation. In the case of automatic suspension of DNR orders, informed consent requires that the physician outlines for the patient the hospital policy, including the duration and context of the suspension. Such clarity minimally offers the patient the opportunity to factor the implications of such a policy into the decision-making process about surgery. Organizational policies that support automatic suspension ideally also incorporate an option for the patient to select another provider, with the recognition that this can have its own complicating factors. In the case of automatic suspension, policies should identify which medical service informs the patient or surrogate. In addition, clear and timely communication should occur with post-anesthesia providers as to the duration of the suspension as the patient progresses from Phase I to Phase III levels of care.

As previously indicated, patients, surrogates, and clinicians alike have raised concern regarding the ethical appropriateness of automatic suspensions of DNR orders in the perioperative period, even with the provision of informed discussion. The argument is that such suspension of orders is a violation of a patient's right to self determination and fails adherence to the principle of patient autonomy.[33-40] This position has obvious ethical implications for providers. It requires intentional dialogue with patients or surrogates regarding the options and implications of maintaining or suspending the DNR order during surgery. Organizational policies can mandate such communication and documentation of the conversation, but the ethical challenge to informed consent remains in the details of it. Informed consent in this instance implies that patients or surrogates are offered information about their procedures, including potential risks and benefits, alternative treatment, and the potential implications of foregoing the intervention. Discussion of how resuscitation would be managed in the perioperative period is an essential but complicated discussion. Conversation within this context, as in other informed consent discussions, should be conducted without coercion, in a language that is understandable to patients or surrogates, and with sufficient time to allow questions and concerns to lead to an informed decision.

Even clear and consistent communication does not readily resolve the complexities of management of a DNR order in the perioperative period.[41] Following the adoption of required reconsideration, discussion of the pragmatics of managing the DNR order in the perioperative period is reflected in two approaches highlighted in the literature. Both support the ethical obligation to respect patient autonomy. One position supports a means or procedure-directed approach that examines routine resuscitative actions and determines which interventions would be offered in the perioperative period. The second position supports an ends-oriented approach that examines the goals of the patient as related to the present procedure. Both options suggest a limited resuscitation approach during the perioperative period, as distinct from the two extreme options of suspension of DNR orders with unrestrained resuscitative efforts or maintenance of current DNR orders limiting all interventions not immediately associated with routine anesthesia care. The limited resuscitation approaches should be considered special within the hospital context because they might otherwise conflict with the established medical and ethical practice of considering a menu of interventions related to resuscitation or the exercising of slow codes.

The procedure-directed approach provides a specific checklist of specific provider interventions.[42] The application of this approach requires consideration of each optional intervention (i.e., those not associated with routine anesthesia care) individually between the patient or surrogate and the surgeon or anesthesia provider.[37] The advantages of procedure-directed orders are the reduction of ambiguity and the consistency of application from one clinician to another throughout intraoperative resuscitation management. The limitations to procedure-directed orders include an expectation that anything but the most likely problems would be anticipated in advance and of the lack of flexibility offered the clinician in response to a temporary and readily reversible event.

The goal-oriented approach seeks to incorporate the patient's values as the primary consideration in determination of the extent of resuscitation.[43] Patients offer guidance as to preferred outcomes but leave specific interventions to the discretion of the provider. Although this approach supports patient autonomy, it also provides a larger role for the provider. The advantage to this approach is that it offers flexibility to the clinician to act in accordance with a broad understanding of patient preferences should an unanticipated event occur in the operating room setting.[42] The limiting argument for this position has been that it risks putting unanticipated decision-making power back in the hands of the physician.

Keys to success for either of these approaches are communication and documentation. The complexity of this issue underscores the significant ethical obligations of the perioperative nurse. The obligation to act in the patient's best interest demands that the nurse be knowledgeable and informed, beginning with having a clear understanding of the organization's DNR policy and its specific application to the perianesthesia period.[44] Equally important is that the nurse have knowledge of the DNR status of the patient during that period, including any documentation regarding limited resuscitation and knowledge of the timeframe in the case of temporarily suspended DNR orders.

## Privacy and Confidentiality

Maintenance of the privacy and confidentiality of patients remains a challenge for health care organizations and clinicians. Privacy and confidentiality are complementary rather than synonymous concepts.[45] *Privacy* suggests that a patient has the right to control general access and distribution of personal information about one's health and implies that boundaries that protect a patient's personal space are respected within a clinical setting. *Confidentiality* relates to the personal trust that intimate information shared by a patient with a clinician is only used for the patient's medical benefit. As such, information is shared with those members of the interdisciplinary team on a need-to-know basis. Information should be shared with third parties only with permission of the patient except in the cases of an identified surrogate for the patient who lacks the decision-making capacity. The ethical responsibility to maintain privacy and confidentiality proceeds from the principle of respect for persons. Such responsibility is particularly critical for the most vulnerable of patients, including those under the effects of anesthesia.

One of the most significant challenges to patient privacy during the perioperative period is the physical setting of the postanesthesia care unit (PACU). More often than not, the PACU is configured as a large room where patients are held in close proximity separated only by a curtain and thus is an area ripe for compromise. Private communications between patients and clinicians are subject to being overheard by other patients or even visitors. Staff not directly involved in the care of particular patients may encounter neighbors and friends who are recovering from surgery and would have preferred to remain unnoticed. One particular conflict that may emerge stems from the rights of parents who wish to be present when a minor child awakens from surgery. Although sensitivity to the needs of children is shown, the presence of parents in the PACU can compromise the privacy obligated to other patients.

How does the PACU nurse observe multiple patients while ensuring privacy? The typical PACU nurse monitors more than one patient, thus exposing patients to potential violations of personal space in the interest of patient safety. A further challenge to the nurse can be finding the appropriate way to respond to the physician who performs examinations without properly drawing the curtain or who engages in intimate conversations with patients without proper discretion as to volume and content.

Teaching hospitals carry additional potential dilemmas in maintenance of patient privacy. The parameters of what is ethically permissible or appropriate relative to observation or examination by students or others in training of patients who are anesthetized remains ethically ambiguous. Should examination itself, the type of examination, the number of students observing, the nature and extent of the consent process, or some combination of these factors drive the parameters of ethical appropriateness? Should informed consent include details regarding these parameters? What is the extent of ethical obligation on the perianesthesia nurse to speak up as a patient advocate?

The professional responsibility to maintain confidentiality and privacy is clearly required from the perianesthesia nurse. The exchange of privileged patient information should follow the organization's policies on confidentiality and the code of ethical conduct of the appropriate professional organization, which would include at a minimum the sharing of information on a need-to-know basis and the proper collection of patient data for research purposes.

## Patient Safety

The ethical responsibility for all clinicians and health care providers to act in the best interest of patients is no more evident than in the obligation to ensure patient safety. The significance of this obligation on perianesthesia nurses is both organizational and personal. Minimally, this obligation stems from the ethical principle of nonmaleficence. Organizational obligation includes responsibility to ensure that the environment is safe for patients. Critical to patient safety is the requirement that a clinician at any given point in the treatment process has shown appropriate competencies for the level of care being provided. Competency implies possession of the knowledge, skills, attitudes, and behavior to deliver the appropriate level of care on a consistent basis.[46] Clinicians are obligated to know and to function within the standard of care of their professional role and the professional standards of practice within their discipline.[47] This responsibility can be particularly challenging for nurses in the PACU, an environment frequently characterized by overcrowding because of limited intensive care unit (ICU) beds and staffing shortages and where nurses might be asked to provide care outside the unit's scope of care.[48]

The principle of beneficence speaks to the perianesthesia nurse's responsibility to a wide range of ethical obligations. Ethical dilemmas that face clinicians may include how to respond to a colleague who appears impaired in some way, what to do regarding the reporting of a medical error, or how to respond to a situation in which a colleague is engaged in deceptive practice or illegal behavior, all situations that impact maintenance of a safe environment and adherence to ethical practice and organizational guidelines. Responsibility extends to the nurse's obligation to follow best practice processes and to take initiative to eliminate errors, such as calling "time out" if guidelines such as those designed to ensure correct site surgery are not properly followed.[49]

The transfer of the patient from the operating room (OR) to the PACU has the potential to introduce a number of ethical dilemmas related to patient safety. One common dilemma faced by the perianesthesia nurse in the PACU setting is the obligation regarding unintended intraoperative awareness. The responsibilities of the nurse in this instance can be multiple. With an interview of the patient who is emerging from the influence of anesthesia to determine whether any recollection of events exists or whether the patient experienced pain during the surgical procedure, the nurse must make an initial assessment. If the finding is affirmative, the nurse must then determine how to communicate the information. Clear documentation of the patient's response and notification of the surgeon and the anesthesia provider are critical. Equally important is communication of the patient's experience to the ICU or floor nurse who will assume care for the patient and who can identify resource personnel who could be available to support the patient who has experienced such trauma. The level of ethical dilemma becomes more complicated should the perianesthesia nurse discover that a pattern of unintended intraoperative awareness emerge as the result of care by a specific anesthesiologist, anesthetist, or surgeon.

The hand off from the OR to the PACU can be complicated by the pressure of time. What essential information needs to be passed from the OR nurse or the nurse anesthetist to the PACU nurse? How should the transfer of a patient whose condition is marginally stable or the one whose condition is hemodynamically stable but in pain be handled between the nurse anesthetist and the PACU nurse? How could this situation be compromised by a demanding OR schedule that anticipates a speedy return to the OR by the anesthetist? Minimal responsibility in this instance includes documentation of the patient's status on arrival, information on the surgical/anesthesia course, and collaboration in the care of the patient until the PACU nurse accepts responsibilities.[58] The assessment and management of pain in the postoperative period remains a critical ethical obligation and can be a source of tension between the transferring anesthetist and the receiving PACU nurse. This process can be particularly complicated for the pediatric patient or the geriatric patient with cognitive impairment because clinicians may need knowledge and specialized training for these populations.[50] In such cases, a tendency can be seen to underestimate the level of pain severity and undertreat the patient. The safe transfer of care should be extended again when the patient moves from the PACU to another care setting. Although guidelines for the safe transfer of care have been identified by both the American Society of PeriAnesthesia Nurses and the American Society of Anesthesiologists, successful patient outcomes in these situations are facilitated with clear and proper communication skills.

A corollary of the ethical principle of respect for persons and the obligation to ensure patient safety is truth telling. The ethical responsibility to tell the truth in medicine exists at both organizational and individual patient levels. Organizationally, the perianesthesia nurse needs to determine the ethical course of action in disclosing potential safety problems under the pressure to move patients efficiently through the system. At an individual patient level, the perianesthesia nurse is challenged to determine the ethical course of action in facilitating disclosure of a medical error, even one seemingly inconsequential.[51]

At one point or another, all health care professionals encounter a case that conflicts with their own personal value system or that creates significant emotional discomfort. Perianesthesia nurses are no different. Nursing professionals should make every effort to anticipate in advance such potential conflicts and reference any organizational personnel policies that address this conflict. Generally speaking, refusal of anticipated conflicts of moral conscious is ethical provided no compromise to patient safety exists.

## RESOURCES FOR RESOLVING ETHICAL DILEMMAS

Clear and consistent communication between clinicians and patients and among clinicians continues to be the backbone of good ethical practice. Despite the most diligent practice, ethical dilemmas continue to challenge clinicians. The ethical responsibility for the perianesthesia nurse can become particularly burdensome in the perioperative environment, where issues of power and politics are never far away. Identification of resources to support staff who seek resolution of ethical conflicts can relieve the burden. Managers and supervisors should not be overlooked as resources for assistance. Supervisors should be dependable sources for accessing organizational policies or for support in dealing with colleagues in other disciplines. Staff access to organizational and departmental policies has been enhanced with the use of an institution's Intranet postings. In addition, the Code of Ethics for nearly all relevant professional nursing organizations is available through Internet web sites. Questions regarding ethical practices related to release of patient information, business practice, or even professional behavior can be referred to ever-expanding Corporate Compliance programs.

### Ethics Committees and Consultation Services
The Standards of The Joint Commission (TJC), formerly known as the Joint Commission on the Accreditation of Healthcare Organizations, require that hospitals have an identifiable process for the resolution of ethical dilemmas. Subsequently, most hospital-established ethics committees are charged with three functions: the development of policies to address recurrent difficult situations, such as DNR or withdrawal of care orders; education to the organization that addresses issues faced by the organization or its specialty disciplines; and consultation to patients, families, and staff for the mediation of conflicts or exploration of treatment options. Although guidelines to determine the functioning of ethics committees can vary from organization to organization, generally speaking, access to the ethics committee is available to any individual with standing in a case. This access includes patients or surrogates and staff involved in the care of the patient. Consultation services are generally provided by a subcommittee of the membership that possesses some training in clinical ethics. Consultations, whether by the committee as a whole or by subcommittee, serve as nonbinding recommendations that identify the ethically appropriate options of care available to the physician and patient.

Consultation provided by members of the ethics committee can be a critical resource for the perianesthesia nurse who is uncertain about the appropriate ethical course in a given clinical situation. The goal of ethics consultation is the improvement of patient outcomes through a process of reasoned decision making. Consultation typically takes the form of facilitation and dialogue to ensure that the key ethical issues and the essential perspectives of persons with standing in a case are provided adequate voice. The value of ethics consultation is the availability and timely response of a neutral resource to assist staff in the exploration of ethically appropriate alternatives to a situation that lacks consensus. The reality that an ethics consultation, like a medical consultation, is a resource, not a final decision, may disappoint clinicians who seek a quick resolution for a complex situation or an ally to advance a particular position.

### Ethics Case Review Methodology
The struggle around ethical dilemmas for most clinicians occurs when a clinical situation creates a conflict of personal values or when the rights of individual patients appear to not be respected. The use of a pragmatic tool to examine a moral problem is a valuable resource for the novice and the experienced clinician. Thoughtful case analysis requires a reasoned methodology that ensures that a reasoned approach is followed and that influential factors are given appropriate consideration. The use of a case-based methodology can facilitate responsible reflection with an objective theoretic

framework while attending to the specifics of a particular situation. Detailed case-based approaches are available.[52] In general, the literature points to five common elements for the case review process: assessment/gathering, establishment of ethical questions, identification and analysis of alternatives, selection and implementation, and evaluation.

**Assessment/Gathering.** This stage begins with identification and gathering of the medical facts of the case. What is the patient's condition? What treatment options are available? What is the patient's prognosis with and without treatment? What is the patient's capacity to make an informed decision? What are the patient's preferences regarding alternatives to care and quality of life factors? For the patient without capacity, were any preferences previously expressed, either verbally or in the form of a written advance directive? If not, what are the preferences expressed by the surrogate? Do any cultural or social factors come into play for the patient or surrogate, such as individual beliefs or values? Identification of potential resources within the organization that could assist in resolving the dilemma is also a key component of assessment/gathering.

**Ethical Questions.** At this point, identification of the ethical issue or problem should be clarified. What points of conflict are raised by the case? Differentiation of facts and feelings and bracketing of personal agendas are important. Identification of which ethical principles are relevant to the case, and why, becomes the group task.

**Identification and Analysis of Alternatives.** Difficult ethical situations are often characterized by more than one morally justifiable course of action. Each alternative should be examined within the context of the medical situation and the patient or surrogate preferences and analyzed with attention to institutional issues and third-party interests. Case history, whether prominent in the literature or particular to the organization, also serves as a resource to assist in the consistent treatment of like ethical situations.

**Selection and Implementation.** The selection and implementation of a particular course of action is often driven by the medical indications of the case and, when known, the patient or surrogate preferences. In the absence of clear preferences, the *best interest standard* should be factored into the decision. The decision should be defensible by one or more ethical principles. Any treatment alternative selected in an ethically ambiguous situation should be consistent with the goals of a comprehensive plan of care for the patient. Rationale for the selection of an alternative should be communicated to involved parties. At this point, any legal considerations ought to be incorporated before final implementation.

**Evaluation.** The implementation of any medical decision includes an element of ongoing evaluation. Consideration of the benefit of any intervention and the goals of treatment should be subject to periodic and regular review. Often accomplished through retrospective case review, this consideration includes assessment of desired outcomes and identification of unanticipated complications. On final resolution of a case, final outcomes and any new learning should be communicated to the multiple constituents.

# SUMMARY

Clinical ethics continue to develop into a mature field with established acceptance among health care professionals. Codes of Professional Ethics are now the norm for nursing organizations. A growing literature is found on ethical issues in perianesthesia nursing. Evolving technology and increased emphasis on patient rights presents ever-increasing options for care and considerations for decision making within the medical community. In addressing these issues, the perianesthesia nursing professional has much to contribute. Development of the competencies and skills to be effective clinicians who possess the critical assessment tools necessary to negotiate difficult situations in an environment of culturally diverse values is crucial.

# REFERENCES

1. *American Heritage Dictionary of the English Language*, ed 3, 1996, Houghton Mifflin Company, Boston, MA.
2. Beauchamp TL, Childress JF: *Principles of biomedical ethics*, ed 5, 2001, Oxford University Press, New York, NY.
3. Fletcher JC, Miller FG, Spencer EM: Clinical ethics: history, content, and resources. In Fletcher JC, Lombardo PA, Marshall MF, et al, editors: *Introduction to clinical ethics*, ed 2, 1997, University Publishing Group, Hagerstown, MD.
4. Rothman DJ: *Strangers at the bedside: a history of how law and bioethics transformed medical decision making*, 1991, Basic Books, New York, NY.
5. Jonsen AR: *The birth of bioethics*, 1998, Oxford University Press, New York, NY.
6. Alexander L: Medical science under dictatorship, *N Engl J Med* 241:39-47, 1949.
7. Jones JH: *Bad blood*, 1993, The Free Press, New York, NY.

8. Heller J: Syphilis victims in U.S. study went untreated for 40 years, *NY Times*, July 26, 1972.

9. National Research Act of 1974, Pub. L. 93-348.

10. The National Commission for the Protection of Human Subjects of Biomedical and Behavioral Research: *The Belmont report: ethical principles and guidelines for the protection of human subjects of research*, 1979. available at www.hhs.gov/ohrp/humansubjects/guidance/belmont.htm. Accessed on 10/25/2006.

11. In the matter of Karen Quinlan, an alleged incompetent, 70 NJ 10, 355 A.2d 647 (1976).

12. The Multi-Society Task Force on PVS: Medical aspects of the persistent vegetative state—first of two parts, *N Engl J Med* 330:1499-1508, 1994.

13. Cruzan versus Director, Missouri Department of Health, 497 US 261, 11 S. Ct. 2841 (1990).

14. Patient Self-Determination Act, 42 USCA, section 1395 (a) (1) (Q).

15. Meisel A, Snyder L, Quill T: Seven legal barriers to end-of-life care: myths, realities, and grains of truth, *JAMA* 284:2495-2501, 1996.

16. Upadya A, Muralidharan V, Thorevska N, et al: Patient, physician, and family member understanding of living wills, *Am J Respir Crit Care Med* 166:1430-1435, 2002.

17. Gostin LO: Ethics, the Constitution, and the dying process: the case of Theresa Marie Schiavo, *JAMA* 293:2403-2407, 2005.

18. Wolfson J: Erring on the side of Theresa Schiavo: reflections of the special guardian ad litem, *Hastings Center Report* 35(3):16-19, 2005.

19. Thogmartin JR: Medical examiner, district six of the state of Florida: *Report of autopsy for Schiavo, Theresa*, case #505439, June 13, 2005.

20. Shalowitz D, Garrett-Mayer E, Wendler D: The accuracy of surrogate decision makers, *Arch Intern Med* 166:493-497, 2006.

21. American Nurses Association: *Code of Ethics for Nurses*, available at www.ana.org/ethics/code. Accessed 11/26/2006.

22. Wood J: Ethical decision making, *J PerAnesth Nurs* 16(1):6-10, 2001.

23. American Medical Association, available at www.ama-assn.org. Accessed 11/26/2006.

24. Boyle RS: The process of informed consent. In Fletcher JS, Spencer ES, Lombardo PA, editors: *Fletcher's introduction to clinical ethics*, ed 3, 2005, University Publishing Group, Hagerstown, MD.

25. Galenti GA: Applying cultural competence to perianesthesia nursing, *J PerAnesth Nurs* 21(2):97-102, 2006.

26. Sullivan EE: Issues of informed consent in the geriatric population, *J PerAnesth Nurs* 19(6):430-432, 2004.

27. American Association of Perianesthesia Nurses available at www.aspan.org, Accessed 9/12/2006.

28. American College of Surgeons available at www.facs.org, Accessed 11/26/2006.

29. American Society of Anesthesiologists available at www.asahq.org, Accessed 11/26/2007.

30. Association of Operating Room Nurses available at www.aorn.org, Accessed 9/30/2006.

31. American Association of Nurse Anesthetists available at www.aana.com. Accessed 9/30/2006.

32. Mohr M: Ethical conflicts during anesthesia "Do not resuscitate" orders in the operating room, *Anesthetist* 46(4):267-274, 1997.

33. Walker RM: DNR in the OR resuscitation as an operative risk, *JAMA* 266(17):2407-2412, 1991.

34. Cohen CB, Cohen PJ: Required reconsideration of "do not resuscitate" orders in the operating room and certain other treatment settings, *Law Med Health Care* 20(4):354-363, 1992.

35. Igoe S, Cascella S, Stockdale K: Ethics in the OR: DNR and patient autonomy, *Nurs Manage* 24(9):112A,D,H, 1993.

36. Golanowski M: Do-not-resuscitate: informed consent in the operating room and postanesthesia care unit, *J Post Anesth Nurs* 10(1):9-11, 1995.

37. Craig DB: Do not resuscitate orders in the operating room, *Can J Anaesth* 43(8):840-851, 1996.

38. Clemency MV, Thompson NJ: Do not resuscitate orders in the perioperative period: patient perspectives, *Anesth Analgesia* 84(4):859-864, 1997.

39. Lonchyna VA: To resuscitate or not...in the operating room: the need for hospital policies for surgeons regarding DNR orders, *Ann Health Law* 6:209-227, 1997.

40. Goldberg S: Do-not-resuscitate orders in the OR—suspend or enforce? *AORN J* 75(2):296-299, 2002.

41. Ewanchuk M, Brindley PG: Perioperative do-not-resuscitate orders—doing 'nothing' when 'something' can be done, *Crit Care* 10(4):219, 2006.

42. Guarisco KK: Managing do-not-resuscitate orders in the perianesthesia period, *J PerAnesth Nurs* 19(5):300-307, 2004.

43. Truog RD, Waisel DB, Burns JP: DNR in the OR: a goal-directed approach, *Anesthesiology* 90(1):281-295, 1999.

44. Keffer MJ, Keffer HL: The do-not-resuscitate order: moral responsibilities of the perioperative nurse, *AORN J* 59(3):648-650, 1994.

45. DeRenzo EG: Privacy and confidentiality. In Fletcher JS, Spencer ES, Lombardo PA, editors: *Fletcher's introduction to clinical ethics*, ed 3, 2005, University Publishing Group, Hagerstown, MD.

46. Burden N, Saufl N: Why ethical standards? An introduction to the Perianesthesia standards for ethical practice, *J PerAnesth Nurs* 16(1):2-5, 2001.

47. Mamaril ME: Standards of perianesthesia nursing practice: advocating patient safety, *J Perianesth Nurs* 18(3):168-172, 2003.

48. Iacono MV: Perianesthesia staffing...thinking beyond numbers, *J Perianesth Nurs* 21(5): 346-352, 2006.

49. Odom-Forren J: A tragedy unfolds: lessons to learn, *J Perianesth Nurs* 21(5):367-369, 2006.

50. Schroeter K: Pain management: ethical issues for the perianesthesia nurse, *J Perianesth Nurs* 14(6):393-397, 1999.

51. Espin S, Levinson W, Regehr G, et al: Error or "act of God"? A study of patients' and operating room team members' perceptions of error definition, reporting, and disclosure, *Surgery* 139: 6-14, 2006.

52. Spencer EM: A case method for consideration of moral problems. In Fletcher JS, Spencer ES, Lombardo PA, editors: *Fletcher's introduction to clinical ethics*, ed 3, 2005, University Publishing Group, Hagerstown, MD.

# 9

# RESEARCH: EVIDENCE-BASED CLINICAL PRACTICE

*Chuck J. Biddle, PhD, CRNA*

Clinical research seeks to resolve, refine, and clarify the issues involved in the care and management of patients. Each day, perianesthetic nurses (PANs) are faced with a host of common and uncommon patient scenarios that demand thoughtful, efficient decision making and resultant interventions. How they come to decide what course of action to take is, in many cases, as important as the action itself. Decisions that involve the care of patients should be evidence based, a process of considerable complexity that involves judging sources of information, evaluating the quality and relevance of information, recognizing the contextual elements that may alter the application of that information in a particular setting, and assessing its impact on the patient.

Today PANs have an enormous amount of information and experience (personal, collegial, published) from which to draw. The purpose of this chapter is to encourage and empower PANs to:

- Read and understand clinical research.
- Use research-driven information in patient interventions.
- Encourage and mentor colleagues in use of best-evidence approaches to care.
- Critically reflect on outcomes associated with research-driven interventions.

## DEFINITIONS

**Blinding:** Whoever receives or assesses the treatment/intervention does not know which treatment has been received. Single blinding implies that the patient does not know what intervention they have received. Double blinding implies that neither patient nor assessor/observer knows. Triple blinding implies that the final data analysis is carried out in ignorance of which interventions subjects have received, in addition to the subjects and observers being unaware of what treatment was applied to whom.

**Controlled Clinical Trial:** Patients are randomly assigned to a control (receiving the standard treatment or placebo) or intervention group (receiving the new or experimental treatment) and the outcome is measured and compared. Such trials are considered the most reliable and impartial method of determination of treatment effectiveness.

**Evidence-based Practice:** The conscientious, explicit, and judicious use of current best evidence in making decisions about the care of individual patients, integrating individual expertise with the best available external evidence from systematic research.

**Metaanalysis:** The statistical combination of the results of at least two, and usually many more, studies to produce a single estimate of the effect of an intervention.

**Prospective Study:** Follows patients forward in time, with use of carefully defined protocols to determine an outcome that is unknown beforehand. This powerful type of study allows one to determine cause-and-effect relationships.

**Retrospective Study:** Looks backward in time, usually with use of medical records or existing databases. This type of study is weaker than a prospective study and only permits one to determine the nature of association between a treatment and outcome.

## THE PROCESS OF EVIDENCE-BASED CLINICAL PRACTICE

What health care providers do in a given circumstance is often more a matter of entrenched belief than a course of action firmly grounded in research. The published series, *Clinical Evidence*, the international source of best available evidence related to common clinical interventions in various disease states, reveals that of 2404 treatments reviewed, 360 (15%) were rated "beneficial," 538 (22%) were "likely to be beneficial," 180 (7%) were "a trade off between benefit and harm," 115 (5%) were "unlikely to be beneficial," 89 (4%) were "likely to be ineffective or harmful," and 1122 (47%) had "unknown effectiveness."[1] One might interpret these results in many ways, but clearly the results point to the theme that many treatment decisions are inadequately grounded in firm scientific rationale.

The fundamentals of medicine and nursing have evolved from a time when the teaching and practice of authoritative figures (sages) were simply passed down and applied to patients uncritically. Advances came with clinical evolution but primarily in the form of case reports, case series, editorials, and other publications that were too often based on preconceived notions and deliberate or unintentional bias. The advent of the randomized controlled clinical trial (RCT) some six decades ago set the stage for a new era in patient care. In the RCT, patients are randomized to treatment strategies, the effects of outside influences on outcome are considered, and methodologic precision is not only employed with regard to the interventions applied to patients but also to how outcomes are measured. Despite advances, practitioners, and nurses in particular, are often resistant about bringing research advances to the bedside. In one study, investigators in the early 1990s revealed that only 21% of 1200 practicing nurses had implemented a new research finding in the previous 6 months.[2]

One historic example of the uncritical acceptance and application of an intervention is bloodletting. One modern example is the uncritical acceptance and widespread application of episiotomy, which has now been challenged by a number of clinical trials, including a recent metaanalysis.[4]

Evidence-based clinical practice (EBCP) involves a series of five consecutive, somewhat overlapping steps that include the following:

1. Asking a clinical question that deserves an answer
2. Seeking out the best evidence that applies
3. Judging the nature and quality of the evidence
4. Assessing whether the evidence applies to a particular patient
5. Evaluating the effect of the intervention

### Step 1: Asking a Question that Deserves an Answer

Should a child with an upper respiratory infection on the day of a scheduled procedure undergo anesthesia and the elective surgery? What fluid and glucose management strategy should be used in the patient with diabetes who is recovering from a major peripheral vascular procedure? Is use of ketorolac safe in the patient with a fresh tonsillectomy? What can be done to minimize the risk of ventilator-acquired pneumonia in the postoperative patient who is undergoing mechanical ventilation? What limits should be placed on family visits in the postanesthesia care unit (PACU)? Should all patients recovering from general anesthesia receive supplemental oxygen in the PACU? Should the patient with obstructive sleep apnea with significant pulmonary hypertension who is recovering from general anesthesia receive continuous positive airway pressure (CPAP) in the PACU? Such questions are common in practice and merit careful consideration in terms of intervention-related outcome, but relevant questions also apply to diagnosis, prognosis, and the potential for harm. It may seem like word play, but the answers to our questions are more likely to be important and valid if the questions posed are good. Questions should be focused to the extent that they are applicable to the patients that are cared for and can be researched.

### Steps 2 and 3: Searching for Relevant Evidence and Judging its Worth

Once a question is at hand, the search for information begins, a process that can be both time consuming and challenging. Seeking evidence to address the question, "What is the best antiemetic for the postoperative patient," is much different than seeking to address, "Is isopropyl alcohol inhalation more effective than ondansetron in the management of post–general anesthesia nausea in the postpartum patient undergoing tubal ligation?"

Although providers usually have an opinion about care-related questions, EBCP demands that we critically evaluate researchable and meaningful information sources to best address a particular patient's care. *Index Medicus* and *Medline* are familiar and excellent sources but are not applicable in all circumstances, especially if time is of the essence. A particularly valuable database specifically related to EBCP is the Cochrane Collaboration, a collection of well-conducted clinical trials that are organized into specific topics. Established web sites, well-regarded (peer-reviewed, authoritative) textbooks, or even colleagues with a robust knowledge base are also good sources. But the level of confidence bestowed on a colleague, database, or book must be contingent on whether the information is evidence based. The phrase "garbage in, garbage out" has particular application here.

Definitions of EBCP abound, but Sackett's description, "it is the conscientious, explicit and judicious use of current best evidence in making decisions about the care of individual patients, integrating individual expertise with the best available external evidence from systematic research"[4] is preferred for its practicality

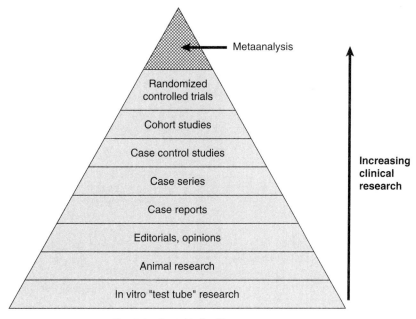

**Fig. 9-1** Pyramid of evidence.

and relevance. Recognition is important that not all evidence that is retrieved or brought to bear on a question has the same value. The pyramid of evidence shown in Fig. 9-1 shows that the randomized double-blind controlled clinical trial has greater worth than the editorial or case report. This hierarchy of value is case and issue sensitive because not all questions have relevant or applicable RCTs. On the other hand, when a number of RCTs are directed towards a similar issue, these can sometimes be combined, with rigorous methodology and a common set of statistical proceduring, to produce what is known as a metaanalysis (or quantitative systematic review). Recent examples of anesthesia-related and PACU-related metaanalyses are noted.[5-7]

This chapter is not meant to be an exhaustive review of how to critically review published papers; rather it presumes a certain level of sophistication on the part of the reader in terms of critically appraising the literature. One should point out that the three rather arbitrary levels of research design are namely:

- *Explorative*: When little is known beforehand, the research helps form questions.
- *Descriptive*: Patient/intervention relationships are identified and explored.
- *Predictive*: Theory is tested in laboratory or clinical trials.

The nature of the clinical question at hand suggests which research design is most relevant. Whatever type of research design is examined, certain key points need to be considered when

one reviews and considers a particular paper's worth (see Box 9-1).

### Step 4: Determining Whether the Evidence Applies to a Particular Patient

Translation of knowledge into practice is the next critical step. Once the evidence is deemed valid and important, the next step involves determination of its application to the patient's care. EBCP then becomes an ongoing process of inquiry, with the asking of "why do it this way" and "what compelling reasons are there to do it differently to achieve a better outcome?" The factors that influence these decisions are complex. Ultimately, the decision to implement a treatment or intervention is a blend of experience and science (evidence) combined with assessment of the value the evidence has in the context and setting of a particular patient. What is meant by context? Box 9-2 illustrates a few of the contextual factors that PANs must consider as they engage in EBCP decision making.

### Step 5: Evaluating the Effect (Outcome) of the Evidence-Based Intervention

Absolutely vital to the process of EBCP is evaluation. In this step, one determines whether the evidence has altered the usual practice pattern and, if so, whether it has been associated with improved efficiency and health outcome and has maintained the quality of care. Evaluation allows not only for deciding whether the intervention works but also for determining whether

---

**Box 9-1    A Guide for Researchers\* and Clinicians† in Evaluation of Research Reports**

**PROBLEM**

Is it lucid, researchable, justified, and practical?

**HYPOTHESIS OR RESEARCH QUESTION**

Is it clear, with the variables under consideration identified and logically related to each other?

**DEFINITIONS**

Are terms adequately defined and put into their appropriate context?

**LITERATURE CITED**

Is it relevant, current, and organized? Is it logical, and does it justify the study?

**METHODS**

Is the sample representative of the population being considered? Is it large enough?
Are the interventions, controls, and measurement tools described and are they valid?
Is the design compatible with the problem and the hypothesis or research question?
Does any evidence exist of drift from established procedures (did they do what they said they planned)?
Are the data-gathering procedures defined?
Is enough information provided for replication of the study, if desired?
Are the statistical procedures described and appropriate?

**RESULTS**

Are they presented clearly, concisely, and without bias?
Are they organized and displayed logically in tables or figures?
Are they relevant to the problem or hypothesis?

**DISCUSSION**

Is it logically based on the results and related to the initial problem, hypothesis, or question?
Have the authors gone too far; that is, have they overgeneralized their findings?
Is the writing impartial and scientific?
Can this study be used in the practice setting, and what are the risks of implementing it?

---

\*Researchers should benefit by critically asking whether they have included answers to these questions in their report.
†Clinicians should benefit by judging the report on the basis of completeness, utility, and relevance to the question at hand.

---

variations arise (e.g., dosing, timing, duration, complications, unexpected occurrences, etc). With this evaluation, a kind of living evolving document arises that can be used for purposes of assessment of efficacy, quality assurance, and risk.

## SUMMARY

Many of the research questions that pertain to perianesthesia nursing can largely be compartmentalized into three fundamental areas: pain, critical care, and clinical anesthesia. Respective example questions might be "How might the pain of a 5-year-old who has undergone a tonsillectomy be best treated?" "What vasopressor is best for the patient for femoral-popliteal bypass with a

poor ejection fraction from a recent myocardial infarction?" and "What are the patient risks of retrobulbar anesthesia versus general anesthesia for detached retina surgery with a cause of long-standing diabetes?"

Evidence-based clinical practice is a process that affords the opportunity to explore, implement, and assess interventions that are applied to the patient. At the heart of EBCP is the RCT. A brief checklist is noted in Box 9-3 to help in judging the value of a particular RCT. EBCP represents a shift in the culture of providing health care away from basing decisions exclusively on opinion, past practice, and precedent and towards making more use of science, research, and evidence to guide clinical decision

---

**Box 9-2 Example of Contextual Considerations in the Process of EBCP**

**CONSIDERATIONS IN WEIGHING THE APPLICATION OF A THERAPY IN A PARTICULAR PATIENT:**

- Age and gender
- Hydration status
- Smoking history
- Current drug therapy
- Duration of illness
- Severity of symptoms
- Cost of therapy
- Side effects
- Inpatient or outpatient
- Coexisting conditions
- Physician and staff familiarity and experience with intervention
- The degree of technical mastery that is necessary to perform the intervention
- Staff makeup (specialists, generalists)
- Type of hospital (community, medical center, urban, rural)
- Support personnel
- Reasonable follow-up available for assessment of the intervention's outcome

---

This list is partial and is meant only to stimulate thinking regarding how factors may influence the application and outcome of a particular intervention.

---

**Box 9-3 Checklist for Evaluation of the Randomized Controlled Trial**

- Is a clear objective for the study stated?
- Is the sample size adequate?
- Is the study population well described?
- Are the interventions clearly described?
- Are randomization and blinding procedures adequate?
- Are valid and reliable outcome measures used?
- Is attrition (dropouts) considered in the analysis?
- Are the statistical methods appropriate?
- Are both clinical and statistical significance reported?
- Are the results generalizable to clinical practice?

---

making. This train has definitely left the station. All are invited to step aboard.

## REFERENCES

1. Tovey D: Clinical guidance. www.clinical evidence.com/uhf. Winter, 2005.
2. Bostrom J, Suter WN: Research utilization: making the link to practice, *J Nurs Staff Devel* 9:28-34, 1993.
3. Hartman K, et al: Outcomes of routine episiotomy, *JAMA* 293:2141-2148, 2005.
4. Sackett D: Evidence-based medicine: what it is and what it isn't, *Br Med J* 312:71-72, 1996.
5. Biddle C: Metaanalysis of the effectiveness of nonsteroidal anti-inflammatory drugs in a standardized pain model, *AANA J* 70:111-118, 2002.
6. Schreiber JU, et al: Prevention of succinylcholine-induced fasciculation and myalgia: a metaanalysis of randomized trials, *Anesthesiology* 103:877-884, 2005.
7. Lee A, Done ML: Use of nonpharmacologic techniques to prevent postoperative nausea and vomiting: a metaanalyis, *Anesth Analg* 88:1362-1369, 1999.

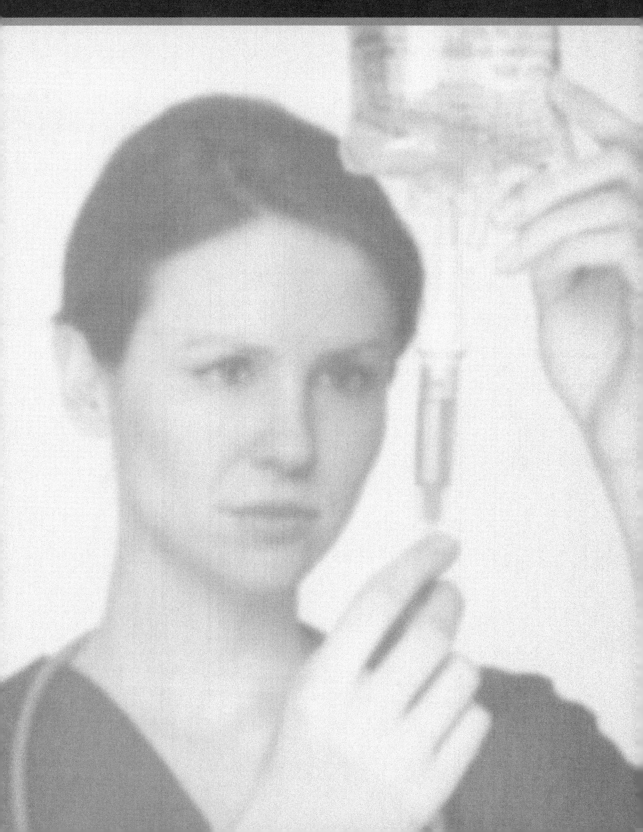

# 10

## THE NERVOUS SYSTEM

*Cecil B. Drain, PhD, RN, CRNA, FAAN, FASAHP*

The essence of physiology is regulation and control. The nervous system is not only affected by surgery performed on the patient but also is affected directly by general inhalational anesthetics, intravenous anesthetics, and regional anesthetics. Hence, most patients in the postanesthesia care unit (PACU) have some alteration in central nervous system (CNS) function. Consequently, the perianesthesia nurse must have an understanding of some of the basic anatomic and physiologic principles that are operative in the CNS. This chapter provides the perianesthesia nurse with a comprehensive review of both the anatomy and the physiology of the central and peripheral nervous system.

## DEFINITIONS

**Afferent:** Carrying sensory impulses toward the brain.

**Autoregulation:** An alteration in the diameter of the resistance vessels to maintain a constant perfusion pressure during changes in blood flow.

**Cistern:** A reservoir or cavity.

**Commissure:** White or gray matter that crosses over in the midline and connects one side of the brain or spinal cord with the other side.

**Decussate:** Refers to crossing of parts.

**Dorsal:** Posterior.

**Efferent:** Carrying motor impulses away from the brain.

**Estrus:** The cycle of changes in the female genital tract produced as a result of ovarian hormonal activity.

**Inferior:** Beneath; also used to indicate the lower portion of an anatomic part.

**Lower Motor Neurons:** Neurons of the spine and cranium that directly innervate the muscles (e.g., those found in the anterior horns or anterior roots of the gray matter of the spinal cord).

**Metabolic Regulation:** A change in blood flow in response to the metabolic requirements of tissues.

**Neuroglia:** The supporting structure of nervous tissue that consists of a fine web of tissue made up of modified ectodermal elements. It encloses branched cells known as neuroglia or glia cells but lacks nerve fibers itself. It performs less specialized functions of the nerve network.

**Oculogyric:** A paroxysm in which the eyes are held in a fixed position, usually up and sideways, for minutes or several hours.

**Plexus:** A network of nerves.

**Postural Reflexes:** Reflexes that are basically proprioceptive, concerned with the position of the head in relation to the trunk and with adjustments of the extremities and eyes to the position of the head.

**Proprioception:** Sensory input from joints, tendons, and muscles that underlies posture, movement, and changes in equilibrium.

**Ramus (rami):** The primary division of a nerve.

**Righting Reflexes:** Reflexes that maintain the head in an upright position in relation to the environment, through use of the eyes, vestibular apparatus, and muscles of the neck and trunk.

**Upper Motor Neurons:** Neurons in the brain and spinal cord that activate the motor system (e.g., the descending fibers of the pyramidal and extrapyramidal tracts).

**Ventral:** Anterior.

## CENTRAL NERVOUS SYSTEM

The CNS comprises the brain and spinal cord and is exceedingly complex, both anatomically and physiologically. None of the structures in the CNS function in an isolated manner. Neural activity at any level of the CNS always modifies or is modified by influences from other parts of the system, which accounts for the unique nature and extreme complexity of the CNS, much of which remains to be clearly understood.

### The Brain

The human brain serves both structurally and functionally as the primary center for control and regulation of all nervous system functions. As such, it is the highest level of control and integration of sensory and motor information in the entire body.

The brain (encephalon) is divided into the following three large areas based on its embryonic development: (1) the forebrain (prosencephalon) contains the telencephalon (cerebrum) with its hemispheres and the diencephalon; (2) the midbrain (mesencephalon) contains the cerebral peduncles, the corpora quadrigemina, and the cerebral aqueduct; and (3) the hindbrain (rhombencephalon) comprises the medulla oblongata, the pons, the cerebellum, and the fourth ventricle.

### The Forebrain

**The Telencephalon (Cerebrum).** The cerebrum is the largest part of the brain. It fills the entire upper portion of the cranial cavity and consists of billions of neurons that synapse to form a complex network of neural pathways.

The cerebrum consists of two hemispheres interconnected by a large band of white fiber tracts known as the corpus callosum. Each hemisphere is further subdivided into four lobes that correspond in name to the overlying bones of the cranium. These lobes are the frontal, parietal, temporal, and occipital lobes (Fig. 10-1). Both hemispheres consist of an external cortex of gray matter, the underlying white matter tracts, and the basal ganglia (cerebral nuclei). Each

hemisphere also contains a lateral ventricle, which is an elongated cavity concerned with the formation and circulation of cerebrospinal fluid (CSF).

**The Cerebral Cortex.** The cerebral cortex has an elaborate mantle of gray matter and is the most highly integrated area in the nervous system. It is arranged in a series of folds that dip down into the underlying regions. These folds greatly expand the surface area of the gray matter within the limited confines of the skull. Each fold is known as a convolution or gyrus. Grooves exist between these convolutions. A shallow groove is known as a sulcus, whereas a deeper one is known as a fissure.

The cerebral hemispheres are separated from each other anteroposteriorly by the longitudinal fissure. The transverse fissure separates the cerebrum from the cerebellum beneath it.

Each hemisphere has three sulci between the lobes. The central sulcus (also known as the fissure of Rolando) separates the frontal and parietal lobes. The lateral sulcus (the fissure of Sylvius) lies between the frontal and parietal lobes above and the temporal lobe below. The small parietooccipital sulcus is located between its corresponding lobes (Fig. 10-2; see Fig. 10-1).

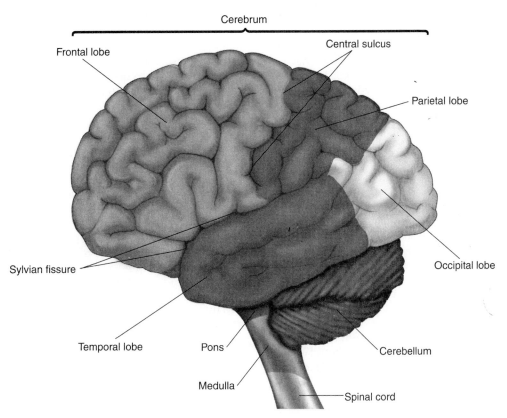

**Fig. 10-1** Left lateral view of brain, showing principal divisions of brain and four major lobes of cerebrum.

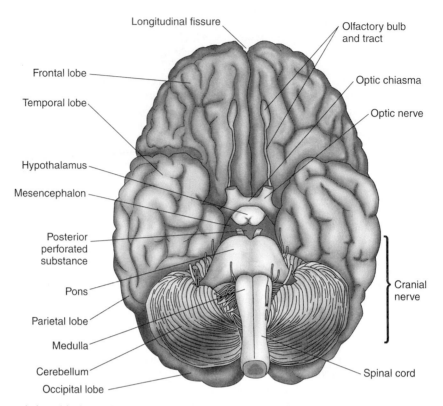

**Fig. 10-2** Basal view of brain. (*Redrawn from Guyton AC:* Basic neuroscience: anatomy and physiology, *ed 2, Philadelphia, 1991, Saunders.*)

The white matter of the cerebrum is situated below the cortex and is composed of three main groups of myelinated nerve fibers arranged in related bundles or tracts. The commissural fibers transmit impulses between the hemispheres. The largest of these fibers is the corpus callosum. The projection fibers ascend and descend to transmit impulses from one level of the CNS to another. A notable example is the internal capsule that surrounds most of the basal ganglia and, in part, connects the thalamus and the cerebral cortex. Finally, the association fibers disseminate impulses from one part of the cortex to another within the same hemisphere.

**Basal Ganglia (Cerebral Nuclei).** A cerebral nucleus is a group of neuron cell bodies within the CNS. Four of these deep-lying masses of gray matter are located within the white matter of each hemisphere and are collectively known as the basal ganglia (Fig. 10-3). These masses are the caudate nucleus, the lentiform nucleus (divided into the putamen and the globus pallidus), the amygdala, and the claustrum. Together, they exert a steadying influence on muscle activity. Along with that portion of the internal capsule that lies between them, the caudate and lentiform nuclei compose the corpus striatum, the most significant functional unit of

the basal ganglia. The basal ganglia are an important part of the extrapyramidal motor pathway that connects nuclei with each other, with the cortex, and with the spinal cord. The ganglia also connect with areas in the hindbrain (the red nucleus and the substantia nigra) to assist in the role of smoothing and coordinating muscle movements. Disturbances in these ganglia result in tremor, rigidity, and loss of expressive and walking movements, as seen in Parkinson's syndrome.

**Functional Aspects of the Cerebrum.** Nearly every portion of the cerebral cortex is connected with subcortical centers, and no areas in the cortex are exclusively motor (expressive) or exclusively sensory (receptive) in nature. However, some regions are primarily concerned with the expressive phase of cortical functioning, whereas others are primarily receptive in nature. The activities of these areas are integrated by association fibers that compose the remainder of the cerebral cortex. Association fibers play important roles in complex intellectual and emotional processes.

**Motor Areas.** No single area of motor control exists within the brain because the integration and control of muscle activity depends on the harmonious activities of several areas, including

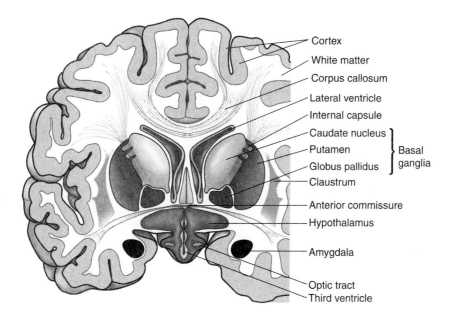

**Fig. 10-3**   Coronal section of cerebrum in front of thalamus, showing especially basal ganglia. (*Redrawn from Guyton AC:* Basic neuroscience: anatomy and physiology, *ed 2, Philadelphia, 1991, Saunders.)*

the cerebral cortex, the basal ganglia, and the cerebellum.

*Primary Motor Area.* The primary motor area of the cerebral cortex is located in the precentral gyrus of the frontal lobe, just anterior to the central sulcus, and is concerned mainly with the voluntary initiation of finely controlled movements, such as those of the hands, fingers, lips, tongue, and vocal cords. Skeletal muscles responsible for these discrete movements are largely represented by neurons in the motor cortex. Muscles of the arms, legs, and trunk are served by a comparatively small group of neurons, so that this part of the motor cortex controls larger groups of muscles and produces grosser movements (Fig. 10-4).

The axons of the pyramidal cell bodies in the primary motor area descend through the internal capsule, midbrain, and pons to the medulla, where most of them decussate, or cross, to the opposite side and continue down into the spinal cord. These fibers constitute the crossed pyramidal or lateral corticospinal tracts. Fibers that have not crossed are known as the uncrossed pyramidal or ventral corticospinal tracts. Most of these fibers eventually decussate at lower levels within the cord. Pyramidal cell axons also connect within the brain with the basal ganglia, the brainstem, and the cerebellum. All of the complex connections of the pyramidal cells play important roles in the overall coordination and control of skeletal muscle activity.

*Premotor Area.* The premotor area of each hemisphere is located in the cortex immediately anterior to the precentral gyrus in the frontal lobe. On the whole, this area is concerned with movement of the opposite side of the body, especially with control and coordination of skilled movements of a complex nature. In addition to its subcortical connections with the primary motor area, its neurons also have direct connections with the basal ganglia and related nuclei in the brainstem, for example, the reticular formation. Many of the axons from these subcortical centers cross to the opposite side before descending as extrapyramidal tracts in the spinal cord. Collectively, the connections from the premotor area to these related nuclei make up the extrapyramidal system, which coordinates gross skeletal muscle activities that are largely automatic in nature. Examples are postural adjustments, chewing, swallowing, gesticulating, and associated movements that accompany voluntary activities. Certain portions of the extrapyramidal tract also have an inhibitory effect on spontaneous movements initiated by the cerebral cortex and serve to prevent tremors and rigidity. Complete structural and functional separation of the pyramidal and extrapyramidal systems is impossible because they are so closely connected in the harmonious work of executing complex coordinated movements (see Fig. 10-3).

Of interest to the PACU nurse is that drugs used to produce neuroleptanesthesia may cause

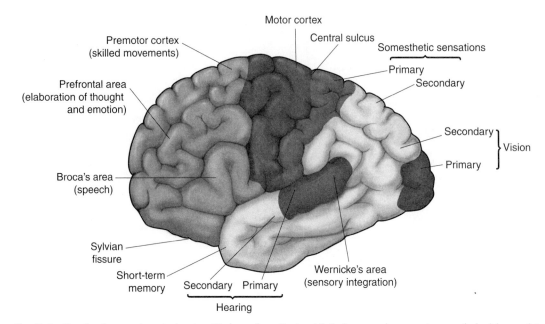

**Fig. 10-4** Functional areas of cerebral cortex. (*Redrawn from Guyton AC:* Basic neuroscience: anatomy and physiology, *ed 2, Philadelphia, 1991, Saunders.*)

extrapyramidal reactions. More specifically, the neuroleptics, such as the phenothiazines (of which chlorpromazine is the prototypal drug), and the butyrophenones, as typified by droperidol (Inapsine) and haloperidol (Haldol), are known to produce extrapyramidal reactions. The following four types of extrapyramidal reaction exist: drug-induced parkinsonism, akathisia, acute dystonic reactions, and tardive dyskinesia.

Drug-induced parkinsonism, which can occur 1 to 5 days after the administration of the neuroleptic drug, is typified by a generalized slowing of automatic and spontaneous movements (bradykinesia), with a masklike facial expression and a reduction in arm movements. The most noticeable signs of the drug-induced parkinsonism syndrome are rigidity and oscillatory tremor at rest. Treatment is with antiparkinsonian agents, such as levodopa, trihexyphenidyl, and benztropine.

*Akathisia*, which can occur 5 to 60 days after the administration of a neuroleptic drug, is a term that refers to a subjective feeling of restlessness accompanied by a need on the part of the patient to move about and pace back and forth. Treatment requires a reduction in the dosage of the responsible drug.

Acute dystonic reactions may occur after the administration of some psychotropic drugs and are characterized by torsion spasms, such as facial grimacing and torticollis. These reactions are occasionally seen when a phenothiazine is first administered and are associated with

oculogyric crises. Acute dystonic reactions may be mistaken for hysterical reactions or seizures and may usually be reversed with anticholinergic antiparkinsonian drugs, such as benztropine or trihexyphenidyl.

Tardive dyskinesia is a late-appearing neurologic syndrome that is characterized by stereotypic, involuntary, rapid, and rhythmically repetitive movements, such as continual chewing movements and darting movements of the tongue. Treatment is not always satisfactory because antiparkinsonian drugs sometimes exacerbate tardive dyskinesia. Tardive dyskinesia often persists despite discontinuation of the responsible drug.

Two important structural aspects of the premotor area are worth noting for those who care for neurosurgical patients. First, the fibers from both the primary motor and the premotor areas are funneled through the narrow internal capsule as they descend to lower areas of the CNS. This action is significant because the internal capsule is a common site of cerebrovascular accidents. Second, lesions within one side of the internal capsule result in paralysis of the skeletal muscles on the opposite side of the body because of the crossing of fibers within the medulla.

*Motor Speech Area.* This area is only one point in the complicated network needed to form spoken and written words. The motor speech area lies at the base of the motor area and slightly anterior to it in the inferior frontal gyrus and is also known as Broca's area (see Fig. 10-4). In right-handed people (most of the population), the language and speech areas are usually located in the left hemisphere. In those who are left-handed, these areas may lie within the right or the left hemisphere.

*Prefrontal Area.* This area of the frontal lobe lies anterior to the premotor area, has extensive connections with other cortical areas, and is believed to play an important role in complex intellectual activities, such as mathematic and philosophic reasoning; abstract and creative thinking; learning; judgment and volition; and social, moral, and ethical values. The prefrontal area also influences certain autonomic functions of the body with the conduction of impulses directly or indirectly through the thalamus to the hypothalamus, which makes possible certain physiologic responses to feelings such as anger, fear, and lust.

**Sensory Areas.** Sensory information from one side of the body is received by the general sensory (or somesthetic) area of the opposite hemisphere, which is located in the parietal lobe in the area of the postcentral gyrus. Crude sensations of pain, temperature, and touch can be experienced at the level of the thalamus, but true discrimination of these sensations is a function of the parietal cortex. The activities of the general sensory area allow for proprioception; for the recognition of the size, shape, and texture of objects; and for the comparison of stimuli as to intensity and location.

The auditory area lies in the cortex of the superior temporal lobe. Each hemisphere receives impulses from both ears. The visual area is located in the posterior occipital lobe, where extremely complex transformations in the signals conveyed by the optic nerve occur. The right occipital cortex receives impulses from the right half of each eye, and the left occipital cortex receives impulses from the left half of each eye. The olfactory area (sense of smell) is believed to be located in the medial temporal lobe, and the gustatory area (sense of taste) is located nearby at the base of the postcentral gyrus.

**Association Areas.** Large areas of the cortex remain for which no discrete function is known. These areas are called association areas. They play a major role in the integration of the sensory and motor phases of cortical function by providing complex connections between them.

**Limbic System.** The principal structural and functional units of the limbic system are the two rings of limbic cortex and a number of related subcortical nuclei, the anterior thalamic nuclei, and portions of the basal nuclei (Fig. 10-5). The terms *limbic system, limbic lobe,* and *rhinencephalon* are often used interchangeably. In general, the limbic system is concerned with a wide variety of autonomic somatosensory and somatomotor responses, especially those involved with emotional states and other behavioral responses. Within the limbic system, the

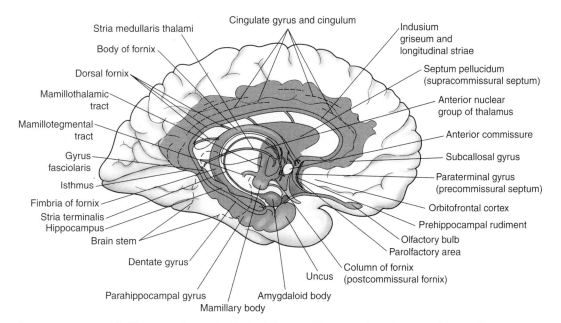

**Fig. 10-5** Anatomy of limbic system, illustrated with *shaded areas* of figure. (*Redrawn from Warwick R, Williams PL:* Gray's anatomy, *ed 35, Philadelphia, 1973, Saunders.*)

benzodiazepine and opiate receptors have been identified (see Chapters 19 and 20).

The limbic system, which acts in close concert with the hypothalamus, can evoke a variety of autonomic responses, including changes in heart rate, blood pressure, and respiratory rate. This system plays an intimate role in the genesis of emotional states, particularly anxiety, fear, and aggression. Stimulation of the limbic system also evokes complex motor responses directly related to feeding behavior. The limbic system has been shown to have major relationships with the reticular formation of the brainstem and is presumed to have a role in the alerting or arousal process. The system is also implicated in the hypothalamic regulation of pituitary activity and may be associated somehow with the memory process for recent events as well. In addition, it is intimately concerned with complex phenomena, such as the control of various biologic rhythms, sexual behavior, and motivation.

**The Diencephalon.** The second major division of the forebrain is the diencephalon (Fig. 10-6), which consists of the thalamus, the epithalamus, the subthalamus, and the hypothalamus. The diencephalon also contains the third ventricle

and is almost completely covered by the cerebral hemispheres. This portion of the brain has a primary role in sleep, emotion, thermoregulation, autonomic activity, and endocrine control of ongoing behavioral patterns.

The thalamus consists of right and left egg-shaped masses, which make up the greatest bulk of the diencephalon and form the lateral wall of the third ventricle. Each thalamus serves as a relay center for all incoming sensory stimuli, except for taste. These impulses are then grouped and transmitted to the appropriate area of the cerebral cortex. Because of its interconnections with the hypothalamus, the limbic system, and the frontal, temporal, and parietal lobes, this structure is also integrally involved with emotional activities, instinctive responses, and attentive processes.

The epithalamus contains the pineal body (or gland), which is known to secrete melatonin. Melatonin inhibits gonadal development and regulates estrus. Its most important function is to slow maturation. Melatonin is believed to have its greatest effect on brain tissue rather than on the gonads themselves.

The subthalamus is situated below the thalamus and above the midbrain and serves as a

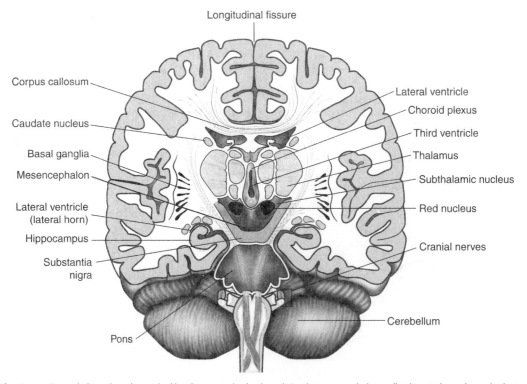

**Fig. 10-6** Coronal view of cerebrum, looking from anterior backward. Section was made immediately anterior to lower brainstem and through middle of thalamus. (*Redrawn from Guyton AC:* Basic neuroscience: anatomy and physiology, *ed 2, Philadelphia, 1991, Saunders.*)

correlation center for the optic and vestibular impulses. Stimulation of centers in or around the subthalamic nuclei produces the excitation of appropriate patterns of action in the brainstem and spinal cord, which results in rhythmic motions of forward progression necessary in the act of walking. Damage to the subthalamic nuclei on one side is known to cause violent involuntary movements of the limbs on the opposite side of the body. These movements are brought about by contractions of the proximal muscles.

The hypothalamus is a group of bilateral nuclei that forms the floor and part of the lateral walls of the third ventricle. Extremely complex in function, the hypothalamus has extensive connections with the autonomic nervous system and with other parts of the CNS. It also influences the endocrine system by virtue of direct and indirect connections with the pituitary gland and the release of its own hormones. In association with these other structures, the hypothalamus participates in the regulation of appetite, water balance, carbohydrate and fat metabolism, growth, sexual maturity, body temperature, pulse rate, blood pressure, sleep, and aspects of emotional behavior. Because of the connection of the hypothalamus with the thalamus and cerebral cortex, emotions can influence visceral responses on certain occasions.

***The Midbrain.*** The midbrain, or mesencephalon, is a short narrow segment of nervous tissue that connects the forebrain with the hindbrain (Fig. 10-7). The midbrain is vital as a conduction pathway and as a reflex control center. Passing through the center of the midbrain is the cerebral aqueduct, a narrow canal that serves to connect the third ventricle of the diencephalon with the fourth ventricle of the hindbrain for the circulation of CSF.

The cerebral peduncles are located in the anterior portion of the midbrain and consist of multiple projection fibers that connect the cerebral cortex with other structures in the brainstem. Their dorsal aspect (the tegmentum) contains the motor nuclei of the oculomotor, trigeminal, and trochlear nerves. The ventral aspect contains the red nucleus, a part of the reticular formation, and the origin of a portion of the extrapyramidal system.

The corpora quadrigemina are structures that are quite complex as they are major multisensory integrative structures. The structures are a group of cells divided in the midline and transversely to form four distinct areas, or colliculi. The inferior colliculi are vital components of the auditory pathway and are responsible for complex acoustic reflexes. The superior colliculi are optic reflex centers.

The centers for postural and righting reflexes are found in the midbrain. The dorsal, or posterior, portion of the midbrain is concerned with visual and auditory reflexes, such as movement of the eyes in accordance with changes in head position, the pupillary light reflex, and turning of the head in the direction of a noise. Key structures of the reticular formation also originate in this area. Also, cranial nerves III (oculomotor) and IV (trochlear) originate in the ventral aspect of the midbrain.

***The Hindbrain.*** The hindbrain, or rhombencephalon, consists of the pons, the medulla oblongata, the cerebellum, and the fourth ventricle (Fig. 10-8).

***The Pons.*** The pons is literally the bridge between the midbrain and the medulla oblongata as it lies in front of the fourth ventricle and separates it from the cerebellum. It receives many ascending and descending fibers en route to other points in the CNS. The pons also contains the motor and sensory nuclei of cranial nerves V (trigeminal), VI (abducens), VII (facial), and VIII (acoustic). The pontine nuclei of the pons are composed of gray matter. White fiber tracts connect the medulla

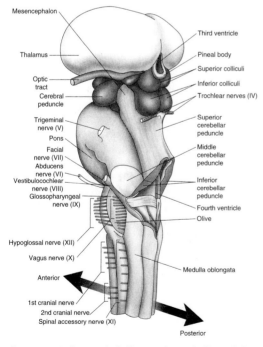

**Fig. 10-7** Brainstem, including portions of diencephalon, midbrain, and hindbrain. (*Redrawn from Guyton AC: Basic neuroscience: anatomy and physiology, ed 2, Philadelphia, 1991, Saunders.*)

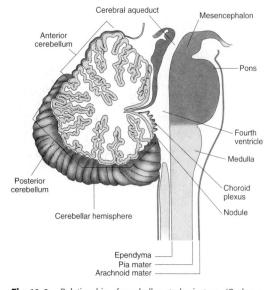

**Fig. 10-8**    Relationship of cerebellum to brainstem. (*Redrawn from Guyton AC:* Basic neuroscience: anatomy and physiology, *ed 2, Philadelphia, 1991, Saunders.*)

below with the cerebrum above. These are the so-called corticospinal tracts. White fiber (cortico-bulbar) tracts also connect the cerebellum with the pons. The roof of the pons contains a portion of the reticular formation, and the lower pons assists in the regulation of respiration.

**The Medulla Oblongata.** The medulla oblongata is an expanded continuation of the spinal cord and is located between the foramen magnum and the pons. It is anatomically complex and not usually amenable to surgery. Many of the white fiber tracts between the brain and spinal cord decussate as they pass through the medulla. Centers for many complex reflexes are located in the medulla oblongata and include those for swallowing, vomiting, coughing, and sneezing. The originating nuclei of cranial nerves IX (glossopharyngeal), X (vagus), XI (accessory), and XII (hypoglossal) are found in the medulla oblongata (Table 10-1; see Fig. 10-7). Because of these originating nuclei, the medulla plays an essential role in the regulation of cardiac, respiratory, and vasomotor reflexes. Injuries to the medulla, such as those that accompany basal skull fracture, often prove fatal.

**The Cerebellum.** The cerebellum comprises two hemispheres and a constricted central portion. It overlaps the pons and the medulla oblongata dorsally and is located just below the occipital lobes of the cerebrum. The cerebellum is separated from the cerebrum by the tentorium above it and has a bilayered cortex composed of gray

matter. Beneath the gray matter are white fiber tracts that extend like branches of a tree to all parts of the cerebellar cortex. Deep within the white matter are masses of gray matter called the cerebellar nuclei. These connect the cerebellar hemispheres with each other and with areas in the cerebrum, the hindbrain, and the spinal cord.

The cerebellum has no sensory function and does not initiate movement as the cerebrum does. Functionally, it does coordinate muscle tone and voluntary movements through important connections via the spinal cord with the proprioceptor endings in skeletal muscles, tendons, and joints. In addition, the cerebellum is involved in reflexes necessary for the maintenance of equilibrium and posture, through its connections with the vestibular apparatus of the inner ear. The cerebellum also receives optic and acoustic information, but the specifics of the anatomic pathways involved have not yet been discerned.

Damage to the cerebellum does not result in paralysis or sensory loss. The outcome of damage depends on which portion of the structure is involved. Damage to one part may result in loss of balance, nystagmus, and a reeling gait (cerebellar ataxia). Damage to another area may cause disturbances in the postural reflexes. Posterior lobe disturbances result in changes in voluntary movements, such as discrepancies in force, direction, and range of movements; lack of precision in movements; and, possibly, intention tremors.

**The Fourth Ventricle.** The fourth ventricle is a diamond-shaped space located between the cerebellum posteriorly and the pons and medulla oblongata anteriorly. The ventricle contains CSF.

**The Brainstem.** Authors disagree to some extent as to what structures collectively constitute the brainstem. All agree that it includes the midbrain, the pons, and the medulla oblongata. Some believe that the diencephalon rightly belongs in the group. Whichever grouping is used, all functions of each structure within it may be considered to be basic activities of the brainstem. All of the cranial nerves are attached to the brainstem (if the diencephalon is included), with the exception of the olfactory nerve and the spinal portion of the accessory nerve.

**The Reticular Formation.** The reticular formation lies within the brainstem (including the diencephalon). An important function of the reticular formation is its action as an intermediary between the upper and lower motor neurons of the extrapyramidal system. In this way, the reticular formation facilitates or augments reflex activity and voluntary movements. Its motor neurons can be excitatory or inhibitory in action. For example,

## Table 10-1    Cranial Nerves and Their Functions

| Number | Name | Type | Function |
|---|---|---|---|
| I | Olfactory | Sensory | Smell |
| II | Optic | Sensory | Vision |
| III | Oculomotor | Mixed: mainly motor | Motion of eye up, in, and down<br>Raising of eyelid<br>Constriction of pupil<br>Accommodation of pupil to distance<br>Proprioceptive impulses |
| IV | Trochlear | Mixed: mainly motor | Motion of eye down<br>Proprioceptive impulses |
| V | Trigeminal:<br>Ophthalmic branch<br>Maxillary branch<br>Mandibular branch | Mixed | Motor: muscles of mastication<br>Sensory: face, nose, and mouth<br>Proprioceptive impulses from teeth sockets and jaw muscles |
| VI | Abducens | Mixed: mainly motor | Outward motion of eye<br>Proprioception from eye muscles |
| VII | Facial | Mixed: mostly motor, some sensory and autonomic | Motor: movement of facial muscles, ear, nose, and neck<br>Sensory: taste and anterior two thirds of tongue<br>Autonomic: secretion of saliva and tears |
| VIII | Acoustic:<br>Cochlear branch<br>Vestibular branch | Sensory | Cochlear: hearing<br>Vestibular: maintenance of equilibrium and posturing of head |
| IX | Glossopharyngeal | Mixed: motor, sensory, and autonomic | Motor: muscles of swallowing<br>Sensory: taste, posterior third of tongue, and sensation from pharynx<br>Autonomic: impulses to parotid glands and decrease blood pressure and pulse |
| X | Vagus | Mixed: motor, sensory, and autonomic | Motor, sensory, and autonomic: information to and from larynx, pharynx, trachea, esophagus, heart, and abdominal viscera |
| XI | Spinal accessory | Mixed: mostly motor | Cranial portion: motor and sensory information to and from voluntary muscles of pharynx, larynx, and palate (swallowing)<br>Spinal portion: motor information to sternocleidomastoid and trapezius muscles<br>May form components of cardiac branches of vagus |
| XII | Hypoglossal | Mixed: mostly motor | Motor and sensory information to and from tongue muscles<br>Position sense |

with inhibition of extensor muscles, it facilitates the action of flexor muscles.

Every pathway that carries information to the brain also contributes afferent fibers to the reticular formation, so that it is kept well informed about conditions of both the outside world and the internal organs. Efferent impulses that leave the reticular formation travel to the cerebral cortex and to the spinal cord. By virtue of its location in and connections with the brainstem and diencephalon, the reticular formation participates integrally in their activities.

Another important function of the reticular formation is the activation and regulation of those brain activities related to attention arousal and consciousness. For this reason, it is often called the reticular activating system (RAS).

Damage to the reticular formation results in greatly decreased levels of consciousness. When the cerebral cortex is isolated from the RAS by disease or injury of the upper portion of the midbrain, decerebrate rigidity occurs. This abnormal posturing results from the dominant effect of the extensor muscles and a lack of inhibition from opposing motor neurons and flexor muscles. The rigidity is accompanied by a profoundly reduced level of consciousness.

**Protection of the Brain.** The brain is protected by the cranial bones, the meninges, and the CSF (Figs. 10-9 and 10-10).

**The Cranial Bones.** Eight cranial bones encase the brain and support and protect it from most ordinary bumps and jarring. In the adult, immovable fibrous joints, or sutures, fuse these bones together to form the rigid walls of the box known as the cranium. The base of the cranium is both thicker and stronger than its roof or walls.

The bones of the cranium are the frontal, right and left parietal, occipital, sphenoid, ethmoid, and right and left temporal bones. The frontal bone forms the anterior roof of the skull and the forehead. Within the frontal bone are the frontal sinuses, which communicate with the nasal cavities. The parietal bones form much of the top and sides of the cranium. The occipital bone forms the back and a large portion of the base of the skull. The two temporal bones are complicated and form part of the sides and a part of the base of the skull. Their inner surfaces are not as smooth and regular as the bones previously mentioned. Parts of the temporal bones articulate with the condyles of the lower jaw, and air cells in the mastoid portions of the temporal bones communicate with the middle ear. The sphenoid bone occupies a central portion of the floor of the skull. It alone articulates with each of the other cranial bones. Its middle portion contains the sphenoid sinuses, which open into the nasal cavity. The upper portion of the sphenoid bone has a marked saddle-like depression, the sella turcica, which holds the pituitary gland. The ethmoid bone is light and has a spongy structure. It is located between the orbital cavities and is a cribriform plate that forms the roof of the nasal cavity

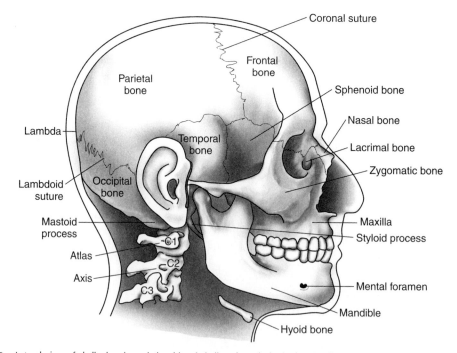

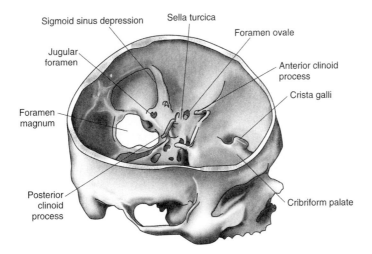

**Fig. 10-10** Interior of cranial cavity.

and part of the base of the cranium. The ethmoid sinuses open into the nasal cavities.

Several features of the cranial bones are particularly noteworthy for the PACU nurse. Among these features is the fact that the air cells in the mastoid portion of the temporal bone may become infected from otitis media or after surgery on the middle or inner ear. This mastoiditis may cause severe complications if it extends through the thin plate of bone that separates it from the cranial meninges. Another point of interest is that surgical access to the pituitary gland is commonly accomplished through the sphenoid bone via the nostrils; one example is transsphenoidal hypophysectomy. Finally, nasal suctioning is absolutely contraindicated in the patient with cranial surgery because of the danger of

perforation of the cribriform plate of the ethmoid bone, which results in leakage of CSF and permits direct access to the brain by infectious organisms.

One main opening is located at the base of the skull and is called the foramen magnum. It marks the point at which the brainstem changes structure and becomes identified inferiorly as the spinal cord. Many smaller openings in the skull allow the cranial nerves and some blood vessels to pass through it to and from the face, the jaw, and the neck. The atlas of the vertebral column (the first cervical vertebra) supports the skull and forms a moveable joint with the occipital bone.

**The Meninges.** The meninges (Fig. 10-11) are three fibrous membranes between the skull and the brain and between the vertebral column and the spinal cord. The outer membrane is the dura

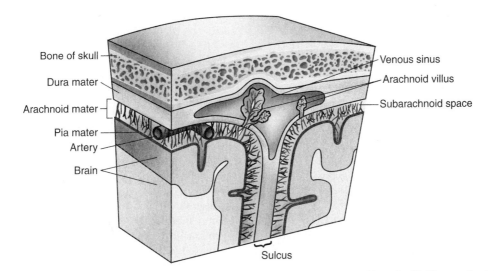

**Fig. 10-11** Expanded view of meninges covering section of brain. Note also venous sinus with arachnoid villi protruding into it. (*Redrawn from Guyton AC:* Basic neuroscience: anatomy and physiology, *ed 2, Philadelphia, 1991, Saunders.*)

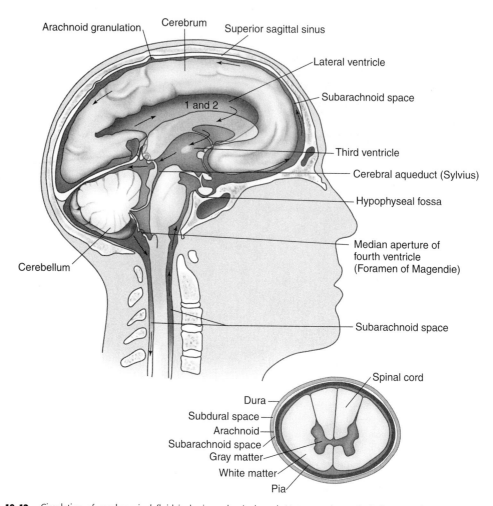

**Fig. 10-12**   Circulation of cerebrospinal fluid in brain and spinal cord. Note superior sagittal sinus. (*Redrawn from Jacob SW, Francone CA, Lossow WJ: Structure and function in man, ed 5, Philadelphia, 1982, Saunders.*)

mater and the inner is the pia mater; between them lies the arachnoid mater.

*The Dura Mater.* The dura mater is a shiny tough inelastic membrane that envelops and supports the brain and spinal cord and, by various folds, separates parts of the brain into adjoining compartments. The portion within the skull differs from the dura of the spinal cord in three ways. First, the cranial dura is firmly attached to the skull. The spinal dura has no attachment to the vertebrae. Second, the cranial dura consists of two layers; it not only covers the brain (meningeal dura) but also lines the interior of the skull bones (periosteal dura). Third, the two layers of the cranial dura are in contact with each other in some places but separate in others where the inner layer dips inward to form the protective partitions between parts of the brain. Also, the spaces or channels formed by these separations of dural layers are filled with

venous blood that is leaving the brain; these spaces are called cranial venous sinuses and are an elaborate network unique to the brain (Fig. 10-12; see Fig. 10-11).

Three major partitioning folds of the meningeal dura exist. The falx cerebri separates the right and left hemispheres of the cerebrum. The tentorium cerebelli supports and separates the occipital lobes of the cerebrum from the cerebellum. The falx cerebelli separates the two cerebellar hemispheres. The tentorium separates the posterior cranial chamber from the remainder of the cranial cavity and serves as a line of demarcation for describing the site of a surgical procedure or a lesion as either supratentorial or infratentorial.

Encased between the two dural layers are two major groups of venous channels that drain blood from the brain. None of these vascular channels possesses valves, and their walls are extremely thin because of the absence of muscular tissue.

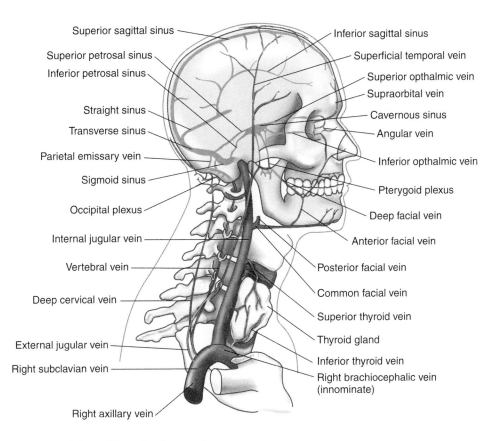

Superior sagittal sinus
Superior petrosal sinus
Inferior petrosal sinus
Straight sinus
Transverse sinus
Parietal emissary vein
Sigmoid sinus
Occipital plexus
Internal jugular vein
Vertebral vein
Deep cervical vein
External jugular vein
Right subclavian vein
Right axillary vein

Inferior sagittal sinus
Superficial temporal vein
Superior opthalmic vein
Supraorbital vein
Cavernous sinus
Angular vein
Inferior opthalmic vein
Pterygoid plexus
Deep facial vein
Anterior facial vein
Posterior facial vein
Common facial vein
Superior thyroid vein
Thyroid gland
Inferior thyroid vein
Right brachiocephalic vein
(innominate)

**Fig. 10-13** *Venous drainage of brain, head, and neck.*

The superior-posterior group consists of one paired and four unpaired sinuses. The anterior-inferior group consists of four paired sinuses and one plexus. The sinuses function to drain venous blood into the internal jugular veins, which are the principal vessels responsible for the return of the blood from the brain to the heart (Fig. 10-13).

*The Arachnoid.* The arachnoid is a fine membrane between the dura mater and the pia mater. Between the arachnoid and the dura is the subdural space, a noncommunicating space filled with CSF. The cerebral blood vessels that traverse this space have little supporting structure, which makes them particularly vulnerable to insult at this point.

The arachnoid forms a type of roof over the pia mater, to which it is joined by a network of trabeculae in the subarachnoid space. It does not follow the depressions of the surface architecture. The arachnoid sends small tuft-like extensions through the meningeal layer of the dura into the cranial venous sinuses. These extensions are called the arachnoid granulations or arachnoid villi. The arachnoid villi serve as a pathway for the return of CSF to the venous blood system. Subarachnoid CSF is most abundant in

the grooves between the gyri, particularly at the base of the brain, where the more freely communicating compartments form six subarachnoid cisternae, or reservoirs.

*The Pia Mater.* The inner layer of the meninges, the pia mater, is a fine membrane rich in blood (choroid) plexuses and mesothelial cells. This layer is closely associated with the arachnoid and covers the brain intimately, following the invaginations and convolutions of the brain surface. The veins of the brain lie between threadlike trabeculae in the subarachnoid space. Branches of the cortical arteries in the subarachnoid space are carried with the pia mater and enter the brain substance itself (Fig. 10-14).

**The Cerebrospinal Fluid System.** The CSF is a clear colorless watery fluid with a specific gravity of 1.007. A principal function of this fluid is to act as a cushion for the brain. Because both brain tissue and CSF have essentially the same specific gravity, the brain literally floats within the skull. CSF also serves as a medium for the exchange of nutrients and waste products between the blood stream and the cells of the CNS.

Cerebrospinal fluid is found within the ventricles of the brain, in the cisterns that

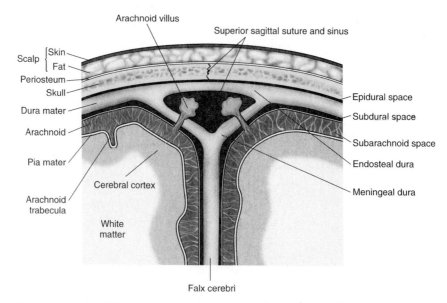

**Fig. 10-14**   Coronal section of skull, brain, meninges, and superior sagittal sinus. (*Redrawn from Jacob SW, Francone CA, Lossow WJ: Structure and function in man, ed 5, Philadelphia, 1982, Saunders.*)

surround it, and in the subarachnoid spaces of both the brain and the spinal cord (Figs. 10-15 and 10-16). The largest of the cisterns is the cisterna magna, which is located beneath and behind the cerebellum.

Although some CSF is formed by filtration through capillary walls throughout the brain's vascular bed, its primary site of formation is in the choroid plexuses within the ventricles. This formation is achieved with a system of secretion and diffusion. The choroid plexuses are highly vascular tufted structures composed of many small granular pouches that project into the ventricles of the brain. CSF is formed continuously and is reabsorbed at a rate of approximately 750 mL per day. The net pressure of the CSF is regulated in part by a balance between formation and reabsorption.

The four ventricles of the brain communicate directly with each other. The first and second (lateral) ventricles are elongated cavities that lie within the cerebral hemispheres. The third ventricle is a slit-like cavity beneath and between the two lateral ventricles. The fourth ventricle is a diamond-shaped space between the cerebellum posteriorly and the pons and medulla oblongata anteriorly.

The circulation of CSF is as follows. Each lateral ventricle contains a large choroid plexus that forms CSF. From the lateral ventricles, the fluid passes through an interventricular foramen (foramen of Monro) into the third ventricle. Together with the additional fluid formed there, the CSF travels posteriorly through the cerebral aqueduct (aqueduct of Sylvius) into

the fourth ventricle, where more fluid is produced. The combined CSF volumes then pass through three openings that lead from the fourth ventricle to the cranial subarachnoid space of the cisterna magna. These openings are the two lateral foramina of Luschka and the medial foramen of Magendie. From the cisterna magna, CSF flows freely within the entire subarachnoid space of the brain and spinal cord.

The main route of reabsorption of excess CSF is through the arachnoid villi that project from the subarachnoid spaces into the venous sinuses of the brain, particularly those of the superior sagittal sinus. The arachnoid villi provide highly permeable regions that allow free passage of CSF, including protein molecules and some small particulate matter contained within it. The process of osmosis is believed to be mainly responsible for the reabsorption of the fluid.

**Blood-brain and Blood–cerebrospinal Fluid Barriers of the Central Nervous System.** Throughout the body, the constancy of the composition of the extracellular fluid is maintained by multiple homeostatic mechanisms. Because of the exquisite sensitivity of the neurons in the CNS, additional mechanisms are necessary to prevent the far-reaching consequences that even minor fluctuations in their chemical environment cause. In health, the unique blood-brain and blood-CSF barriers present in most regions of the CNS have evolved to accomplish this task. The development of the blood-brain barrier occurs gradually during the first several years of childhood.

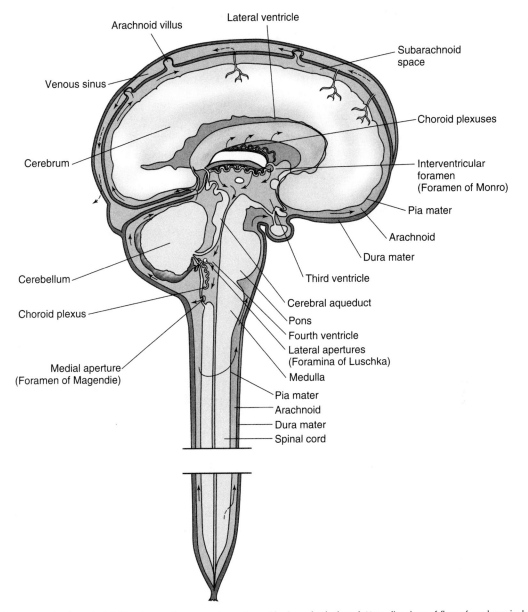

**Fig. 10-15**   Cerebrospinal fluid system and meningeal coverings of brain and spinal cord. Note directions of flow of cerebrospinal fluid indicated by *arrows*. (*Redrawn from Guyton AC:* Basic neuroscience: anatomy and physiology, *ed 2, Philadelphia, 1991, Saunders.*)

The site of the blood-brain barrier is not at the surface of the neurons themselves. Rather, it is located between the plasma within the capillaries and the extracellular space of the brain. The exchange of many physiologically important substances within the capillaries of the CNS is generally believed to be slowed or practically prohibited by several anatomic factors rather than by any single factor alone. These structures likely also form a sequence of morphologic barriers that act in concert to prevent the rapid transport of substances from the blood to the nervous tissue.

These barriers include the tight intercellular junctions between the epithelial cells of the capillaries that appear to effectively reduce permeability. A substantial basement membrane surrounds the capillaries, and an external membrane is provided by the end-feet of the astrocytes between the neurons and the capillaries. These appear to have a major role in retarding or preventing the passage of foreign substances into the brain tissue.

Despite the uncertainty as to the ultimate site of the blood-brain barrier, a firmly established fact is that the rapidity with which substances

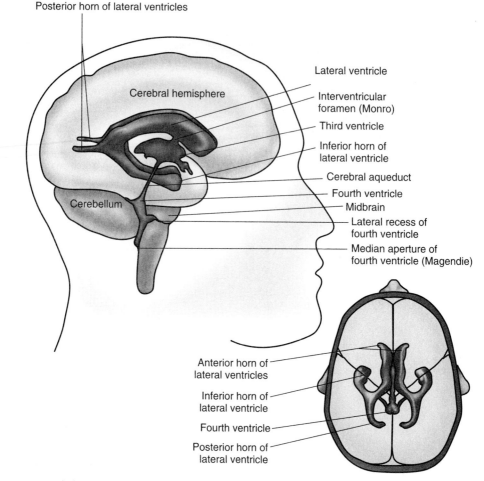

Posterior horn of lateral ventricles

Cerebral hemisphere

Lateral ventricle

Interventricular foramen (Monro)

Third ventricle

Inferior horn of lateral ventricle

Cerebral aqueduct

Fourth ventricle

Midbrain

Lateral recess of fourth ventricle

Median aperture of fourth ventricle (Magendie)

Cerebellum

Anterior horn of lateral ventricles

Inferior horn of lateral ventricle

Fourth ventricle

Posterior horn of lateral ventricle

**Fig. 10-16**   Ventricular system, lateral and superior views.

penetrate brain tissue is inversely related to their molecular size and directly related to their lipid solubility. Only water, carbon dioxide, and oxygen cross the blood-brain barrier rapidly and readily, whereas glucose crosses more slowly and by a facilitated transport mechanism. Water-soluble compounds, electrolytes, and protein molecules generally cross slowly. Most general anesthetics effectively cross the blood-brain barrier because of their high lipid solubility.

Of critical clinical importance is the fact that the effectiveness of the blocking mechanism of the blood-brain barrier may break down in areas of the brain that are infected, traumatized, or irradiated or that contain tumors. As effective as the blood-brain barrier is, no substance is completely excluded from reaching the central neurons. Instead, the rate of transport of substances through the barrier is of major significance in maintenance of the constancy of the internal environment of the brain.

A limited number of structures in the brain have unique capillaries and are not restricted by

the blood-brain barrier. These organs appear to function as chemoreceptors and as such must be in intimate contact with the chemical substances within the blood. The posterior pituitary gland is one of these structures. The blood-CSF barrier is located at the choroid plexus. As in the case of the blood-brain barrier, the rate of transport of substances across the blood-CSF barrier is controlled by molecular size and lipid solubility.

The routes whereby substances leave the CSF are different from those by which they enter. They may leave rapidly via the arachnoid villi, regardless of their molecular size or lipid solubility. Alternatively, the bulk circulation of the CSF throughout the brain enhances the direct removal of certain lipid-soluble substances across the blood-brain barrier.

***Arterial Blood Supply to the Brain.*** The entire arterial blood supply to the brain, with the exception of a small amount that flows in the anterior spinal artery to the medulla, is carried through the neck by four vessels: the two

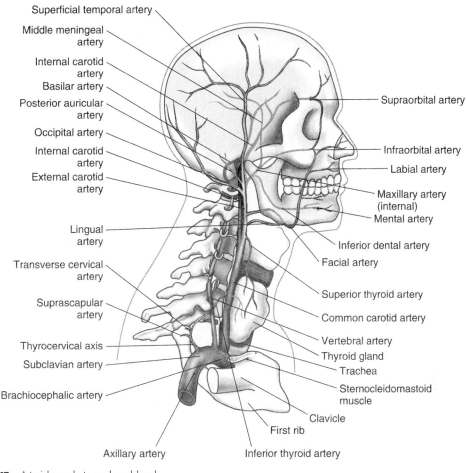

**Fig. 10-17** Arterial supply to neck and head.

vertebral arteries and the two carotid arteries (Figs. 10-17 and 10-18).

The two vertebral arteries supply the posterior portion of the brain. They ascend in the neck through the transverse foramina on each side of the cervical vertebrae, enter the skull through the foramen magnum, and anastomose near the pons to form the basilar artery of the hindbrain. A relatively small volume of the total blood flow to the brain is carried by the vertebral or basilar artery. The circle of Willis, in turn, is formed by the union of the basilar artery and the two internal carotid arteries. Before they join the circle of Willis, these arteries send essential branches to the brainstem, cerebellum, and falx cerebelli.

The circle of Willis is a ring of blood vessels that surrounds the optic chiasm and the pituitary stalk. The following three pairs of large arterial vessels that supply the cerebral cortex originate from the circle of Willis: the anterior, the middle, and the posterior cerebral arteries. Each pair of arteries supplies specific areas of the brain: (1) the anterior cerebral arteries supply about half of the frontal and parietal

lobes, including much of the corpus callosum; (2) the middle cerebral arteries perfuse most of the lateral surfaces of the hemispheres and send off branches to the corpus striatum and the internal capsule; and (3) the posterior cerebral arteries supply the occipital lobes and the remaining portions of the temporal lobes that are not supplied by the middle cerebral arteries.

***Regulation of Cerebral Blood Flow.*** The CNS has a complex and structurally diverse system for facilitation of appropriate cerebral blood flow. With the advent of positron emission tomography (PET) and magnetic resonance imaging (MRI), studies are being conducted to investigate these most specialized vascular beds.

**Intracranial Pressure Dynamics.** Intracranial pressure (ICP) is that pressure exerted against the skull by its contents: CSF, blood, and brain. The volumes of these contents may fluctuate slightly, but, despite variations, the total volume and ICP remain nearly constant. Compensatory mechanisms account for this stability in the overall ICP.

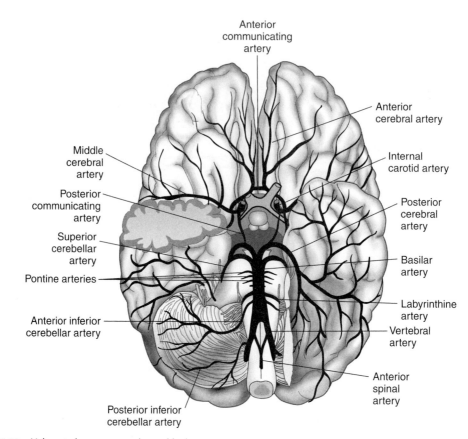

**Fig. 10-18**    Major arteries as seen on base of brain.

In health, the CSF pressure system is dynamic and allows the pressure to vary only slightly by means of a compensatory mechanism that shunts CSF into the spinal subarachnoid space. The spinal dura covers the cord loosely and does not adhere to the vertebrae, which allows it to expand, whereas the cranial dura cannot. When CSF pressure becomes too great within the cranium because of an increase in volume of any of its contents, CSF is shunted out of the cranium, thus decreasing cranial volume and CSF pressure. In addition, CSF may be absorbed at an increased rate, which further aids in maintenance of normal pressure.

Autoregulation of cerebral blood volume is a compensatory mechanism responsible for maintenance of cerebral perfusion pressure (CPP) at a constant level. It is an alteration in the diameter of the resistance vessels aimed at maintaining a constant perfusion pressure during changes in blood flow. When autoregulation is intact, vasodilatation occurs in response to moderate degrees of hypercapnia, hypoxia, hyperthermia, and increased ICP. The normal ICP ranges from 4 to 15 mm Hg. Normal CPP is 100 to 90 mm Hg.

In normal conditions, CPP and resultant blood flow are determined by the difference between the inflow and the outflow pressures. Inflow pressures are represented by the mean systemic arterial pressure (MSAP), and in normal conditions, the mean outflow pressure is equivalent to the mean venous pressure. In situations in which ICP is greater than venous pressure, the following equation applies:

$$CPP = MSAP - ICP$$

That any increase in ICP or reduction in MSAP reduces CPP and the resulting cerebral blood flow is readily apparent.[1]

Autoregulation is capable of maintaining a constant CPP only until the finite limit of CSF compensation is reached (Fig. 10-19). The spinal subarachnoid space is capable of holding only a limited amount of fluid, and, despite its inability to hold any additional displaced fluid, autoregulation continues. In this event, autoregulation ceases to be beneficial or effective in prevention of further increases in ICP.

## Spinal Cord
### *Protection of the Spinal Cord*
**Bones of the Spine.** The spine is composed of a series of irregular bony vertebrae "stacked" one atop the other to form a strong but flexible

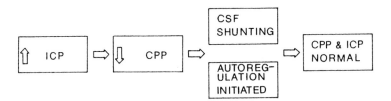

**Fig. 10-19** Cerebrospinal fluid shunting and autoregulation as effective compensatory mechanisms. *ICP,* Intracranial pressure; *CPP,* cerebral perfusion pressure; *CSF,* cerebrospinal fluid.

column. They are joined by a series of ligaments and intervening cartilages and have two primary functions. Together these structures support the head and trunk. The spine also protects the spinal cord and its 31 pairs of spinal nerve roots by encasing them in a long canal formed by openings in the center of each vertebra. This vertebral canal extends the entire length of the spine and conforms to the various spinal curvatures and to the variations in size of the spinal cord itself.

Seven cervical, 12 thoracic, and five lumbar vertebrae exist. In the adult, the sacrum consists of five vertebrae fused to form one bone. Similarly, the coccyx results from the fusion of four or five rudimentary vertebrae.

Despite variations in their structure, all but two vertebrae share certain anatomic and functional aspects. With the exception of C1 and C2, all have a solid drum-shaped body that serves anteriorly as the weight-bearing segment. The posterior segment of the vertebra is called the arch, and each one comprises two pedicles, two laminae, and seven processes (four articular, two transverse, and one spinous). Projecting from the upper part of the body of each vertebra is a pair of short thick pedicles. The concavities above and below the pedicles are the four intervertebral notches. When the vertebrae are articulated, the notches in each adjacent pair of bones form the oval intervertebral foramina, which communicate with the vertebral canal and transmit the spinal nerves and blood vessels.

Arising from the pedicles are two broad plates of bone, the laminae, which meet and fuse at the midline posteriorly to form an arch. Projecting backward and downward from this junction is the spinous process, a knobby projection easily palpated under the skin of the back. Lateral to the laminae, near their junction with the pedicles, are paired articular processes, which facilitate movement of the vertebral column. The two superior processes of each vertebra articulate with the inferior processes of the vertebra immediately above it. The small surfaces where they articulate are called facets. The transverse processes are located somewhat anterior to the junction of the pedicles and the laminae. They are

between the superior and inferior articular processes. These and the spinous processes provide sites for the attachment of muscles and ligaments. The hollow opening formed by the body of the vertebra and the arch is termed the *vertebral foramen,* a protected space through which the spinal cord passes.

Between each of the vertebrae and atop the sacrum is an intervertebral disk composed of compressible tough fibrous cartilage concentrically arranged around a soft pulpy substance called the nucleus pulposus. Each disk acts as a cushion-like shock absorber between the vertebrae. When the intervertebral disk is ruptured, the soft nucleus pulposus may protrude into the vertebral canal, where it can exert pressure on a spinal nerve root and cause disturbances in motor and sensory functions. This herniated nucleus pulposus may require surgical excision through a laminectomy, if the herniation is severe enough.

Many important variations exist among the regional vertebrae. For example, the first cervical vertebra, or atlas, is ring-shaped and supports the cranium. It has no body or spinous process and allows for nodding motion of the head. The second cervical vertebra, or axis, is most striking because of the odontoid process, or dens, that arises perpendicularly to articulate with the atlas and allows rotation of the head. The cervical spine as a whole is extremely mobile and is therefore particularly susceptible to acceleration-deceleration and torsion injuries that hyperflex or hyperextend the neck. Also, the spinal cord is relatively large in this area and therefore sustains damage fairly easily after injury to the cervical spine (Fig. 10-20).

The 12 thoracic vertebrae increase in size as they approach the lumbar area. They are distinctive in that they have facets on their transverse processes and bodies for articulation with the ribs. The thoracic spine is fixed by the ribs, but the lumbar spine is not, which creates a vulnerability that is responsible for an increased incidence rate of fracture-dislocation at T12, L1, and L2. These injuries are typically found in motor vehicle accident victims who were wearing lap seatbelts without shoulder restraints.

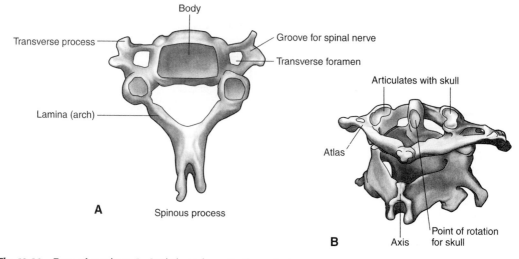

**Fig. 10-20**   Types of vertebrae. **A,** Cervical vertebrae; **B,** atlas and axis.

The five lumbar vertebrae are large and massive because of their prominent role in weight bearing. They have no transverse foramina. The sacrum, with its five fused vertebrae, is large, triangular, and wedge-shaped. It forms the posterior wall of the pelvis and articulates with L5, the coccyx, and the iliac portions of the hips. The triangular coccyx is formed by four small segments of bone, the most rudimentary part of the vertebral column.

**Spinal Meninges.** In addition to the bony vertebral column, the spinal cord is covered and protected by the continuous downward projection of the three meninges that perform the same protective function for the brain. The dura mater is the outermost membrane and is a strong but loose and expandable sheath of dense fibrous connective tissue that ends in a blind sac at the end of the second or third segment of the sacrum and protects the cord and the spinal nerve roots as they leave the cord. The dura does not extend beyond the intervertebral foramina. As noted previously, the spinal dura differs from the cranial dura in that the spinal dura is not attached to the surrounding bone, consists of only one layer, and does not send partitions into the fissures of the cord.

The epidural space is located between the outer surface of the dura and the bones of the vertebral canal. It contains a quantity of loose areolar connective tissue and a plexus of veins. The subdural space is a potential space that lies below the inner surface of the dura and the arachnoid membrane. It contains only a limited amount of CSF.

The middle meningeal layer is the arachnoid membrane, which is thin, delicate, and nonvascular; it is continuous with the cranial arachnoid and follows the spinal dura to the end of the dural sac. For the most part, the dura and arachnoid are unconnected, although they are in contact with each other.

The arachnoid is attached to the pia mater by delicate filaments of connective tissue. The considerable space between these two meningeal layers is called the subarachnoid space. It is continuous with that of the cranium and is largest at the lower end of the spinal canal, where it encloses the masses of nerves that form the cauda equina. The spinal subarachnoid space contains an abundant amount of CSF and is capable of expansion to the point of completely filling the entire space included in the dura mater. It plays a vital role in the regulation of ICP by allowing for the shunting of CSF away from the cranium. When spinal anesthesia is used, the local anesthetic agent is deposited into the subarachnoid space. Because the CSF in the subarachnoid space bathes the spinal nerves before they exit, the local anesthetic effectively blocks spinal nerve conduction.

The third and innermost meningeal layer of the spine is the delicate pia mater. Although it is continuous with the cranial pia mater, it is less vascular, thicker, and denser in structure than the pia mater of the brain. The pia mater intimately invests the entire surface of the cord, and, at the point where the cord terminates, it contracts and continues down as a long slender filament (central ligament) through the center of the bundle of nerves of the cauda equina and anchors the cord at the base of the coccyx.

*Lumbar Puncture.* The examination of CSF and determination of CSF pressure are frequently of great value in the diagnosis of neurologic and neurosurgical conditions. The collection of CSF is ordinarily accomplished through the insertion of a long spinal needle between L3 and L4 or L4 and L5, through the dura and arachnoid into the subarachnoid space. Because the spinal cord in adults ends at the level of the disk between L1 and L2, danger of injuring the cord with this procedure is minimal. In children, the spinal cord may extend below L3 so that the subarachnoid space is usually safely entered in the areas between L4 and L5. In both adults and children, flexion of the spine raises the cord superiorly somewhat farther, thus minimizing the risk of damage to the cord. Because the most superior points of the iliac crests are at the level of the upper border of the spine of L4, they are used as anatomic reference points in selection of the site for lumbar puncture. For a complete description of spinal and epidural anesthesia, please see Chapter 25.

*Structure and Function of the Spinal Cord and the Spinal Nerve Roots.* The lowest level of the functional integration of information in the CNS takes place in the spinal cord. Here, information is received in the form of afferent (sensory) nerve impulses from the periphery of the body. This information may be processed locally within the cord but more often is relayed to higher brain centers for additional processing and modification, thus resulting in sophisticated and elaborate motor (efferent) responses. A discussion of the spinal cord primarily involves the consideration of its function as a relay system for both afferent and efferent impulses.

The spinal cord is the elongated slightly ovoid mass of central nervous tissue that occupies the upper two thirds of the vertebral canal. In the adult, it is approximately 45 cm (17 in) long, although this length varies somewhat from individual to individual depending on the length of the trunk. The cord is actually an inferior extension of the medulla oblongata and begins at the level of the foramen magnum of the occipital bone.

From that point, the cord continues downward to the upper level of the body of L2, where it narrows to a sharp tip called the conus medullaris. From the end of the conus, an extension of the pia mater known as the filum terminale continues to the first segment of the coccyx, where it attaches (Fig. 10-21).

The small central canal of the spinal cord contains CSF. This cavity extends the entire length of the cord and communicates directly

PHYSIOLOGIC CONSIDERATIONS IN THE PACU

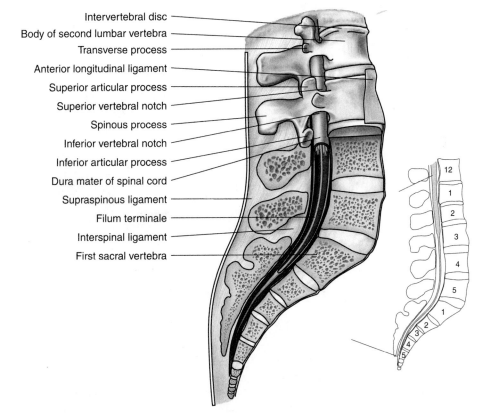

Intervertebral disc
Body of second lumbar vertebra
Transverse process
Anterior longitudinal ligament
Superior articular process
Superior vertebral notch
Spinous process
Inferior vertebral notch
Inferior articular process
Dura mater of spinal cord
Supraspinous ligament
Filum terminale
Interspinal ligament
First sacral vertebra

**Fig. 10-21**  Vertebral column showing structure of vertebrae, filum terminale, and termination of dura mater.

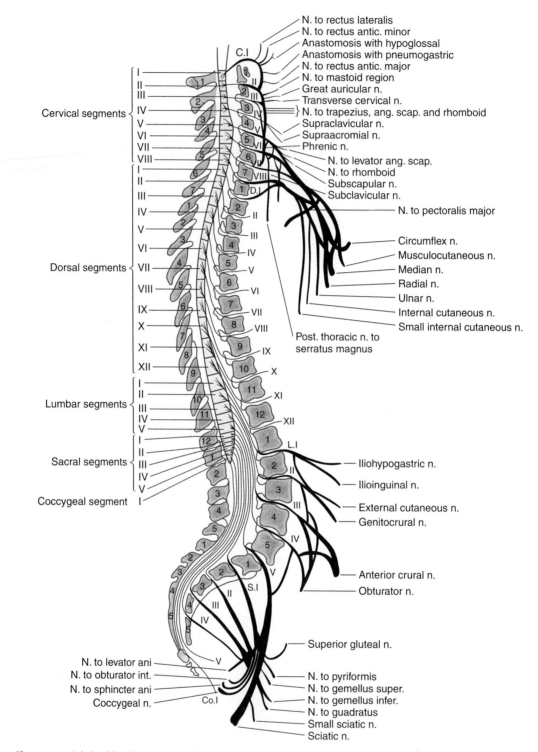

**Fig. 10-22**  Relationship of segments of spinal cord and their nerve roots to bodies and spinous processes of vertebrae.

with the fourth ventricle of the medulla oblongata.

The spinal cord (Fig. 10-22) is composed of 31 horizontal segments of varying lengths. It comprises 10 cervical, 12 thoracic, 5 lumbar, 5 sacral, and 1 coccygeal segment, each with a corresponding pair of spinal nerves attached.

During the growth of the fetus and young child, the spinal cord does not continue to lengthen as the vertebral column lengthens.

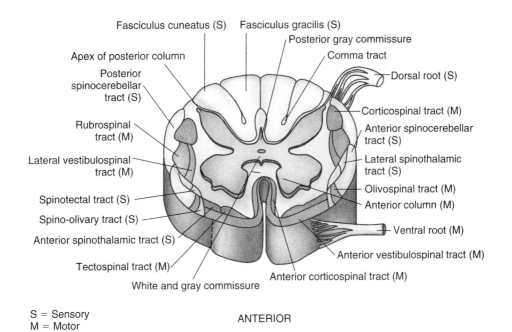

Fasciculus cuneatus (S)   Fasciculus gracilis (S)

Posterior gray commissure

Comma tract

Apex of posterior column

Posterior spinocerebellar tract (S)

Dorsal root (S)

Rubrospinal tract (M)

Corticospinal tract (M)

Anterior spinocerebellar tract (S)

Lateral vestibulospinal tract (M)

Lateral spinothalamic tract (S)

Olivospinal tract (M)

Spinotectal tract (S)

Anterior column (M)

Spino-olivary tract (S)

Anterior spinothalamic tract (S)

Ventral root (M)

Tectospinal tract (M)

Anterior vestibulospinal tract (M)

White and gray commissure

Anterior corticospinal tract (M)

S = Sensory
M = Motor

ANTERIOR

**Fig. 10-23**   Major ascending and descending tracts of spinal cord.

PHYSIOLOGIC CONSIDERATIONS IN THE PACU

Consequently, the cord segments, from which spinal nerves originate, are displaced upward from their corresponding vertebrae. This discrepancy becomes greater with each downward segment. For example, the cervical and thoracic nerve roots take an almost horizontal course as they leave the spinal cord and emerge through the intervertebral foramina. The lumbar and sacral nerve roots, however, are extremely long and take an oblique downward course before finally emerging from their appropriate lumbar or sacral intervertebral foramina. The large bundle of nerves lying within the inferior vertebral canal is called the cauda equina for its resemblance to a horse's tail (see Fig. 10-22). Several longitudinal grooves divide the spinal cord into regions. The deepest of these grooves is the anterior median fissure. Opposite this, on the posterior surface of the cord, is the posterior median fissure. These divide the cord into symmetric right and left halves that are joined in the central midportion (Fig. 10-23).

Like the brain, the spinal cord comprises areas of gray matter and areas of white matter. Unlike the locations in the brain, the gray matter of the cord is situated deep in its center, whereas the white matter is on the surface. The gray matter of the cord is composed of large masses of nerve cell bodies, along with dendrites of association and efferent neurons and unmyelinated axons, all embedded in a framework of neuroglia cells. The gray matter is also rich in blood vessels. The gray matter has two main functions: 1, synapses within the gray matter relay signals between the periphery and the brain, sometimes via the white matter of the cord; and 2, nuclei in the gray matter also function as centers for all spinal reflexes and even integrate some motor activities within the cord itself (such as the "knee-jerk" stretch reflex).

The white matter of the cord completely invests the gray matter. It consists primarily of long myelinated axons in a network of neuroglia and blood vessels. Its fibers are arranged into bundles called tracts, columns, or pathways that pass up and down, linking various segments of the cord and connecting the spinal cord with the brain, thus integrating and coordinating sensory and motor functions to or from any level of the CNS.

When viewed in cross section, the gray matter of the cord looks like the letter H, two crescent-shaped halves joined together by the gray commissure surrounded by white matter. For descriptive purposes, the four segments of the H are called right and left anterior (ventral) and posterior (dorsal) horns. The anterior motor (efferent) neurons lie within the anterior (ventral) gray horns and send fibers through the spinal nerves to the skeletal muscle. The nerve cell bodies that make up the posterior (dorsal) gray horns receive sensory (afferent) signals from the periphery via the spinal nerve roots. The lateral gray horns project from the intermediate portion of the H. The nerve cells in these horns (called preganglionic autonomic neurons) give rise to fibers that lead to the autonomic nervous system.

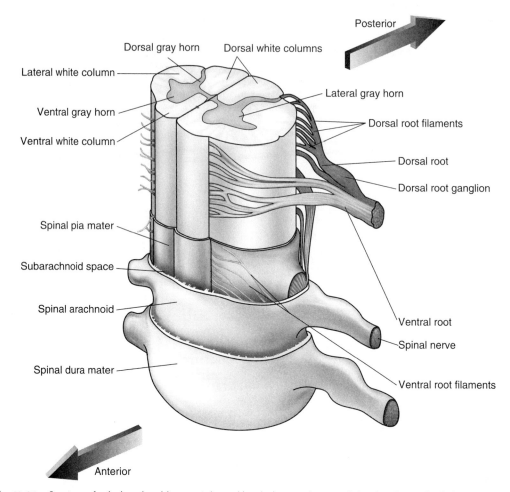

**Fig. 10-24**    Structure of spinal cord and its connections with spinal nerves by way of dorsal and ventral spinal roots. Note also spinal pia mater, spinal arachnoid, and spinal dura mater, which are known as meninges, or coverings of spinal cord. (*Redrawn from Guyton AC:* Basic neuroscience: anatomy and physiology, *ed 2, Philadelphia, 1991, Saunders.*)

The white matter of each half of the cord is divided into the following three columns (or funiculi): the ventral, the lateral, and the dorsal. Each column is subdivided into tracts, which are large bundles of nerve fibers that are arranged in functional groups. The ascending or sensory projection tracts transmit impulses to the brain, and the descending or motor projection tracts transmit impulses away from the brain to various levels of the spinal cord. Some short tracts travel up or down the cord for only a few segments of the cord. These propriospinal (association or intersegmental) tracts connect and integrate separate cord segments of gray matter with one another and consequently have important roles in the completion of various spinal reflexes.

The 31 pairs of spinal nerves are symmetrically arranged. Each nerve contains several types of fibers and arises from the spinal cord by two roots: a posterior (dorsal) and an anterior (ventral) root (Fig. 10-24). The axons that make up the fibers in the anterior roots originate from the cell bodies and dendrites in the anterior and lateral gray horns. The anterior (ventral) root is the motor root, which conveys impulses from the CNS to the skeletal muscles. The posterior (dorsal) root is known as the sensory root. Sensory fibers originate in the posterior root ganglia of the spinal nerves. Each ganglion is an oval enlargement of the root that lies just medial to the intervertebral foramen and contains the accumulated cell bodies of the axons that make up the sensory fibers. One branch of the ganglion extends into the posterior gray horn of the cord. The other branch is distributed to both visceral and somatic organs and mediates afferent impulses to the CNS. The cutaneous (skin) area innervated by a single posterior root is called a dermatome. Knowledge of dermatome levels is useful clinically in determination of the level of anesthesia after spinal or regional anesthesia (see Chapter 25).

The lateral gray horns of the spinal cord give rise to fibers that lead into the autonomic nervous system, which controls many of the internal (visceral) organs. Sympathetic fibers from the thoracic and lumbar cord segments are distributed throughout the body to the viscera, blood vessels, glands, and smooth muscle. Parasympathetic fibers, present in the middle three sacral nerves, innervate the pelvic and abdominal viscera. Hence, the ventral (anterior) root of the spinal nerve is often called the motor root, although it is also responsible for the preganglionic output of the autonomic nervous system.

The anterior and posterior roots extend to the intervertebral foramen that correspond to their spinal cord segment of origin. As they reach the foramen, the two roots unite to form a single mixed spinal nerve that contains both motor and sensory fibers. As the nerve emerges from the foramen, it gives off a small meningeal branch that turns back through the same foramen to innervate the spinal cord membranes, blood vessels, intervertebral ligaments, and spinal joint surfaces. The spinal nerve then branches into two divisions that are called rami. Each ramus contains fibers from both roots. The posterior rami supply the skin and the longitudinal muscles of the back. The larger anterior rami supply the anterior and lateral portions of the trunk and all of the structures of the extremities. However, the anterior rami (except those of the 11 thoracic nerves) do not go directly to their destinations. Instead, they are first rearranged without intervening synapses to form intricate networks of nerve fibers called plexuses.

The five major plexuses are the cervical, brachial, lumbar, sacral, and pudendal. Peripheral nerves emerge from each plexus and are named according to the region that they supply.

The cervical plexus comprises the first four cervical spinal nerves. The phrenic nerve is the most important branch of the cervical plexus because it supplies motor impulses to the diaphragm. Any injury to the spinal cord above the origin of the phrenic nerve (C4) results in paralysis of the diaphragm and death. Selective anesthesia of the brachial or pudendal plexuses is often used in regional anesthesia. With the local anesthetic deposited at or near the brachial plexus, the musculocutaneous, median, ulnar, and radial nerves can be anesthetized, thereby allowing painless surgery from the elbow to the fingers. The pudendal nerve, which supplies motor and sensory fibers to the perineum, can be anesthetized with a pudendal plexus block. This type of nerve block is effective in relieving some of the pain of childbirth. Among the nerves given off by the lumbar plexus are the ilioinguinal, genitofemoral, obturator, and femoral nerves. Among those given off by the sacral plexus are the superior and the inferior gluteal nerves.

Anterior rami from the thoracic area do not form a plexus but lead instead to the skin of the thorax and to the intercostal muscles directly. The thoracic and upper lumbar spinal nerves also give rise to white rami (visceral efferent branches), or preganglionic autonomic nerve fibers. Parts of this ramus join the spinal nerves to the sympathetic trunk. The gray ramus is present in all spinal nerves.

The term *final common pathway* is often seen in literature. It refers to the motor neurons in the anterior gray horns. All excitatory or inhibitory impulses that control movement, from the cerebral cortex to the proprioceptors, influence the motor neurons of the anterior horn either directly or indirectly. Thus, all neural impulses that arise in receptors—and in the brain and spinal cord—must ultimately converge in this area before movement of skeletal muscle can be integrated. Hence, the term final common pathway.

*Vascular Network of the Spinal Cord.* The spinal cord derives its rich arterial blood supply from the vertebral arteries and from a series of spinal arteries that enter the cord at successive levels. Segmentally, the spinal arteries that enter the intervertebral foramina are given off by the intercostal vessels and by the lateral sacral, iliolumbar, inferior thyroid, and vertebral arteries.

The venous supply inside and outside the entire length of the vertebral canal is derived from a series of venous plexuses (Fig. 10-25) that anastomose with each other and end in intervertebral veins. The intervertebral veins leave the cord through the intervertebral foramina with the spinal nerves.

## AUTONOMIC NERVOUS SYSTEM

The autonomic nervous system is made up of the sympathetic and parasympathetic nervous systems. These two divisions of the autonomic nervous system function to regulate and control the visceral functions of the body. In their regulation and control function, they usually work in opposition to each other. However, recent evidence suggests that these two divisions are as well defined as excitatory or inhibitory, but physiologic regulation and control of these systems by

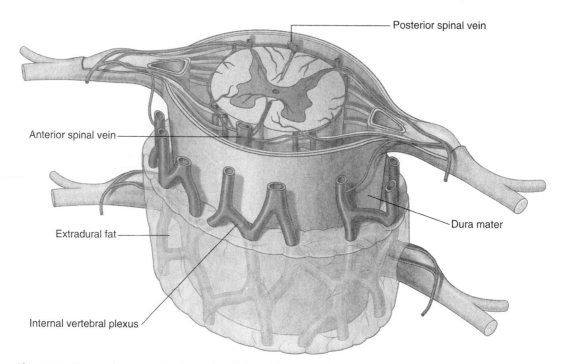

Posterior spinal vein

Anterior spinal vein

Dura mater

Extradural fat

Internal vertebral plexus

**Fig. 10-25**   Venous plexus are veins that drain spinal cord from a number of longitudinal channels that drain into internal vertebral plexus in epidural space of vertebral canal, which then ultimately drains into segmentally arranged vessels that connect with major systemic veins. (*From Drake R, Vogl W, Mitchell A:* Gray's anatomy for students, *Philadelphia, 2005, Churchill Livingstone.*)

virtue of a balance between these two systems does occur.

### Sympathetic Nervous System

The sympathetic nervous system originates from the thoracolumbar (T1 to L2) segments of the spinal cord. This system is mainly excitatory in physiologic function; however, research indicates that some inhibitory function in the sympathetic nervous system does exist. Because the sympathetic nervous system involves the cardiovascular system and cardiovascular drugs, it is discussed in detail in Chapter 11.

### Parasympathetic Nervous System

The parasympathetic nervous system basically functions as an inhibitor of the sympathetic nervous system. It originates in the cranium via cranial nerves III, V, VII, IX, and X. Cranial nerve X, or the vagus nerve, is the most important nerve because it carries about 75% of the parasympathetic nerve impulses. The parasympathetic nervous system also originates in the sacral portion of the spinal cord. Consequently, the parasympathetic nervous system uses the craniosacral outflow tracts. Because of the pharmacologic implications of the parasympathetic nervous system, it is discussed in detail in Chapters 11 and 23.

## SUMMARY

This chapter demonstrates the physiologic concept of regulation and control. The nervous system is quite complex, with both central and peripheral components working in concert. It has electric and chemical neurotransmitters that in many ways functions best in a homeostatic environment. Should the body suffer injury or change in fluid status or temperature, to name a few examples, the nervous system does not function appropriately. Consequently, evaluation of the nervous system by the perianesthesia nurse is an important component of nursing care in the PACU.

## BIBLIOGRAPHY

Aitkenhead A, Smith G, Rowbotham D: *Textbook of anaesthesia,* ed 5, Philadelphia, 2007, Churchill Livingstone.

Alspach J: *Core curriculum for critical care nursing,* ed 6, Philadelphia, 2005, Saunders.

Atlee J: *Complications in anesthesia,* ed 2, Philadelphia, 2007, Saunders.

Barash P, Cullen B, Stoelting R: *Clinical anesthesia,* ed 5, Philadelphia, 2001, Lippincott Williams & Wilkins.

Benumof J, Saidman L: *Anesthesia & perioperative complications*, ed 2, St Louis, 1999, Mosby.

Brunton L, Lazo J, Parker K: *Goodman and Gilman's the pharmacological basis of therapeutics*, ed 11, New York, 2005, McGraw-Hill Professional.

Cote C, Todres I, Goudsouzian N, et al: *A practice of anesthesia for infants and children*, ed 3, Philadelphia, 2001, Saunders.

Cottrell J, Smith D: *Anesthesia and neurosurgery*, ed 4, St Louis, 2001, Mosby.

Drake R, Vogl W, Mitchell A: *Gray's anatomy for students*, Philadelphia, 2005, Churchill Livingstone.

Estafanous F, Barash P, Reves J, editors: *Cardiac anesthesia: principles and clinical practice*, ed 2, Philadelphia, 2001, Lippincott Williams & Wilkins.

Evers A, Maze M: *Anesthetic pharmacology: physiologic principles and clinical practice*, Philadelphia, 2004, Churchill Livingstone.

Fisher L: *Benumof's anesthesia and uncommon diseases*, ed 5, Philadelphia, 2007, Saunders.

Gallager C, Issenberg B: *Simulation in anesthesia*, Philadelphia, 2007, Saunders.

Ganong W: *Review of medical physiology*, ed 22, New York, 2005, McGraw-Hill Medical.

Guyton A, Hall J: *Textbook of medical physiology*, ed 11, Philadelphia, 2006, Saunders.

Kaplan J, editor: *Thoracic anesthesia*, ed 2, New York, 1991, Churchill Livingstone.

Kier L, Dowd C: *The chemistry of drugs for nurse anesthetists*, Chicago, 2004, AANA Publishing, Inc.

Lake C, Hines R, Blitt C: *Clinical monitoring: practical applications for anesthesia and critical care*, Philadelphia, 2001, Saunders.

Longnecker D, Murphy F: *Dripps, Eckenhoff, Vandam introduction to anesthesia*, ed 9, Philadelphia, 1997, Saunders.

Longnecker D, Tinker J, Morgan G: *Principles and practice of anesthesiology*, ed 2, St Louis, 1991, Mosby.

Miller R, editor: *Anesthesia*, ed 5, Philadelphia, 2000, Churchill Livingstone.

Murray J, Nadel J: *Textbook of respiratory medicine*, ed 2, Philadelphia, 1994, Saunders.

Nagelhout J, Zaglaniczy K: *Nurse anesthesia*, ed 3, St Louis, 2005, Saunders.

Shorten G, Browne J, Carr D, et al: *Postoperative pain management: an evidence-based guide to practice*, Philadelphia, 2006, Saunders.

Stoelting R: *Pharmacology and physiology in anesthetic practice*, ed 3, Philadelphia, 1999, Lippincott-Raven.

Stoelting R, Miller R: *Basics of anesthesia*, ed 4, Philadelphia, 2000, Churchill Livingstone.

Townsend C, Beauchamp R, Evers B, et al: *Sabiston textbook of surgery: the biological basis of modern surgical practice*, ed 17, Philadelphia, 2004, Saunders.

PHYSIOLOGIC CONSIDERATIONS IN THE PACU

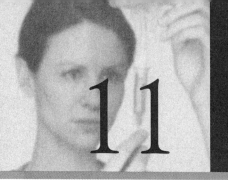

# 11

# THE CARDIOVASCULAR SYSTEM

*Cecil B. Drain, PhD, RN, CRNA, FAAN, FASAHP*

The cardiovascular system has a significant impact on the patient recovering from anesthesia. A most helpful aspect of the cardiovascular system is the many ways we have to monitor its status. This system also reflects the status of the patient in the postanesthesia care unit (PACU). More specifically, a return to normal values by the cardiovascular system is a good indicator of the progression of emergence of the patient from anesthesia.

Also, many drugs used for anesthesia depend on the cardiovascular system to produce their effects. Many of the same drugs also have effects on the cardiovascular system. Therefore, the perianesthesia nurse must understand the physiologic principles that relate to the cardiovascular status of the patient in the PACU who has received an anesthetic.

The basic anatomy of certain structures of the cardiovascular system is not covered completely in this chapter because basic nursing texts provide ample material on this subject. However, the clinical correlation between the physiology of the cardiovascular system and perianesthesia nursing care is provided throughout the chapter.

## DEFINITIONS

**Adrenergic:** A term that describes nerve fibers that liberate norepinephrine.

**Afterload:** The impedance to left ventricular ejection. The afterload is expressed as total peripheral resistance (TPR).

**Angina Pectoris:** Chest pain caused by myocardial ischemia.

**Arrhythmia:** An abnormal rhythm of the heart, also referred to as dysrhythmia.

**Arteriosclerosis:** Degenerative changes in the arterial walls that result in thickening and loss of elasticity.

**Automaticity:** The ability of the cardiac pacemaker cells to undergo depolarization spontaneously.

**Bathmotropic:** Affecting the response of cardiac muscle (or any tissue) to stimuli.

**Bigeminy:** A premature beat along with a normal heart beat.

**Bradycardia:** A heart rate of 60 bpm or less.

**Cardiac Arrest:** Ventricular standstill.

**Cardiac Index:** A "corrected" cardiac output used to compare patients with different body sizes. The cardiac index (CI) equals the cardiac output (CO) divided by the body surface area (BSA).

**Cardiac Output:** The amount of blood pumped to the peripheral circulation per minute.

**Cholinergic:** Describes nerve fibers that liberate acetylcholine.

**Chronotropic:** Affecting the rate of the heart.

**Conduction:** Movement of cardiac impulses through specialized conduction systems of the heart that facilitate coordinated contraction of the heart.

**Cor Pulmonale:** Pulmonary hypertension as a result of obstruction of the pulmonary circulation that causes right ventricular hypertrophy.

**Cyanosis:** Bluish discoloration, seen especially on the skin and mucus membranes, as a result of a reduced amount of oxygen in the hemoglobin.

**Diastole:** The period of relaxation of the heart, especially of the ventricles.

**Dromotropic:** Affecting the conductivity of a nerve fiber, especially the cardiac nerve fibers.

**Ectopic:** Located away from a normal position; in the heart, a beat that arises from a focus outside the sinus node.

**Ectopic Pacemaker:** Focus of ectopic pacemaker shown as premature contractions of the heart that occur between normal beats.

**Electrolyte:** An ionic substance found in the blood.

**Embolism:** A blood clot or other substance, such as lipid material, in the blood stream.

**Excitability:** The ability of cardiac cells to respond to a stimulus with depolarization.

**Exsanguinate:** To deprive of blood.

**Fibrillation:** An ineffectual quiver of the atria or ventricles.

**Flutter:** A condition, usually atrial, in which the atria contract 200 to 400 bpm.

**Heart Block (complete):** A condition that results when conduction is blocked by a lesion at any level in the atrioventricular junction.

**Hypertension:** Persistently elevated blood pressure.

**Hypervolemia:** An abnormally large amount of blood in the circulatory system.

**Infarction:** A necrotic area as a result of an obstruction of a vessel.

**Inotropic:** Affecting the force of contraction of muscle fibers, especially those of the heart.

**Ischemia:** Local tissue hypoxia from decreased blood flow.

**Leukocytosis:** Increased number of white blood cells; a white blood cell count higher than 10,000 per $mm^3$.

**Leukopenia:** Decreased number of white blood cells; a white blood cell count lower than 5000 per $mm^3$.

**Murmur:** An abnormal heart sound heard during systole, diastole, or both.

**Myocardium:** The muscular middle layer of the heart between the inner endocardium and the outer epicardium.

**Normotensive:** With a normal blood pressure.

**Occlusion:** An obstruction of a blood vessel by a clot or foreign substance.

**Pacemaker:** The area in which the cardiac rate commences, normally at the sinoatrial node.

**Palpitation:** A patient's abnormal rate, rhythm, or fluttering of the heart.

**Paroxysmal Tachycardia:** A period of rapid heart beats that begins and ends abruptly.

**Pericarditis:** An inflammation of the pericardium.

**Peripheral Resistance:** Resistance to blood flow in the microcirculation.

**Polycythemia:** An excessive number of red blood cells, which is reflected in an abnormally high hematocrit level.

**Preexcitation Syndrome:** When the atrial impulse bypasses the atrioventricular node to produce early excitation of the ventricle.

**Preload:** The left ventricular end-diastolic volume (LVEDV).

**Pulse Deficit:** The difference between the apical and radial pulses.

**Reentry (circus movement):** Reexcitation of cardiac tissue by the return of the same cardiac impulse via a circuitous pathway.

**Syncope:** Fainting, giddiness, and momentary unconsciousness, usually caused by cerebral anoxia.

**Systole:** The period of contraction of the heart, especially the ventricles.

**Thrombosis:** The formation of a clot (thrombus) inside a blood vessel or a chamber of the heart.

# THE HEART

## The Cardiac Cycle

The heart is a four-chambered mass of muscle that pulsates rhythmically and pumps blood into the circulatory system. The chambers of the heart are the atria and the ventricles. The atria, which are pathways for blood into the ventricles, are thin walled, have myocardial muscle, and are divided into the right and left atria by a partition. During each cardiac cycle, approximately 70% of the blood flows from the great veins through the atria and into the ventricles before the atria contract. The other 30% is pumped into the ventricles when the atria contract. On contraction of the right atrium, the pressure in the heart is 4 to 6 mm Hg. The contraction of the left atrium produces a pressure of 6 to 8 mm Hg.

Three pressure elevations are produced by the atria, as depicted on the atrial pressure curve. They are termed the a, c, and v waves (Fig. 11-1). The a wave is a result of atrial contraction. The c wave is produced by both the bulging of atrioventricular (AV) valves and the pulling of the atrial muscle when the ventricles contract. The v wave occurs near the end of the ventricular contraction as the amount of blood in the atria slowly increases and the AV valves close.

The ventricles receive blood from the atria and then act as pumps to move blood through the circulatory system. During the initial third of diastole, the AV valves open and blood rushes into the ventricles. This phase is called the period of rapid filling of the ventricles. The middle third of diastole is referred to as diastasis, during which a small amount of blood moves into the ventricles. During the final third of diastole, the atria contract and the other 30% of the ventricles fills. As the ventricles contract, the AV valves contract and then close, thereby preventing blood from flowing into the ventricles from the atria.

As the ventricles begin to contract during systole, the pressure inside the ventricles increases, but no emptying of the ventricles occurs. During this time, called the period of isometric contraction, the AV valves are closed. As the right ventricular pressure rises to more than 8 mm Hg and the left ventricular pressure exceeds 80 mm Hg, the valves open to allow the blood to leave the ventricles. This period, termed the period of ejection, consumes the first three quarters of systole. The remaining fourth quarter is referred to as protodiastole, when almost no blood leaves the ventricles yet the ventricular muscle remains contracted. The ventricles then relax, and the

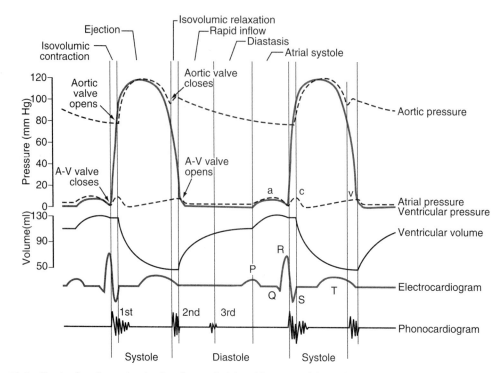

**Fig. 11-1**   Events of cardiac cycle, showing changes in left atrial pressure, left ventricular pressure, aortic pressure, ventricular volume, electrocardiogram, and phonocardiogram. (*From Guyton A, Hall J:* Textbook of medical physiology, *ed 10, Philadelphia, 2000, Saunders.*)

pressure in the large arteries pushes blood back toward the ventricles, which forces the aortic and pulmonary valves to close. This phase is the period of isometric relaxation.

At the end of diastole, each ventricle usually contains approximately 120 mL of blood–the end-diastolic volume. During systole, each ventricle ejects 70 mL of blood, which is the stroke volume. The blood that remains in the ventricle at the end of systole is end-systolic volume and amounts to approximately 50 mL.

### Cardiac Output

Cardiac output is the amount of blood ejected from the left or right ventricle in 1 minute. In the normal adult with a heart rate of 70 bpm, the cardiac output is approximately 4900 mL. This estimate can be derived with taking the rate of 70 times the stroke volume of 70 mL. User-friendly sophisticated equipment is now available to monitor a patient's cardiac output in the PACU. The information derived from serial measurements of the cardiac output can be helpful in assessment of the general status of the cardiovascular system and in determination of the appropriate amount and type of fluid therapy for the patient.

The cardiac output is measured with a variety of techniques. Kaplan suggests that the thermodilution method, which uses the Swan-Ganz catheter, is the clinical method of choice. For a higher degree of reproducibility, Kaplan recommends a technique of standardization in which the injectate temperature and volume, and the speed of injection, are carefully controlled and duplicated. The most reproducible results have been obtained with injections of 10 mL of cold (1° C to 2° C) 5% dextrose in water. One should remember that the thermodilution technique measures right-sided cardiac outputs. Hence, measurements of cardiac output with the thermodilution technique are usually unreliable for patients with intracardiac shunts.

Other methods of calculation of the cardiac output are the Fick and Stewart techniques. The Fick technique involves calculations of the amount of blood needed to carry oxygen taken up from the alveoli per unit of time. This technique is said to be accurate within a 10% margin of error. In the Stewart technique, a known quantity of dye is injected and its concentration is measured after the dye is dispersed per unit of time.

Cardiac output can be influenced by venous return. As the Frank-Starling law of the heart states, "The heart pumps all the blood that it receives so that damming of the blood does not occur." If the heart receives an extra amount of blood from the veins (↑ preload), the cardiac muscle becomes stretched and the stretched muscle contracts with an increased force to pump the extra blood out of the heart. If the heart receives less blood than normal (↓ preload), according to the Frank-Starling law of the heart, it contracts with less force. This concept is important to the perianesthesia nurse. For example, if a patient is undergoing mechanical ventilation and too much positive endexpiratory pressure is overinflating the lungs, the increased pressure on the inferior vena cava impedes the venous return to the heart, thereby decreasing blood pressure. The blood pressure is derived from the following interacting factors: the force of the heart, the peripheral resistance, the volume of blood, the viscosity of blood, and the elasticity of the arteries. Thus, cardiac output can be seen to play a major role in the maintenance of a normal blood pressure.

### Arterial Blood Pressure

The arterial blood pressure consists of the systolic and diastolic arterial pressures. The systolic blood pressure is the highest pressure that occurs within an artery during each contraction of the heart. The diastolic blood pressure is the lowest pressure that occurs within an artery during each contraction of the heart. The mean arterial pressure is the average pressure that pushes blood through the systemic circulatory system. Methods of assessment and monitoring of the arterial blood pressure in the PACU are discussed in Chapter 27.

Some factors that affect the arterial blood pressure are the vasomotor center, the renal system, vascular resistance, the endocrine system, and chemical regulation. The vasomotor center, located in the pons and the medulla, has the greatest control over the circulation. This center picks up impulses from all over the body and transmits them down the spinal cord and through vasoconstrictor fibers to most vessels of the body. These impulses may be excitatory or inhibitory. One type of pressoreceptor that sends impulses to the vasomotor center is the baroreceptor. The baroreceptors are located in the walls of the major thoracic and neck arteries, in particular, the arch of the aorta. When these vessels are stretched by an increased blood pressure, they send inhibitory impulses to the vasomotor center, which lowers the blood pressure. The aortic and carotid bodies located in the bifurcation of the carotid arteries and along the aortic arch can increase systemic pressure when stimulated by a low partial pressure of oxygen in arterial blood ($PaO_2$).

The renal regulation of arterial pressure occurs through the renin-angiotensin-aldosterone mechanism (see Chapter 13).

The vascular resistance of the systemic vascular system can alter systemic pressure. As the total cross-sectional area of an artery decreases, the systemic vascular resistance increases. Therefore, as the blood flows out of the aorta, a decrease in the arterial pressure in each portion of the systemic circulation is directly proportional to the amount of vascular resistance. This principle is the reason that the arterial pressure in the aorta is much higher than the pressure in the arterioles, which have a small cross-sectional area.

The nervous system, when stimulated with exercise or stress, elevates the arterial pressure via sympathetic vasoconstrictor fibers throughout the body.

When the radial artery is to be cannulated for direct monitoring of blood pressure and sampling of arterial blood gases in the PACU, an Allen test should be performed. This test is used for assessment of the risk of hand ischemia if occlusion of the cannulated vessel should occur. The Allen test is performed with the patient making a tight fist, which partially exsanguinates the hand. The nurse then occludes both the radial and the ulnar arteries with digital pressure. The patient is asked to open the hand, and the compressed radial artery is then released. Blushing of the palm (postischemic hyperemia) should be observed. After about a minute, the test should be repeated on the same hand with the nurse now releasing the ulnar artery while continuing to compress the radial artery. If the release of pressure over the ulnar artery does not lead to postischemic hyperemia, the contralateral artery should be similarly evaluated. The results of the Allen test should be reported as "refill time" for each artery.

### Valves of the Heart

The semilunar valves are the aortic and pulmonary valves. They consist of three symmetric valve cusps, which can open to the full diameter of the ring yet provide a perfect seal when closed. During diastole, they prevent backflow from the aorta and pulmonary arteries into the ventricles.

The AV valves are the tricuspid and mitral valves. These valves prevent blood from flowing back into the atria from the ventricles during systole.

Attached to the valves are the chordae tendineae, which are attached to the papillary muscles, which in turn are attached to the endocardium of the ventricles. When the ventricles contract, so do the papillary muscles, thus

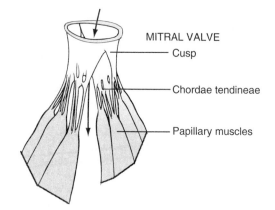

**Fig. 11-2**   Mitral valve and its attachments. (*From Guyton A, Hall J:* Textbook of medical physiology, *ed 10, Philadelphia, 2000, Saunders.*)

pulling the valves toward the ventricles to prevent bulging of the valves into the atria (Fig. 11-2).

## Heart Muscle

The heart muscle comprises three major muscle types: atrial muscle, ventricular muscle, and excitatory and conductive muscle fibers. The atrial and ventricular muscles act much like skeletal muscles. The excitatory and conductive muscles function primarily as an excitatory system for the heart and a transmission system for conduction of impulses throughout the heart.

The cardiac muscle fibers are arranged in a latticework; they divide and then rejoin. The constriction of the cardiac muscle fibers facilitates action potential transmission. The muscle is striated, and the myofibrils contain myosin and actin filaments. Cardiac muscle cells are separated by intercalated disks, which are actually the cardiac cell membranes that separate the cardiac muscle cells from one another.

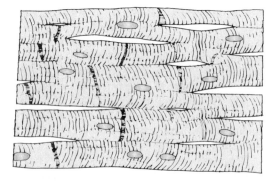

**Fig. 11-3**   "Syncytial" nature of cardiac muscle. (*From Guyton A, Hall J:* Textbook of medical physiology, *ed 10, Philadelphia, 2000, Saunders.*)

The intercalated disks do not hinder conductivity or ionic transport between cardiac muscle cells to any great extent. When the cardiac muscle is stimulated, the action potential spreads to excite all the muscles, which is called a functional syncytium (Fig. 11-3). This functional syncytium can be divided into atrial and ventricular syncytia, which are separated by fibrous tissue. However, an impulse can be transmitted throughout the atrial syncytium and then via the AV bundle to the ventricular syncytium. The "all-or-none" principle is in effect: when one atrial muscle fiber is stimulated, all the atrial muscle fibers react if the action potential is met. This principle applies to the entire ventricular syncytium as well.

The main properties of cardiac muscle are excitability (bathmotropism), contractility (inotropism), rhythmicity and rate (chronotropism), and conductivity (dromotropism). When cardiac muscle is excited, its action potential is reached and the muscle contracts. Certain chemical factors alter the excitability and contractility of cardiac muscle (Box 11-1).

## Conduction of Impulses

Not only does the heart have a special system for generating rhythmic impulses, but this system is able to conduct these impulses throughout the heart. This system for providing rhythmicity and conductivity consists of the sinoatrial (SA) node, the AV node, the AV bundle, and the Purkinje's fibers (Fig. 11-4). The SA node is situated at the posterior wall of the right atrium and just below the opening of the superior vena cava. The SA node generates impulses with self excitation, which is produced by the interaction of sodium and potassium ions. The SA node provides a rhythmic excitation approximately 72 times per minute in the adult at rest. The action potential then spreads throughout the atria to the AV node.

The AV node is located at the base of the wall between the atria. Its primary function is to delay the transmission of the impulses to the ventricles, which allows time for the atria to empty before the ventricles contract. The impulses then travel through the AV bundle, sometimes called the bundle of His. The AV node is able to discharge impulses 40 to 60 times per minute if not stimulated by an outside source.

The Purkinje's fibers originate at the AV node, form the AV bundle, divide into the right and left bundle branches, and spread downward around the ventricles. The Purkinje's fibers can transmit the action potential rapidly, thus allowing immediate transmission of the

## Box 11-1 Chemical Factors that Affect Cardiac Muscle Excitability and Contractility

**CAUSING INCREASE**
High pH
Alkalosis
High calcium concentration

**CAUSING DECREASE**
High potassium concentration
High lactic acid concentration
Acidosis

cardiac impulse throughout the ventricles. The Purkinje's fibers are able to discharge impulses between 15 and 40 times per minute if not stimulated by an outside source.

The parasympathetic nerve endings are distributed mostly at the SA and AV nodes, over the atria, and, to a lesser extent, over the ventricles. If stimulated, they produce a decrease in the rate of rhythm of the SA node and slow the excitability at the AV node. The sympathetic nerves are distributed at the SA and AV nodes and all over the heart, especially the ventricles. Sympathetic stimulation increases the SA node rate of discharge, increases cardiac excitability, and increases the force of contraction.

### Coronary Circulation

The coronary arteries furnish the heart with its blood supply. The main coronary arteries are on the surface of the heart, but smaller arteries

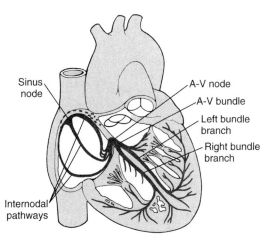

**Fig. 11-4** Sinoatrial node and Purkinje's system of heart. (*From Guyton A, Hall J:* Textbook of medical physiology, *ed 10, Philadelphia, 2000, Saunders.*)

penetrate the heart muscle to provide it with nutrients. The inner surface of the heart derives its nutrition directly from the blood in its chambers.

The coronary arteries originate at two orifices just above the aortic valve. The right coronary artery descends by the right atrium and ventricle and usually terminates as the posterior descending coronary artery. The left coronary artery is usually about 1 cm in length and divides into the anterior descending and circumflex arteries. The anterior descending artery usually terminates at the apex of the heart and anastomoses with the posterior descending artery. The anterior descending artery supplies part of the left ventricle, the apex of the heart, and most of the interventricular septum.

The left circumflex artery descends posteriorly and inferiorly down to and terminates in the left marginal artery or communicates with the posterior descending coronary artery. Venous drainage is with superficial and deep circuits. The superficial veins empty into either the coronary sinus or the anterior cardiac veins, both of which drain into the right atrium. The deep veins drain into the thebesian or sinusoidal channels.

The regulation of coronary blood flow is determined primarily with the oxygen tension of the cardiac tissues. The most powerful vasodilator of the coronary circulation is hypoxemia. Other factors that may affect coronary blood flow are carbon dioxide, lactate, pyruvate, and potassium, all of which are released from the cardiac muscle. Coronary artery steal occurs when collateral perfusion of the myocardium is significantly reduced by an increase in blood flow to a portion of the myocardium that is normally perfused. More specifically, drug-induced vasodilatation of normal coronary arterioles can then divert or steal blood flow from potentially ischemic areas of the myocardium perfused by the vessels that have increased resistance (atherosclerotic vessels). Coronary artery steal can occur when arteriolar-vasodilating drugs, such as nitroprusside and isoflurane (Forane), are administered. This situation is especially likely to occur in people who are "stealprone"; they constitute about 23% of the patients with coronary artery disease, especially those patients who have significant stenosis and occlusions to one or more coronary arteries.

Stimulation of the parasympathetic nervous system causes an indirect decrease in coronary blood flow. Direct stimulation is slight because of the sparse amount of parasympathetic nerve fibers to the coronary arteries. The sympathetic nervous system serves to increase coronary blood

## Box 11-2   Functional Classification of Cardiac Cases

*Class I*: No limitation. Ordinary physical activity does not cause undue fatigue, dyspnea, palpitation, or angina.

*Class II*: Slight limitation of physical activity. Such patients are comfortable at rest. Ordinary physical activity results in fatigue, palpitation, dyspnea, or angina.

*Class III*: Marked limitation of physical activity. Less than ordinary activity leads to symptoms. Patients are comfortable at rest.

*Class IV*: Inability to carry on any physical activity without discomfort. Symptoms of congestive failure or angina are present even at rest. With any physical activity, increased discomfort is experienced.

Modified from Perloff JK: The clinical manifestations of cardiac failure in adults, *Hospital Practice* 5:43, 1970.

flow both directly (as a result of the action of acetylcholine and norepinephrine) and indirectly (caused by a change in the activity level of the heart). The coronary arteries have both alpha and beta receptors in their walls (see p. 157, Adrenergic and Cholinergic Receptors).

Because so much cardiac disease involves the coronary arteries, the anesthetic risk rate increases in patients with cardiac disease. A functional classification of cardiac cases is based on the ability to perform physical activities (Box 11-2). Patients in classes III and IV have a significant risk for surgery and anesthesia and should undergo complete monitoring when they receive care in the PACU.

### Effect of Anesthesia on the Heart

Research now shows that cardiac dysrhythmias are observed in about 60% of all patients who undergo anesthesia. The inhalation anesthetics, such as halothane, enflurane, and isoflurane, can evoke nodal rhythms or increase ventricular automaticity or both. These anesthetics also slow the rate of SA node discharge and prolong the bundle of His-Purkinje and ventricular conduction times. Along with these changes in rhythm, alterations in the balance of the autonomic nervous system between the parasympathetic and sympathetic systems caused by drugs such as anticholinergics and catecholamines or by light anesthesia can initiate cardiac dysrhythmias. Hence, in the immediate postoperative period, cardiac dysrhythmias are likely because of light anesthesia during emergence or because of the administration of drugs that alter sympathetic activity. Consequently, continuous monitoring of cardiac rate and rhythm is mandated in the PACU.

### Myocardial Infarction

Acute myocardial infarction is a commonly encountered medical emergency that can occur in the PACU. The objectives in the management of a patient with an acute myocardial infarction are pain relief, control of complications, salvaging of ischemic myocardium, and a return to a productive life. The diagnosis of myocardial infarction is made on the basis of clinical findings, and therapy should be instituted immediately when suspected. (Cardiopulmonary resuscitation is discussed in Chapter 57.) An electrocardiogram performed in the PACU may reveal an injury pattern, but normal electrocardiographic results certainly do not exclude a diagnosis of myocardial infarction.

Physical assessment for a suspected myocardial infarction may include the following subjective findings: (1) pain or pressure, which is usually substernal but may be manifested in the neck, shoulder, jaws, arms, or other areas; (2) nausea; (3) vomiting; (4) diaphoresis; (5) dyspnea; and (6) syncope. The onset of pain may occur with activity but may also occur at rest. The duration may be prolonged, from 30 minutes to several hours. Objective findings may include hypotension, pallor, and anxiety. The blood pressure, pulse, and heart sounds may be normal with an acute myocardial infarction. On auscultation of the chest, the abnormal cardiac findings may include atrial gallop, ventricular gallop, paradoxic second heart sound ($S_2$), friction rub, and abnormal precordial pulsations.

The electrocardiographic pattern may vary by the location and extent of the infarction, but myocardial damage may occur without changes in the electrocardiogram. Some typical features of a transmural infarction are acute ST-segment elevation in leads that reflects the area of injury, abnormal Q waves, and T-wave inversion.

The laboratory data usually reflect an elevated sedimentation rate and white blood cell count. The levels of enzymes serum glutamic-oxaloacetic transaminase, lactic dehydrogenase (LDH), and creatine phosphokinase (CPK) may be elevated. Results of enzymatic studies with acute myocardial infarction do not indicate a specific cause because other conditions and disease states may affect these enzyme levels. LDH and CPK isoenzyme studies may be necessary to differentiate the various disease abnormalities. Intramuscular injections may significantly elevate the level of CPK and therefore should be avoided. Also, surgical procedures that involve major trauma to muscle cause a postoperative increase in the CPK level. Because of the increase in the CPK level associated with surgical trauma, the perianesthesia nurse should use good judgment in evaluation of enzyme studies in patients in whom acute myocardial infarction is suspected.

Research studies have shown that patients who have had a myocardial infarction within 6 months before surgery have a recurrence rate of 54.5% for a myocardial infarction that could occur during or after the surgical procedure. If the myocardial infarction occurred between 6 months and 2 years before surgery, the rate of recurrence of infarction is between 20% and 25%. Between the second and third years, the incidence rate of reinfarction is about 5%. Most studies indicate that 3 years after the original myocardial infarction, the recurrence rate is about 1%, which equals the normal rate of myocardial infarction in the general population. Hence, the chance of a patient having an acute myocardial infarction in the PACU can be considered significant. This chance is especially true for patients in the PACU who have had a myocardial infarction within the last 3 years, who have a documented myocardial infarction risk factor (such as angina, hypertension, and diabetes), or who have some combination of the previous factors.

## Perianesthesia Nursing Care

The perianesthesia nurse should be constantly alert for complications such as anxiety, arrhythmias, shock, left ventricular failure, and pulmonary and systemic embolisms. Pain and apprehension may be relieved with treatment with morphine sulfate or meperidine hydrochloride (Demerol). Oxygen should be administered with nasal prongs because a face mask may increase the patient's apprehension. Continuous cardiac monitoring should be instituted, and the patient should be kept in a quiet area. Drugs such as atropine, lidocaine, digitalis, quinidine, sodium nitroprusside (SNP), phentolamine, and nitroglycerin should be available. A machine for countershock also should be immediately available. Fluid therapy and urine output should be monitored completely for prevention of fluid overload. A Swan-Ganz catheter

or central venous pressure (CVP) monitor may be used for determination of fluid replacement in patients with reduced intravascular volume and hypotension (see discussion of CVP catheters in the following section). A benign myocardial infarction does not exist; all patients with a diagnosed myocardial infarction need constant competent perianesthesia care.

***Central Venous Pressure Monitor.*** The CVP monitor enhances the assessment of venous return and hypovolemia. More specifically, the CVP monitor is used to assess the adequacy of central venous return, blood volume, and right ventricular function. The actual pressure reading obtained from this monitor reflects the pressure in the great veins when blood returns to the heart.

The left ventricular end-diastolic pressure (LVEDP) serves as a good indicator of left ventricular preload. With a patient with a good ejection fraction, the CVP measurement serves as an approximate value for the LVEDP. However, one should remember that the CVP has limited value in assessment of left ventricular hemodynamics.

In the immediate postoperative setting, the CVP remains an excellent parameter for indication of the adequacy of blood volume. In the hypovolemic state, the CVP is decreased. The administration of appropriate fluids and blood to expand the intravascular space increases the CVP toward the patient's baseline reading. In the clinical setting, no absolute predetermined normal value for a CVP reading exists. The best use of this particular monitoring mode is for serial measurements for assessment of cardiovascular performance. See Chapter 27 for a complete discussion of the CVP monitor.

***Pulmonary Artery Catheter.*** The pulmonary artery catheter is used to monitor the central venous, pulmonary artery, and pulmonary capillary wedge pressures. This balloon-tipped catheter with four or five ports is discussed in detail in Chapter 27.

In the immediate postoperative period, the pulmonary artery catheter is usually used for patients with clinical shock, compromised ventricular function, and severe cardiac or pulmonary disease. Also, patients who have had extensive surgical procedures or major cardiovascular surgery can benefit from this monitor. Accurate monitoring of left-sided and right-sided preload along with the rapid determination of cardiac output makes this monitor an excellent parameter for determination of mechanical and pharmacologic therapy, with the intended outcome of enhanced cardiac performance and tissue perfusion.

## CIRCULATORY SYSTEM

### Red Blood Cells

The healthy red blood cell (RBC) is in the form of a biconcave disk that can change its shape to move through the microcirculation. The major function of the RBC is the transport of oxygen to the tissue cells; it is also an important factor in carbon dioxide transport. The RBC is responsible for approximately 70% of the buffering power of whole blood in the maintenance of acid-base balance.

The RBCs are produced by the bone marrow. The normal rate of production is sufficient to form about 1250 mL of new blood per month. This rate is also the normal rate of destruction. The average life span of an RBC is 120 days. The hematocrit value is the percentage of RBCs in the blood. The optimal range in adults is between 30% and 42%. When the hematocrit level is reduced to lower than 30%, the oxygen-carrying capacity declines steeply. Moreover, when the hematocrit level rises higher than 55%, the oxygen-carrying capacity declines because the increase in blood viscosity causes increased work for the heart and decreased cardiac output. The normal amount of hemoglobin in the RBC ranges from 10 to 13.5 g. Indeed, the amount and type of hemoglobin determine the oxygen-carrying capacity. Recent evidence indicates that the cutoff value for risk of reduced oxygen-carrying capacity and blood volume is a hemoglobin level of 11 g, a hematocrit of 27%, or both. Transfusion with blood or blood products to raise the level of hemoglobin should be strongly considered for any patient with values lower than the cutoff values.

### White Blood Cells

White blood cells (WBCs), or leukocytes, are the body's major defense against infection. The two primary types of circulating leukocytes are polymorphonuclear leukocytes (PMNs) and lymphocytes. The role of the PMNs in combating infection is to migrate to the infectious site in large numbers and phagocytize the invading microbe. The role of the lymphocytes is to mediate immunoglobulin production and act in the delayed hypersensitivity in the type IV reaction (see Chapter 17). Evaluations of the WBC count should focus on the number of PMNs. When the PMN level is lower than 1000 per mm$^3$, the incidence rate of infections is increased. Postanesthesia patients with a PMN level of 500 to 100 per mm$^3$ are at great risk of infection. Some of the major clinical situations that cause a reduction in PMN levels (leukopenia) are viral infections, including human immunodeficiency virus, and cancer chemotherapy.

### Blood Platelets

Normal hemostasis requires a proper interaction between blood vessels, platelets, and coagulation proteins. Any dysfunction in any one of the three components has a profound effect on hemostasis. When a tissue injury occurs, the vessel wall vasoconstricts and activates the extrinsic pathway for coagulation proteins. Platelet adhesion and aggregation occur along with the activation of the intrinsic and extrinsic pathways for the coagulation proteins. The result of this interaction is a hemostatic plug.

Clinical evaluation for proper coagulation focuses on the following four tests: bleeding time (BT), platelet count (PC), prothrombin time (PT), and partial thromboplastin time (PTT). The BT and PC are tests for evaluation of platelet function, and the PT and PTT are tests for evaluation of the coagulation system.

A prolongation of the BT and surgically related hemorrhage seem to be correlated. The normal BT is between 2 and 11 minutes. The test results are considered abnormal when the BT is longer than 12 minutes. The template procedure should be used when the BT is performed because it is more sensitive than older methods. The normal platelet count is between 200,000 and 450,000 per mm$^3$. More specifically, the patient usually tolerates surgery and the postanesthesia phase quite well in regard to hemostasis with a platelet count of 100,000 per mm$^3$ or higher. Patients with a platelet count of 50,000 to 100,000 per mm$^3$ may have ecchymoses from tissue trauma. If the platelet count is lower than 50,000 per mm$^3$, many alterations in bleeding may occur. These patients need constant evaluation and therapy in the postoperative period.

The PTT is a test for evaluation of the intrinsic and common coagulation pathways of the coagulation system. It is most commonly used for monitoring of heparin therapy. Normal results are considered to be 25 to 32 seconds, depending on the reagent. Abnormal results are considered to be longer than 35 seconds. The PT is used to examine the extrinsic coagulation system for evaluation of oral anticoagulant therapy. Normal results are based on laboratory control for interpretation. Usually, the control is normal in patients with an appropriately functioning extrinsic coagulation system. When the value is more than 3 seconds above the control, the test results are considered to be abnormal.

Postoperative bleeding can occur when the patient's preoperative or intraoperative coagulation study results are abnormal. Bleeding tendencies are enhanced by the presence of post-operative hypertension. In addition, when hemostasis is lacking at the suture line or extensive surgical tissue trauma exists, the like-lihood of postoperative bleeding is increased. Finally, the use of antibiotics during and after surgery can also increase bleeding tendencies. Therefore, the perianesthesia nurse should eval-uate the patient's preoperative and intraopera-tive coagulation study results and examine the surgical incision for bleeding during initial assessment. Certainly, the postoperative trauma patient who has undergone extensive surgical trauma should be constantly monitored for bleeding tendencies, especially if intraoperative antibiotics were administered. If the patient is undergoing anticoagulant therapy, continued monitoring of the anticoagulant activity is mandated. Finally, in the patient with a demon-strated bleeding tendency, maintenance of a normal arterial blood pressure must be ensured. For a complete review of the fluid and electro-lyte administration see Chapter 14.

### Blood Vessels

The circulatory system can be divided into the systemic and the pulmonary circulation. The systemic or peripheral circulation comprises arteries, arterioles, capillaries, venules, and veins. The walls of the blood vessels, except the capillaries, are composed of three distinct coats: the tunica adventitia, the tunica media, and the tunica intima. The outer layer, the tunica adventitia, consists of white fibrous connective tissue, which gives strength to and limits the distensibility of the vessel. The vasa vasorum, which supplies nourishment to the larger vessels, is in this layer. The middle layer, the tunica media, consists of mostly circularly arranged smooth muscle fibers and yellow elastic fibers. The innermost layer, the tunica intima, is a fine transparent lining that serves to reduce resistance to the flow of blood. The valves of the veins are formed by the foldings of this layer. The capillaries consist of a single layer of squamous epithelial cells, which is a continua-tion of tunica intima.

The arteries are characterized by elasticity and extensibility. The veins have a poorly devel-oped tunica media and are therefore much less muscular and elastic than arteries.

### Microcirculation

Microcirculation is the flow of blood in the finer vessels of the body. It involves the arterioles, capillaries, and venules. The arteries subdivide to the last segment of the arterial system, the arteriole. The arteriole consists of a single layer

of smooth muscle in the shape of a tube for conducting blood to the capillaries. As the arte-rioles approach the capillaries, they lack the coating of smooth muscle and are termed metar-terioles. At the point at which the capillaries originate from the metarterioles, a smooth muscle fiber, the precapillary sphincter, encircles the capillary. At the other end of the capillary is the venule, which is larger but has a much weaker muscular coat than the arteriole.

The capillaries are usually no more than 4 to 9 μm in diameter, which is barely large enough for corpuscles to pass through in single file. Blood moves through the capillaries in intermit-tent flow, caused by the contraction and relaxa-tion of the smooth muscle of the metarterioles and the precapillary sphincter. This motion is termed *vasomotion*. The metarterioles and pre-capillary sphincter open and close in response to oxygen concentration in the tissues—a form of local autoregulation.

The microcirculation serves three major func-tions: (1) transcapillary exchange of nutrients and fluids; (2) maintenance of blood pressure and volume flow; and (3) return of blood to the heart and regulation of active blood volume.

## ADRENERGIC AND CHOLINERGIC RECEPTORS

The cardiovascular system and the concept of adrenergic and cholinergic receptors are closely related. The perianesthesia nurse must understand the pharmacodynamics of these receptors.

### Functional Anatomy: The Mediators

*Cholinergic* is a term used to describe the nerve endings that liberate acetylcholine. The cho-linergic neurotransmitter, acetylcholine, is pres-ent in all preganglionic parasympathetic fibers, all preganglionic sympathetic fibers, all postgan-glionic parasympathetic fibers, and all somatic motor neurons. Two exceptions to the general rule are postganglionic sympathetic fibers to the sweat glands and to the vasculature of skeletal muscle. These fibers are considered sympathetic anatomically but cholinergic in terms of their neurotransmitter (i.e., they release acetylcholine as their neurotransmitter).

The term *adrenergic* is used to describe nerves that release norepinephrine as their neuro-transmitter. Epinephrine may be present in the adrenergic fibers in small quantities, usually representing less than 5% of the total amount of both epinephrine and norepinephrine. The ad-renergic fibers are the postganglionic sympathetic fibers, with the exception of the postganglionic

## Box 11-3    Cholinergic and Adrenergic Nerves

**MEDIATOR: ACETYLCHOLINE–CHOLINERGIC NERVES**
*Effects*
All preganglionic parasympathetic fibers
All preganglionic sympathetic fibers
All postganglionic parasympathetic fibers
All somatic motor neurons
Postganglionic sympathetic fibers to sweat glands
Postganglionic sympathetic vasodilator fibers innervating skeletal muscle vasculature

**MEDIATOR: NONEPINEPHRINE–ADRENERGIC NERVES**
*Effects*
All postganglionic sympathetic fibers (except those to sweat glands and efferent fibers to skeletal muscle)

Modified from Drain CB: Current concepts on the pharmacodynamics of adrenergic and cholinergic receptors, *AANA J* 44:272, 1976.

sympathetic fibers to the sweat glands and to the efferent fibers to the skeletal muscle (Box 11-3).

The adrenal medulla should be considered separately because it is innervated by a preganglionic sympathetic fiber that liberates the neurotransmitter acetylcholine and because the postganglionic portion is the adrenal medulla, which behaves much like a postganglionic sympathetic fiber. The adrenal medulla is therefore stimulated by acetylcholine, which causes the release of both epinephrine and norepinephrine from its chromaffin cells. As opposed to the usual finding of a preponderance of norepinephrine at the postganglionic nerve fiber terminals,

the distribution in the adrenal medulla is 80% epinephrine and 20% norepinephrine. Therefore, the neurotransmitter of the adrenal medulla is epinephrine.

***Cholinergic Neurotransmitter: Biochemistry.***
The neurotransmitter acetylcholine is synthesized from choline and acetate through the enzymatic activity of choline acetylase to form acetylcholine (Box 11-4); it is then stored in vesicles. When acetylcholine is released from a preganglionic fiber, it may then act on the membrane of the preganglionic fiber with a positive feedback mechanism, thus enhancing the release of acetylcholine. The calcium ion facilitates this additional release of acetylcholine. This process is called excitation-secretion coupling through calcium.

***Adrenergic Neurotransmitter: Biochemistry.***
The adrenergic neurotransmitter, epinephrine, begins in the body as phenylalanine, which is hydroxylated to tyrosine, which is again hydroxylated to form L-dopa, an amino acid. This process is probably the weakest step in the biosynthetic chain and may be a possible site of action of an autonomic drug. A soluble enzyme, L-dopa decarboxylase, acts on L-dopa to form dopamine, which, in turn, is synthesized to norepinephrine. In the adrenal medulla, norepinephrine may be methylated in the cell to form the final product, epinephrine. This reaction is catalyzed by the enzyme phenylethanolamine-N-methyltransferase (see Box 11-4).

The storage site of norepinephrine in the adrenergic nerves appears to be in the intracellular granules. Depletion of the total content of norepinephrine through continued nerve stimulation is difficult, but with continuous chronic drug administration, a clinical hypotensive state may be caused by the decreased sympathetic vasomotor tone.

## Box 11-4    Synthesis of Neurotransmitters

**CHOLINERGIC**
Choline + Acetate $\xrightarrow{\text{Choline acetylase}}$ Acetycholine

**ADRENERGIC**

Phenylalanine $\longrightarrow$ Tyrosine $\xrightarrow{\text{Tyrosine hydrolase}}$ L-dopa $\xrightarrow{\text{L-dopa decarboxylase}}$

Dopamine $\xrightarrow{\text{Dopamine beta oxidase}}$ Norepinephrine $\xrightarrow{\text{Phenylethanolamine-N-methyltransferase}}$ Epinephrine

Modified from Drain CB: Current concepts on the pharmacodynamics of adrenergic and cholinergic receptors, *AANA J* 44:272, 1976.

The mechanism of release of norepinephrine from the adrenergic fibers and epinephrine from the adrenal medulla appears to be that of reverse pinocytosis. Pinocytosis is a mechanism by which the membrane engulfs substances in the extracellular fluid. With the influence of the appropriate stimuli, an opening is created through which the soluble contents of a portion of the storage granules are released. The major means of inactivation of norepinephrine is through a mechanism known as uptake, in which the released neurotransmitter is recaptured into the neuronal system by the neuron that released it or by neurons adjacent to it and, in some instances, by neurons associated with tissues some distance from the original site of release.

The norepinephrine that is not recaptured is metabolized eventually to vanillylmandelic acid. Epinephrine also undergoes a number of steps in its biodegradation to vanillylmandelic acid. An increase in vanillylmandelic acid concentration in the urine is useful in the diagnosis of conditions such as pheochromocytoma and neuroblastoma (Fig. 11-5).

When a patient is administered a drug that is a monoamine oxidase inhibitor—such as isocarboxazid (Marplan), pargyline (Eutonyl), phenelzine sulfate (Nardil), or tranylcypromine sulfate (Parnate)—a buildup of epinephrine or norepinephrine can occur and lead to sympathetic hyperactivity. This occurrence is especially likely when substances or drugs such as tyramine or indirect-acting vasopressors such as ephedrine are administered.

## Cholinergic Receptors
The pharmacologic and physiologic actions of acetylcholine are apparently mediated by its combination with specific cholinergic receptors. The actions of acetylcholine and drugs that mimic acetylcholine are mediated through two types of cholinergic receptors: nicotinic and muscarinic (see Chapter 23).

When the nicotinic receptors are stimulated, the following responses are observed:
1. Stimulation of autonomic ganglia, both parasympathetic and sympathetic.

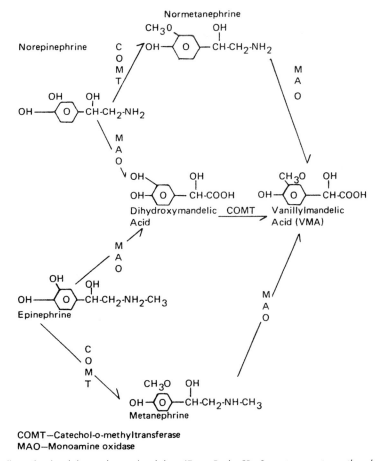

**Fig. 11-5** Metabolism of epinephrine and norepinephrine. (*From Drain CB: Current concepts on the pharmacodynamics of adrenergic and cholinergic receptors, AANA J 44:272, 1976.*)

2. Stimulation of the adrenal medulla, which results in the release of both epinephrine and norepinephrine.
3. Stimulation of skeletal muscle at the motor endplate.

The muscarinic responses elicited by muscarine and acetylcholine are the following:
1. Stimulation or inhibition of smooth muscle in various organs or tissues.
2. Stimulation of exocrine glands.
3. Slowing of cardiac conduction.
4. Decrease in myocardial contractile force.

Nicotinic responses in terms of antagonism can be blocked with drugs such as ganglionic or neuromuscular blocking agents, or both, whereas muscarinic responses are blocked with the class of drugs best typified by atropine.

Muscarine is a specific agonist at muscarinic receptors, whereas nicotine is a specific agonist at nicotinic receptors. However, acetylcholine is capable of stimulating both receptor types (Table 11-1).

A series of compounds is specific in its ability to combine with acetylcholinesterase and inhibit its activity through competitive inhibition.

The prototype compounds in this category are neostigmine (Prostigmin), physostigmine salicylate (Antilirium), pyridostigmine (Regonol, Mestinon), and edrophonium (Tensilon, Enlon).

Belladonna alkaloids such as atropine have adverse effects that are peculiar to the PACU phase of the surgical experience. More specifically, belladonna alkaloids that cross the blood-brain barrier can cause disorientation, violent behavior, or somnolence. Physostigmine salicylate, an anticholinesterase that is capable of penetrating the blood-brain barrier, has been shown to be useful in reversing the adverse effects of belladonna alkaloids on the central nervous system (CNS). Physostigmine salicylate is also useful in reversing the disorientation or somnolence caused by drugs such as diazepam, the phenothiazines, the tricyclic antidepressants, the antiparkinsonian drugs, promethazine, droperidol, and, in some instances, halothane. Patients in the PACU who may benefit from treatment with physostigmine are those who have received a belladonna alkaloid or neuroleptic type of agent either before or during surgery, who have had disorientation or

### Table 11-1  Cholinergic Receptors

| Organ Stimulated by Cholinergic Agonist | Response | Type of Cholinergic Receptor Response |
|---|---|---|
| **Heart** | | |
| SA node | Negative chronotropic effect | Muscarinic |
| Atria | Decreased contractility and increased conduction velocity | Muscarinic |
| AV node and conduction system | Decrease in conduction velocity—AV block | Muscarinic |
| **Eye** | | |
| Sphincter muscle of iris | Contraction (miosis) | Muscarinic |
| **Lung** | | |
| Bronchial muscle | Contraction | Muscarinic |
| Bronchial glands | Stimulation | Muscarinic |
| **Exocrine Glands** | | |
| Salivary glands | Profuse watery secretion | Muscarinic |
| Lacrimal glands | Secretion | Muscarinic |
| Nasopharyngeal glands | Secretion | Muscarinic |
| Adrenal medulla | Catecholamine secretion | Nicotinic |
| Autonomic ganglia | Ganglion stimulation | Nicotinic Muscarinic |
| **Skeletal Muscle** | | |
| Motor endplate | Stimulation | Nicotinic (motor endplate receptor) |

Modified from Drain CB: Current concepts on the pharmacodynamics of adrenergic and cholinergic receptors, *AANA J* 44:272, 1976.

restlessness or both for more than 30 minutes after anesthesia, and who are difficult to arouse over an appropriate period. Patients with any one of these dysfunctions qualify for treatment and can be given 1-mg increments of physostigmine intravenously at 15-minute intervals until they are conscious and oriented to time, place, and person. Once treatment has begun, the perianesthesia nurse should monitor the blood pressure and pulse immediately before and 5 minutes after the administration of physostigmine. Also, some patients may have side effects from physostigmine, such as nausea, pallor, sweating, and bradycardia. Because glycopyrrolate (Robinul) does not cross the blood-brain barrier, treatment of the side effects of physostigmine is especially helpful. Finally, patients who have undergone treatment with physostigmine probably should remain in the PACU for about 1 hour after the administration of the anticholinesterase.

### Adrenergic Receptors

The stimulation of the sympathetic nervous system can be both inhibitory and excitatory, which has caused considerable confusion. Originally, theories were postulated that this phenomenon handled the release of two different compounds. The variation in the effects of stimulation was later found to be related not to the differences in chemical release but rather to a difference in the receptors' responses to the transmitter.

The adrenergic receptors, which respond to catecholamines, can be subdivided into three main types: the dopaminergic, the alpha, and the beta. The dopaminergic receptors are primarily in the CNS and the mesenteric and renal blood vessels. The agonist for these receptors is dopamine. The alpha receptors can be further divided into alpha$_1$ and alpha$_2$ receptors. The postsynaptic alpha$_1$ receptors are excitatory in action, except in the intestine. Stimulation of the alpha$_1$ receptors causes smooth muscle contraction, which results in a vasoconstriction or pressor response. Hence, the alpha$_1$ receptor is activated by the release of norepinephrine, and this released norepinephrine also activates the presynaptic alpha$_2$ receptors to inhibit the further release of norepinephrine. Thus, the alpha$_1$ receptor is activated by the release of norepinephrine, and the released norepinephrine in turn stimulates the alpha$_2$ receptor, thus producing inhibition of the release of norepinephrine and resulting in a negative feedback loop (Fig. 11-6).

The drug clonidine (Catapres) is believed to stimulate the alpha$_2$ receptors, which lower the

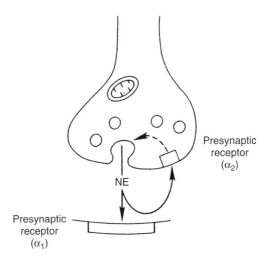

**Fig. 11-6** Presynaptic and postsynaptic alpha receptors at ending of norepinephrine-secreting neuron. (*Adapted from Ganong WF:* Review of medical physiology, *ed 20, New York, 2001, Lange Medical Books/McGraw-Hill Medical Publications Division.*)

sympathetic outflow of norepinephrine and ultimately lead to a hypotensive effect. In addition to lowering catecholamine levels, clonidine can reduce the plasma renin activity. This antihypertensive drug enjoys a significant degree of popularity, but it can have a negative impact on the patient in the PACU. More specifically, the clonidine withdrawal syndrome has been reported when the drug has been stopped abruptly. The sequelae of the syndrome resemble pheochromocytoma in that shortly after the withdrawal of the clonidine the patient can have hypertension, tachycardia, and increased blood levels of catecholamines. Treatment of this syndrome usually involves a reinstitution of the clonidine therapy and alpha-adrenergic blocking agents such as phentolamine.

Stimulation of the beta receptor causes vascular smooth muscle relaxation, which then leads to a decrease in blood pressure through a decrease in peripheral resistance. The beta receptor can be divided into two types: beta$_1$ and beta$_2$. Beta$_1$-subtype receptors are found in all cardiac tissue except the coronary vasculature and are responsible for characteristic effects noted after stimulation of the heart with epinephrine, including the following effects: (1) increase in heart rate; (2) increase in contractile force; (3) increase in conduction velocity; and (4) shortening of the refractory period. Beta$_1$-subtype receptors mediate effects elicited by catecholamines (Table 11-2).

The physiology of the beta receptor has many implications for the care of the PACU patient.

## Table 11-2 Adrenergic Receptors

| Response | Type of Adrenergic Receptor |
|---|---|
| **Heart** | |
| Positive inotropic effect | Beta$_1$ |
| Positive chronotropic effect | Beta$_1$ |
| Cardiac arrhythmias | Beta$_1$ |
| Positive dromotropic effect | Beta$_1$ |
| **Vascular** | |
| Arterial and arteriolar constriction | Alpha$_1$ |
| Coronary artery constriction | Alpha$_1$ |
| Coronary artery dilatation | Beta$_1$ |
| Arteriolar relaxation | Beta$_2$ |
| **Gastrointestinal Tract** | |
| Intestinal relaxation | Alpha$_1$, beta$_1$ |
| Sphincter contraction (usually) | Alpha$_1$ |
| **Urinary Bladder** | |
| Bladder relaxation (detrusor) | Beta$_2$ |
| Bladder contraction (trigone and sphincter) | Alpha$_1$ |
| **Eye** | |
| Contraction (mydriasis) | Alpha$_1$ |
| Ciliary muscle of iris | Beta$_2$ |
| **Metabolic** | |
| Liver glycogenolysis (hyperglycemia) | Alpha$_1$, beta$_2$ |
| Muscle glycogenolysis | Beta$_1$ |
| Lipolysis | Beta$_1$ |
| Oxygen consumption (increases) | Beta$_1$, beta$_2$ |
| **Other Smooth Muscle** | |
| Bronchial (relaxation) | Beta$_2$ |
| Spleen (contraction) | Alpha$_1$ |
| Ureter (contraction) | Alpha$_1$ |
| Uterus (contraction) | Alpha$_1$ |
| Uterus (relaxation)—nonpregnant condition | Beta$_2$ |

Modified from Drain CB: Current concepts on the pharmacodynamics of adrenergic and cholinergic receptors, *AANA J* 44:272, 1976.

Once the beta receptor has been activated by *first messengers*, endogenous catecholamines or exogenous beta agonists such as isoproterenol, certain biochemical events occur (Fig. 11-7). The enzyme adenylate cyclase, which is located on the plasma membrane, is stimulated with beta-receptor activation. Then, within the cell, adenosine triphosphate (ATP) is broken down to 3',5'-adenosine monophosphate (cyclic AMP). The cyclic AMP is then released into the cytoplasm of the cell and acts to modulate cellular activities. Hence, the cyclic AMP is considered to be the *second messenger*. Cyclic AMP is inactivated to 5-AMP by the enzyme phosphodiesterase.

Clinically, isoproterenol or terbutaline may be administered to increase the cyclic AMP levels in the beta$_2$ receptors in the bronchial airways with the intended result of bronchodilatation. Another way to increase the cyclic AMP levels is inhibition of the action of phosphodiesterase. Caffeine and the methylxanthines, such as aminophylline, are inhibitors of the enzyme phosphodiesterase and can be used alone or in combination (for synergistic effects) with the beta agonists to produce the desired bronchodilatation in the patient. One should remember that other catecholamine effects are produced by the increase in cyclic AMP levels. Consequently, although aminophylline is considered a bronchodilator, it increases the myocardial contractility and heart rate of the patient, thus mandating that the perianesthesia nurse monitor both respiratory and cardiac function when methylxanthines are administered.

The coronary arteries contain alpha$_1$ and beta$_1$ receptors and therefore also have the ability to vasoconstrict and vasodilate (see Table 11-2). The endogenous catecholamines, norepinephrine and epinephrine, are capable of stimulating both the alpha and the beta receptors.

### Site of Action of Autonomic Drugs

Methyldopa (Aldomet; the alpha-methylated analogue of L-dopa) is an antihypertensive drug. Methyldopa reduces the sympathetic nerve stimulation through the production of a selective agonist, alpha methylnorepinephrine.

Guanethidine has the ability to prevent nerve stimulation and thus inhibit norepinephrine release. Guanethidine interferes with the storage of norepinephrine and, if given chronically, results in a decrease in the amount of norepinephrine stored in adrenergic nerves. Reserpine also shares this latter action with guanethidine. Thus, chronic use of guanethidine and reserpine results in a relative depletion of the norepinephrine content from sympathetic nerves (Table 11-3).

The calcium channel blockers have been found to have considerable value in the treatment of supraventricular tachycardias, angina pectoris, and myocardial infarction. The prototype calcium channel blockers are verapamil (Isoptin), nifedipine (Procardia, Adalat), and diltiazem (Cardizem). All three drugs depress calcium entry into conduction tissue and cardiac

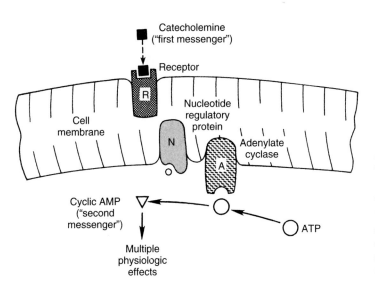

**Fig. 11-7** Catecholamine (first messenger) binds to beta-receptor protein, which activates enzyme adenylate cyclase via nucleotide regulatory protein, which binds guanosine monophosphate. Via adenylate cyclase, ATP is broken down to cyclic AMP. Cyclic AMP, or second messenger, then activates protein kinase, which ultimately produces variety of physiologic effects. (*Modified from Catt KJ, Harwood JP, Clayton RN, et al: Regulation of peptide hormone receptors and gonadal steroidogenesis,* Recent Prog Horm Res 36:557-662, 1980.)

muscle, which results in a depression of conduction and leads to a reduction of the circus movements. These calcium entry blockers produce hypotension with different mechanisms. Nifedipine, like SNP, decreases the systemic vascular resistance with a compensatory tachycardia, and verapamil and diltiazem lower the cardiac output by exerting a negative dromotropic effect. The effects of the calcium channel blockers may be enhanced with inhalation anesthesia agents such as halothane. Consequently, in the PACU, patients who received an inhalation of anesthetic and are undergoing treatment with a calcium channel blocker may have some hypotension. Hence, the perianesthesia nurse should vigorously monitor the cardiovascular parameters of these patients and report any confirmed hypotension to the attending physician.

Dopamine is a naturally occurring biochemical catecholamine precursor of norepinephrine. It exerts a positive inotropic effect and a minimal chronotropic effect on the heart. Therefore, the contractility of the heart is increased without a change in the afterload (total peripheral resistance), which leads to an increase in cardiac output. The increase is in the systolic and pulse pressures, with virtually no effect on the diastolic pressure. Dopamine is not associated with tachyarrhythmias and produces less of an

| Table 11-3 | Drugs That Interfere with Specific Steps in Process of Chemical (Neurohumoral) Transmission | |
|---|---|---|
| | **Adrenergic Nerves** | **Cholinergic Nerves** |
| Synthesis of mediator | Methyldopa | Hemicholinium |
| Storage of mediator | Reserpine | — |
| Release of mediator | Guanethidine | Botulinus toxin |
| Combination of mediator with its receptor | Phenoxybenzamine (alpha receptor) Propranolol (beta receptor) | Atropine (muscarinic) Nicotine (nicotinic) |
| Enzymatic destruction of mediator | Pyrogallol (COMT inhibitor) Tranylcypromine (MAO inhibitor) | Physostigmine (cholinesterase inhibitor) |
| Prevention of inactivation of mediator (blocks uptake) | Cocaine | — |
| Repolarization of postsynaptic membrane (persistent depolarization) | — | Succinylcholine |

From Drain CB: Current concepts on the pharmacodynamics of adrenergic and cholinergic receptors, AANA J 44:272, 1976.
COMT, Catechol-O-methyl transferase.

increase in myocardial oxygen consumption than does isoproterenol. Blood flow to peripheral vascular beds may decrease while mesenteric flow increases. One of the major reasons for the increase in the use of dopamine clinically is its dilatation of the renal vasculature. This action is the result of the inotropic effect and decreased peripheral resistance. Therefore, the glomerular filtration rate is increased along with the renal blood flow and sodium excretion.

Dobutamine (Dobutrex) is synthetically derived from the catecholamine isoproterenol. Consequently, it produces a positive inotropic effect with specificity to the beta$_1$ receptors, thus resulting in an increase in cardiac output with minimal effects on blood pressure, heart rate, and systemic vascular resistance. The drug is usually administered intravenously in a dose range of 2 to 10 μg/kg/min and is especially useful for patients who are recovering from cardiopulmonary bypass surgery. Dobutamine is sometimes combined with a vasodilator to reduce afterload in an effort to optimize the cardiac output.

## Hypotension Therapy

Hypotension in the immediate postoperative period is of great concern and deserves the prompt attention of the perianesthesia nurse. When hypotension is detected in the postanesthesia patient, the nurse should first reaffirm the measurements. An incorrectly placed or sized blood pressure cuff or malfunction of the stethoscope can yield incorrect measurements (see Chapter 27). If an arterial catheter transducer system is used, it should be appropriately zeroed and calibrated and the air bubbles removed to ensure that artificially low readings are not observed. Also, if the patient is hypothermic or receiving alpha-adrenergic agonists such as phenylephrine (Neosynephrine), the patient may have low blood pressures in the radial and brachial arteries, whereas the central blood pressure may be higher. This difference is because of the peripheral vasoconstriction produced by the alpha-adrenergic drugs.

If the hypotension is confirmed, hypovolemia should be considered as a possible cause. The clinical signs of hypotension from hypovolemia include cold, pale, clammy, or diaphoretic skin; rapid thready pulse; shallow rapid respirations; disorientation, restlessness, or anxiety; decreased CVP; and oliguria. The nursing assessment of the patient with hypotension should include an inspection of the dressings for excessive bleeding and an evaluation for the clinical signs of hypovolemia. If the patient's circulating blood

volume is reduced by more than 15% to 20%, hypotension can ensue. This condition usually happens when the patient has not received appropriate fluid volume replacement during surgery. Other factors in the development of postoperative hypovolemia are ongoing internal or external hemorrhage, sweating, insensible losses, and third-space losses. Third-space losses occur when an exudation of fluid into the tissues occurs (see Chapter 14). Other causes of hypotension include a high alveolar-inflating pressure when a patient is undergoing mechanical ventilation, ventricular dysfunction, myocardial ischemia, and cardiac dysrhythmias. If the hypotension is 30% less than the preoperative baseline blood pressure readings or one or more of the clinical signs of hypovolemia is present, the attending physician should be notified.

Usual therapy for hypotension in the PACU includes the administration of a high fractional concentration of oxygen, fluid infusion, reversal of residual anesthetic depressant effects, repositioning of the patient to facilitate venous return, reduction in ventilator airway pressures, and administration of vasopressors or anticholinergics or both, such as glycopyrrolate or atropine, as indicated. More specifically, the first line of defense is to return the patient's condition to normovolemia and, in this instance, administer a bolus of crystalloid solution of about 300 to 500 mL. The anticholinergics are indicated if sinus bradycardia accompanies the hypotension. The vasopressors exert their effect either directly or indirectly. The direct-acting vasopressor exerts its effect directly on the receptor. Conversely, the pharmacologic action of an indirect vasopressor facilitates the release of norepinephrine from its storage vesicles (primarily the terminal sympathetic nerve fibers), which stimulates the adrenergic receptor to achieve the desired effect. Therefore, a direct-acting vasopressor is probably necessary to achieve a response in patients who are depleted of catecholamines by drugs such as reserpine and guanethidine (Table 11-4).

Another area of consideration in selection of a vasopressor is the cardiotonic action desired. Metaraminol (Aramine), with its action of norepinephrine release, causes improved cardiac function as a result of its beta-receptor activity. Conversely, phenylephrine and methoxamine (Vasoxyl) possess little or no cardiac effect and exert a pressor action with pure alpha stimulation. The alpha-adrenergic agonists are useful especially for patients who have received a "high" spinal or epidural anesthetic. High levels of regional anesthetics are associated with peripheral vasodilatation and bradycardia because of a sympathetic blockade. Consequently,

| Table 11-4 | Adrenergic Drugs According to Action |
|---|---|
| **Generic Name** | **Tradename** |
| **Direct-Acting Adrenergic Amines** | |
| Epinephrine | Adrenalin |
| Norepinephrine | Levophed |
| Dopamine | Intropin |
| Dobutamine | Dobutrex |
| Isoproterenol | Isuprel |
| Methoxamine | Vasoxyl |
| Phenylephrine | Neosynephrine |
| **Indirect-Acting Adrenergic Amines** | |
| Metaraminol | Aramine |
| Mephentermine | Wyamine |
| Ephedrine | Ephedrine |

an alpha-adrenergic agonist produces peripheral vascular vasoconstriction, or a mixed-action alpha and beta drug such as ephedrine can be administered.

A new category of drugs that combat hypotension is the cardiac inotropic agents. This class of drugs produces positive inotropic and vasodilating effects and can be considered to be related to digitalis in regard to pharmacologic effects. The major pharmacologic actions of these drugs include increased cardiac output and decreased LVEDP. These drugs are of benefit for the short-term management of congestive heart failure, especially in patients with congestive heart failure who do not have adequate responses to digitalis, diuretics, or vasodilators. Also, the inotropic agents may be valuable in the treatment of cardiogenic shock. This class of drugs can be considered as an alternative to catecholamines for the treatment of low cardiac output in the postoperative period. Drugs in this category include amrinone (Inocor) and milrinone. As with other vasopressors, constant monitoring of the patient's vital signs is warranted when inotropic agents are administered.

### Hypertension Therapy

A hypertensive emergency may occur in the PACU. The patient may arrive in a hypertensive state or may become hypertensive during the postanesthesia phase. If the diastolic blood pressure rises to about 120 to 140 mm Hg and the patient has a headache, blurred vision, and papilledema along with disorientation, the physician should be notified immediately.

Before any intervention can be instituted, the cause of the postoperative hypertension must be determined. First, the evaluation should focus on the equipment used to determine the blood pressure; it may not be functioning correctly. For example, the blood pressure cuff may be too narrow; the transducer may not be calibrated correctly; or transducer overshoot may be seen. Next, the evaluation should focus on preexisting diseases. More specifically, the patient may have essential hypertension, and the blood pressure readings may be normal for that patient.

Increased sympathetic nervous system activity causes postoperative hypertension. More specifically, pain, stimulation with an endotracheal tube, bladder distention, and preeclampsia are some of the clinical phenomena that may lead to hypertension. Postoperative pain should be assessed because it can cause a significant degree of hypertension. Pain can be eliminated as a causative factor with determination of whether adequate analgesia exists. If the patient has a significant amount of pain, an analgesic should be administered immediately. In addition, if the hypertension is caused by acute anxiety, the use of sedatives may dramatically reduce the blood pressure. Hypoxemia along with hypercarbia from hypoventilation is also a common cause of postoperative hypertension. Hence, during the evaluation of the patient, the patient's rate and depth of ventilation should be assessed. If the patient has hypoventilation, prompt use of the stir-up regimen is mandated. Another assessment tool in the evaluation of postoperative hypertension is the amount and degree of hypothermia. More specifically, if the patient is shivering, an accompanying increase in blood pressure is seen. Prompt interventions to increase the patient's core temperature to reduce shivering is warranted (see Chapter 53). An assessment of the patient's fluid volume status should be made to determine whether hypervolemia exists because fluid overload can cause postoperative hypertension. Also, if the patient has acute pulmonary edema caused by hypertensive heart disease, correction of the pulmonary edema usually reduces the blood pressure to acceptable limits. Certainly, a determination should be made to see whether a hypertensive emergency exists; if it does, treatment must be started promptly.

If pharmacologic antihypertensive therapy is deemed necessary by the physician, the drugs listed in Table 11-5 usually are instituted. For severe postoperative hypertension, SNP is probably the drug of choice. While the SNP is prepared, nifedipine (Adalat, Procardia) can be given sublingually. Nifedipine reduces the blood pressure and enhances coronary blood flow,

**Table 11-5　Drugs Used for Treatment of Hypertensive Crisis**

| Drug* | Route | Initial Dose | Onset of Action (min) | Duration of Action | Comment |
|---|---|---|---|---|---|
| Diazoxide (Hyperstat) | IV | 3-5 mg/kg slow bolus | 3-5 | 5-12 h | |
| Sodium nitroprusside (Nipride, Nitropress) | IV | 0.25-0.5 µg/kg/min | 1-2 | < 5 min | Titrate dose for desired effect |
| Nitroglycerin (Tridil, Nitrol IV, Nitrostat IV) | IV | 0.25-3 µg/kg/min | 2-5 | < 5 min | |
| Phentolamine (Regitine) | IV | 5-15 mg bolus; 200-400 mg/L infusion | Immediate | < 15 min | Titrate dose for desired effect |
| Hydralazine (Apresoline) | IV | 5-10 mg | 15-20 | 4-6 h | Given slowly when IV |
| | IM | 10-40 mg | 30 | | |
| Trimethaphan camsylate (Arfonad) | IV | 10-20 µg/kg/min | 1 | 2-4 min | |
| Propranolol (Inderal, Ipran) | IV | 0.1-0.5 mg slowly, up to 2 mg | 10 | 4-6 h | May repeat dose |
| Esmolol (Brevibloc) | IV | 50-300 µg/kg/min | 5 | 20 min | Avoid concentration > 10 mg/mL |
| Labetalol (Normodyne, Trandate) | IV | 0.25 mg/kg | 10 | 4-6 h | Give slowly |
| Nifedipine (Procardia, Adalat) | SIV | 10 mg | 3 | 7 h | SIV dose while nitroglycerin is prepared |
| | IV | 10 mg (slow) | 5-10 | | |
| Verapamil (Calan, Isoptin) | IV | 2.5-5 mg | 2-5 | 4-6 h | |

*IV*, Intravenous; *IM*, intramuscular; *SIV*, slow intravenous infusion.
*Listed by generic name, with trade name in parentheses.

especially in the presence of ischemic heart disease. Also, the use of nifedipine may preclude the use of a central venous catheter that is required when SNP is given. For sublingual administration of nifedipine, a 10-mg capsule is punctured with a pin in several places and the contents are squeezed under the tongue. Should SNP be necessary, the dose is 0.25 to 0.5 µg/kg/min. Once the patient's condition is stabilized, hydralazine 5 to 10 mg and propranolol 0.2 to 0.5 mg may be given in repeated intravenous doses to wean the patient off SNP. Propranolol should be titrated to maintain the heart rate at about 100 bpm. Other beta blockers, such as labetalol, metoprolol, and esmolol, may be used intravenously. Esmolol may be the drug of choice because of its short duration of action and rapid onset. The hydralazine can be given as intravenous boluses every 20 to 30 minutes to keep the patient's condition normotensive. Because these drugs are extremely potent and have their own complications, they are discussed briefly in the following sections.

**Diazoxide.** Diazoxide (Hyperstat) is avidly bound to and inactivated by serum proteins and thus must be given as a rapid (within 15 seconds) intravenous bolus of 3 to 5 mg/kg every 5 minutes. After three bolus administrations, if the desired response is still not obtained, use of SNP should be considered. That diazoxide cannot be titrated in accordance with the patient's response is the major disadvantage of diazoxide as compared with SNP. The onset of action of this drug is within 3 to 5 minutes, and its duration is between 5 and 12 hours. Its action is immediate and is achieved through its direct vasodilating effects. Because the drug has more effect on the resistance vessels than the capacitance vessels, it decreases the afterload and has no effect on the preload. Concurrent administration of a loop diuretic, such as furosemide (40 to 80 mg intravenously), is usually advantageous especially if the patient's condition is edematous as a result of either cardiac or renal failure.

**Sodium Nitroprusside.** A compound of unusual chemical structure, SNP (Nipride) is immediately effective in all cases of severe hypertensive crises, including those resistant to diazoxide. Its action is thought to result from the peripheral arteriolar dilatory effect of the drug. Because it can lower blood pressure rapidly, careful intravenous administration with constant bedside arterial pressure monitoring is required. The drug is extremely light sensitive and must be administered through bottles and tubing that are wrapped and protected from the light. Only fresh solutions should be used. Solutions that are more than 4 hours old should be discarded because they may form thiocyanates. Treatment is started with a solution of 250 mL of 5% dextrose in water and 50 mg of SNP (200 µg/mL) with use of an infusion pump to ensure a precise flow rate. A dose of 1 to 2 µg/kg/min usually produces a prompt decrease in blood pressure, which returns to control levels within 5 minutes after the drug is stopped. Acute postoperative hypertension can be treated with a one-time single intravenous injection of 50 to 100 µg of SNP. The onset of action of this drug is 1 or 2 minutes, and its duration of action is 2 to 5 minutes. Because of its unique chemical structure, cyanide is released into the blood stream when the drug is used. The cyanide is quickly converted to thiocyanate by the liver. Thiocyanate toxicity (fatigue, nausea, anorexia, muscle spasms, and disorientation) may result from prolonged use or from high dosages; therefore, monitoring of serum thiocyanate levels is advised when the drug is used longer than 24 hours. Toxic symptoms appear with serum thiocyanate levels of 5 to 10 mg/dL, and the compound can be rapidly removed with peritoneal dialysis. As with diazoxide, once blood pressure has been brought to control levels, concomitant use of an oral medication such as guanethidine or methyldopa allows the gradual tapering and discontinuance of SNP.

**Phentolamine.** Phentolamine mesylate (Regitine), an alpha-receptor blocker, is specifically indicated for management of hypertensive crises associated with increased circulating catecholamines. These crises may result from pheochromocytoma or the sudden release of tissue catecholamine stores caused by certain drugs or foods that contain tyramine in patients receiving monoamine oxidase (MAO) inhibitors (pargyline derivatives, primarily Eutonyl). The antipressor effect of a single intravenous injection is short lived, usually lasting less than 15 minutes. Therefore, administration of phentolamine with intravenous infusion (200 to 400 g/L) is desirable, along with titration of the dosage to achieve the desired pressure level after the blood pressure has been controlled initially with a rapid intravenous dose of 2 to 15 mg. Because the drug blocks only alpha receptors, beta-mediated effects of the circulating

catecholamine on the heart must be controlled with the specific beta blocker, propranolol hydrochloride.

With rare exception, these three drugs (diazoxide, SNP, and phentolamine) can be considered the mainstays of modern therapy in acute hypertensive crises. The other drugs discussed here should be considered second-line drugs. Their primary disadvantages include slower onset of action, rapid development of tachyphylaxis, and marked central nervous system depressant effects. In most instances, they should be used to supplement and initiate long-term control once the acute crisis is resolved with the primary drugs.

**Hydralazine.** Hydralazine (Apresoline) is not effective in hypertensive encephalopathy–complicating acute or chronic glomerulonephropathy; it is used in encephalopathy that has chronic essential hypertension as an underlying cause. Blood pressure is reduced through vasodilatation, which reduces vascular resistance and results in a marked increase in cardiac output and heart rate that can aggravate underlying angina and cardiac failure. The determining factor in this situation is the net change in myocardial oxygen consumption achieved with lowering the elevated afterload. On the other hand, a decrease in blood pressure produced with hydralazine is not accompanied by a commensurate decrease in renal blood flow, so the drug is especially suited for management of hypertensive emergencies associated with renal insufficiency. The initial intravenous dose of 5 to 10 mg should be given. The onset of action of this drug is 15 to 20 minutes, and the duration is about 4 to 6 hours. Alternatively, the drug dosage may be increased in 5-mg increments up to 20 mg. The maintenance dose depends on patient response but is generally 5 to 10 mg intravenously every 4 to 6 hours.

**Trimethaphan Camsylate.** Trimethaphan (Arfonad) is a ganglionic vasodepressor that blocks both the sympathetic and parasympathetic systems at the autonomic ganglia. The effect is primarily orthostatic; therefore, large doses must be used to reduce blood pressure in supine patients. The head of the bed should be elevated (reverse Trendelenburg's position), if possible, to augment the antipressor action. The dose of this drug is 10 to 20 µg/kg/min. The onset of action is about 1 minute, and the duration of action is 2 to 4 minutes. The 500-mg ampule of trimethaphan is mixed in 250 mL of normal saline solution, which results in a strength of 2 mg/mL. Complications of such ganglionic blockade include atony of the bowel and bladder and paralytic ileus, especially when the drug is used longer than 24 hours. Because of the commensurate decrease in the glomerular filtration rate when the blood pressure is lowered with the use of this agent, use is not recommended in patients for whom renal insufficiency complicates the hypertensive crisis. The drug's major disadvantage is that it rapidly loses effectiveness after 24 to 72 hours and another agent must be substituted. The drug requires extremely close monitoring by the perianesthesia nurse.

**Nitroglycerin.** Nitroglycerin is a potent vasodilator that produces relaxation of both arterial and venous smooth muscles. The pharmacologic effects of nitroglycerin are mainly on the venous circulation. It produces an increase in venous capacitance, which leads to a reduction in venous return and a decrease in right atrial and pulmonary capillary wedge pressures. Therefore, the main effect of nitroglycerin is a reduction in the preload. Also, the myocardial oxygen demand is decreased because of the decrease in myocardial wall tension.

Intravenous nitroglycerin may be indicated for treatment of myocardial ischemia, control of hypertension, relief of angina pectoris, and production of vasodilatation for patients with severe congestive heart failure.

When intravenous nitroglycerin is administered in the PACU, an automated infusion pump should be used. The usual dosage is between 0.25 and 3 μg/kg/min. The onset of action for this drug is 2 to 5 minutes, and the duration of action is between 3 and 5 minutes. The patient should be continuously monitored for hypotension. Should hypotension occur, an alpha agonist, such as methoxamine, may be used to ensure that the patient's coronary perfusion pressure is maintained. Nitroglycerin migrates into plastic; hence, the perianesthesia nurse should periodically change the plastic tubing on the automated infusion pump and also ensure that only glass bottles are used for dilution.

**Propranolol.** Propranolol (Inderal, Ipran) is the prototype beta-blocking drug; consequently, all drugs in this class are compared with propranolol. This drug is known to be nonselective because it blocks both beta$_1$ and beta$_2$ receptors. After administration of this drug, decreased heart rate, contractility, and cardiac output occur. The drug can be administered in single intravenous doses of 0.1 to 0.5 mg, with a maximum dose of about 2 mg.

**Esmolol.** Esmolol (Brevibloc) is a cardioselective ultrashort-acting beta-blocking agent with a rapid onset and short duration of action. Because it is cardioselective, esmolol does not appear to affect bronchial or vascular tone at the doses required to reduce the heart rate. This drug has also been shown to blunt the response to endotracheal intubation and can be effective in treatment of postoperative hypertension. In the treatment of postoperative hypertension, a loading dose of 500 μg/kg should be administered over a 1-minute period. Then, a continuous infusion of 50 to 300 μg/kg/min should be started. The peak response of esmolol occurs in 5 minutes, with a duration of action of about 20 minutes.

**Labetalol.** Labetalol (Normodyne, Trandate) is a drug that possesses antagonist activity at both the alpha and beta receptors. With intravenous administration, it is about seven times more potent on the beta receptors than on the alpha receptors. More specifically, this drug is an alpha$_1$ antagonist and has antagonist activities on both the beta$_1$ and beta$_2$ receptors. For treatment of postoperative hypertension, a loading dose of 0.25 mg/kg should be administered over a 2-minute period. After this initial dose, intravenous titration to effect should be done at 10-minute intervals to a total of 300 mg. If a continuous infusion is needed, a dose of 2 mg/min can be used.

**Metoprolol.** Metoprolol (Lopressor) is a beta blocker that can be used in patients with reactive and obstructive lung disease because this drug selectively blocks the beta$_1$ effects and consequently blocks the inotropic and chronotropic responses. This selective beta-adrenergic effect is dose related; at high doses, both beta$_1$ and beta$_2$ receptors become blocked and airway resistance may increase. For treatment of postoperative hypertension, an intravenous dose of 2 to 5 mg should be used.

## SUMMARY

The anatomy and physiology of the cardiovascular system has been presented in depth. Various methods included invasive and noninvasive techniques. The electrocardiogram and the electrical activity of the heart were presented, and all the excellent texts mentioned in the bibliography should help the perianesthesia nurse gain expertise in this area. Also, the myocardial infarction was presented and the various cardiovascular drugs that are currently used were described in detail. One area of medical research is in discovery of new drugs to enhance cardiovascular function. The reader is also recommended to seek the current literature in this area as new methods and drugs continue to be introduced.

# BIBLIOGRAPHY

Aitkenhead A, Smith G, Rowbotham D: *Textbook of anaesthesia*, ed 5, Philadelphia, 2007, Churchill Livingstone.

Alspach J: *Core curriculum for critical care nursing*, ed 6, Philadelphia, 2005, Saunders.

Atlee J: *Complications in anesthesia*, ed 2, Philadelphia, 2007, Saunders.

Barash P, Cullen B, Stoelting R: *Clinical anesthesia*, ed 5, Philadelphia, 2001, Lippincott Williams & Wilkins.

Benumof J, Saidman L: *Anesthesia & perioperative complications*, ed 2, St Louis, 1999, Mosby.

Brunton L, Lazo J, Parker K: *Goodman and Gilman's the pharmacological basis of therapeutics*, ed 11, New York, 2005, McGraw-Hill Professional.

Drake R, Vogl W, Mitchell A: *Gray's anatomy for students*, Philadelphia, 2005, Churchill Livingstone.

Estafanous F, Barash P, Reves J, editors: *Cardiac anesthesia: principles and clinical practice*, ed 2, Philadelphia, 2001, Lippincott Williams & Wilkins.

Evers A, Maze M: *Anesthetic pharmacology: physiologic principles and clinical practice*, Philadelphia, 2004, Churchill Livingstone.

Fisher L: *Benumof's anesthesia and uncommon diseases*, ed 5, Philadelphia, 2007, Saunders.

Gallager C., Issenberg B: *Simulation in anesthesia*, Philadelphia, 2007, Saunders.

Ganong W: *Review of medical physiology*, ed 22, New York, 2005, McGraw-Hill Medical.

Guyton A, Hall J: *Textbook of medical physiology*, ed 11, Philadelphia, 2006, Saunders.

Kier L, Dowd C: *The chemistry of drugs for nurse anesthetists*, Chicago, 2004, AANA Publishing, Inc.

Lake C, Hines R, Blitt C: *Clinical monitoring: practical applications for anesthesia and critical care*, Philadelphia, 2001, Saunders.

Longnecker D, Murphy F: *Dripps, Eckenhoff, Vandam's introduction to anesthesia*, ed 9, Philadelphia, 1997, Saunders.

Longnecker D, Tinker J, Morgan G: *Principles and practice of anesthesiology*, ed 2, St Louis, 1998, Mosby.

Miller R, editor: *Anesthesia*, ed 5, Philadelphia, 2000, Churchill Livingstone.

Murray J, Nadel J: *Textbook of respiratory medicine*, ed 2, Philadelphia, 1994, Saunders.

Nagelhout J, Zaglaniczy K: *Nurse anesthesia*, ed 3, St Louis, 2005, Saunders.

Smartt S: The pulmonary artery catheter: gold standard or redundant relic, *J PeriAnesthesia Nurs* 20(6): 373–379, 2005.

Stoelting R: *Pharmacology and physiology in anesthetic practice*, ed 3, Philadelphia, 1999, Lippincott-Raven.

Stoelting R, Miller R: *Basics of anesthesia*, ed 4, Philadelphia, 2000, Churchill Livingstone.

Townsend C, Beauchamp R, Evers B, et al: *Sabiston textbook of surgery: the biological basis of modern surgical practice*, ed 17, Philadelphia, 2004, Saunders.

PHYSIOLOGIC CONSIDERATIONS IN THE PACU

# 12

# THE RESPIRATORY SYSTEM

Cecil B. Drain, PhD, RN, CRNA, FAAN, FASAHP

For the past few years, no new inhalation anesthetic agent has been introduced. This lack of a new agent is the result of a variety of factors, but the bottom line is that the inhalational agents presently in use possess positive characteristics and researchers are unable to develop a significant improvement to the agents already on the market. The good news of this situation is that a significant amount of research can be performed on these time-tested agents and the result of all this is enhanced patient safety.

The inhalation anesthetic agents depress respiratory function. They also depend largely on the respiratory system for removal during emergence from anesthesia. The other anesthetic agents, such as intravenous agents, also depress respiration. Much of the morbidity and mortality that occurs in the postanesthesia care unit (PACU) can be attributed to an alteration in lung mechanics and a dysfunction in airway dynamics. In fact, 70% to 80% of the morbidity and mortality that occur in the PACU is postulated to be associated with some form of respiratory dysfunction. Consequently, a detailed discussion of the many facets of respiratory anatomy and physiology is presented in this chapter. If the perianesthesia nurse incorporates this information into clinical practice, care of the surgical patient in the immediate postoperative period will be enhanced.

## DEFINITIONS

**Acidemia:** Lower than normal blood pH (increased hydrogen ion concentration).
**Acidosis:** The process that leads to an increase in hydrogen ion concentration in the blood.
**Adventitious Sounds:** Abnormal noises that may be heard superimposed on a patient's breath sounds.
**Alkalemia:** Higher than normal blood pH (decreased hydrogen ion concentration).
**Alkalosis:** The process that leads to a decrease in hydrogen ion concentration in the blood.

**Apnea:** The absence of breathing.
**Apneustic Breathing:** Prolonged inspiratory efforts interrupted by occasional expirations.
**Atelectasis:** Collapse of the alveoli.
**Bradypnea:** Respiratory rate, in the adult, that is lower than 8 breaths per minute.
**Bronchiectasis:** Dilatation of the bronchi.
**Bronchospasm:** Constriction of the bronchial airways caused by an increase in smooth muscle tone in the airways.
**Central Sleep Apnea:** A cessation of breathing during sleep as a result of transient abolishment of the drive to the respiratory muscles.
**Cheyne-Stokes Respirations:** Periods of apnea alternating with rhythmic, shallow, and progressively deeper and then shallower respirations that are associated with brain damage, heart or kidney failure, or drug overdose.
**Compliance (lung):** A measure of distensibility of the lungs; the amount of change in volume per change in pressure across the lung.
**Cyanosis:** A sign of poor oxygen transport, characterized by a bluish discoloration of the skin, produced when more than 5 g of hemoglobin per deciliter of arterial blood are in the deoxygenated, or reduced, state.
**Dyspnea:** A patient's perception of shortness of breath.
**Epistaxis:** Hemorrhage from the nose.
**Hypercapnia:** Increased tension of carbon dioxide ($PaCO_2$) in the blood.
**Hyperoxemia:** Increased tension of oxygen ($PaO_2$) in the blood.
**Hyperpnea:** Increased rate of respirations.
**Hyperventilation:** Overventilation of the alveoli in relation to the amount of carbon dioxide produced by the body.
**Hypocapnia:** Decreased $PaCO_2$ in the blood.
**Hypoventilation:** Underventilation of the alveoli in relation to the amount of carbon dioxide produced by the body.
**Hypoxemia:** Decreased $PaO_2$ in the blood.
**Hypoxia:** Inadequate tissue oxygen levels.
**Kussmaul Respirations:** Rapid deep respirations associated with diabetic ketoacidosis.

**Methemoglobin:** Hemoglobin that has the iron atom in the ferric state.
**Minute Ventilation ($V_E$):** The volume of air expired during a period of 1 minute.
**Orthopnea:** Severe dyspnea that is relieved when the patient elevates the head and chest.
**Oxyhemoglobin:** Hemoglobin that is fully oxygenated.
**Paroxysmal Nocturnal Dyspnea (PND):** A sudden onset of severe dyspnea when the patient is lying down.
**Partial Pressure:** The pressure exerted by each individual gas when mixed in a container with other gases.
**Periodic Breathing:** A regular waxing and waning of ventilation as a result of fluctuations in central respiratory drive.
**Polycythemia:** Increased number of red blood cells (RBCs) in the blood.
**Rales:** Short discontinuous explosive adventitious sounds, usually called crackles.
**Reduced Hemoglobin:** Hemoglobin in the deoxy state (not fully saturated with oxygen).
**Respiration:** The process by which oxygen and carbon dioxide are exchanged between the outside atmosphere and the cells in the body.
**Rhonchi:** Continuous musical adventitious sounds.
**Sleep Apnea:** Repeated absence of breathing during sleep, sometimes hundreds of times during the night and often for a minute or longer.
**Torr:** Units of the Torricelli scale, the classic mercury scale, which is used to express the same value as millimeters of mercury (mm Hg).
**Ventilation:** The mechanical movement of air in and out of the lungs.
**Wheeze:** A high-pitched sibilant rhonchus usually produced on expiration.

## RESPIRATORY SYSTEM ANATOMY

### The Nose

The nose, the first area in which inhaled air is filtered (Fig. 12-1), is lined with ciliated epithelium. Cilia move mucus and particles of foreign matter to the pharynx to be expectorated or swallowed (Fig. 12-2). Other functions of the nose include humidification and warming

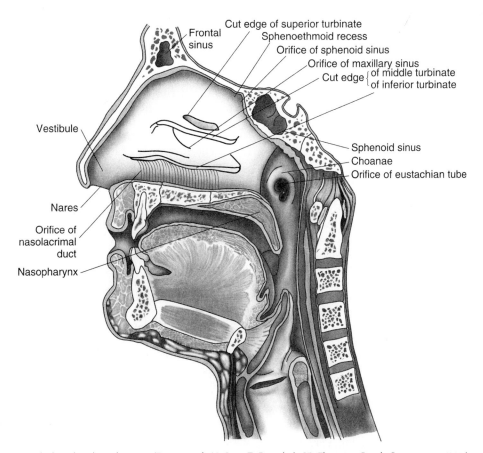

**Fig. 12-1** Sagittal section through nose. *(From Lough M, Boat T, Doershuk CF: The nose, Respir Care 20:844, 1975.)*

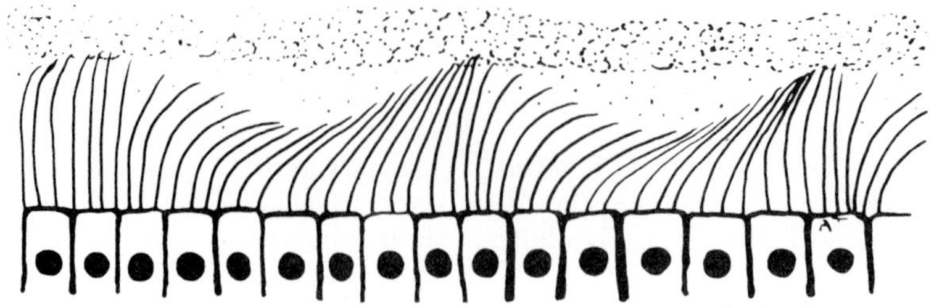

**Fig. 12-2**   Mucus blanket of nasal airways. Outer (gel-like) layer rests on tips of beating cilia, and inner (water) layer bathes cilia. Particles are trapped on sticky outer blanket and carried posteriorly into nasopharynx by organized beating of cilia. *(From Lough M, Boat T, Doershuk CF: The nose,* Respir Care *20:845, 1975.)*

of the inhaled air and the olfactory function of smell.

Dry gases are often administered during anesthesia. These gases dry the mucus membranes and slow the action of the cilia. The administration of moist gases in the PACU with various humidification and mist therapy devices keeps this physiologic filter system viable.

A tracheostomy precludes the functions of the nose, and proper tracheostomy care, including the administration of humidified oxygen, must be instituted.

The blood supply to the nose is provided by the internal and external maxillary arteries, which are derived from the external carotid artery, and by branches of the internal carotid arteries. The venous plexus of the nasal mucosa is drained into the common facial vein, the anterior facial vein, the exterior jugular vein, or the ophthalmic vein. A highly vascular plexus of vessels is located in the mucosa of the anterior nasal septum. This plexus is called Kiesselbach's plexus or Little's area. In most instances, this area is the source of epistaxis.

Epistaxis may occur in the PACU after trauma to the nasal veins from nasotracheal tubes or to nasal airways during anesthesia. If epistaxis occurs, prompt action should be taken to prevent aspiration of blood into the lungs. The patient should be positioned with the head up and flexed forward toward the chest. Cold compresses applied to the bridge of the nose and neck may be effective in slowing or stopping the bleeding. If the bleeding is profuse, the oral cavity should be suctioned carefully and the attending physician notified. A nasal pack or cautery with silver nitrate or electric current may be necessary to stop the bleeding.

## The Pharynx

The pharynx originates at the posterior aspect of the nasal cavities and is called the nasopharynx until it reaches the soft palate, where it becomes the oropharynx. The oropharynx extends to the level of the hyoid bone, where it becomes the laryngeal pharynx, which extends caudally to below the hyoid bone.

## The Larynx

The larynx, or voice box (Fig. 12-3), is situated anterior to the third, fourth, and fifth cervical vertebrae in the adult male. It is situated higher in women and children. Nine cartilages held together with ligaments and intertwined with many small muscles constitute the larynx. The thyroid cartilage, the largest, is V-shaped; its protruding prominence is commonly referred to as the Adam's apple. The thyroid cartilage is attached to the hyoid bone by the hyothyroid membrane and to the cricoid cartilage. The cricoid cartilage is situated below the thyroid cartilage and anteriorly forms a signet-shaped ring. The signet lies posteriorly as a quadrilateral lamina joined in front by a thin arch. The inner surface of the cricoid cartilage is lined with a mucus membrane. In children younger than 12 years of age, the cricoid cartilage is the smallest opening to the bronchi of the lungs.

The epiglottis, a cartilage of the larynx, is an important landmark for tracheal intubation that serves to deflect foreign objects away from the trachea. This cartilage is leaf-shaped and projects outward above the thyroid cartilage over the entrance to the trachea. The lower portion is attached to the thyroid lamina, and the anterior surface is attached to the hyoid bone and thereby to the base of the tongue. The valleys on either side of the glossoepiglottic fold are termed the valleculae.

The arytenoid cartilages are paired and articulate with the lamina of the cricoid through the articular surface on the base of the arytenoid. The anterior angle of the arytenoid cartilage projects forward to form the vocal process. The medial surface of the cartilage is covered by a mucus membrane to form the lateral portion of the rima glottis—that is, the split between the vocal cords. The rima glottis is completed anteriorly by the thyroid cartilage and posteriorly by the cricoid cartilage.

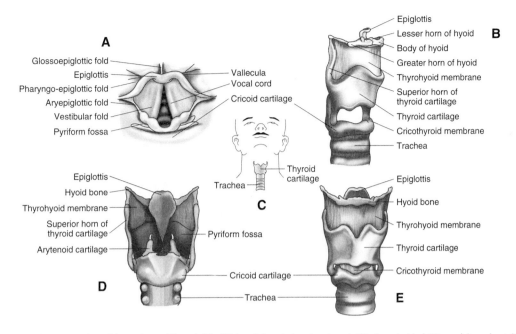

**Fig. 12-3** Larynx as viewed from above (**A**) and side (**B**) in relation to head and neck (**C**), from behind (**D**), and from front (**E**). (**A** to **E**, Redrawn from Jacob SW, Francone CA, Lossow WJ: Structure and function in man, ed 5, Philadelphia, 1982, Saunders.)

The corniculate cartilages are two small nodules that are located at the apex of the arytenoid. The cuneiform cartilage is a flake of cartilage within the margin of the aryepiglottic folds. It probably serves to stiffen the folds.

The larynx has nine membranes and extrinsic or intrinsic ligaments. Extrinsic ligaments connect the thyroid cartilage and the epiglottis with the hyoid bone and the cricoid cartilage with the trachea. Intrinsic ligaments connect the cartilages of the larynx with each other.

The fissure between the vocal folds, or true cords, is termed the rima glottidis or glottis. In the adult, this opening between the vocal cords is the narrowest part of the laryngeal cavity. Any obstruction in this area leads to death via suffocation if not promptly relieved. The rima glottidis divides the laryngeal cavity into two main compartments: (1) the upper portion is the vestibule, which extends from the laryngeal outlet to the vocal cords and includes the laryngeal sinus, sometimes called the middle compartment; and (2) the lower compartment, which extends from the vocal cords to the lower border of the cricoid cartilage and thereafter is continuous with the trachea.

The muscles of the larynx are also either intrinsic or extrinsic. The intrinsic muscles control the movements of the laryngeal framework. They open the cords on inspiration, close the cords and the laryngeal inlet during swallowing, and alter the tension of the cords during speech.

The extrinsic muscles are involved in the movements of the larynx as a whole, such as in swallowing.

The nerve supply to the larynx is from the superior and recurrent laryngeal nerves of the vagus. The superior laryngeal nerve passes deep to both the internal and the external carotid arteries and divides into a small external branch that supplies the cricothyroid muscles that tense the vocal ligaments. The larger internal branch pierces the thyrohyoid membrane to provide sensory fibers to the mucosa of both sides of the epiglottis and the larynx above the cords.

The recurrent laryngeal nerve on the right side exits from the vagus as it crosses the right subclavian artery and ascends to the larynx in the groove between the trachea and esophagus (Fig. 12-4). Once the nerve reaches the neck, it assumes the same relationships as on the right. This nerve provides the motor function to the intrinsic muscles of the larynx, with the exception of the cricothyroid, and also provides sensory function to the laryngeal mucosa below the vocal cords.

Laryngospasm, a spasm of the laryngeal muscle tissue, may be complete (with complete closure of the vocal cords) or incomplete (with partial closure of the vocal cords). Patients with partial or complete airway obstruction, such as laryngospasm, usually have a paradoxic rocking motion of the chest wall. This motion can be misinterpreted as normal abdominal breathing. Hence, the perianesthesia nurse should always

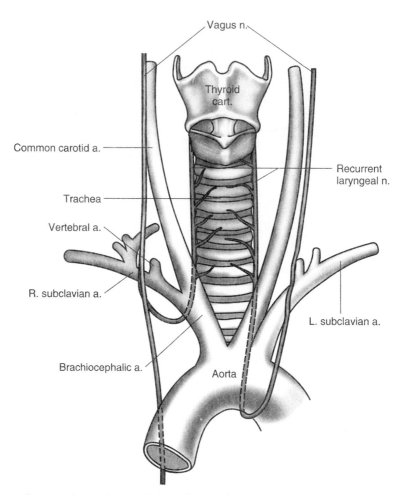

**Fig. 12-4**  Course of recurrent laryngeal nerve. *(Redrawn from Jacob SW, Francone CA, Lossow WJ: Structure and function in man, ed 5, Philadelphia, 1982, Saunders.)*

auscultate the patient's lungs to determine the degree of ventilation and should not rely on just a visual assessment of the motion of the chest.

When a laryngospasm occurs in the PACU, prompt emergency treatment is necessary to save the patient's life. The perianesthesia nurse should have someone on the PACU staff summon the anesthetist or anesthesiologist when laryngospasm is suspected. Treatment consists of mask ventilation with sustained moderate pressure on the reservoir bag. This maneuver usually helps to overcome the partial laryngospasm. Complete laryngospasm not relieved with positive pressure within at least 1 minute necessitates more aggressive treatment. Intravenous (0.5 mg/kg) or intramuscular (1 mg/kg) succinylcholine may be administered to relax the smooth muscle of the larynx. Endotracheal intubation may be necessary. The nurse must remember that ventilation of the patient should be continued until complete respiratory functioning has returned.

## The Trachea

The trachea is a musculomembranous tube surrounded by 16 to 20 incomplete cartilaginous rings. These C-shaped rings prevent the collapse of the trachea and thereby maintain free passage of air. The trachea is lined with ciliated columnar epithelium, which aids in the removal of foreign material.

The area at the distal end of the trachea at the point of bifurcation into the right and left main stem bronchi is called the carina (Fig. 12-5). The carina contains sensitive pressoreceptors, which on stimulation (i.e., with an endotracheal tube) cause the patient to cough and "buck." The angle created at the point of bifurcation into the right and left main stem bronchi is clinically significant to the perianesthesia nurse. This angle varies according to the age and gender of the patient (Table 12-1). The angle at the right main stem bronchus is smaller than the angle at the left main stem bronchus. Foreign material can easily enter the

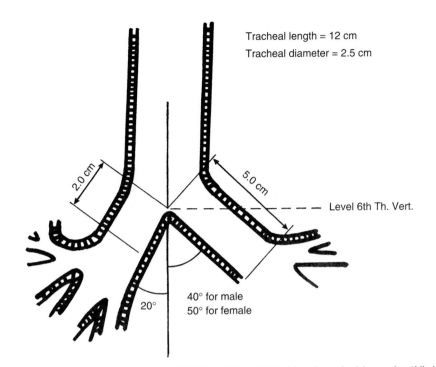

Tracheal length = 12 cm

Tracheal diameter = 2.5 cm

2.0 cm

5.0 cm

Level 6th Th. Vert.

20°

40° for male
50° for female

**Fig. 12-5** Bifurcation of trachea into main stem bronchi. *(From Collins VJ:* Principles of anesthesiology, *ed 2, Philadelphia, 1976, Lea & Febiger.)*

right main stem bronchus at this point. Endotracheal tubes, if advanced too far, usually enter the right main stem bronchus and thereby occlude the left main stem bronchus. Thus, the left lung cannot be ventilated. Signs of this complication include decreased or absent breath sounds in the left side of the chest, tachycardia, and uneven expansion of the chest on inspiration and expiration.

### The Bronchi and Lungs

Each primary bronchus supplies a number of lobar bronchi (Fig. 12-6). Humans have an upper, middle, and lower lobe bronchus on the right and only an upper and lower lobe bronchus on the left. Within each pulmonary lobe, a lobar (secondary) bronchus soon divides into tertiary branches that are remarkably constant as to number and distribution within the lobe.

| Table 12-1 | Variations of Bronchial Bifurcation Angles in Adults and Children | |
|---|---|---|
| | Right Bronchus (Degrees) | Left Bronchus (Degrees) |
| Newborn | 12-35 | 30-65 |
| Adult male | 20 | 40 |
| Adult female | 19 | 51 |

The segment of a lobe aerated by a tertiary bronchus is usually well delineated from adjoining segments by complete planes of connective tissue. These areas of the lung are well defined; therefore, pulmonary diseases may be limited to a particular segment or segments of a lobe.

The bronchi bifurcate 22 or 23 times from the main stem bronchus to the terminal bronchi. These bronchi have connective tissue and cartilaginous support. The terminal bronchi branch to the bronchioles with a diameter of 1 mm or smaller and lack cartilaginous support. Bronchioles have thin highly elastic walls composed of smooth muscle, which is arranged circularly. When the circular smooth muscle is contracted, the bronchiolar lumen is constricted. This circular smooth muscle is innervated by the parasympathetic nervous system (vagus nerve), which causes constriction, and the sympathetic nervous system, which causes dilatation. The patency of the terminal bronchioles therefore is determined by the tonus of the muscle produced by a balance between the two components of the nervous system. Bronchospasm occurs when the smooth muscles constrict or experience spasm, ultimately leading to airway obstruction.

The terminal bronchioles divide into the respiratory bronchioles in which actual gas exchange first occurs. The respiratory

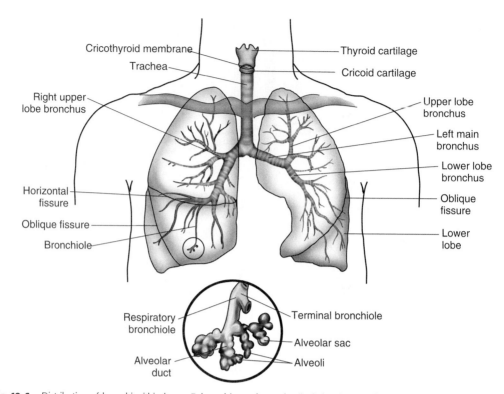

**Fig. 12-6** Distribution of bronchi within lungs. Enlarged inset shows detail of alveolus. *(Redrawn from Jacob SW, Francone CA, Lossow WJ: Structure and function in man, ed 5, Philadelphia, 1982, Saunders.)*

bronchioles bifurcate to form alveolar ducts, and these, in turn, terminate in spherical enclosures called the alveolar sac. The sacs enclose a small but variable number of terminal alveoli.

The number of alveoli in an average adult's lungs is estimated to be about 750 million. The surface area available for gas exchange is approximately 125 m². Alveoli are shaped like soap bubbles in a glass. The interalveolar septum has a supporting latticework composed of elastic collagenous and reticular fibers. The capillaries are incorporated into and supported by the fibrous lattice. The capillary networks in the lungs are the richest in the body.

The lungs receive unoxygenated blood from the left and right pulmonary arteries, which originate from the right ventricle of the heart. The divisions of the pulmonary artery tend to follow the bifurcations of the airway. Typically, two pulmonary veins exit from each lung, and all four veins empty separately into the left atrium. The blood that arrives in the rich pulmonary capillary network from the pulmonary arteries provides for the metabolic needs of the pulmonary parenchyma. Other portions of the lungs, such as the conducting vessels and airways, need their own private circulation. The bronchial arteries, which arise from the aorta, provide the oxygenated blood to the

lung tissue. The blood of the bronchial arteries returns to the heart by way of the pulmonary veins.

Each lung is contained in a thin elastic membranous sac called the visceral pleura, which is adherent to the external surface of the lung. Another membrane, the parietal pleura, lines the chest wall. These two membranes normally are quite close to each other. A few milliliters of viscous fluid are secreted between them for lubrication. The visceral pleura continuously absorbs this fluid.

## RESPIRATORY SYSTEM PHYSIOLOGY

### Lung Volumes and Capacities

Perianesthesia care of the patient is largely based on knowledge of the physiology and pathophysiology of the respiratory system. Dysfunction in lung volumes and capacities that occurs in the patient after surgery is the compelling reason for institution of the stir-up regimen in the PACU. Accordingly, the physiology of the lung volumes and capacities and lung mechanics are described in detail. Table 12-2 provides the definition and normal value for each lung volume and capacity. As shown in Table 12-2 and Fig. 12-7, a lung capacity comprises two or more lung volumes.

## Table 12-2  Lung Volumes and Capacities

| Terminology | Definition | Healthy Male* (mL) | Healthy Female* (mL) |
|---|---|---|---|
| Tidal volume (V$_T$) | Volume of air inspired or expired at each breath | 660 (230) | 550 (160) |
| Inspiratory reserve volume (IRV) | Maximal volume of air that can be inspired after normal inspiration | 2240 (—) | 1480 (—) |
| Expiratory reserve volume (ERV) | Maximal volume of air that can be expired after normal expiration | 1240 (412) | 730 (300) |
| Residual volume (RV) | Volume of air remaining in lungs after maximal expiration | 2120 (520) | 1570 (380) |
| Vital capacity (VC) | Maximal volume of air that can be expired after maximal inspiration | 4130 (750) | 2760 (540) |
| Total lung capacity (TLC) | Total volume of air contained in lungs at maximal inspiration | 6230 (830) | 4330 (620) |
| Inspiratory capacity (IC) | Maximal volume of air that can be inspired after normal expiration | 2900 (—) | 2030 (—) |
| Functional residual capacity (FRC) | Volume of gas remaining in lungs after normal expiration | 3330 (680) | 2300 (490) |

*Data are mean values, with the standard in milliliters deviation in parentheses.
Adapted from Wylie WB, Churchill-Davidson HC, editors: *A practice of anaesthesia*, ed 4, London, 1978, Lloyd-Luke Medical Books.

**The Lung Volumes.** The tidal volume (V$_T$) represents the amount of air moved into or out of the lungs during a normal ventilatory excursion. Monitoring of this lung volume is important when the patient is receiving ventilatory support. Because the V$_T$ measurement is highly variable, it is not an extremely helpful parameter in pulmonary function tests. Clinically, the V$_T$ can be estimated at 7 mL/kg. For example, a man who weighs 70 kg has a V$_T$ of approximately 490 mL (7 × 70 = 490).

The expiratory reserve volume (ERV) is the maximal amount of air that can be expired from the resting position after a normal spontaneous expiration. The ERV reflects muscle strength, thoracic mobility, and a balance of forces that determine the resting position of the lungs and chest wall after a normal expiration. This lung volume is usually decreased in patients who are morbidly obese (see Chapter 48). This lung volume also is decreased in the immediate postoperative period in patients who have undergone an upper abdominal or thoracic operation.

The residual volume (RV) is the volume of air that remains in the lungs at the end of a maximal expiration. This lung volume represents the balance of forces of the lung elastic forces and thoracic muscle strength. Patients with skeletal muscle relaxant that was not adequately reversed at the end of the anesthetic period may have an elevated RV because

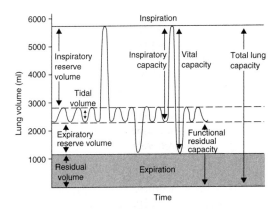

**Fig. 12-7** Graphic representation of normal lung volumes and capacities. *(From Guyton A, Hall J: Textbook of medical physiology, ed 12, Philadelphia, 2000, Saunders.)*

enough muscle strength cannot be generated to force all the air out of the lungs. As the RV increases, more air remains in the lungs so that the air does not participate adequately in gas exchange and becomes dead-space air. As the dead-space volume of air increases, it can impinge on the $V_T$ and hypoxemia can ensue. The importance of the RV is that it allows for continuous gas exchange throughout the entire breathing cycle by providing air to most of the alveoli and that it aerates the blood between breaths. Consequently, the RV prevents wide fluctuations in oxygen and carbon dioxide concentrations during inspiration and expiration.

The inspiratory reserve volume (IRV) reflects a balance of the lung elastic forces, muscle strength, and thoracic mobility. The IRV is the maximal volume of air that can be inspired at the end of a normal spontaneous inspiration. Physiologically, the IRV is available to meet increased metabolic demand at a time of excess physical exertion. It assists in moving a larger volume of air into the alveoli through each ventilatory cycle to increase the overall performance and efficiency of the respiratory system.

**The Lung Capacities.** The inspiratory capacity (IC) is the maximal volume of air that can be inspired from the resting expiratory position. The IC is the sum of the $V_T$ and the IRV.

The functional residual capacity (FRC) represents the previously mentioned resting position. The FRC is the volume of air that remains in the lungs at the end of a normal expiration when no respiratory muscle forces are applied. At FRC, the mechanical forces of the lung and thorax are at rest and no air flow is present. Because the FRC is usually reduced in patients who are recovering from anesthesia, this particular lung capacity is of great importance to the perianesthesia nurse when intensive nursing care is rendered to such patients. For this reason, breathing maneuvers, such as the sustained maximal inspiration (SMI), are instituted in the PACU to raise the FRC (see the next section on lung mechanics). The FRC represents the sum of the ERV and the RV. A severe increase in the FRC is often associated with pulmonary distention, which is technically a state of hyperinflation of the lung. This state of hyperinflation can be caused by two abnormal conditions: airway obstruction and loss of elasticity. Airway obstruction is exemplified by an episode of acute bronchial asthma; a loss of lung elasticity is usually associated with emphysema. A severe decrease in FRC is associated with pulmonary fibrosis and can be the sequela of postoperative atelectasis.

The vital capacity (VC) is the amount of air that can be expired after the deepest possible inspiration. The VC is the sum of the $V_T$, the ERV, and the IRV. The VC measures many factors that simultaneously affect ventilation, including activity of respiratory centers, motor nerves, and respiratory muscles, and thoracic maximum, airway and tissue resistance, and lung volume.

The total lung capacity (TLC) is simply the total amount of air in the lung at a maximal inspiration. The TLC is the sum of the VC and the RV.

Clinical measurements of the TLC, FRC, and RV are difficult because these values include a gas volume that cannot be exhaled. Therefore, the measurements require sophisticated pulmonary function testing equipment with gas dilution techniques or plethysmography. As will be seen, measurements of lung volumes and capacities are useful in the evaluation of lung function.

### Lung Mechanics

*Mechanical Features of the Lungs.* Mechanical forces of the respiratory system actually determine the lung volumes and capacities. For an understanding of how these lung volumes and capacities are determined and how they are affected by anesthesia and surgery, the perianesthesia nurse should become familiar with the balance of forces concept of the respiratory system (see the section on the combined mechanical properties of the lungs and chest wall. The PACU stir-up regimen is designed to increase the postoperative patient's lung volumes and capacities with enhancement of the mechanical forces of the respiratory system.

The lungs and chest wall are viscoelastic structures, one within the other. Because they are elastic, the lungs always want to collapse or recoil to a smaller position. Therefore, as can be seen in the pressure-volume (P-V) curve of the lungs alone (Fig. 12-8), at less than RV, the lungs are collapsed and no pressure is transmitted across the lungs (i.e., no transpulmonary pressure). When the lungs are inflated to a volume halfway between RV and TLC, the lungs seek to recoil or collapse back to the resting position at or actually less than RV, which is reflected by an increase in transpulmonary pressure. When the lungs are fully inflated at TLC, a maximal transpulmonary pressure is also exhibited. By analogy, when a balloon is completely deflated, the pressure measured at the mouth of the balloon is zero. When the balloon is partially inflated, the pressure increases as the elastic forces of the balloon try to make the balloon recoil to its resting position. If the balloon is maximally inflated, the elastic recoil of the balloon is greater, as is the pressure measured at the mouth of the balloon.

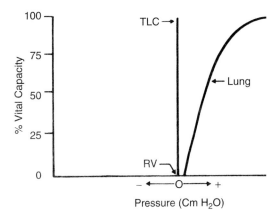

**Fig. 12-8** Static deflation pressure-volume curve for lung. Positive pressures represent pressures that tend to decrease lung volume. *TLC,* Total lung capacity; *RV,* residual volume. *(From Drain C: Physiology of the respiratory system related to anesthesia,* CRNA: Clin Forum Nurse Anesthetists *7(4):163-180, 1996.)*

## Pulmonary Hysteresis

Inflation and deflation paths of the P-V curve of the lung are not aligned on top of each other (Fig. 12-9). The path of deformation (inspiration) to TLC is different from the path followed when the force is withdrawn (expiration) from TLC to RV. This phenomenon is known as pulmonary hysteresis. The following factors contribute to pulmonary hysteresis: (1) properties of the tissue elements (a minor factor); (2) recruitment of lung units; and (3) the surface tension phenomenon (surfactant).

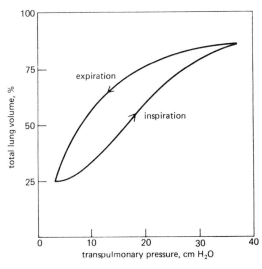

**Fig. 12-9** Inflation and deflation paths of pressure-volume curve of lungs. *(From Levitzky M: Pulmonary physiology, ed 5, New York, 1999, McGraw-Hill.)*

**Elastic Properties of the Lung.** The elastic properties of the lung tissue contribute only a small part to the phenomenon of hysteresis.

**Recruitment of Lung Units.** Recruitment of lung units has an important part in pulmonary hysteresis. For an understanding of recruitment of lung units, the nurse must be familiar with the concept of airway closure. An apex-to-base gradient of alveolar size exists in the lung (Fig. 12-10). This gradient occurs because of the weight of the lung, which tends to "pull" the lung toward its base. As a result, the pleural pressure is more negative at the apex than at the base of the lung. Ultimately, at low lung volumes, the alveoli at the apex are inflated more than the alveoli at the base. At the base of the lungs, some alveoli are closed to ventilation because the weight of the lungs in that area causes the pleural pressure to become positive. Airways open only when the critical opening pressure is achieved during inflation and the lung units peripheral to them are recruited to participate in volume exchange. This process is called radial traction or a tethering effect on airways. An analogy of a nylon stocking may aid in explanation of this concept. When no traction is applied to the nylon stocking, the holes in the stocking are small. As traction is applied to the stocking from all sides, each nylon filament pulls on the others, which spreads apart all the other filaments; and the holes in the stocking enlarge. Similarly, as one airway opens, it produces radial traction on the next airway and pulls the next airway open; in other words, it recruits airways to open. The volume of air in the alveoli behind the closed airways is termed the closing volume (CV). The CV plus the RV is termed the closing capacity (CC). The CC normally occurs at less than the FRC.

During the early emergence phase of anesthesia, patients usually have low lung volumes, which can lead to airway closure. Consequently, a postoperative breathing maneuver that has a maximal alveolar inflating pressure, a long alveolar inflating time, and high alveolar inflating volume, such as the SMI or yawn maneuver, should be used to facilitate the maximal recruitment of lung units. With the recruitment of lung units, the FRC could be raised out of the closing volume range and ultimately hypoxemia could be reduced.

**Surface Tension Phenomenon.** The surface tension phenomenon relates to the action of surfactant on lung tissue. Surfactant is a phospholipid rich in lecithin that is produced by the type II alveolar cells. Surfactant lines the alveolus as a thin surface-active film. This film has a

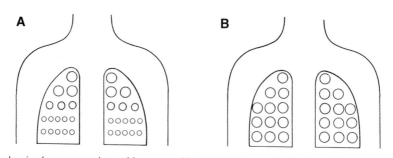

**Fig. 12-10**    Alveolar size from apex to base of lungs, as subject inhales from residual volume **(A)** to total lung capacity **(B)**.

physiologic action of reducing the surface tension of the alveoli and terminal respiratory airways. If the surfactant were not present, the surface tension would be fixed and greater pressure would be needed to keep the alveolus open. As a result, small alveoli would empty into larger ones; atelectasis would regularly occur at low lung volumes; and large expanding pressures would be necessary to reopen collapsed lung units. Surfactant is also an important factor in alveolar inflation because it provides uniformity in the inflation of lung units. In these ways, surfactant helps impart stability to alveoli in the normal lung. In addition to a major role in pulmonary hysteresis, surfactant also contributes to lung recoil and reduces the workload of breathing.

### Lung Compliance

Several other terms that relate to the P-V curve of the lung deserve attention. One term is lung compliance ($C_L$), which is defined as the change in volume for a given change in pressure or the pressure needed for maintenance of a given volume of inflation. The normal value for $C_L$ is 0.1 L per cm $H_2O$.

$$CL = \frac{\Delta V}{\Delta P}$$

with $V$ representing volume and $P$ representing pressure.

Lung compliance is a measure of the distensibility of the lungs during breathing. According to convention, $C_L$ means the slope on the static deflation portion of the P-V curve over the $V_T$ range. Therefore, $C_L$ can be said to be the slope of the P-V curve, and it may remain unchanged even if marked changes in lung elastic properties cause a shift of the P-V curve to the left or right. Hence, clinical measurement of the compliance of the lung is done over the $V_T$ range, during deflation. Measurement of the $C_L$ over any other portion of the P-V curve may result in an inaccurate reading as compared with a normal value. Lung elastic recoil ($Pst_L$) is the pressure exerted by the lung (transpulmonary pressure) because of

its tendency to recoil or collapse to a smaller resting state. At low lung volumes, the $Pst_L$ is low; at high lung volumes, the $Pst_L$ is high. This elastic retractive force ($Pst_L$) is the result of the overall structural elements of the lung combined with the lung surface tension forces. As mentioned previously, the $C_L$ represents the slope of the P-V curve and the $Pst_L$ represents the points along the P-V curve. Changes in $C_L$ and $Pst_L$ have dramatic implications in the alteration in lung volumes that occurs in the immediate postoperative period (see the section on postoperative lung volumes).

***The Equal Pressure Point.*** The equal pressure point (EPP) has many clinical implications to perianesthesia practice. More specifically, intraoperative and postoperative mechanical ventilations, along with pursed lips and abdominal breathing of the patient with compliant airways, are based on this concept.

One can imagine the alveoli and airways as a balloon in a box (Fig. 12-11). Flow out of the balloon is facilitated by the recoil of the balloon, which forces the air out of the balloon through the neck and out into the atmosphere. Addition of pressure all over the box forces the air out of the balloon at a higher rate of flow. Physiologically, the balloon recoil is analogous to the alveolar recoil pressure (Palv). The pressure pushing down on the balloon and its neck corresponds to a positive pleural pressure (Ppl) that is generated on a forced expiratory maneuver. For the air to move out of the alveoli, the alveolar pressure must exceed the pressure at the mouth (Pao). The pressure inside the neck of the balloon corresponds to the intraluminal airway pressure. Consequently, the alveolar pressure comprises the recoil pressure of the alveoli and the plural pressure. Also, the pressure to generate air flow decreases down the airway to the mouth (see Fig. 12-11). During a forced expiratory maneuver, the plural pressure pushes down on the alveoli and the airways. If the alveolar recoil pressure is 30 and the plural pressure is 20, the alveolar pressure is 50. The pressure inside the airway (intraluminal pressure)

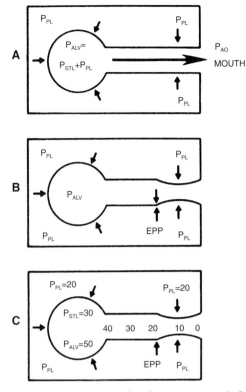

**Fig. 12-11** EPP during forced expiratory maneuver. **A,** Bag-in-box concept. **B,** Equal pressure point added to model. **C,** Conceptual numbers used to illustrate concept of EPP. *Palv*, Alveolar pressure; *Pst$_L$*, elastic recoil pressure; *Ppl*, plural pressure; *Pao*, pressure at mouth. *(From Traver G: Respiratory nursing: the sience and the art, New York, 1982, John Wiley & Sons.)*

decreases progressively downstream toward the mouth. The EPP occurs when the intraluminal pressure is equal to the plural pressure ($20 = 20$); from that point on, the plural pressure exceeds the intraluminal pressure and dynamic compression of the airway occurs. Total collapse of the airways from the EPP and the mouth does not normally occur because of the compliance of the airways. Physiologically, the dynamic compression reduces the airways radius and thus results in an increase in flow rates in the compressed area that aids physiologic mechanisms, such as the cough maneuver, to sheer and expel secretions and mucus out of the airways.

In the patient with highly compliant airways (i.e., with chronic obstructive pulmonary disease), the dynamic compression can completely close the airways. The air that is trapped increases the FRC and becomes dead space. The harder the patient tries to expel air, the greater the plural pressure becomes and more dynamic compression occurs; thus, a vicious cycle ensues. Interventions

to help these patients move air out of the lungs are focused on a reduction of the amount of dynamic compression on the airways. The interventions are to increase the expiratory time and provide physiologic PEEP. Lengthening of the expiratory time aids in reduction of the amount of positive plural pressure on the airways, and physiologic PEEP enhances the airway's intraluminal pressure in the highly compliant airways. In the awake patient with highly compliant airways, abdominal breathing prolongs the expiratory time and pursed lips breathing provides physiologic PEEP. In the patient who is anesthetized, prolonging the expiratory time (i.e., inspiration:expiration [I:E] ratio of 1:3) on the ventilator and use of physiologic PEEP (i.e., 5 cm/$H_2O$) aids in moving air out of the airways.

***The Pulmonary Time Constant.*** The pulmonary time constant is similar to the half-life used in assessment of the pharmacokinetic activity of drugs. A time constant represents the amount of time necessary for flow to decrease by a rate equal to one half the initial flow. A time constant equals the resistance multiplied by the compliance. Therefore, the time necessary to reach each time constant depends on the individual values of resistance and compliance. In normal conditions, the decrease in flow at the first time constant is about 37% of the initial flow, or about 63% of the total volume added or removed from the lungs. The first time constant represents the time necessary for removal or addition of 63% of the total volume of air in the lungs. The decrease in flow rate at the second time constant is about 14%, and the percent volume of air added or removed from the lungs is 86%. The decrease in flow at the third time constant is 5%, with a corresponding 95% volume added or removed. Hence, the higher the time constant, the more air removed or added to the lungs.

The clinical implications of time constants are extremely important in the perianesthesia care of patients who have received an inhalation anesthetic. Patients who have increased airway resistance or increased $C_L$, or both, have a prolonged time necessary for filling and emptying of the lungs. The lung units in this situation are referred to as slow lung units. The patient with slow lung units usually has chronic obstructive pulmonary disease. Patients with a significant amount of increased secretions also have some slow lung units. Consequently, patients with slow lung units usually have a slow emergence from inhalation anesthesia. Patients with a low $C_L$, such as patients with pulmonary fibrosis, have fast lung units. Hence, these patients can fill or empty the lungs rather rapidly and have a rapid emergence from inhalation anesthesia.

### Mechanical Features of the Chest Wall.
Because of its elastic properties, the chest wall always springs out or recoils outward, seeking a larger resting volume. The resting volume of the lungs alone is less than RV, and the resting volume of the chest wall is about 60% of the VC.

The action of the chest wall can be illustrated with the analogy of a wire screen attached around a balloon. The wire screen tends to spring outward; so at lower balloon volumes, the screen pulls the balloon open. A measure of the pressure at the mouth of the balloon reflects a negative number. At about 60% of the total capacity of the balloon, the screen no longer tends to spring outward. At that point, the addition of air causes the screen to push down on the balloon—a reflection of a positive pressure at the mouth of the balloon. The screen around the balloon can be likened to the chest wall. As shown in Fig. 12-12, at lower lung volumes, the chest wall clearly is inclined to recoil outward, thus creating a negative pressure; and at about 60% of the VC, the chest wall starts to push down on the lungs, thus creating a positive pressure. The result of the interplay between the chest wall's strong tendency to spring outward and the lung's strong tendency to recoil inward is the subatmospheric pleural pressure.

Pleural pressure can become positive during a cough or other forced expiratory maneuvers. Pneumothorax can occur when the chest wall is opened or when air is injected into the pleural cavity. With this occurrence, the lungs collapse because they naturally recoil to a smaller position; the ribs flare outward because of their natural inclination to recoil outward. Clinically, inspection of a patient with a pneumothorax may reveal protuding ribs on the affected side.

The two types of pneumothorax are open (simple) and closed (tension). Simple pneumothorax occurs when air flow into the pleural space results in a positive pleural pressure. The lungs collapse because the recoil pressure is not counterbalanced with the negative pleural pressure. Treatment for a pneumothorax can be conservative or more aggressive, depending on the type and amount of pneumothorax. Aggressive treatment consists of the insertion of chest tubes into the pleural space to recreate the negative pleural pressure. This maneuver reestablishes normal ventilatory excursions. In most instances, the air leak between the lung and the pleural space seals after the chest tubes have been removed. If air continues to

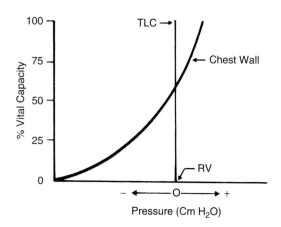

**Fig. 12-12**   Pressure-volume curve of chest wall during deflation going from TLC to RV. Positive pressures of chest wall represent pressures that tend to decrease lung size, and negative pressures represent pressures that tend to increase lung volume because of outward recoil tendency of chest wall at about 60% of vital capacity or less. *TLC*, Total lung capacity; *RV*, residual volume. *(From Drain C: Physiology of the respiratory system related to anesthesia, CRNA: Clin Forum Nurse Anesthetists 7(4):163-180, 1996.)*

flow into the intrapleural space but cannot escape, the intrapleural pressure continually increases with each succeeding inspiration. Like a one-way valve, pressure increases and a tension pneumothorax develops. In a brief period, as the intrapleural pressure increases, the affected lung is compressed and puts a great amount of pressure on the mediastinum. Hypoxemia and reduction in cardiac output result, and if treatment is not instituted immediately, the patient may die. Treatment consists of immediate evacuation of the excess air from the intrapleural space with either chest tubes or a large-bore needle. A tension pneumothorax is truly a medical emergency.

### Combined Mechanical Properties of the Lungs and Chest Wall.
The combined P-V characteristics of the lungs and the chest wall have many implications for the perianesthesia nurse. The combined P-V curve is the algebraic sum of the individual P-V curves of the lungs and chest wall. When no muscle forces are applied to the respiratory system, the FRC is determined by a balance of elastic forces between the lungs and the chest wall (Fig. 12-13). Any pathophysiologic or pharmacologic process that affects the elasticity of either the lungs or the chest wall affects the FRC.

### Alterations in the Balance of Pulmonary Forces in the Perianesthesia Patient.
During the induction of anesthesia, the shape of the P-V curve of

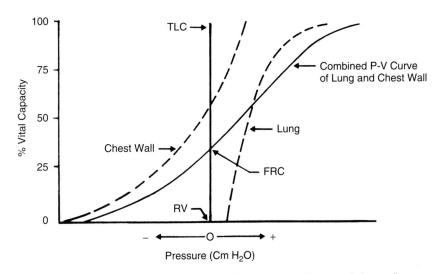

**Fig. 12-13** Combined P-V curves of lungs and chest wall. Individual P-V curves of lungs and chest wall are represented with *dashed lines.* They are transposed from static deflation P-V curves of lungs (see Fig. 12-8) and chest wall (see Fig. 12-12). Combined P-V curve is algebraic sum of deflation curves of lungs and chest wall. In combined P-V curve, FRC can be seen to be determined by balance of elastic forces of lungs and chest wall when no respiratory muscles are applied. *P-V,* Pressure-volume; *TLC,* total lung capacity; *RV,* residual volume; *FRC,* functional residual capacity. *(From Drain C: Physiology of the respiratory system related to anesthesia,* CRNA: Clin Forum Nurse Anesthetists *7(4):163-180, 1996.)*

the chest wall is altered. This agent-independent phenomenon is probably the result of loss of chest wall elasticity. Thus, the P-V curve of the chest wall of a patient with normal lung function is shifted to the right, the balance of forces occurs sooner, and the FRC decreases (Fig. 12-14). This shift to the right affects the P-V curve of the lung; it also shifts to the right, and secondary changes occur in the lung. More specifically, the changes consist of an increase in lung recoil ($\uparrow Pst_L$) and a decrease in $C_L$ ($\downarrow C_L$). Ultimately, the lung becomes stiffer, and the FRC decreases and may drop into the closing capacity range. Hence, during tidal ventilation, some airways are closed to ventilation and ventilation-perfusion mismatching occurs ($\downarrow$ alveolar ventilation/perfusion [$\downarrow V_A/Q_C$]), which ultimately leads to hypoxemia. Research indicates that this phenomenon, coupled with sighless breathing patterns in the PACU, can cause patients to have hypoxemia in the recovery phase of the anesthetic (see section on postoperative lung volumes).

## Pulmonary Circulation

The basic functions of the pulmonary circulation are exchanging gas, providing a reservoir for the left ventricle, furnishing nutrition, and protecting the lungs.

*Gas Exchange.* The major aspects of gas exchange are discussed in the section on blood gas transport. However, because of the implications for perianesthesia nursing care, the concepts of transit time and pulmonary vascular resistance are presented here.

Of the 5 L of blood that flows through the lungs every minute, only 70 to 200 mL are active in gas exchange at any one time. The time an RBC takes to cross the pulmonary capillary bed is 0.75 seconds, yet the RBC takes only 0.25 seconds to become saturated with oxygen—that is, until all the oxygen-bonding sites on the hemoglobin molecule are occupied. Because the transit time is 0.75 seconds and the saturation time is only 0.25 seconds, the body has a tremendous back up of 0.5 seconds for hemoglobin saturation with oxygen. If the RBCs move across the pulmonary capillary bed at an accelerated pace (decreased transit time), the amount of time available for oxygen to saturate the RBCs is decreased; during stress or exercise, however, the complete saturation of the hemoglobin can still be accomplished because the transit time of a RBC rarely decreases at less than 0.25 seconds.

However, this process is not true for patients with interstitial fibrosis who have a thickened respiratory exchange membrane. These patients may have a normal $PaO_2$ at rest, but exercise or exertion of surgery increases the cardiac output and decreases the RBC transit time. Therefore, the hemoglobin does not become completely

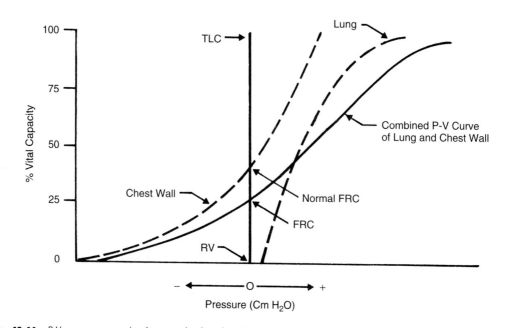

**Fig. 12-14** P-V curve representing lung mechanics of patient in immediate postoperative period who has undergone upper abdominal or thoracic surgical procedure. This patient has loss of chest wall elastic recoil that causes lungs to become less compliant. Consequently, combined P-V curve shifts to right, thus leading to decline in FRC because balance of forces occurs at lower lung volumes. *P-V*, Pressure-volume; *FRC*, functional residual capacity; *TLC*, total lung capacity; *RV*, residual volume. *(From Drain C: Pathophysiology of the respiratory system related to anesthesia,* CRNA: Clin Forum Nurse Anesthetists *7(4):181-192, 1996.)*

saturated during its passage through the pulmonary capillary bed. This phenomenon occurs because more time is needed for oxygen to pass through the diseased membrane. For these patients, the lower limit for complete saturation may be 0.5 seconds, not 0.25 seconds. Hence, patients with disorders of the respiratory exchange membrane can have a lower oxygen saturation ($SaO_2$) on the pulse oximeter with any exertion that could decrease RBC transit time. Clinically, this phenomenon is sometimes called desaturation on exercise. Thus, patients in the PACU who are suspected of having this problem should be given low-flow oxygen and be closely monitored for desaturation via a pulse oximeter. Because of the possibility of desaturation, the low-flow oxygen administration should not be discontinued until the patient's condition stabilizes, which may indicate continued administration after the patient is discharged from the PACU. Measures should be started to reduce the extrinsic factors, such as stress, elevated body temperature, and anxiety, which increase the cardiac output.

The pulmonary and systemic circulations have the same pump—the heart. The pulmonary system receives the same cardiac output as the systemic circulation, approximately 5 L/min. The pulmonary circulation, in comparison with the systemic circulation, is a low-pressure system with low resistance to flow, distensible vessels with extremely thin walls, and a small amount of smooth muscle. Many stimuli affect pulmonary vascular resistance. Probably the most potent vasoconstrictor of the lung is alveolar hypoxia. Research indicates that neuroendothelial bodies, which respond to a low $PaO_2$, may exist close to the pulmonary vascular bed. Also, the neuroendothelial bodies may liberate prostaglandins or histamine, or both, when alveolar hypoxia is present. Pulmonary vascular resistance does not seem to be affected by the volatile anesthetics such as halothane, enflurane, and isoflurane. However, nitrous oxide can increase pulmonary vascular resistance, especially in patients with preexisting pulmonary hypertension. Neonates who may or may not have preexisting pulmonary hypertension are prone to development of increased pulmonary vascular resistance when nitrous oxide is administered. If a patient in the PACU is prone to development of increased pulmonary vascular resistance, the effect of nitrous oxide on pulmonary vascular resistance is almost dissipated as a result of the rapid excretion from the lungs of nitrous oxide because of its low blood-gas coefficient.

In the postoperative period, if a patient has atelectasis in some portion of the lungs, the

$PaO_2$ in that particular area of the lungs is reduced. As a result, the neuroendothelial bodies are stimulated to produce increased pulmonary vascular resistance in that area of the lungs. Eventually, the blood is redirected or shunted to areas of the lungs that are adequately ventilated. So, the $SaO_2$ in a patient with atelectasis may indicate hypoxemia (<90%). After about 5 to 12 minutes, the $SaO_2$ may be slightly improved because of the increased pulmonary vascular resistance in the area of atelectasis. Therefore, the perianesthesia nurse should continue to use an aggressive stir-up regimen on a patient with atelectasis, even though the patient's $SaO_2$ values indicate a slight improvement.

*Reservoir for the Left Ventricle.* In regard to functioning as a reservoir for the left ventricle, the pulmonary veins are considered extensions of the left ventricle.

*Nutrition.* The pulmonary circulation can be divided into the bronchial circulation and the actual pulmonary circulation. The bronchial circulation carries nutrients and oxygen down to the respiratory bronchioles in the lungs. The bronchial circulation empties its deoxygenated blood via the pulmonary veins to the left heart. The pulmonary circulation carries nutrients to the respiratory bronchioles and the alveoli.

*Protection.* The role of the lungs in protection is vital for the preservation of the human organism. For example, on the surface of the pulmonary epithelium are invaginations called caveoli.

Bradykinin and angiotensin I are enzymatically converted on the surface of the caveoli. Ninety percent of the bradykinin is deactivated in the caveoli during each pass through the lungs, and angiotensin I is converted to angiotensin II with angiotensin-converting enzyme in the lungs. In the presence of hypoxia, the conversion of angiotensin I to angiotensin II is inhibited. Also, in the hypoxemic state, less than 12% of the bradykinin is deactivated by the lungs. In the hypoxemic state, the liberated bradykinin then become prostaglandins. Interestingly, the inappropriate levels of prostaglandins as a result of hypoxemia in the chronic state are thought to produce the clubbing of the fingers in patients with long standing chronic hypoxemia. Finally, the pulmonary epithelium also deactivates norepinephrine and serotonin. Serotonin plays an important part in platelet aggregation. Increased levels of serotonin from decreased lung function caused by hypoxia or lung disease lead to a high risk for venous thrombus. The implications for PACU care are that patients who are immobile and hypoxemic ($SaO_2$ < 90%) should be monitored for pulmonary and systemic thromboemboli.

### Water Balance in the Lung

The alveoli stay dry with a combination of pressures and lymph flow (Fig. 12-15). The forces that tend to push fluid out of the pulmonary capillaries are the capillary hydrostatic pressure ($P_{cap}$) minus the interstitial fluid hydrostatic pressure ($P_{is}$). The forces that tend to pull fluid

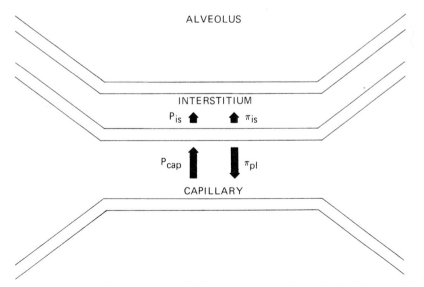

**Fig. 12-15**    Illustration of factors that affect movement of fluid from pulmonary capillaries. *$P_{cap}$,* Capillary hydrostatic pressure; *$P_{i,s}$,* interstitial hydrostatic pressure (assumed to be negative); *$p_{pl}$,* plasma colloid pressure; *$p_{is}$,* interstitial colloid osmotic pressure. *(From Levitzky M: Pulmonary physiology, ed 5, New York, 1999, McGraw-Hill.)*

into the pulmonary capillaries are the colloid osmotic pressure of the proteins in the plasma of the pulmonary capillaries ($\pi_{pl}$) minus the colloid osmotic pressure of the proteins in the interstitial fluid ($\pi_{is}$). The Starling equation describes the movement of fluid across the capillary endothelium:

$$Q_f = K_f (P_{cap} - P_{is}) - \sigma_f (\pi_{pl} - \pi_{is})$$

in which

$Q_f$ is the net flow of fluid; $K_f$ is the capillary filtration coefficient, which describes the permeability characteristics of the membrane to fluids; and $\sigma_f$ is the reflection coefficient, which describes the ability of the membrane to prevent extravasation of solute particles.

Thus, the membrane is permeable to fluid; and in normal circumstances, $\sigma_f$ is equal to 1.0 in the equation.

With substitution of normal values into the Starling equation,

$$Q_f = K_f[10 \, torr - (-3 \, torr)]$$
$$- \sigma_f (25 \, torr - 19 \, torr)$$

in which $K_f$ and $\sigma_f$ are dropped from the equation because they are considered normal and do not affect the outcome of the example; therefore:

$$Q_f = (13 \, torr) - (6 \, torr)$$
$$Q_f = + 7 \, torr$$

Thus, the pressure favors flow out of the capillaries to the interstitium of the alveolar wall tracts through the interstitial space to the perivascular and peribronchial spaces to facilitate transport of the fluid to the lymph nodes. Hence, a net pressure of 7 torr pushes fluid to the interstitial space. The lymph flow draining the lungs is about 20mL/h in rate of flow. So, the lungs depend on a continuous net fluid flux to remain in a consistently "dry" state.

Pulmonary edema, defined as increased total lung water, is associated with dysfunction of any parameter of the Starling equation. Examples of conditions that produce an overwhelming amount of fluid to be drained by the lymphatic system are elevated pulmonary capillary pressure (from left-sided heart failure), decreased capillary colloid osmotic pressure (from hypoproteinemia or overadministration of intravenous solutions), and extravasation of fluid through the pulmonary capillary membrane (from adult respiratory distress syndrome). The earliest form of pulmonary edema is characterized by engorgement of the peribronchial and perivascular

spaces and is known as interstitial edema. If interstitial edema is allowed to continue, alveolar pulmonary edema develops.

Pulmonary edema is difficult to assess in the early stages. As the fluid volume increases in the interstitium that surrounds the blood vessels and airways, reflex bronchospasm may occur. A chest radiograph at this time reveals Kerley's B lines, which denote fluid in the interstitium. Once the lymphatics become completely overwhelmed, fluid enters the alveoli. In the beginning of this pathophysiologic process, fine crackles are heard on auscultation. As pulmonary edema progresses into the alveoli, coarse crackles are heard, especially at the base of the lungs. Because of the direct stimulation of the J receptors in the interstitium, the patient has a tachypneic ventilatory pattern. Initial arterial blood gas values show a low $PaO_2$ and $PaCO_2$. As the pulmonary edema progresses, the $PaCO_2$ increases because hyperventilation (tachypnea) is not able to counterbalance the rise in the carbon dioxide in the blood. Finally, when the pulmonary edema becomes fulminant, the sputum becomes frothy and blood-tinged.

Treatment of pulmonary edema is based on the Starling equation. If edema is cardiogenic, the focus of the treatment is a lowering of the hydrostatic pressures within the capillaries. Noncardiogenic pulmonary edema is usually treated with the infusion of albumin to increase the osmotic forces. Diuretics and dialysis also may be used in noncardiogenic edema in an effort to lower the vascular pressures. Positive end-expiratory or continuous positive airway pressure is used with high oxygen concentrations to correct the hypoxemia.

## Blood Gas Transport

Respiration is the gas exchange between cellular levels in the body and the external environment. The three phases of respiration are: (1) ventilation, the phase of moving air in and out of the lungs; (2) transportation, which includes diffusion of gases in and out of the blood in both pulmonary and systemic capillaries, reactions of carbon dioxide and oxygen in the blood, and circulation of blood between the lungs and the tissue cells; and (3) gas exchange, in which oxygen is used and carbon dioxide is produced. Blood gas transport is the important link in the carrying of gas to or from the cell.

At sea level, the barometric pressure is 760 torr. Air contains approximately 21% oxygen, which exerts a partial pressure of 159 torr. As described by Dalton's law of partial pressure, the total pressure of a given volume of a gas mixture is equal to the sum of the separate or partial pressures that each gas would exert if that gas alone occupied the entire volume. Therefore, the total pressure is equal to the sum of the partial pressures of the major gases in the atmosphere. For example:

$$P_{TOTAL} = PN_2 + PO_2$$

in which $P_{TOTAL}$ is total atmospheric pressure, $PN_2$ is partial pressure of nitrogen, and $PO_2$ is partial pressure of oxygen. If the actual numeric quantities then are substituted into the formula, 760 torr = 601 torr + 159 torr.

As expressed in percentages, 100% (total atmospheric pressure) is equal to 79.07% (nitrogen) plus 20.93% (oxygen). Thus, nitrogen is 601 torr ($0.7907 \times 760$), and oxygen is 159 torr ($0.2093 \times 760$). In the lower airways, water vapor exerts a pressure that can be accounted for with Dalton's law. At the body temperature of 37° C, the water vapor pressure in the lower airways is 47 torr. Because the water vapor pressure affects the partial pressures of both nitrogen and oxygen, it is subtracted from the atmospheric pressure of 760 torr, which results in a pressure of 713 torr (760 torr – 47 torr = 713 torr). For determination of the $PO_2$ in the lower airways, the percent oxygen (20.93) is multiplied by 713 torr, with a resultant $PO_2$ of 149.2 torr. The respiratory exchange ratio can be used to understand how the alveolar partial pressure of oxygen is determined. This ratio represents carbon dioxide production divided by oxygen consumption. The normal respiratory exchange ratio is 0.8. Theoretically, then, for every 12 torr of carbon dioxide that is added to the alveolus, 12 torr of oxygen is displaced. Therefore, with no respiratory pathophysiology present, if the $PaCO_2$ is 40 torr, 48 torr of oxygen is removed from the alveolus, in which: $4 \times 10 = 40$ torr (carbon dioxide) and thus $4 \times 12 = 48$ torr (oxygen).

The result is a $PaO_2$ of 101 torr (149 torr – 48 torr = 101 torr), which is called the 12-10 concept and is helpful in assessment of arterial blood gas determinations in the PACU (see section on causes of hypoxemia).

As oxygen diffuses across the pulmonary membrane, the $PO_2$ is further decreased to 95 torr by a venous admixture. This effect occurs because of vascular shunts that normally redirect 1% or 2% of the total cardiac output either to nonaerated areas in the lungs themselves or directly through the heart, bypassing the lungs.

## Oxygen Transport

Oxygen is carried in the blood in combination with hemoglobin or in simple solution. About 98% of oxygen transported from the lungs to the cells is carried in combination with hemoglobin in the RBC, a reversible chemical combination. The remaining 2% is dissolved in the plasma and in the cytoplasm of the RBC. The amount of oxygen transported in both forms is directly proportional to the $PO_2$.

When the blood passes through the lungs, it does not normally become completely saturated with oxygen. Usually, the hemoglobin becomes about 97% saturated. Hemoglobin that is saturated with oxygen is called oxyhemoglobin.

Normally, the oxygen content of the arterial blood is 19.8 mL/dL of blood. This total oxygen content in the arterial blood ($CaO_2$) is equal to the oxygen-carrying capacity of hemoglobin, which is 1.34 times the number of grams of hemoglobin. That number divided by 100 is the oxygen content carried by the hemoglobin. For determination of the total amount of oxygen in the blood, the oxygen content that is dissolved in the plasma must be added to the oxygen content of the hemoglobin. The amount of oxygen dissolved in the plasma is determined with multiplication of the $PaO_2$ by the solubility coefficient for oxygen in plasma, which is 0.003.

Therefore, the equation for the total oxygen content in the blood is:

$$CaO_2 = Hb \times 1.34 \times \%Hb \text{ saturation} + (PaO_2 \times 0.003)$$

in which $Hb$ is hemoglobin. If the normal values of Hb are 15 g, percent Hb saturation as 97 and $PaO_2$ as 95 torr are substituted into the equation:

$$CaO_2 = \frac{(15 \times 1.34 \times 97)}{100} + (95 \times 0.003)$$

$$CaO_2 = 19.497 + 0.285$$

$$CaO_2 = 19.782 \text{ mL of oxygen per dL of blood}$$

One must remember that oxygen content is different from oxygen partial pressures. Content refers only to the amount of oxygen carried by the blood, not to its partial pressure ($PO_2$).

In the lungs, venous blood is oxygenated or arterialized. The oxygen bond with hemoglobin is loose and reversible. The bond is also $PO_2$-dependent—that is, the higher the $PaO_2$, the more oxygen saturation of the hemoglobin. However, the hemoglobin cannot be supersaturated. When all the bonding sites on the hemoglobin molecule are occupied by oxygen, no matter how much more oxygen is presented to

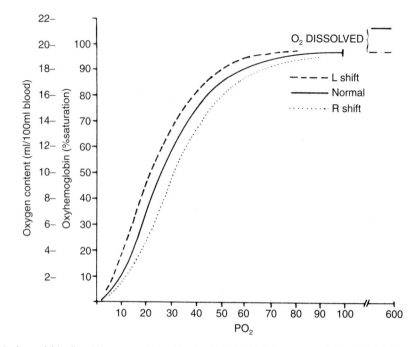

**Fig. 12-16**   Oxyhemoglobin dissociation curve. *(From Guenter C, Welch M:* Pulmonary medicine, *Philadelphia, 1977, Lippincott.)*

the hemoglobin, the oxygen is not able to bond to the hemoglobin.

The oxygen-hemoglobin dissociation curve relates the percentage of oxygen saturation of hemoglobin to the $PaO_2$ value. Note in Fig. 12-16 that the curve is sigmoid in shape with a steep portion between the 10-torr and 50-torr $PaO_2$ range, with a leveling off above 70 torr. The flat portion of the curve indicates the capacity to oxygenate most of the hemoglobin despite wide variations in the $PO_2$ (70 to 98 torr). This flat portion of the curve can be called the association portion of the curve, and it corresponds to the external respiration that is taking place in the lungs. The steep portion of the curve indicates the capacity to unload large amounts of oxygen in response to small tissue $PO_2$ changes. This part of the curve is called the dissociation portion of the oxygen-hemoglobin dissociation curve.

As discussed, the normal oxygen content at the association portion of the curve is about 19.8 mL of oxygen per dL of blood. At the venous dissociation portion of the curve, the content of oxygen is 15.2 mL of oxygen per dL of blood. The following formula is used to derive the content of oxygen in the mixed venous blood ($CvO_2$):

$$CvO_2 = \frac{Hb \times 1.34 \times \%Hb \text{ saturation}}{100}$$
$$+ (PvO_2 \times 0.003)$$

in which $PvO_2$ is pressure of oxygen in the mixed venous blood.

With substitution of normal values for mixed venous blood of Hb as 15 g, percent Hb saturation as 75, and $PvO_2$ as 40 into the formula:

$$CvO_2 = \frac{(15 \times 1.34 \times 75)}{100} + (40 \times 0.003)$$

$$CvO_2 = 15.08 + 0.12$$

$CvO_2 = 15.20$ mL of oxygen per dL of blood

Therefore, in this example, the net delivery of oxygen to the tissues is 4.6 mL of oxygen per dL of blood (19.8 − 15.2 = 4.6).

***Factors that Affect Oxygen Transport.*** The association portion of the oxygen-hemoglobin dissociation curve is not necessarily a fixed line determined solely by the $PaO_2$. The height and the slope of the curve are dependent on many factors, including pH and temperature. Generally, a decrease in pH (an increase in hydrogen ions) or an increase in body temperature causes a shift of the curve to the right, which leads to a decrease in the height and slope of the curve. Ultimately, less saturation (loading) of the hemoglobin is found for a given $PaO_2$. Hence, patients who have a low pH or high temperature, or both, probably benefit from a higher fraction of inspired oxygen ($FiO_2$) than normal for facilitation of an appropriate level of saturation of hemoglobin. However, before changes in the FiO$_2$ are made, arterial blood gas determinations should be analyzed.

At the dissociation portion of the oxygen-hemoglobin dissociation curve, the same is true. This portion is not a fixed line because it also changes position in response to physiologic processes. At the tissue level, metabolically active tissues produce more carbon dioxide and more acid ($\downarrow$ pH) and have an elevated temperature. All of these products of metabolism shift the curve to the right. The curve shifts far more in response to physiologic processes in the dissociation portion than in the association part. Metabolically active tissues produce more carbon dioxide and need more oxygen. The effect of carbon dioxide on the curve is closely related to the fact that deoxyhemoglobin binds hydrogen ions more actively than does oxyhemoglobin. As a result, at the tissue level, increased carbon dioxide decreases the affinity of hemoglobin for oxygen. Thus, the dissociation portion of the curve is shifted to the right and more oxygen is given to the tissue. This effect of carbon dioxide on oxygen transport is called the Bohr effect.

2,3-Diphosphoglycerate (2,3-DPG) regulates the release of oxygen to the tissue. It is a glycolytic intermediary metabolite that is more concentrated in the RBC than anywhere else in the body. High concentrations of 2,3-DPG shift the oxyhemoglobin dissociation curve to the right, which makes oxygen more available to the tissues. Lower concentrations of 2,3-DPG cause a shift of the curve to the left, which ultimately leads to the release of less oxygen to the tissues. The clinical implications of these observations involve the administration of outdated whole blood. Whole blood stored longer than 21 days has low levels of 2,3-DPG. Therefore, if outdated blood is administered to a patient, the tissues do not receive an appropriate amount of oxygen because of the shift to the left of the oxygen-hemoglobin dissociation curve.

**Pulse Oximetry and the Oxygen Dissociation Curve.** Oxygen delivered to the tissues is determined by the cardiac output and the CaO$_2$. Most of the oxygen is bound to the hemoglobin, and the percentage of the oxygen bound to the hemoglobin is expressed as the SaO$_2$. The amount of oxygen that is dissolved in simple solution in the arterial blood is the PaO$_2$. A gradient is set from the lung to the tissues in regard to oxygen delivery and is represented by the oxygen dissociation curve. A normal curve, without any shifts left or right, is determined by the PaCO$_2$, pH, body temperature, and hemoglobin and 2,3-DPG levels. A normal curve is

therefore set at values of PaCO$_2$ of 40 torr, pH of 7.4, temperature of 37°C, and hemoglobin of 15 g/dL. With the oxygen dissociation curve (see Fig. 12-16), the PaO$_2$ can be determined with the SaO$_2$ reading on the pulse oximeter. For example, an SaO$_2$ of 90% corresponds to a PaO$_2$ of 60 torr. With the curve, at less than an SaO$_2$ of 90%, the PaO$_2$ drops rapidly (the dissociation portion of the curve). Clinically, an SaO$_2$ of 90% can be considered hypoxemia, and severe hypoxemia occurs when the PaO$_2$ is less than 40 torr or the SaO$_2$ is 75%.

### Carbon Dioxide Transport

The transport of carbon dioxide begins within each cell in the body. Carbon dioxide is a main byproduct of the energy-supplying mechanisms of the cell. Approximately 200 mL/min of carbon dioxide is produced within the body at rest. Carbon dioxide is 20 times more soluble in water than oxygen; therefore, it traverses the fluid compartments of the body rapidly. The intracellular partial pressure of carbon dioxide is 46 torr. A 1-torr gradient exists between the cell and the interstitial fluid. Carbon dioxide diffuses out of the cell to the interstitial fluid and has a new partial pressure of 45 torr. When the tissue capillary blood enters the venules, the partial pressure of the carbon dioxide is 45 torr.

Carbon dioxide is transported in the blood in three forms: (1) physically dissolved in solution; (2) as carbaminohemoglobin; and (3) as bicarbonate ions.

**Carbon Dioxide in Simple Solution.** About 12% of the total amount of carbon dioxide transported in the body is physically dissolved in solution.

**Carbaminohemoglobin.** Approximately 30% of carbon dioxide is transported as carbaminohemoglobin, a chemical combination of carbon dioxide and hemoglobin that is reversible because the binding point on the hemoglobin is on the amino groups and is a loose bond. This chemical bonding of carbon dioxide with hemoglobin can be graphically described with the use of the carbon dioxide dissociation curve. Two differences are found between the carbon dioxide dissociation curve (Fig. 12-17) and the oxygen-hemoglobin dissociation curve. First, over the normal operating range of blood the partial pressure of carbon dioxide (PCO$_2$) from 47 (venous or PvCO$_2$) to 40 (arterial or PaCO$_2$) torr, the slope of the carbon dioxide dissociation curve is nearly linear and not sigmoid like the oxygen-hemoglobin dissociation curve. Second, the total carbon dioxide content is about twice the total oxygen content. Oxygen

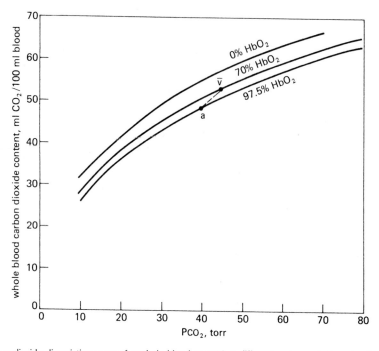

**Fig. 12-17**  Carbon dioxide dissociation curves for whole blood at 37°C at different oxyhemoglobin saturations. *a*, Arterial point (code; am); $\bar{v}$, mixed venous point. *(From Levitzky M:* Pulmonary physiology, *ed 5, New York, 1999, McGraw-Hill.)*

has a definite effect on carbon dioxide transport. On the upper curve, or venous portion of the carbon dioxide curve, note that the point for the $PvCO_2$ is 47 and the $PvO_2$ is 40. On the lower curve, or arterial carbon dioxide curve, observe the points for the $PaCO_2$ of 40 torr and the $PaO_2$ of 100 torr. Notice how the venous carbon dioxide curve is shifted to the left and is above the arterial curve. This description is the effect of oxygen on carbon dioxide transport, or the Haldane effect. In terms of physiologic significance, the Haldane effect plays a more important role in gas transport than does the Bohr effect. Specifically, in the lungs, the binding of oxygen with hemoglobin tends to displace carbon dioxide from the hemoglobin (oxyhemoglobin is more acidic than deoxyhemoglobin). At the tissue level, oxygen is removed from the hemoglobin (as the result of a pressure gradient), which reduces the acidity of the hemoglobin and enables it to bind more carbon dioxide. In fact, because the hemoglobin is in the reduced state (deoxygenated), the hemoglobin can carry 6 volumes percent more carbon dioxide than the amount of carbon dioxide that could be carried by oxyhemoglobin.

**Bicarbonate.**  Sixty-five percent of carbon dioxide is transported as bicarbonate, which is the product of the reaction of carbon dioxide with water. When the carbon dioxide and

water join, they form carbonic acid. Almost all the carbonic acid dissociates to bicarbonate and hydrogen ions, as seen in the following equation:

$$CO_2 + H_2O \xrightarrow{\text{Carbonic anhydrase}} H_2CO_3 \rightarrow$$
$$H^+ + HCO_3$$

This reaction occurs mostly within the RBCs because carbonic anhydrase accelerates the hydration of carbon dioxide to carbonic acid 220 to 300 times faster than if carbon dioxide and water were joined without this enzymatic catalyst.

When the bicarbonate produced in this reaction in the RBCs exceeds the bicarbonate ion level in the plasma, it diffuses out of the cell. The positively charged hydrogen ion tends to remain within the RBC and is buffered by hemoglobin. Because of ionic imbalance, chloride, a negatively charged ion that is abundant in the plasma, diffuses into the RBC to maintain electric balance. This movement is called the chloride shift. Because of the increase in osmotically active particles within the cell, water from the plasma diffuses into the RBC. This process explains why the RBCs in the venous side of the circulation are slightly larger than the arterial RBCs (Fig. 12-18).

As the venous blood enters the pulmonary capillaries, the carbon dioxide in simple solution

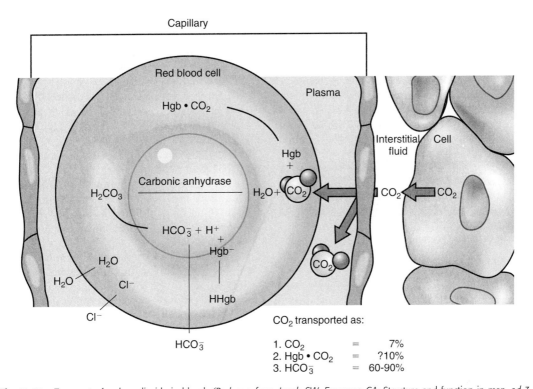

**Fig. 12-18** Transport of carbon dioxide in blood. *(Redrawn from Jacob SW, Francone CA: Structure and function in man, ed 3, Philadelphia, 1974, Saunders.)*

freely diffuses to the alveoli. The carbaminohemoglobin reverses to free the carbon dioxide, which diffuses across the alveoli and is then expired. The hydrogen and the bicarbonate combine to form carbonic acid, which is rapidly broken down by carbonic anhydrase to form carbon dioxide and water. The carbon dioxide then diffuses through the alveoli and is expired.

Not all carbon dioxide is eliminated with pulmonary ventilation. Other buffer systems that remove excess carbon dioxide are acid-base buffers and urinary excretion by the kidneys. The respiratory system can adjust to rapid fluctuations in carbon dioxide, whereas the kidneys may need hours for restoration of a normal carbon dioxide tension.

### Acid-base Relationships

A buffer is a substance that causes a lesser change in hydrogen ion concentration to occur in a solution on addition of an acid or base than would have occurred had the buffer not been present. The buffers can respond in seconds to fluctuations in carbon dioxide tension. Buffers include the carbonic acid–bicarbonate system, the proteinate-protein system, and the hemoglobinate-hemoglobin system.

The pH is a measure of alkalinity or acidity and depends on the concentration of hydrogen ions. Acidic solutions have more hydrogen ions, and alkaline solutions have fewer hydrogen ions. The pH is described in logarithmic form. Acid solutions have more hydrogen ions and a lower pH, which indicates acidity. If, on the other hand, the hydrogen ion concentration is low, then the pH is high, which indicates alkalinity. The pH range is from 1 to 14, with 7 as the equilibrium (pK). The normal pH value in extracellular fluid is 7.35 to 7.45, which is slightly alkaline.

The normal bicarbonate level in the extracellular fluid is 24 mEq. Base excess is used to describe alkalosis or acidosis. If a positive base excess number is noted, more base in the extracellular fluid is indicated. If a negative number is reported, the base is being used to neutralize the acid to a point of encroaching on the amount of available base, which is shown with a negative value for the base excess (acidosis).

***Respiratory Acid-base Imbalances.*** Respiratory acidosis is characterized by a $PaCO_2$ above the normal range of 36 to 44 torr. All other primary processes that tend to cause acidosis are metabolic. Some common causes of carbon dioxide retention and respiratory acidosis are summarized in Box 12-1.

Respiratory alkalosis is characterized by a reduced $PaCO_2$. Hyperventilation frequently causes this disorder. Common causes of excessive carbon dioxide elimination and respiratory alkalosis are summarized in Box 12-2.

In respiratory alkalosis or acidosis, a linear exchange takes place between the carbon dioxide and bicarbonate concentrations, which is summarized as follows:

1. In acute respiratory acidosis, bicarbonate concentration is approximately 1 mEq/L for each 12-torr change in $PaCO_2$.
2. In chronic respiratory acidosis, the change in actual bicarbonate concentration is approximately 2 mEq/L for each 12-torr change in $PaCO_2$.
3. The change in actual bicarbonate concentration with a chronic change in $PaCO_2$ above the range of 40 torr change is approximately 4 mEq/L for each 12-torr change in $PaCO_2$. This rule holds true for 1 or 2 days after the onset of the disorder because of the slow renal buffer system.

Another rule of thumb for determination of whether the acid-base disorder is entirely respiratory in origin is that an acute increase in $PaCO_2$ by 12 torr produces a corresponding decrease in pH by 0.07 pH units. In chronic hypercapnia, each increase in $PaCO_2$ by 12 torr results in a corresponding decrease in pH by 0.03 pH units. $PaCO_2$ and pH changes that deviate significantly from these standards suggest that the acid-base disorder is not completely respiratory in origin. For example, if a patient who is recovering from a spinal anesthetic in the PACU has blood gases (room air) of $PaO_2$ of 92 torr, $PaCO_2$ of 30 torr, and pH of 7.47 as compared with preoperative arterial blood gas values (room air) of $PaO_2$ of 80 torr, $PaCO_2$ of 40 torr, and pH of 7.40, the rule of thumb can be applied. Because the $PaCO_2$ decreased by 12 torr and the pH increased by 0.07 pH units, the patient clearly has respiratory alkalosis, not a metabolic disorder. Moreover, with the 12-12 concept, one can determine that this patient probably has acute hyperventilation because the $PaCO_2$ decreased by 12 and thus, the $PaO_2$ should increase by 12, or from 80 to 92 torr.

***Metabolic Acid–base Imbalances.*** Metabolic acidosis usually results with an increase in nonvolatile acids or a loss of bases from the body. The usual result is a deficit in buffer, base excess, and bicarbonate. Because acidosis stimulates respiration, the $PaCO_2$ usually decreases. The magnitude of the ventilatory response usually differentiates between acute and chronic metabolic acidosis. Some of the common causes of metabolic acidosis are summarized in Box 12-3.

Metabolic alkalosis is produced by an excessive elimination of nonvolatile acids (such as in vomiting, gastric aspiration, and hypokalemic alkalosis) or by an increase in bases (such as in alkali administration or hypochloremic alkalosis caused by some diuretics). A summary of blood

---

**Box 12-1   Common Causes of Carbon Dioxide Retention and Respiratory Acidosis (Hypoventilation)**

**NORMAL LUNGS**
Anesthesia
Sedative drugs (overdose)
Neuromuscular disease
Poliomyelitis
Myasthenia gravis
Guillain-Barré syndrome
Obesity (pickwickian syndrome)
Brain damage
Cardiac arrest
Pneumothorax
Pulmonary edema
Bronchospasm
Laryngospasm

**ABNORMAL LUNGS**
Chronic obstructive pulmonary disease (chronic bronchitis, asthma, and emphysema)
Diffuse infiltration pulmonary disease (advanced)
Kyphoscoliosis (severe)

---

**Box 12-2   Common Causes of Excessive Carbon Dioxide Elimination and Respiratory Alkalosis (Hyperventilation)**

**NORMAL LUNGS**
Anxiety
Fever
Drugs (aspirin)
Central nervous system lesions
Endotoxemia

**ABNORMAL LUNGS**
Pneumonia
Diffuse infiltrative pulmonary disease (early)
Acute bronchial asthma (early)
Pulmonary vascular disease
Congestive heart failure (early)

| Box 12-3 | Common Causes of Metabolic Acidosis |
|---|---|

Increased nonvolatile acids
Diabetes mellitus
Uremia
Severe exercise
Hypoxia
Shock
Idiopathic
Methyl alcohol ingestion (formic acid)
Aspirin ingestion (salicylic acid)
Excessive loss of bases (usually $NaCO_3$ from lower gastrointestinal tract)
Severe diarrhea (e.g., cholera, diarrhea in infants)
Fistulas (e.g., pancreatic, biliary)

gas discrepancies in each condition is provided in Table 12-3.

## Matching of Ventilation to Perfusion

*Distribution of Ventilation.* A gravity dependent gradient of pleural pressure in the upright lung exists at resting lung volumes. The weight of the lung tends to pull the lung tissue toward the base of the lung. As a result, the intrapleural pressure is more negative at the apex of the lung in comparison with the intrapleural pressure at the base and over the $V_T$ range (the alveoli at the apex being more fully inflated as compared with the alveoli at the base). Consequently, the alveoli at the base have a greater capacity for volume change during inspiration, whereas the alveoli at the apex are already "stretched," or distended. In a healthy subject who breathes out to RV and then inspires in small steps, the initial inspired air (a small portion) goes to the apex and the base remains completely underventilated. After a certain lung volume is attained, the base of the lung receives almost all of the air because of the capacity of the alveoli at the base of the lung for volume change. Therefore,

| Table 12-3 | Summary of Blood Gas Discrepancies in Acidosis and Alkalosis | | |
|---|---|---|---|
| Condition | $HCO_3^-$ | $PCO_2$ | pH |
| Metabolic acidosis | ↓ | ↓ | ↓ |
| Respiratory acidosis | ↑ | ↑ | ↓ |
| Metabolic alkalosis | ↑ | ↑ | ↑ |
| Respiratory alkalosis | ↓ | ↓ | ↓ |

because of the mechanical properties of the lung, the greatest volume change during inspiration from RV to TLC occurs near the base of the lungs.

*Distribution of Perfusion.* A gravity-dependent gradient for perfusion in the lungs exists; approximately 80% to 90% of blood flow occurs from the middle portion to an area near the base of the lungs. Therefore, the blood flow per unit of lung volume increases down the lung from the apex to the base.

*Matching.* Matching of alveolar ventilation ($\dot{V}_A$) to perfusion ($\dot{Q}_C$) is defined in terms of a certain volume of alveolar gas that is necessary for arterialization of a given volume of mixed venous blood. The normal alveolar ventilation ratio is:

$$\frac{\dot{V}_A}{\dot{Q}_C} = \frac{4000 \text{ mL/min}}{5000 \text{ mL/min}} = 0.8$$

If blood and gas were matched equally throughout the lung, the $\dot{V}_A/\dot{Q}_C$ would be 1. However, in the healthy lung, the matching of ventilation to perfusion is not proportional, which results in varying $\dot{V}_A/\dot{Q}_C$ throughout the lung. More specifically, ventilation at the apex is high as opposed to perfusion, and perfusion is higher than ventilation at the base of the lung. Finally, if all the $\dot{V}_A/\dot{Q}_C$ relationships were added together, the mean ratio would be 0.8.

## Causes of Hypoxemia

*Hypoventilation.* The $PaO_2$ and $PaCO_2$ are determined with the balance between the addition of oxygen and the removal of carbon dioxide by the alveolar ventilation and the removal of oxygen and the addition of carbon dioxide by the pulmonary capillary blood flow. If the alveolar ventilation is decreased (with no other lung pathologic changes present), the $PaO_2$ decreases and the $PaCO_2$ increases. In fact, the $PaO_2$ decreases almost proportionally to the increase in the $PaCO_2$. Recall the calculations made in the 12-12 concept. At any specific inspired oxygen tension, a 12-torr increase in the $PaCO_2$ causes an approximate 12-torr decrease in the arterial oxygen tension. For example, if the normal $PaCO_2$ is equal to 40 torr and the $PaO_2$ is equal to 95 torr and the patient's alveolar ventilation decreases because of narcotics given in the PACU, the $PaCO_2$ increases to 60 torr. The new $PaO_2$ should be 71 torr (change of 20 torr in the $PaCO_2$, so 12 + 12 = 24 − 95 = 71). Therefore, with assessment of blood gas data and with the 12-10 relationship determined to be present, hypoventilation should be suspected. One should remember that the 12-10 relationship does not have to be exact, but if the numbers are close to the 12-10 relationship, hypoventilation is the probable cause. An increased $FiO_2$ value affects the 12-10 relationship. However, most patients in the PACU undergo low-flow oxygen therapy, and therefore, the $FiO_2$ is usually between 25% and 50%. Consequently, if the values seem to change proportionally, hypoventilation can still be suspected. Hypoventilation is the most common cause of hypoxemia in the PACU. Nursing interventions should include administration of a higher $FiO_2$ via low-flow oxygen therapy; stimulation of the patient; use of an aggressive stir-up regimen; and possible pharmacologic reversal of narcotics or muscle relaxants.

***Ventilation/Perfusion Mismatching.*** If the 12-10 relationship is not present during the analysis of the arterial blood gases, $\dot{V}_A/\dot{Q}_C$ mismatching is probably the cause. However, determination of whether the mismatching problem is the result of increased or decreased $\dot{V}_A/\dot{Q}_C$ is difficult. As seen in Fig. 12-19 normal $\dot{V}_A/\dot{Q}_C$ exists when appropriate matching of ventilation to perfusion occurs. Decreased $\dot{V}_A/\dot{Q}_C$ occurs when the matching ventilation is reduced in comparison with perfusion of the alveoli, and increased $\dot{V}_A/\dot{Q}_C$ is caused by increased ventilation as compared with perfusion.

***Decreased Ventilation to Perfusion.*** Reduced ventilation, in comparison with perfusion, ($\downarrow\dot{V}_A/\dot{Q}_C$) may be caused by excessive secretions or partial bronchospasm. When atelectasis or airway closure occurs, intrapulmonary shunting results. In these situations, oxygen cannot diffuse properly across to the pulmonary capillary blood. In decreased $\dot{V}_A/\dot{Q}_C$, some oxygen diffuses across from the alveoli to the pulmonary capillary blood. Thus, the alveolar-arterial oxygen difference ($PAO_2 - PaO_2$) is slightly reduced. If a large gradient exists in the $PAO_2 - PaO_2$ value, intrapulmonary shunting is probably present. For a patient who is breathing room air, the normal $PAO_2 - PaO_2$ value is

between 5 and 15 torr. When a patient is breathing oxygen at a $FiO_2$ of 0.5 (50%), the $PAO_2 - PaO_2$ value should be about 50 torr. A gradient greatly in excess of 50 torr suggests $\dot{V}_A/\dot{Q}_C$ mismatching. The focus of the nursing interventions for improvement of decreased $\dot{V}_A/\dot{Q}_C$ is on airway clearance, reinflation of alveoli, and enhanced patency of the airways. The newly advocated stir-up regimen of turn, cascade cough, and SMI should improve the decreased $\dot{V}_A/\dot{Q}_C$. Percussion or vibration, or both, may also need to be instituted to facilitate secretion clearance. Also, if partial bronchospasm (expiratory wheeze) is suspected, the attending physician should be consulted about institution of appropriate bronchodilator therapy.

At this point, a clarification of terms used to describe decreased $\dot{V}_A/\dot{Q}_C$ and shunt is in order. Basically, intrapulmonary shunts result in the mixing of venous blood that has not been properly oxygenated into the arterial blood (pulmonary vein). Anatomic shunts, which occur normally, are attributed to the 2% or 3% of the cardiac output that bypasses the lungs. The shunted unoxygenated venous blood comes mainly from the bronchial circulation, which empties into the pulmonary veins, and from the thebesian vessels that drain the myocardium into the left heart. Intrapulmonary shunts occur when mixed venous blood does not become oxygenated when it passes by underventilated, unventilated, or collapsed alveoli. Absolute intrapulmonary shunts, sometimes called true shunts, are associated with totally unventilated or collapsed alveoli. Shuntlike intrapulmonary shunts are the areas of low $\dot{V}_A/\dot{Q}_C$ in which blood draining the partially obstructed alveoli has a lower arterial oxygen content than the alveolar capillary units that are well matched. As a result, the presence of anatomic shunts is normal. Abnormal shunts can be classified as physiologic shunts. Physiologic shunts are made up of the anatomic shunts plus intrapulmonary shunts (absolute and shuntlike intrapulmonary shunts).

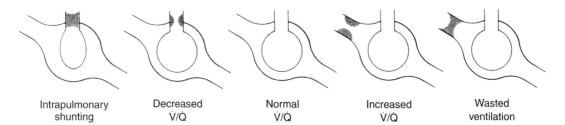

| Intrapulmonary shunting | Decreased $\dot{V}/\dot{Q}$ | Normal $\dot{V}/\dot{Q}$ | Increased $\dot{V}/\dot{Q}$ | Wasted ventilation |

**Fig. 12-19** Graphic representation of normal and abnormal matching of ventilation ($V_A$) to perfusion ($Q_C$). *(From Harper R: A guide to respiratory care: physiology and clinical applications, Philadelphia, 1981, Lippincott.)*

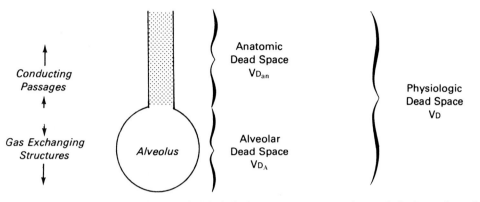

**Fig. 12-20**  Graphic representation of dead space. Physiologic dead space represents sum of anatomic dead space in conducting passages (*shaded area*) and alveolar dead space in alveoli (*circle*). *(From Harper R:* A guide to respiratory care: physiology and clinical applications, *Philadelphia, 1981, Lippincott.)*

***Increased Ventilation to Perfusion.*** According to Fig. 12-20, compromise of the circulation to the individual alveolocapillary unit creates an excess of ventilation in comparison with perfusion. If the flow of blood in the pulmonary capillary is partially obstructed, increased $\dot{V}_A/\dot{Q}_C$ results. If the flow of blood is completely obstructed, such as with a pulmonary embolus, only ventilation continues and produces wasted or dead space. Wasted ventilation is the total amount of inspired gas that does not contribute to carbon dioxide removal; it is also known as physiologic dead space ($V_D$physio). $V_D$physio is that volume of each breath that is inhaled but does not reach functioning terminal respiratory units. $V_D$physio has two components: alveolar and anatomic dead space. Alveolar dead space ($V_D$alv), as depicted in Fig. 12-20, is that volume of air contributed by all those terminal respiratory units that are overventilated relative to their perfusion. Anatomic dead space ($V_D$anat) consists of the volume of air in the conducting airways that does not participate in gas exchange. This category includes all air down to the respiratory bronchioles. The following formula depicts $V_D$physio:

$$V_D\text{physio} = V_D\text{alv} + V_D\text{anat}$$

Normally, $V_D$physio consists mainly of $V_D$anat, with the $V_D$alv component being minute, which explains why the normal $V_D$physio volume in milliliters is approximately equal to the weight of a person in pounds. For example, a person who weighs 150 lb has a $V_D$physio of 150 mL. When alveoli become overventilated in comparison with perfused, the $V_D$alv increases, which in turn increases the $V_D$physio.

The amount of $V_D$physio can be determined with the Bohr equation. Clinically, the Bohr equation is commonly referred to as the $V_D/V_T$. The ratio of dead space ($V_D$) to $V_T$ can be used in determination of whether obstruction to pulmonary capillary blood flow is partial ($\dot{V}_A/\dot{Q}_C$) or complete (wasted ventilation). The $V_D/V_T$ can be derived from the following equation:

$$\frac{V_D}{V_T} = \frac{PaCO_2 - P_ECO_2}{P_ECO_2}$$

in which the *PaCO$_2$* is the arterial carbon dioxide partial pressure and the *P$_E$CO$_2$* is the partial pressure of the expired carbon dioxide.

The $V_D/V_T$ ratio is normally 0.3. If the $V_D/V_T$ increases to 0.6, more than half of the $V_T$ is dead space. The minute ventilation ($V_E$) can double in most patients, but beyond that amount, the effort is too exhausting and a $V_D/V_T$ ratio of more than 0.6 usually mandates that the patient's ventilation be assisted mechanically.

**Implications for Perianesthesia Care**

In the early postoperative period (including the transport of the patient from the operating room to the PACU), the patient should be considered to have a reduced FRC and hypoventilation and to have some ventilation-perfusion mismatch. All these factors lead to a reduction in arterial oxygenation as reflected by low $SaO_2$ and $PaO_2$ values. Research now shows that hypoxemia exists during transport to the PACU. Consequently, all patients should receive supplemental oxygenation during transport to the PACU and certainly throughout their stay there. In addition, because these respiratory alterations occur in almost all patients in recovery from anesthesia, pulse oximetry should be used on each patient during transport and in the PACU.

## REGULATION OF BREATHING

In the past, medullary control of breathing was thought to be a function of reciprocal inhibition between the inspiratory and expiratory centers. Research now indicates a more discrete regulatory process that occurs at two levels: the sensors and the controllers. Patients with altered regulation and control of breathing present a significant challenge to the perianesthesia nurse. Also, anesthesia, surgery, and medications administered in the PACU can have a profound impact on the patient's regulatory processes of breathing.

### The Sensors

*Peripheral Chemoreceptors.* The carotid and aortic bodies are the peripheral chemoreceptors and are located at the bifurcation of the common carotid arteries and at the arch of the aorta, respectively. The carotid and aortic bodies are responsible for the immediate increase in ventilation as a result of lack of oxygen. These peripheral chemoreceptors are made up of highly vascular tissue and glomus cells. The carotid and aortic bodies monitor only the $PaO_2$, not the $CaO_2$ of the hemoglobin. Therefore, the receptors are not stimulated in conditions such as anemia and carbon monoxide and cyanide poisoning.

The carotid bodies are much more important physiologically than are the aortic bodies. The carotid bodies respond, in order of degree of response, to low $PaO_2$, high $PaCO_2$, and low pH. The carotid bodies respond to a low $PaO_2$, and the response is augmented by a high $PaCO_2$, a low pH, or both. The physiologic responses to the stimulation of the carotid sinus are hyperpnea, bradycardia, and hypotension. The aortic bodies, on the other hand, respond to a low $PaO_2$ and to a high $PaCO_2$ but not to pH. The results of stimulation of the aortic bodies are hyperpnea, tachycardia, and hypertension.

The carotid and aortic bodies mainly respond to a low $PaO_2$. This response is commonly called the hypoxic or secondary drive. The impulse activity in these chemoreceptors begins at a $PaO_2$ of about 500 torr. A rapid increase in impulses occurs at a $PaO_2$ lower than 100 torr. The impulses are greatly increased as the $PaO_2$ falls to a value less than 60 torr. At less than 30 torr, the impulse activity from the chemoreceptors decreases because of the direct oxygen

deficit in the glomus cells. In addition, these peripheral arterial chemoreceptors are stimulated by low arterial blood pressure and increased sympathetic activity.

*Central Chemoreceptors.* The central chemoreceptors lie near the ventral surface of the medulla. Specifically, these chemosensitive areas are near the choroid plexus (venous blood) and next to the cerebrospinal fluid (CSF). The central chemoreceptors respond indirectly to carbon dioxide because the blood-brain barrier allows lipid-soluble substances (e.g., carbon dioxide, oxygen, and water) to cross the barrier, whereas water-soluble substances (e.g., sodium, potassium, hydrogen ion, and bicarbonate) pass through the membrane at very slow rates. Bicarbonate requires active transport to cross the barrier. Therefore, carbon dioxide enters the CSF and is hydrated to form carbonic acid. The carbonic acid rapidly dissociates to form hydrogen ion and bicarbonate. The hydrogen ion concentration in the CSF parallels the arterial $PCO_2$. Actually, the hydrogen ion concentration stimulates ventilation via hydrogen receptors located in the central chemoreceptor area. In summary, carbon dioxide has little direct effect on the stimulation of the receptors in the central chemoreceptor area but does have a potent indirect effect. This indirect effect is the result of the inability of hydrogen ions to easily cross the blood-brain barrier. For this reason, changes in hydrogen ion concentration in the blood have considerably less effect in stimulating the chemoreceptor area than do changes in carbon dioxide. Consequently, the central chemoreceptor area precisely controls ventilation and therefore the $PaCO_2$. For that reason, the index to the adequacy of ventilation is the $PaCO_2$.

Bicarbonate is the only major buffer in the CSF. The pH of the CSF is a result of the ratio between bicarbonate and carbon dioxide in the CSF. Carbon dioxide is freely diffusible in and out of the CSF via the blood-brain barrier. However, bicarbonate is not freely diffusible and requires active or passive transport to enter or leave the CSF. When an acute increase in the $PaCO_2$ occurs, carbon dioxide enters the CSF and is hydrated, and hydrogen ions and bicarbonate are formed. The hydrogen ion stimulates the chemoreceptors, and the bicarbonate decreases the pH of the CSF. The resultant hyperpnea lowers the blood $PaCO_2$ and thus creates a gradient that favors the diffusion of carbon dioxide out of the CSF. The blood $PaCO_2$ and pH are corrected immediately, but the pH in the CSF requires some time to reestablish a normal carbon dioxide–bicarbonate level because of the poor diffusibility of bicarbonate. This process is usually not a problem with normal respiratory function. However, for the patient with chronic carbon dioxide retention (chronic hypercapnia) who has hyperventilation to a "normal" $PaCO_2$ of 40 torr, serious deleterious effects may occur. Patients with a chronically elevated $PaCO_2$ have a higher amount of carbon dioxide and bicarbonate in the CSF, but the ratio is maintained in a chronic situation. In this instance, the patient is breathing at a higher set point. That is, instead of maintenance at 40 torr, the normal $PaCO_2$ for this patient might be maintained at 46 torr and near-normal sensitivity to changes in the $PaCO_2$ may be present. If this patient underwent aggressive ventilation in the PACU with the goal of lowering the $PaCO_2$ to 40 torr, significant negative repercussions could occur. With a lower $PaCO_2$, the carbon dioxide in the CSF diffuses out and the bicarbonate remains because of its inability to diffuse out of the CSF. Thus, an excess of bicarbonate in comparison with carbon dioxide ($\uparrow$ bicarbonate pool) exists in the CSF and causes the primary stimulus to ventilation to cease. Because the patient's condition is hyperventilation, the $PaCO_2$ decreases and the $PAO_2$ increases (because of the 12-10 concept). Therefore, the secondary (hypoxic) drive may also become extinguished and this patient may have no effective drive for ventilation. If patients with chronic hypercapnia are acutely hyperventilated, they must be monitored for apnea once the accelerated ventilation is discontinued. A more appropriate technique is maintenance of the $PaCO_2$ at the level that is normal for that patient to avoid an apneic situation. Thus, for the patient with chronic carbon dioxide retention who is emerging from anesthesia, an overaggressive stir-up regimen (hyperventilation) should be avoided. The patient should perform the sustained maximal inspiration (SMI) at normal intervals, and the arterial blood gas values should be closely monitored.

In some patients with chronic carbon dioxide retention (chronic hypercapnia), the sensitivity to hydrogen ions via the carbon dioxide may be effectively decreased to the point at which the primary stimulus to ventilation becomes the low $PaO_2$ at the carotid and aortic bodies. The low $PaO_2$ becomes an effective stimulus to ventilation, especially when the $PaCO_2$ is elevated. The high $PaCO_2$ augments the response to the low $PaO_2$ with the peripheral chemoreceptors. For this reason, the patient breathes via the hypoxic drive. Because the carotid bodies are the major peripheral chemoreceptors, patients who use the hypoxic drive may also have bradycardia and hypotension. For that reason, patients

with abnormally high preoperative $PaCO_2$ values who have bradycardia and hypotension should be suspected of using the hypoxic drive as the primary drive to ventilation. In the PACU, patients suspected of primary use of this drive should be monitored closely and given oxygen to attain adequate oxygen content (a hemoglobin saturation of between 80% and 90%). The primary goal is to keep the patient oxygenated without extinguishing the main control of ventilation. High-flow techniques that use a Venturi mask that works on the Venturi principle to ensure precise $FiO_2$ values (i.e., 24% to 50%) can be used with these patients.

***The Response to Carbon Dioxide.*** Carbon dioxide is the primary stimulus to ventilation. The carbon dioxide response test is used for assessment of the ventilatory response to carbon dioxide. In this test, the subject inhales carbon dioxide mixtures (with the $PaO_2$ held constant) so that the inspired $PaCO_2$ gradually increases. Normally, the $V_E$ increases linearly as the $PaCO_2$ increases (Fig. 12-21). Some disease states and drugs cause the carbon dioxide response curve to shift to the left or the right. If the curve shifts to the left, the subject is more responsive to carbon dioxide. Factors such as thyroid toxicosis, aggressive personality, salicylates, and ketosis shift the curve to the left. A decreased ventilatory response to carbon dioxide occurs when the curve is shifted to the right and is called a blunted response. Patients who have a blunted response to carbon dioxide need intensive perianesthesia nursing care. The ventilatory response to an increased concentration of inspired carbon dioxide is blunted by hypothyroidism, mental depression, aging, general anesthetics, barbiturates, and narcotics. Many patients in the PACU either have these conditions or have received these drugs during

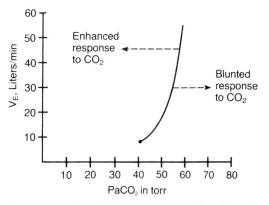

**Fig. 12-21** Carbon dioxide response curve. *(From Traver G: Respiratory nursing: the science and the art, New York, 1982, John Wiley & Sons.)*

surgery. This blunted response to carbon dioxide is one of the main justifications for supplemental oxygen administration to all patients who are emerging from anesthesia in the PACU. This response is also the rationale behind the need for critical perianesthesia nursing care that includes frequent assessment and interventions such as the stir-up regimen for prevention of respiratory depression.

***Upper Airways Receptors.*** Receptors that are sensitive to mechanical stimulation and chemical agents and have afferent pathways via the trigeminal and olfactory nerves are located in the nose. Activation of these receptors can cause apnea, bradycardia, and, most commonly, a sneeze. When a patient is to undergo nasal intubation, the perianesthesia nurse should monitor for bradycardia and apnea and be prepared for necessary interventions. Atropine or glycopyrrolate (Robinul) may be necessary for the vagolytic effect; succinylcholine may facilitate the intubation. Finally, for provision of positive-pressure ventilation, a bag-valve-mask system should be immediately available should apnea occur.

Receptors located in the epipharynx are sensitive to mechanical stimulation. Their activation is associated with the sniff or aspiration reflex. Mechanical stimulation of these receptors causes deep inspiration, bronchodilatation, and hypertension. This reflex is a protective reflex that allows material in the epipharynx to be brought down to the pharynx, clearing the nasal airways. In the larynx are irritant receptors that respond to both mechanical and chemical stimulation. Afferent pathways from these receptors travel along the internal branch of the superior laryngeal nerve. Stimulation invokes many responses, including coughing, slow deep breathing, apnea, bronchoconstriction, and hypertension. In addition, the trachea possesses irritant receptors. Stimulation of these receptors can cause responses such as coughing, bronchoconstriction, and hypertension.

During any procedure that involves the intubation of the trachea, the perianesthesia nurse should be prepared to assess the appropriate cardiorespiratory parameters and implement nursing care as necessary.

***Lung Receptors.*** Pulmonary stretch receptors (PSRs) lie within the smooth muscle of the small airways. These receptors are activated by marked distention or deflation (atelectasis) of the lungs. On marked inflation of the lungs, the activation of the PSR leads to a slowing of inspiratory frequency because of an increase in expiratory time. Bronchodilatation and tachycardia also may result from activation of these receptors. The

PSRs are thought to be part of the Hering-Breuer reflex. The low threshold for the PSR is present for approximately the first 3 months of life; after that, the threshold is high throughout adulthood. Hence, for the adult, the Hering-Breuer reflex is not important in the control of ventilation except in the anesthetized state. When an adult is administered general anesthesia and ventilation with prolonged maximal lung inflations, a prolonged expiratory time can result because of activation of the PSR.

Of great interest in regard to the pathogenesis of asthma are the irritant receptors that lie between the airway epithelial cells. These receptors respond to chemical irritants (e.g., histamine) and mechanical irritants (e.g., small particles and aerosols) that irritate the pulmonary epithelium. The irritant receptors are mediated by vagal afferent fibers, and on receptor stimulation, bronchoconstriction and hyperpnea occur. The pathogenesis of asthma is suggested to revolve around the sequence of histamine release, which stimulates the irritant receptors and ultimately leads to bronchoconstriction mediated via the vagus nerve.

The J-receptors, or juxtapulmonary capillary–receptors, are located in the wall of the pulmonary capillaries. Like the irritant receptors, J-receptors' afferent impulses are transmitted to the central nervous system by the vagus nerve. Normal stimuli of the J-receptors include pneumonia, pulmonary congestion, and increased interstitial fluid pressure. Stimulation of these receptors by interstitial or pulmonary edema results in tachypnea, bradycardia, and hypotension. Therefore, in assessment of patients who are at risk for development of pulmonary edema, the nurse should always evaluate the rate of ventilation. With the knowledge that interstitial edema usually precedes pulmonary edema and that increased interstitial congestion stimulates the J-receptors, the nurse should consider a rapid shallow breathing pattern to be a danger signal and report it to the attending physician.

Located in the walls of the large systemic arteries, especially in the aortic and carotid sinuses, are stretch receptors called baroreceptors. These receptors help to control the systemic blood pressure. They also affect ventilation. When the systemic blood pressure increases, a reflex hypoventilation occurs because of stimulation of the baroreceptors. On the other hand, a low systemic blood pressure causes the baroreceptors to produce a reflex hyperventilation. Hence, if a patient in the PACU has a significant amount of hypertension or hypotension, a reflex ventilatory response usually occurs because of the stimulation of the baroreceptors in the large systemic arteries.

## The Controllers

The controllers of breathing are located in the central nervous system and comprise two functionally and anatomically separate components. Voluntary breathing is controlled in the cortex of the brain. Automatic breathing is controlled by structures within the brainstem. The spinal cord functions to integrate the output of the brainstem and the cortex. The cortex can override the other controllers of breathing if voluntary control is desired. Examples of voluntary control include voluntary hyperventilation and breath holding.

***The Brainstem.*** Located bilaterally in the upper pons is the pneumotaxic center. This center functions to fine-tune the respiratory pattern with modulating the activity of the apneustic center and regulating the respiratory system's response to stimuli such as hypercarbia, hypoxia, and lung inflation. Near the pontomedullary border is the apneustic center. This center is probably the site of the inspiratory cutoff switch that terminates inspiration. In fact, apneusis, which consists of prolonged inspirations with occasional expirations, results when the apneustic center has been deactivated. Consequently, the apneustic center is also a fine-tuner of the rhythm of breathing.

Located in the medullary center, above the spinal cord, are two groups of neurons: the dorsal respiratory group (DRG) and the ventral respiratory group (VRG). The DRG is composed of inspiratory neurons and is the initial intracranial processing site for many reflexes that affect breathing. It is probably the site of origin of the rhythmic respiratory drive. The DRG sends motor fibers via the phrenic nerve to the diaphragm. It sends inspiratory fibers to the VRG, which is also part of the medullary center. However, the VRG does not send fibers to the DRG; therefore, the reciprocal inhibition theory of the regulation of breathing seems unlikely. The VRG is made up of both inspiratory and expiratory cells. The VRG neurons are driven by the cells of the DRG; thus, respiratory rhythmicity and the processing of sensory inputs do not occur initially within the VRG. The major function of the VRG is to project impulses to distant sites and to drive either the spinal respiratory motor neurons (primary intercostal and abdominal) or the auxiliary muscles of breathing innervated by the vagus nerve.

The DRG receives information from almost all the chemoreceptors, the baroreceptors, and the other sensors in the lung. In turn, the DRG generates a breathing rhythm that is fine-tuned by the apneustic center (inspiratory cutoff switch) and the pneumotaxic center. The inspiratory motor impulses are sent to the diaphragm and to the VRG. The VRG then drives spinal respiratory neurons (innervating the intercostal and abdominal muscles) or the auxiliary muscles of respiration innervated by the vagus nerve. Again, the cerebral cortex can override these centers if voluntary control of breathing is desired. Also, the vagus nerve has a profound effect on many aspects of the control of breathing because the afferent pathways of the vagus nerve from the stretch receptors, J-receptors, and irritant receptors serve to modulate the rhythm of breathing. Thus, any dysfunction that includes transection of the vagi results in irregular breathing patterns, depending on the level of dysfunction (pons or medulla).

## Sleep Apnea

The regulation of breathing has been described in detail, and obviously, multiple effects stimulate many levels of receptors to facilitate breathing. Yet, sleep apnea has become a major health issue and certainly a major concern in the perianesthesia setting. More than 12 million Americans are estimated to have some form of sleep apnea.

Sleep apnea has three forms: obstructive, central, and mixed. Obstructive sleep apnea (OSA) is caused by an obstruction or blockage of the airway. This obstruction usually occurs in the posterior pharynx, with soft tissue collapse leading to obstruction of the airway. Central sleep apnea is not a single disease entity but rather includes several disorders in which the definitive event is the withdrawal of effective central drive to the respiratory muscles. The mixed type of sleep apnea is a combination of obstructive and central components. Consequently, sleep apnea can be the result of a variety of pathophysiologic disorders, such as underlying defects in the respiratory controller or neuromuscular systems to include soft tissue collapse.

The clinical manifestations of sleep apnea are variable because of the different mechanisms that can produce the syndrome. Fig. 12-22 schematically shows the physiologic responses and clinical features that result from sleep apnea. The risk factors for the development of sleep apnea are presented in Box 12-4 and the presenting symptoms that can be evaluated before surgery at the preoperative interview are presented in Box 12-5.

Management of the patient with sleep apnea begins with a good preoperative screening.

PRIMARY EVENTS

PHYSIOLOGICAL
CONSEQUENCES

CLINICAL FEATURES

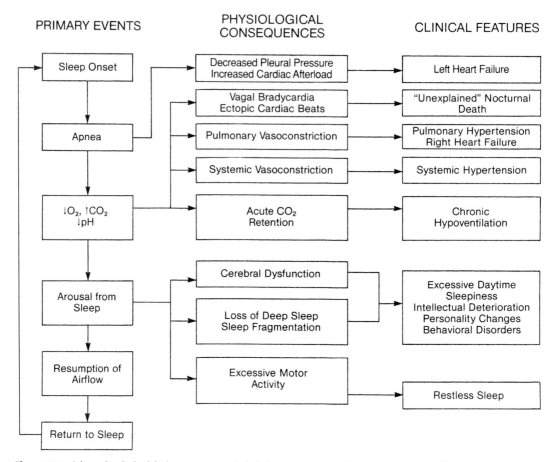

**Fig. 12-22**   Schematic of physiologic responses and clinical features that result from sleep apnea. *(From Murray J, Nadel J: Textbook of respiratory medicine, ed 2, Philadelphia, 1994, Saunders.)*

Questions that should be asked should include, "Do you snore?" and "Do you ever fall asleep easily or sometimes inappropriately?" Other key questions can include, "Do you feel tired or groggy when you wake up?," "Do you have headaches in the morning?," "Do you recall waking frequently during the night?," and "Do any of your family members have sleep apnea?"

If obstructive sleep apnea occurs in a patient in the PACU, basic airway care should be given. Certainly sedation is not in the best interest of the patient, as a difficult airway is often present

---

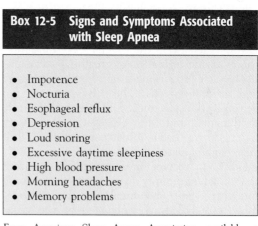

| Box 12-4 | Risk Factors Associated with Sleep Apnea |
| --- | --- |

- Family history of sleep apnea
- Excess weight
- Large neck
- Recessed chin
- Male gender
- More than 60 years of age
- Consumption of alcoholic beverages
- History of chronic smoking
- Abnormal structure of the upper airway

From American Sleep Apnea Association, available at *www.sleepapnea.org/info/practitioner/painandsleepapnea.html*, accessed March 13, 2007.

| Box 12-5 | Signs and Symptoms Associated with Sleep Apnea |
| --- | --- |

- Impotence
- Nocturia
- Esophageal reflux
- Depression
- Loud snoring
- Excessive daytime sleepiness
- High blood pressure
- Morning headaches
- Memory problems

From American Sleep Apnea Association, available at *www.sleepapnea.org/info/practitioner/painandsleepapnea.html*, accessed March 13, 2007.

in the PACU. Many times, these patients come to the PACU after a tracheostomy is performed during surgery. Pediatric patients many times have a tonsillectomy and adenoidectomy for treatment of sleep apnea. Airway management should include: avoidance of the supine position, especially in adults; repositioning of the airway; supplemental oxygen; provision for a patent airway; and then application of continuous positive airway pressure (CPAP) via a nose mask, in that order of level of nursing interventions (see Chapter 30). CPAP has been shown to be effective in patients with central sleep apnea associated with congestive heart failure and facilitates a more appropriate emergence from anesthesia or sedation.

## POSTOPERATIVE LUNG VOLUMES

Postoperative pulmonary complications are the most common single cause of morbidity and mortality in the postoperative period. The reported incidence rate of postoperative pulmonary complications ranges from 4.5% to 76%.

### Patients with Abnormal Pulmonary Function
When patients undergo anesthesia and surgery, certain risk factors predispose them to the development of postoperative pulmonary complications. Patients at the highest risk are those with preexisting pulmonary problems with abnormal pulmonary function before surgery. The other major risk factors associated with postoperative pulmonary complications are chronic cigarette smoking, obesity, and advanced age.

***Preexisting Pulmonary Disease.*** Patients with preexisting pulmonary disease can have clinical or subclinical manifestations of the disease state. Consequently, preoperative pulmonary function tests are valuable in assessment of the presence or absence of pulmonary pathophysiology and in determination of operative risk. Obstructive lung disease (i.e., asthma, emphysema, and chronic bronchitis), the most common category of lung disease, can be assessed with flow-volume measurements. Most pulmonary researchers suggest that a maximal voluntary ventilation that is less than 50% of what is predicted, a maximal expiratory flow rate below 220 L/min, or a forced expiratory volume in 1 second below 1.5 L indicates an increased operative risk for pulmonary complications. These flow-volume measurements are valuable predictors of the patient's ability to generate an adequate cough, which is a pulmonary defense mechanism rendered ineffective in the immediate postoperative period by anesthesia and surgery. Consequently, these patients need vigorous informed nursing care in

the immediate postoperative period. Priorities of nursing care should include frequent use of the stir-up regimen of turn, cascade cough, and SMI, along with the use of appropriate nursing interventions designed to enhance secretion clearance, which ensure airway patency.

Patients with restrictive lung disease (i.e., pulmonary fibrosis and morbid obesity) represent a significant risk for postoperative pulmonary complications when pulmonary function test results reveal a VC or a diffusion capacity of less than 50% of predicted values or exercise arterial blood gas values that show slight hypoxemia on exertion. In the PACU, these patients need a vigorous stir-up regimen with attention to tissue oxygenation via monitoring for hypoxemia. This regimen is needed because, during the surgical experience and in the PACU, physiologic stress can occur. One of the major products of physiologic stress is an increase in cardiovascular parameters, which reduces the transit time of the RBCs across the respiratory gas exchange membrane. Because of the pathologic changes in the respiratory membrane, patients with restrictive lung disease can have desaturation on exertion, such as in the stress reaction.

***Cigarette Smoking.*** Chronic cigarette smoking has been shown to increase the incidence rate of postoperative pulmonary complications as demonstrated in my research. Patients who smoke only 12 cigarettes a day have a six-fold increase in pulmonary morbidity rates in the postoperative period. The incidence rate of pulmonary embolism is higher in the smoker because of increased coagulability produced by chronic cigarette smoking. The ciliated epithelium of the lungs is damaged by chronic cigarette smoking. This damage can cause some blockage of the mucociliary transport system, which finally results in bronchiolar obstruction, infection, and atelectasis. Patients who smoke should be encouraged to stop smoking for at least 2 weeks before surgery to allow the mucociliary transport system to return to a nearly normal level of function. The focus of nursing care for the active chronic cigarette smoker should be similar to the interventions discussed for the patient with obstructive lung disease.

***Obesity.*** The patient who is markedly overweight has a significant chance of development of postoperative pulmonary complications caused by the altered lung volumes and capacities from the excess adipose tissue. Expansion of the lungs is hindered by an enlarged abdomen, which elevates the diaphragm and adds weight on the chest wall, thereby hindering the outward recoil of the chest wall. This hindrance leads to decreased thoracic wall compliance and ulti-mately to a reduced FRC. Finally, these compli-cations result in hypoxemia from increased airway closure and $\dot{V}_A/\dot{Q}_C$ abnormalities (see Chapter 48). The goal of nursing interventions in the PACU is prevention of further airway closure. Thus, a vigorous stir-up regimen, includ-ing early ambulation, should help prevention of further reduction in the FRC. That measure reduces the amount of airway closure, alleviates the hypoxemia, and ultimately improves the out-come of the patient.

***Advanced Age.*** Patients of advanced age (older than 70 years of age) have a slightly higher risk of development of postoperative pul-monary complications. A greater decrease in the FRC after surgery in patients of advanced age has been shown. Because the closing volume increases with age, significant airway closure can occur after surgery during tidal ventilation. Although advanced age is not associated with the same degree of risk as the factors previously discussed, it can increase the danger of the other risk factors. However, patients of advanced age should receive a vigorous stir-up regimen in the PACU if only because of the alterations in lung mechanics.

### Physiology of Perianesthesia Pulmonary Nursing Care

Because of the change in the mechanical proper-ties of the lungs and chest wall, patients emerging from anesthesia have a decrease in lung volumes and capacities (Fig. 12-23). This decrease is espe-cially true of the patient who has undergone a thoracic or upper abdominal surgical procedure. In the PACU, a further reduction in lung volumes and capacities may be seen. The major factor that contributes to this reduction in lung volumes in the patient after surgery is a shallow monotonous sighless breathing pattern that is caused by general inhalation anesthesia, pain, and narcotics. Sighless ventilation may result in an uneven distribution of surfactant and a loss of stability of the small airways and alveoli, which can then lead to alveolar collapse and ultimately to atelectasis. Normally, adults breathe regularly and rhythmically, spontaneously performing a maximal inspiration that is held for about 3 seconds at the peak of inspiration. This physio-logic process, or SMI, is commonly called a sigh or a yawn.

In normal lungs, the closing volume is less than the resting lung volume (i.e., the FRC), and airways remain open during tidal breathing. In the immediate postoperative period, patients who have a sighless monotonous low-$V_T$ venti-latory pattern usually have a reduced FRC.

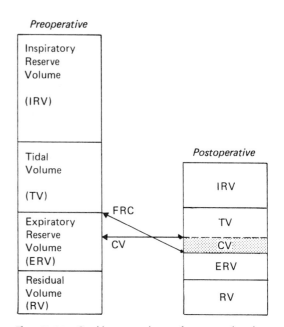

**Fig. 12-23** Graphic comparison of preoperative lung volumes to probable lung volumes in immediate postoperative period in patient who has undergone upper abdominal surgi-cal procedure. *FRC,* Functional residual capacity; *CV,* closing volume. *(From Drain C: Pathophysiology of the respiratory system related to anesthesia,* CRNA: Clin Forum Nurse Anesthetists *7(4):181-192, 1996.)*

When the FRC plus $V_T$ is within the closing volume range, the airways that lead to depen-dent lung zones may be effectively closed throughout tidal breathing (see Fig. 12-23). Inspired gas then is distributed mainly to the upper or nondependent lung zones. Perfusion continues to follow the normal gradi-ent, with higher flows to the dependent areas of the lung.

In the immediate postoperative period, as airway closure occurs, gas is trapped behind closed airways. This sequestered air can become absorbed, and the alveoli then become airless (atelectasis). The atelectasis, as it becomes more widespread, leads to a decrease in ventilation as compared with perfusion (low $\dot{V}_A/\dot{Q}_C$), which results in a widening of the $PAO_2 - PaO_2$ value and ultimately to hypoxe-mia. In addition, atelectatic areas in the lung provide an excellent culture medium in which pneumonia can develop.

Various investigators have shown a decrease in lung volumes in the postoperative period. Patients who have undergone an upper abdom-inal surgical procedure have an immediate postoperative decrease in the FRC from hour 1 to hour 2 (Fig. 12-24). The FRC then seems to return to near the baseline value by about the fourth postoperative hour. A second

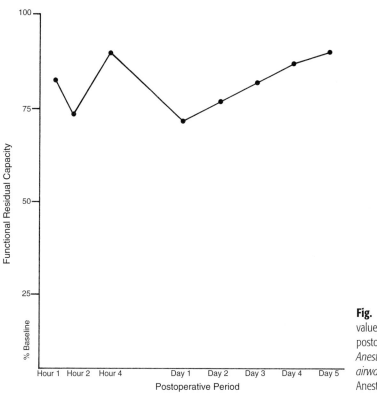

**Fig. 12-24** Composite curve of mean values of functional residual capacity in postoperative period. *(From Drain C: Anesthesia care of the patient with reactive airways disease,* CRNA: Clin Forum Nurse Anesthetists *7(4):207-212, 1996.)*

subsequent decrease in the FRC is then seen after hour 4, and baseline values are not restored until 5 days after surgery. A possible explanation of the "peaks and valleys" in the FRC during the postoperative period may be that the first reduction in the FRC is associated with anesthesia and the latter reduction may be from pain. General inhalation anesthesia and pain can dampen the physiologic sigh mechanism. Consequently, all patients who have undergone a surgical procedure, especially those who have incision sites near the thorax or diaphragm, should be strongly encouraged to perform the SMI maneuver both in the PACU and on the surgical unit. The incentive spirometer, a device designed to use positive feedback to encourage the patient to perform the SMI maneuver, can be used by the patient on the surgical unit.

## OXYGEN ADMINISTRATION IN THE POSTANESTHESIA CARE UNIT

Administration of oxygen to the patient in the PACU is an important facet in the emergence phase of anesthesia. Oxygen is given to the patient in the PACU primarily because of the blunted or depressed response to carbon dioxide and low lung volumes. Administration of supplemental oxygen during the recovery phase of anesthesia is especially important for the patient who has received a general or spinal anesthetic. The methods of oxygen administration are summarized in Chapter 27.

### Perianesthesia Nursing Care

A patent airway must be maintained throughout the administration of oxygen. The patient should be encouraged to cascade cough, perform the SMI, and change positions according to the stir-up regimen discussed in this chapter and in Chapter 27. If a nasal catheter is used, the catheter should be removed every 6 hours for cleansing and reinsertion into the other nostril. Also, the nasal mucosa should be inspected periodically for dryness when a nasal catheter or prongs are used. Oxygen given in the dry gas form can cause drying and irritation of the mucosa, impair the ciliary action, and thicken secretions; therefore, oxygen should always be administered with humidity.

The perianesthesia nurse must receive a report from the anesthesiologist or anesthetist or both as to the patient's preoperative pulmonary status. Whether the patient has a history of chronic retention of carbon dioxide, as occurs in chronic obstructive pulmonary disease, is especially important to ascertain. As described in this chapter, the patient with carbon dioxide retention who receives oxygen in the PACU should be monitored carefully for any signs of hypoventilation, confusion, or semicomatose condition. If any of these signs appear, the surgeon and anesthesiologist or anesthetist should be notified immediately.

### Oxygen Toxicity

When excessive concentrations of inspired oxygen (>60%) are administered to patients for a prolonged period, the eyes, lungs, and central nervous system can be damaged.

***Eyes.*** Premature infants who have a high $PaO_2$ longer than 24 hours are at risk for development of retrolental fibroplasia, which is caused by vasoconstriction of the blood vessels of the retina as a result of high oxygen concentrations in the blood. Retrolental fibroplasia presents in an acute form as vascular retinopathy at the developing edge of blood vessels in the premature infant's eye. This presentation is followed by perivascular exudation, tissue hyperplasia, and scar tissue that exerts traction on the retina and leads to retinal detachment and destruction of the infant's vision. Research indicates that the incidence rate of acute retrolental fibroplasia is inversely proportional to birth weight. Most of the clinical research indicates that for minimization of the risk of development of retrolental fibroplasia, the infant's $PaO_2$ should be maintained between 60 and 90 torr. Perianesthesia nurses should use their best-informed judgment when caring for these infants. As with the adult, the infant who needs a high-inspired oxygen concentration to provide adequate oxygenation should not be denied oxygen because of fear of complications.

***Lungs.*** Concentrations of oxygen higher than 60% damage the lungs within 3 or 4 days. A 120% oxygen concentration administered for 24 to 48 hours also causes pulmonary damage, the signs of which are manifested by type II cell dysfunction in the lung. The type II cells secrete surfactant, and the lack of surfactant in the alveoli leads to alveolar collapse. The hyperoxic environment also stops the ciliary action in the lungs. The early symptoms of this disorder include cough, nasal congestion, sore throat, reduced VC, tracheobronchitis, and substernal discomfort. The early signs of airway irritation may appear when a patient has received 80% to 120% oxygen continuously for 8 hours or longer. The lung appears to indefinitely tolerate oxygen concentrations lower than 40%.

***Central Nervous System.*** Headache is an early indicator of oxygen toxicity. As oxygen toxicity continues to develop, the patient has some confusion. When a patient is receiving a high concentration of oxygen and has these signs and symptoms, the attending physician should be notified. Convulsions usually are not seen in the PACU but may occur when oxygen is delivered in above-normal atmospheric pressure, such as in hyperbaric oxygen chambers.

## SUMMARY

The inhalation agents continue to see a significant amount of use in the operating room. They are now time tested and possess excellent qualities that do not have a significant impact on the patient. More specifically, the agents used today are more rapid, do not have a significant impact on the major organ systems, and are easily removed, if the patient undergoes appropriate emergence. Nursing research has been performed in this area, with the PACU for the clinical trial. Based on research, use of the modified stir-up regime as opposed to the deep-breathing maneuver in recovery of patients during the immediate postoperative period is so important, especially in the clinical world of evidence-based practice.

## BIBLIOGRAPHY

Aitkenhead A, Smith G, Rowbotham D: *Textbook of anaesthesia*, ed 5, Philadelphia, 2007, Churchill Livingstone.

Alspach J: *Core curriculum for critical care nursing*, ed 6, Philadelphia, 2005, Saunders.

Atlee J: *Complications in anesthesia*, ed 2, Philadelphia, 2007, Saunders.

Barash P, Cullen B, Stoelting R: *Clinical anesthesia*, ed 5, Philadelphia, 2001, Lippincott Williams & Wilkins.

Benumof J, Saidman L: *Anesthesia & perioperative complications*, ed 2, St Louis, 1999, Mosby.

Brunton L, Lazo J, Parker K: *Goodman and Gilman's the pharmacological basis of therapeutics*, ed 11, New York, 2005, McGraw-Hill Professional.

Cote C, Todres I, Goudsouzian N, et al: *A practice of anesthesia for infants and children*, ed 3, Philadelphia, 2001, Saunders.

Drain C: Anesthesia care of the patient with reactive airways disease, *CRNA: Clin Forum Nurse Anesthetists* 7(4):207-212, 1996.

Drain C: Pathophysiology of the respiratory system related to anesthesia, *CRNA: Clin Forum Nurse Anesthetists* 7(4):181-192, 1996.

Drain C: Physiology of the respiratory system related to anesthesia, *CRNA: Clin Forum Nurse Anesthetists* 7(4):163-180, 1996.

Drain C, Robinson S: The pharmacology of respiratory disorders related to anesthesia, CRNA: *Clin Forum Nurse Anesthetists* 7(4):193-199,1996.

Drake R, Vogl W, Mitchell A: *Gray's anatomy for students*, Philadelphia, 2005, Churchill Livingstone.

Estafanous F, Barash P, Reves J, editors: *Cardiac anesthesia: principles and clinical practice*, ed 2, Philadelphia, 2001, Lippincott Williams & Wilkins.

Evers A, Maze M: *Anesthetic pharmacology: physiologic principles and clinical practice*, Philadelphia, 2004, Churchill Livingstone.

Fisher L: *Benumof's anesthesia and uncommon diseases*, ed 5, Philadelphia, 2007, Saunders.

Gallager C, Issenberg B: *Simulation in anesthesia*, Philadelphia, 2007, Saunders.

Ganong W: *Review of medical physiology*, ed 22, New York, 2005, McGraw-Hill Medical.

Guyton A, Hall J: *Textbook of medical physiology*, ed 11, Philadelphia, 2006, Saunders.

Kaplan J, editor: *Thoracic anesthesia*, ed 2, New York, 1991, Churchill Livingstone.

Lake C, Hines R, Blitt C: *Clinical monitoring: practical applications for anesthesia and critical care*, Philadelphia, 2001, Saunders.

Longnecker D, Murphy F: *Dripps, Eckenhoff, Vandam introduction to anesthesia*, ed 9, Philadelphia, 1997, Saunders.

Longnecker D, Tinker J, Morgan G: *Principles and practice of anesthesiology*, ed 2, St Louis, 1998, Mosby.

Miller R, editor: *Anesthesia*, ed 5, Philadelphia, 2000, Churchill Livingstone.

Moos D, Cuddeford D: Implications of obstructive sleep apnea syndrome for the perianesthesia nurse, *J PeriAnesthesia Nurs* 21(2):103-118, 2006.

Murray J, Nadel J: *Textbook of respiratory medicine*, ed 2, Philadelphia, 1994, Saunders.

Nagelhout J, Zaglaniczy K: *Nurse anesthesia*, ed 3, St Louis, 2005, Saunders.

Passannante A, et al: Anesthestic management of patients with obesity and sleep apnea, *Anesthesiol Clin North Am* 23:479-490, 2005.

Shorten G, Browne J, Carr D, et al: *Postoperative pain management: an evidence-based guide to practice*, Philadelphia, 2006, Saunders.

Stoelting R: *Pharmacology and physiology in anesthetic practice*, ed 3, Philadelphia, 1999, Lippincott-Raven.

Stoelting R, Miller R: *Basics of anesthesia*, ed 4, Philadelphia, 2000, Churchill Livingstone.

PHYSIOLOGIC CONSIDERATIONS IN THE PACU

# 13

# THE RENAL SYSTEM

Cecil B. Drain, PhD, RN, CRNA, FAAN, FASAHP

The renal system is becoming more and more an important factor in the assessment and care of the patient in the PACU because the kidneys excrete ... in that the kidneys excrete many drugs unchanged or excrete the byproduct of the metabolism of a particular drug. Homeostasis is maintained with proper kidney function because the kidneys regulate the balance of acid-base, electrolyte, and fluid volumes and remove waste materials and toxic substances from the body. The kidneys also play a part in the regulation of the cardiovascular system. Hence, the kidneys are significant in the physiologic regulation and control of the body.

Proper kidney function is imperative to ensure positive outcomes for the patient recovering from anesthesia in the postanesthesia care unit (PACU). When kidney function is reduced, anesthetic drugs do not get metabolized as they normally would, which leads to a prolonged emergence. When this process is coupled with changes in cardiac function, the emergence phase of the anesthetic can be difficult. With the profound impact the kidneys have on the patient's recovery and with the advent of kidney transplants, assessment of kidney function is one of the key factors in the assessment of the perianesthesia patient. Assessment of kidney function is sometimes difficult in the PACU, especially in the patient who is not catheterized. In patients who have urinary catheters in place after surgery, assessment of kidney function should be part of the perianesthesia nursing care. On this basis, an understanding of renal anatomy and physiology is important for facilitation of the outcomes of all perianesthesia patients recovering from anesthesia.

## DEFINITIONS

**Acetonuria:** The appearance of acetone in the urine. Acetonuria is present when excessive fats are consumed or when an inadequate amount of carbohydrates is metabolized.

**Albuminuria:** The presence of protein in the urine, also called proteinuria. Albumin is the most common protein found in the urine. This condition usually indicates a malfunction in glomerular filtration.

**Azotemia:** The presence of nitrogenous products in the blood, usually because of decreased kidney function.

**Cystitis:** An inflammation of the bladder.

**Dysuria:** Painful or difficult urination.

**Enuresis:** Involuntary discharge of urine.

**Glycosuria:** The presence of glucose in the urine.

**Hematuria:** The presence of blood in the urine.

**Nephritis:** Inflammation of the kidney; called Bright's disease.

**Nephrosis:** Degeneration of the kidney without the occurrence of inflammation.

**Oliguria:** A decrease in the normal amount of urine formation.

**Pyelitis:** An inflammation of the renal pelvis and calices.

**Stricture:** An abnormal narrowing; in the urinary tract, a narrowing of the ureter or urethra.

**Uremia:** The toxic condition usually caused by renal insufficiency and retention of nitrogenous substances in the blood.

**Urinary Incontinence:** The inability to retain urine in the bladder.

**Urinary Retention:** Failure to expel urine from the bladder.

## ANATOMY OF THE KIDNEYS

The kidneys are two bean-shaped organs in the retroperitoneal spaces near the upper lumbar area. The right kidney is at a slightly lower level than the left. Each kidney weighs approximately 150 g. The notched portion of the kidney is called the hilum, which is where the ureter, the renal vein, and the renal artery enter the kidney (Fig. 13-1).

The ureter opens into a large cavity called the pelvis. From the pelvis, two to five major calices project deeper into the kidney. The major calices branch out to form six to 10 minor

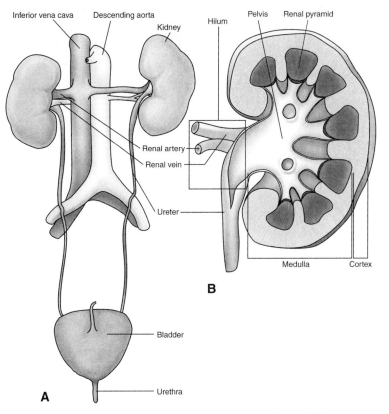

Inferior vena cava   Descending aorta
Kidney
Hilum   Pelvis   Renal pyramid
Renal artery
Renal vein
Ureter
Medulla   Cortex
**B**
Bladder
Urethra
**A**

**Fig. 13-1**  Anatomy of renal and urinary systems. **A,** Urinary system. **B,** Cross section of a kidney.

calices. The ends of the minor calices are capped by the renal papillae.

The medulla is the inner portion of the kidney. It comprises several pyramids, which correspond to the number of minor calices. The base of the pyramid projects toward the outer portion of the kidney, which is termed the cortex. The apex of the pyramid forms the papillae, which cap each minor calix.

Blood is supplied to the kidney by the renal artery. The rate of blood flow through both kidneys of a man who weighs 70 kg is about 1200 mL/min, or about 21% of the cardiac output. As the renal artery enters the kidney at the hilum, it divides into the interlobar arteries in the medulla; then, as the arteries enter the cortex, they divide into the arciform (arcuate) arteries. The afferent arteries project from the interlobar arteries and go to the nephron, where they divide into capillaries. The capillaries form the efferent arterioles, which then divide to form the peritubular capillaries, which help supply the nephron, a portion of the tubular capillaries, and the vasa recta, which descend around the loop of Henle, in the case of juxtamedullary nephrons. These nephrons, which are close to the renal medulla, have a long extended

loop of Henle that dips deep into the medulla. They then return to the venules, as do the tubular capillaries (Figs. 13-2 and 13-3).

The nephron is the functional unit of the kidney. The two kidneys contain approximately 2.4 million nephrons. Each nephron can be divided into three major portions: the renal

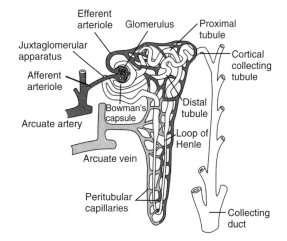

Efferent arteriole   Glomerulus   Proximal tubule
Juxtaglomerular apparatus
Afferent arteriole
Cortical collecting tubule
Bowman's capsule   Distal tubule
Arcuate artery
Loop of Henle
Arcuate vein
Peritubular capillaries
Collecting duct

**Fig. 13-2**  Functional nephron. *(From Guyton A, Hall J: Textbook of medical physiology, ed 10, Philadelphia, 2000, Saunders.)*

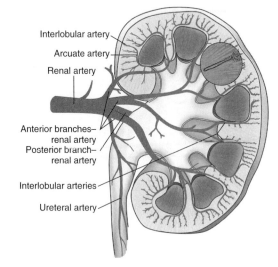

| Table 13-1 | Measure of Reabsorption by the Kidney Excreted | | |
|---|---|---|---|
| Substance | Filtered (mEq/24 h/ 170 L) | Reabsorbed (mEq/24 h/ 169 L) | Excreted (mEq/24 h/ 45 L) |
| Sodium | 24,500 | 24,350 | 150 |
| Chloride | 17,800 | 17,700 | 150 |
| Bicarbonate | 4,900 | 4,900 | 1 |
| Potassium | 700 | 600 | 24 |
| Glucose | 780 | 780 | 0 |
| Urea | 870 | 460 | 410 |
| Creatinine | 12 | 0 | 12 |

**Fig. 13-3** Arterial supply to kidney. Soon after entering hilum of kidney, renal artery divides into several anterior and posterior branches. Branches divide into interlobar arteries, which course between medullary pyramids. Interlobar arteries then give off arcuate arteries, which course between cortex and medulla. From this arcuate complex arise interlobar arteries, which give off afferent arterioles to glomeruli.

corpuscle, the renal tubule, and the collecting ducts. The blood enters the afferent arteriole and goes into the glomerulus in the cortex, which consists of a network of 50 parallel capillaries encased in Bowman's capsule. This structural component is the renal capsule.

The renal tubules begin in Bowman's capsule. A pressure gradient forces fluid to leave the glomerulus and enter Bowman's capsule. The fluid then flows into the proximal tubule, which is still in the cortex of the kidney, and then into the loop of Henle. The loop of Henle is at first thick-walled but becomes thin-walled at the distal segment in the medulla of the kidney. The fluid then flows into the distal tubule, located in the cortex of the kidney, and passes into the collecting ducts, which go from the cortex to the medulla where they form papillary ducts (ducts of Bellini) and into the renal pelvis by way of the renal calices. At this point, the fluid in the renal pelvis is termed urine.

## RENAL PHYSIOLOGY

The constituents of urine are formed by filtration, reabsorption, and secretion. Filtration occurs as the blood passes through the glomerulus. The force of filtration is a pressure gradient that pushes fluid through the glomerular membrane. Approximately 180 L of water every 24 hours is filtered out of plasma with other

substances (Table 13-1). Blood cells and colloidal substances are usually retained in the blood because they are too large to pass through the epithelium. The presence of red blood cells or protein in the urine usually indicates a pathologic process in the kidney.

Reabsorption occurs in the proximal and distal tubules. Approximately 99% of the water is reabsorbed. Many substances in the water are reabsorbed with active or passive transport. Active transport requires energy for movement of the substance across the membrane. Passive transport can be regarded as simple diffusion that is devoid of energy.

Substances such as glucose, amino acids, sodium, potassium, calcium, and magnesium—those that are important constituents of body fluids—are almost entirely reabsorbed. Certain substances are reabsorbed in limited quantities and consequently appear in the urine in considerable amounts. Some of these substances are urea, creatinine, and the phosphates.

The last mechanism in the formation of urine is secretion. Various substances, including hydrogen and potassium ions, are secreted directly into the tubular fluid through the epithelial cells that line the renal tubules.

## REGULATION OF KIDNEY FUNCTION

The formation of urine and the retention of substances needed for proper body function are aided by three physiologic mechanisms: the countercurrent mechanism, autoregulation, and hormone control.

### Countercurrent Mechanism

The countercurrent mechanism is used by the kidneys to concentrate urine. This mechanism is aided by the anatomic arrangement of the loops of Henle of the juxtamedullary nephrons,

which go deep into the medulla, and the peritubular capillaries, which are called the vasa
recta. The osmolality of the interstitial fluid
increases as it moves more deeply into the
medulla; this greater osmolality results in
active transport of solutes into the interstitial
fluid. This countercurrent mechanism is useful
when the body needs to excrete a large amount
of waste products yet reabsorb the normal
amount of solutes. This mechanism is also
useful when the water in the body needs to be
conserved, as in conditions of inadequate water
supply, in which water is conserved while waste
products are eliminated.

## Autoregulation

Autoregulation helps to keep the glomerular filtration at a near normal rate, despite fluctuations
in arterial pressure. In fact, within the blood pressure range of 60 to 160 torr, little change in either
renal plasma flow or glomerular filtration rate
occurs. Consequently, as the arterial pressure
increases, the sympathetic innervation to the
afferent arterioles causes constriction, thus keeping the glomerular filtration rate constant. The
reverse is also true. When the arterial pressure is
low, dilatation of the afferent arterioles serves to
keep the glomerular filtration rate constant.

## Hormone Control

The antidiuretic hormone (ADH) is secreted by
the posterior pituitary gland. The secretion of
this hormone is influenced by plasma osmolality.
If hypertonicity of the blood occurs, ADH is
secreted and water is retained by the kidneys.
If the blood is hypotonic, less ADH is formed
and the kidneys release water. This hormone
acts on the distal tubule and collecting tubules
by altering their permeability to water.

The juxtaglomerular apparatus is located just
before the glomerulus. If the sodium concentration is low, if the pressure in the afferent
arteriole is low, or if a reduced glomerular filtration rate or increased sympathetic stimulation
exists, an enzyme, renin, is released from the
juxtaglomerular cells.

Renin probably plays an important role in
conservation of sodium in hypotensive states
and control of fluid volume excretion. Renin,
when released in the blood, catalyzes the splitting
of angiotensin I from a renin substrate. As angiotensin I passes through the lungs, it is converted
to angiotensin II (Fig. 13-4). Angiotensin II is a
highly effective pressor agent and a major stimulus to the secretion of aldosterone. Aldosterone, a
mineralocorticoid, appears to act on the distal
tubule and the thick segment of the ascending
loop of Henle. When secreted, aldosterone

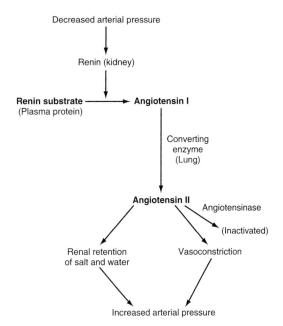

**Fig. 13-4** Renin-angiotensin-vasoconstrictor mechanism for arterial pressure control. *(From Guyton A, Hall J:* Textbook of medical physiology, *ed 10, Philadelphia, 2000, Saunders.)*

controls the reabsorption of some of the sodium
and water. Because the renin-angiotensin system
causes this reabsorption of water and sodium,
it plays a role in the control of arterial blood
pressure.

## RENAL ROLE IN REGULATION OF BODY HOMEOSTASIS

The kidneys play a role in regulation of body
fluids. For the most part, they determine the
adjustment of blood volume, extracellular fluid
volume, and osmolality of the extracellular
fluids, electrolytes, and ions; they remove waste
products and toxic substances; and they maintain the acid-base balance.

The kidneys regulate blood volume in the following manner. When the circulating blood
volume is excessive, the cardiac output and arterial pressure increase, thus causing stimulation of
volume receptors located in the left and right
atria and the baroreceptors located in the carotid,
aortic, and pulmonary regions. The net effect is
an increase in urine formation, with a return of
blood volume to a normal range. Aldosterone and
ADH also have a role in improvement of the
economy of blood volume and electrolytes.

If the patient's condition is hypovolemic,
the kidneys conserve fluid and thus return the
blood volume to normal limits.

The normal intake of water into the body
in 24 hours is 2500 mL. Of this, 1200 mL are

| Table 13-2 | Average Water Loss per 24 Hours at Average Temperature and Humidity | |
|---|---|---|
| Route | | Amount (mL) |
| Through the skin | | 500 |
| Through the lungs | | 350 |
| Through the kidneys | | 1500 |
| Through the feces | | 150 |

| Table 13-3 | Principal Constituents of Urine | |
|---|---|---|
| Constituents | | Amount (g/L) |
| **Organic** | | |
| Urea | | 20-300 |
| Uric acid | | 0.6-0.75 |
| Creatinine | | 1.5 |
| Others | | 2.6 |
| **Inorganic** | | |
| Sodium chloride | | 9.0 |
| Potassium chloride | | 2.5 |
| Sulfuric acid | | 1.8 |
| Phosphoric acid | | 1.8 |
| Ammonia | | 0.5-15 |
| Calcium | | 0.2 |
| Magnesium | | 0.2 |

ingested liquids and 1000 mL are water in solid food. The remaining 300 mL are water derived from oxidation of food in the tissue cells. Table 13-2 shows the avenues by which water is lost in a 24-hour period.

The extracellular fluid volume is controlled by the kidneys as they control the blood volume. The relative ratio of the extracellular fluid volume to blood volume depends on the physical properties of the circulation and of the interstitial spaces, including compliances and dynamics.

The kidney maintains the osmolality of the extracellular fluid mainly by regulating the extracellular sodium concentration. Extracellular sodium controls 90% to 95% of the effective osmotic pressure of extracellular fluid.

The kidneys also control the extracellular concentration of other electrolytes, such as potassium, calcium, magnesium, and phosphate ions.

## COMPONENTS OF URINE

The end product of excretion by the kidneys is urine, which is 95% water and 5% solids. The solids, which account for approximately 60 g/L of urine, are listed in Table 13-3. Urea is derived mostly from the catabolism of amino acids. Creatinine is thought to be derived from creatine, a nitrogenous substance found in muscle tissue. Because it is not reabsorbed by the tubular mechanism of the kidney, creatinine level is a good indicator of kidney function. Creatinine and sulfates are considered nonthreshold substances because they are excreted in their entirety. Uric acid is an end product of purine metabolism, formed from purines ingested as food and from those formed in the body.

High-threshold substances are almost entirely reabsorbed in the kidney. They are an important portion of the blood and are excreted only if they are in an excess concentration. Some of the high-threshold substances are glucose, potassium, calcium, and magnesium. Low-threshold substances, such as urea, uric acid,

and phosphates, are only minimally reabsorbed by the kidney.

In consideration of the substances found in urine, knowledge of the characteristics of normal urine is useful. Normal urine should be amber in color because of the pigment urochrome and should also be clear and transparent. It usually is acidic, with a pH of about 6, because of the presence of sodium acid phosphate. The specific gravity is between 1.003 and 1.025. The volume of urine excreted every 24 hours is about 1500 mL.

## ACID-BASE BALANCE

The kidneys play a major role in acid-base balance. Although they are the most powerful acid-base regulators, they need several hours to 1 day to return the hydrogen ion concentration to a normal range. The buffer systems (bicarbonate, phosphate, and protein) can react within a fraction of a second to alterations in hydrogen ion concentration. In contrast, the respiratory system usually takes 1 to 3 minutes to react.

The pH is a negative logarithmic expression of the hydrogen ion concentration in the body fluids (see Chapter 14). Bicarbonate and carbon dioxide are also factors. The bicarbonate is mainly under renal control, whereas the carbon dioxide is under respiratory control. The 20:1 ratio exists because approximately 20 times more bicarbonate than carbon dioxide is in the plasma. Thus, any change in the 20:1 ratio affects the pH. Any change that negates the functioning of the kidneys or the rest of the body may affect the bicarbonate portion of the ratio and is a metabolic problem. Conversely, any change in the function of the lungs, which usually affects the carbon dioxide portion of the ratio, is a respiratory problem.

If, for example, a large amount of a bicarbonate solution is rapidly infused into a patient and ventilation does not change ($PCO_2$ stays constant), the result is a higher value for the bicarbonate and no change in the $PCO_2$. The net result is a higher pH, which constitutes alkalosis, in this case termed metabolic alkalosis. On the other hand, if an acid is infused, the ratio becomes smaller and the pH falls, indicating acidosis, which is termed metabolic acidosis.

Respiratory acidosis occurs when the $PCO_2$ is increased, as in acute hypoventilation, for example. The pH is lowered because the ratio becomes smaller. Conversely, if the patient has hyperventilation, the $PCO_2$ drops and the ratio rises, thus increasing the pH and producing respiratory alkalosis.

The kidneys regulate pH by increasing or decreasing the bicarbonate ion concentration in the body fluid. This regulation is done with a complex series of reactions, which begins with hydrogen ions being secreted into the tubular fluid. Carbon dioxide, an end product of tubular cell metabolism, combines with water to form carbonic acid ($H_2CO_3$). The carbonic acid dissociates to form hydrogen (H) and bicarbonate ($HCO_3$). The hydrogen ion is taken via active transport to the renal tubule and usually exchanges in the tubule with sodium. Via active transport, the sodium moves to the extracellular fluid, where it combines with the bicarbonate that was reabsorbed into the extracellular fluid to form sodium bicarbonate ($NaHCO_3$). In the tubules, the hydrogen ion that was actively transported to the tubule combines with the filtrate bicarbonate to form carbonic acid. The carbonic acid dissociates to form carbon dioxide and water. The carbon dioxide is reabsorbed into the extracellular fluid and eventually excreted by the lungs; the water is excreted as part of the urine.

The kidneys correct alkalosis by decreasing the bicarbonate in the extracellular fluid, which occurs because fewer hydrogen ions enter the tubules because of a low carbon dioxide concentration and because a high bicarbonate concentration exists in the tubules. The bicarbonate cannot be reabsorbed without first combining with the hydrogen; therefore, the excess bicarbonate ions are lost to the urine as are other positive ions such as sodium and hydrogen. Cellular potassium may exchange with the sodium instead of the cellular hydrogen to conserve the hydrogen, which may help return the pH to normal limits.

Renal correction of acidosis is achieved by increasing the amount of bicarbonate in the extracellular fluid. An excess of hydrogen ions in comparison with the bicarbonate filtration into the tubules exists. The excess hydrogen ions are secreted into the tubules, where they combine with the phosphate or the ammonia buffer systems. The sodium ions in the tubules move via active transport to the extracellular fluid and combine with the bicarbonate ion to form sodium bicarbonate, which helps correct the acidosis. The urine is acidic because the kidney is excreting the excess hydrogen ions.

## DIURETIC THERAPY IN THE PACU

In the PACU, diuretics are commonly used for reduction of brain size and intracranial pressure, treatment of hypervolemia, prevention of oliguria, or help in diagnosis of the cause of the oliguria. The major side effects of diuretic therapy are related to the contraction of the extracellular fluid volume and the alterations in potassium concentrations. Diuretics are categorized according to the site of action on renal tubules and the mechanism of altering the secretion of urine. The major categories of diuretics are osmotic diuretics, thiazide diuretics, potassium-sparing diuretics, loop diuretics, aldosterone antagonists, and carbonic anhydrase inhibitors. Because the use of diuretics is so important in the PACU, a brief review of the major types of diuretics is presented.

### Osmotic Diuretics

Osmotic diuretics are used for evaluation of the cause of oliguria, reduction of intracranial pressure and brain size, and protection of the kidneys against the development of acute renal failure. Urea is an effective osmotic diuretic; however, this drug does have some disadvantages that limit its use as compared with mannitol. The major disadvantage of urea is that it causes a significant amount of rebound increase in intracranial pressure and a high incidence rate of venous thrombosis. Mannitol, a six-carbon sugar, is the prototype of the osmotic diuretics. This high–molecular-weight drug, when given intravenously, increases the plasma osmolality, with a resulting expansion of the intravascular volume by means of drawing fluid from the intracellular space into the extracellular space. In the kidneys, mannitol's osmotic effect on the tubules leads to a diuretic effect. The major concern with mannitol therapy is an increased extracellular fluid volume, which can be of grave consequence in patients with impending pulmonary edema. Hence, the perianesthesia nurse should frequently assess the pulmonary parameters in patients who receive mannitol and in whom pulmonary edema is possible. An early sign of pulmonary edema is wheezing. Wheezing usually indicates interstitial edema. If wheezing is detected in a patient who is nonasthmatic, the attending physician should be notified immediately. As the edema formation progresses, wet basilar rales or crackles may be heard during auscultation of the chest. The crackles become coarser as the pulmonary edema worsens.

## Thiazide Diuretics

Thiazide diuretics are mainly used in the treatment of hypertension, edema, and diabetes insipidus. These diuretics are secreted in the proximal convoluted tubule and have their major effect in the loop of Henle, where chloride reabsorption is inhibited. This reabsorption results in diluting defects and increased distal delivery of salt and water. Patients on long-term thiazide diuretic therapy can have increased urinary losses of water, sodium, chloride, and potassium and some loss of bicarbonate. Hence, these patients are particularly susceptible to hypochloremic hypokalemic metabolic alkalosis. Some of the common thiazide diuretics are chlorothiazide (Diuril), benzthiazide (Exna), and hydrochlorothiazide (Esidrix, HydroDiuril, Oretic).

The most common untoward effect of thiazide diuretics is hypokalemia. Hypokalemia, which is a reduced serum potassium level, can cause paralytic ileus, severe weakness or flaccid paralysis, hypotension, atrial and ventricular dysrhythmias, and potentiation of digitalis toxicity. If treatment for hypokalemia should be instituted, intravenous potassium replacement may be given in the PACU. If the infusion rates of the potassium replacement exceed 40 mEq/h or if the concentration of potassium in the individual intravenous container is greater than 40 mEq/L, continuous electrocardiographic (ECG) monitoring should be instituted for detection of any dysrhythmias. Also, if potassium chloride is added to solutions in flexible plastic bags in the PACU, the nurse should ensure that it is properly mixed in the infusion solution to prevent the patient from receiving an inadvertent bolus of potassium chloride. Other untoward side effects of thiazide diuretics are dermatitis, bone marrow depression, and reduced liver function.

## Potassium-sparing Diuretics

This class of diuretics acts on the distal convoluted tubule. The product of their actions is an increased urinary output without potassium loss. The most popular potassium-sparing diuretics include triamterene (Dyrenium) and amiloride (Midamor). A fixed-dose combination of triamterene and hydrochlorothiazide, which is marketed under the trade name of Dyazide, can also be considered to be in this category of diuretics. The major side effect of this class of diuretics is hyperkalemia, which can occur because of excess usage along with overusage of potassium supplementation. The symptoms of hyperkalemia include muscular weakness, conduction defects, ventricular dysrhythmias, and ileus. For a reduction in the effects of hyperkalemia, calcium gluconate or calcium chloride may be administered. Also, for a reduction in the high potassium levels, sodium bicarbonate, glucose, or insulin in combination with glucose may be given.

## Loop Diuretics

The loop diuretics, of which ethacrynic acid (Edecrin), bumetanide (Bumex), and furosemide (Lasix) are the prototype drugs, are used primarily in the treatment of pulmonary edema and general edema and in the diagnosis of acute renal failure. The loop diuretics are secreted into the tubule and have their major action on the medullary concentrating segment where chloride transport is inhibited. Consequently, they interfere with the concentrating and diluting mechanisms of the kidneys, which results in the production of isotonic urine. In addition, because of the increased delivery of salt with these drugs, potassium secretion is increased. Hence, the major problems with these drugs are in the realm of deafness (caused by ethacrynic acid), hepatic dysfunction, hypokalemia, alkalosis, extracellular fluid volume contraction, and electrolyte imbalance. Because of their high potency and their ability to act rapidly, loop diuretics are usually the diuretic of choice when indicated for the patient in the PACU. The two major concerns when one of these drugs is administered are hypokalemia and hypovolemia. The effects and treatment of hypokalemia were discussed in the section on thiazide diuretics. The objective findings that indicate hypovolemia (contraction of the extracellular fluid volume) are hypotension, tachycardia, and low right-ventricular and left-ventricular filling pressures. Treatment can include repositioning the patient with the legs elevated or the administration of intravenous salt-containing solutions, or both.

## Aldosterone Antagonists

Drugs in this category, of which spironolactone (Aldactone) is the prototype drug, act on the aldosterone receptors in the conducting ducts. Spironolactone acts to antagonize the effects of aldosterone. Aldosterone enhances the reabsorption of sodium and chloride and increases the excretion of potassium in the renal tubules. Consequently, when spironolactone is administered, sodium and chloride reabsorption are increased and potassium excretion is decreased. Because of this decrease in potassium excretion in the conducting ducts, hyperkalemia, especially when renal dysfunction is present, is a serious side effect of the drug. Spironolactone is indicated for patients with fluid overload from cirrhosis of the liver, nephrotic syndrome, and congestive heart failure.

### Carbonic Anhydrase Inhibitors

Drugs in this class bind to the carbonic anhydrase enzyme in the proximal renal tubules. The outcome is inhibition of the actions of carbonic anhydrase, which results in the diminished excretion of hydrogen ions and increased excretion of bicarbonate with an ionic exchange with potassium and sodium. The net result is a diuresis of alkaline urine. The prototype drug in this category is acetazolamide (Diamox). This drug is indicated for the reduction of intraocular pressure and the management of seizures. If this drug is administered to a patient with chronic obstructive pulmonary disease, careful monitoring of the patient's rate of ventilation and $PaCO_2$ level is mandated because excessive bicarbonate is lost in the urine and because hypercarbia can result, which can ultimately lead to central nervous system (CNS) depression.

## EFFECTS OF ANESTHESIA ON RENAL FUNCTION

In patients with normal renal function who receive general inhalation anesthesia, some depression of renal function occurs. This effect arises because all of the general anesthetics depress functions such as glomerular filtration rate, renal blood flow, and urinary flow. The depression in renal function is the result of direct and indirect effects of the general anesthetic agents. In regard to the vascular effects during general anesthesia, the renal blood flow may be depressed because of renal vasoconstriction, systemic hypotension, or both. Of interest is that droperidol, which is a tranquilizer, has the smallest effect on the changes in renal function. In most instances, the renal depression caused by the anesthetic agents is completely reversible at the end of the operative procedure.

Patients who undergo anesthesia in lighter planes may have some manifestations of the stress response. One of the hormones that is released in response to a stressor is ADH. This hormone is the most important regulator of urine volume. When ADH is released, it promotes an increase in tubular reabsorption of water, which results in a decrease in urine volume and an increase in urine concentration. Other biochemical products of the stress response, namely epinephrine, norepinephrine, and the renin-angiotensin system, also affect the renal system. More specifically, when these amines are liberated, renal blood flow is decreased. Because some patients can undergo a stress response with anesthesia, the perianesthesia nurse must monitor renal function during the emergent phase of the anesthesia. Patients who have undergone major abdominal or thoracic surgery commonly have some diuresis during the immediate postoperative period. Hence, urine volume and concentration should be monitored in all patients who: (1) have undergone a major surgical procedure; (2) have received general anesthesia for more than 2 hours; (3) have a compromised cardiovascular or renal system, or both; and (4) have had a significant blood volume replacement during the preoperative or intraoperative phase of the anesthetic experience.

## EFFECTS OF DRUGS IN PATIENTS WITH COMPROMISED RENAL FUNCTION

Patients with severe renal disease usually have anemia, body fluid relocation, abnormal cell membrane activity, and alterations in blood albumin and electrolyte levels. In addition, patient conditions are usually debilitated; and, if uremia exists, CNS depression is usually present. Drugs that are not metabolized in the body and are therefore excreted unchanged by the kidneys should be avoided in patients with severe renal disease. Hence, the long-acting barbiturates barbital and phenobarbital and the skeletal muscle relaxants decamethonium and gallamine, along with digoxin and lanatoside C, should be avoided in these patients. Because about half of the administered dose of the belladonna alkaloids atropine and hyoscyamine is excreted unchanged, the dosage should be modified by the degree of severity of the renal impairment. When CNS depression is present in the patient with renal impairment, the actions of narcotics are intensified and prolonged. Also, diazepam, which has a 24-hour half-life, is probably not a good choice because of its additive effect on the CNS depression. In patients with mild to moderate renal dysfunction, all inhalation anesthetics, except methoxyflurane and possibly enflurane, can be used in the usual clinical dose range. Because thiopental depends on redistribution for the termination of its action, it may be used in patients with renal impairment. However, the sleeping time is increased in proportion to the degree of uremia. The skeletal muscle relaxants succinylcholine, curare, and pancuronium are also acceptable for use in the patient with compromised kidney function. Neuroleptanalgesia, which derives from the combination of a narcotic and a tranquilizer, when achieved with nitrous oxide and oxygen, is an acceptable technique for the patient with uremia. If a patient has received Innovar, which is the prototype neuroleptanalgesic drug, the perianesthesia nurse should monitor the patient for prolonged depressant effects of the drug. More specifically, the tranquilizer component of Innovar, droperidol, has a long half-life; therefore, its prolonged effects, coupled with CNS depression from the uremia, may cause the patient to be slow to arouse in the immediate postoperative emergence phase. Consequently, airway patency and the cardiovascular parameters should be monitored closely for an extended period when droperidol has been administered to the patient in either the preoperative or the intraoperative phase of the anesthetic experience.

### RENAL SHUTDOWN OR FAILURE

Acute renal failure can occur in the PACU for a variety of reasons, such as hemorrhage and circulatory failure from trauma or extensive surgery, acute glomerulonephritis, vascular occlusions, or toxicity from drugs.

The most common cause of acute renal failure is acute tubular necrosis. Oliguria produces the clinical setting in which renal cell necrosis may develop. Persistent oliguria, less than 25 mL of urine per hour for more than 2 hours, constitutes a medical emergency, and the surgeon should be notified immediately. The urine volume may be abnormally high in conditions in which the glomerular filtration rate is reduced to the point of renal failure, and the increased urine volume represents a supplemental failure of tubular function. In patients with mild to moderate renal dysfunction, enflurane may potentially cause nephrotoxicity because enflurane is metabolized to inorganic fluoride. However, clinical studies have not been able to show this possibility. Nephrotoxicity is characterized by polyuria and azotemia. Therefore, the accurate and continuous measurement of urine volume is essential in the postoperative nursing care of the patient with suspected renal failure.

Creatinine clearance is a laboratory test that provides an excellent index for measurement of the quantity of glomerular filtrate. Creatinine is a component of urine not reabsorbed with tubular mechanisms. Hence, every milliliter of glomerular filtrate should contain precisely the same quantity of creatinine as 1 mL of plasma.

Measurement of urinary sodium yields information about sodium absorption. The urine plasma osmolar ratio provides an index of water reabsorption in the collecting tubules and is an excellent measurement of tubular function. The quality rather than the quantity of the urine provides useful information about the renal state of the patient (Fig. 13-5).

### PERIANESTHESIA NURSING CARE

Perianesthesia nursing care centers on recognition and care of the patient in impending renal failure. Urinary output should be monitored with an indwelling urethral catheter. This monitoring provides moment-to-moment information concerning urine output and its constituents that can be measured. Modern collecting devices provide a closed system between the catheter and a graduated measuring flask that can be emptied from the bottom without disconnecting the catheter. In this way, the danger of gross contamination is minimized and the necessary monitoring facility is still provided.

Continuous ECG monitoring should be done because the patient in acute renal failure probably has hyperkalemia, which can lead to cardiac arrest. The ECG changes indicative of hyperkalemia are initially high-peaked T waves and depressed S-T segments. If ECG interpretation indicates hyperkalemia, the addition of the rapid short-term treatment of hyperkalemia with the administration of $Ca^{++}$, $HCO_3$, dextrose, and insulin to drive the potassium back into the cell is necessary. One should note that a subsequent disappearance of T waves, heart block, and diastolic cardiac arrest occur with increasing levels of potassium (Fig. 13-6).

Osmotic diuretics, such as mannitol, or one of the loop diuretics, such as ethacrynic acid and furosemide, may be used in the treatment of tubular necrosis. A central venous pressure monitor may be inserted for measurement of blood volume. If renal failure continues, dialytic therapy is probably necessary.

## SUMMARY

The anatomy and physiology of the renal system has been presented in detail in an effort to apprise the perianesthesia nurse of the complex physiology of this system and also to show how

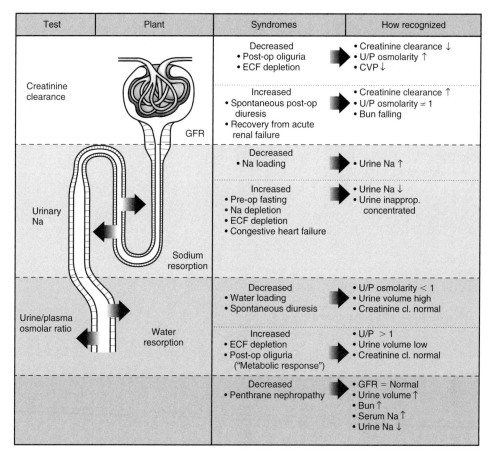

| Test | Plant | Syndromes | How recognized |
|---|---|---|---|
| Creatinine clearance | GFR | Decreased<br>• Post-op oliguria<br>• ECF depletion | • Creatinine clearance ↓<br>• U/P osmolarity ↑<br>• CVP ↓ |
| | | Increased<br>• Spontaneous post-op diuresis<br>• Recovery from acute renal failure | • Creatinine clearance ↑<br>• U/P osmolarity ≈ 1<br>• Bun falling |
| Urinary Na | Sodium resorption | Decreased<br>• Na loading | • Urine Na ↑ |
| | | Increased<br>• Pre-op fasting<br>• Na depletion<br>• ECF depletion<br>• Congestive heart failure | • Urine Na ↓<br>• Urine inapprop. concentrated |
| Urine/plasma osmolar ratio | Water resorption | Decreased<br>• Water loading<br>• Spontaneous diuresis | • U/P osmolarity < 1<br>• Urine volume high<br>• Creatinine cl. normal |
| | | Increased<br>• ECF depletion<br>• Post-op oliguria ("Metabolic response") | • U/P > 1<br>• Urine volume low<br>• Creatinine cl. normal |
| | | Decreased<br>• Penthrane nephropathy | • GFR = Normal<br>• Urine volume ↑<br>• Bun ↑<br>• Serum Na ↑<br>• Urine Na ↓ |

**Fig. 13-5**   Alterations in renal function that result from normal kidney acting to correct or preserve abnormal internal environment. Quantity and quality of urine are appropriate for preserving entire organism, but alterations, if uncorrected, may result in renal damage. *GFR,* Glomerular filtration rate; *ECF,* extracellular fluid; *U/P,* urine/plasma; *CVP,* central venous pressure; *BUN,* blood urea nitrogen; *CL,* clearance; *VOL,* volume. *(Redrawn from Kinney JM, Egdahl RH, Zuidema GD: Manual of preoperative and postoperative care, ed 2, Philadelphia, 1971, Saunders.)*

the renal system regulates and controls body systems. The renal system is, along with the lungs, the key system that maintains the acid-base homeostatis in the body. Because diuretics are such key pharmacologic agents in the perioperative period, their actions were presented in detail. With all this in mind, an overview of the perianesthesia nursing care was presented with a focus on the renal system. A more in-depth discussion of the care of the patient for genitourinary surgery to include renal transplantation is presented in Chapter 41.

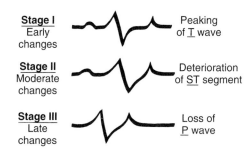

**Stage I**
Early changes — Peaking of T wave

**Stage II**
Moderate changes — Deterioration of ST segment

**Stage III**
Late changes — Loss of P wave

**Fig. 13-6**   Stages of electrocardiographic evidence of hyperkalemia. *(From Kinney JM, Egdahl RH, Zuidema GD: Manual of preoperative and postoperative care, ed 2, Philadelphia, 1971, Saunders.)*

## BIBLIOGRAPHY

Aitkenhead A, Smith G, Rowbotham D: *Textbook of anaesthesia,* ed 5, Philadelphia, 2007, Churchill Livingstone.

Alspach J: *Core curriculum for critical care nursing,* ed 6, Philadelphia, 2006, Saunders.

Atlee J: *Complications in anesthesia,* ed 2, Philadelphia, 2007, Saunders.

Barash P, Cullen B, Stoelting R: *Clinical anesthesia,* ed 5, Philadelphia, 2001, Lippincott Williams & Wilkins.

Benumof J, Saidman L: *Anesthesia & perioperative complications,* ed 2, St Louis, 1999, Mosby.

Brunton L, Lazo J, Parker K: *Goodman and Gilman's the pharmacological basis of therapeutics*, ed 11, New York, 2005, McGraw-Hill Professional.

Cote C, Todres I, Goudsouzian N, et al: *A practice of anesthesia for infants and children*, ed 3, Philadelphia, 2001, Saunders.

Drake R, Vogl W, Mitchell A: *Gray's anatomy for students*, Philadelphia, 2005, Churchill Livingstone.

Evers A, Maze M: *Anesthetic pharmacology: physiologic principles and clinical practice*, Philadelphia, 2004, Churchill Livingstone.

Fisher L: *Benumof's anesthesia and uncommon diseases*, ed 5, Philadelphia, 2007, Saunders.

Ganong W: *Review of medical physiology*, ed 22, New York, 2005, McGraw-Hill Medical.

Guyton A, Hall J: *Textbook of medical physiology*, ed 11, Philadelphia, 2006, Saunders.

Kier L, Dowd C: *The chemistry of drugs for nurse anesthetists*, Chicago, 2004, AANA Publishing, Inc.

Lake C, Hines R, Blitt C: *Clinical monitoring: practical applications for anesthesia and critical care*, Philadelphia, 2001, Saunders.

Longnecker D, Murphy F: *Dripps, Eckenhoff, Vandam introduction to anesthesia*, ed 9, Philadelphia, 1997, Saunders.

Longnecker D, Tinker J, Morgan G: *Principles and practice of anesthesiology*, ed 2, St Louis, 1998, Mosby.

Miller R, editor: *Anesthesia*, ed 5, Philadelphia, 2000, Churchill Livingstone.

Nagelhout J, Zaglaniczy K: *Nurse anesthesia*, ed 3, St Louis, 2005, Saunders.

Stoelting R: *Pharmacology and physiology in anesthetic practice*, ed 3, Philadelphia, 1999, Lippincott-Raven.

Stoelting R, Miller R: *Basics of anesthesia*, ed 4, Philadelphia, 2000, Churchill Livingstone.

Townsend C, Beauchamp R, Evers B, et al: *Sabiston textbook of surgery: the biological basis of modern surgical practice*, ed 17, Philadelphia, 2004, Saunders.

Walsh S, Retik A: *Campbell's urology*, ed 8, Philadelphia, 2002, Saunders.

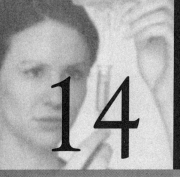

# 14

## FLUID AND ELECTROLYTES

*Cecil B. Drain, PhD, RN, CRNA, FAAN, FASAHP*

Many improvements have been made in the methods and types of fluids and electrolytes that are administered to patients in the perioperative period. The maintenance of appropriate concentrations of body fluid and electrolytes is essential to normal physiologic function of all body systems. A clear understanding of the basic physiology in this area along with a brief introduction to the many types and regimes of fluid management of the patient is presented. Also, this chapter uses the most current method of reporting concentrations of the electrolytes and of presentation of clinical laboratory data. Hence, the current International System of Units (SI) of millimole (mmol) as opposed to mEq and millimole per liter (mmol/L) as opposed to mEq per liter are used.

## DEFINITIONS

**Anions:** Ions that carry a negative charge and migrate to the anode (terminal) in an electric field.

**Autologous:** Originating within the same person, such as an autotransfusion.

**Cations:** Ions that carry a positive charge and migrate to the cathode (terminal) in an electric field.

**Chvostek's sign:** An abnormal spasm of the facial muscles elicited by light taps on the facial nerve that indicates hypocalcemia.

**Colloids:** Compounds such as red blood cells (RBCs), albumin, or dextran that, because of size, are retained within a specific fluid compartment and increase the oncotic pressure of that compartment.

**Cryoprecipitate:** A preparation rich in factor VIII needed to restore normal coagulation in hemophilia. The preparation is collected from fresh human plasma that has been frozen and thawed.

**Crystalloids:** Balanced electrolyte solutions that are in isotonic solutions of water or dextrose and can move between the intravascular and interstitial compartments.

**Edema:** Accumulation of fluid in the interstitial spaces.

**Hemolysis:** A disruption of the integrity of the red cell membrane that causes release of cell contents to include hemoglobin.

**Hemostasis:** The arrest of bleeding by the interaction of the platelet with the blood vessel wall and the formation of the platelet plug.

**Hypercalcemia:** Increased plasma concentration of calcium (> 5.6 mmol/L).

**Hyperkalemia:** Greater than 6 mmol/L blood concentration of potassium.

**Hypermagnesemia:** An increase in the plasma concentration of magnesium (> 2.6 mmol/L).

**Hypernatremia:** An increase in sodium in the plasma of more than 145 mmol/L.

**Hypertonic Solutions (hyperosmotic):** Solutions that have an osmolality greater than that of plasma.

**Hypocalcemia:** Reduced plasma concentration of calcium (< 4.4 mmol/L).

**Hypokalemia:** Less than 3 mmol/L blood concentration of potassium.

**Hypomagnesemia:** A decrease in the plasma concentration of magnesium (< 1.6 mmol/L).

**Hyponatremia:** A decrease of sodium in the plasma of less than 135 mmol/L.

**Hypotonic Solutions (hypoosmotic):** Solutions that have an osmolality less than that of plasma.

**Isotonic Solutions:** Solutions that have the same osmolality as plasma.

**Milliequivalent (mEq):** Replaced with the SI units millimole (mmol); mEq/L has been replaced by mmol/L.

**Osmolality:** A physical property of a solution, one that is dependent on the number of dissolved particles in the solution.

**Tetany:** A condition characterized by cramps, muscle twitching, sharp flexion of the wrist and ankle joints, and convulsions.

**Third Space:** Losses of fluid and electrolytes from the extracellular fluid (ECF) to a nonfunctional space, an acute sequestered space that accompanies surgery.

**Trousseau's Sign:** A test for latent tetany in which carpal spasm is induced with inflation of a sphygmomanometer cuff on the upper arm to a pressure that exceeds systolic blood pressure for 3 minutes.

## BODY FLUID BALANCE

Water is the most abundant component of the body. It represents approximately 60% of adult body weight and as much as 75% to 77% of body weight in infants less than 1 month of age. By approximately age 17 years, the adult percentage is attained; and in a 154-lb or 70-kg person, the total body water is about 42 L. Because women have higher fat content in their bodies and because fat is essentially water-free, they have a lower water content than men do. Older adults and obese individuals also have a lower proportion of water in their bodies. Water is essential to the body. It is the medium within which metabolic reactions take place to facilitate the ionization of electrolytes; it acts as a reagent in many chemical reactions; it transports nutrients to cells and removes waste products; and its high specific heat and heat of vaporization make it especially suitable as a temperature regulator.

The total amount of body water remains stable, as its intake usually equals its output. Water intake includes not only the water consumed in beverages but also the fluids obtained from the metabolism of solid foods. The water taken in by beverages and food is referred to as exogenous water. Although variance does occur on a day-to-day basis, overall, the average adult in a moderate climate with a mixed diet consumes about 2500 to 3000 mL daily. Approximately 1000 mL is obtained from beverages and 1500 mL from solid and semisolid foods. The water formed during metabolism of organic foodstuffs is called endogenous water. Because metabolism varies with body temperature, the amount of exercise performed, and other factors, the amount of endogenous water available also varies on a day-to-day basis. In a healthy adult who performs a moderate amount of exercise, an average of 300 to 350 mL of endogenous water is available daily. Intake is influenced by the thirst center in the hypothalamus. If the fluid volume inside the cells decreases, salivary secretion is reduced, thereby causing a dry mouth and the sensation of thirst. In normal circumstances, an individual then drinks and restores the fluid volume (Box 14-1).

Water output also remains quite stable and usually approximates the total body water intake. Removal or output of water from the body is through four types of excretion: the lungs, gastrointestinal tract, skin, and kidney.

---

### Box 14-1  Normal Intake and Output of Water Per Day

**INTAKE**
Water: 1000 mL
Endogenous water: 1500 mL

*Total water intake: 2500 mL*

**OUTPUT**
Insensible loss: 250 mL
Skin: 250 mL
Respiratory tract: 400 mL
Urine: 1500 mL
Feces: 100 mL

*Total water output: 2500 mL*

---

### Lungs

Expired air is nearly saturated with water. The amount lost through the lungs varies with the humidity and the temperature of inspired air and with the rate and depth of respiration. As a rule, about 300 to 400 mL of water is thus lost daily. This loss of water via the respiratory tract is termed insensible loss of water, so named because one is not aware of this loss. The water content of inhaled gases decreases as the ambient temperature decreases. Consequently, the insensible water loss from the lungs is higher in cold environments. Hence, patients with respiratory dysfunction need a greater water intake to offset the increased insensible water loss when they are in cold environments. Also, an increase in the respiration rate can increase the water loss to as much as 2000 mL, which is significant in patients with chronic obstructive pulmonary disease (see Chapter 48).

### Gastrointestinal Tract

The amount of water lost via the feces averages to be about 100 mL daily. However, with vomiting or diarrhea, this loss may be greatly increased. Up to 7000 mL can be lost with diarrhea and 6000 mL with vomiting. The implications to the perianesthesia nurse are great because this condition can significantly impact the volume status of the patient who is actively vomiting. In such cases, fluids should be increased in rate and the anesthesia practitioner should be notified.

### Skin

Water lost via the skin can be considered in two categories: insensible perspiration and sensible perspiration. The skin is not impervious to water, and a constant diffusion of moisture from its deeper layers to the dry surface where the water evaporates occurs. Insensible loss depends largely on environmental humidity. Sensible perspiration refers to loss of water with production of sweat. Sweating is an emergency mechanism for regulation of body temperature when the heat produced by metabolic processes is excessive. The amount of sweat therefore varies with exercise and with body temperature. In a moist atmosphere, sweat may be more visible than in a dry atmosphere, but the amount of water lost is the same. Despite its role as a safety factor, sweating can become a hazard when body water supplies are low because the body continues to lose sweat to maintain its temperature. In the healthy adult who performs moderate exercise in a comfortable environment, approximately 500 mL of water is lost in both sensible and insensible perspiration.

### Kidneys

Water loss via the kidneys varies with the supply of body water. The kidneys are able to concentrate the urine, and the specific gravity may approach 1.040. On the other hand, if the amount of excess water is great, such as might occur when a large quantity is administered intravenously, the kidneys excrete dilute urine, the specific gravity of which might approach 1.002. In normal conditions, the kidneys excrete about 1.5 L per day. In patients who are vomiting or have diarrhea, less water is available, and the kidneys respond promptly to curtail most of the water loss via urine. The two hormones responsible for control of the volume of urine are antidiuretic hormone (ADH) from the posterior pituitary and aldosterone from the adrenal cortex. ADH, by increasing the permeability of the renal distal convoluted tubule and collecting ducts, increases the amount of water reabsorbed and thus decreases the urine volume. Aldosterone increases the renal reabsorption of sodium and of water secondarily. Both hormones are secreted in response to lowered blood volume and serve to control output to balance intake. However, a minimal loss of fluids is obligatory. Therefore, monitoring of fluid balance is critical.

## DISTRIBUTION OF BODY FLUIDS

The fluids in the body can be divided into two compartments along with a potential third compartment. The total body water is equal to about 60% of the total body weight, or about 42 L in the average 70-kg man. The two compartments are normally divided relative to the location of the cell membrane: intracellular (inside the cell) and extracellular (outside the cell). The intracellular fluid (ICF) is estimated to be about 40% of the body weight, or about 28 L of fluid, and represents about two thirds of the total body water. It provides a medium for all intracellular activities. The other compartment, the ECF, is approximately 20% of the body weight and ranges from 12 to 14 L of fluid. The extracellular fluid compartment includes the blood plasma or intravascular fluid, the interstitial fluid (ISF) that bathes the cells, the lymph, the cerebrospinal fluid (CSF), and the transcellular fluids. The transcellular fluids include the synovial fluid, peritoneal fluid, digestive fluids, and fluids of the eye and ear. The lymph, CSF, and the transcellular fluids normally constitute only about 1% of the body mass. Blood constitutes 4% of the body weight, and the interstitial fluid 15.7%.

The third compartment, which is commonly called the third space, is a concept that is defined as a compartment that includes the interstitial spaces that are swollen by local responses to tissue trauma and hormonal influx from the stress of surgery. This third space can occur even when patients have undergone massive surgical procedures and the fluid loss, to include insensible loss, is appropriately replaced. This accumulation of fluid in the third space compartment usually occurs during and immediately after the surgical procedure and is difficult to clinically differentiate from actual blood loss. Clinically, the signs of hypovolemia reflect third space loss and actual blood loss. The treatment includes infusion of fluids in the range of 3 to 10 mL/kg/h and is usually adequate along with establishment of the underlying cause. The third space loss usually resolves in several postoperative days, and the nurse on the unit that receives the patient after the postanesthesia care unit (PACU) should be alert for signs of possible fluid overload as the fluid returns after surgery to the ECF.

Fluid balance involves not only maintenance of the total amount of body water but also the maintenance of a relatively constant distribution of that water in the different compartments. Circulation of fluid between compartments depends on the relative hydrostatic and osmotic pressures in each compartment. Hydrostatic pressure is the force that pushes fluid from one compartment to the other. For example, if the hydrostatic pressure in the capillaries (blood pressure) exceeds the pressure in the interstitial space, fluid moves from the capillary into the interstitial space. Osmotic pressure is the "pull" of fluids into the compartment.

It is a function of the number of dissolved molecules in the solution and is not influenced by weight or size of the molecule. Because of the relatively large quantities, the electrolytes are the major contributors to the osmotic pressure of the fluids. The electrolytes are a group of compounds that dissociate in solution to form ions. These ions carry an electric charge. The cations are positively charged electrolytes and include sodium, potassium, calcium, and magnesium. The anions are negatively charged ions and include chloride, bicarbonate, phosphate, sulfate, and ions of inorganic acids such as lactate. Protein also carries a negative charge at physiologic pH. Each of the fluid compartments of the body contains electrolytes, and although the concentration and specific composition of electrolytes in each compartment vary, the number of cations in each compartment balances the number of anions to maintain electric neutrality.

The major ions found in the extracellular fluid are sodium and chloride, whereas potassium and phosphate are predominately intracellular ions. The preponderance of sodium outside the cell and potassium inside the cell is the result of a cell membrane "pump" that exchanges sodium and potassium ions. This active transport mechanism requires energy from adenosine triphosphate (ATP). Sodium represents almost half the osmotic strength of the plasma.

The major difference between the two major compartments that make up the extracellular fluid is the much higher protein content in the plasma than in the interstitial fluid. Because capillary membranes are not selectively permeable to small particles, ions and small molecules can exchange rapidly between the plasma and the ISF. However, because proteins are too large to cross the capillary barrier, they remain in the plasma. As a result, the electrolyte composition differs slightly from the plasma and the interstitial fluid. Specifically, the sodium concentration in plasma is slightly greater, whereas the chloride concentration is slightly less than in the interstitial fluid and the sum of the diffusible ions. Thus, the osmotic pressure in the plasma is greater. The osmotic pressure caused by plasma colloids is called the colloid osmotic pressure (COP) or oncotic pressure. Protein molecules are responsible for the COP or oncotic pressure. The proteins that exert a COP help to retain the plasma water in the intravascular compartment. Albumin is the major protein in the plasma that contributes to the COP.

The extracellular fluid is regulated carefully by the kidneys to facilitate the cells being bathed in fluid that contains appropriate concentrations of electrolytes to include sodium, potassium, and nutrients. A patient with major abdominal surgery usually excretes about 100 mmol of potassium during the first 48 postoperative hours and about 25 mmol each day thereafter. As a result, the potassium is usually administered intravenously in the immediate postoperative period. One should note that plasma potassium measurements do not exactly predict total body potassium because potassium is primarily an intracellular ion. From a clinical chemistry point of view, the international standard unit is called a millimole (mmol), commonly called the milliequivalent (mEq). The clinical implications for the perianesthesia nurse is that patients who undergo major surgery should routinely have potassium levels checked and evaluated before surgery for determination of whether they are receiving any non–potassium-sparing diuretics (see Chapter 13).

## EDEMA

A delicate balance of pressures keeps fluids passing between compartments. A dynamic equilibrium exists between the plasma and the interstitial fluid because proteins are too large to cross the capillary barrier, which creates a colloid osmotic pressure between the two components. The hydrostatic pressures of the blood and the interstitial fluid tend to oppose each other, which is called the effective filtration pressure. Similarly, the colloid osmotic (or oncotic) pressure is the opposition between the blood and the interstitial fluid. The final common pathway is that these pressures result in a pulling in opposite directions when in appropriate physiologic equilibrium that does not allow fluid to accumulate into the interstitial spaces. Edema then results when either of the two pressures are in dysfunction.

## ELECTROLYTES

The electrolytes, which only constitute a small fraction of the body weight, are essential for facilitation of normal body function. The electrolytes maintain electroneutrality and chemical conditions in the body fluids, equilibrium between ECF and ICF, and regulation of neuromuscular activity. Monitoring of electrolyte concentrations is usually analyzed before and after surgery, many times in the PACU.

### Sodium
Sodium, a cation, is primarily found in the extracellular fluid. The blood plasma sodium averages about 142 mmol/L and usually does not vary

more then 5 mmol/L. Variations greater than this can affect many physiologic activities; thus, mechanisms for regulation of sodium concentration are of prime importance in maintenance of balance. Basically, the body regulates sodium with conservation mechanisms when the sodium is low; and if body stores of sodium are high, the body excretes sodium via sweat, feces, and, in large part, the kidneys.

The body fluids are maintained in an isotonic state with regulation of the concentration of sodium and its most abundant anion, chloride. Concentration of sodium and chloride in the fluids is maintained primarily with loss or retention of water. Loss of salt is accompanied by loss of water and retention of salt by retention of water. Hence, one could say that water moves into areas where salt is in higher concentration, which is why patients are often placed on a low salt diet in an effort to reduce fluid overload on the heart and other major organs. However, patients who receive magnesium sulfate do have impaired fluid excretion.

Of clinical interest is that patients who have undergone urologic surgery and need the use of irrigation fluids in the bladder are susceptible to hyponatremia. The most common surgical procedure that can have this complication is a transurethral resection of the prostate (TURP). The irrigation fluids typically consist of sorbitol and mannitol in 100 mL of water, called Cytal, and, also commonly, glycine in a 1.5% solution. The amount of irrigation solution absorbed through the venous sinuses in the bladder averages about 10 to 30 mL per minute of resection time. For this reason, the resection time is usually limited to less than an hour. This absorption of the irrigating fluid results in the fluid entering the vascular system, which leads to volume overload and ultimately to dilutional hyponatremia.

The resulting lowering of the serum sodium concentrations can cause serious cardiac and neurologic consequences. Concentrations of sodium at 140 mmol/L are usually associated with the development of cardiac dysrhythmias and progressive neurologic symptoms such as restlessness, confusion, nausea, vomiting, coma, and convulsions.

Hypernatremia is most often caused by a loss of body fluids that results in sodium excess. The clinical signs of this condition resemble the signs of hypovolemia, and many times edema is also present because of the sodium excess.

### Potassium

Potassium is the most important intracellular ion. Measurement of intracellular potassium is difficult; therefore, only extracellular potassium is measured. The normal values are between 3.5 and 5.5 mmol/L. Potassium is important in the maintenance of cardiac rhythm, deposition of glycogen in liver cells, and transmission and conduction of nerve impulses. It also contributes to cellular energy production. Overall, abnormal potassium concentrations can have serious effects on the contractility of the heart, resulting in arrhythmias and possibly cardiac arrest.

Potassium depletion may or may not be accompanied by changes in plasma potassium concentration. True depletion develops only with a net loss of potassium, whereas a decrease in plasma potassium, hypokalemia, may occur with a shift of potassium from the ECF to the ICF. Decreased intake can cause a mild deficit because the mechanisms for potassium conservation are not as efficient as those for sodium. Severe depletion results from abnormal losses rather than decreased intake. Most common causes of severe potassium loss are usually associated with diuretics (see Chapter 13), acute blood loss, and lack of replacement over time (e.g., nothing by mouth (NPO) plus a long surgical procedure). Cardiac arrhythmias and weakness of skeletal muscle are commonly observed in mild hypokalemia, which reflects potassium's role in neuromuscular function. Severe depletion can cause widespread damage to cell function and structure.

If the patient has a low potassium level, a serum level between 3.5 and 2.6 mmol/L, the rate of potassium infusion is usually about 40 mmol/h. Treatment of hypokalemia for potassium concentrations of less than 2.5 mmol/L requires the administration of 0.5 mmol/kg of potassium chloride. This treatment usually raises the serum potassium concentration by 0.6 mmol/L. If the patient is receiving catecholamine drugs, the increase is only about 0.1 mmol/L; if the patient is receiving beta-adrenergic antagonists, the serum concentration increases by about 0.9 mmol/L. One should note that correction of hypomagnesemia may be needed to avoid the increased loss of potassium by the kidneys.

Hyperkalemia is associated with situations in which cells are injured or destroyed. Other causes of hyperkalemia include renal failure and crush injuries, burn victims, and newborns who receive relatively large transfusions. Usually, the administration of succinylcholine, a depolarizing skeletal muscle relaxant, can produce hyperkalemia (as discussed in Chapter 23). However, accidental lethal doses have been administered to patients with rapid intravenous infusion in the PACU. Cases have been recorded in which death occurred within 5 minutes of the rapid injection of just 25 mmol of potassium. Hence, in no circumstance should the perianesthesia nurse administer potassium chloride intravenous (IV) push.

## Calcium

Calcium is deposited in the bone tissue as crystalline salts composed primarily of calcium and phosphate; the remainder is in the plasma, ISF, and soft tissues. The major fraction of calcium that accounts for its physiologic effects is the ionizable calcium in plasma, of which the normal plasma concentration is maintained between 1.0 to 1.2 mmol/L. The remainder is bound to protein and other substances in nonionizable form. Calcium has an important function in neuromuscular transmission, skeletal muscle contraction, blood coagulation, and exocytosis necessary for release of neurotransmitters and autocoids. Also, the balance of the appropriate calcium concentration is controlled by the parathyroid hormone, calcitonin, and vitamin D. Calcium also has a reciprocal relationship with phosphate ions.

When the calcium ion concentration in the plasma becomes reduced, the reduction can be severe enough to cause extreme immediate effects. The nervous system becomes progressively more irritable as the membrane becomes increasingly permeable to sodium, and at a certain critical level of calcium, the nerve fibers become so irritable that they begin to discharge spontaneously. Impulses pass to skeletal muscles and cause severe tetanic spasms called tetany. Severe hypocalcemia rarely gives rise to other acute responses because the tetany may be rapidly fatal. An increased secretion of parathyroid hormone, most commonly caused by a parathyroid tumor, can cause hypercalcemia. In this situation, nervous system depression results in reduced reflex activity, and depression of muscle contractility results in skeletal muscle weakness, constipation, and loss of appetite. Because some calcium is excreted in the urine, a mild hypercalcemia can induce kidney stones as the calcium combines with phosphate or other anions and precipitates.

Hypocalcemia occurs when the serum calcium concentration is lower than 4.5 mmol/L and is usually the result of hypoparathyroidism, pancreatitis, or renal failure. In this case, the neuromuscular function becomes impaired and decreased myocardial contractility, increased central venous pressure, and hypotension are seen. Because the skeletal muscle spasms, laryngospasm is quite possible (see Chapter 27). Hence, when caring for patients with hypocalcemia, the perianesthesia nurse should have appropriate airway equipment readily available for resuscitation.

## Phosphate

Inorganic phosphate ions normally range from about 0.85 to 1.45 mmol/L for adults and 0.75 to 1.52 mmol/L for children. However, the major portion of phosphate ions are found within the cells, and these ions regulate phosphate function. They are, in fact, the major anions in the ICF and probably represent the single most important mineral constituent in cellular activity. Phosphates serve many functions, including forming RBCs and acting as an intermediary in the metabolism of carbohydrates, proteins, and fats. Phosphate promotes deposition of calcium in the bone and is essential for the delivery of oxygen via the RBCs to body tissues. The small number of phosphate ions in the plasma is important in acid-base balance by way of the phosphate buffer system. Phosphate is also important in regulation of energy metabolism, in the form of adenosine triphosphate (ATP).

## Magnesium

Magnesium is an essential element that is found primarily in muscle and bone. It apparently has an effect on tissue irritability and is a cofactor in various enzyme reactions. Magnesium has a large impact on cardiac cell membrane ion transport and is essential for activation of many enzyme systems. Magnesium is an essential regulator of calcium within cells and is the natural physiologic antagonist of calcium. In regard to skeletal muscle contraction, the presynaptic release of acetylcholine (ACh) depends on the actions of magnesium. The current reference values for magnesium are 0.7 to 1.11 mmol/L.

Hypomagnesemia is many times overlooked as an electrolyte deficiency; chronic alcoholics, persons with poor diets, patients with high renal loss of magnesium, and patients with protracted vomiting or diarrhea may have this syndrome. Subsequently, patients who have undergone cardiopulmonary bypass surgery may be susceptible because of the dilutional effects of the pump-priming solutions. Symptoms of acute hypomagnesemia may include Chvostek's and Trousseau's signs, carpopedal spasm, stridor, skeletal muscle weakness, seizures, and coma. In the perianesthesia period, ventricular dysrhythmias are usually the most common symptom of hypomagnesemia. Treatment for this syndrome is magnesium 1 to 2 g IV over 5 to 60 minutes or a continuous infusion of magnesium at 0.5 to 1.0 g/h. With severe life-threatening hypomagnesemia, an infusion of magnesium of 10 to 20 mg/kg is usually administered over 10 to 20 minutes.

Hypermagnesemia is a rare clinical phenomena. The most common cause of hypermagnesemia is the parenteral administration of magnesium as a treatment for pregnancy induced hypertension. Symptoms of hypermagnesemia include sedation, myocardial depression, relaxed skeletal muscles and, when severe, paralysis of the muscles of ventilation. Treatment of the life-threatening hypermagnesemia is with calcium gluconate, 10 to 15 mg/kg given intravenously followed by increased fluid loading to produce diuresis in an effort to enhance the excretion of the excess magnesium.

## PERIOPERATIVE BLOOD AND FLUID REPLACEMENT

Because of many factors such as NPO, insensible fluid loss, and the surgical stresses of hemostatic function; fluid status, medical/surgical history; and medication regimens should be assessed. If problems with hemostasis are envisioned, coagulation function should be assessed before surgery to ensure appropriate intraoperative and postoperative coagulation. Of interest is the fact that a patient can lose up to 75% red cell volume if the total blood volume of 5000 mL is maintained with the administration of colloid or crystalloid solutions. However, if the red cells are not replaced, the result is a loss in oxygen-carrying capacity because RBCs carry approximately 90% of the oxygen in the blood. In the situation of massive transfusions, many complications can arise in the PACU, such as dilutional coagulopathy, acidosis, electrolyte abnormalities, and other long-term consequences as described in Chapter 29.

### Assessment of Coagulation

The coagulation function for hemostasis is usually viewed in two separate events. The first event is platelet function, which includes aggregation, adhesion, and release of platelet contents and the coagulation cascade of events, which results in the deposition of a fibrin network to form a clot.

Routine screening tests are commonly performed before surgery and particularly for any patient with a history of bleeding problems. These tests include the platelet count and bleeding time for assessment of platelet function and the prothrombin time (PT) and partial thromboplastin time (PTT) for assessment of the coagulation cascade.

The normal platelet count is 130 to $370 \times 10^9$/L. Interestingly, patients with hemostatic stress of a major surgical procedure begin to have bleeding during the operation when the platelet counts become less than $100 \times 10^9$/L. Moreover, certain drugs, such as aspirin, Plavix, and the nonsteroidal antiinflammatory drugs (NSAIDs), potentially increase surgical bleeding.

Bleeding times are used to measure the primary phase of hemostasis. On the basis of the standardized method, the normal bleeding time is 3 to 10 minutes. This time is elevated in individuals with qualitative platelet abnormalities. In this instance, patient bleeding times are helpful diagnostically in that they provide data for determination of whether to proceed with procedures that involve bleeding into closed spaces. A bleeding time greater than 1.5 times the normal predicts significant hemostatic abnormality.

The prothrombin time (PT) and the activated partial thromboplastin time (APTT) tests are reliable and accurate. The PT evaluates the extrinsic system of coagulation (requiring a tissue factor to initiate clotting) and is sensitive to defects in fibrinogen and to the clotting factors V, VII, and X. The APTT evaluates the intrinsic system of coagulation (all factors found in the circulation) and is sensitive to defects in fibrinogen; prothrombin; and the factors V, VIII, IX, X, XI, and XII. The PT is evaluated during management of coumadin therapy. The APTT monitors heparin therapy. The normal PT values are between 11 to 13.2 seconds, and the normal APTT is between 22.5 to 32.2 seconds.

Another test, fibrinogen, is also helpful in the prediction of coagulation problems—particularly disseminated intravascular coagulation (DIC). The normal value for this test is 195 to 365 mg/dL.

Disseminated intravascular coagulation (DIC) is discussed in detail in Chapter 29. As an overview, it is an uncontrolled activation of the coagulation system, with consumption of platelets and clotting factors. Diagnosis is based on such factors as the presence of thrombocytopenia, prolongation of the prothrombin time and partial thromboplastin time, and increased circulating concentrations of fibrin degradation products in the presence of diffuse hemorrhage. Treatment is focused on removal of the cause, such as hemolytic transfusion reactions, low cardiac output, hypovolemia, and sepsis. The other parameters of treatment include the administration of platelet concentrates and fresh frozen plasma.

## CRYSTALLOID AND COLLOID ADMINISTRATION

The use of crystalloid or colloid fluid administration in the PACU is usually based on the purpose of the fluid therapy and replacement, an attempt to maintain the patient's condition as normally volemic as possible during and after the surgical procedure. Research on these two types of fluid administration cites many advantages and disadvantages for each type. However, no definitive data seem to support significant differences in outcomes. Hence, the choice of fluid type should be based on the immediate short-term needs of the patient and not on personal preferences and availability of the particular fluid. Some of the factors on which to base the decision are the amount of volume loss, the type of loss amount, and whether the patient has autologous blood available.

Crystalloid fluids are electrolyte solutions dissolved in water or dextrose and water. These electrolytes are impermeable to the cellular membrane, and dextrose crosses cell membranes. However, crystalloids are freely permeable to the vascular membranes. Crystalloid solutions help determine the total osmotic pressure or osmolality that helps balance water between the extracellular and the intracellular compartments. Osmolality reflects the number of dissolved particles in solutions. An isotonic solution has the same osmolality as plasma, whereas a hypertonic solution has an elevated concentration of particles and a hypotonic solution has fewer dissolved particles than plasma does. Administration of hypertonic solutions promotes movement of water from the cells into the plasma and shrink the brain, whereas hypotonic solutions expands the brain.

Isotonic crystalloid solutions have a sodium concentration of between 130 to 150 mmol/L and an osmolality of 280 to 310 mOsm/L. The isotonic fluids remain in the extracellular fluid, and the sodium-free solutions are distributed throughout the total body water. Hypertonic crystalloid solutions have a sodium concentration of greater than 150 mmol/L and an osmolality of greater than 310 mmol/L.

The amount of crystalloid needed to replace 1 mL of blood loss is about 5 mL of saline or Ringer's solution. The ratios certainly depend on the circumstances. For example, in patients with major hemorrhage, the ratio can be 1 mL of blood volume replaced with 1 mL of Ringer's solution. The ratio can go as high as 10 mL of Ringer's to 1 mL of blood volume in the patient with massive trauma who has received large amounts of fluid.

The advantages of crystalloid use are that crystalloids are inexpensive, promote urinary flow, and restore third-space losses. The disadvantages of crystalloid use are that crystalloids can dilute plasma proteins, decrease the colloid pressure, and lead to a filtration from the intravascular to the interstitial compartment, which could result in interstitial pulmonary edema. However, crystalloids are an excellent choice for use as maintenance fluids for compensation for insensible losses, as replacement for body fluid deficits, and for special replacements of specific fluids and electrolytes.

Colloids are solutions that contain natural or synthetic molecules that are usually impermeable to the vascular membrane. Hence, they remain predominately in the intravascular space. By doing so, colloids determine the colloid oncotic pressure that helps to balance the water distribution between the intravascular and interstitial spaces. Albumin is the prototype natural colloid and accounts for about two thirds of the plasma oncotic pressure. Dextrans 40 and 70, along with hetastarch 6% with an osmolality of 310 mmol/L, are the major synthetic colloids in clinical use. The advantages of colloid use are that the solution tends to remain in the intravascular compartment, thus causing less peripheral edema and rapidly restoring the circulating volume. Also, smaller volumes of colloids as compared with crystalloids can be used for fluid resuscitation, and the colloids restore the patient volume status sooner and create a sustained increase in plasma volume. Finally, because colloids increase the plasma colloid oncotic pressure, they prevent pulmonary edema. Some of the disadvantages with colloid use include the expense, the potential to cause coagulation problems and anaphylactic reactions, and the interference with blood-typing and cross-matching procedures. Although colloids improve the circulating volume, they redistribute into the third space and can exacerbate edema after 24 hours.

### Perioperative Replacement for Crystalloid and Colloid Administration

An intravenous line is started before surgery, and maintenance fluids are infused to replace the insensible loss from the last intake of oral fluids. The usual rate is 2 mL/kg/h. During surgery, the insensible loss rate of 2 mL/kg/h is continued along with an increase in rate according to the surgical trauma. For minimal trauma, 4 mL/kg/h is added. For moderate trauma, 6 mL/kg/h is added, and for severe trauma, 8 mL/kg/h. A colloid solution is added if the blood loss is greater than 20% of the patient's total blood volume. Total blood volume is equal to approximately 5000 mL. PACU monitoring to ensure appropriate fluid support should include vital signs and urine output.

## BLOOD COMPONENT THERAPY

Blood is a viscous fluid medium that contains white blood cells (leukocytes), RBCs (erythrocytes), platelets, and plasma. The RBCs are biconcave disks that contain hemoglobin, which transports oxygen and acts as a buffer to help maintain acid-base balance. The membrane of the RBC has antigens, and the plasma contains circulation antibodies. The ABO and Rh classification systems are two of the common blood group systems. ABO/Rh blood typing is extremely important for prevention of incompatibility between donor and recipient. A person with blood type AB is termed a universal recipient because AB blood has no A or B antibodies in the plasma. An individual with type O is termed a universal donor because no A or B antigens are present on the RBCs. During the screening process for compatibility, the ABO/Rh blood typing normally is performed; then an antibody screen is performed to detect the presence of the various antibodies in the recipient's and the donor's blood. The last test is the cross match, in which a trial transfusion is simulated.

Donated blood can be stored as whole blood or centrifuged and separated into RBCs, leukocytes, platelets, and plasma. Whole blood less than 24 hours old is considered fresh whole blood. A unit of blood contains 450 mL of blood and 63 mL of anticoagulant. If the blood is more than 24 hours old, it contains no viable platelets and a reduced content of factors V and VIII. Also, a decrease is seen in RBC adenosine triphosphate and 2,3-diphosphoglycerate levels, which usually resolves with dilution with the patient's blood during transfusion. Blood lactate increases the longer the blood is stored, which can be problematic if multiple blood transfusions are given. Usually sodium bicarbonate is administered to offset the lactate (acid). The patient's potassium also should be monitored because the potassium can be released off the RBC. The patient's pH and $PCO_2$ are used for evaluation of the need for the sodium bicarbonate. Normal blood storage does not exceed 35 days. Red blood cells should be administered via a large-gauge needle, and a blood filter and warmer should be used. A standard blood filter removes degenerated platelets, leukocytes, and fibrin accumulation. The standard filter has

pores between 170 to 230 μm and can be used for up to 2 to 4 units.

The use of autologous blood for transfusions is popular because it reduces the chances for disease transmission and incompatibility and saves the use of banked blood. In this case, the patient donates his or her own blood within 21 to 42 days of operation, depending on the anticoagulant used in the blood storage. The autologous patients are usually given iron supplements and erythropoietin in an effort to keep hemoglobin levels within normal limits.

Another type of autologous blood transfusion is the use of acute isovolemic hemodilution during the operative procedure. In this situation, a portion of the allowable blood loss is collected with a large-bore intravenous cannula. Usually an equal amount of crystalloid is administered to dilute and subsequently reduce the number of RBCs during the operation. Near the end of the operation, the autologous blood is reinfused to provide more RBCs and fresh platelets.

The last type of autologous blood transfusion is the use of intraoperative blood collection systems that collect the blood lost from the operation, which is then reinfused into the patient. Commercial products are available for this collection and collecting. They use anticoagulants and either provide washed RBCs or the entire blood products back to the patient. Because of the risk of reinfusion of bacteria or tumor cells, this procedure is not used on patients who are having surgical procedures performed on the bowel or on malignancies.

The role of the perianesthesia nurse in the administration of blood and blood products is critical to the well being of the patient. The importance of the nurse's checking and rechecking the blood and following all hospital procedures on the appropriate administration of blood or blood products cannot be overstated.

### Perioperative Fluid Therapy: An Example
Usually, for most healthy patients, blood loss is replaced with crystalloid in which for every mL of blood lost, 3 mL of crystalloid is administered. If a colloid solution is chosen, the blood loss is replaced milliliter for milliliter. That is, for each milliliter of blood loss, 1 mL of colloid solution is administered. If the anemia from blood loss continues, the administration of blood therapy may need to be started.

With the serious consequences of HIV and other blood-borne diseases, the basis for the determination of when to administer blood has been revised. Formerly, if a patient had a hematocrit level of 30 or less or a hemoglobin level of less than 10 g/dL, blood was usually administered. Now, the major factor in the determination of the administration of blood is the hemoglobin. When a patient has a hemoglobin of 7 g/dL or less, blood is usually administered. The formula used in calculation of the approximate allowable loss of blood is that the allowable loss (AL) is equal to the estimated blood volume (EBV) times the preanesthesia hemoglobin ($Hb_{initial}$) minus the target hemoglobin ($Hb_{target}$), which is divided by the $Hb_{initial}$.

$$AL = EBV \times \frac{Hb_{initial} - Hb_{target}}{Hb_{initial}}$$

For example, for a 70-kg male patient, the estimated blood volume is 5180 mL. For adult men, the total blood volume is equal to 74 mL times the weight in kg. In adult women, total blood volume is 70 mL times the weight in kg. Our adult male in this example has a hemoglobin level before anesthesia of 13 g/dL. Determination was that the patient should not have the hemoglobin level drop to less than 7 g/dL before blood should be administered. Hence, the target hemoglobin value is 7.0 g/dL. Therefore, the equation is the following:

$$AL = 5180 \, mL \times \frac{13_{g/dL} - 13_{g/dL}}{13_{g/dL}}$$

Thus, this adult male patient's acceptable blood loss is 2391 mL. The first 2391 mL of blood loss could be replaced with crystalloid or colloids. After that, blood or blood component therapy is usually instituted.

## TYPES OF BLOOD COMPONENT THERAPY

### Red Blood Cells

These RBCs can be described as units derived from a unit of whole blood that has been centrifuged with most of the plasma removed. In addition, red blood cell units may be diluted with saline solution, but not in normal conditions. This dilution is indicated in older adults, patients with increased oxygen demand, and patients that do not have compensation with an increased cardiac output. The RBCs help to restore oxygen transport but do not facilitate blood coagulation. Also, no medications or other blood products should be added to the RBCs before or during administration. The potential for fluid overload exists during the administration of RBCs, especially in older adults. The perianesthesia nurse should monitor the respiratory status of these patients. Respiratory dysfunction in this situation may include dyspnea and arterial hypoxemia.

### Fresh Frozen Plasma

Fresh frozen plasma (FFP) is used for treatment of bleeding or documented coagulation problems. It should not be used for volume expansion or for replacement of large deficiencies in coagulation factors. FFP is separated from whole blood usually within 8 hours of collection. It can be stored for up to 1 year. One should note that various plasma products are now available that do not meet the preparation requirements for FFP, including plasma, liquid plasma, thawed plasma, and plasma frozen within 24 hours after phlebotomy.

### Platelets

Platelet concentrate is usually suspended in 50 mL of plasma. It is indicated for thrombocytopenia primarily from massive blood transfusion and for thrombocytopathies that are usually drug induced. One unit of platelets usually increases the platelet concentration in the adult by $5000/mm^3$ to $10,000/mm^3$ and in the newborn by $75,000/mm^3$ to $100,000/mm^3$. The platelets are administered via a large-gauge needle with a filter (170-$\mu$m to 220-$\mu$m) that is in line.

### Cryoprecipitate

Cryoprecipitate is produced with thawing fresh frozen plasma and collecting the precipitate. It can be frozen and stored for up to a year. Cryoprecipitate is used for the specific treatment of bleeding associated with deficiencies in fibrinogen, factor XIII, von Willebrand's factor, and factor VIII. The cryoprecipitate should be administered within 6 hours after thawing through a standard blood or special component infusion set with an inline 170-$\mu$m filter.

### Albumin

Albumin is used for acute volume expansion and is considered a colloid. It does not contain any cellular products and is available in 5% or 25% solutions in saline. Albumin is heat treated, which eliminates the possibility of transmission of hepatitis and other diseases.

## TRANSFUSION REACTIONS

First, the appropriate procedures for obtaining the blood sample for type and cross match should be followed. The patient who is receiving the blood should be identified by name and hospital number. Then, the unit of blood should be checked against that patient by checking the name of the patient and hospital number as written on the unit of blood. Two PACU nurses should conduct this identification process.

During the administration of the blood or blood products, the patient should be monitored for acute hemolytic reactions. Although the symptoms of a transfusion reaction may be masked by the depressant effects of the anesthetic, usually an acute hemolytic transfusion reaction is signaled by cardiovascular instability, such as severe hypotension. If a transfusion reaction is suspected, blood should be drawn and sent to the laboratory to have the direct antiglobulin test (DAT) which indicates whether a hemolytic transfusion reaction has occurred. This test is the first test performed by the blood bank (or Transfusion Medicine) once a transfusion reaction is suspected. Another excellent parameter for which to monitor is any unexplained bleeding at the operative site. Other signs include pain at the infusion site, anxiety, chills, headache, an increase in temperature, and decreased renal function. If the reaction is an allergic transfusion reaction, the patient has signs of urticaria, stridor, hypotension, and pruritus. A delayed type of hemolytic transfusion reaction may be seen in the PACU. The signs and symptoms include fever and malaise. Laboratory tests that reflect this condition include increased direct bilirubin, decreasing hematocrit, and increased urine urobilinogen levels.

If a hemolytic transfusion reaction is suspected, the PACU nurse should stop the transfusion immediately and attach normal saline solution to the intravenous catheter. The attending physician and the blood bank should be notified, and a specimen of blood should be drawn and sent to the blood bank along with the blood unit and administration set. A specimen of urine should be obtained to send to the laboratory for evaluation for hemoglobin content. Finally, the other units of blood for that patient should be rechecked.

## VOLUME STATUS ASSESSMENT OF THE PATIENT IN THE POSTANESTHESIA CARE UNIT

Assessment of hypovolemia in the PACU can be difficult because vasoconstriction from such things as surgical stress, intraoperative catecholamine administration, and hypothermia can sometimes compensate for the hypovolemia. Other assessment tools include poor skin perfusion, such as cool, pale, and clammy skin particularly in the feet; oliguria; hypotension; tachycardia; and tachypnea. Also, the estimated blood loss and the type and amount of replacement fluids recorded on the anesthesia record should be evaluated for excessive blood loss. Once these symptoms are seen, the PACU nurse should check the patient for excess bleeding and the IV infusion sites for infiltration. The nurse should also notify the attending physician immediately.

## SUMMARY

The intent of this chapter was to provide a broad scope view of the complex topic of fluid and electrolytes. The major electrolytes were presented along with the area of fluid replacement and fluid loss. Coagulation is presented in regard to the normal cascade of the various factors and the various laboratory tests that can be used for assessment of coagulation from both the intrinsic and extrinsic components. Finally, one of the assessment parameters in the PACU is the assessment for hypovolemia.

## BIBLIOGRAPHY

Aitkenhead A, Smith G, Rowbotham D: *Textbook of anaesthesia,* ed 5, Philadelphia, 2007, Churchill Livingstone.

Alspach J: *Core curriculum for critical care nursing,* ed 6, Philadelphia, 2006, Saunders.

Atlee J: *Complications in anesthesia,* ed 2, Philadelphia, 2007, Saunders.

Barash P, Cullen B, Stoelting R: *Clinical anesthesia,* ed 5, Philadelphia, 2001, Lippincott Williams & Wilkins.

Benumof J, Saidman L: *Anesthesia & perioperative complications,* ed 2, St Louis, 1999, Mosby.

Brunton L, Lazo J, Parker K: *Goodman and Gilman's the pharmacological basis of therapeutics,* ed 11, New York, 2005, McGraw-Hill Professional.

Evers A, Maze M: *Anesthetic pharmacology: physiologic principles and clinical practice,* Philadelphia, 2004, Churchill Livingstone.

Fisher L: *Benumof's anesthesia and uncommon diseases,* ed 5, Philadelphia, 2007, Saunders.

Gallager C, Issenberg B: *Simulation in anesthesia,* Philadelphia, 2007, Saunders.

Ganong W: *Review of medical physiology,* ed 22, New York, 2005, McGraw-Hill Medical.

Guyton A, Hall J: *Textbook of medical physiology,* ed 11, Philadelphia, 2006, Saunders.

Kier L, Dowd C: *The chemistry of drugs for nurse anesthetists,* Chicago, 2004, AANA Publishing, Inc.

Lake C, Hines R, Blitt C: *Clinical monitoring: practical applications for anesthesia and critical care,* Philadelphia, 2001, Saunders.

Litwack K: Perioperative fluid administration: colloid or crystalloid, *J PeriAnesth Nurs* 8(2):15-18, 1997.

Longnecker D, Murphy F: *Dripps, Eckenhoff, Vandam introduction to anesthesia,* ed 9, Philadelphia, 1997, Saunders.

Longnecker D, Tinker J, Morgan G: *Principles and practice of anesthesiology*, ed 2, St Louis, 1998, Mosby.

Miller R: *Anesthesia*, ed 5, Philadelphia, 2000, Churchill Livingstone.

Murray J, Nadel J: *Textbook of respiratory medicine*, ed 2, Philadelphia, 1994, Saunders.

Nagelhout J, Zaglaniczy K: *Nurse anesthesia*, ed 3, St Louis, 2005, Saunders.

Rose B, Post T: *Clinical physiology of acid-base and electrolyte disorders*, ed 5, New York, 2001, McGraw-Hill Professional.

Stoelting R: *Pharmacology and physiology in anesthetic practice*, ed 3, Philadelphia, 1999, Lippincott-Raven.

Stoelting R, Miller R: *Basics of anesthesia*, ed 4, Philadelphia, 2000, Churchill Livingstone.

Townsend C, Beauchamp R, Evers B, et al: *Sabiston textbook of surgery: the biological basis of modern surgical practice*, ed 17, Philadelphia, 2004, Saunders.

Weiskopf R: The rational perioperative use of blood and blood components, *Anesthesia Today* 8(2):7-10, 1997.

# 15

# THE ENDOCRINE SYSTEM

*Cecil B. Drain, PhD, RN, CRNA, FAAN, FASAHP*

The great professor of physiology always began his lecture with, "The essence of physiology is regulation and control." So true is that statement of the endocrine system. It is regarded as one of the two physiologic regulating and control systems: the nervous system and the endocrine system. Many interrelationships exist between the endocrine and the nervous systems. Dysfunction of the endocrine system is associated with overproduction or underproduction of a single hormone or multiple hormones. This dysfunction may be the primary reason for surgery, or it may coexist in patients who need surgery on other organ systems. To ensure appropriate nursing interventions for the patient with endocrine dysfunction in the postanesthesia care unit (PACU), the perianesthesia nurse must understand the physiology and pathophysiology of the endocrine system.

## DEFINITIONS

**Endocrine Gland:** A group of hormone-secreting and hormone-excreting cells.
**Gluconeogenesis:** The conversion of amino acids into glucose.
**Glycogenesis:** The deposition of glycogen in the liver.
**Hormone:** A biochemical substance secreted by a specific endocrine gland and transported in the blood to distant points in the body for regulation of rates of physiologic processes.
**Lipolysis:** The mobilization of deposited fat.
**Releasing Factor (RF):** A hormone of unknown chemical structure secreted by the hypothalamus.
**Releasing Hormone (RH):** A hormone secreted from the hypothalamus.
**Stress:** A chemical or physical disturbance in the cells or tissues produced by a change either in the external environment or within the body that necessitates a response to counteract the disturbance.
**Target Organ:** A gland whose activities are regulated by tropic hormones.

**Tropic Hormone:** A hormone that regulates the blood level of a specific hormone secreted from another endocrine gland.

## MEDIATORS OF THE ENDOCRINE SYSTEM: THE HORMONES

A hormone is a biochemical substance synthesized in an endocrine gland and secreted into body fluids for regulation or control of physiologic processes in other cells of the body. Biochemically, hormones are either proteins (or derivatives of proteins or amino acids) or steroids.

Protein hormones, such as the releasing hormones, catecholamines, and parathormone, fit the fixed-receptor model of hormone action. In this model, the stimulating hormone, called the first messenger, combines with a specific receptor for that hormone on the surface of the target cell. This hormone-receptor combination activates the enzyme adenylate cyclase in the membrane. That portion of the adenylate cyclase that is exposed to the cytoplasm causes the immediate conversion of cytoplasmic adenosine triphosphate into cyclic adenosine monophosphate (AMP). The cyclic AMP then acts as a second messenger and initiates any number of cellular functions.

In the mobile receptor model, a steroid hormone, because of its lipid solubility, passes through the cell membrane into the cytoplasm, where it binds with a specific receptor protein. The combined receptor protein-hormone either diffuses or is transported through the nuclear membrane and transfers the steroid hormone to a smaller protein. In the nucleus, the hormone activates specific genes to form the messenger ribonucleic acid (RNA). The messenger RNA then passes out of the nucleus into the cytoplasm, where it promotes the translation process in the ribosomes to form new proteins. Hormones that fit the fixed-receptor model produce an almost instantaneous response on the part of the target organ. In contrast, because of their action on the genes to cause protein synthesis, when the steroid hormones are secreted, a characteristic delay in

229

the initiation of hormone response varies from minutes to days.

## PHYSIOLOGY OF THE ENDOCRINE GLANDS

### The Pituitary Gland

The pituitary gland rests in the sella turcica of the sphenoid bone at the base of the brain. This gland is divided into anterior and posterior lobes. Because of its glandular nature, the anterior lobe is called the adenohypophysis; the posterior lobe is an outgrowth of a part of the nervous system, the hypothalamus, and is called the neurohypophysis. The pituitary gland receives its arterial blood supply from two paired systems of vessels: (1) the right and left superior hypophyseal arteries from above; and (2) the right and left inferior hypophyseal arteries from below. However, the anterior lobe receives no arterial blood supply. Instead, its entire blood supply is derived from the hypophyseal portal veins. This rich capillary system facilitates the rapid discharge of releasing hormones that have target cells in the anterior hypophysis.

Although the pituitary gland is called the master gland, it is actually regulated by other endocrine glands and by the nervous system. The secretion of the hormones of the anterior hypophysis is primarily influenced and controlled by the higher centers in the hypothalamus. Releasing hormones are secreted by the hypothalamic nuclei through the infundibular tract to the portal venous system of the pituitary gland to their respective target cells of the adenohypophysis. Consequently, the hypothalamus brings about fine regulation of the action of the anterior pituitary, and still higher nervous centers apparently further modulate the production of the releasing factors. Hence, the many influences that enter the brain and central nervous system impinge on the anterior pituitary gland either to enhance or to dampen its activity.

Hormonal control of the pituitary involves certain feedback systems. For example, corticotropin-releasing hormone stimulates the production and release of adrenocorticotropin (ACTH). The increased concentration of ACTH causes the hypothalamus to decrease its production of corticotropin-releasing hormone, which in turn reduces ACTH production and ultimately reduces the blood level of ACTH. Therefore, when exogenous corticoids are administered chronically, ACTH secretion decreases and the adrenal cortex atrophies. On the other hand, the removal of endogenous corticoids with a bilateral adrenalectomy can result in a tumor of the pituitary gland because of the absence of the feedback depression of the corticotropin-releasing hormone.

The posterior lobe of the pituitary gland has an abundant nerve supply. Nerve cell bodies in the posterior lobe produce two neurosecretions (antidiuretic hormone and oxytocin), which are stored as granules at the site of the nerve cell bodies. When the hypothalamus detects a need for either neurohypophyseal hormone, nerve impulses are sent to the posterior lobe and the hormone is released by granules into the neighboring capillaries. Consequently, the hormonal function of the posterior lobe is under direct nervous system regulation.

### Hormones of the Adenohypophysis

***Growth Hormone, or Somatotropin.*** The growth hormone is unique because it stimulates no target gland but acts on all tissues of the body. Its primary functions are maintenance of blood glucose levels and regulation of the growth of the skeleton. Growth hormone conserves blood glucose by increasing fat metabolism for energy. It enhances the active transport of amino acids into cells, increases the rate of protein synthesis, and promotes cell division. In addition, growth hormone enhances the formation of somatomedin, which acts directly on cartilage and bone to promote growth. The active secretion of growth hormone is regulated in the hypothalamus via growth hormone–releasing hormone. Stimuli such as hypoglycemia, exercise, and trauma cause the hypothalamus to secrete growth hormone–releasing hormone, which is transported to the anterior lobe of the pituitary gland and released into the blood. Secretion of growth hormone can be inhibited by somatostatin, also called growth hormone–inhibiting hormone, which is secreted by the hypothalamus and the delta cells of the pancreas.

Hyposecretion of the growth hormone before puberty leads to dwarfism, or failure to grow. After puberty, growth hormone hypofunction may result in the condition known as Simmonds' disease. This disease is characterized by premature senility, weakness, emaciation, mental lethargy, and wrinkled dry skin. Giantism is the result of growth hormone hyperfunction before puberty. After puberty, when the epiphyses of the long bones have closed, growth hormone hyperfunction leads to acromegaly. In this disease, the face, hands, and feet become enlarged. Patients with acromegaly are prone to airway obstruction caused by protruding lower jaws and enlarged tongues. Hence, in the PACU, constant vigilance to the respiratory status of these patients is essential.

***Thyroid-stimulating Hormone, or Thyrotropin.*** The follicular cells of the thyroid are the target for thyroid-stimulating hormone (TSH). This hormone promotes the growth and secretory activity of the thyroid gland. Production of TSH is regulated in a reciprocal fashion by the blood levels of thyroid hormone and the formation of thyrotropin-releasing hormone in the hypothalamus.

**Adrenocorticotropin.** Adrenocorticotropin promotes glucocorticoid, mineralocorticoid, and androgenic steroid production and secretion by the adrenal cortex. This hormone is released in response to stimuli such as pain, hypoglycemia, hypoxia, bacterial toxins, hyperthermia, hypothermia, and physiologic stress. More specifically, the hypothalamus monitors for these various stressors, and on excitation, corticotropin-releasing hormone (CRH) is secreted, which stimulates ACTH secretion from the adenohypophysis. Levels of adrenocortical hormones in the blood regulate secretion of ACTH with a hypothalamic feedback mechanism.

**Gonadotropic Hormones.** Gonadotropic hormones regulate the growth, development, and function of the ovaries and testes. The gonadotropic hormones are the follicle-stimulating hormone and the luteinizing hormone. Secretion of the gonadotropic hormones is stimulated by gonadotropin-releasing hormone; the hormones are secreted by the hypothalamus.

**Lactogenic Hormone, or Prolactin.** Prolactin stimulates postpartum lactation. Unlike other pituitary hormones, the hypothalamic control of prolactin secretion is predominantly inhibitory.

**Melanocyte-stimulating Hormone.** Melanocyte-stimulating hormone exerts its effect on the melanin granules in pigmented skin.

### Hormones of the Neurohypophysis

**Antidiuretic Hormone, or Vasopressin.** During normal activities of daily living, antidiuretic hormone (ADH) is secreted in small amounts into the blood stream for promotion of reabsorption of water by the renal tubules, which leads to a decreased excretion of water by the kidneys. When ADH is secreted in large quantities, vasoconstriction of the smooth muscles occurs and ultimately elevates the blood pressure. The pressor effects of ADH are produced only with large doses that are not in the usual physiologic range. The secretion of ADH is regulated by several feedback loops, one of which involves plasma osmolality. Within the hypothalamus are osmoreceptors, whose function is secretion of ADH when plasma osmolarity is increased. On the other hand, dilution of plasma inhibits ADH secretion. The second feedback loop or major stimulus of ADH secretion is the volume or stretch receptors located in the left atrium. These receptors are activated when the extracellular fluid volume is increased; with this activation, ADH secretion is inhibited. The baroreceptors, which are located in the carotid sinus and aortic arch, are the receptors for the third feedback loop. A decrease in the arterial blood pressure stimulates the baroreceptors, which in turn stimulate a release of ADH. Both the stretch receptors and the baroreceptors transmit neuronal input to the brain via the vagus nerve.

Lack of ADH leads to a condition called diabetes insipidus. This condition is characterized by the output of a large volume of dilute sugar-free urine.

**Oxytocin.** Oxytocin produces contraction of uterine muscle at the end of gestation and has a role in milk excretion—that is, in stimulation of the contraction of the surrounding myoepithelial cells of the mammary glands.

### Pituitary Dysfunction

Hyperfunction rarely involves more than one endocrine gland. On the other hand, hypofunction does usually involve more than one endocrine gland, although instances of isolated deficiencies have been reported. A common cause of pituitary hypofunction is compression of glandular cells by the expansion of a functional or nonfunctional tumor. In this situation, an excess of one hormone may coexist with a deficiency of another.

### The Pineal Gland

The pineal gland is situated in the diencephalon just above the roof of the midbrain. This gland is considered an intricate and highly sensitive biologic clock because the secretory activity of the pineal gland is greatest at night. The pineal gland secretes melatonin, which affects the size and secretory activity of the ovaries and other organs. The production and release of melatonin are regulated by the sympathetic nervous system. In fact, the pineal gland is considered a neuroendocrine transducer because it converts nervous system input into a hormonal output.

### The Thyroid Gland

The thyroid gland is located in the anterior middle portion of the neck immediately below the larynx. The gland consists of two lobes that are attached by a strip of tissue called the isthmus. Structurally, this gland is made up of tiny sacs called follicles. Each follicle is formed by a single layer of epithelial cells that surround a cavity that contains a secretory product known as colloid. This colloid fluid consists mainly of a glycoprotein-iodine complex called thyroglobulin.

On stimulation with TSH, thyroid hormones are produced in the following steps: (1) iodide trapping; (2) oxidation and iodination; (3) storage of the hormones in the colloid as part of the thyroglobulin molecules; and (4) proteolysis, which can be inhibited by iodide, and release of the hormones. The two hormones released from the thyroid gland are triiodothyronine ($T_3$) and thyroxine ($T_4$). $T_4$ represents more than 95% of the circulating thyroid hormone and is considered to be relatively inactive physiologically in comparison with $T_3$. Consequently, although $T_3$ has a relatively low concentration, it passes out of the blood stream faster than $T_4$, has a more rapid action, and is probably the major biologically active thyroid hormone. After these hormones are secreted by the thyroid gland, they are transported to all parts of the body by means of plasma proteins, in the form of protein-bound iodinated compounds. Hence, the laboratory test for protein-bound iodine is useful in determination of the amount of circulating thyroid hormone in the blood.

Triiodothyronine and $T_4$ regulate the metabolic activities of the body. More specifically, they regulate the rate of cellular oxidation. Also, they are essential for the normal growth and development of the body. Other metabolic activities that are influenced by $T_3$ and $T_4$ are promotion of protein synthesis and breakdown, increase of glucose absorption and utilization, facilitation of gluconeogenesis, and maintenance of fluid and electrolyte balance. The thyroid hormones are also involved in a feedback mechanism. The concentration of $T_3$ and $T_4$ in the blood regulates the secretion of TSH by the anterior pituitary gland. TSH regulates the growth and secretory activity of the thyroid gland.

The thyroid gland also secretes thyrocalcitonin, or calcitonin, for maintenance of the proper level of calcium in the blood. More specifically, calcitonin decreases the serum concentration of calcium by counteracting the effects of parathormone and inhibiting the resorption of calcium from the bones.

### The Parathyroid Glands

The parathyroid glands are located on the posterior portion of the thyroid gland. In most instances, one parathyroid gland is present on each of the four poles of the thyroid gland. The parathyroid glands release a polypeptide hormone called parathormone. This hormone is the principal regulator of the calcium concentration in the body. Parathormone· is released into the circulation by a negative feedback mechanism that depends on the serum concentration of calcium. Hence, a high serum concentration of calcium suppresses the synthesis and release of parathormone and a low serum calcium concentration stimulates the release of the hormone. Normal serum calcium concentrations depend on the regulatory mechanisms, which include parathormone, calcitonin, phosphorus, magnesium, and vitamin D. In fact, the serum calcium concentration is maintained by these regulatory mechanisms within narrow and constant limits. The normal serum calcium level is 9 to 10.3 mg/dL for men and 8.9 to 10.2 mg/dL for women. Serum levels of calcium expressed in milliequivalents per liter are one half the value given in milligrams per deciliter.

Parathormone influences the rate at which calcium is transported across membranes in the bone, the gastrointestinal tract, and the kidneys. More specifically, calcium release from bone is facilitated by parathormone-induced stimulation of osteoclastic activity. The absorption of calcium by the gastrointestinal tract is enhanced by the parathormone-induced synthesis of vitamin D. Parathormone activates the synthesis of vitamin D and leads to increased tubular reabsorption of calcium and enhanced renal tubular clearance of phosphorus, which results in more calcium entering the circulation.

### The Adrenal Glands

The adrenal glands are located on the apex of each kidney. Each gland consists of an outer portion called the cortex and an inner portion called the medulla. The medulla is responsible for the secretion of catecholamines (see Chapter 11). The preganglionic fibers of the sympathetic nervous system provide the stimulation that facilitates the liberation of the catecholamines by the medullary cells. The cortex makes up the bulk of the adrenal gland and is responsible for the secretion of the steroids. The cortex is divided anatomically and physiologically into three zones: the zona glomerulosa, the zona fasciculata, and the inner zona reticularis. These zones are the sites of secretion of the three major steroid hormones: the mineralocorticoids, the glucocorticoids, and the androgens, respectively.

The mineralocorticoids are responsible for the maintenance of fluid and electrolyte balance. Aldosterone is, physiologically, the most important mineralocorticoid. The basic action of aldosterone is promotion of the reabsorption of sodium with stimulation of cellular sodium pumps in the target tissue. Overall, aldosterone causes increased tubular reabsorption of sodium and excretion of potassium, which decreases urinary excretion of sodium and chloride and increases urinary secretion of potassium, consequently expanding the extracellular fluid compartment. Aldosterone secretion is increased by ACTH, a depletion in sodium, and an increase in potassium. The secretion of aldosterone is also regulated by the renin-angiotensin system. Thus, when the blood supply to the kidneys is low, the juxtaglomerular cells are stimulated to release renin. Renin, which is an enzyme, enters the blood and converts the plasma protein angiotensinogen to angiotensin I. In the lungs and elsewhere, angiotensin I is converted enzymatically to the physiologically active form, angiotensin II. One of the basic actions of angiotensin II is stimulation of the adrenal cortex for secretion of aldosterone. Thus, aldosterone secretion is regulated by the blood pressure and volume; and because it causes retention of sodium and a rise in blood pressure, aldosterone also acts as a feedback mechanism to shut off the further release of renin.

The glucocorticoids are secreted in the zona fasciculata. Cortisol (hydrocortisone) constitutes about 95% of the total glucocorticoid activity, with corticosterone and cortisone making up the remaining 5%. These hormones function to preserve the carbohydrate reserves of the body with promotion of gluconeogenesis, glycogenesis, lipolysis, and oxidation of fat in the liver. Because they conserve carbohydrates, these hormones serve as functional antagonists to insulin. Finally, these hormones possess an excellent antiinflammatory action. The major regulator of their secretion is ACTH, which is secreted by cells in the anterior pituitary gland. ACTH is, in turn, modulated by CRH, which is secreted by the hypothalamus. Cortisol serves as a negative feedback mechanism for inhibition of both ACTH and CRH production. Physical and mental stresses stimulate the release of CRH from the hypothalamus. Hence, in addition to the catecholamines, cortisol and ACTH are considered to be the major stress hormones.

The androgens, or sex hormones, are actively involved in the preadolescent growth spurt and the appearance of axillary and pubic hair.

## The Pancreas
Islet of Langerhans cells are scattered throughout the pancreas. The three islet cell types, alpha, beta, and delta, secrete glucagon, insulin, and somatostatin, respectively. Glucagon has several functions that are diametrically opposed to those of insulin. Glucagon is commonly referred to as the hyperglycemic factor, and its most important function is to increase the blood glucose level.

This increased glucose level in the blood is the result of the effects of glucagon on glucose metabolism—that is, glycogenolysis (in the liver) and increased gluconeogenesis. When the blood glucose concentration decreases lower than 70 mg/dL, the alpha cells secrete glucagon to protect against hypoglycemia. Also, amino acids enhance the secretion of glucagon. In this instance, the glucagon helps prevent the hypoglycemia that can result because amino acids stimulate insulin release, which tends to reduce the blood glucose concentration. The secretion of glucagon appears to be inhibited by the release of somatostatin from the delta cells of the pancreas, and because it is a polypeptide, glucagon is rapidly destroyed by proteolytic enzymes.

Insulin is a protein secreted by the beta cells of the islets of Langerhans in response to elevated levels of blood glucose. Its secretion is inhibited by low blood glucose levels and somatostatin. In addition, insulin secretion can be inhibited by epinephrine, glucocorticoids, and thyroxine. When insulin is secreted by the beta cells, a metabolic state that favors the storage of nutrients is set into action. These physiologic actions include: (1) retention of glucose by the liver; (2) slowing of hepatic glucose release; (3) increase in uptake of glucose by muscle (stored as glycogen) and adipose tissue (stored as triglycerides); (4) translocation of amino acids and neutral fats into muscle and adipose tissue; and (5) retardation of lipolysis and proteolysis. Hence, insulin seems to "open the door" of most of the cell membranes of the body to facilitate the movement of glucose, amino acids, and fatty acids into the cells. Diabetes mellitus, which is a disease that involves the synthesis, storage, and release of insulin, is discussed in detail in Chapter 48.

## The Gonads
The hormone testosterone is produced in the interstitial cells of the testes. The synthesis and secretion of this hormone are regulated by luteinizing hormone, which is secreted by the anterior pituitary gland. Testosterone regulates the development and maintenance of the male secondary sexual characteristics and produces some metabolic effects on bone and skeletal muscle. Another action of this hormone is the modulation of male behavior with limbic system stimulation. Estrogen, another gonadal hormone, is secreted by the ovarian follicles in response to the follicle-stimulating hormone and the luteinizing hormone of the anterior pituitary gland and is responsible for the development and maintenance of the secondary

sexual characteristics in the female. Estrogen, along with progesterone, which is produced by the cells of the corpus luteum, plays an important role in the menstrual cycle.

## SELECTED SYNDROMES AND DISEASES ASSOCIATED WITH THE ENDOCRINE SYSTEM

### Hypoadrenocorticism

A reduction in function of the hormones associated with the pituitary-adrenal axis can develop as a result of: (1) the destruction of the adrenal cortex by degenerative disease, neoplastic growth, or hemorrhage; (2) a deficiency of ACTH; or (3) prolonged administration of corticosteroid drugs. Primary adrenal insufficiency (Addison's disease) results from destruction of the adrenal cortex. At present, most cases of Addison's disease are caused by idiopathic atrophy that is probably the result of an autoimmune disease. Other causes include tuberculosis, histoplasmosis, bilateral hemorrhage from anticoagulation therapy, surgical removal of the adrenal glands, tumor chemotherapy, metastasis to the adrenal glands, and sepsis.

A deficiency of ACTH is associated with panhypopituitarism. Patients who have been administered frequent "bursts" of exogenous steroid preparations such as prednisone can have a suppression of output of endogenous corticosteroids because of augmentation of the feedback mechanism to the anterior pituitary gland. Concern about the development of hypoadrenocorticism should be shown in the case of any patient who has received 20 mg of prednisone per day for more than 2 weeks in the preceding 12 months (although author opinions vary on dosage and length of time). The recovery of the normal function of the pituitary-adrenal axis may be as long as 12 months after the discontinuation of steroid therapy. Patients who are even remotely suspected to have hypoadrenocorticism are usually administered steroids before, during, and after surgery.

This perioperative steroid coverage is needed because infection, injury, operation, or other stressors activate the pituitary-adrenal axis. If this axis is suppressed (i.e., hypoadrenocorticism), acute adrenal insufficiency (Addisonian crisis) can develop, which is a life-threatening situation that requires prompt action by the PACU nurse. Clinical manifestations of the Addisonian crisis include dehydration, nausea and vomiting, muscular weakness, and hypotension, followed by fever, marked flaccidity of the extremities, hyponatremia, hyperkalemia, azotemia, and shock. Therefore, the PACU nurse

should monitor patients who are even remotely likely to have the Addisonian crisis develop. If some of the signs and symptoms appear, the attending physician should be notified immediately. The severely ill patient must be treated while the diagnosis is being confirmed. Two to 4 mg of dexamethasone is usually administered intravenously along with intravenous therapy of 5% dextrose in normal saline solution. Dexamethasone is the drug of choice because it does not interfere with the diagnostic tests and yet does provide the needed glucocorticoid. If dexamethasone is not available, administration of a single 100-mg intravenous dose of hydrocortisone is advantageous to obtain both the glucocorticoid and the mineralocorticoid activity. This dose can be followed by 50 to 100 mg of hydrocortisone administered parenterally every 6 hours. During the administration of the treatment, the PACU nurse should continuously monitor the patient's cardiorespiratory status.

### Syndrome of Inappropriate Secretion of Antidiuretic Hormone

The syndrome of inappropriate secretion of antidiuretic hormone (SIADH) occurs in the event of continued secretion of ADH in the presence of serum hypoosmolality. More specifically, the feedback loops that regulate ADH secretion and inhibition fail. Usually, both dilution and expansion of the blood volume serve to stimulate a suppression of the release of ADH. However, in SIADH, the feedback loops do not respond appropriately to the osmolar or volume change, and a pathologic positive feedback loop continues, thus resulting in continued production of ADH.

When hemorrhage and trauma occur during a surgical procedure, ADH secretion is appropriately elevated; and in this situation, SIADH can be induced as a result of overzealous fluid administration. Because of the urinary sodium loss that occurs along with the water retention, the syndrome of acute water intoxication may be seen in the PACU. The symptoms of water intoxication derive from increased brain water, inoperative sodium pump, and hyponatremia. The symptoms begin with headache, muscular weakness, anorexia, nausea, and vomiting and lead to confusion, hostility, disorientation, uncooperativeness, drowsiness, and terminal convulsions or coma. These symptoms usually do not occur if the serum sodium level is higher than 120 mEq/L. Therefore, in patients who have had major vascular surgery, trauma, or hemorrhage, the perianesthesia nurse should assess frequently for the symptoms of SIADH and notify the attending physician if the symptoms become evident. The focus of treatment for SIADH is fluid restriction, diuresis with mannitol or furosemide, and administration of sodium chloride. Also, the perianesthesia nurse should frequently assess the neurologic signs and cardiorespiratory status of the patient with SIADH and measure and record accurately the intake and output of all fluids.

## SUMMARY

The hormones secreted by the endocrine system along with the nervous system provide regulation and control of the body. Dysfunction of the production of any one of the hormones can have disastrous effects on the body. Surgery is performed on many of the glands or organs where the secreting endocrine gland is located. Of particular significance to the perianesthesia nurse are the parathyroid glands. One of the adverse outcomes of thyroid surgery is the accidental removal of one or more of the parathyroid glands. This complication is one of many that perianesthesia nurses need to assess when the site of surgery is located near an endocrine gland. The hormone insulin was briefly described, with a more detailed discussion of insulin and diabetes in Chapters 27, 29, and 48.

## BIBLIOGRAPHY

Aitkenhead A, Smith G, Rowbotham D: *Textbook of anaesthesia*, ed 5, Philadelphia, 2007, Churchill Livingstone.

Alspach J: *Core curriculum for critical care nursing*, ed 6, Philadelphia, 2005, Saunders.

Atlee J: *Complications in anesthesia*, ed 2, Philadelphia, 2007, Saunders.

Barash P, Cullen B, Stoelting R: *Clinical anesthesia*, ed 5, Philadelphia, 2001, Lippincott Williams & Wilkins.

Benumof J, Saidman L: *Anesthesia & perioperative complications*, ed 2, St Louis, 1999, Mosby.

Brunton L, Lazo J, Parker K: *Goodman and Gilman's the pharmacological basis of therapeutics*, ed 11, New York, 2005, McGraw-Hill Professional.

Cote C, Todres I, Goudsosuzian N, et al: *A practice of anesthesia for infants and children*, ed 3, Philadelphia, 2001, Saunders.

Coursin DB, Coursin DB, Unger B: Endocrine complications in intensive care unit patients, *Semin Anesth Perioperative Med Pain* 21(1):59-74, 2002.

Degroot LJ, Jameson L: *Endocrinology*, ed 5, Philadelphia, 2006, Saunders.

DeManicor N: Primary hyperparathyroidism: a case study, *J Perianesth Nurs* 19(5):334-343, 2004.

Drake R, Vogl W, Mitchell A: *Gray's anatomy for students*, Philadelphia, 2005, Churchill Livingstone.

Estafanous F, Barash P, Reves J, editors: *Cardiac anesthesia: principles and clinical practice*, ed 2, Philadelphia, 2001, Lippincott Williams & Wilkins.

Evers A, Maze M: *Anesthetic pharmacology: physiologic principles and clinical practice*, Philadelphia, 2004, Churchill Livingstone.

Fisher L: *Benumof's anesthesia and uncommon diseases*, ed 5, Philadelphia, 2007, Saunders.

Gallager C, Issenberg B: *Simulation in anesthesia*, Philadelphia, 2007, Saunders.

Ganong W: *Review of medical physiology*, ed 22, New York, 2005, McGraw-Hill Medical.

Guyton A, Hall J: *Textbook of medical physiology*, ed 11, Philadelphia, 2006, Saunders.

Kaplan J, editor: *Thoracic anesthesia*, ed 2, New York, 1991, Churchill Livingstone.

Kier L, Dowd C: *The chemistry of drugs for nurse anesthetists*, Chicago, 2004, AANA Publishing, Inc.

Lake C, Hines R, Blitt C: *Clinical monitoring: practical applications for anesthesia and critical care*, Philadelphia, 2001, Saunders.

Larsen P, Kronenberg H, Melmed S: *Williams textbook of endocrinology*, ed 10, Philadelphia, 2003, Saunders.

Longnecker D, Murphy F: *Dripps, Eckenhoff, Vandam introduction to anesthesia*, ed 9, Philadelphia, 1997, Saunders.

Longnecker D, Tinker J, Morgan G: *Principles and practice of anesthesiology*, ed 2, St Louis, 1998, Mosby.

Mazzaferri E: *Year book of endocrinology*, St Louis, 2007, Mosby.

Miller R, editor: *Anesthesia*, ed 5, Philadelphia, 2000, Churchill Livingstone.

Murray J, Nadel J: *Textbook of respiratory medicine*, ed 2, Philadelphia, 1994, Saunders.

Nagelhout J, Zaglaniczy K: *Nurse anesthesia*, ed 3, St Louis, 2005, Saunders.

Noble K: Thyroid storm, *J PeriAnesth Nurs* 21(2):119-425, 2006.

Shorten G, Browne J, Carr D, et al: *Postoperative pain management: an evidence-based guide to practice*, Philadelphia, 2006, Saunders.

Stoelting R: *Pharmacology and physiology in anesthetic practice*, ed 3, Philadelphia, 1999, Lippincott-Raven.

Stoelting R, Miller R: *Basics of anesthesia*, ed 4, Philadelphia, 2000, Churchill Livingstone.

Townsend C, Beauchamp R, Evers B, et al: *Sabiston textbook of surgery: the biological basis of modern surgical practice*, ed 17, Philadelphia, 2004, Saunders.

# 16

# THE HEPATOBILIARY AND GASTROINTESTINAL SYSTEM

*Cecil B. Drain, PhD, RN, CRNA, FAAN, FASAHP*

Because so many surgical procedures involve the gastrointestinal tract, the perianesthesia nurse in the postanesthesia care unit (PACU) must understand some functions of the organs of this system. This chapter discusses the overall function of each organ and the possible postoperative complications that may involve the gastrointestinal tract. Of specific interest to the reader is the section on nausea and vomiting. This section is intended to provide a starting point with use of the anatomy and physiology of these systems for understanding one of the most serious complications in perianesthesia nursing: postoperative nausea and vomiting (PONV). Also, the concept of a full stomach is presented. These complications not only are serious and necessitate informed perianesthesia nursing intervention (see Chapter 29), but they also can be an issue in a medical malpractice case. Therefore, the reader is encouraged to review Chapter 7 which deals with legal issues and the importance of documentation of the incident that occurs in the PACU.

## DEFINITIONS

**Achalasia:** A condition in which the lower esophageal sphincter fails to relax during the swallowing mechanism and food transmission from the esophagus to the stomach is impeded or prevented. This condition is also called megaesophagus.

**Achlorhydria (Hypochlorhydria):** A condition in which hydrochloric acid is not secreted by the stomach.

**Biliary:** Pertaining to the gallbladder and bile ducts.

**Cholelithiasis:** The presence of a common bile duct stone. Also called chronic cholangitis.

**Chyme:** Food that has become mixed with the secretions of the stomach and is passed down the gut.

**Deglutition:** The act of swallowing.

**Diarrhea:** Rapid movement of fecal matter through the large intestine.

**Enteric System:** The gastrointestinal tract.

**Gastritis:** Inflammation of the gastric mucosa.

**Lithotripsy:** A procedure for treatment of upper urinary tract stones.

**Nausea:** Conscious recognition of subconscious excitation in an area of the medulla closely related to the vomiting center.

**Oxyntic Glands:** Gastric glands that secrete hydrochloric acid, pepsinogen, intrinsic factor, and mucus.

**Pancreatitis:** Inflammation of the pancreas.

**Peptic Ulcer:** An excoriated area of the mucosa caused by the digestive action of gastric acid; frequently located in the first few centimeters of the duodenum.

**Pyrosis:** Heartburn, of which gastroesophageal reflux is usually the cause.

**Vomiting:** A method for the gastrointestinal tract to rid itself of its contents when almost any part of the upper gastrointestinal tract becomes overirritated, distended, or excitable. The physical act of vomiting results when the muscles of the diaphragm and abdomen contract so that the gastric contents can be expelled.

## THE ESOPHAGUS

The esophagus is a muscular tube that extends from the pharynx to the stomach (Fig. 16-1). It is located behind the trachea and in front of the thoracic aorta and traverses the diaphragm to enter the esophagogastric junction, sometimes called the cardia. Approximately 5 cm above the junction with the stomach is the gastroesophageal sphincter, which functions to prevent the reflux of stomach contents into the esophagus. The resting pressure is normally about 30 torr. This pressure is maintained by the vagus nerve and by the nervous system. Ordinarily, the sphincter remains constricted except in the act of swallowing. Anticholinergic drugs, such as atropine, and pregnancy decrease the resting pressure of the lower esophagus. Drugs that increase the lower esophageal pressure include metoclopramide (Reglan) and antacids. Another factor that prevents reflux of gastric

Hiatal hernia can occur where the esophagus traverses the diaphragm. Ultimately, a lower esophageal stricture may occur that can cause symptoms such as heartburn, pain, and vomiting. Patients with a hiatal hernia need constant observation for active and passive vomiting during the emergent phase of anesthesia. This monitoring is especially important if the surgery was performed on an emergency basis when the patient had a full stomach.

## THE STOMACH

The stomach can be anatomically divided into the following three sections: the fundus, the body, and the pyloric portion (Fig. 16-2). The fundus is the dome of the stomach, where peptic juice is secreted. The body is the middle portion of the stomach and is lined with parietal cells that secrete hydrochloric acid. The pH of the solution as secreted is approximately 0.8, which is extremely acidic. The total gastric secretion on a 24-hour basis is about 2 L. This volume normally has a pH of about 1 to 3.5. Histamine has a major role in hydrochloric acid production by the parietal cells in the stomach, which is an effect mediated by histamine$_2$ (H$_2$) receptors, vagal stimulation, and the hormone gastrin. Activation on any one of these receptors potentiates the response of the other to stimulation. Blockade of the activated receptor produces a reduction in acid response because the potentiating effect of the stimulation is reduced. The third portion of the stomach is the pyloric portion, sometimes called the pyloric antrum. Here, a thick viscous mucus and the hormone gastrin are secreted. At the end of the antrum

Physiologic Considerations in the PACU

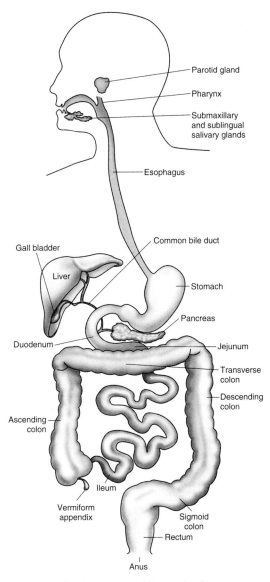

**Fig. 16-1** Digestive system and its associated structures.

contents into the esophagus is physiologic compression by intraabdominal pressure on the esophagus just below the diaphragm. This mechanism is referred to as a flutter valve closure. The main function of the esophagus is to conduct ingested material to the stomach. The innervation of the esophagus appears to originate from the vagus.

### Disorders of the Esophagus
Esophageal achalasia, a disease of unknown origin, is characterized by an absence of peristalsis in the esophagus and by constriction of the cardiac sphincter. The patient with this disorder usually has hypermotility and diffuse spasms of the esophagus.

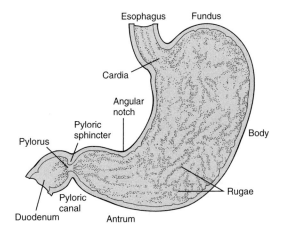

**Fig. 16-2** Anatomy of stomach. *(From Guyton A, Hall J: Textbook of medical physiology, ed 10, Philadelphia, 2000, Saunders.)*

is the pylorus, an opening surrounded by a strong band of sphincter muscle that controls the amount of gastric contents that enter the duodenum.

The vagus nerve (parasympathetic nervous system) provides the nerve supply to the stomach. Stimulation of the vagus causes increased motility of the stomach and the secretion of acid, pepsin, and gastrin. Thus, a vagotomy is sometimes performed during gastric surgery to decrease gastric motility and acid production. However, that the $H_2$ receptor is a major pathway for stimuli of acid secretion should be stated.

Nervous and hormonal stimulation have profound effects on gastric volume and pH. More specifically, stimulation of the parasympathetic nervous system causes increased gastric secretion, and stimulation of the sympathetic nervous system causes decreased gastric secretion. Consequently, pain and fear, which activate the sympathetic nervous system, decrease gastric emptying. In addition, the administration of opioids and active labor prolong gastric emptying. Food, depending on the type and amount, passes through the stomach at a variable rate. For example, foods rich in carbohydrates pass through the stomach in a few hours, whereas proteins exit more slowly. The emptying time for fats is the slowest. Fluids, on the other hand, pass through the stomach rather rapidly. In fact, 90% of 750 mL of ingested saline solution exits the stomach within 30 minutes. Also, 150 mL of fluids taken 1 or 2 hours before induction of anesthesia stimulates peristalsis and facilitates gastric emptying. Consequently, the small sips of water taken with the preoperative oral medications may in fact contribute to lower intraoperative and postoperative gastric volumes. Finally, a prolonged period of fasting does not ensure that the stomach is completely empty of fluids or food.

### Effect of Pregnancy on Gastric Motility and Secretions

During pregnancy, many alterations occur as a result of the enlarged uterus and altered hormonal state. Because of the enlarged uterus, the stomach and intestine are moved cephalad and the axis of the stomach is shifted to a more horizontal position. The gastric emptying time is increased in women who are at least 34 weeks pregnant. In regard to the gastric volume and pH, no difference between pregnant and nonpregnant states seems to exist. Consequently, pregnant patients who have had nothing by mouth (NPO) for elective surgery do not have any additional risk of aspiration pneumonitis

than do nonpregnant patients. However, research does suggest that pregnant patients who have pyrosis (heartburn) may be at greater risk for regurgitation and subsequent development of aspiration pneumonitis. In addition, if intramuscular narcotics are given during labor, gastric emptying time is substantially delayed. Epidural anesthesia with local anesthetics does not seem to affect gastric volume or pH; however, if narcotics are introduced into the epidural space, a delay in gastric emptying occurs.

### Postoperative Nausea and Vomiting

This section serves as an introduction into a most serious complication that can occur in the PACU. During the early days of anesthesia described in Chapter 29, the incidence rate of postoperative nausea and vomiting (PONV) was estimated at around 80%. Despite major advances in anesthesia and surgical techniques, the rate for adult surgical patients is between 20% and 30% and, depending on the definition of PONV, the incidence rates vary between 14% and 80%. Vomiting with subsequent aspiration of gastric contents into the airways and lungs is an important cause of morbidity and mortality in the PACU. Various reports have indicated a 4% to 27% risk of this phenomenon. Patients with a gastric pH lower than 2.5 and a gastric volume of more than 25 mL are at high risk of serious pulmonary complications if they have vomiting and regurgitation with subsequent aspiration. Many new research studies indicate that this concept of less than 2.5 pH and more than 25 mL may not be as predictive as suggested. However, the concept still serves as a "marker" on the possible morbidity of the patient if aspiration occurs. The two most common predictors of increased morbidity rate after aspiration are the pH and whether medium to large particles were part of the aspirated matter.

Various methods for increasing the pH and decreasing the volume of the gastric contents can be used. Anticholinergic agents, such as atropine and glycopyrrolate, inhibit the production of gastric juice, but only to a highly variable degree. These drugs also have side effects of tachycardia, reduced gastric sphincter tone, and delayed gastric emptying. Antacid prophylaxis with the administration of oral antacids has had mixed success because the subsequent aspiration of the antacid particles, which are nonabsorbable, can have devastating effects on the lungs. The oral antacid sodium citrate (Bicitra) has become popular because it has soluble particles that produce less severe hypoxia and lung abnormalities if aspirated. This drug has been used with great success in patients who need cesarean section.

Histamine$_2$ receptor–blocking drugs have met with some success in the treatment of gastric hypersecretory states. Cimetidine (Tagamet) is an H$_2$ receptor–blocking agent that is used as a premedication regimen for control of gastric acid production before the induction of anesthesia. The length of action of this drug is 3 hours, with a peak action of about 60 to 90 minutes. Cimetidine does not change the lower esophageal pressure, the rate of gastric emptying, or the volume of gastric juice. Cimetidine can cause a dose-related neuropsychiatric disturbance that is characterized by confusion, slurred speech, hallucinations, delirium, and coma. These symptoms dissipate once the blood level of cimetidine is reduced to 1.5 µg/mL or lower. Because cimetidine inhibits the metabolism of any drug that is biotransformed by the cytochrome P-450 microsomal enzyme system in the liver, drugs such as propranolol, metoprolol, lidocaine, bupivacaine, diazepam, midazolam, theophylline, and warfarin are potentiated when given in conjunction with cimetidine. Hence, cimetidine can prolong the length of action of these drugs.

Ranitidine (Zantac) is an H$_2$ receptor–blocking agent that is gaining wide popularity as a premedication. With its H$_2$ receptor–blocking actions, ranitidine inhibits gastric secretion in response to acetylcholine, histamine, and gastrin. This drug is more potent than cimetidine and is administered in about half the dose of cimetidine, with a peak of 90 minutes and a length of action of about 10 hours. Ranitidine is usually given orally about 1 hour before anesthesia. The usual dose is 150 mg. Ranitidine has a small clinically insignificant effect on the cytochrome P-450 system. Two new H$_2$-receptor antagonists, famotidine and nizatidine, have been introduced into clinical practice. These drugs are similar to cimetidine and ranitidine. Unlike cimetidine, neither drug binds to the cytochrome P-450 system; hence, they do not interfere with the hepatic metabolism of other drugs.

Metoclopramide (Reglan) is a drug that is often included in the premedication regimen. This drug is a dopamine antagonist that increases the lower esophageal sphincter pressure; speeds gastric emptying, thereby reducing the gastric volume; and prevents or alleviates nausea and vomiting. Metoclopramide can be given orally in a 10-mg dose as part of a premedication regimen. It also can be given intravenously at 0.15 mg/kg to produce its antiemetic properties. Metoclopramide has minimal side effects.

A problem for which every perianesthesia nurse should watch is regurgitation after anesthesia. When a patient is under the influence of a general anesthetic, the swallowing mechanism is abolished. Foodstuffs or fluids can be passively or actively vomited. The vomitus may then be aspirated into the trachea and lungs. In some instances, this type of aspiration is called Mendelson's syndrome. Inspiration of vomitus can lead to aspiration pneumonia. This condition can occur during the induction of anesthesia, during the operation, or in the immediate PACU phase as the patient emerges from anesthesia.

A great deal of research on PONV over the past few years has yielded drugs that have certainly improved the outcomes of the patient in regard to PONV. The 5-HT3 antagonists, such as ondansetron, tropisetron, granisetron, and dolasetron, competitively antagonize the effect of 5-HT at the 5-HT$_3$ receptor site. Other drug therapies being used are the antihistamines (promethazine and dimenhydrinate), anticholinergics (scopolamine), neuroleptics (droperidol and triflupromazine), and glucocorticoids, such as dexamethasone. The pathophysiology and pharmacology of PONV is discussed at length in Chapter 29.

The basics of care for vomiting in the PACU setting indicate that the patient should be placed in a head-down position and given oxygen immediately. The purpose of the head-down position is to allow fluid to flow *away* from the lungs rather than *into* the lungs. Consequently, if at all possible, the patient should be placed in this position if aspiration is suspected. Fluid should be suctioned rapidly while administration of oxygen continues. If the patient's airway is obstructed by large particles, finger or forceps should be used to clear the debris and then oxygen should be administered. The physician or anesthesia provider should be notified immediately. Once the acute situation is over, documentation of actions should be done. If possible, notes should be taken during the process to aid with accurate documentation (see Chapter 7).

Further treatment may include intubation and instillation of a weak solution of bicarbonate or saline through the endotracheal tube to aid in the neutralization of acidic gastric fluid in the respiratory tract. Steroids and antibiotics may also be administered.

A patient in recovery from a general anesthetic should be assessed for possible passive regurgitation, especially if the patient was not intubated during surgery. Clinical signs include dyspnea, cyanosis of varying degrees, and tachycardia. On auscultation of the lungs, abnormal sounds are usually heard. If the assessment indicates the possibility of this syndrome, oxygen should be administered and the physician notified at once.

Patients who had a full stomach at induction of anesthesia, who underwent intestinal or emergency surgery, or who have a suspected hiatal hernia have a higher incidence rate of this syndrome. The best treatment is prevention. These patients should have a complete return of consciousness before the endotracheal tube is removed. If the endotracheal tube is to be removed in the PACU, the patient should be placed in a lateral position with the head down. Oxygen should be administered, and suction should be available for immediate use before the extubation is performed.

## THE INTESTINE

The duodenum, which is a part of the small intestine, arises at the pylorus of the stomach and ends at the duodenojejunal junction. The duodenum is divided into the following four segments: superior, descending, transverse, and ascending. The common bile duct and the main pancreatic duct empty into the descending duodenum. The main function of the stomach and the first portion of the duodenum is to alter the form of food and to supply enzymes for digestion.

The jejunum begins at the descending duodenum at the duodenojejunal angle. It constitutes the first two fifths of the small intestine, and the ileum occupies the distal three fifths of the small intestine. The mesentery, which contains blood vessels, nerves, lymphatics, lymph nodes, and fat, stabilizes the small bowel and prevents it from twisting and constricting its blood supply.

The digestive glands secrete large quantities of water to aid in the digestive process. Between 5 and 10 L of water are estimated to enter the small intestine, and only about 500 mL leave the ileum and enter the colon. Among the important materials absorbed from the small intestine are sodium, bicarbonate, chloride, calcium, iron, carbohydrates, fats, and amino acids.

Sodium is absorbed by the small intestine at a rate of 25 to 35 g per day. This absorption accounts for approximately 16% of all the sodium in the body. When a patient has extreme diarrhea, sodium can be depleted to a lethal level within a few hours.

## THE COLON AND RECTUM

At the end of the small intestine is the ileocecal valve, which functions to prevent backflow of fecal material from the colon into the small intestine.

The colon is divided anatomically into the cecum, ascending colon, transverse colon, and descending and sigmoid colon. The functions of the colon are the absorption of water and electrolytes, which occurs principally in the proximal half of the colon, and the storage of fecal material, which occurs in the distal colon. The contents of the cecum are mainly liquid, as compared with the solid material contained in the sigmoid colon. Therefore, if a patient has undergone a colostomy, knowledge of the portion of the colon from which the stoma originates is important for determination of whether the excreted fecal material has the normal amount of water content.

Of surgical importance is the appendix, which arises from the cecum at its inferior tip. The appendix represents a special type of intestinal obstruction when it becomes inflamed by hyperplasia of submucosal lymphoid follicles, fecaliths, foreign bodies, or tumors.

The rectum functions entirely as an excretory canal and has no digestive function. It begins anatomically at the distal end of the sigmoid colon and ends at the anus. It is tubular and has two layers. The innermost layer is the lumen of the intestinal tract, and the outermost layer is skeletal muscle of the pelvic floor. The muscle is innervated by the parasympathetic nervous system.

## THE ANUS

The anus is the termination of the alimentary canal. It is encircled by striated muscle and innervated by somatic sympathetic and parasympathetic fibers. Because of the parasympathetic innervation of the rectum and anus, parasympathetic stimulation may occur during a rectal examination or surgical procedure. This parasympathetic reflex can also occur when a patient is recovering from a general anesthetic. If a physician deems a rectal examination necessary, the perianesthesia nurse should be prepared to monitor the patient for bradycardia and laryngospasm because they may result from stimulation of the anus and rectum.

## THE LIVER

The importance of the liver is generally underestimated. In Chinese medicine, the liver is considered the most important organ of the body. It is one of the basic homeostatic organs because it maintains the consistency of the blood on a minute-to-minute basis.

The liver is located in the right upper quadrant of the abdomen. It has a dual blood supply that consists of the hepatic artery and the portal vein. Both carry oxygen and nutrients to the liver for assimilation. The sinusoids, which surround the hepatocytes (liver cells), empty into a venous system that eventually forms the hepatic vein and empties into the inferior vena cava. About 1600 mL of blood per minute flow through the liver; this amount is about 30% of the cardiac output. The hepatocytes absorb nutrients from the portal venous blood; store and release proteins, lipids, and carbohydrates; excrete bile salts; synthesize plasma proteins, glucose, cholesterol, and fatty acids; and metabolize exogenous and endogenous compounds. Also, hepatocytes have alpha$_1$-adrenergic, alpha$_2$-adrenergic, and beta$_2$-adrenergic receptors on their plasma membranes. The preponderance of adrenergic receptors seems to be alpha$_1$, and, an increase in intracellular calcium ions has been shown on stimulation of these receptors.

The liver is the body's most important storage organ. It is able to absorb glucose in the form of glycogen, and it maintains a normal glucose concentration in the body. The liver also stores amino acids, iron, and vitamins. The liver can store up to 400 mL of blood in the sinusoids. If a person loses an appreciable amount of blood, the liver can release stored blood into the circulation to replace what was lost.

The liver performs many vital physiologic functions that have a significant impact on the pharmacologic actions of many of the drugs used in the perioperative period. More specifically, the liver performs biotransformation of drugs with the cytochrome P-450 microsomal enzyme system. Consequently, knowledge of bilirubin metabolism, protein synthesis, and drug biotransformation is of critical importance to the perianesthesia nurse.

### Bilirubin Metabolism
Bilirubin is made from one of the byproducts of red blood cell hemolysis: hemoglobin. The reticuloendothelial system converts hemoglobin to unconjugated bilirubin. The bilirubin is transported to the liver via serum albumin. In the liver, the bilirubin is then removed from the albumin and is conjugated with glucuronic acid. Conjugated bilirubin is highly water soluble and easily excreted in the urine. The other type of bilirubin, unconjugated bilirubin, is lipid soluble and not excreted in the urine. Conditions such as sickle cell disease, thalassemia minor, drug-induced hemolysis, and breakdown of red blood cells (RBCs) after massive transfusions can increase unconjugated bilirubin levels.

This increase eventually leads to an increase in bilirubin production. Jaundice, a yellowish tint to the body tissues, can be caused by a high concentration of bilirubin in the extracellular fluids. Consequently, diseases that are considered prehepatic cause an increase in unconjugated bilirubin and eventually lead to what is known as hemolytic jaundice. Obstructive jaundice occurs when the outflow of bile is blocked by an obstruction such as gallstones, stricture, or compression from external masses. In this instance, the conjugated bilirubin level increases in the serum. The third type of jaundice, toxic jaundice, usually follows damage to the liver cells. Use of chloroform can cause this type of jaundice, as can use of carbon tetrachloride.

### Protein Synthesis
The liver is responsible for the synthesis of most of the proteins found in the plasma. Albumin is the most notable of the plasma proteins synthesized by the liver. Albumin synthesis is regulated by the state of nutrition; therefore, a nutritional deficit results in reduced albumin production. Because many drugs used in anesthesia are protein-bound, a reduction in the albumin level can have a significant impact on the pharmacologic action of the drugs. Because the protein-binding sites are reduced, the unbound fraction of the drug is increased, which ultimately leads to an increased sensitivity to the drug or a prolonged action. This condition is particularly true for the highly protein-bound barbiturates. Hence, in the PACU, patients with hyponatremia who have received thiopental during surgery should be closely monitored for respiratory and cardiovascular depression from the prolonged action of the ultra–short-acting barbiturate. The liver also synthesizes the enzyme pseudocholinesterase (plasma cholinesterase). This protein is the principal enzyme in the metabolism of succinylcholine and the ester-type local anesthetics. Succinylcholine, which is the principal depolarizing skeletal muscle relaxant in use, has an inverse correlation between duration of action and pseudocholinesterase levels. Therefore, any patient with suspected liver dysfunction who has received succinylcholine during surgery should be closely monitored for respiratory depression in the immediate postoperative period. Finally, the liver produces a large proportion of the protein substances used in coagulation.

### Drug Biotransformation
The enzymes needed for oxidation and conjugation in the liver are called the microsomal enzymes. These enzymes are part of the cytochrome P-450 microsomal system. Exposure to

certain drugs, including barbiturates and some anesthetics, can lead to an increase in the microsomal enzymes. This process is commonly called enzyme induction. Enzyme induction increases the rate of drug biotransformation. Patients with severe liver disease may have reduced microsomal activity in the liver. Hence, drugs such as thiopental, diazepam, and meperidine have a prolonged action caused by a decreased rate of drug biotransformation by the microsomal enzymes. Consequently, patients with severe hepatic disease should be closely monitored for respiratory and cardiovascular depression in the PACU phase of the anesthetic experience.

## Acute Hepatic Failure

Acute hepatic failure is a rare syndrome that may be seen if the patient has undergone a period of severe hypotension (40 mm Hg systolic) during anesthesia. Because of the hypotension, the liver cells die and the patient appears lethargic and drowsy after surgery. Persistent oliguria, which leads to anuria within 24 to 48 hours, is the cardinal symptom of this syndrome. The signs of liver damage ensue and include headache, anorexia, malaise, vomiting, and pyrexia. The syndrome leads to persistent vomiting, and by the end of the first week, jaundice may be present. The final stages of this disease are marked by delirium, coma, and death.

Treatment of this syndrome is entirely symptomatic and includes maintenance of fluid and electrolyte balance, treatment of the anuria, and a high carbohydrate diet.

## THE GALLBLADDER

The gallbladder is a thin-walled pear-shaped organ attached to the inferior surface of the liver (Fig. 16-3). It is 7 to 10 cm long and 3 to 5 cm wide. The gallbladder has a capacity of 30 to 60 mL of fluid. Anatomically, it is divided into the fundus; the distal tip; the corpus (body), the middle body portion; the infundibulum, a pouch-like structure; and the neck, which leads to the cystic duct. The cystic duct joins the common hepatic duct to form the common bile duct. The common bile duct and the main pancreatic duct of Wirsung usually join at the choledochoduodenal junction, which is a passageway through the duodenal wall. The muscle of the choledochoduodenal junction is the sphincter of Oddi, which regulates the flow of bile into the duodenum. Many common narcotic analgesics can produce spasm of the sphincter of Oddi and the duodenum and can increase the pressure in the biliary tree.

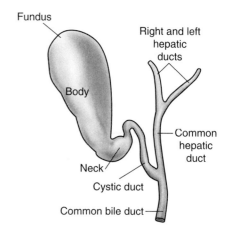

**Fig. 16-3**  Gallbladder showing right and left hepatic ducts coming from liver, common hepatic duct, cystic duct, and common bile duct. (*Redrawn from Jacob S, Francone C, Lossow WJ: Structure and function in man, ed 5, Philadelphia, 1982, Saunders.*)

Cholelithiasis is a common occurrence in patients with chronic gallbladder disease. As many as 20 million people have some form of cholelithiasis. Gallstones are composed of cholesterol, which is almost insoluble in pure water. The causes of gallstones include an excess of cholesterol in the bile, chronic inflammation of the epithelium, excessive absorption of bile acids from the bile, and excessive absorption of water from the bile. A new surgical procedure called biliary lithotripsy offers distinct advantages over cholecystectomy. The advantages include no surgical incision, less pain, a shorter postoperative period, and a reduction in costs to the patient. Consequently, the patient has a 50% reduction in postoperative pulmonary complications because of this new procedure. Formerly, a cholecystectomy was performed; that procedure was associated with a 50% reduction in the vital capacity on the first postoperative day. In fact, in the immediate postoperative period, the total lung capacity, vital capacity, and functional residual capacity all tend to decrease, thus causing a closure of the small airways and atelectasis. With the advent of biliary lithotripsy, the gallstones are broken into small fragments and the patient receives either local anesthesia and sedation or general anesthesia. Complications of this procedure are associated with the type of anesthetic technique and its inherent complications and from the shock wave therapy used during the procedure. The most common problems from this procedure include nausea, vomiting, abdominal pain, hemoptysis, and diarrhea. Perianesthesia nursing care for a patient recovering from biliary lithotripsy should include the normal peri-anesthesia care of a patient for upper abdominal surgery (see Chapter 40).

## THE PANCREAS

The pancreas is situated in the upper abdomen behind the stomach. It is a slender organ that consists of a head, a body, and a tail (Fig. 16-4). Its main duct, through which pass the pancreatic enzymes, runs the entire length of the gland and opens into the duodenum along with the common bile duct. Scattered throughout the pancreas are small clusters of cells called the islets of Langerhans. They are responsible for the production and secretion of hormones that they empty directly into the blood stream; therefore, the islets of Langerhans are considered an endocrine gland. The following three types of cells are found in the islets of Langerhans: alpha, beta, and delta. The alpha cells are associated with the production of the hormone glucagon, and the beta cells are associated with insulin. The physiologic significance of the delta cells has not been determined.

Insulin is secreted in response to an increase in the concentration of glucose. The secretion of insulin is inhibited when a low concentration of glucose exists. Glucagon is frequently called hyperglycemic factor because it causes hyperglycemia by stimulating the breakdown of liver glycogen with consequent release of glucose into the circulation. It also stimulates gluconeogenesis, which is the formation of glucose from noncarbohydrate sources.

The pancreas excretes juice for digestion of all three major types of food: carbohydrates, fats, and proteins. The pancreatic juice also contains large amounts of bicarbonate ions, which help neutralize the acidic chyme as it passes into the duodenum from the stomach.

### Pancreatitis

Acute pancreatitis is a serious complication of surgery on the biliary tract. It can occur as a result of common duct exploration during gallbladder surgery. Acute postoperative pancreatitis should be suspected with excessive pain, vomiting, fever, tachycardia, persistent ileus, or jaundice. The perianesthesia nurse should be aware of these symptoms, which, if detected, should be reported to the surgeon. Treatment of this disorder may include nasogastric suction, anticholinergic drugs, antibiotics, and replacement of fluids and electrolytes.

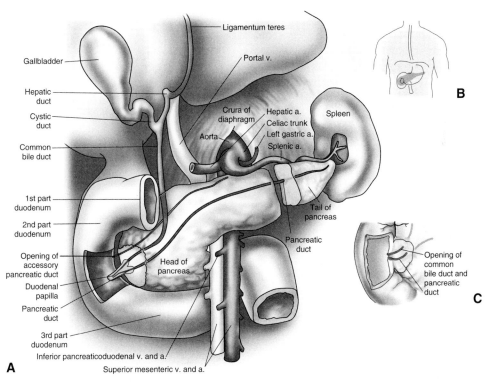

**Fig. 16-4 A**, Relationship of pancreas to duodenum, showing pancreatic and bile ducts joining at duodenal papilla. Section has been removed from pancreas to expose pancreatic duct. **B**, Anatomic position of pancreas. **C**, Common variation. *(Redrawn from Jacob S, Francone C, Lossow WJ: Structure and function in man, ed 5, Philadelphia, 1982, Saunders.)*

## THE SPLEEN

Because of its anatomic location, not its physiologic functions, the spleen is discussed here (see Chapter 40).

The spleen is an oval organ located in the upper left quadrant of the abdominal cavity. Its physiologic functions include the filtering of blood and foreign material, hematopoiesis, and, in some instances, the production of lymphocytes and antibodies.

The spleen is a highly vascular organ, and approximately 350 L of blood normally flow through it daily. The spleen acts as a reservoir of blood. It can store so many RBCs that splenic contraction can cause the hematocrit of the systemic blood to increase as much as 3% or 4%.

Normal health is possible after splenectomy because other tissues can assume the functions the spleen normally performs. Splenectomy is usually performed for the cure or alleviation of hematologic disease or because of its traumatic rupture. Because the spleen is friable and vascular, blood loss from a splenectomy can be high. Therefore, the perianesthesia nurse must assess the blood loss and the cardiovascular status of the patient during the recovery phase.

## SUMMARY

The hepatobiliary and gastrointestinal systems are certainly multidimensional, and the understanding of the anatomy and physiology of these systems is essential to the perianesthesia nurse. The pathophysiologies of some disorders that pertain to perianesthesia care were presented. Problems such as PONV (see Chapter 29), changes during pregnancy, and drug biotransformation were introduced. A complete overview of the care of the gastrointestinal, abdominal, and anorectal surgical patient is presented in Chapter 40.

## BIBLIOGRAPHY

Aitkenhead A, Smith G, Rowbotham D: *Textbook of anaesthesia*, ed 5, Philadelphia, 2007, Churchill Livingstone.

Alspach J: *Core curriculum for critical care nursing*, ed 6, Philadelphia, 2005, Saunders.

Atlee J: *Complications in anesthesia*, ed 2, Philadelphia, 2007, Saunders.

Barash P, Cullen B, Stoelting R: *Clinical anesthesia*, ed 5, Philadelphia, 2001, Lippincott Williams & Wilkins.

Benumof J, Saidman L: *Anesthesia & perioperative complications*, ed 2, St Louis, 1999, Mosby.

Brunton L, Lazo J, Parker K: *Goodman and Gilman's the pharmacological basis of therapeutics*, ed 11, New York, 2005, McGraw-Hill Professional.

Carter S: Redefining the surgical team's management of postoperative ileus, *J PeriAnesth Nurs (Suppl)* 21(2A):S1-S29, 2006.

Couture D, Maye J, O'Brien D, et al: Therapeutic modalities for the prophylactic management of postoperative nausea and vomiting, *J PeriAnesth Nurs* 21(6):398-403, 2006.

Drake R, Vogl W, Mitchell A: *Gray's anatomy for students*, Philadelphia, 2005, Churchill Livingstone.

Evers A, Maze M: *Anesthetic pharmacology: physiologic principles and clinical practice*, Philadelphia, 2004, Churchill Livingstone.

Fisher L: *Benumof's anesthesia and uncommon diseases*, ed 5, Philadelphia, 2007, Saunders.

*Review of medical physiology*, ed 22, New York, 2005, McGraw-Hill Medical.

Golembiewski J, Tokumaru S: Pharmacological prophylaxis and management of adult postoperative/postdischarge nausea and vomiting, *J PeriAnesth Nurs* 21(6):385-397, 2006.

Guyton A, Hall J: *Textbook of medical physiology*, ed 11, Philadelphia, 2006, Saunders.

Hiley M, Giesecke A: The patient with a full stomach, *Semin Anesth* 9(3):204-210, 1990.

Jacobs B, Swift C, Dubow H, et al: Time required for oral ranitidine to decrease gastric fluid acidity, *Anesth Analg* 73:787-789, 1991.

Kier L, Dowd C: *The chemistry of drugs for nurse anesthetists*, Chicago, 2004, AANA Publishing, Inc.

Lake C, Hines R, Blitt C: *Clinical monitoring: practical applications for anesthesia and critical care*, Philadelphia, 2001, Saunders.

Longnecker D, Murphy F: *Dripps, Eckenhoff, Vandam introduction to anesthesia*, ed 9, Philadelphia, 1997, Saunders.

Longnecker D, Tinker J, Morgan G: *Principles and practice of anesthesiology*, ed 2, St Louis, 1998, Mosby.

Mamaril M, Windle P, Burkard J: Prevention and management of postoperative nausea and vomiting: a look at complementary techniques, *J PeriAnesth Nurs* 21(6):404-410, 2006.

Miller R, editor: *Anesthesia*, ed 5, Philadelphia, 2000, Churchill Livingstone.

Murphy M, Hooper V, Sullivan E, et al: Identification of risk factors for postoperative nausea and vomiting in the perianesthesia adult patient, *J PeriAnesth Nurs* 21(6):377-384, 2006.

Nagelhout J, Zaglaniczy K: *Nurse anesthesia*, ed 3, St Louis, 2005, Saunders.

Odom-Forren J, Fetzer S, Moser D: Evidence-based interventions for post discharge nausea and vomiting: a review of the literature, *J PeriAnesth Nurs* 21(6):411-430, 2006.

Palmer A, Waugaman W, Conklin K, et al: Does the administration of oral bicitrate before elective cesarean section affect the incidence of nausea and vomiting in the parturient? *Nurse Anesth* 2(3):126-133, 1991.

Roberts A: Post anesthesia care of the biliary lithotripsy patient, *J PostAnesth Nurs* 56:392-396, 1990.

Shorten G, Browne J, Carr D, et al: *Postoperative pain management: an evidence-based guide to practice*, Philadelphia, 2006, Saunders.

Stoelting R: *Pharmacology and physiology in anesthetic practice*, ed 3, Philadelphia, 1999, Lippincott-Raven.

Stoelting R, Miller R: *Basics of anesthesia*, ed 4, Philadelphia, 2000, Churchill Livingstone.

Townsend C, Beauchamp R, Evers B, et al: *Sabiston textbook of surgery: the biological basis of modern surgical practice*, ed 17, Philadelphia, 2004, Saunders.

Vila P: Acid aspiration prophylaxis in morbidly obese patients: famotidine versus ranitidine, *Anesthesia* 46:967-969, 1991.

PHYSIOLOGIC CONSIDERATIONS IN THE PACU

# 17

# THE INTEGUMENTARY SYSTEM

Cecil B. Drain, PhD, RN, CRNA, FAAN, FASAHP

The integumentry system is the body's first line of defense against many pathologic substances. Certainly, in the hospital setting, patients are at risk for many unwanted infections caused by pathogens that continue their viability in the building and its contents. Chapter 5 provides an in depth discussion of infection control in the postanesthesia care unit (PACU). The intent of this chapter is to provide the reader with the anatomy and physiology of the integumentary system for a basis of understanding of infection control and aseptic technique and an overview of the patient with thermal injury (see also Chapter 45). The integumentary system performs many functions that influence the perianesthesia nursing interventions in the PACU. A firm understanding of the integumentary system facilitates the perianesthesia nursing care provided to the patient with a compromised first line of defense: the integumentary system.

## DEFINITIONS

**Chilblain:** Trauma caused by exposure to cold temperatures above freezing and associated with high humidity.

**Desquamation:** The process by which dead cells are shed at a fairly constant rate.

**Frostbite:** Trauma caused by the crystallization of tissue fluids in the skin or subcutaneous tissue.

**Immersion Foot:** Trauma that occurs when the skin of the foot is exposed to water that is below 10° C (50° F) for a long period.

## INTEGUMENTARY SYSTEM ANATOMY

The skin, or integument, provides a boundary between the internal and external environments of the body. The surface area covered by the skin is about 1.8m$^2$ in the average male and 1.6 m$^2$ in the average female and accounts for 15% of the total body weight. The skin is divided into two major layers: the epidermis and the dermis, which includes the hypodermis.

## The Epidermis

The epidermis consists of stratified squamous epithelium and has no blood vessels. The cells of the innermost, or basal, layer (stratum basale or stratum germinativum) of the epidermis are constantly dividing and producing cells of the outer layers. Basal cell cancer develops from this layer. The prickly layer, or stratum spinosum, which is located immediately above the basal layer, consists of cells that are connected by intercellular bridges. Squamous cell cancer arises from this layer (Fig. 17-1).

The granular layer, or stratum granulosum, contains three or four layers of cells. Squamous epithelial cells are converted in this layer into hard material with a process called cornification. The next layer, the stratum lucidum, develops only on the palms of the hands and the soles of the feet. The outermost epidermal layer, called the horny layer or stratum corneum, comprises dead cells, keratin, surface lipids, and dirt. Dead cells are shed at a fairly constant rate with a process called desquamation. The epidermis also has keratinizing and glandular appendages. Keratinizing appendages comprise the hair and the nails, and glandular appendages include the sweat, scent, and sebaceous glands.

## The Dermis

The dermis, or corium, lies below the epidermis and consists of collagenous, elastic, and reticular fibers. It also contains blood vessels, nerves, lymphatics, and smooth muscle.

## The Hypodermis

The hypodermis functions as a shock absorber and heat insulator. Located under the dermis, it comprises fat, smooth muscle, and areolar tissue.

## INTEGUMENTARY FUNCTIONS

The skin has many important functions, the most important of which is to act as a barrier between the internal and external environments. In addition, skin plays an important

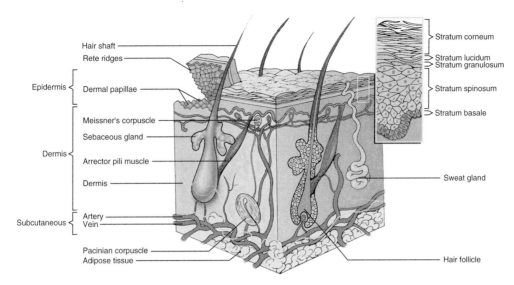

**Fig. 17-1** Layers of epidermis. *(From Monahan FD, Sands, J, Neighbors M, et al:* Medical-surgical nursing health and illness perspectives, *ed 8, St Louis, 2007, Mosby.)*

part in body temperature and fluid regulation, excretion, secretion, vitamin D production, sensation, appearance, and many other functions that have yet to be identified.

### Thermoregulation

Skin, subcutaneous tissue, and fat in the subcutaneous tissue provide heat insulation for the body. Heat is lost from the body to the surroundings by radiation, conduction, convection, and evaporation (Fig. 17-2). Radiation of heat from the body accounts for about 60% of the total heat loss. In this mechanism, heat is lost in the form of infrared heat waves. Conduction of heat to objects represents about 3% of the total heat loss, whereas conduction of heat to the air represents about 15% of the total heat loss. When water is carried away from the skin by air currents, convection of heat occurs. Evaporation constitutes about 22% of the heat loss. Even without sweating, water still evaporates from

the skin and the lungs. This insensible loss is about 600 mL per day.

The skin regulates body temperature by conserving heat in a cold environment. Sweating can lower the body temperature in hot environments. The sweat glands are innervated by the sympathetic and parasympathetic nervous systems. When the anterior hypothalamus in the preoptic area is stimulated by excess heat, impulses are sent from this area by way of the autonomic pathways to the spinal cord. From the spinal cord through the sympathetic outflow tracts, the impulses go to the skin all over the body. The sweat glands are innervated by sympathetic nerve fibers. However, in these specific fibers, the neurotransmitter is acetylcholine. Consequently, these fibers are actually sympathetic cholinergic nerve fibers and are stimulated by epinephrine or norepinephrine.

The sweat gland consists of two portions: a deep subdermal coiled portion that secretes the sweat and a duct portion that conducts the sweat to the skin. Sweat has a pH of 3.8 to 6.5 and contains sodium, chloride, potassium, calcium, lactic acid, and urea. Therefore, sweating is an act of excretion and secretion.

### Protection

The skin protects the body from injurious physical, chemical, electric, thermal, or biologic stimuli. Of particular importance to the perianesthesia nurse is the presence of bacteria on the skin that may cause sepsis when a patient's skin barrier is broken. Normal flora of the skin include gram-positive cocci and rods. Diphtheroids are also widely distributed on the

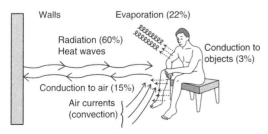

**Fig. 17-2** Major mechanisms of heat loss from body. *(From Guyton A, Hall J:* Textbook of medical physiology, *ed 11, Philadelphia, 2006, Saunders.)*

skin, especially in moist areas. The normal pH of the skin is 4 to 6, from lactic acid and amino acid residues of keratinization.

When intact, the skin stops pathogenic organisms from entering the body and at the same time prevents the loss of water, electrolytes, and proteins to the external environment. Once the skin is broken (e.g., with surgical incision or venipuncture), the barrier between the internal and external environments is broken, which is why aseptic technique is important whenever opening of the skin is anticipated or has occurred.

## IMPORTANCE OF ASEPTIC TECHNIQUE

Because all skin has pathogenic organisms on it, skin can never be sterile. Precautions should be taken to reduce the number of pathogenic organisms that may be introduced into a wound. Handwashing technique is most important. This technique should be accomplished before care is given to the patient. A good mechanical scrub with a skin antiseptic, such as a soap that contains iodine, should be done.

The surgical wound site should be kept clean, and the dressings should remain sterile. If any question arises about sterility because of excess bleeding, fluid, or physical contamination, the dressing should be changed. Special precautions to reduce the introduction of pathogenic organisms should be taken with patients who are prone to infection. This group includes patients who are obese, anemic, or debilitated; those with vascular insufficiency, chronic obstructive pulmonary disease, and diabetes mellitus; and those with an immune deficiency, including patients who are undergoing chemotherapy or chronic steroid therapy or who have acquired immunodeficiency syndrome (AIDS). Aseptic technique in wound care for these patients should include the wearing of a surgical mask and the use of sterile gloves and drapes.

### Universal Precautions in the Postanesthesia Care Unit

The Centers for Disease Control (CDC) developed the "Universal Precautions for Prevention of Transmission of the Human Immunodeficiency Virus (HIV) and Hepatitis B Virus (HBV) in Healthcare Settings," and the Occupational Health and Safety Administration's (OSHA) universal standards are presented as a supplement to the CDC precautions. These two documents are discussed in Chapter 5 with more complete information on the universal precautions in the PACU along with the OSHA's most current document.

### Sterile Technique for Intravenous Therapy

Establishment of an intravenous infusion should be accomplished with sterile technique. The site chosen for cannula (needle) placement should be prepared in a suitable fashion. An excellent method uses 1% iodine in 70% isopropyl alcohol. After at least 30 seconds of drying time, the iodine solution should be washed off with 70% isopropyl alcohol. Both agents should be applied with friction, from the center of the field to the periphery. An iodophor skin preparation may be substituted in patients with sensitive skin but should not be washed off with alcohol because its antibacterial action may depend in part on the sustained release of free iodine. In the rare instance in which iodine preparations cannot be tolerated at all, vigorous prolonged (more than 1 minute) washing with 70% isopropyl alcohol is acceptable.

After the intravenous administration route is established, the cannula (needle) should be securely anchored to prevent irritating to-and-from motion and to avoid potential transport of cutaneous bacteria into the puncture wound. Although evidence is not conclusive, additional protection from infectious complications may follow topical antimicrobial applications to the infusion site. Because study results have shown that antibiotic ointments may actually favor the selective growth of fungi, the use of topical antiseptic iodophor ointment should be considered. The intravenous site should be covered with a sterile dressing.

### Burn Injuries

The postoperative care of the patient with burn injury can be most challenging to the perianesthesia nurse. These patients usually have a complex array of pathophysiologic difficulties, from deranged fluid and electrolyte balance, respiratory complications, and disrupted temperature regulation to psychologic disturbances. A burn, no matter how small, represents a total body assault.

Infection is the most common and the most dreaded complication after a burn injury; therefore, aseptic skin care is of primary importance. Nursing care of the patient with a burn injury is complex; the reader should refer to Chapter 45 for discussion of specific pathophysiologic processes, assessment, and nursing interventions for the patient with burn injury in the PACU.

The four main types of burn injuries include cold, chemical, electric, and thermal. A cold injury is trauma caused by exposure to cold. Conditions such as frostbite, chilblain, immersion foot, and trench foot are the result. Frostbite results from the crystallization of tissue fluids in the skin or subcutaneous tissue. Chilblain results from exposure to cold temperatures above freezing associated with high humidity. Immersion foot occurs when the skin of the foot is exposed to water that is below 10° C for a long period.

Chemical burns are produced by caustic agents, either acid or base. These burns are devastating because without appropriate emergency treatment, the agents continue to cause destruction of fascia, fat, muscle, and bone.

Electric burns, which result from direct contact with electric voltage, are deceiving in appearance. Although only the entrance and exit wounds may be visible, massive damage is often sustained as the high-energy sources follow conductive muscle and nerves. Damage may necessitate amputation of extremities. Thermal injury often occurs in addition to the electric burn from the heat of arcing currents or ignited clothing.

The most common type of burn injury is the thermal burn, which is caused by excessive heat. Metabolic derangement and problems in maintenance of thermal control develop. Unless otherwise indicated, this discussion refers to thermal burns. The terms partial thickness, deep dermal, and full thickness are commonly used in the classification of burn injuries. The terms first degree, second degree, third degree, and sometimes fourth degree are based on the characteristics and surface appearance of the burn wound.

A partial-thickness burn heals without grafting. Grafting occurs when only part of the skin has been damaged or destroyed but enough epithelial cells remain in the skin to provide new epidermis, which includes hair follicles and sweat glands. The partial-thickness burn can also be referred to as a first-degree or second-degree burn. Partial-thickness burns can be divided into three categories: (1) superficial burns, in which partial skin loss is seen but no dermal death and therefore no slough; (2) intermediate partial-thickness burn, typically characterized by healing from the level of the hair follicles; and (3) deep partial-thickness burn, which typically heals from the level of the sweat ducts.

A deep-dermal burn is a partial-thickness burn that can heal without grafting. However, if the burn is complicated by infection or mechanical trauma, it is likely to be converted into a full-thickness burn.

Full-thickness burns cause destruction of all the skin. No viable epithelial elements are present, and destruction of the subcutaneous tissue, muscles, and bones may be seen. The wound must be grafted because the skin does not regenerate. The full-thickness burn is equivalent to the third-degree burn. Destruction of the full-thickness burn that extends to the structures underneath the skin to include the bone is called a fourth-degree burn.

## SUMMARY

The anatomy and physiology of the integumentary system was presented in detail. Also, an overview was presented on the subjects of aseptic technique, universal precautions, and burn injuries. In light of all the possible invasive pathogens such as HIV and hepatitis B, the perianesthesia nurse must have a firm understanding of the basics of the integumentary system as presented here. For a more comprehensive description of PACU infection control, see Chapter 5 for aseptic technique; and for care of the patient with burn injury, see Chapter 45.

## BIBLIOGRAPHY

Aitkenhead A, Smith G, Rowbotham D: *Textbook of anesthesia*, ed 5, Philadelphia, 2007, Churchill Livingstone.

Alspach J: *Core curriculum for critical care nursing*, ed 6, Philadelphia, 2005, Saunders.

Atlee J: *Complications in anesthesia*, ed 2, Philadelphia, 2007, Saunders.

Barash P, Cullen B, Stoelting R: *Clinical anesthesia*, ed 5, Philadelphia, 2001, Lippincott Williams & Wilkins.

Benumof J, Saidman L: *Anesthesia & perioperative complications*, ed 2, St Louis, 1999, Mosby.

Drake R, Vogl W, Mitchell A: *Gray's anatomy for students*, Philadelphia, 2005, Churchill Livingstone.

Evers A, Maze M: *Anesthetic pharmacology: physiologic principles and clinical practice*, Philadelphia, 2004, Churchill Livingstone.

Fisher L: *Benumof's anesthesia and uncommon diseases*, ed 5, Philadelphia, 2007, Saunders.

Ganong W: *Review of medical physiology*, ed 22, New York, 2005, McGraw-Hill Medical.

Graham-Brown R, Bourke J: *Mosby's color atlas and text of dermatology*, ed 2, St Louis, 2007, Mosby.

Guyton A, Hall J: *Textbook of medical physiology*, ed 11, Philadelphia, 2006, Saunders.

Habif T, et al: *Skin disease: diagnosis and treatment*, ed 2, St Louis, 2005, Mosby.

Nagelhout J, Zaglaniczy K: *Nurse anesthesia*, ed 3, St Louis, 2005, Saunders.

Stoelting R: *Pharmacology and physiology in anesthetic practice*, ed 3, Philadelphia, 1999, Lippincott-Raven.

Stoelting R, Miller R: *Basics of anesthesia*, ed 4, Philadelphia, 2000, Churchill Livingstone.

Townsend C, Beauchamp R, Evers B, et al: *Sabiston textbook of surgery: the biological basis of modern surgical practice*, ed 17, Philadelphia, 2004, Saunders.

# 18

## THE IMMUNE SYSTEM

Cecil B. Drain, PhD, RN, CRNA, FAAN, FASAHP

During the past three decades, a virtual explosion of information about the immune system has occurred. Diseases once believed to be based in other physiologic systems are now found, as a result of medical research, to have bases in the immune system. For example, myasthenia gravis was once thought to be a neuromuscular disease; however, research has shown the origin of the disease to be in the immune system. Today, in the postanesthesia care unit (PACU), perianesthesia nurses must treat patients with immunosuppression or hypersensitivity reaction or patients who have immune diseases such as acquired immunodeficiency syndrome (AIDS). An informed appreciation of the physiology and pathophysiology of the immune system is essential for the appropriate perianesthesia care of the surgical patient.

## DEFINITIONS

**Acquired Immunity:** The ability of the human body to develop an extremely powerful specific immunity against most invading agents.

**Active Acquired Immunity:** Immunity that develops when a person comes into direct contact with a pathogen either by contracting the disease produced by the pathogen or by vaccination against the disease.

**Antibody:** A globulin molecule with the potential to attack agents that are foreign to the host.

**Antigen:** A protein, large polysaccharide, or large lipoprotein complex that stimulates the process of acquired immunity.

**B Lymphocytes or Bursa-Dependent Cells:** Immunocompetent lymphocytes that are named for the preprocessing that occurs in the bursa of Fabricius of birds and is responsible for humoral immunity.

**Cellular or Cell-Mediated Immunity:** A type of acquired immunity that uses sensitized lymphocytes as the primary defense.

**Clone:** A group of cells that originate from a single parent cell.

**Hapten:** A substance that has a low molecular weight and combines with an antigenic substance to elicit an immune response.

**Humoral Immunity:** A type of acquired immunity that uses antibodies as the primary defense.

**Immunity:** The ability of the human body to resist almost all types of organisms or toxins that can damage tissues and organs.

**Immunodeficiency Disease:** Immunosuppression that results from a deficiency of a single humoral antibody group or from a combined deficiency of both T-cell and B-cell systems.

**Immunosuppression:** A state of nonresponsiveness of the immune system to antigenic challenge.

**Innate Immunity:** General processes in the human body, other than those of acquired immunity, that are responsible for protection against organisms and toxins.

**Lymphopenia:** Decreased function of the lymphoid organs.

**Passive Acquired Immunity:** Immunity that results when a person receives immune cells or immune serum produced by someone else.

**Phagocytosis:** The envelopment and digestion of bacteria or other foreign substances.

**Sensitized Lymphocytes:** Lymphocytes that are made competent by processing to facilitate immunologic activity, such as attachment to and destruction of a foreign agent.

**Stem Cells:** Unspecialized cells that give rise to specific specialized cells such as T and B lymphocytes.

**T Lymphocytes:** Sensitized lymphocytes that are responsible for cellular immunity.

## PHYSICAL AND CHEMICAL BARRIERS

The body's first line of immunologic defense is the mechanical barrier provided by the epithelial surface. Some parts of the epithelium have extensions from their surface, such as the cilia and the mucus in the respiratory system. These extensions provide not only an additional physical barrier to the entrance of foreign substances but also an efficient removal system. In the stomach, hydrochloric acid, which is thought to have bactericidal action, is secreted. As an additional defense, the skin produces chemicals that inactivate bacteria. The surfaces of the boundary tissues also have specific defenses in the form of secretory antibodies. Consequently, surgical incisions, intravenous cannulation, and many other invasive procedures can cause major breaks in the first line of defense. Hence, the perianesthesia nurse should use good aseptic or sterile technique for prevention of an overwhelming bacterial invasion through the boundary tissues.

## INNATE IMMUNITY

Innate or nonspecific immunity is the body's second line of immunologic defense against foreign material. In this type of immunity, activation occurs during each exposure to an invading substance. Recognition does occur at the level of distinguishing between self and nonself; however, the mechanisms of innate immunity cannot identify the specific invader.

Phagocytosis is the primary mechanism of innate immunity. The cells in the body that carry out the phagocytic functions of innate immunity are monocytes, which are macrophages, and neutrophils (polymorphonuclear leukocytes), which are microphages. The overall immunologic functions of phagocytes are to localize the antigen and to destroy, inactivate, or process it for handling by other components of the immune system. The process of phagocytosis can be enhanced with the combination of an antigen and a plasma protein called opsonin, a substance associated with the immune system. Finally, phagocytosis gives transitory protection to the body so that it is not overwhelmed by foreign materials before the immune system (acquired immunity) is activated.

## ACQUIRED IMMUNITY

Acquired or adaptive immunity is the body's third line of immunologic defense. Acquired immunity is mediated by the capability of specific antibodies or sensitized lymphocytes to recognize and to react to antigens from the offending agent. The following two closely allied types of acquired immune mechanisms occur in the body: humoral immunity and cellular (cell-mediated) immunity.

### Humoral Immunity
Humoral immunity is conferred by circulating antibodies that are found in the globulin fraction of blood proteins and are therefore called immunoglobulins (Ig). The processing that is involved

in production of the immunoglobulin begins with the lymphocytic stem cells in the bone marrow. These stem cells, which are incapable of forming antibodies, make pre–B lymphocytes that are taken up by the lymph nodes and processed in the as yet unidentified "bursa-equivalent" tissue to become mature immunocompetent B lymphocytes. These processed B lymphocytes are then released into the blood, where they become entrapped in the lymphoid tissue. On stimulation with an antigen, the B lymphocyte specific for that antigen enlarges, divides, and differentiates into plasma cells that have specificity for that antigen. The plasma cells then produce and secrete an antibody or sensitized lymphocyte. During the first exposure to the antigen, lymphocytes from one specific type of lymphoid tissue form clones. The clones are responsive only to the antigen responsible for initial development. On the second stimulation by the same antigen, the clones proliferate rapidly, thus leading to the formation of a large amount of antibody. Some cells in this clone mature to form plasma cells, whereas other cells of the clone become B lymphocyte memory cells. When the immune system responds to the first presentation of the antigen, the immune system remembers the antigen by means of the B lymphocyte memory cell. The immune system can remember the antigen for years. In other words, on the first stimulation by an antigen, the plasma cells produce antibodies (immunoglobulins) as the primary response. The primary response is usually evident about 4 to 10 days after the initial exposure to the antigen. On the second stimulation by the same antigen, a second response occurs. This secondary response, in which a massive amount of antibody specific to the antigen is produced within 1 or 2 days, lasts for months. The secondary response is more rapid, stronger, and more persistent than the primary response because of the memory cells and clones that are produced by the initial exposure to the antigen. If the T lymphocytes are activated by the same antigen, the T-lymphocyte helper cells enhance the response of the B lymphocytes. Therefore, because of this cooperative effort, the total number of lymphocytes in the lymphoid tissue increases markedly. On second exposure to an antigen, the same plasma cell can produce the particular antibody needed and can convert from one type of antibody secretion to another as needed. Once the specific antibodies from the plasma cells are no longer needed, further production of the antibodies is suppressed by the antibodies themselves or by T-lymphocyte suppressor cells (Fig. 18-1).

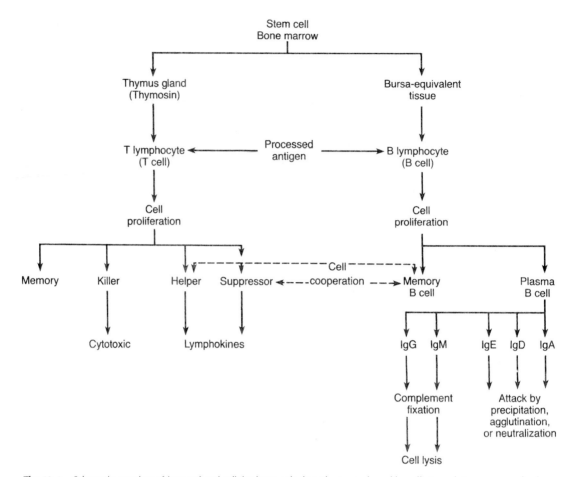

**Fig. 18-1**   Schematic overview of humoral and cellular immunologic pathways and resulting effector substances or mechanisms of activity.

The immunoglobulins are large proteins with specific structural arrangements of polypeptide chains with specific amino acid sequences. The immunoglobulins are divided into five primary classes on the basis of structural arrangements: IgA, IgD, IgE, IgG, and IgM.

Immunoglobulin A is a small molecule that constitutes about 15% of the total immunoglobulins and is present in most body secretions. This antibody activates complement through the alternate properidin pathway. Also, secretory immunity is mediated by IgA. The secretory antibodies are found on the mucosal surfaces of the oral cavity, the lungs, and the intestinal and urogenital tracts and in mammary secretions. This secretory IgA differs from other antibodies in that it has a protein molecule, called a secretory piece, attached to it. Secretory IgA is effective against viruses and some bacteria.

Immunoglobulin D constitutes about 1% of the total immunoglobulins. The exact function of IgD is unknown. However, this

immunoglobulin may be involved with the differentiation of the B lymphocytes, and a relationship has been suggested between IgD and antibody activity directed toward insulin, penicillin, milk proteins, diphtheria toxoid, thyroid antigens, and the products of abnormal tissue growth.

Immunoglobulin E is present in minute quantities (about 0.002% of total serum immunoglobulins) and is associated with type I immediate hypersensitivity reaction.

Immunoglobulin G is the smallest antibody and constitutes about 75% of the total plasma antibodies. IgG is the only antibody that can cross the placental barrier and thus confer passive immunity to the fetus. IgG is the primary antibody involved in the secondary response. It is active against many bloodborne infectious agents such as bacteria, viruses, parasites, and some fungi.

Immunoglobulin M is the largest antibody; it constitutes about 10% of plasma antibody.

IgM is the main antibody involved in the primary antibody response, and it fixes complement.

Antibodies, once secreted by the plasma cells, protect the body against invading agents with the following three mechanisms of action: (1) attacking the antigen; (2) activating the complement system, which results in cell lysis; and (3) activating the immediate hypersensitivity reaction, which localizes the invader and may negate its virulence. More specifically, antibodies can inactivate the invading antigen with precipitation, agglutination, neutralization, or complement fixation. Precipitation occurs when an insoluble antibody forms a complex with a soluble antigen (such as tetanus toxin) and the resulting antigen-antibody complex becomes insoluble and precipitates. When antigens are bound together and react with an antibody, agglutinated aggregates occur. Neutralization is achieved when antibodies cover the toxic sites of an antigenic agent or when antibodies counteract toxins released by bacteria. Rarely are the potent antibodies able to attack a cell membrane directly and cause lysis. However, one of the powerful effects of the binding of the antigen-antibody complex is the activation of complement, which serves to amplify this interaction. More specifically, when IgG or IgM binds to an antigen, the complement system is activated and a cascade system of nine different enzyme precursors (C1 through C9) reacts sequentially. The final result of the activation of the complement system is puncture of the antigen's cell membrane (cell lysis) and thus rupture of its cellular agents.

### Cellular Immunity

Cellular immunity is the second type of specific immunity; it uses T lymphocytes and macrophages. Some specific functions of the cellular immunity system are protection against most viruses, slow-acting bacteria, and fungal infections; mediation of cutaneous delayed hypersensitivity reactions; rejection of foreign grafts; and immunologic surveillance.

The T lymphocytes, like the B lymphocytes, originate from primitive stem cells and go through stages of maturation (see Fig. 18-1). Once the immature lymphocyte leaves the bone marrow, it migrates to the thymus gland, where it is acted on by the hormone thymosin. The T lymphocyte then becomes mature and immunocompetent. Thus, it is a thymus-dependent, or T lymphocyte. These mature T lymphocytes can circulate in the blood and lymph, or they may come to rest in the inner cortex of the lymph nodes, where they may form subgroups of T lymphocytes.

These T lymphocytes function overall in the immune system by serving in regulatory, effector, and cytotoxic capacities. The regulatory T lymphocytes are the helper or suppressor T lymphocytes. These lymphocytes amplify or suppress responses of other T lymphocytes or responses of B lymphocytes. The helper T lymphocytes produce a soluble factor that is necessary, in some instances, for antibody formation by B lymphocytes. This helper action is most important for IgE and IgG production. The underproduction of helper cells is associated with AIDS. The suppressor T lymphocytes appear to regulate or suppress the activity of B lymphocytes in the production of antibodies. Evidence indicates that the suppressor T lymphocytes can become pathologically active against helper T lymphocytes and other aspects of cellular immunity. For this reason, these suppressor T lymphocytes may have a role in immune tolerance and in the development of autoimmune disease, such as myasthenia gravis. Effector T lymphocytes are probably responsible for the delayed hypersensitivity reactions, the rejection of foreign tissue grafts and tumors, and the elimination of viral-infected cells. Effector T lymphocytes have antigen receptors on their surfaces that are significant in the initiation of cellular immunity. When an antigen enters the body, it undergoes processing by the phagocytes. The antigen then travels to the regional lymph node, which drains the area of antigen invasion. In this lymph node, the T lymphocyte recognizes the antigen, binds to the antigen, and proliferates. The T lymphocyte becomes sensitized when it comes into contact with the antigen. In addition, memory T lymphocytes result from this interaction. Hence, on a second exposure to the antigen, a more intense, efficient, and rapid cellular immunity results. This contact also results in the release of lymphokines by the T lymphocyte. Some of the lymphokines are: (1) chemotactic factor, which recruits phagocytes into the area; (2) migration inhibitory factor, which prevents the migration of phagocytes away from the area; (3) transfer factor, which induces noncommitted T lymphocytes to form T lymphocytes of the same antigen-specific clone as the original cells; (4) lymphotoxin, which is a nonspecific cellular toxin; and (5) interferon, which inhibits the replication of viruses.

The direct cellular cytotoxicity that is mediated by cellular immunity involves cytotoxic lymphocytes, or killer cells, and macrophages. The role of these cytotoxic T lymphocytes is not well established; however, they are believed to be involved in nonspecific killing of viruses, rejection of allografts, and immune surveillance of malignant diseases.

## HYPERSENSITIVITY REACTIONS

The immune system serves mainly as protection from harmful substances. However, in some instances, the activation of the immune system can cause deleterious effects, which is termed allergic response or hypersensitivity reaction. Briefly, this response represents a magnified or inappropriate reaction by the host to an antigenic substance; it can result in immunologic disease. Hypersensitivity reactions are divided into four major categories called type I through type IV hypersensitivity reactions (Table 18-1).

### Type I Hypersensitivity Reaction (Anaphylactic, Immediate)
Type I hypersensitivity reaction occurs in persons who were previously sensitized to a specific antigen. The antibodies formed against that antigen are of the IgE classification. The term reagins is used to describe these IgE antibodies. Reaginic antibodies bind to mast cells in tissues that surround the blood vessels and to blood basophils. When the previously sensitized host is reexposed to the same antigen, the antigen reacts with the reaginic antibody that is attached to the cell and an immediate swelling and then rupture of the basophil or mast cell results in a release of chemical mediators into the local environment. These chemical mediators include: (1) histamine, which causes local

vasodilatation and increased permeability of the capillaries; (2) slow-reacting substance of anaphylaxis, which causes prolonged contraction of some smooth muscle, such as that of the bronchi; (3) chemotactic factor, which draws neutrophils and macrophages into the area of the antigen-antibody reaction; and (4) lysosomal enzymes, which elicit a local inflammatory reaction. These chemical mediators act on the "shock organs," such as the mucosa, skin, bronchi, and heart. The resulting clinical manifestations of the type I reaction include urticaria, allergic rhinitis, allergic asthma, and, in severe cases, systemic anaphylaxis.

### Type II Hypersensitivity Reaction (Cytotoxic)
In the type II hypersensitivity reaction, the antigen and the antibody complex react, thereby injuring the cell membrane or a surface tissue with direct destruction by antibody of cellular elements. The antibodies involved in the type II reaction are either IgG or IgM, and the reaction is enhanced by complement. Hemolytic anemia is an example of a type II reaction that affects the red blood cells (RBCs). For example, when penicillin is absorbed on the RBC membrane, the interaction of antipenicillin antibody, penicillin, and complement causes a reaction that results in the lysis of RBCs.

### Type III Hypersensitivity Reaction (Arthus)
The type III hypersensitivity reaction involves the formation of immune complexes of antigen and antibody (IgG or IgM). These immune complexes precipitate in and around small vessels

**Table 18-1   Categories of Hypersensitivity Reactions**

| Type | Mechanism | Outcome | Reaction Time | Examples |
|---|---|---|---|---|
| I (Anaphylactic) | Antigen-IgE reaction at surface of mast cells and basophils | Release of mediators | Immediate | Asthma Hay fever Systemic anaphylaxis |
| II (Cytotoxic) | Binding of IgM or IgG with antigens on surface of cell; enhanced by complement fixation | Cell lysis and tissue damage | Variable | Hemolytic anemia Goodpasture's disease |
| III (Arthus) | Microprecipitation of immune complex formed by antigen and IgM or IgG; enhanced by complement fixation | Tissue damage and release of vasoactive substances | 4-18 h | Serum sickness Farmer's lung Allergic alveolitis Glomerulonephritis SLE |
| IV (Delayed) | Direct interaction of antigen with sensitized T lymphocytes | Release of mediators and tissue damage | 24-48 h | Contact dermatitis Tuberculosis |

*SLE*, Systemic lupus erythematosus.

and damage the target tissue by activating complement. Also involved in this process is an inflammatory reaction that is initiated by the gathering of inflammatory cells and the release of vasoactive amines from platelets. As this process continues, polymorphonuclear leukocytes phagocytize the immune complexes and cause inflammation and necrosis of the blood vessels and surrounding tissue because of the release of lysosomal enzymes. Serum sickness and systemic lupus erythematosus are clinical examples of type III hypersensitivity reactions.

### Type IV Hypersensitivity Reaction (Delayed or Cell-Mediated)

Type IV hypersensitivity reaction is the only hypersensitivity reaction that does not involve antibodies. In the type IV reaction, the exposure to an antigen and the subsequent binding of the antigen with antigen-specific reactive T lymphocytes initiate the production of lymphokines from the T lymphocytes, with tissue damage as the end result. The antigen responsible for the type IV reaction can be bacterial, fungal, protozoan, or viral. Contact dermatitis, allograft rejection, and delayed response in tuberculin skin tests are examples of delayed hypersensitivity reactions.

## LATEX ALLERGY

The prevalence rate of confirmed allergic reactions among health care workers ranges from 5% to 10%. Moreover, recent studies indicate that about 8% to 12% of the health care population become sensitized to latex. Since 1987, when universal precautions were instituted to prevent the spread of human immunodeficiency virus (HIV), hepatitis viruses, and other infectious agents, health care workers have routinely worn latex gloves as a protective barrier. Also, the Occupational Safety and Health Administration (OSHA) instructed health care workers to wear protective material as a barrier. A great demand then occurred for surgical gloves, and hence, the accounts of the amount of latex proteins found in surgical gloves varied.

Many products contain latex; at home, these products include rubber bands, some carpets, earphones, and mouse pads. In the hospital setting, tourniquets, pressure cuff tubing, and urinary catheters often contain latex. In the perianesthesia area, possible routes of exposure include contact with mucosa, direct contact of particles with an open surgical wound, and aerosolized particles that are bound to the powder in the latex article. Interestingly, these particles can stay suspended for up to 5 hours.

The degree of reactions to latex varies; irritant contact dermatitis is basically a nonallergic reaction. Symptoms such as dry, itchy, or irritated areas that may be red and cracked usually occur within the first 6 to 24 hours after exposure. The reaction can be caused by exposure to powders added to the gloves, repeated hand washing and drying, or the use of cleaners and sanitizers. Because this reaction is not a true allergy, it usually clears up after the irritant is removed.

Allergic contact dermatitis is also a nonallergic reaction. Symptoms, which usually occur within 24 to 48 hours, include erythema, vesicles, papules, pruritus, blisters, and crusting of the area that touched the latex. This type of response is caused by the chemical additives that are used in the manufacture of latex and are usually thiurams or carbamates.

Of major concern is the type I immediate hypersensitivity, which is the IgE-mediated response. This response usually occurs within minutes of exposure to the latex; however, it can occur within a few hours in some cases. A mild reaction is characterized by skin redness, urticaria, and itching. Severe reactions can produce acute rhinorrhea, sneezing, angioedema, bronchospasm, and anaphylactic shock.

Many organizations are investigating latex allergies, and the American Society of Anesthesiologists (ASA) has a task force that can be found on the Internet at www.asahq.org/ProfInfo/latexallergy.html. Also, the American Association of Nurse Anesthetists has an excellent web site on latex allergies at www.aana.com/crna/prof/latex.asp. Other helpful sites are the National Institute for Occupational Safety and Health at www.cdc.gov/niosh/latex-alt.html, the Latex Allergy Home Page at www.netcom.com/~nam1/latex_allergy.html, and "How to manage a latex-allergic patient" at www.anes.com/lair/latex/manage.html.

The best treatment for a latex allergic response is avoidance. Patients who are at risk for an allergic reaction caused by latex are listed in Box 18-1. Health care personnel with known sensitivity should carry their own nonlatex gloves, usually made of vinyl or neoprene. They also should use nonlatex tourniquets and latex-free or glass syringes and should use stopcocks to inject drugs. Intravenous line tubing should have no latex ports, or if the latex ports exist, they should be taped. Box 18-2 summarizes the various recommendations for patients with known or risk of latex allergic reactions.

If a reaction to latex develops in the patient in the PACU, the first intervention is removal of the patient from ongoing exposure to the latex. The reactions can vary from mild

| Box 18-1 | Patients Who Should Be Strongly Considered at Risk for an Allergic Reaction to Latex |
|---|---|

- A complete medical history is the most reliable screening examination for prediction of a reaction to latex
- History of atopic immunologic reactions
- History of contact dermatitis
- A history of documented immunologic reactions during a medical or surgical procedure of unknown etiology
- A history of allergies to food products, including fruits, nuts, bananas, avocados, celery, figs, chestnuts, and papayas
- Neural tube defects, including spina bifida, myelomeningocele/meningocele, and lipomyelomeningocele
- Multiple operations in the past
- Chronic bladder catheterizations

respiratory reactions that can be treated on a symptomatic level; to hives, which can occur immediately to several hours after exposure; to a type I hypersensitivity anaphylactic reaction.

Treatment for the type I reaction should consist of first carefully looking for the latex allergen, such as rubber drains in the wound, inadvertent use of latex gloves, latex that contains urinary draining tubes, or intravenous (IV) tubing. One should remove all latex from the patient bedside; change gloves; discontinue antibiotics and blood administration; maintain the airway; administer 100% oxygen; intubate the trachea if necessary; and maintain intravascular volume support. Once the diagnosis of type I IgE-mediated anaphylaxsis has been confirmed, epinephrine should be administered intravenously in doses of 0.1 mg/kg and titrated to effect. These small doses stabilize the patient's condition and avoid ventricular tachycardia and malignant arrhythmias.

## IMMUNOSUPPRESSION

With the advent of organ transplantation, patients often arrive in the PACU in an

| Box 18-2 | Summary of the Recommendations for Perianesthesia Care of Patients with Known or Risk of Latex Allergic Reactions |
|---|---|

### PREOPERATIVE AND INTRAOPERATIVE CARE
- Remove all latex products from the operating room.
- Use a latex-free reservoir bag on anesthesia machine, oral airways, endotracheal tubes, and laryngeal mask airways.
- Use a latex-free breathing circuit with plastic mask and bag.
- Anesthesia ventilator must have a latex-free bellows.
- Place all monitoring devices, cords, and tubes (oximeter, blood pressure cuffs, electrocardiograph wires) in stockinet and secure with tape to prevent direct skin contact.
- Cover all rubber injection ports on IV bags with tape and label "Do not inject fluid through ports."
- Use intravenous tubing without latex ports or cover with tape.
- Use nonlatex gloves.
- Use nonlatex tourniquets.
- Draw medication directly from opened multidose vials.
- Draw up medications immediately before the beginning of the case.
- Use latex-free or glass syringes.
- Use stopcocks to inject drugs.

### POSTANESTHESIA PHASE OF CARE
- Place a sign on the door and flag the chart of the patient to alert personnel to the hypersensitivity.
- Ensure that patient recovers in a private area.
- Use good handwashing techniques.
- Use only latex-free syringes and gloves.
- Use ampules or remove stoppers from vials before use.
- Cover injection ports on minibags and use latex-free tubings.
- Remain alert for signs and symptoms (hypotension, tachycardia, and bronchospasm) of a latex allergy response and have appropriate emergency drugs and equipment available.

immunosuppressed state. Consequently, the perianesthesia nurse must have a basic knowledge of the forms of immunosuppression and the appropriate nursing care measures that can be implemented for the patient with immunosuppression.

## Forms of Immunosuppression

The nonresponsive state of the immune system may be caused by a natural tolerance to self-antigens, to a pathologic state, or to induced immunosuppression. Researchers are attempting to understand immunosuppression by artificially manipulating the immune system to produce a natural tolerance to self-antigens. Pathologic states such as lymphoma and leukemia are examples of the second form of immunosuppression, in which the immune system becomes unresponsive because of the pathologic changes in the immunocompetent cells. Induced immunosuppression can be accomplished with the administration of an antigen, antisera, or antibody; hormones and cytotoxic drugs; radiation; or surgery. For the most part, induced immunosuppression is used for tissue and organ transplants.

For patients with allergies, the administration of low-dose antigen provides relief in some instances from the antigen-antibody reaction. This desensitizing process produces antibodies that block the interaction between the antigen and the antibody-producing cells. Another method of provision of tolerance to self-antigens is with the administration of antisera or antibody in an attempt to coat the antigenic sites. The object is to prevent immunocompetent cells from combining with the antigen. This method of immunosuppression is 100% effective in prevention of Rh sensitization and ultimately erythroblastosis fetalis. Corticosteroids produce immunosuppression by reducing the amount of T and B lymphocytes that circulate in the blood, by blocking lymphokine release, and by decreasing the number of monocytes. Cytotoxic drugs are used in the treatment of cancer and autoimmune diseases. The most popular drugs are azathioprine and cyclophosphamide. These drugs suppress immune system function by killing unstimulated lymphocytes. X irradiation suppresses most of the immunocompetent cells with the induction of a profound lymphopenia. Surgical removal of the thymus gland, spleen, or lymph nodes may alter the immune response with removal of tissue needed for the maturation of both the cellular and the humoral immune systems.

## Perianesthesia Care of the Patient with Immunosuppression

The major responsibilities of the perianesthesia nurse who cares for the patient with immunosuppression are prevention of infection and early diagnosis and treatment of infection. Opinions differ in regard to placement of the patient who is nonleukopenic in protective isolation. However, if the peripheral leukocyte count is less than 2000 cells/mm$^3$, the patient probably will benefit from protective isolation. Before the patient is admitted to the PACU, sources of cross contamination should be eliminated. Blood pressure cuffs and other equipment that are to be used directly on the patient should be cleaned and disinfected with appropriate solutions. Aseptic technique should be followed at all times. In addition, needle puncture sites and surgical wounds should be cleaned and dressed with appropriate cleaners and ointments. If Foley catheters are used, open skin should be monitored closely for the beginning signs of infection. Patients with immunosuppression may not show the classic symptoms of infection. The temperature of the patient with immunosuppression should be closely monitored, and if it rises above 38° C, the attending physician should be notified immediately. Rectal thermometers should be avoided because they can cause mucosal injury and contamination.

## SUMMARY

The physiology of the immune system has been presented. This area of medical physiology has been enhanced in its degree of research and treatment with the onset of AIDS and the organ transplant surgeries that depend on drugs and such for suppression of the immune system. Many new pathophysiologic processes will be discovered in the near future that are related directly to the immune system.

## BIBLIOGRAPHY

American Association of Nurse Anesthetists: Latex allergy protocol, *J Am Assoc Nurs Anesthetists* 61:223-224, 1993.

Atlee J: *Complications in anesthesia*, Philadelphia, 1999, Saunders.

Barash P, Cullen B, Stoelting R: *Clinical anesthesia*, ed 3, Philadelphia, 1997, Lippincott.

Benumof J: *Anesthesia and uncommon diseases*, ed 4, Philadelphia, 1998, Saunders.

Benumof J, Saidman L: *Anesthesia & perioperative complications*, ed 2, St Louis, 1999, Mosby.

Floyd P: Latex allergy update, *J Perianesth Nurs* 15(1):26-30, 2000.

Gorringe-Moore R: Immunology and the lung. In Traver G, editor: *Respiratory nursing: the science and the art*, New York, 1982, John Wiley & Sons.

Grass J, Harris A: Postcesarean section analgesia, *Wellcome Trends Anesth* 9(6):3-8, 1991.

Groenwald S: Physiology of the immune system, *Heart Lung* 9(4):645-650, 1980.

Guyton A, Hall J: *Textbook of medical physiology*, ed 10, Philadelphia, 2000, Saunders.

Hardman J, Limbird L: *Goodman and Gilman's the pharmacological basis of therapeutics*, ed 9, New York, 1996, McGraw-Hill.

Holzman R: Managing the latex-allergic and latex-sensitive patient, *Audio-Digest Anesth* 42(11):1-2, 2000.

Jacobsen W: *Manual of perianesthesia care*, Philadelphia, 1992, Saunders.

Jocius M: Immunohematology and transfusion reaction, *AANA J* 50(1):42-48, 1982.

Katzung B: *Basic and clinical pharmacology*, ed 2, Los Altos, Calif, 1984, Lange Medical Publications.

Longnecker D, Tinker J, Morgan G: *Principles and practice of anesthesiology*, ed 2, St Louis, 1998, Mosby.

McIntosh L: *Essentials of nurse anesthesia*, New York, 1997, McGraw-Hill.

Miller R: *Anesthesia*, ed 3, New York, 1990, Churchill Livingstone.

Murray J: *The normal lung*, ed 2, Philadelphia, 1986, Saunders.

Nagelhout J, Zaglaniczny K: *Nurse anesthesia*, ed 2, Philadelphia, 2001, Saunders.

Paskawicz J, Chatwani A: Latex allergy: a concern for anesthesia personnel, *Am J Anesth* 28:435-441, 2001.

Rana A, Luskin A: Immunosuppression, autoimmunity, and hypersensitivity, *Heart Lung* 9(4): 651-657, 1980.

Spindler J, Mehlisch D, Brown C: Intramuscular ketorolac and morphine in the treatment of moderate to severe pain after major surgery, *Pharmacotherapy* 10:51S-58S, 1990.

Stites D, Stobo J, Fudenberg A, et al: *Basic and clinical immunology*, Los Altos, Calif, 1984, Lange Medical Publications.

Stoelting R: *Pharmacology and physiology in anesthetic practice*, ed 3, Philadelphia, 1999, Lippincott.

Stoelting R, Miller R: *Basics of anesthesia*, ed 4, New York, 2000, Churchill Livingstone.

Vance D: Interferon, *J Post Anesth Nurs* 2(1):43-44, 1987.

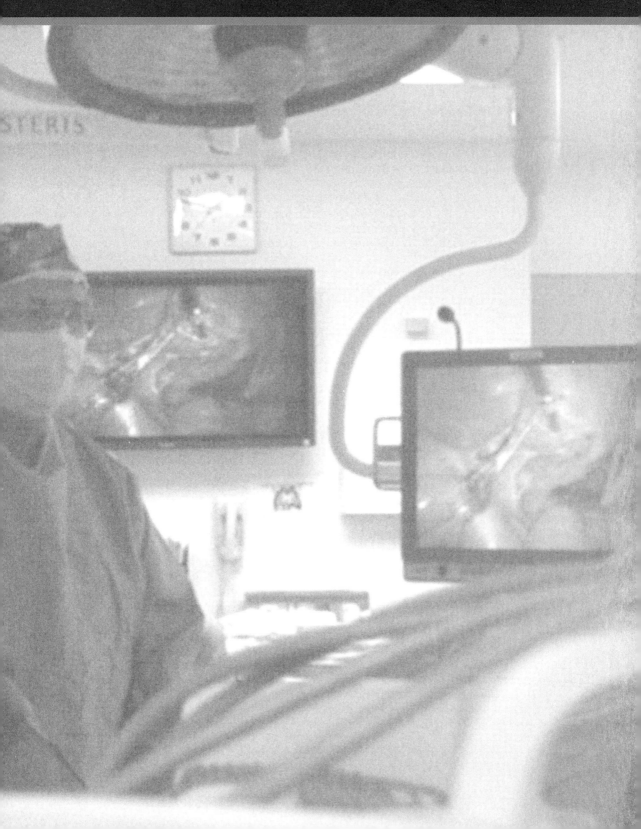

Section III

# CONCEPTS IN ANESTHETIC AGENTS

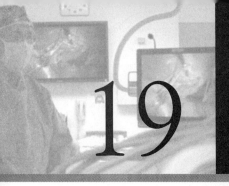

# 19

# BASIC PRINCIPLES OF PHARMACOLOGY

*Cecil B. Drain, PhD, RN, CRNA, FAAN, FASAHP*

The pharmacokinetics and pharmacodynamics of the drugs used in perianesthesia care are ever changing. Consequently, a complete review of the principles and concepts of pharmacology is presented in this chapter. The specific pharmacologies of drugs related to perianesthesia care are discussed in the physiology chapters in Section II, as are the concepts of anesthetic agents in the chapters in Section III. The pharmacology of the individual drug can be best understood in relation to the functions of the physiologic system that is most impacted by the particular drug or classification of drugs. Also, a discussion of the possible drug-drug interactions is presented in detail.

The final portion of this chapter provides an overview of drug interactions between anesthetic and nonanesthetic drugs and includes the herbal agents that can be purchased over the counter and herbal preparations. These concepts are discussed in detail because they are increasingly relevant to the perianesthesia nurse. Clinically, at least 10% of the patients for perianesthesia are taking some form of herbal preparation. With the growth of interest in the fields of drug interaction, drug surveillance, and clinical pharmacology, knowledge of drug actions is important in the care of the patient for perianesthesia. Consequently, knowledge of the principles of pharmacology becomes a meaningful and useful tool in the delivery of nursing care to the patient in the postanesthesia care unit (PACU).

## DEFINITIONS

**Additive Effect:** Occurs when a second drug with properties similar to the first is added to produce an effect equal to the algebraic sum of the effects of the two individual drugs.

**Agonists:** Drugs such as dopamine that attach and activate specific receptors.

**Antagonists:** Drugs such as Narcan that attach to a specific receptor and do not activate the receptor and that prevent the agonist from stimulating the receptor.

**Competitive Antagonist:** When the concentration of the antagonist is higher than the agonist concentration, which remains constant, with the result of antagonism of the agonist. This process is described in detail in regard to the pharmacology of the neuromuscular blocking drugs in Chapter 23.

**Cross Tolerance:** The result of two drugs with similar actions administered to a patient in whom tolerance has developed to that category of drugs (i.e., narcotics). The amount of each individual drug must be increased to achieve the desired effect. An example of cross tolerance is a patient with a heroin addiction who receives high-dose narcotics in the PACU for maintenance of minimal analgesia.

**Efficacy of a Drug:** Refers to the maximum effect that can be produced by a drug.

**Hyperreactivity:** An abnormal reaction to an unusually low dose of a drug. For example, patients with Addison's disease, myxedema, or dystrophia myotonica have hyperreactivity to unusually low doses of barbiturates.

**Hypersensitivity (Anaphylaxis):** Refers to a drug-induced antigen-antibody reaction. The particular hypersensitivity reaction can be either a type I immediate (anaphylactic) or a type IV delayed reaction. Hypersensitivity reactions can occur with succinylcholine, antibiotics, and many other drugs that are administered in the PACU (see Chapter 18).

**Hyporeactivity:** An indication that a person needs excessively large doses of a drug to obtain a therapeutic or desired effect.

**Idiosyncrasy:** An unusual drug effect, regardless of the dose, in a patient whose condition is particularly susceptible. These patients usually have hypersensitivity or genetic dysfunction.

**Metareactivity:** Unusual drug side effects unrelated to the dosage strength. Metareactivity is also referred to as an idiosyncratic reaction, such as the occurrence of skeletal muscle pain and increased intraocular pressure with administration of succinylcholine.

**Pharmacodynamics:** The study of the mechanisms of action of drugs and other biochemical and physiologic effects on the body.

**Pharmacokinetics:** The study of the movement of drugs throughout the body, including the processes of absorption, distribution, localization in tissues, biotransformation, and excretion.

**Potency of a Drug:** The dose necessary of a particular drug to produce a specific effect that is designated as the effective dose (ED). Similarly, when that effect is achieved in a particular percentage of patients, it is called $ED_{50}$ for 50% of the patients and $ED_{95}$ for 95% of the patients who show an effect to the drug.

**Receptors:** That portion on a cell at which attachment of drugs leads to a physiologic response. The receptors are selective in that they only recognize and bind to specific pharmacologic or physiologic agents.

**Synergistic Effect:** Addition of a second drug to a drug with properties similar to the first that results in an effect greater than the algebraic sum of the effects of the two individual drugs.

**Tachyphylaxis:** An acute drug tolerance—for example, succinylcholine administered by intravenous drip. Over time, a higher drip rate is needed to achieve the necessary response.

**Tolerance:** A type of hyporeactivity that is acquired during chronic exposure to a drug in which unusually large doses are needed to reach a desired effect. A prime example is a person who has become dependent to narcotics and needs larger than normal doses to elicit the desired therapeutic response.

## DRUG RESPONSES

Drugs are administered via a certain route of administration at a certain dosage with the expectation of a desired response. Many factors affect the time of onset, the intensity, and the duration of action of a particular drug. The perianesthesia nurse must be aware of the basic principles of drug interaction with the biologic system. Hence, a review of the basic concepts of drug responses is presented, with particular emphasis on the patient in the PACU.

### Dose-response Relationships

The response of a drug in the changing of a physiologic state may be either quantal or graded. The quantal response is the final intended response, such as sleep, that is intended with the drug. The quantal data are usually plotted on a dose-response curve of log-dose distribution. The dose of the drug is plotted against the frequency of response to the drug. The

median effective dose is the $ED_{50}$ and represents the point on the slope of the curve when 50% of the subjects report a quantal response to the drug. The therapeutic index represents the relative safety of a drug and is the ratio between the toxic dose ($TD_{50}$) and the $ED_{50}$. The margin of safety is another method of measurement of the safety of a drug; it is the ratio between the time when 5% of the subjects have toxic effects ($TD_5$) and the dose at which 95% have the quantal or desired response ($ED_{95}$).

The graded response uses multiple evaluations of the response of the drug. A continuous scale that ranges from no response to maximum response is used. An example of graded response criteria is the train-of-four, which is used in measurement of the response to muscle relaxants (see Chapter 23). Usually, the percentage of skeletal muscle function represents the percentage of occupancy of the receptors by the drug being evaluated.

### Pharmacokinetic Actions

Pharmacokinetics comprise the absorption, distribution, and elimination of a drug in the body. Consequently, pharmacokinetics can be viewed as what the body does to a drug.

The pharmacokinetic models for the distribution of drugs are based on either a physiologic or a compartmental model. The physiologic model for drug distribution quantifies a drug according to its distribution in various anatomic and physiologic compartments. For example, parameters such as tissue mass, blood volume and flow, partition coefficients, diffusion, and active transport mechanisms are considered in identification of the distribution of a drug. An example of the physiologic model is seen with a description of the distribution of the anesthetic drug thiopental. After thiopental is injected intravenously, it goes through various anatomic and physiologic organ systems. With redistribution from the brain, the drug is dissipated and its anesthetic actions consequently are terminated. Because of the difficulty in obtaining human data for the physiologic model of drug distribution, this model is rarely used.

The compartmental model has replaced the physiologic model for determination of drug distribution. This model is used in the mathematic prediction of a drug's concentration in blood or plasma. A compartment represents a theoretic space. A mathematic model can be used to describe the pharmacokinetics of the disposition of a drug. A two-compartment model is usually used in depiction of a central compartment and a peripheral compartment. The central compartment includes plasma and blood cells and

CONCEPTS IN ANESTHETIC AGENTS

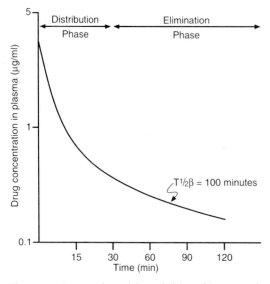

**Fig. 19-1**  Concentrations of drug administered intravenously plotted on logarithmic scale over time.

highly perfused tissues such as the heart, lungs, brain, liver, and kidneys. The peripheral compartment represents all other fluids and tissues in the body. With this two-compartment model, a drug can be introduced into the central compartment, move into the peripheral compartment, and then return to the central compartment where removal from the body occurs. The two-compartment model is constructed with the serum concentration versus time and is called the plasma concentration curve. From this curve, the distribution and elimination half-times of the drug can be determined with logarithms. The resulting curve (Fig. 19-1) can be divided into two phases: the distribution (alpha) phase and the elimination (beta) phase.

Elimination clearance quantifies the ability of the body to remove the drug. The major mechanisms for eliminaton of a drug from the body are hepatic clearance and renal clearance. The half-life (T½) of a drug is the time at which 50% of the total amount of the drug has been eliminated from the body. The elimination half-life (T½$_B$) is the time that the plasma concentration is at 50% of the elimination phase; the T½$_B$ is directly proportional to the volume distribution of the drug and inversely proportional to the drug clearance. Consequently, when the T½$_B$ for a particular drug is known, a large initial dose called a loading dose of a drug can be given to achieve a therapeutic concentration. The drug can then be given via infusion or in multiple doses at calculated intervals, based on the T½$_B$, for a steady-state plasma concentration.

In addition, the time necessary for elimination of a particular dose of a drug can be predicted with the T½$_B$. Usually, 95% of the drug can be eliminated in five half-lives.

### Systemic Absorption by Routes of Administration

***Oral Route of Administration.*** When a drug is administered orally, it is absorbed in the small intestine, which has a large surface area. A drug must be lipid soluble to cross the gastrointestinal lining. After such absorption, the drug passes to the liver by way of the portal veins before it can enter the systemic circulation. The liver extracts and metabolizes some of the drug, a process termed the first-pass hepatic effect. The drugs that are particularly subject to this effect are lidocaine and propranolol; thus, these drugs are administered in much higher doses orally than intravenously.

Oral administration of drugs in the PACU has some distinct disadvantages. For example, nausea and vomiting may occur and may reduce the amount of the drug available for absorption by the small intestine. Also, because the gastric volume and pH are altered either by preoperative drugs or anesthesia and surgery, the absorption process can be affected.

***Sublingual Route of Administration.*** The sublingual route of administration has several important advantages over the oral route because the sublingual route bypasses the first-pass hepatic effect. This route can be particularly favorable in the PACU for drugs such as nifedipine and nitroglycerin.

***Subcutaneous and Intramuscular Routes of Administration.*** These routes of administration require simple diffusion from the site of injection into the systemic circulation. Consequently, the routes do not provide a reliable rate of systemic absorption, which is particularly true in the PACU when patients are hypothermic and hypotensive and usually have some peripheral vasoconstriction. In addition, if a patient with a hypothermic condition in the PACU is administered a drug either subcutaneously or intramuscularly, the drug probably will not produce the desired effects. However, when the patient undergoes rewarming, a significant amount of the drug can be rapidly liberated from the injection site, thus causing a large concentration of the drug in the systemic circulation. This large concentration can be dangerous when narcotics are administered.

***Intravenous Route of Administration.*** This route of administration facilitates the delivery of a desired concentration of a drug in a rapid and precise fashion. In the PACU, because patients generally have a certain amount of hypothermia, hypotension, delirium, and unconsciousness, the intravenous route is most acceptable for administration of drugs.

***Aerosolized Medications to the Respiratory Tract.*** This route of administration facilitates direct delivery from inhaled aerosols to a targeted organ, which reduces the systematic drug exposure and side effects. Many aerosol delivery devices can be used for administration of bronchoactive inhaled aerosols. The most commonly used method of administration in the PACU is the aerosolized nebulizer, in which a specific amount of drug is administered in a solution of normal saline and is nebulized with a ventilator or oxygen delivery devices. Other devices for delivery of the drug either orally or nasally via inhalation are the metered dose inhaler (MDI) with or without a holding chamber or spacer device, the small volume nebulizer (SVN), and the dry powder inhaler (DPI). The MDI, SVN, and the DPI devices deliver about the same percentage of the drug to the target organ, the lungs, with the MDI increasing the patient flow rates better than the SVN and the DPI. Table 19-1 presents some of the drugs that activate the lung adrenergic and anticholinergic receptors in regard to onset, peak, and duration. Table 19-2 summarizes the major drug groups and their intended outcome in respiratory care.

## Removal of Drugs from the Systemic Circulation

Drugs are principally cleared from the systemic circulation via the hepatic, biliary, and renal systems. The hepatic system has a high blood flow and can extract many lipid-soluble drugs from the systemic circulation. In the liver, drugs undergo biotransformation and become pharmacologically inactive. Enzyme induction or a decrease in protein binding enhances the hepatic clearance of some drugs (see Chapter 16). After they have been metabolized in the liver, drugs can be transported to the biliary system for excretion. Also, some drugs, such as the glucuronides, are actively transported to the bile and excreted in an inactive form.

The kidneys secrete many water-soluble drugs in their unchanged form. Renal excretion of drugs depends on the following major physiologic processes that occur in the kidneys: glomerular filtration, active tubular secretion, and passive tubular reabsorption. Appropriate renal function is needed for facilitation of many of the drugs administered in the perioperative period. Consequently, concern about renal function should merit creatinine clearance or serum creatinine level tests because these laboratory tests correlate well with renal drug elimination.

## Effects of Physiologic Dysfunction on Pharmacologic Action

***Renal Disease.*** Kidney disease reduces the effectiveness of drug clearance. Indirectly, it also reduces hepatic clearance with a resultant production of exaggerated effects and a prolongation in the action of the drugs that have a reduction in renal clearance. In renal drug clearance, the laboratory test of creatinine clearance, for measurement of glomerular filtration (see Chapter 13), can be used for prediction of the degree of a drug's renal clearance. In patients who are anephric or in patients with severe kidney disease, the elimination clearance is decreased and the $T\frac{1}{2}_B$ is increased, thus prolonging the effects of the drugs, especially when they are administered at particular dosing intervals. However, a single dose of these nondepolarizing neuromuscular blocking agents is usually unaffected in the patient who is anephric.

***Hepatic Disease.*** Patients with hepatic diseases such as cirrhosis and ascites may have difficulty in clearance of some anesthetic drugs from the body. Liver function testing is unreliable in prediction of the level of impairment in hepatic clearance. Any patient with documented liver disease should be considered at risk for decreased clearance of drugs. Therefore, in patients with documented hepatic disease, all drugs administered in the PACU should be titrated to desired effect for an appropriate pharmacologic outcome.

***Cardiovascular Disease.*** Cardiovascular diseases that cause a reduction in tissue perfusion have a significant impact on drug distribution and clearance. For example, when lidocaine is administered to patients with congestive heart failure, the dose should be reduced by one half because of changes in volume distribution and clearance. Patients who have undergone cardiopulmonary bypass surgery can have a hemodilution of drugs. However, this change in the central compartment is transitory because the plasma drug concentration is compensated in the peripheral tissue compartment.

## DRUG-DRUG INTERACTIONS

When a patient simultaneously receives two or more drugs, the drugs may or may not interact to cause a toxic reaction. Patients are often given drugs other than the ones associated with anesthesia and surgery. Thus, the potential for a drug-drug interaction is present in these patients (Table 19-3). These interactions are divided into two broad categories: pharmacokinetic and pharmacodynamic.

*Text continued on p. 271.*

## Table 19-1  Drugs Used in the PACU: Perianesthesia Drug List

| Drug | Route | Onset | Peak | Duration of Action | Classification |
|---|---|---|---|---|---|
| Adenosine (Adenocard) | IV | <20 s | 20-30 s | 1 min | Antiarrhythmic |
| Albuterol (Proventil, Ventolin) | INH | <5 min | 0.5-2 h | 3-6 h | Bronchodilator |
| Alfentanil (Alfenta) | IV | 1-2 min | 1-2 min | 10-60 min | Opioid agonist |
|  | Epidural | 5-15 min | 30 min | 30 min - 1 h |  |
| Aminocaproic acid (Amicar) | IV | 1-2 h |  | 8-12 h | Hemostatic agent |
| Aminophylline | IV | 1-2 min | 30-60 min | 4-10 h | Bronchodilator |
|  | PO | <30 min | 1-5 h | 4-8 h |  |
| Amrinone (Inocor) | IV | 2-5 min | 10 min | 30 min - 2 h | Positive inotrope |
| Atenolol (Tenormin) | IV | 5 min | 5 min | 12-24 h | β-blocker |
|  | PO | 30-60 min | 2-4 h | 24 h |  |
| Atracurium (Tracrium) | IV | 2-5 min | 3-5 min | 20-35 min | NMB |
| Atropine | IV, cardiac | 30-60 s | 1-2 min | 15-30 min | Anticholinergic |
|  | IV, dry | 30-60 min | 60-90 min | 4 h |  |
|  | OS |  |  |  |  |
|  | ETT | 10-20 s |  |  |  |
|  | IM | 5-40 min | 20-60 min | 2-4 h |  |
|  | INH | 3-5 min | 15-90 min | 3-6 h |  |
| Bretylium (Bretylol) | IV/IM | 1-5 min | 20 min - 2 h | 6-24 h | Antiarrhythmic |
| Bumetanide (Bumex) | IV | 1-5 min | 15-30 min | 4 h | Loop diuretic |
| Bupivacaine (Marcaine) | Epidural | 4-7 min | 30-45 min | 2-7 h | Local anesthetic |
|  | Infiltration | 2-10 min | 30-45 min | 3-7 h |  |
|  | Spinal | <1 min | 15 min | 2-4 h |  |
| Butorphanol (Stadol) | IV | 1-2 min | 5-10 min | 3-4 h | Analgesic (agonist-antagonist combination) |
|  | IM | 10-15 min | 30-60 min | 3-4 h |  |
| Captopril (Capoten) | PO | <15 min | 1-2 h | 2-6 h | ACE inhibitor |
| Chloroprocaine (Nesacaine) | Epidural | 6-12 min | 10-20 min | 30-60 min | Local anesthetic; not to be used for spinal anesthesia |
| Cimetidine (Tagamet) | IV | 30-45 min | 60-90 min | 4-5 h | H₂-receptor antagonist |
|  | PO | 15-45 min | 1-2 h | 2-4 h |  |
| Cisatracurium (Nimbex) | IV | 1-4 min | 2-7 min | 22-65 min | Nondepolarizing NMB |
| Clonidine (Catapres, Dixarit) | PO | 30-60 min | 2-4 h | 6-8 h | Antihypertensive |
|  | IV | 30-60 min | 2-4 h | 6-10 h |  |
| Epidural |  | <15 min | 3-4 h |  |  |
|  | Spinal |  |  |  |  |
| Cocaine HCl | Topical | <1 min | 2-5 min | 30-120 min | Topical anesthetic; vasoconstrictor |
|  | PO | 30-60 min |  | 2-4 h |  |
|  | IM | 20-60 min |  | 2-3 h | Opioid agonist |
| Cyclosporine (Sandimmune) | PO | 1-6 h | 8-12 h | 1-4 d | Immunosuppressant |
| Dantrolene (Dantrium) | IV | <5 min | 60 min | 3 h | Skeletal muscle relaxant; for treatment of malignant hyperthermia |
|  | PO | 1-2 h | 4-6 h | 8-12 h |  |

**Table 19-1  Drugs Used in the PACU: Perianesthesia Drug List—cont'd**

| Drug | Route | Onset | Peak | Duration of Action | Classification |
|---|---|---|---|---|---|
| Desflurane (Suprane) | INH | 1-2 min | | Emergence in 8-9 min | Inhalational anesthetic agent |
| Desmopressin (DDAVP) | IV | 30 min | 1.5-3 h | 8-20 h | Synthetic vasopressin analogue |
| | Intranasal | <60 min | 1-5 h | 8-20 h | |
| Dexmedetomidine (Precedex) | IV | 1-3 min | 5-10 min | Effects last about 3-5 min after discontinuance of IV infusion | $\alpha_{2b}$-receptor agonist sedative agent |
| Dexamethasone | IV | <8 h | 12-24 h | 36-54 h | Long-acting corticosteroid |
| (Decadron) | IM | <8 h | 1-2 h | 72 h | |
| (Respihaler) | INH | <20 min | 2-4 h | 12 h | |
| (Turbinaire) | Intranasal | <15 min | | 12-24 h | |
| Diazepam (Valium) | IV | 1-5 min | 4-8 min | 15-60 min | Benzodiazepine |
| | IM | 15-30 min | | 3-6 h | |
| | PO | 30-60 min | 1-2 h | 3-6 h | |
| Digoxin (Lanoxin) | IV | 5-30 min | 1-5 h | 3-4 d | Inotropic agent |
| | IM | 30 min | 4-6 h | 3-4 d | |
| | PO | 30 min - 2 h | 6-8 h | 3-4 d | |
| Diltiazem (Cardizem) | IV | 1-3 min | 2-7 min | 1-3 h | Calcium channel blocker |
| | PO | 30 min | 2-3 h | 4-6 h | |
| | PO, extended | 1-3 h | 4-11 h | 18-24 h | |
| Diphenhydramine (Benadryl) | IV | <3 min | 1-2 h | 3-6 h | Antihistamine |
| | PO | 1 h | 1-2 h | 4-6 h | |
| Dobutamine (dobutamine) | IV | 2 min | 1-10 min | 5-10 min | Vasopressor (adrenergic agonist) |
| Dopamine (Intropin) | IV | 2-4 min | 5 min | <10 min | Catecholamine |
| Doxapram (Dopram) | IV | 20-40 s | 1-2 min | 5-12 min | Respiratory and cerebral stimulant |
| Droperidol (Inapsine) | IV/IM | 3-10 min | 30 min | 8-16 h | Tranquilizer |
| Edrophonium (Enlon, Tensilon) | IV | 30-60 s | 1-5 min | 5-20 min | Anticholinesterase |
| | IM | 2-10 min | 5-10 min | 10-40 min | |
| Enalapril (Vasotec) | PO | 1 h | 4-6 h | 12-24 h | ACE inhibitor |
| Enalaprilat (Vasotec IV) | IV | 10-15 min | 1-4 h | 6 h | ACE inhibitor |
| Enoxaparin (LMW heparin) | SQ | 20-60 min | 3-5 h | 12 h | Anticoagulant |
| Ephedrine | IV | <30 s | 2-5 min | 10-60 min | Sympathomimetic |
| | IM | 1-3 min | <10 min | 30-60 min | |
| Epinephrine (Adrenalin) | IV | <30 s | 2-3 min | 5-10 min | Catecholamine |
| | ETT | 15-30 s | 15-25 min | | |
| | INH | 1 min | 1-5 min | 1-3 h | |
| | SQ | 5-15 min | 20 min | 1-3 h | |
| Esmolol (Brevibloc) | IV | 1-2 min | 5-6 min | 10-20 min | Cardioselective blocker |

*Continued*

## Table 19-1    Drugs Used in the PACU: Perianesthesia Drug List—cont'd

| Drug | Route | Onset | Peak | Duration of Action | Classification |
|---|---|---|---|---|---|
| Ethacrynic acid (Edecrin) | IV | 5-15 min | 30 min | 2 h | Loop diuretic |
| Etidocaine (Duranest) | Infiltration | 3-5 min | 5-15 min | 2-3 h | Local anesthetic |
| | Epidural | 5-15 min | 15-20 min | 3-5 h | |
| Etomidate (Amidate) | IV | 30-60 s | 1 min | 5-14 min | Nonbarbiturate hypnotic |
| Famotidine (Pepcid) | IV | <30 min | 30 min | 8-12 h | Histamine (H₂) antagonist |
| | PO | 20-45 min | 1-3 h | 8-12 h | |
| Fenoldopam (Corlopam) | IV (continuous infusion) | 5 min | 15 min | Rapidly metabolized after discontinued | Antihypertensive |
| Fentanyl (Sublimaze) | IV | <30 s | 3-7 min | 30-60 min | Opioid agonist |
| | Epidural/spinal | 4-10 min | <30 min | 3-8 h | |
| | IM | <8 min | 20-30 min | 1-2 h | |
| | Transdermal | 12-18 h | 1-3 d | 3 d | |
| Flumazenil (Romazicon) | IV | 1-2 min | 6-10 min | 45-90 min | Benzodiazepine-receptor antagonist |
| Furosemide (Lasix) | IV | 2-5 min | 20-30 min | 2 h | Loop diuretic |
| | PO | 30-60 min | 1-2 h | 4-8 h | |
| Glucagon | IV/IM | 5 min | 2-20 min | 10-30 min | Antihypoglycemic |
| Glipizide (Glucotrol) | PO | 60-90 min | 2-3 h | 10-24 h | Hypoglycemic |
| Glycopyrrolate (Robinul) | IV | 1-3 min | 3-5 min | 2-3 h | Anticholinergic |
| | IM | 15-30 min | 30-45 min | 2-7 h | |
| Granisetron (Kytril) | IV | 2-4 min | 5-8 min | 24 h | Serotonin receptor antagonist |
| Haloperidol (Haldol) | IV | 5-30 min | 1 h | 6-8 h | Long-acting tranquilizer |
| Heparin (Liquaemin, Panheparin) | IV | Immediate | Dose-dependent | Dose-dependent | Anticoagulant |
| | SQ | 20-30 min | 2-4 h | 12-16 h | |
| Hetastarch (Hespan) | IV | 15-30 min | 1 h | 24-48 h | Plasma expander |
| Hyaluronidase (Wydase) | SQ | Immediate | | 30-60 min | Enzyme to increase absorption |
| Hydralazine (Apresoline) | IV | 5-20 min | 10-60 min | 2-4 h | Direct-acting arterial vasodilator |
| | IM | 10-30 min | 30-80 min | 2-8 h | |
| | PO | 30-120 min | 2 h | 2-8 h | |
| Hydrocortisone sodium succinate (Solu-Cortef) | IV/IM | 5 min | | 30-36 h | Corticosteroid |
| Hydromorphone (Dilaudid) | IV | <60 s | 5-20 min | 2-4 h | Opioid (mixed) |
| | IM/PO | 15-30 min | 30-60 min | 4-6 h | |
| Ibutilide fumarate (Covert) | IV | Immediate | 10 min | 10-30 min | Antiarrhythmic |
| Insulin, Lente | SQ | 1-4 h | 7-15 h | 18-26 h | Antidiabetic agent |
| Insulin, NPH | SQ | 1-2 h | 4-12 h | 18-26 h | |
| Insulin, Regular | SQ | 30-60 min | 1-5 h | 5-8 h | |
| Insulin, Semilente | SQ | 1-3 h | 4-10 h | 12-16 h | |
| Insulin, Ultralente | SQ | 4-8 h | 14-24 h | 28-36 h | |

## Table 19-1  Drugs Used in the PACU: Perianesthesia Drug List—cont'd

| Drug | Route | Onset | Peak | Duration of Action | Classification |
|------|-------|-------|------|--------------------|----------------|
| Insulin, NPH 70/ Regular 30 | SQ | 30 min | 2-12 h | 24 h | |
| Ipratropium (Atrovent, Itrop) | INH | 15-30 min | 1-2 h | 4-5 h | Cholinergic blocker for reactive airways disease |
| Isoflurane (Forane) | INH | 1-2 min | | 15 min after discontinued | Inhalational general anesthetic |
| Isoproterenol (Isuprel) | IV | Immediate | 1 min | 1-5 min | Sympathomimetic |
| Ketamine (Ketalar) | IV | 30-60 s | 1 min | 5-15 min | Dissociative |
| | IM | 3-4 min | 5-8 min | 12-25 min | anesthetic |
| Ketorolac (Toradol) | IV | <1 min | 30 min | 4-6 h | Nonsteroidal |
| | IM | <10 min | 45-60 min | 4-6 h | antiinflammatory |
| | PO | 30-60 min | 1-3 h | 3-7 h | |
| Labetalol (Normodyne, Trandate) | IV | 1-3 min | 5-15 min | 0.25-2 h | Adrenergic |
| | PO | 20-40 min | 1-4 h | 4-12 h | antagonist |
| Lansoprazole (Prevacid) | PO | 1 h | 2 h | > 24 h | Proton pump inhibitor |
| Levobupivacaine (Chirocaine) | SQ | 2-10 min | 30-45 min | 200-400 min | Local anesthetic |
| | Epidural | 4-7 min | 30-45 min | 200-400 min | |
| | Spinal | <1 min | 15 min | 200-400 min | |
| Lidocaine (Xylocaine) | IV | 45-90 s | 1-2 min | 10-20 min | Local anesthetic |
| | Epidural | 5-15 min | 20-30 min | 60-120 min | |
| | Infiltration | <60 s | 20-30 min | 30-120 min | |
| | Spinal | <60 s | <10 min | 60-90 min | |
| Lorazapam (Ativan) | IV | 1-5 min | 20-40 min | 4-6 h | Benzodiazepine |
| | PO | 20-30 min | 2 h | 10-20 h | |
| Magnesium sulfate | IV | Immediate | 2-3 min | 30 min | Anticonvulsant |
| Mannitol (Osmitrol) | IV, diuresis | 15-60 min | 1-3 h | 3-8 h | Osmotic diuretic |
| | IV to lower: ICP | <15 min | 60 min | 3-8 h | |
| | IOP | 30-60 min | 1-2 h | 4-6 h | |
| Meperidine (Demerol) | IV | 1-3 min | 5-20 min | 2-4 h | Synthetic |
| | IM | 5-10 min | 30-50 min | 2-4 h | opioid |
| | PO | 10-45 min | 60 min | 2-4 h | agonist |
| Mepivacaine (Carbocaine) | Epidural | 5-15 min | 15-45 min | 3-5 h | Local anesthetic |
| | Infiltration | 3-5 min | 15-45 min | 45-90 min | |
| Metaproterenol (Metaprel) | INH | <60 s | 60 min | 1-4 min | Bronchodilator |
| Methadone (Dolophine) | IV | 1-3 min | 15 min | 6 h | Synthetic opioid |
| | IM | 3-60 min | 30 min | 6 h | |
| | PO | 30-60 min | 45 min | 6 h | |
| Methohexital (Brevital Sodium) | IV | <30 s | 30-120 s | 5-10 min | Ultra short-acting barbiturate |
| | Rectal | 5-7 min | 5-10 min | 45-90 min | |
| Methylene Blue (Urolene Blue) | IV | <1 min | <1 h | Varies | Antidote for methemo-globinemia |
| Methylergonovine (Methergine) | IV | Immediate | 5-10 min | 45 min | Oxytocic |
| | IM | 2-5 min | 30 min | 3 h | |

*Continued*

**Table 19-1    Drugs Used in the PACU: Perianesthesia Drug List—cont'd**

| Drug | Route | Onset | Peak | Duration of Action | Classification |
|------|-------|-------|------|--------------------|----------------|
| Metoclopramide (Reglan) | IV | 1-3 min | 30-60 min | 1-2 h | Dopamine-receptor antagonist-antiemetic |
|  | IM | 10-15 min | 30-60 min | 1-2 h |  |
|  | PO | 30-60 min | 1-2 h | 1-2 h |  |
| Metoprolol (Toprol) | IV | <5 min | 20 min | 5-8 h | β-blocker |
|  | PO | <15 min | 90 min | 12-19 h |  |
| Midazolam (Versed) | IV | 1-5 min | 2-5 min | 15-90 min | Benzodiazepine |
|  | IM | 10-15 min | 30-60 min | 1-3 h |  |
|  | PO | 10-15 min | 30-60 min | 2-6 h |  |
| Milrinone (Primacor) | IV | 2 min | 15 min | 2 h | Inotropic agent |
| Morphine | IV | <1 min | 20 min | 2-7 h | Opioid agonist |
| Morphine (Duramorph) | Epidural | 60 min | 90 min | 6-18 h | Opioid agonist |
|  | IM | 1-5 min | 30-60 min | 3-7 h |  |
|  | PO | 15-60 min | 30-60 min | 3-7 h |  |
|  | PO extended | 60-90 min | 1-4 h | 6-12 h |  |
|  | Spinal | <60 min | 1-2 h | 12-24 h |  |
| Nalmefene HCl (Revex) | IV | 2 min | 5 min | 4-6 h | Opioid antagonist |
|  | IV | 2-3 min | 15-30 min | 3-6 h |  |
|  | IM | 15 min | 30-60 min | 3-6 h |  |
| Naloxone (Narcan) | IV | 1-2 min | 5-15 min | 1-4 h | Opioid antagonist |
|  | IM | 2-5 min | 5-15 min | 1-4 h |  |
| Naltrexone (ReVia, Trexan) | PO | 5 min | 1 h | 24-72 h | Opioid antagonist |
| Neostigmine (Prostigmin) | IV | <3 min | 7 min | 45-60 min | Anticholinesterase |
| Nicardipine (Cardene) | IV | 1 min | 15 min | 3 h | Calcium channel blocker |
|  | PO | <30 min | 0.5-1 h | 3 h |  |
| Nifedipine (Procardia) | PO | 15-20 min | 30-120 min | 4-12 h | Calcium channel blocker |
|  | PO, extended | 20-30 min | 6 h | 24 h |  |
|  | SL | 5 min | 20-45 min | 4-12 h |  |
| Nitroglycerin | IV | 1-2 min | 1-5 min | 3-5 min | Peripheral vasodilator |
|  | Ointment | 20-60 min | 3-6 h |  |  |
|  | SL | 1-3 min | 30-60 min |  |  |
|  | Transdermal | 40-60 min | 18-24 h |  |  |
| Nitroprusside (Nipride, Nitropress) | IV | 30-60 s |  | 1-10 min | Peripheral vasodilator |
| Nitrous oxide (N$_2$O) | INH | 1-5 min |  | 5-10 min after discontinued | General inhalation anesthetic |
| Nizatidine (Axid) | PO | 30-60 min | 0.5-3 h | 8-12 h | H$_2$-receptor antagonist |
| Norepinephrine (Levophed) | IV | <60 s | 1-2 min | 2-10 min | Catecholamine |
| Omeprazole (Prilosec) | PO | 1 h | 2 h | 72 h | Proton pump inhibitor |
| Ondansetron (Zofran) | IV | <30 min | 1-1.5 h | 12-24 h | Serotonin (5-HT$_3$) receptor antagonist 5-HT$_3$ |
| Oxazepam (Serax) | PO | 30 min | 2 h | 8-12 h | Benzodiazepine |

**Table 19-1  Drugs Used in the PACU: Perianesthesia Drug List—cont'd**

| Drug | Route | Onset | Peak | Duration of Action | Classification |
|---|---|---|---|---|---|
| Oxytocin (Pitocin) | IV<br>IM | <30 s<br>3-5 min | 20-40 min<br>40 min | 60 min<br>2-3 h | Oxytocic |
| Pancuronium (Pavulon) | IV | 1-3 min | 3-5 min | 40-90 min | Nondepolarizing skeletal muscle relaxant |
| Phentolamine (Regitine) | IV<br>IM | 1-2 min<br>5-20 min |  | 10-15 min<br>30-45 min | α-adrenergic blocker |
| Pentobarbital (Nembutal) | IV | Immediate | 1-2 min | 15 min | Barbiturate |
| Phenylephrine (Neo-Synephrine) | IV<br>Nasal | <30 s<br>0.5-4 h | 1 min | 15-20 min | α-adrenergic agonist |
| Phenytoin (Dilantin) | IV | 3-5 min | 1-2 h | 22 h | Anticonvulsant |
| Physostigmine (Antilirium) | IV | 3-8 min | 5-10 min | 0.5-5 h | Anticholinesterase |
| Pipecuronium (Arduran) | IV | 2-3 min | 3-6 min | 45-120 min | Long-acting NMB agent |
| Prilocaine (Citanest) | SQ<br>Epidural | 1-2 min<br>5-15 min | <30 min<br><30 min | 0.5-1.5 h<br>1-3 h | Local anesthetic |
| Procainamide (Pronestyl) | IV | Immediate | 5-15 min | 2.5-5 h | Antiarrhythmic |
| Procaine (Novocain) | SQ<br>Spinal<br>Epidural | 2-5 min<br>2-5 min<br>5-25 min | <30 min<br><30 min<br><30 min | 0.25-0.5 h<br>0.5-1.5 h<br>0.5-1.5 h | Local anesthetic |
| Prochlorperazine (Compazine) | IV<br>IM<br>PO<br>Rectal | 3-5 min<br>10-20 min<br>30-40 min<br>60 min | 15-30 min<br>15-30 min<br>2-4 h<br>3-4 h | 3-4 h<br>3-4 h<br>3-4 h | Antiemetic, antipsychotic |
| Promethazine (Phenergan) | IV<br>IM | 3-5 min<br>20 min | 1-2 h<br>1-2 h | 2-8 h<br>2-8 h | Phenothiazine, H₁-receptor antagonist |
| Propofol (Diprivan) | IV | 30-60 s | 1 min | 5-20 min | Nonbarbiturate anesthesia induction agent |
| Propanolol (Inderal) | IV<br>PO | <2 min<br>30 min | 1 min<br>60-90 min | 1-6 h<br>8-12 h | α-adrenergic receptor antagonist |
| Protamine sulfate | IV | 30-60 s | <5 min | 2 h | Heparin antagonist |
| Ranitidine (Zantac) | IV<br>PO | <15 min<br><30 min | 1-2 h<br>2-3 h | 6-8 h<br>8-12 h | H₂-receptor antagonist |
| Remifentanil (Ultiva) | IV | 1-5 min |  | Opiate effect ceases 18 min after discontinued | Opioid |
| Ritodrine HCl (Yutopar) | IV | Immediate |  | 3-6 h | α₂-adrenergic agonist; tocolytic agent |
| Rocuronium (Zemuron) | IV | 45-90 s | 1-3 min | 30-120 min | Nondepolarizing NMB agent |

*Concepts in Anesthetic Agents*

*Continued*

## Table 19-1   Drugs Used in the PACU: Perianesthesia Drug List—cont'd

| Drug | Route | Onset | Peak | Duration of Action | Classification |
|------|-------|-------|------|--------------------|----------------|
| Ropivacaine HCl (Naropin) | SQ Epidural | 1-5 min 5-13 min | | 2-6 h 3-5 h | Amide local anesthetic |
| Salmeterol (Serevent) | INH | 10-20 min | 30 min | 12 h | $\alpha_2$-adrenergic agonist |
| Scopolamine (Transderm-Scop) | IV IM Transdermal | Immediate 30 min 4 h | | 30-60 min 4-6 h 72 h | Anticholinergic |
| Sodium citrate (Bicitra) | PO | 2-10 min | 60 min | 60-90 min | Nonparticulate neutralizing buffer |
| Somatostatin (Zecnil) | IV | 5-10 min | 45 min | 1 h | Synthetic somatostatin |
| Sotalol HCl (Betapace) | PO | 1 h | 2.5-4 h | 4-6 h | Antiarrhythmic |
| Sodium bicarbonate | IV | 2-10 min | 10-30 min | 30-60 min | Neutralizing buffer |
| Sodium citrate | PO | <60 s | 3-4 min | 2 h | Neutralizing buffer |
| Sodium nitroprusside | IV | 30-60 s | 1-2 min | 1-10 min | Antihypertensive |
| Succinylcholine (Anectine, Quelicin) | IV IM | 30-60 s 2-3 min | 1 min 10-30 min | 4-6 min | Depolarizing skeletal muscle relaxant |
| Sufentanil (Sufenta) | IV Epidural/spinal | 1-3 min 4-10 min | 3-5 min <30 min | 20-45 min 2-4 h | Opioid agonist |
| Terbutaline (Brethine) | INH PO SQ | 5-30 min 30 min 15 min | 1-2 h 2-3 h 30-60 min | 3-4 h 4-8 h 1.5-4 h | $\alpha_2$-adrenergic agonist |
| Tetracaine (Pontocaine) | Spinal | <10 min | 15-60 min | 1.25-3 h | Local anesthetic |
| Thiamylal (Surital) | IV | Immediate | | 10-30 min | Ultra short-acting barbiturate |
| Thiopental (Pentothal) | IV | 30-60 s | 20-40 s | 5-15 min | Ultra short-acting barbiturate |
| Torsemide (Demadex, Presaril) | IV | 10 min | 1-2 h | 6-8 h | Loop diuretic |
| Vancomycin (Vancocin) | IV | 15-30 min | 4-6 h | 8-12 h | Antimicrobial agent |
| Vasopressin (Pitressin) | IV | 15-30 min | 30-60 min | 2-8 h | Antidiuretic hormone |
| Vecuronium (Norcuron) | IV | 2-3 min | 3-5 min | 25-40 min | Nondepolarizing NMB agent |
| Verapamil (Isoptin) | IV PO IM, IV, SQ PO | 2-5 min 30 min 1-3 h Up to 5-7 d | <10 min 1-2 h | 30-60 min 3-7 h 6-48 h 2-5 d after therapeutic dose reached | Calcium channel blocker Water-soluble vitamin Anticoagulant |

*DDAVP,* 1-Deamino-8-D-arginine vasopressin; *LMW,* low–molecular weight; *NPH,* neutral protamine Hagedorn; *IV,* intravenous; *INH,* inhalation; *PO,* oral; *OS,* osseous; *ETT,* endotracheal tube; *IM,* intramuscular; *SQ,* subcutaneous; *ICP,* intracranial pressure; *IOP,* intraocular pressure; *SL,* Sublingual; *NMB,* nondepolarizing neuromuscular blocker; *ACE,* angiotensin-converting enzyme; *5-HT,* serotonin. Adapted from Nagelhout J, Zaglaniczny K, Haglund V: *Handbook of nurse anesthesia,* ed 2, Philadelphia, 2001, Saunders; and Waugaman W, Foster S, Rigor B: *Principles and practice of nurse anesthesia,* ed 3, Norwalk, Conn, 1999, Appleton & Lange.

## Table 19-2 Major Drug Groups and Intended Outcome in Respiratory Care

| Drug Group | Intended Physiologic Response | Generic Agent (Tradename) |
|---|---|---|
| Adrenergic agents | α-adrenergic stimulation produces bronchial relaxation to reduce airway resistance and improve flow rates in patients with obstructive lung disease | Epinephrine<br>Isoproterenol (Isuprel)<br>Isoetharine (Bronkosol)<br>Terbutaline (Brethine)<br>Metaproterenol (Metaprel)<br>Albuterol (Ventolin)<br>Pirbuterol (Maxair)<br>Bitolterol (Tornalate)<br>Salmeterol (Serevent)<br>Procaterol (Mescalcin) |
| | α-adrenergic stimulation produces bronchial relaxation, peripheral vascular vasoconstriction, and nasal decongestion | Ephedrine<br>Phenylephrine (Neo-Synephrine) |
| Anticholinergic agents | Relaxation of cholinergic (vagal)-induced bronchoconstriction to improve flow rates in patients with obstructive lung disease | Ipratropium (Atrovent) |
| Mucoactive agents | Modification of properties of respiratory tract mucus to facilitate clearance of secretions | Acetylcystine (Mucomist)<br>Dornase alfa (Pulmozyme) |
| Corticosteroids | Reduce inflammation in respiratory tract | Dexamethasone (Decadron)<br>Beclomethasone (Vanceril)<br>Triamcinolone (Kenalog)<br>Flunisolide (Aerobid)<br>Fluticasone (Flonase/Flovent)<br>Budesonide (Rhinocort) |
| Antiasthmatic agents | Inhibits chemical mediators of inflammation to help prevent onset of asthma attack | Cromolyn (Intal)<br>Nedocromil (Tilade)<br>Zafirlukast (Accolate)<br>Zileuton (Zyflo)<br>Montelukast (Singulair) |
| Antiinfective agents | Inhibits or stops specific infective agents, such as *P. carinii* (pentamidine) or respiratory syncyial virus (ribavirin), or for management of *P. aeruginosa* in cystic fibrosis (tobramycin) | Pentamidine<br>Ribavirin (Rebetron)<br>Tobramycin (TOBI) |
| Exogenous surfactants | Enhances lung compliance by reducing surface tension<br>Approved for direct intratracheal instillation | Colfosceril (Exosurf)<br>Beractant (Survanta) |

Adapted from Rau J: Recent developments in respiratory care pharmacology, *J Perianesth Nurs* 13(6):362, 1998.

## Pharmacokinetic Interactions

Interactions of a second drug that produce alterations in absorption, distribution, metabolism, or excretion of the first drug are known as pharmacokinetic interactions. Hence, when one drug alters any pharmacokinetic parameter of another, with a resultant alteration in the concentration of the drug at the receptor site, a pharmacokinetic interaction has taken place. In other words, the absorption, distribution, or elimination of the drug concentration at the receptor site is changed, which results in an altered pharmacologic response from the person.

**Absorption.** The absorption of one drug may be enhanced or inhibited by another drug. With the addition of epinephrine to solutions of local

*Text continued on p. 276.*

## Table 19-3 Drug-Drug or Drug-Induced Interactions in PACU

| Drug(s) | Interactions | Result | Mechanism |
| --- | --- | --- | --- |
| **Antihypertensive Drugs** | | | |
| Reserpine | Inhalation anesthetics | Hypotension | Inhibits synthesis and storage of norepinephrine in sympathetic nerve endings |
| Propranolol | Inhalation anesthetics | Bradycardia, hypotension | Additive effect |
| Verapamil | Halothane | Enhancement of A-V block | Additive inhibitor effect |
| | | Potentiates all skeletal muscle relaxants | |
| Clonidine | Inapsine | Rebound hypertension | Sudden inhibition of cardiovascular and vasoconstrictor centers |
| Diuretics | Halothane | Hypotension | Reduced extracellular sodium and water, which is compensated for by vasoconstriction |
| | | | Halothane dilates constricted vascular beds |
| Propranolol | Lidocaine | Enhanced negative inotropic effect | Propranolol reduces liver blood flow and lidocaine clearance |
| Lidocaine | d-Tubocurarine | Increased duration of neuromuscular blockade | Synergistic effect |
| Procainamide | | | |
| Bretylium | | | |
| Phenytoin | | | |
| Disopyramide | | | |
| Digitalis | Succinylcholine | Arrhythmias | Direct effect or caused by hyperkalemia that can be induced by succinylcholine |
| Quinidine | Digitalis (digoxin) | Can produce digitalis intoxication | Decreases digitalis clearance and increases concentration of digitalis |
| Propranolol | Heparin | Myocardial depression | Heparin increases free fatty acids, which displace propranolol from plasma protein binding sites, leading to increased free propranolol |
| Quinidine | Myasthenia gravis plus skeletal muscle relaxants | Postoperative respiratory depression | Blockade of acetylcholine receptors at neuromuscular postsynaptic membrane |
| Digitalis | Thiazide diuretics | Increased potassium excretion by kidneys | Combined effect of two drugs on kidneys promotes potassium excretion |

| | | | |
|---|---|---|---|
| **Antibiotics** | | | |
| Neomycin | Nondepolarizing skeletal muscle relaxants | Potentiates nondepolarizing muscle relaxants, respiratory depression | Neuromuscular blockade caused by reduction in amplitude of end-plate potential |
| Streptomycin | | | |
| Dihydrostreptomycin | | | |
| Polymyxin A | | | |
| Polymyxin B | | | |
| Colistin | | | |
| Viomycin | | | |
| Paromomycin | | | |
| Kanamycin | | | |
| Lincomycin | | | |
| Gentamicin | | | |
| Tetracycline | | | |
| **Narcotics** | | | |
| Morphine | Inhalation anesthetics | Potentiation, respiratory, and cardiovascular depression | Depressant effects of inhalation anesthetics and narcotics are additive |
| Meperidine | | | |
| Sublimaze | | | |
| Sufentanil | | | |
| Meperidine | Enovid | Birth control pill potentiates meperidine | Excess female sex hormones with oral contraceptive therapy, which may slow metabolism of meperidine |
| | Norinyl | | |
| | MAOI | | |
| Meperidine | MAOI | MAOI interacts with meperidine metabolite | Type I: seizures<br>Type II hypotension |
| **Sympathomimetic Amines** | | | |
| Epinephrine | Halothane | Cardiac arrhythmias | Anesthetic agents sensitize myocardium to endogenous and exogenous catecholamines |
| | Enflurane | | |

A-V, Atrioventricular.

Continued

CONCEPTS IN ANESTHETIC AGENTS

## Table 19-3   Drug-Drug or Drug-Induced Interactions in PACU—cont'd

| Drug(s) | Interactions | Result | Mechanism |
|---|---|---|---|
| **Electrolytes** | | | |
| Increased extracellular potassium | Skeletal muscle relaxants | Increased resistance to depolarization and greater sensitivity to nondepolarizing muscle relaxants | Acute increase in extracellular potassium increases end-plate transmembrane potential, thus causing hyperpolarization |
| Decreased extracellular potassium | Skeletal muscle relaxants | Increased effects of depolarizing muscle relaxants and increased resistance to nondepolarizing muscle relaxants | Acute decrease in extracellular potassium lowers resting end-plate transmembrane potential |
| Increased calcium levels | Nondepolarizing skeletal muscle relaxants | Decreased response | Calcium increases quantal release of acetylcholine and enhances excitation-contraction coupling mechanism |
| Magnesium ions | Muscle relaxants | Potentiation | Magnesium ions cause partial muscle relaxation by blocking release of acetylcholine |
| Calcium chloride | Digitalis | Additive effect on heart | High concentrations of calcium inhibit positive inotropic actions of digitalis and potentiate digitalis toxicity |
| **Miscellaneous** | | | |
| Echothiophate iodide | Succinylcholine | Prolonged apnea | Echothiophate is cholinesterase inhibitor, and succinylcholine is destroyed by pseudocholinesterase |
| Tolbutamide | Dicumarol | Intensification of the effects of tolbutamide, leads to hypoglycemia | Dicumarol displaces tolbutamide from its binding site on plasma proteins and makes more tolbutamide available in free form |
| Succinylcholine | d-Tubocurarine | Prolonged apnea | Both drugs act at acetylcholine receptor, thus causing synergistic effect on myoneural junction |
| Procaine Nesacaine Pontocaine | Succinylcholine | Prolonged apnea | All these drugs are metabolized by enzyme pseudocholinesterase |
| Furosemide | Nondepolarizing skeletal muscle relaxants | Intensified neuromuscular block | Concomitant use of these drugs may reduce effective plasma concentration of enzyme |
| Thiazide Ethacrynic acid | | | Electrolyte imbalance (hypokalemia) |

| Drug | Interacting agent | Effect | Mechanism |
|---|---|---|---|
| Aminophylline | d-Tubocurarine | Antagonized neuromuscular blockade | End-plate effect is antagonized by increase in neurotransmitter |
| Procaine | Pancuronium — Nondepolarizing and depolarizing skeletal muscle relaxants | Enhanced neuromuscular blockade | Decreased end-plate potential |
| Lidocaine Lithium | Pancuronium — Succinylcholine | Potentiated neuromuscular blockade | Lithium ions are substituted for sodium ions at presynaptic level |
| Chlorpromazine | Nondepolarizing skeletal muscle relaxants | Enhanced neuromuscular blockade | Potentiation of neuromuscular blockade |
| All inhalation anesthetics | Nondepolarizing skeletal muscle relaxants | Augment block in dose-dependent manner in following decreasing order of potency: isoflurane and enflurane, halothane, nitrous oxide | Central nervous system depression or presynaptic inhibition of acetylcholine |
| Insulin | Corticosteroids, oral contraceptives, loop and thiazide diuretics | Reduction in effects | Insulin antagonizes effects |
| Diethylstilbestrol (Stilphostrol) | Succinylcholine | Prolonged neuromuscular blockade | Decreased plasma cholinesterase |
| Hydrocortisone Dexamethasone Prednisolone | Phenobarbital | Decreased effects of the steroids | Increased metabolism |

CONCEPTS IN ANESTHETIC AGENTS

anesthetics, the absorption of the anesthetic is prolonged through the vasoconstrictive action of epinephrine. The local vasoconstriction produced by epinephrine delays the systemic absorption of the local anesthetic, and the effect of the local anesthetic ultimately is prolonged. When a patient has been administered a preoperative aluminum-containing antacid and then is administered tetracycline in the late postoperative period, absorption of the tetracycline is reduced.

**Distribution.** Pharmaceutical incompatibility is one type of pharmacokinetic distribution interaction. This situation occurs, for example, when one drug reacts chemically with another. In this situation, when one drug (e.g., aspirin) displaces another drug (e.g., phenytoin) from plasma protein-binding sites, the blood concentration of the free drug is increased, which may result in toxic blood levels. When a large dose of thiopental is administered to an obese patient who also receives halothane, the anesthetic action may be prolonged considerably and last well into the PACU phase. This reaction is caused by the prolonged retention of thiopental in the adipose tissue because of the circulatory depressant action of halothane. Hence, at the end of the period of anesthesia, the redistribution and subsequent elimination of thiopental are delayed, which causes a prolonged hypnotic effect.

### Elimination

**Biotransformation.** When patients are administered enzyme-inducing agents, such as barbiturates and the antibiotic rifampin, the activity of the enzyme systems of the liver is increased. This increase results in a more rapid metabolism and excretion of drugs that are metabolized by a particular liver enzyme system. For example, if a barbiturate is administered to a patient who is on a stabilized dose of the anticoagulant warfarin, the warfarin blood level may be reduced, which may result in a lowered prothrombin time. If this situation occurs (stabilization with an anticoagulant and administration of an enzyme-inducing agent) and the barbiturate is discontinued, the nurse must monitor the patient for the potentially more serious problem of excessive anticoagulation and hemorrhage.

The drug cimetidine (Tagamet) is sometimes administered before surgery for a reduction in the amount of gastric secretion and for an increase in the gastric pH. Cimetidine is a potent inhibitor of drug metabolism and can slow the elimination of antipyrine, warfarin, diazepam, and propranolol. This effect results in an increased drug concentration and enhanced pharmacologic effect of the latter drugs.

**Excretion.** The pharmacokinetic parameters of concern in excretion relate to one drug facilitating or hindering the excretion of another. An example occurs when probenecid is administered together with penicillin. The outcome of this interaction is that the pharmacologic actions of penicillin are prolonged because of the slower T½ produced by probenecid. Certainly, this effect can be considered a desirable drug-drug interaction.

### Pharmacodynamic Interactions

Pharmacodynamic interactions occur when one drug alters the pharmacologic effects of another drug. For example, when a patient is treated with an antibiotic such as an aminoglycoside or polymyxin and receives a skeletal muscle relaxant such as curare, a prolonged neuromuscular blockage may result. Another example is a patient who receives thiazide diuretic therapy and has resultant hypokalemia. If the patient is administered digitalis, digitalis toxicity may result. Also, if the patient undergoing thiazide therapy is administered a nondepolarizing muscle relaxant, the neuromuscular blockade is intensified.

## DRUG-DRUG INTERACTIONS AND THE PACU

### Antibiotics

Aminoglycoside and polymyxin antibiotics have been reported to interact with some anesthetic agents and with skeletal muscle relaxants. Streptomycin and the other aminoglycoside antibiotics produce a partial neuromuscular blockade by inhibiting the release of acetylcholine from the presynaptic membrane and by stabilizing the postsynaptic membrane. The order of decreasing potency of aminoglycosides for causing a partial neuromuscular blockade is neomycin, kanamycin, amikacin, gentamicin, and tobramycin. When a nondepolarizing skeletal muscle relaxant such as curare or pancuronium is administered to a patient who receives an aminoglycoside antibiotic, the neuromuscular blockade is intensified and pharmacologic reversal is difficult. Studies indicate that the aminoglycoside neuromuscular blockade can sometimes be partially reversed with calcium and neostigmine, whereas the neuromuscular blockade produced by polymyxin B is enhanced with neostigmine and not reversed with calcium. The antibiotics that prolong the actions of the nondepolarizing skeletal muscle relaxants are neomycin, streptomycin, dihydrostreptomycin, kanamycin, gentamicin, polymyxin A, polymyxin B, colistin, lincomycin, and tetracycline. The antibiotics that enhance the pharmacologic actions of the depolarizing skeletal relaxant succinylcholine include neomycin, streptomycin, kanamycin, polymyxin B, and colistin. These drugs must usually be given for at least 2 weeks before any clinically significant depression in the neuromuscular transmission occurs; such a depression may produce only slight muscular weakness in the patient. Antibiotics that have no skeletal muscle relaxant properties are penicillin, chloramphenicol, and the cephalosporins.

## Sympathomimetic Amines

The volatile inhalation anesthetics, particularly halothane, can sensitize the heart to sympathomimetic amines, such as epinephrine, and thus produce cardiac arrhythmias. Patients in recovery from halothane anesthesia in the PACU still have a significant amount of halothane in the body. Consequently, epinephrine or other sympathomimetic amines should not be administered. If epinephrine must be used for hemostasis or for vasoconstriction in a local anesthetic, the epinephrine concentration should not be greater than 1:100,000 to 1:200,000, and the total adult dose should not be greater than 10 mL of 1:100,000 solution in 10 minutes; that is, the total dose should not exceed 30 mL of 1:100,000 solution in 1 hour.

## Antihypertensives

Estimates suggest that 1 to 2 million patients with hypertension receive anesthesia each year in the United States. Anesthetic agents have been reported to produce changes in cardiac output, peripheral resistance, and regional blood flow patterns in patients with normotensive and hypertensive conditions.

Hypertension is treated by lowering systemic vascular resistance, by reducing cardiac output, or both. Antihypertensive drugs alter the circulatory hemostasis, strongly influence the activity of pressor amines, and may alter the response to muscle relaxants and narcotic analgesics. Antihypertensive drugs can produce systemic conditions that may result in a hypotensive crisis during anesthesia and in the immediate postoperative period. Therefore, patients in the PACU who have been on long-term antihypertensive medication therapy and who have received a 100% potent inhalation anesthetic should be specifically monitored for cardiac dysrhythmias and hypotension. If a hypotensive crisis occurs in the PACU, the patient should have the legs elevated, and oxygen and, if necessary, vasopressors should be administered. The anesthesiologist and surgeon should be notified immediately so that specific treatment can be instituted.

## Narcotics

Probably the most significant and dangerous drug-drug interaction that can occur in the perianesthesia period is the interaction between meperidine (Demerol) and monoamine oxidase inhibitors (MAOIs). The presumed physiologic dysfunction is that the MAOI decelerates the breakdown of meperidine because of N-demethylase inhibition by the MAOI. The result of the interaction between these two drugs is either a type I response that includes seizures, agitation, rigidity, and hyperpexia or a type II response that is depressive in nature and characterized by hypotension, respiratory depression, and coma.

Every perianesthesia nurse has probably observed the drug-drug interaction between narcotics administered in the PACU and the inhalation anesthetic agents administered in the operating room. If the anesthetic agent has not been completely eliminated and the patient is administered a narcotic, a synergistic effect between the two drugs occurs. The outcome of this interaction is usually respiratory depression because both drugs are respiratory depressants.

If the two drugs have interacted in this way, a narcotic (opioid) antagonist, such as naloxone (Narcan), can be administered to reverse the respiratory depression produced by the narcotic. However, naloxone does not reverse respiratory depression produced by the inhalation anesthetic agents such as enflurane (Ethrane) or isoflurane (Forane).

Naloxone reverses respiratory depression and analgesia produced by an opioid. In the PACU, reversal of the respiratory depression and preservation of some postoperative analgesia with nalbuphine (Nubain) are usually advantageous. The pharmacology of nalbuphine is discussed in detail in Chapter 22.

## Steroids

Although the case of exogenous steroids administered to a patient with steroid dependency is not actually an interaction of two drugs that alters one of the pharmacokinetic parameters, the problems that result from this circumstance are presented.

Patients with adrenocortical insufficiency cannot withstand the stress of anesthesia and surgery. For example, if a patient with chronic obstructive pulmonary disease has been treated with long-term steroids, usually some degree of adrenocortical insufficiency exists. Hence, because of the alteration in the receptor site, the patient may react to surgery and anesthesia with hypotension, respiratory depression, or

CONCEPTS IN ANESTHETIC AGENTS

**Table 19-4  Drugs Commonly Used in PACU for Sedation**

Dexmedetomidine
Fentanyl
Lorazapam
Midazolam
Haloperidol
Propofol

delayed recovery. For prevention of a hypotensive crisis during the perioperative period, these patients are usually maintained on corticosteroids before, during, and after the surgical procedure.

If these symptoms appear in a patient in the PACU who did not receive this steroid coverage, the preferred treatment is hydrocortisone (see Chapter 15).

## SPECIAL CONSIDERATIONS IN PHARMACOLOGY ASSOCIATED WITH PERIANESTHESIA CARE

### Sedative Drugs for PACU Patients
Patients in the PACU sometimes need sedation for a variety of reasons, most commonly fear, loss of control, confusion, and noise, lights, and alarms. These stimuli can cause a stress response that is experienced by some patients in the PACU; sedative drugs are sometimes used to prevent the adverse physiologic effects of stress, such as increased oxygen consumption, tachycardia, hypertension, and exacerbated hyperglycemia. The drugs that are most commonly used for sedation in the PACU are listed in Table 19-4. The institution of drugs for promotion of sedation is a difficult task in the PACU because the patient may have

residual effects of the intraoperative anesthetic agents still active in the body. Hence, a bedside sedation scoring system is helpful in determination of the degree of sedation and in prediction of when concerns about oversedation should be realized. Although many sedation scoring systems are available, the Ramsay Sedation Scoring System appears to be quite appropriate for assessment of drug-induced sedation. The Ramsay Scale consists of six scoring levels. The first three levels (Table 19-5) are usually administered while the patient is awake, and levels 4 through 6 are assessed during varying degrees of sleep. Drakulavic and associates in 1999 used univariate analysis to show that a Ramsay level of 4 or greater was associated with increased risk for nosocomial pneumonia. Because oversedation is associated with increased risk of edema, thromboemboli, gastric regurgitation, and aspiration, to name a few, patients in the PACU should have Ramsay Sedation levels in the range of 3 or less.

### Herbal Medicinals
During the past few years, usage of an herbal product has escalated to the point that more than 24 million Americans use at least one herbal product. The industry has annual sales of more than $12 billion and is projected to only increase because of the ongoing dissatisfaction with conventional medicine and the health care system in general. Most concerning to the health care practitioner is that of the Americans who use alternative forms of therapy, including herbal products, more than 60% of patients do not inform family physicians of the drugs or therapies that they use.

Because of the rapid onset in popularity of the use of herbal products, research in this area is lacking, particularly in the area of the

**Table 19-5  Ramsay Sedation Scoring System**

| Ramsay Score | Clinical Parameters for Bedside Assessment of Sedation | Global Degree of Sedation |
|---|---|---|
| 1 | Anxious, restless, perhaps agitated | |
| 2 | Cooperative and oriented | Varying degrees of awake state |
| 3 | Easily arousable, responds appropriately | |
| 4 | Brisk response to light glabellar tap or loud auditory stimulus | |
| 5 | Sluggish response to glabellar tap or auditory stimulus | Varying degrees of asleep state |
| 6 | Asleep, does not respond to previous stimuli | |

From Prielipp R, Young C: Current drugs for sedation of critically ill patients, *Semin Anesthesia Perioperative Med Pain* 20(2):85-94, 2001.

## Table 19-6  Herbal Drugs and Possible Interactions with Anesthesia

| Herbal | Actions | Key Component | Untoward Effects |
|---|---|---|---|
| Aristolochia | Aphrodisiac and anticonvulsant | Aristolochic acid | Nephrotoxic and cardiogenic |
| Ephedra | Weight loss, stimulant, ergogenic | Ephedrine | Adrenergic stimulant; hypertension, bronchodilatation, diuresis, tachycardia |
| Feverfew | Temperature reduction, migraine prophylaxis, treatment of rheumatoid arthritis | Parthenolide | Risk of bleeding, insomnia, anxiety (should be discontinued 1 week before surgery) |
| Garlic | Reduction in blood pressure, decrease in total cholesterol | Allicin | Risk of postoperative bleeding (should be discontinued 1 week before surgery) |
| Ginger | Decreases platelet aggregation, antiemetic, motion sickness | Oleoresins | Risk of postoperative bleeding (should be discontinued 1 week before surgery) |
| Ginkgo | Decreases RBC aggregation, memory loss, improved cognitive function, chronic venous insufficiency | GBE | Significant risk of postoperative bleeding (should be discontinued 1 week before surgery) |
| Ginseng | Stress reduction, increased physical performance, improved cardiovascular function, anticancer properties, antioxidant | Ginsenosides | Insomnia, irritability, and mania; interactions with digoxin, warfarin, and lithium (should be discontinued 1 week before surgery) |
| Golden Seal | Laxative, antiinflammatory, antiemetic | Berberine; hydrastine | Seizures, respiratory depression, hypertension, electrolyte imbalance |
| Kava | Anxiolytic, analgesic, muscle relaxant, anticonvulsant, local anesthetic properties | Kavapyrones | MAOI, platelet aggregation inhibition, potentiate anesthetics (should be discontinued 1 week before surgery) |
| St. John's Wort | Antidepressant, sedative/hypnotic | Hypericin, pseudohypericin | Should not be coadministered with other antidepressants; potential to interact with amphetamines and adrenergic stimulants; prolongs effects of anesthesia. Because antidepressants may be used in perioperative period, should be discontinued 1 week before surgery. |
| Valerian | Sedative, muscle relaxant | Valerianic acid | Potentiates sedatives, including anesthetics |

*RBC*, Red blood cell; *GBE*, ginkgo biloba extract.

impact on postoperative outcomes. In response, the American Society of Anesthesiologists (ASA) has issued a statement cautioning patients who take herbal products to refrain from those medications at least 2 weeks before surgery. Hence, because of the possible negative perianesthesia outcome caused by herbal products, a brief overview of the more popular herbal products is presented in Table 19-6.

### Drugs Used in the Postanesthesia Care Unit
Because of all the possible drugs used in the PACU, Table 19-1 presents most of the drugs that may be used in the perianesthesia care of the surgical patient.

## SUMMARY

The intent of this chapter is to provide the perianesthesia nurse with a review of the drugs that are currently used in the perianesthesia period. An overview of the pharmacodynamics and pharmacokinetics was presented, and the common drugs were presented in table form along with the drug-drug interactions and an overview of the drugs used in sedation. Finally, because many people take some form of herbal drugs, a brief overview is present on this area of pharmacology.

## BIBLIOGRAPHY

Adv Anesthetic Pharmacol, Audio-Digest Anesthesiol 49(3):1-4, 2007.

Aitkenhead A, Smith G, Rowbotham D: Textbook of anesthesia, ed 5, Philadelphia, 2007, Churchill Livingstone.

Alspach J.: Core curriculum for critical care nursing, ed 6, Philadelphia, 2005, Saunders.

Assemi M: Herbal preparations: concerns for operative patients, Anesthesia Today 10(3):19-23, 2000.

Atlee J: Complications in anesthesia, ed 2, Philadelphia, 2007, Saunders.

Barash P, Cullen B, Stoelting R: Clinical anesthesia, ed 5, Philadelphia, 2001, Lippincott Williams & Wilkins.

Benumof J, Saidman L: Anesthesia & perioperative complications, ed 2, St Louis, 1999, Mosby.

Brunton L, Lazo J, Parker K: Goodman and Gilman's the pharmacological basis of therapeutics, ed 11, NewYork, 2005, McGraw-Hill Professional.

Cote' C, Todres I, Goudsouzian N, et al: A practice of anesthesia for infants and children, ed 3, Philadelphia, 2001, Saunders.

Drakuloviv M, Torres A, Bauer T, et al: Supine body postion as a risk factor for nosocomial pneumonia in mechanically ventilated patients: a randomized trial, Lancet 354:1851-1858, 1999.

Estafanous F, Barash P, Reves J, editors: Cardiac anesthesia: principles and clinical practice, ed 2, Philadelphia, 2001, Lippincott Williams & Wilkins.

Estafanous F: Opioids in anesthesia, II, Boston, 1991, Butterworth-Heinemann.

Evers A, Maze M: Anesthetic pharmacology: physiologic principles and clinical practice, Philadelphia, 2004, Churchill Livingstone.

Farmer W, Silverman D: Potential effects of herbal medicinals on perioperative care, Semin Anesthesia Perioperative Med Pain 20(2):110-119, 2001.

Fisher L: Benumof's anesthesia and uncommon diseases, ed 5, Philadelphia, 2007, Saunders.

Gallager C, Issenberg B: Simulation in anesthesia, Philadelphia, 2007, Saunders.

Ganong W: Review of medical physiology, ed 22, New York, 2005, McGraw-Hill Medical.

Guyton A, Hall J: Textbook of medical physiology, ed 11, Philadelphia, 2006, Saunders.

Kier L, Dowd C: The chemistry of drugs for nurse anesthetists, Chicago, 2004, AANA Publishing, Inc.

Longnecker D, Murphy F: Dripps, Eckenhoff, Vandam introduction to anesthesia, ed 9, Philadelphia, 1997, Saunders.

Longnecker D, Tinker J, Morgan G: Principles and practice of anesthesiology, ed 2, St Louis, 1998, Mosby.

Miller R, editor: Anesthesia, ed 5, Philadelphia, 2000, Churchill Livingstone.

Mueller R, Lundberg D: Manual of drug interactions for anesthesiology, ed 3, New York, 1996, Churchill Livingstone.

Murray J, Nadel J: Textbook of respiratory medicine, ed 4, Philadelphia, 2005, Saunders.

Nagelhout J: Drug interactions: introduction, Anesthesia Today 1(4):1-5, 1990.

Nagelhout J, Zaglaniczy K: Nurse anesthesia, ed 3, St Louis, 2005, Saunders.

Prielipp R, Young C: Current drugs for sedation of critically ill patients, Semin Anesthesia Perioperative Med Pain 20(2):85-94, 2001.

Rau J: Recent developments in respiratory care pharmacology, J Perianesth Nurs 13(6):359-369, 1998.

Shorten G, Browne J, Carr D, et al: Postoperative pain management: an evidence-based guide to practice, Philadelphia, 2006, Saunders.

Stoelting R: Pharmacology and physiology in anesthetic practice, ed 3, Philadelphia, 1999, Lippincott.

Stoelting R, Miller R: Basics of anesthesia, ed 4, Philadelphia, 2000, Churchill Livingstone.

White P: Perioperative drug manual, ed 2, Philadelphia, 2005, Saunders.

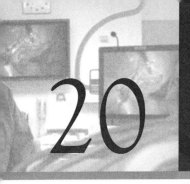

# 20

# INHALATION ANESTHESIA

Cecil B. Drain, PhD, RN, CRNA, FAAN, FASAHP

The inhalational anesthetic agents in use today have survived the many examinations of research, and clinically, they have been proven to add significant safety factors and improved outcomes for the perianesthesia patient. For anticipation of a patient's reaction on emergence from an inhalation anesthetic in the postanesthesia care unit (PACU), the perianesthesia nurse should have a thorough understanding of the pharmacologic concepts of inhalation anesthesia. Although the complexity of these agents, coupled with drug interactions and the various levels of physical health, makes prediction of the exact nature of each patient's emergence from inhalation anesthesia difficult, an understanding of some general principles prepares the perianesthesia nurse for the most commonly expected outcomes.

## DEFINITIONS

**Adjustable Positive-Pressure Relief (APR) Valve:** Used for release of excessive gas on the circle system of an anesthesia machine.

**Amnesia:** A component of anesthesia in which the patient is unable to recall the events that occurred during the administration of the inhalational anesthetic.

**Analgesia:** A component of anesthesia in which the patient is unable to experience pain.

**$CO_2$ Absorption Canisters:** Located in a circle system on an anesthesia machine that clears rebreathed gas that contains carbon dioxide by passing through a canister that contains a chemical carbon dioxide ($CO_2$) absorbent.

**Delirium:** A portion of a stage of anesthesia in which the patient has a transient disturbance during loss of consciousness accompanied by a change in cognition that has a fluctuating course.

**Diffusion Hypoxia:** Sometimes referred to as the "Fink phenomenon"; refers to the rapid exit of nitrous oxide and thus partial reduction of the percentage of oxygen that can be inhaled during the immediate (first 4 to 5 minutes) emergence phase of recovery from anesthesia. Supplemental oxygen and the use of the modified stir-up regime negate this effect of nitrous oxide on emergence.

**Effective Dose (ED):** The dose of a drug necessary to produce a certain effect in a certain percentage of patients. For example, the $ED_{50}$ is the term for when a drug produces a particular effect in 50% of the patients.

**Hypnosis:** A component of anesthesia in which the patient becomes unconscious.

**Inhalation Anesthesia:** Anesthetic substances, in either volatile or gaseous form, that are inhaled via an anesthesia machine.

**Lacrimation:** Tears from the lacrimal glands on the medial side of the tissue surrounding the eyes.

**Minimal Alveolar Concentration (MAC):** A measure of potency of inhalational anesthetic agents; occurs when the equilibrium end-tidal anesthetic concentrations, expressed as a fraction of 1 atm, prevent movement in response to surgical skin incision in 50% of human subjects.

**Muscle Relaxation:** A component of anesthesia in which the patient has reduced tension of the skeletal muscle.

**Nociception:** A component of anesthesia in which the patient is unable to sense pain.

**Scavenger System:** Used to reduce exposure to escaping gases from the anesthesia machine; a waste gas suction tube (scavenger) is connected to the APR valve and anesthesia ventilator relief valve, and the gases are then vented to the outside atmosphere via an operating room suction system.

**Solubility Coefficient:** The ratio of the concentration of an anesthetic in blood or other tissue to that in a gas phase when the two are in equilibrium.

**Sympatholysis:** A component of anesthesia in which the patient is blocked from having an autonomic response to nociceptive stimuli.

**Vaporizer:** A device on the anesthesia machine that converts liquid anesthetics into metered amounts of vapor that are added to the fresh gas mixture to produce a known concentration of the vaporized form of the inhalational anesthetic agent.

## BASIC CONCEPTS

### Evolution of the Signs and Stages of Anesthesia

The five components of anesthesia are hypnosis, analgesia, muscle relaxation, sympatholysis, and amnesia. In the past, when diethyl ether was the primary general anesthetic, assessment of anesthetic depth with the signs and stages of anesthesia was quite simple; the patient could be monitored with assessment of the pupils, respiratory activity, muscle tone, and various reflexes. The ether signs and stages were devised to give some means of assessment of the depth of anesthesia. The first three stages were described by Plomley in 1847; a year later, John Snow added a fourth stage: overdose. During World War I, Guedel more accurately defined and described the signs and stages of anesthesia. A graphic representation of these signs and stages is provided in Fig. 20-1.

With the advent of modern anesthesia, which included the addition of fluorinated inhalation anesthetic agents, muscle relaxants, and various pharmacologic adjuncts, the usual predictable signs and stages as described by Guedel were abolished. Even now in the PACU, many of these pharmacologic adjuncts have an impact on the "prediction" of the depth of anesthesia. The classic signs and stages provide some help in the assessment and care of the patient after surgery. Many times in today's anesthesia practice, these signs and stages provide a "language" for description of the level of anesthesia during and

after surgery. Consequently, a brief description, including the incorporation of some of the pharmacology of the modern anesthetics, is given.

Stage I begins with the initiation of anesthesia and ends with the loss of consciousness. It is commonly called the stage of analgesia. This stage has been described as the lightest level of anesthesia and represents sensory and mental depression. Stage I is the level of anesthesia used with nitrous oxide. Patients are able to open their eyes on command, breathe normally, maintain protective reflexes, and tolerate mild painful stimuli.

Stage II starts with the loss of consciousness and ends with the onset of a regular pattern of breathing and the disappearance of the lid reflex. This is also called the stage of delirium. This stage is characterized by excitement, and so many untoward responses such as vomiting, laryngospasm, and even cardiac arrest may take place during this stage. With the use of anesthetic agents that act much more rapidly than ether, this stage is passed rather quickly. In addition, the induction of anesthesia is usually facilitated with short-acting barbiturates that expedite a short duration of stage II.

Stage III is the stage of surgical anesthesia. With ether anesthesia, this stage is defined as lasting from the onset of a regular pattern of breathing to the cessation of respiration. At this stage of anesthesia, response to surgical incision is absent. The modern concept of MAC is predicated in part with the signs and stages of

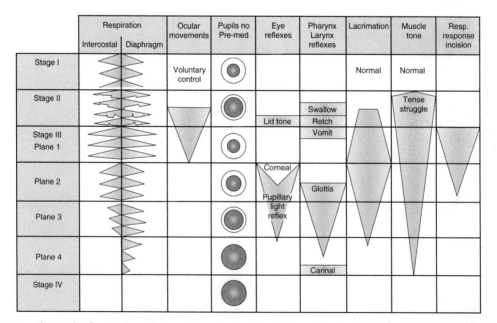

**Fig. 20-1** Signs and reflex reactions of stages of anesthesia. (Adapted from Gillespie NA: Signs of anesthesia, *Anesth Analg* 22:275, 1943.)

surgical anesthesia. MAC is exceeded by a factor of 1.3 in stage III because most patients do not respond to surgical incision at this level of anesthesia. Patients who receive 1.3 MAC anesthesia have a depression in all elements of nervous system function—that is, sensory depression, loss of recall, reflex depression, and some skeletal muscle relaxation. From this point, with the modern anesthetics, increased MAC results in further respiratory, cardiovascular, and central nervous system (CNS) depression. The difficulty is that each of the newer agents affects the clinical signs, such as blood pressure, differently. Consequently, monitoring of the level of anesthesia depends on the particular properties of each agent.

Most surgical procedures in which ether anesthesia was used were performed at this stage of anesthesia, which is divided into four planes. Plane 1 is entered when the lid reflex is abolished and respiration becomes regular. During this plane, the vomiting reflex is gradually abolished. The nurse working in the PACU must know that swallowing, retching, and vomiting reflexes tend to disappear in that order during induction and reappear in the same order during emergence from anesthesia.

Plane 2 lasts from the time the eyeballs cease to move and become concentrically fixed to the beginning of a decrease of activity of the intercostal muscles, or thoracic respiration. The reflex of laryngospasm disappears during this plane. Plane 3 is entered when intercostal activity begins to decrease. Complete intercostal paralysis occurs in lower plane 3, and respiration is produced solely by the diaphragm. Plane 4 lasts from the time of paralysis of the intercostal muscles to the cessation of spontaneous respiration.

Tracheal tug often appears in association with deep anesthesia and intercostal paralysis. This effect represents an unopposed action of the diaphragm, which displaces the hilum of the lung and thereby increases traction on the trachea.

Stage IV lasts from the time of cessation of respiration to failure of the circulatory system. This level of anesthesia is considered the stage of overdose.

When ether is used as the sole inhalation agent, these signs and stages are seen in reverse order on emergence from the anesthetic. No one clinical sign can be considered a reliable indicator of anesthetic depth by itself. All clinical signs must be viewed in the context of the patient's status along with the particular characteristics of the individual anesthetic agent used.

Some of the more reliable indicators of depth of anesthesia for the more modern inhalation anesthetics include changes in breathing pattern, eye movement, lacrimation, and muscle tone. Because the ventilation is under autonomic control, it is the most sensitive indicator of depth of anesthesia. In the PACU, a patient who uses diaphragmatic ventilation without the intercostal muscles should be considered to be in surgical anesthesia. As the ventilatory pattern returns to a more normal rate, rhythm, and pattern, the patient can be considered to be in light anesthesia and about to have total emergence. Eye movement as opposed to pupillary size is a good indicator of anesthetic depth. Light anesthesia is present with eye movement. Deeper anesthesia is present when the eyes are close together in a cross-eyed position. Lacrimation does not occur during surgical anesthesia when a patient receives desflurane (Suprane), isoflurane (Forane), or sevoflurane (Ultane). Conversely, if a patient received one of those drugs and has tearing, light anesthesia can be considered to be present. As the depth of anesthesia is increased, the amount of muscle tone decreases. Therefore, if a patient in the PACU lacks muscle tone, especially in the jaw and abdomen, the patient should be considered to be in a surgical depth of anesthesia. With the assessment of the degree of muscle tone, the perianesthesia nurse must critically assess the degree of reversal of skeletal muscle relaxants (see Chapter 23) before determining the depth of anesthesia with the criterion of muscle tone. Finally, because the determinants of anesthesia depth have such a high degree of variability, all possible assessment tools should be incorporated into the care of the patient in the PACU. It goes without saying that the bottom line is constant vigilance of the patient's physiologic parameters during emergence from anesthesia and the institution of appropriate nursing interventions based on an ongoing assessment.

## Pharmacokinetics of Inhalation Anesthetics

The pharmacokinetics of inhalation anesthetics involve uptake, distribution, metabolism, and elimination. Basically, this involves a series of partial pressure gradients starting in the anesthesia machine to the patient's brain for induction, and vice versa for emergence. The object of anesthesia is a constant and optimal partial pressure in the brain. The key to attainment of anesthesia is the alveolar partial pressure (PA) in equilibrium with the arterial (Pa) and brain (Pbr) partial pressure of the inhaled anesthetic. The partial pressure of an inhalation anesthetic in the brain is used to determine the depth of anesthesia. The more potent the anesthetic, the lower the partial pressure of the agent needed to produce a certain depth of anesthesia.

***Movement of Inhalation Anesthetic from Anesthesia Machine to Alveoli.*** The determinants of the PA are the inspired partial pressure of the inhalation anesthetic, the characteristics of the anesthesia machine's delivery system, and the patient's alveolar ventilation. The inhaled partial pressure (PI) is the concentration of the inhalation anesthetic that is delivered from the anesthesia machine. The impact of the PI on the rate of increase in the PA is called the concentration effect. The higher the inhaled concentration, the more rapid the induction of anesthesia. The anesthesia machine's delivery system has an impact on the depth of anesthesia and the speed of induction and emergence. For example, the rate of uptake of an anesthetic agent administered via inhalation can be reduced with the diffusion of the anesthetic agent into the rubber tubing of the anesthesia machine, the small losses of anesthetic agent from the body via diffusion across skin and mucous membranes, and, to a lesser extent, the metabolism of the agents by the body.

Alveolar ventilation plays the primary role in delivery of the anesthetic gas. It is determined in large part by the minute ventilation ($V_E$). If the $V_E$ is high, the anesthetic concentration increases quickly in the alveoli, as does the concentration in the arterial blood. This concept is important to understand because the reverse also is true. In the emergence phase of anesthesia, a good $V_E$ is important to ensure elimination of the anesthetic agent.

***Movement of Inhalation Anesthetic from Alveoli to Arterial Blood.*** The movement of the inhalation anesthetic agent from the alveoli to the arterial blood depends on the blood-gas partition coefficient and the cardiac output. The rate at which the anesthetic is taken up by the blood and tissues is governed in part by the solubility of the agent in blood. This is expressed as the blood-gas partition coefficient,

or the Oswald solubility coefficient, and is defined as the ratio of the concentration of an anesthetic in blood to that in a gas phase when the two are in equilibrium (Table 20-1). This concept is difficult to understand because the more soluble the anesthetic agent is, the slower the agent is in producing anesthesia. This effect is because the blood serves as a reservoir and a large volume of the agent must be introduced to attain an equilibrium between the blood partial pressure and the partial pressure in the lungs.

The blood conveys the anesthetic agent to the tissues. Consequently, a normal cardiac output is needed for facilitation of the movement of the inhalation anesthetic through the tissues to the brain. The partial pressure increases most rapidly in the tissues with the highest rates of blood flow. Of interest is the great variation in blood perfusion of certain tissues in the body. The body tissue compartments can be divided into the following major groups:

1. The vessel-rich group, which consists of the heart, brain, kidneys, hepatoportal system, and endocrine glands.
2. The intermediate group of perfused tissues, which consists of muscle and skin.
3. The fat group, which includes marrow and adipose tissue.
4. The vessel-poor group, which has the poorest circulation per unit volume and comprises tendons, ligaments, connective tissue, teeth, bone, and other avascular tissue.

The vessel-rich group of tissues receives 75% of the cardiac output; thus, the brain becomes saturated rapidly with an anesthetic agent administered via inhalation. On termination of the anesthetic, the reverse takes place, and the agent is rapidly removed from the brain.

The tissue tensions of the inhaled anesthetic increase and approach the arterial blood tension and ultimately the PA. One of the tissue groups that affects both the induction and the emergence from anesthesia is the fat group. The oil-gas partition coefficient best exemplifies the

## Table 20-1  Properties of Inhalant Anesthetic Agents

| Alveolar Agent | PARTITION COEFFICIENT | | | Minimal Concentration (% in Oxygen) |
| --- | --- | --- | --- | --- |
| | Blood-Gas | Oil-Gas | Blood-Brain | |
| Isoflurane (Forane) | 0.97 | 93.7 | 1.6 | 1.15 |
| Desflurane (Suprane) | 0.42 | 20.7 | 1.3 | 6.58 |
| Sevoflurane (Ultane) | 0.69 | 53.4 | 1.7 | 1.71 |
| Nitrous oxide | 0.47 | 1.4 | 1.1 | 104.0 |

process involved with the affinity of anesthesia agents to adipose tissue and ultimately the emergence from anesthesia. The oil-gas partition coefficient is defined as the ratio of the concentration of the anesthetic agent in oil (adipose tissue) to that in a gaseous phase when the two are in equilibrium (see Table 20-1). The oil-gas partition coefficients seem to parallel anesthetic requirements. In fact, one can calculate the MAC by knowing the oil-gas partition coefficient. With the constant of 150, the calculated MAC for an anesthetic with an oil-gas partition coefficient of 100 is 1.5%.

Because some anesthetic agents are highly fat soluble, they tend to be readily absorbed by the adipose tissue. This characteristic affects uptake of the anesthetic agent, but of more importance is the prolonged recovery phase that usually ensues with a high oil-gas partition coefficient, such as in the case of halothane. Because adipose tissue is poorly perfused by blood, the adipose tissue releases the agent slowly to the blood at the termination of the anesthesia. Redistribution then takes place; some of the agent is eliminated by the lungs, which are vessel rich, and some is distributed to the brain. The recovery period becomes significantly extended when, to allow for complete saturation of the adipose tissue, the administration time of the anesthetic agent is prolonged.

Halothane (Fluothane) was the classic inhalational anesthetic from the 1960s to the 1990s. Inclusion of halothane in the discussion is helpful because all the inhalational anesthetic agents today have almost the same partition coefficients. Halothane has an oil-gas partition coefficient that is about twice that of isoflurane, desflurane, or sevoflurane. Hence, with use of halothane as the marker, the newer inhalational agents are twice as fast during induction and emergence as before. All three of the inhalational anesthetics today are used in a variety of settings, and all possess a blood-gas partition coefficient less than one (see Table 20-1).

***Movement of Inhalation Anesthetic from Arterial Blood to the Brain.*** The transfer of the inhalation anesthetic from the arterial blood to the brain depends on the blood-brain partition coefficient of the agent and the cerebral blood flow. The blood-brain partition coefficient for most of the inhalation anesthetics is between 1.3 and 2 (see Table 20-1). The concentration gradient during induction of anesthesia is as follows:

$$PA > Pa > Pbr$$

During maintenance of surgical anesthesia, the brain tissue becomes saturated with the anesthetic agent and the brain tissue is in equilibrium with the alveolar and arterial concentration. Consequently,

$$PA = Pa = Pbr$$

## Emergence of Inhalation Anesthesia

When the administration of the anesthetic is terminated, a reverse gradient takes place. In this instance, the PA is almost zero because only oxygen is administered during the emergence phase. The gradient that develops is as follows:

$$PA < Pa < Pbr$$

This gradient favors the removal of the anesthetic agent from the brain tissue. The partial pressure in the tissues declines first and is followed by that in the arterial blood. The agent returns to the lungs and is then eliminated into the atmosphere. The factors that affect the rate of elimination of the agent are the same ones that determine how rapidly an anesthetic agent takes a patient to surgical anesthesia. If a short procedure is performed (< 1 hour), complete equilibrium among PA, Pa, and Pbr might not have occurred, and the recovery from anesthesia is more rapid. The reverse is true; during long procedures in which equilibrium occurs, a prolonged emergence may be anticipated.

## Potency of Inhalation Anesthetic Agents

Potency is determined by factors such as absorption, distribution, metabolism, excretion, and affinity for a receptor. The potency of the anesthetic agent refers to its ability to take the patient through all the stages of anesthesia to respiratory and circulatory arrest without the occurrence of hypoxia or the use of preanesthetic medication. Certainly, circulatory and respiratory arrests are not desired outcomes of the use of anesthetic agents; these features are used merely to describe the potency of anesthetic agents that are used clinically. For example, isoflurane is 100% potent in comparison with nitrous oxide, which is 15% potent. Isoflurane, when administered with oxygen to meet the patient's metabolic needs and when given without premedication, takes the patient to circulatory and respiratory arrest, whereas nitrous oxide administered with oxygen takes the patient only to the first portion of surgical anesthesia and no further. Therefore, clinically speaking, potency of a drug makes little difference as long as the drug that is to be administered has an effective dose for a particular patient., which is why the concept of ED was developed. The ED is the dose of a drug necessary to produce certain effects in a certain percentage of patients. For

## Table 20-2   Factors That Modify Minimum Alveolar Concentration (MAC)

- Factors that increase MAC
  - Young age
  - Hyperthermia
  - CNS stimulation
  - Physostigmine
  - Alcohol dependency
- Factors that decrease MAC
  - Elderly age
  - Hypothermia
  - Acute alcohol ingestion
  - CNS depressants
    - 1.1 Benzodiazepines
    - 1.2 Barbiturates
    - 1.3 Propofol
  - Tranquilizers
  - Narcotics
  - Pregnancy
  - Alpha-2-adrenergic agonists
    - 1.1 Clonidine
    - 1.2 Dexmedetomidine

Modified from Longnecker D, Murphy F: *Dripps/Eckenhoff/Vandam introduction to anesthesia*, ed 9, Philadelphia, 1997, Saunders.

example, an $ED_{50}$ means that a drug produces a particular effect in 50% of the patients.

Another method of determination of potency is with the use of the MAC. The MAC is found with determining the alveolar concentration (at 1 atm) needed for prevention of gross muscular movement in response to painful stimuli in 50% of anesthetized patients. The lower the MAC value, the more anesthetic potency of the inhalation anesthetic. Consequently, the MAC defines the therapeutic effect of inhalational anesthetics as the prevention of movement in response to surgical stimulation.

The potency of an inhalational anesthetic agent with the MAC as the tool of assessment varies with the patient's age, state of health, clinical conditions, and concurrent use of other drugs (with depressant effects). The factors that modify the MAC are presented in Table 20-2. MAC awake is the anesthetic dose at which a patient responds to commands. It is also the dose of anesthetic at which most patients lose consciousness and recall. MAC awake usually corresponds with stage I of anesthesia. Another term used with MAC is MAC-**B**lock **A**drenergic **R**esponse, which is the MAC needed to block the adrenergic and cardiovascular responses to incision; it corresponds to stage III, plane III anesthesia.

## TECHNIQUES OF ADMINISTRATION

The inhalation anesthetics are usually administered by means of an anesthesia machine (Fig. 20-2). The anesthesia machine is essentially a breathing circuit that conveys the agent and oxygen to the patient. It consists of a mask, corrugated tubing, an absorber for removal of expired carbon dioxide, a reservoir bag, unidirectional valves, APR valve, and vaporizers (Fig. 20-3).

### Circle Systems

A variety of techniques can be used to deliver gaseous agents with the anesthesia machine by adding or removing certain features. The most common technique used is the semiclosed circle method, in which some rebreathing of expired gases occurs by opening the APR valve to vent some of the gas to the atmosphere. The closed circle method is used when low gas flows are desired. In this technique, the APR valve is completely closed and complete rebreathing of expired gases occurs. A carbon dioxide absorber is used in both the semiclosed and the closed techniques.

The Bain anesthesia circuit, introduced in 1972, consists of a tube within a tube. The inner noncorrugated tube, which provides fresh

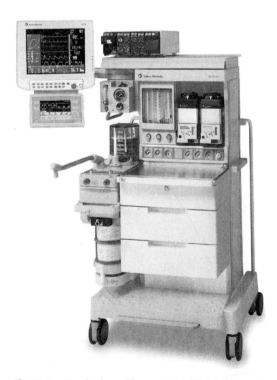

**Fig. 20-2**   Anesthesia machine apparatus. (*Used with permission from Datex-Ohmeda, Madison, Wis.*)

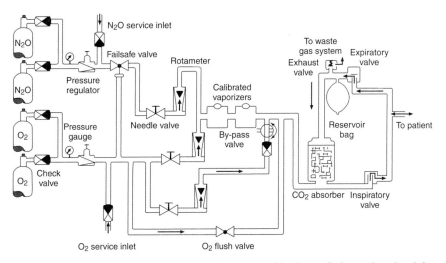

**Fig. 20-3**    Anesthesia machine circuit. Oxygen and nitrous oxide enter machine from cylinders or from hospital service supply. Pressure regulators reduce cylinder pressure to about 3 kg/cm². Check valves to prevent transfilling of cylinders or gas flow from cylinders to service line. Fail-safe valve prevents flow of nitrous oxide if oxygen supply fails. Needle valves in flowmeters control flows to rotameters. Calibrated vaporizers provide preselected concentration of volatile anesthetics. Gases are delivered to circle absorber, where unidirectional valves ensure flow from patient through carbon dioxide absorber. Excess gas is vented through exhaust valve into waste gas scavenger system. Reservoir bag compensates for variations in respiratory demand. *(Adapted from Dripps RD, Eckenhoff JE, Vandam LD: Introduction to anesthesia: the principles of safe practice, ed 7, Philadelphia, 1988, Saunders.)*

gases to the patient, is surrounded by a wider corrugated tube that conveys exhaled gases away from the patient. The circuit attaches to a bag mount that is attached to the anesthesia machine. The bag mount incorporates an exhaust valve and a bag port for attachment of an anesthesia bag or ventilator tubing (Fig. 20-4). The major advantage of this circuit is its versatility; it may be used for both children and adults, it has no directional valves, it is especially useful in surgical procedures that involve the head and neck, and it does not require carbon dioxide absorption (no soda lime) yet patients may be maintained at a normal $PaCO_2$ and pH.

## INHALATION AGENTS

Inhalant anesthetic substances may be divided into the following two groups: volatile and gaseous. Volatile anesthetic agents are chemicals in the liquid state at room temperature that have a boiling point above 20° C. Ethyl chloride, which has a boiling point of 12° C, is also included in this class of anesthetic agents. The volatile inhalation anesthetic agents are divided into two major categories: the halogenated hydrocarbons and the ethers. Examples of the halogenated hydrocarbons are isoflurane, desflurane, and sevoflurane; diethyl ether is an example of the ethers. The gaseous anesthetic agents, such as

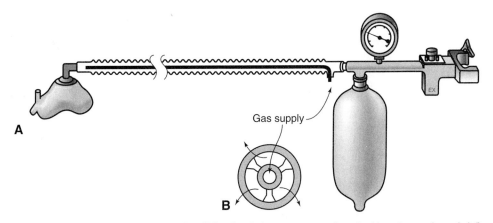

**Fig. 20-4**    Bain system breathing circuit. **A,** Tube-within-tube design. **B,** Cross-section of tubing. *Arrows* show air inflow and outflow. *(From Chu YK, Rah KH, Boyan CP: Is the Bain breathing circuit the future anesthesia system? Anesth Analg 56:84, 1977.)*

nitrous oxide, are in the gaseous state at room temperature. The anesthetic agents currently in use have evolved from the traditional inhalation anesthetics that are not in use today: cyclopropane, chloroform, and diethyl ether.

## Modern Inhalation Anesthetics

*Isoflurane (Forane).* Isoflurane, an analogue of enflurane, is also a halogenated methyl ethyl ether. It produces a dose-related depression of the CNS. But, in contrast with enflurane, this anesthetic agent does not produce convulsive electroencephalographic abnormalities. Isoflurane reduces the systemic arterial blood pressure and total peripheral resistance. However, during isoflurane anesthesia, the heart rate is usually increased and the cardiac output usually remains within normal limits. This agent produces respiratory depression and skeletal muscular relaxation in a dose-related fashion because isoflurane markedly potentiates the actions of the nondepolarizing muscle relaxants. Of interest to the perianesthesia nurse is the fact that isoflurane does not sensitize the myocardium to catecholamines to the same extent as halothane does. Thus, the chance of dysrhythmias is reduced when the patient has received isoflurane anesthesia.

The recovery phase is rapid because of isoflurane's low blood-gas partition coefficient of 0.97. The patient not only awakens promptly but is also quite lucid within 15 to 30 minutes after termination of the anesthetic. However, clinical observation indicates that if the anesthesia time with isoflurane is longer than 45 to 60 minutes, the patient will probably have a slower emergence phase than expected given that the drug has such a low blood-gas partition coefficient.

The lung volumes and capacities, as measured with the Wright respirometer, return to normal in less than 30 minutes along with the ability to raise the head, protrude the tongue, cough on command, and converse clearly. The blood pressure and pulse remain stable. Shivering is seen in 2% of patients, and nausea and vomiting occur only occasionally.

Isoflurane possesses some excellent qualities—that is, a lack of sensitization of the heart to catecholamines, cardiovascular stability, limited biodegradation, good neuromuscular relaxation, and no CNS excitatory effects. Since its introduction into anesthesia practice, isoflurane has enjoyed continuing success among both anesthesia practitioners and perianesthesia nurses.

*Sevoflurane (Ultane).* Sevoflurane is a 100% potent inhalation anesthetic agent that has a blood-gas solubility coefficient of 0.69, which is near nitrous oxide and thus makes it an extremely rapid-acting agent. Consequently, patients emerge from sevoflurane anesthesia in a matter of minutes when they have received this drug as the sole agent. One must remember that a rapid recovery from an inhalation anesthetic usually mandates the need for analgesic drugs in the immediate postoperative period.

The drug is nonirritating to the respiratory tract, and the degree of patient acceptance is high. Sevoflurane can be used in place of halothane for the induction of anesthesia in children. It tends to decrease the blood pressure by decreasing the systemic vascular resistance. Like all other inhalation agents, this drug is a respiratory depressant and blunts the ventilatory response to an increased $PaCO_2$. This drug does undergo some metabolism at about the same degree as does enflurane. The metabolites of sevoflurane include fluoride and hexafluoroisopropanol. On the basis of a number of studies, no evidence of toxicity has been shown in regard to the biodegradation of this agent, probably because of sevoflurane's rapid ventilatory excretion, in which the metabolic byproducts do not seem to be significantly detrimental to the patient.

Like the other ethers, sevoflurane does not sensitize the heart to catecholamines and hence does not predispose to arrhythmias. This inhalation agent does reduce cerebrovascular resistance and can increase intracranial pressure in a dose-related manner. In regard to its effect on skeletal muscle function, it enhances the action of the skeletal muscle relaxants. However, because of the drug's rapid elimination, this characteristic does not have a significant impact on the care of a patient in the PACU who has received sevoflurane during surgery.

Sevoflurane possesses many outstanding qualities. It has great precision and control over anesthetic depth, it does not depress kidney or liver function, it has little effect on heart rate, and, most of all, it is extremely rapid, which speeds up the emergence of the patient in the PACU.

*Desflurane (Suprane).* Desflurane is a fluorinated ether that is similar to isoflurane. This drug has a blood-gas partition coefficient that is the same as cyclopropane (0.42) and even less than nitrous oxide, which makes it extremely rapid acting. As with sevoflurane, patient emergence is extremely rapid and analgesia is needed in the immediate postoperative period. This drug produces a dose-related decrease in blood pressure and cardiac output that is slightly greater than the depression seen with equivalent doses of isoflurane. Because this drug is an ether-type inhalation agent, the incidence rate of cardiac dysrhythmias when epinephrine is administered is extremely low.

The pungency of desflurane irritates the respiratory tract and causes coughing, breath-holding, and laryngospasm. Consequently, the drug is not recommended as an inhalation induction agent, especially in the pediatric age group. This drug depresses respiration in the same fashion as does sevoflurane and thus blunts the response to an increased $PaCO_2$. Because this drug decreases cerebrovascular resistance, it produces in a dose-related fashion. Desflurane also enhances the neuromuscular blockade produced by skeletal muscle relaxants. However, like sevoflurane, this action is not of consequence for the patient in the PACU because of its extremely rapid ventilatory excretion during emergence. Finally, as opposed to sevoflurane, this drug resists biodegradation and is almost totally eliminated by the respiratory system and therefore does not have a negative effect on the kidney or liver.

Desflurane represents a new era in inhalation anesthesia in regard to its impact on the care of the patient in the PACU. More specifically, because of its low solubility, rapid emergence will become quite common and a more rapid release from the PACU and a shorter length of stay in the hospital may be possible.

**Nitrous Oxide.** Nitrous oxide is the only inorganic gas used as an anesthetic agent. It is marketed in blue steel cylinders as a colorless liquid at a pressure of 30 atm. As the pressure is released, nitrous oxide returns to the gaseous state. It is readily soluble in water and heavier than air. Nitrous oxide was probably the first anesthetic agent to be used extensively. The fact that it is still used indicates that, when used properly, it is a valuable and safe anesthetic agent.

Nitrous oxide supports combustion—that is, if a burning match is put into a jar that contains nitrous oxide, it continues to burn. However, this agent is not explosive. Although the nitrous oxide molecule contains oxygen, that oxygen is unavailable for respiration because nitrous oxide does not decompose in the body.

Nitrous oxide is a 15% potent agent; therefore, the maximum depth of anesthesia that can be produced while the patient's metabolic need for oxygen is supplied is the middle of plane 1 of stage III anesthesia. This agent has no side effects unless hypoxia is present. It is nontoxic and nonirritating; however, nitrous oxide can cause postoperative nausea and vomiting, particularly in the ambulatory surgical setting when

the procedure lasts for 1 hour, and quite probably for 2 or more hours. Nitrous oxide is a rapid-acting agent in part because of its blood-gas partition coefficient of 0.47. This agent does not combine with hemoglobin but is carried in physical solution in the blood. It is excreted mostly unchanged by the lungs, although a small fraction is excreted through the skin. It does not sensitize the heart to epinephrine, and it provides a fair amount of analgesia. Even in subanesthetic concentrations, nitrous oxide has an analgesic effect in humans, and 20% concentrations of the gas have been claimed to be as effective as 15 mg of morphine sulfate. If this agent were more potent, it would probably be considered an almost perfect anesthetic.

In current anesthesia practice, nitrous oxide serves an important role because it is administered alone and in combination with various agents. Recently, the balanced technique of anesthesia has been favored because of the number of negative factors associated with some of the more potent volatile inhalation anesthetics. The balanced technique consists of the administration of narcotics that may or may not be in combination with a tranquilizer, a muscle relaxant, nitrous oxide, oxygen, and barbiturates. All the elements of anesthesia or nervous system depression are met: sensory block (analgesia), motor block (muscle relaxation), reflex block, and mental block (narcosis). When nitrous oxide is administered with a potent volatile inhalation anesthetic such as desflurane, it acts as a carrier and also provides an additional analgesic effect. The second gas effect occurs because of nitrous oxide's rapid uptake, after which the potent volatile agent takes the patient to the desired surgical plane. The reverse takes place at termination of the anesthetic.

The solubilities of nitrogen and nitrous oxide differ greatly. Nitrous oxide is 30 times more soluble than nitrogen. An enclosed gas-filled space in the body expands if gas within it is more soluble than the gas respired. For this reason, any enclosed gas-filled cavity in the body expands because of the slow exchange of nitrogen from the cavity for the rapid exchange of large volumes of nitrous oxide from the blood, which is why the use of nitrous oxide is not recommended in surgical procedures for intestinal obstruction or pneumothorax. Nitrous oxide has been shown to dislodge a tympanoplasty graft because of the expansion of the air pocket in the middle ear. Consequently, in surgical procedures that involve the middle ear, the administration of nitrous oxide is usually avoided. Of interest to the perianesthesia nurse is the possible role of nitrous oxide in altering the pressures in the middle ear; nitrous oxide has been suggested to cause nausea and vomiting from the resulting increased pressure in that area.

Diffusion hypoxia after nitrous oxide anesthesia is another area of concern for the perianesthesia nurse. This effect is sometimes called the Fink phenomenon. It occurs when not enough nitrous oxide is removed from the lungs at the end of the surgical procedure. Normally, 100% oxygen is administered at the end of the procedure for removal of the nitrous oxide, which is called nitrous oxide washout. Diffusion hypoxia is directly related to the dilution of alveolar gas by the rapid diffusion of the nitrous oxide out of the blood. This outpouring of nitrous oxide into the alveoli occurs during the first 1 to 5 minutes after the nitrous oxide has been discontinued. Along with this, the rapid movement into the alveoli can cause a dilutional effect of the $PACO_2$ and ultimately a reduction in the stimulus to breathe. Therefore, administration of oxygen via mask to all patients who are admitted to the PACU is highly advisable. This maneuver forestalls the development of severe hypoxia if some unpredicted airway problem occurs. Another measure for avoiding this complication is provision of adequate verbal and physical stimulation to the patient to promote good ventilatory effort. This approach should include encouraging the patient to sigh every 5 minutes to ensure adequate removal of the anesthetic gases.

## ASSESSMENT OF THE EFFECTS OF INHALATION AGENTS IN THE PERIANESTHESIA CARE UNIT

In assessment of the patient's degree of emergence from inhalation anesthesia, the nurse must understand the pharmacologic effects of each anesthetic agent and of the preoperative medications used. Also, the rate of recovery from inhalation anesthesia is predictable based on the solubility of the anesthetic agent, alveolar ventilation, and duration of the anesthetic. Each anesthetic agent is essentially a depressant drug. Certain volatile agents, such as sevoflurane, desflurane, and isoflurane, possess a high degree of myocardial and respiratory depressant properties. One parameter for monitoring of the emergence phase with administration of these agents is the vital signs. Preanesthetic baseline vital sign readings are reliable postoperative indicators of the patient's cardiorespiratory status and can be used in assessment of the patient's stage of recovery. When this assessment is made, however, all other factors of the patient's condition must also be considered.

Total assessment of the patient recovering from anesthesia is discussed in Chapter 27. Most inhalation anesthetics cause some degree of depression of the respiratory system. Consequently, the $PaCO_2$ increases in a dose-related manner, frequency increases, and tidal volume is reduced. Because of the respiratory depression that all patients have after anesthesia and surgery, the perianesthesia nurse must use the stir-up regimen that encourages the patient to perform the sustained maximal inspiration maneuver (see Chapter 27).

To understand the emergence phase of inhalation anesthesia, the nurse also needs a basic understanding of blood-gas and oil-gas partition coefficients. Anesthetic agents are usually administered in combinations, often with nitrous oxide as the carrier gas. The combination of agents usually consists of a 100% potent agent, a carrier agent, and oxygen to meet the metabolic needs of the patient. The agent with the highest blood-gas partition coefficient takes the longest time to be removed from the body. Therefore, if a isoflurane–nitrous oxide–oxygen combination is administered to a patient, the isoflurane, which has the highest blood-gas partition coefficient, is eliminated the most slowly.

Along with the factors attributed to the blood-gas partition coefficient, those attributed to the oil-gas partition coefficient should be considered in an evaluation of length of time of emergence from the anesthetic. When the intraoperative phase is of long duration, an agent with a high oil-gas partition coefficient redistributes into the adipose tissue. As mentioned previously, because the vascular supply to adipose tissue is sparse, the release of the agent to the blood is slow and the emergence is prolonged. Both coefficients must be kept in mind in prediction of the length of the emergence phase from an inhalation anesthetic agent. Isoflurane, for example, has the low blood-gas partition coefficient of 0.97, and one would expect a rapid recovery from its administration. However, isoflurane has a high oil-gas partition coefficient of 93.7, so when it is administered for longer than 2 hours, the adipose tissue is saturated and emergence from the anesthetic agent is prolonged. Nitrous oxide, desflurane, and isoflurane have low blood-gas and oil-gas partition coefficients.

Inhalation agents, because of their depressant effect on the hypothalamus, disrupt the regulation of body temperature that may be manifested by either a reduction or an elevation, depending on the environmental temperature. In the recovery phase, the emerging patient should be monitored for hypothermia or hyperthermia. Serious heat loss may occur in newborns and create difficulties in the reestablishment of adequate ventilatory effort after surgery. Body temperature should be monitored in patients who were febrile before surgery and who received atropine before or during the operative procedure. Agents such as isoflurane that have a direct vasodilatory effect on vascular smooth muscle can cause a temperature drop of $1°$ C in esophageal temperature. Shivering and tremors have been reported during the postoperative period after isoflurane anesthesia, although these phenomena have mostly been associated with a generalized loss of muscle tone during surgery and anesthesia.

Water and electrolyte balance is affected by inhalation anesthesia. Pituitary and adrenocortical systems appear to be affected in such a way that water and sodium retention and potassium loss occur after anesthesia. This balance is also affected, in part, by the stress of surgical trauma. Decreased glomerular filtration, increased tubular reabsorption, and varying degrees of oliguria exist in the recovery phase because of renal vasoconstriction. If renal blood flow is not impaired, glomerular function quickly returns to normal after the operation. The increased tubular reabsorption of water usually persists for 36 to 48 hours but may continue for several days in elderly patients.

## SUMMARY

The inhalation anesthetic agents have moved from the first anesthetic discovered in 1846, ether; to deritives of ether (methoxyflurane); to penthrane that was introduced in the early 1960s; to halothane (fluothane), which was a halogenated hydrocarbon type drug introduced in the late 1960s; to the current inhalational drugs described in this chapter. The armitarium for the anesthesia practitioner has in some ways become simplified, and the current selection of agents offers many advantages to the older drugs. For the perianesthesia nurse, this movement in the use of inhalational anesthetic agents has been very positive. Before, the patient would emerge rather slowly; sometimes it seemed like days. Now, with the current inhalational agents, patients wake up rather quickly. With the advent of these faster acting agents, the perianesthesia nurse is now confronted with new or more profound nursing care issues, such as pain, confusion, and awareness with anesthesia, among others. Consequently, Chapter 31 has been devoted to pain and its physiology, and Chapters 28 and 29 are devoted to the nursing

interventions for the sequelae of confusion and awareness with anesthesia.

The administration of inhalational agents has also become more simplified, and gone is the equipment used through the ether to penthrane days. However, for the assessment of potency, the MAC is still used; and because many practitioners still use the signs and stages first described by Guedel, a description is included in this chapter. Also, the prediction of emergence of the patient recovering from an inhalational anesthetic can be aided with a firm knowledge of the movement of the anesthetic through the various vascular groups along with the various partition coefficients. Finally, an overview of the assessment of a patient recovering from inhalational anesthesia is provided with a detailed discussion presented in Chapter 27.

## BIBLIOGRAPHY

Aitkenhead A, Smith G, Rowbotham D: *Textbook of anesthesia*, ed 5, Philadelphia, 2007, Churchill Livingstone.

Alspach J: *Core curriculum for critical care nursing*, ed 6, Philadelphia, 2005, Saunders.

Atlee J: *Complications in anesthesia*, ed 2, Philadelphia, 2007, Saunders.

Barash P, Cullen B, Stoelting R: *Clinical anesthesia*, ed 5, Philadelphia, 2005, Lippincott Williams & Wilkins.

Benumof J, Saidman L: *Anesthesia & perioperative complications*, ed 2, St Louis, 1999, Mosby.

Brunton L, Lazo J, Parker K: *Goodman and Gilman's the pharmacological basis of therapeutics*, ed 11, New York, 2005, McGraw-Hill Professional.

Chu Y, Rah K, Boyan C: Is the Bain breathing circuit the future anesthesia system? An evaluation, *Anesth Analg* 56:84-87, 1977.

Cote' C, Todres I, Goudsouzian N, et al: *A practice of anesthesia for infants and children*, ed 3, Philadelphia, 2001, Saunders.

Dorsch J, Dorsch S: *Understanding anesthesia equipment*, ed 2, Baltimore, 1989, Williams & Wilkins.

Drake R, Vogl W, Mitchell A: *Gray's anatomy for students*, Philadelphia, 2005, Churchill Livingstone.

Estafanous F, Barash P, Reves J: *Cardiac anesthesia: principles and clinical practice*, ed 2, Philadelphia, 2001, Lippincott Williams & Wilkins.

Evers A, Maze M: *Anesthetic pharmacology: physiologic principles and clinical practice*, Philadelphia, 2004, Churchill Livingstone.

Fisher L: *Benumof's anesthesia and uncommon diseases*, ed 5, Philadelphia, 2007, Saunders.

Gallager C, Issenberg B: *Simulation in anesthesia*, Philadelphia, 2007, Saunders.

Ganong W: *Review of medical physiology*, ed 22, New York, 2005, McGraw-Hill Medical.

Guyton A, Hall J: *Textbook of medical physiology*, ed 11, Philadelphia, 2006, Saunders.

Jones R: Desflurane and sevoflurane: inhalation anesthetics for this decade? *Br J Anaesth* 65:527-536, 1990.

Katoh T, Suguro Y, Nakajima R, et al: Blood concentration of sevoflurane and isoflurane on recovery from anesthesia, *Br J Anaesth* 69:259-262, 1992.

Kier L, Dowd C: *The chemistry of drugs for nurse anesthetists*, Chicago, 2004, AANA Publishing, Inc.

Kulli J, Koch C: Does anesthesia cause loss of consciousness? *Trends Neurosci* 14(1):6-10, 1991.

Lake C, Hines R, Blitt C: *Clinical monitoring: practical applications for anesthesia and critical care*, Philadelphia, 2001, Saunders.

Longnecker D, Murphy F: *Dripps, Eckenhoff, Vandam introduction to anesthesia*, ed 9, Philadelphia, 1997, Saunders.

Longnecker D, Tinker J, Morgan G: *Principles and practice of anesthesiology*, ed 2, St Louis, 1998, Mosby.

Miller R, editor: *Anesthesia*, ed 6, Philadelphia, 2005, Churchill Livingstone.

Murray J, Nadel J: *Textbook of respiratory medicine*, ed 4, Philadelphia, 2005, Saunders.

Nagelhout J, Zaglaniczy K: *Nurse anesthesia*, ed 3, St Louis, 2005, Saunders.

Redai I, Svyatets M, Mets B: Are volatile anesthetics cardioprotective agents? *Semin Anesthesia Perioperative Med Pain* 20(2):95-100, 2001.

Saidman L: The role of desflurane in the practice of anesthesia, *Anesthesiology* 74:399-401, 1991.

Shorten G, Browne J, Carr D, et al: *Postoperative pain management: an evidence-based guide to practice*, Philadelphia, 2006, Saunders.

Stancer-Smiley B, Paradise N: Does the duration of $N_2O$ administration affect postoperative nausea and vomiting? *Nurse Anesth* 2(1):13-20, 1991.

Stoelting R: *Pharmacology and physiology in anesthetic practice*, ed 3, Philadelphia, 1999, Lippincott-Raven.

Stoelting R, Miller R: *Basics of anesthesia*, ed 5, Philadelphia, 2007, Churchill Livingstone.

Townsend C, Beauchamp R, Evers B, et al: *Sabiston textbook of surgery: the biological basis of modern surgical practice*, ed 17, Philadelphia, 2004, Saunders.

Tsai S, Lee C, Kwan W, et al: Recovery of cognitive functions after anesthesia with desflurane or isoflurane and nitrous oxide, *Br J Anaesth* 69:255-258, 1992.

White P, *Perioperative drug manual*, ed 2, Philadelphia, 2005, Saunders.

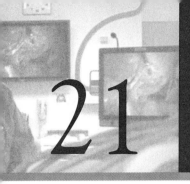

Cecil B. Drain, PhD, RN, CRNA, FAAN, FASAHP

The time-tested use of the inhalation anesthetic agents has proved that the agents possess some definite disadvantages. Because of the biotransformation hazards that have been reported with the halogenated inhalation anesthetics, other techniques have been sought for general anesthesia. Intravenous anesthetics now have a wide range of use in the perioperative period. In fact, in current anesthesia practice, the use of intravenous drugs is now commonplace. Intravenous anesthetics are grouped by primary pharmacologic action into nonopioid and opioid intravenous agents. The nonopioid agents are further grouped into the barbiturates, nonbarbiturates, and sedatives. These drugs can be injected in a rapid intravenous fashion for induction of anesthesia, or they can be used via continuous infusion pump for maintenance of anesthesia. These drugs have certainly found their place in the practice of anesthesia for enhancement of patient outcomes.

## DEFINITIONS

**Agonist:** A drug that has a specific receptor affinity that produces a predictable response.
**Antagonist:** A drug that has the ability to block the effects of an agonist drug at the receptor site.
**Anterograde Amnesia:** The inability to recall events that occur after the onset of amnesia.
**Antianalgesic:** Administration of a drug that partially blocks the analgesic effects of other drugs that produce analgesia.
**Antiemetic:** A drug that prevents or alleviates nausea and vomiting.
**Cardiostimulatory:** Stimulation of the cardiovascular system.
**Dissociative:** Anesthesia that is characterized by analgesia and amnesia without loss of respiratory function.
**Esterases:** A chemical group that breaks down certain enzymes.
**Extrapyramidal:** Effects of the structures outside the cerebrospinal pyramidal tracts of the brain that are associated with movement of the body.

**Gama-Aminobutyric Acid (GABA):** An amino acid that functions as an inhibitory neurotransmitter in the brain and spinal cord.
**Hypertriglyceridemia:** Type I hyperlipoproteinemia.
**Hypovolemia:** Low blood volume.
**Laryngospasm:** Contraction of the vocal cords.
**Neuroleptanalgesia:** A state of profound tranquilization with little or no depressant effect on the cortical centers.
**Parenterally:** Treatment other than through the digestive system.
**Resedation:** Sedation that recurs after clinical signs indicate that the sedation has ceased.
**Sedatives:** Substances that have a calming effect.
**Sympatholytic:** Antiadrenergic effects.
**Sympathomimetic:** A pharmacologic agent that mimics the effects of stimulation of the sympathetic nervous system.
**Thrombophlebitis:** Inflammation of a vein accompanied by the formation of a clot.
**Torsades de Pointes (TdP):** Potentially fatal heart arrhythmia.
**Vagotonic:** Augmenting the parasympathetic activity by stimulating the vagus nerve.

## MECHANISM OF ACTION OF THE NONOPIOID INTRAVENOUS ANESTHETICS

The nonopioid drugs appear to interact with gamma-aminobutyric acid (GABA) in the brain. GABA is an inhibitory neurotransmitter, and activation of the GABA receptors by GABA on the postsynaptic membrane causes inhibition of the postsynaptic neuron. The barbiturates appear to bind to the GABA postsynaptic receptor, with the net result of hyperpolarization of the postsynaptic neuron and inhibition of neuronal activity and, ultimately, loss of consciousness. Conversely, etomidate (Amidate), which is a nonbarbiturate induction agent, probably antagonizes the muscarinic receptors in the central nervous system (CNS) and also acts as an agonist to the opioid receptors. The resultant action of these drugs is a loss of wakefulness.

Sedatives, such as the benzodiazepines, bind to specific receptors in the limbic system. These benzodiazepine receptors use GABA as part of the neurotransmitter system. After the benzodiazepines have bound to the receptor, the action of GABA is enhanced, which leads to the hyperpolarized state and ultimately to inhibition of neuronal activity. The drug flumazenil is a specific benzodiazepine receptor antagonist. Consequently, after the administration of a benzodiazepine agonist, flumazenil can be administered. The pharmacologic actions on the benzodiazepine receptor are reversed, and neuronal activity resumes.

## THE BARBITURATES

Intravenous anesthesia began with barbiturate anesthesia. The long-acting barbiturates were introduced clinically in 1927, but Tovell and Lundy did not begin to use thiopental in clinical anesthesia practice until 1934. Since then, barbiturate anesthesia had great popularity until the late 1990s; and with the advent of propofol, thiopental is used in about 5% of the general anesthetics today.

### Thiopental

Thiopental (sodium pentothal) is most commonly injected intravenously to induce or sustain surgical anesthesia. It is usually used in conjunction with a potent inhalation anesthetic and nitrous oxide–oxygen combinations. The main reason for the use of other anesthetic agents with thiopental is that thiopental is a poor analgesic. For surgical procedures that are short and require minimal analgesia, thiopental and nitrous oxide–oxygen combinations can be used. This technique is commonly called the pentnitrous technique. Thiopental is also used: (1) for maintenance of light sleep during regional analgesia; (2) for control of convulsions; and (3) for rapidly quieting a patient who is too lightly anesthetized during a surgical procedure.

The mode of action of thiopental involves a phenomenon of redistribution. Thiopental has the ability to penetrate all tissues of the body without delay. Because the brain, as part of the vessel-rich group, is highly perfused, it receives approximately 10% of the administered intravenous dose within 40 seconds after injection. The patient usually becomes unconscious at this time. The thiopental then redistributes to relatively poorly perfused areas of the body. In the brain, the level of thiopental decreases to half its peak in 5 minutes and to 1/10 in 30 minutes. Recovery of consciousness usually occurs during this period. Recovery may be prolonged if the induction dose was excessive or if circulatory depression occurs to slow the redistribution phenomenon. Thiopental is metabolized in the body at a rate of 10% to 15% per hour.

Thiopental is a respiratory depressant. The chief effect is on the medullary and pontine respiratory centers. This depressant effect depends on the amount of thiopental administered, the rate at which it is injected, and the amount and type of premedication given to the patient. The response to carbon dioxide is depressed at all levels of anesthesia and is abolished at deep levels of thiopental anesthesia. Therefore, apnea can be an adverse outcome of high-dose thiopental.

Myocardial contractility is depressed and vascular resistance is increased after injection of thiopental. The result is that blood pressure is hardly affected, although it may be transiently reduced when the drug is first administered (when the vessel-rich group is highly saturated).

In addition to being nonexplosive, thiopental has the advantages of: (1) rapid and pleasant induction; (2) reduction of postanesthetic excitement and vomiting; (3) quiet respiration; (4) absence of salivation; and (5) speedy recovery after small doses. The disadvantages of the drug are adverse respiratory actions, including apnea, coughing, laryngospasm, and bronchospasm. Extravenous injection may result in tissue necrosis because of its highly alkaline pH (10.5 to 11).

***Perianesthesia Care.*** Because thiopental may have an antianalgesic effect at low concentrations, some patients who have pain may be irrational, hyperactive, and restless during the initial recovery phase. The patient may exhibit some shivering related to lowered body temperature, which may result from a cold operating suite. Of concern to the perianesthesia nurse is the patient admitted with cold, clammy, and cyanotic skin. This effect occasionally occurs with thiopental and is caused, in part, by the peripheral vasoconstrictive action of the drug.

If the anesthesia time exceeds 1 hour or if the total dose of thiopental exceeds 1 g, patients may have a delayed awakening time because of the redistribution of thiopental. This phenomenon is particularly common in obese patients because the drug is highly fat soluble. At present, no antagonist exists for the barbiturates. Therefore, airway management and monitoring of cardiovascular status are important.

### Methohexital

Methohexital is an ultra–short-acting barbiturate intravenous anesthetic agent. It is usually indicated for short procedures in which rapid complete recovery of the patient is needed. Methohexital is about three times as potent as thiopental, and the recovery time from anesthesia is extremely rapid (4 to 7 minutes) because the drug is redistributed from the CNS to the muscle and fat tissues and a significant portion of the drug is metabolized in the liver. Consequently, the clearance of methohexital is about four times faster than that of thiopental. Methohexital causes about the same degree of cardiovascular and respiratory depression as does thiopental. One should mention, however, that this drug can cause coughing and hiccups and that, after injection, excitatory phenomena, such as tremor and involuntary muscle movements, may appear.

## THE NONBARBITURATES

### Propofol

Propofol (Diprivan) is a rapid-acting nonbarbiturate induction agent. It is administered intravenously as a 1% solution and is the most popular intravenous anesthetic in use today. The dosage for induction is 2 to 2.5 mg/kg. The dosage should be reduced in elderly patients and in patients with cardiac disease or hypovolemia. Also, propofol in combination with midazolam acts synergistically. In fact, the dosage of propofol can be reduced by 50% when it is administered in combination with midazolam. When propofol is used as the sole induction agent, it is usually administered over 15 seconds and produces unconsciousness within about 30 seconds. Emergence from this drug is more rapid than emergence from thiopental or methohexital because propofol has a half-life of 2 to 9 minutes. Hence, the duration of anesthesia after a single induction dose is about 3 to 8 minutes, depending on the dose of the propofol. A major advantage of this drug is its ability to allow the patient a rapid return to consciousness with minimal residual CNS effects. Moreover, the drug's low incidence rate of nausea and vomiting is of particular importance to perianesthesia nursing care. In fact, propofol may possess antiemetic properties.

Propofol decreases the cerebral perfusion pressure, cerebral blood flow, and intracranial pressure. It does produce a reduction in the blood pressure similar in magnitude to or greater than thiopental in comparable doses. The decrease in blood pressure is also accompanied by a reduction in cardiac output or systemic vascular resistance. This reduction in blood pressure is more pronounced in elderly patients and in patients with compromised left-ventricular function. As opposed to the reduction in blood pressure, the pulse usually remains unchanged after the administration of propofol because of a sympatholytic or vagotonic effect of the drug. Therefore, in some patients, bradycardia may be assessed after injection of propofol; in this instance, an anticholinergic drug such as atropine or glycopyrrolate (Robinul) can be administered to reverse the bradycardia.

Propofol has a profound depressant effect on both the rate and depth of ventilation. In fact, after the induction dose is administered, apnea normally occurs. The incidence rate of apnea is greater after propofol than after thiopental and may approach 100%. Consequently, if propofol is administered in the postanesthesia care unit (PACU), the perianesthesia nurse should be prepared to support the patient's ventilation and, if necessary, intubate the patient (see Chapter 30).

Clinically, this drug is useful for intravenous induction of anesthesia, especially for outpatient surgery. The drug is also an excellent choice for procedures that require a short period of unconsciousness, such as cardioversion and electroconvulsive therapy. Also, propofol can be used for sedation during local standby procedures. This drug does not interfere with or alter the effects of succinylcholine because it has such a rapid plasma clearance. Propofol can be used during surgery in a continuous intravenous infusion, and the patients still emerge from anesthesia in a rapid fashion without any CNS depression. This drug can be used in the PACU as a continuous infusion, and the level of sedation can be adjusted by titration to effect. The typical infusion rates for sedation with propofol are between 25 and 100 µg/kg/min.

With administration within 12 hours of intravenous sedation, propofol is characterized by a more rapid recovery from its sedative effects than midazolam. Once propofol is discontinued, extubation can be performed in a short time; propofol is cleared rapidly because of redistribution to fatty tissue and hepatic metabolism to inactive metabolites.

Long-term or high-dose infusions may result in hypertriglyceridemia, which is usually associated with elevated levels of pancreatic enzymes and possibly with pancreatitis. After long infusions, plasma concentrations of propofol gradually increase unless the infusion rate is decreased over time. Current data seem to indicate that the recovery from propofol is less rapid after 12 hours of intravenous sedation. Propofol is contraindicated in patients who are sensitive to soybean oil, egg lecithin, or glycerol and is not recommended for PACU/intensive care unit (ICU) administration in children.

*Perianesthesia Care.* When a patient has received propofol for induction or even via continuous infusion, the perianesthesia nursing care should be based mainly on the other drugs that were used during surgery because propofol is so rapid and has no cumulative effects; its effects are normally dissipated within 8 to 10 minutes. Consequently, the patient usually arrives in the PACU awake and in pain. Therefore, analgesics should be titrated to effect. Titration is recommended in the immediate postoperative period because propofol and opioid analgesics can have a synergistic effect.

Propofol is an excellent addition to clinical anesthesia practice. It offers many advantages and few disadvantages. More specifically, propofol has one major advantage over all the other intravenous induction agents: early awakening. It can be used in the PACU if indicated. The major concern for the perianesthesia care of the patient who has received this drug is the level of postoperative pain. The nursing assessment and appropriate interventions for pain are the most important aspects of care of the patient who has received this drug (see Chapter 28).

## Etomidate

Etomidate (Amidate), which is a derivative of imidazole, is a short-acting intravenous hypnotic that was synthesized in the 1960s by the laboratories of Janssen Pharmaceutica in Beerse, Belgium. It is not related chemically to the commonly used hypnotic agents. This drug is a mere hypnotic and does not possess any analgesic actions. Etomidate is quite safe for administration to patients because it has a high therapeutic index. Metabolism of this drug is accomplished by hydrolysis in the liver and by plasma esterases, with the final metabolite being pharmacologically inactive. The cardiovascular effects of etomidate are minimal; when the drug is injected in therapeutic doses, only a small blood pressure decrease and a slight heart rate increase may be observed. Studies have also shown that etomidate causes a minimal reduction in the cardiac index and the peripheral resistance. This drug does not seem to produce arrhythmias. In regard to the respiratory system, etomidate causes a dose-related reduction in the tidal volume and respiratory frequency, which can lead to apnea. Laryngospasm, cough, and hiccups can occur during injection of this drug; however, the severity of these clinical phenomena can be reduced with an opiate premedication.

Although this drug does cause some pain at the site of injection, it does not appear to cause a release of histamine. Spontaneous involuntary movements and tremor have been observed after the injection of etomidate. These involuntary movements can be reduced with an opiate premedication. Etomidate reduces both intracranial and intraocular pressure and therefore is considered safe for use in patients with intracranial pathologic conditions. This short-acting hypnotic is particularly well suited for the induction of neuroleptanalgesia and inhalation anesthesia. The induction dose ranges from 0.2 to 0.3 mg/kg, which produces sleep in 20 to 45 seconds after injection; the patient wakes within 7 to 15 minutes after induction.

Research has shown that etomidate inhibits steroid synthesis and that patients who receive etomidate via continuous infusion have marked adrenocortical suppression for as long as 4 days. Even when etomidate is administered as a single dose, adrenal function is suppressed for 5 to 8 hours. Consequently, after the administration of etomidate, a decrease is seen in cortisol, 17-alpha-hydroxyprogesterone, aldosterone, and corticosterone levels. Thus, etomidate is administered only to selected patients and is no longer administered via continuous intravenous infusion.

## THE SEDATIVES

### The Benzodiazepines

The benzodiazepines, which are sedatives, have enhanced the anesthetic outcomes of the surgical patient. They depress the limbic system without causing cortical depression. More specifically, they interact with the inhibitory neurotransmitter GABA and thus result in reduced orientation (hypnotic effect), retrograde amnesia, anxiolysis, and relaxing of the skeletal muscle. Opiates and barbiturates enhance the hypnotic action of the benzodiazepines.

*Midazolam.* Midazolam has become a popular drug in anesthesia practice and in the perianesthesia care of the surgical patient. Midazolam can be used for premedication, cardioversion, endoscopic procedures, and induction of anesthesia and as an intraoperative adjunct for inhalation anesthesia. It also is an excellent agent for sedation during regional anesthetic techniques. Midazolam's principal action is on the benzodiazepine receptors in the CNS, particularly on the limbic system, which results in a reduction in anxiety and profound anterograde amnesia. This drug also has excellent hypnotic, anticonvulsant, and muscle-relaxant properties.

The water-soluble midazolam may offer some advantages over diazepam. It causes depression of the CNS by inducing sedation, drowsiness, and, finally, sleep with increasing doses.

Midazolam, in comparison with diazepam, is about three times as potent, has a shorter duration of action, and has a lesser incidence rate of injection pain and postinjection phlebitis and thrombosis. More specifically, this drug has a rapid onset of action, a peak in action between 10 and 30 minutes, and a duration of action between 1 and 4 hours. Midazolam administered at a dose of 0.2 mg/kg produces a decrease in blood pressure, an increase in heart rate, and a reduction in systemic vascular resistance. Midazolam should be used with caution in patients with myocardial ischemia and in those with chronic obstructive pulmonary disease. Postoperative patients who have a substantial amount of hypovolemia should not receive midazolam. Also, midazolam does not affect intracranial pressure. Consequently, this drug can be used safely in neurosurgical patients in addition to patients with intracranial pathophysiology.

This drug can be administered in the PACU, and so the postanesthesia nurse must monitor the patient for respiratory depression after injection because midazolam causes a dose-dependent respiratory depression. Given that every patient in the PACU has received a plethora of depressant drugs during surgery, midazolam can be potentiated quite easily when administered in the PACU. Because of this potentiation factor, any dose of midazolam administered in the PACU should be considered effective enough to cause profound respiratory depression. Therefore, oxygen and resuscitative equipment must be immediately available, and a person skilled in maintaining a patent airway and supporting ventilation should be present. Extra care also should be observed in patients with limited pulmonary reserve and in the elderly and debilitated with reduction of the dosage of midazolam by 25% to 30%.

Midazolam can be given via continuous infusion for patients who need sustained sedation. However, midazolam has a pH-dependent diazepine ring; at physiologic pH, the ring can close, causing CNS penetration. Also, its metabolites are partially active, all of which make midazolam not the drug of choice for long-term sedation. Midazolam is sometimes used in the treatment of critically ill patients who are agitated. The guidelines for use can be found in Box 21-1.

**Diazepam.** Diazepam (Valium) is still a popular drug in anesthesia practice. Because of its ability to allay apprehension, diazepam is indicated for use as a premedicant, as an adjunct to intravenous anesthesia, and as an induction agent. Recovery is usually not prolonged when diazepam is used for the induction of anesthesia.

Diazepam can be used as the sole anesthetic agent for short diagnostic and surgical procedures and can also be used as sedation to make local anesthesia more acceptable to the patient.

Its principal action is depression of limbic system function. Important actions of diazepam are production of anterograde amnesia for as long as 48 hours after surgery, reduction of anxiety, and provision of minimal cardiovascular depressant effects. Clinical doses of diazepam cause a slight degree of respiratory depression; however, when it is combined with an opiate, the chance of respiratory depression, including apnea, is greatly increased.

Diazepam may possess some muscle-relaxant properties. Diazepam has been reported to be antagonistic to depolarizing neuromuscular blocking agents, such as succinylcholine, and the action of the nondepolarizing neuromuscular blocking agents (e.g., vecuronium) are reported to be potentiated. Diazepam has been used clinically for psychomotor and *petit mal* seizures because of its anticonvulsant actions.

Because many patients who undergo cardioversion are debilitated, diazepam may be used as sedation for this procedure. Increments of 2.5 to 5 mg can be given at 30-second intervals until the speech of the patient is slurred or light sleep occurs. At the time of electric discharge, the patient may have brief muscle contraction and slight arousal. When this technique is used, a significant number of the patients have complete amnesia regarding the event. Diazepam can also

CONCEPTS IN ANESTHETIC AGENTS

---

**Box 21-1 Guidelines for the Use of Midazolam for the Treatment of Agitation in the PACU and Critical Care Setting**

**Indications:** For patients with respiratory or cardiac dysfunction; promotes anxiolysis and amnesia

**Onset of action:** 1 to 5 minutes

**Peak of action:** 2 to 5 minutes

**Duration of action:** 15 to 90 minutes

**Dosages:**

**Load:** 1 to 4 mg IV over 2 to 3 minutes

**Maximal load:** 5 mg in 1 hour (without intubation)

10 mg in 1 hour (with intubation)

**Maintenance load:** 1 to 5 mg/h (IV push)

**Intravenous infusions:** 1 to 50 mg/h; no oral form available

**Tapering:** Decrease infusion rate by 10% to 25% of maintenance rate every 24 hours; should be discontinued by day 4

be used to provide anesthesia in endoscopic and dental procedures and to control behavior on emergence from ketamine. Finally, this drug also has strong anticonvulsant activity and can stop generalized seizure activity.

Intramuscularly administered diazepam can be quite painful to the patient. Also, the absorption is often poor. And when diazepam is administered intravenously, thrombophlebitis often occurs. With intravenous administration of diazepam, the drug should be injected slowly, directly into a large vein. The drug should not be mixed with other drugs or diluted. The onset of action of diazepam administered intravenously is immediate, and the duration of action varies from 20 minutes to 1 hour. With intramuscular administration, its onset of action is about 10 minutes, and the duration of action may be as long as 4 hours. Adverse reactions to diazepam include hiccups, nausea, phlebitis at the site of injection, and occasional acute hyperexcited states.

**Lorazepam.** Lorazepam (Ativan), a long-acting benzodiazepine, is used as a premedication in current clinical anesthesia practice and as a long-acting slow-onset benzodiazepine for sedation in the PACU and ICU. This drug has actions similar to those of diazepam but has a slow onset of action from 20 to 40 minutes; the pharmacologic activity may last as long as 24 hours. Lorazepam produces profound anterograde amnesia, tranquilization, and a reduction of anxiety, and the drug provides good cardiovascular and respiratory stability. Therapeutic plasma concentrations are achieved in about 3 hours when the drug is given orally. The drug is well absorbed via the intramuscular route; however, the patient has a significant amount of pain during the injection of the drug. Lorazepam can also be injected intravenously, and the patient may have some burning on injection. Because of its slow onset and long duration, lorazepam is mainly used as a preanesthetic medication. If this drug has been administered in the preoperative period, the effects of lorazepam may last well into the postoperative period because of its prolonged action. If a narcotic is administered in the PACU to a patient who received lorazepam before surgery, the nurse should monitor for increased narcotic sedation and respiratory depression because of the potentiation of the narcotic by lorazepam.

Caution should be taken with use of lorazepam in the PACU for sedation. Lorazepam does not have any active metabolites. This long-acting but slow-onset benzodiazepine is often delivered via intermittent boluses but also may be administered as a continuous infusion. Peak

**Box 21-2   Guidelines for the Use of Lorazepam for the Treatment of Agitation in the PACU and Critical Care Setting**

**Indications:** For patients with respiratory or cardiac dysfunction; promotes anxiolysis and amnesia
**Onset of action:** 1 to 5 minutes
**Peak of action:** 20 to 40 minutes
**Duration of action:** 4 to 6 hours
**Dosages:**
   **Load:** 1 to 2 mg IV over 1 to 2 minutes
   **Maximal load:** 4 mg in 1 hour (without intubation)
   6 mg in 1 hour (with intubation)
   **Maintenance load:** 1 to 3 mg every 1 to 2 hours (IV push)
   **Intravenous infusions:** 1 to 5 mg/h
**Precautions:** Paradoxic effects can occur
   Not dialyzed
   **Tapering:** Decrease infusion rate by 10% to 25% of maintenance rate every 24 hours

effects are not observed for 30 minutes. However, the solvent for lorazepam contains polyethylene glycol 400 and propylene glycol, both of which have been implicated in the development of lactic acidosis, acute tubular necrosis, and hyperosmolar coma when lorazepam is used in prolonged high-dose infusions. However, the toxic threshold for this effect has not been defined; hence, high-dose infusions should be avoided, and monitoring for these side effects should be initiated.

Lorazepam is sometimes used in the treatment of critically ill patients who are agitated. The guidelines for use can be found in Box 21-2.

### The Benzodiazepine Antagonists

**Flumazenil.** Flumazenil (Romazicon), a new benzodiazepine antagonist, was recently introduced into clinical practice in the United States with the trade name Mazicon. However, because the name was similar to the trade name Mavacron (mivacurium chloride), a neuromuscular-blocking agent, the name was changed to Romazicon. This drug antagonizes or reverses the effects of benzodiazepine-induced sedation at the benzodiazepine receptors. Consequently, it reverses the CNS effects of benzodiazepines, such as the sedation and amnesia that are produced by diazepam and midazolam, for example. This drug also reverses the other effects produced by benzodiazepine agonists, including anxiolytic, muscle-relaxant, ataxic, and anticonvulsant actions. However, flumazenil may not be effective in the treatment for benzodiazepine-induced hypoventilation or respiratory failure. This drug is specific for the benzodiazepines and, more specifically, their receptors. Consequently, this drug does not reverse the effects of barbiturates, opiates, and ethanol. Flumazenil should be used with great caution in patients who have a history of epilepsy or chronic benzodiazepine usage because reversal with flumazenil in these patients can result in seizures. The incidence rate of postoperative nausea and vomiting is increased after flumazenil has been administered.

The usual reversal dose for flumazenil is 0.4 mg administered intravenously in 0.1-mg increments. Flumazenil should be administered slowly to avoid the adverse consequences of abrupt wakening. A maximum dose for this drug is 1 mg. The onset of action is usually within 5 minutes, with a duration of action between 1 and 2 hours. Flumazenil has a shorter duration of action than most of the benzodiazepines, and consequently, the risk of resedation can occur after the initial reversal dose was administered. This risk is especially true when high doses of benzodiazepines were previously administered. Therefore, after the administration of flumazenil, the patient should be monitored for resedation and other residual effects of benzodiazepines in the PACU and on the receiving unit. If signs of resedation develop, flumazenil should be given at 20-minute intervals as needed to reverse the sedation. In this situation, no more than 1 mg should be given at any one time, and no more than 3 mg should be given within a 1-hour period. This drug should prove to be a valuable asset in the care of the patient who has received an excessive dose of a benzodiazepine, such as midazolam or diazepam. Consequently, flumazenil is useful during surgery, after surgery, and in the ICU.

*Physostigmine.* In today's perianesthesia care, physostigmine (Antilirium) is an anticholinesterase that crosses the blood-brain barrier. Its action is inhibition of the enzyme acetylcholinesterase, which results in an increase in the availability of acetylcholine at the receptors that are affected by the benzodiazepines in the CNS. The preponderance of acetylcholine counteracts the negative effects of glycine and GABA. Consequently, this drug provides a nonspecific reversal of the CNS side effects of the benzodiazepines scopolamine and ketamine. The dosage is 0.5 to 1 mg, and it should be administered slowly to prevent untoward cholinergic side effects. Because this drug is a nonspecific agent, a number of vagally mediated cholinergic side effects can occur after its administration. These effects include nausea, vomiting, salivation, bradycardia, bronchospasm, and seizures. Hence, because of its nonspecific properties, physostigmine is rarely used for the reversal of the untoward effects of the benzodiazepines.

## The Butyrophenones

The butyrophenones are a class of sedatives that produce a state of profound calm and immobility in which the patient appears to be pain-free and dissociated from the surroundings. They are a potent inhibitor of the chemoreceptor trigger zone–mediated nausea and vomiting. These drugs have some profound side effects but do seem to be useful in anesthesia and postanesthesia care of the surgical patient. The two major butyrophenones used in clinical practice are haloperidol and droperidol.

*Haloperidol.* Haloperidol (Haldol) is a butyrophenone tranquilizer that has limited use in anesthesia practice because of its long duration of action and its high incidence rate of extrapyramidal reactions. However, it has been found to be an excellent antiemetic. The drug is not approved for intravenous use and is usually administered intramuscularly at a dose from 2 to 5 mg. It is used in the treatment of psychoses and as an antiemetic. Haloperidol is sometimes used in the treatment of critically ill patients who are agitated. The guidelines for use can be found in Box 21-3.

*Droperidol.* Droperidol (Inapsine), which was originally investigated by Janssen Pharmaceutica, can be used alone or in combination with fentanyl (Sublimaze) as part of a neuroleptanalgesic technique. Droperidol is rarely used during surgery for purposes of being a component of anesthesia. However, it is administered in small doses for its antiemetic effect after surgery. It produces a state of calm, disinclination to move, and disconnection from surroundings. The drug has an alpha-adrenergic blocking effect, which offers some protection against the vasoconstrictive components of shock; it leads to good peripheral perfusion; and it unmasks hypovolemia. More specifically, when a patient has compensation for a borderline hypovolemic state with activation of the alpha-vasoconstriction mechanisms, vital signs are normal. When a drug such as droperidol is administered to this patient, by virtue of droperidol's alpha-blocking properties, the signs of hypovolemia appear. Hence, the patient's hypovolemia is "unmasked." Droperidol also protects against epinephrine-induced arrhythmias and has an antiemetic

| Box 21-3 | **Guidelines for the Use of Haloperidol for the Treatment of Agitation in the PACU and Critical Care Setting** |
|---|---|

**Indications:** For patients with respiratory or cardiac dysfunction; promotes anxiolysis and amnesia

**Onset of action:** 5 to 30 minutes
**Peak of action:** 1 hour
**Duration of action:** 6 to 8 hours
**Dosages:**
   **Load:** 2.5 to 5 mg IV over 1 to 2 minutes
   **Maximal load:** 20 mg in 1 hour (with and without intubation)
   **Maintenance load:** Once condition is controlled by loading dose, may decrease dose by 50% or by increasing dosing interval
   **Precautions:** Precipitates with heparin
Decreases epinephrine and dopamine activity
Contraindicated in Parkinson's disease
Not dialyzed

effect. In fact, because of its excellent antiemetic properties, droperidol is sometimes administered toward the end of the surgical procedure or in the PACU to reduce the risk of vomiting and aspiration in anxious patients. The antiemetic dose of droperidol is between 1 and 2.5 mg and can be given intravenously. Also, because of its alpha-blocking properties, this drug may be administered in the PACU on a short-term basis to reduce the afterload.

Droperidol is similar to chlorpromazine (Thorazine) in its CNS effects; however, its mechanism of action is different. Droperidol is more selective than chlorpromazine because it provides more tranquility with less sedation and has less effect on the autonomic nervous system. Droperidol has been classified as a neuroleptic and does have some adverse effects that should be assessed throughout the PACU phase. Droperidol may cause hypotension because of its alpha-adrenergic blocking effect and peripheral vasodilatation. It may cause extrapyramidal excitation, such as twitchiness, oculogyric seizures, stiff neck muscles, trembling hands, restlessness, and occasionally, psychologic disturbances (e.g., hallucinations). These can be reversed with atropine or antiparkinsonian drugs such as benztropine mesylate (Cogentin) and trihexyphenidyl hydrochloride (Artane). Clinically, patients who have received droperidol have reported the dichotomy of appearing outwardly

calm while feeling terrified inside and unable to express how they feel. Hence, the perianesthesia nurse should provide emotional support to all patients who have received droperidol.

Droperidol is known to potentiate the action of barbiturates and narcotics. It has a high therapeutic margin of safety with a rapid onset of 10 minutes, and its activity is lessened in 2 to 4 hours, although some effects last as long as 10 to 12 hours.

Droperidol is the prototype neuroleptic drug. A neuroleptic drug is one that reduces motor activity, lessens anxiety, and produces a state of indifference in which the person can still respond appropriately to commands. Neuroleptanalgesia is a state of profound tranquilization with little or no depressant effect on the cortical centers. Therefore, neuroleptanalgesia is achieved with the combination of a neuroleptic such as droperidol and a potent narcotic analgesic such as fentanyl. A step further is neuroleptanesthesia, the combination of a neuroleptanalgesic (droperidol plus fentanyl), a skeletal muscle relaxant, and nitrous oxide and oxygen. The main objective in development of neuroleptanesthesia is provision for all types of operations of a technique that does not depress the metabolic, circulatory, or central nervous systems as severely as do the inhalation anesthetics when used alone. Droperidol is rarely used as the neuroleptic component; other sedatives are used in its place, such as Versed and fentanyl.

The United States Food and Drug Administration (FDA) has strengthened the warnings and precautions in the labeling for droperidol because the drug has been associated with fatal cardiac arrhythmias. More specifically, recent research has shown QT prolongations that indicate delayed recharging of the heart between beats within minutes after injection of droperidol at the upper end of the labeled dose range. Prolonged QT is dangerous because it can cause a potentially fatal heart arrhythmia known as torsades de pointes (TdP). The new warning is intended to facilitate the focus on the potential for cardiac arrhythmias during administration and to urge the practitioner to consider the use of alternative medications in patients at high risk for cardiac arrhythmias.

**Perianesthesia Care.** In the immediate postoperative period, the awakening from neuroleptanesthesia is usually rapid, extremely smooth, and uneventful. A striking feature is the extension of analgesia well into the postoperative period. Explanation is difficult of the mechanism of such a prolonged pain-relieving effect with a drug such as fentanyl, in which the onset is so rapid and the duration of action is so short.

Nursing personnel in the PACU should constantly assess the patient for signs of respiratory depression when droperidol is used, even in small doses for its antiemetic properties. Narcotics should be titrated to effect in patients who have received low dose droperidol. If droperidol was used as the neuroleptic component of the anesthetic, the dosage of narcotic agonists is recommended to be reduced to as little as one fourth to one third the usual dose because of the additive potentiating effects of droperidol.

The patient should be encouraged to cough and perform the sustained maximal inspiration (SMI) maneuver in the PACU (see Chapters 12 and 28). Patients who have received even low dose droperidol can drift back to sleep unless they are encouraged to move about the surroundings. The perianesthesia nurse will find that, because the analgesia extends into the postoperative period, the patient who has received droperidol is more willing to cough and perform the SMI. The perianesthesia nurse should use verbal stimulation with these patients because, if ordered, the patient will be able to take a deep breath; otherwise, respiration may remain slow and shallow, or the patient may even become apneic. Consequently, the perianesthesia nurse must remain with the patient, provide verbal stimulation, and actively monitor for any signs of respiratory depression.

The perianesthesia nurse should monitor for extrapyramidal symptoms; although rare, these symptoms have been detected as long as 24 hours after a single administration of droperidol. Most of the reported extrapyramidal reactions occurred in children younger than 12 years of age. Because of the length of action of droperidol, the perianesthesia nurse is recommended to provide information about the drug to the nursing personnel on the surgical units via hospital in-service education programs even when the drug is given in small doses as an antiemetic.

## NONSTEROIDAL ANTIINFLAMMATORY DRUGS

### Ketorolac

Ketorolac (Toradol) is an analgesic that is classified as a nonsteroidal antiinflammatory drug (NSAID). Its mode of action is inhibition of the prostaglandin synthetase enzyme. Therefore, ketorolac has analgesic, antiinflammatory, and antipyretic actions. An intramuscular dose of 30 mg of this drug is equal to about 12 mg of morphine or 100 mg of meperidine in degree of postoperative pain relief. This drug should not be administered intravenously and so can be administered only via the intramuscular route. When it

is used with supplemental opioids, ketorolac is an excellent postoperative analgesia. For acute postoperative pain, an initial loading dose of 30 mg can be administered intramuscularly. Ketorolac can be administered every 6 hours thereafter at a dose of 15 mg. The duration of analgesia, but not the peak analgesic effect, is increased when the dose is increased beyond its recommended dosage range of 15 to 60 mg. Ketorolac should be given at a lower dose range for patients with renal disease, for the elderly (older than 70 years of age), and for patients who weigh less than 50 kg. Because this drug is an NSAID and not an opioid, its lack of effect on psychomotor activities and on the respiratory system makes it an ideal analgesic for outpatient surgery.

Clinically, for the advantage of the peak effects of ketorolac, the drug is sometimes administered intramuscularly about 1 hour before the end of the surgical procedure. In this instance, the patient usually emerges from anesthesia in an analgesic state that lasts well into the immediate postoperative period. Hence, for an effective analgesic plan in the PACU, the postanesthesia nurse must determine whether ketorolac was given during surgery to avoid analgesic overmedication.

### Other Sedative Medications

***Dexmedetomidine.*** Dexmedetomidine (Precedex) is a new alpha-2 agonist, like clonidine, that is a novel sedative with analgesic properties that controls stress, anxiety, and pain and does not cause respiratory depression. Like clonidine, its mechanism of action is agonism of alpha-2 receptors in certain parts of the brain. Consequently, this drug facilitates patient comfort, compliance, and comprehension by providing sedation along with the ability to rouse the patient.

Dexmedetomidine is seven times more selective for the alpha receptors and has a shorter duration of action and is considered a full agonist for the alpha-2 receptors. Consequently, it is an excellent drug to decrease the amounts of inhalation anesthetics and opioids. It is also an effective drug in attenuating the cardiostimulatory and postanesthetic delirium effects of ketamine. Dexmedetomidine does increase the range of temperatures that do not trigger the thermoregulatory defenses. Hence, it is likely to produce some perioperative hypothermia and to be an effective treatment for postoperative shivering.

With stimulation of the alpha-2 receptors, dexmedetomidine decreases the systolic blood pressure; the systemic vascular resistance is little affected, and the cardiac output, which is initially decreased, returns toward predrug levels. The homeostatic cardiovascular reflexes are

CONCEPTS IN ANESTHETIC AGENTS

maintained; thus, the problems of orthostatic hypotension are avoided.

In the PACU, if dexmedetomidine is administered via intravenous (IV) infusion, the nurse should monitor the patient for significant episodes of bradycardia and hypotension. If intervention is necessary, decreasing or stopping the dexmedetomidine infusion and increasing the rate of intravenous fluid administration along with elevation of the lower extremities may be all that is needed; if the hypotension continues, vasopressor agents may be necessary (see Chapter 11). If the bradycardia continues, the PACU nurse may need to intervene by obtaining a physician order for an anticholinergic such as atropine or glycopyrrolate. A dexmedetomidine infusion is not recommended to last more than 24 hours. Also, because dexmedetomidine resembles the alpha-2 adrenergic agent clonidine, abrupt withdrawal of the drug may result in symptoms associated with abrupt stoppage of clonidine. Consequently, when dexmedetomidine is discontinued, symptoms that include nervousness, agitation, headaches, and a rapid rise in blood pressure should be monitored for and reported to the anesthesia practitioner immediately.

Dexmedetomidine is usually administered with a controlled infusion device. The drug should be titrated to the desired clinical effect, which is usually less than 3 on the Ramsey Sedation Scale (see Table 21-1). Generally, a loading infusion of 1 µg/kg over 10 minutes followed by a maintenance infusion of 0.2 to 0.6 µg/kg/h and the rate of the maintenance infusion can be adjusted to achieve the desired level of sedation.

## THE DISSOCIATIVE ANESTHETICS

### Ketamine

Traditionally, general anesthetic agents achieved control of pain with depression of the CNS. Ketamine, an anesthetic agent that has been introduced has a totally different mode of action. It selectively blocks pain conduction and perception, leaving those parts of the CNS that do not participate in pain transmission and perception free from the depressant effects of the drug. Ketamine is termed dissociative because patients whose conditions are totally analgesic usually do not appear to be asleep or anesthetized but rather disassociated from the surroundings. The drug is nonbarbiturate and nonnarcotic. It is administered parenterally and has a short duration. Early laboratory studies with ketamine suggested that most of the drug's activity is centered in the frontal lobe of the cerebral cortex.

The clinical characteristics of ketamine consist of a state of profound analgesia combined

| Table 21-1 | **Ramsay Level of Sedation Scale** |
|---|---|
| Clinical Score | Level of Sedation Achieved |
| 6 | Asleep, no response |
| 5 | Asleep, sluggish response to light glabellar tap or loud auditory stimulus |
| 4 | Asleep, but with brisk response to light glabellar tap or loud auditory stimulus |
| 3 | Patient responds to commands |
| 2 | Patient cooperative, oriented, and tranquil |
| 1 | Patient anxious, agitated, or restless |

with a state of unconsciousness. The patient usually has marked horizontal and vertical nystagmus. The eyes are usually open and shortly become centered and appear in a fixed gaze. The pupils are moderately dilated and react to light. Respiratory function is usually unimpaired, except after rapid intravenous injection, when it may become depressed for a short time. Ketamine is sympathomimetic in action and is beneficial to patients with asthma because of its bronchodilating effect. When patients receive ketamine, the pharyngeal and laryngeal reflexes remain intact. The tongue usually does not become relaxed, so the airway usually remains unobstructed. Ketamine accelerates the heart rate moderately and increases both the systolic and the diastolic pressure for several minutes, after which the pulse and blood pressure return to preinjection levels. Finally, ketamine increases cerebral blood flow and, consequently, intracranial pressure. Therefore, this drug definitely is contraindicated in patients who are at risk for increased intracranial pressure.

Ketamine can be administered intramuscularly or intravenously. The intramuscular dose is 4 to 6 mg/lb, and the anesthesia lasts from 20 to 40 minutes. The intravenous dose is usually 0.5 to 2 mg/lb, with anesthesia lasting 6 to 10 minutes. Complete recovery from ketamine varies according to the duration of surgery and the amount of ketamine used throughout the procedure. When a single dose of intravenous ketamine is used, recovery time is usually rapid and does not exceed 30 minutes. When supplemental intravenous doses need to be administered, more particularly when supplemental intramuscular doses are necessary, recovery is often markedly prolonged, sometimes as long as 3 hours.

**Perianesthesia Care.** When patients emerge from ketamine anesthesia, they may go through a phase of vivid dreaming, with or without psychomotor activity manifested by confusion, irrational behavior, and hallucinations. The perianesthesia nurse should be aware that such psychic aberrations are usually transient and appear to be preventable by avoiding early verbal or tactile stimulation of the patient, which helps prevent fear and anxiety reactions. Short-acting barbiturates administered intravenously can effectively control the psychic responses sometimes seen after the administration of ketamine. Pediatric patients seem to be less prone to these psychic disturbances. Results of a study revealed that droperidol may be effective in eliminating some of the adverse psychic emergence phenomena of ketamine. Other sedatives such as diazepam have also been found effective in suppression of these phenomena. Also, the drug dexmedetomidine (Precedex) can help suppress this adverse phenomena. Thus, when a patient is admitted to the PACU, the nurse should be aware of any sedatives or whether dexmedetomidine has been administered to the patient.

On arrival in the PACU, the patient should be secluded from auditory, visual, and tactile stimuli and be observed for any signs of respiratory depression. Mechanical airway obstruction, particularly when caused by marked salivation, accounts for most of the instances of respiratory insufficiency after ketamine anesthesia. When the patient does not have adequate respiratory exchange, oxygen should be administered via mask until it is restored. Other important signs to watch for are persistent blood pressure elevation, tachycardia, bradycardia, dreaming, delirium, hallucinations, euphoria, and increased muscle tone. All PACU personnel must know that attempts to rouse patients while they are still unable to see, hear, and orient themselves may set off a chain of anxiety reactions that may ultimately lead to severe psychomotor responses and even more irrational behavior. Should the patient have this augmented psychomotor behavior, dexmedetomidine (Precedex) or one of the benzodiazepine sedation drugs can be administered to facilitate a reduction in the aberrant behavior.

The widespread use of ketamine requires an entirely different approach to perianesthesia nursing care. Certainly, the agent has some deficiencies, but commonly overlooked is the fact that it is one of the safest anesthetics. Its safety justifies its important place in the drugs used by the anesthesiologist. Ketamine appears to be an excellent anesthetic for pediatric patients, as the sole agent for short procedures, for induction of anesthesia in patients at extremely poor risk, and for patients with burns that necessitate surgical treatment. Certain adult orthopedic and diagnostic procedures have also been found suitable for the use of ketamine anesthesia. Ketamine continues to be popular for certain types of anesthetic procedures. Because it is a dissociative agent, its actions should be well understood by the PACU staff to ensure effective informed care of the patient.

## SUMMARY

The nonopioid pharmacologic agents are gaining popularity because they are becoming more opioid-like without the side effects. Also, the induction agents have changed from thiopental to propofol in a short time. The same can be said for the benzodiazepines; diazepam has now been overcome by midazolam. In both cases, the newer drugs offer distinct advantages during surgery, and more importantly, after surgery in the PACU. The many new sedatives also now offer distinct advantages and certainly facilitate positive outcomes for the surgical patient. Finally, the drug ketamine has continued over the years to serve as an excellent anesthetic for specific situations. Also, the PACU stay for the patient who has received ketamine has improved significantly because of the many adjunct drugs that can now be used to prevent the psychic aberrations associated with that drug in the PACU.

## BIBLIOGRAPHY

Aitkenhead A, Smith G, Rowbotham D: *Textbook of anaesthesia*, ed 5, Philadelphia, 2007, Churchill Livingstone.

Alspach J: *Core curriculum for critical care nursing*, ed 6, Philadelphia, 2005, Saunders.

Atlee J: *Complications in anesthesia*, ed 2, Philadelphia, 2007, Saunders.

Barash P, Cullen B, Stoelting R: *Clinical anesthesia*, ed 5, Philadelphia, 2005, Lippincott Williams & Wilkins.

Benumof J, Saidman L: *Anesthesia & perioperative complications*, ed 2, St Louis, 1999, Mosby.

Blouin R, Gross J: Ventilation and conscious sedation, *Semin Anesth* 15(4):335-342, 1996.

Borchardt M: Review of the clinical pharmacology and use of the benzodiazepines, *J Perianesth Nurs* 14(2):65-72, 1999.

CONCEPTS IN ANESTHETIC AGENTS

Brunton L, Lazo J, Parker K: *Goodman and Gilman's the pharmacological basis of therapeutics,* ed 11, New York, 2005, McGraw-Hill Professional.

Drake R, Vogl W, Mitchell A: *Gray's anatomy for students,* Philadelphia, 2005, Churchill Livingstone.

Evers A, Maze M: *Anesthetic pharmacology: physiologic principles and clinical practice,* Philadelphia, 2004, Churchill Livingstone.

Fisher L: *Benumof's anesthesia and uncommon diseases,* ed 5, Philadelphia, 2007, Saunders.

Food and Drug Administration: *FDA strengthens warning for droperidol,* Washington, DC, 2001, FDA Talk Paper.

Gallager C, Issenberg B: *Simulation in anesthesia,* Philadelphia, 2007, Saunders.

Ganong W: *Review of medical physiology,* ed 22, New York, 2005, McGraw-Hill Medical.

Gold M, Sacks D, Grosnoff D et al: Comparison of propofol with thiopental and isoflurane for induction and maintenance of general anesthesia, *J Clin Anesth* 1(4):272-276, 1989.

Guyton A, Hall J: *Textbook of medical physiology,* ed 11, Philadelphia, 2006, Saunders.

Katz R, editor: Propofol: a critical assessment, *Semin Anesth* 6:1-54, 1992.

Kier L, Dowd C: *The chemistry of drugs for nurse anesthetists,* Chicago, 2004, AANA Publishing, Inc.

Korttila K, Ostman P, Faure E et al: Randomized comparison of recovery after propofol-nitrous oxide versus thiopentone-isoflurane-nitrous oxide anaesthesia in patients undergoing ambulatory surgery, *Acta Anaesthesiol Scand* 34:400-403, 1990.

Longnecker D, Murphy F: *Dripps, Eckenhoff, Vandam introduction to anesthesia,* ed 9, Philadelphia, 1997, Saunders.

Longnecker D, Tinker J, Morgan G: *Principles and practice of anesthesiology,* ed 2, St Louis, 1998, Mosby.

Miller R, editor: *Anesthesia,* ed 6, Philadelphia, 2005, Churchill Livingstone.

Nagelhout J, Zaglaniczy K: *Nurse anesthesia,* ed 3, St Louis, 2005, Saunders.

Prielipp R, Young C: Current drugs for sedation of critically ill patients, *Semin Anesthesia Perioperative Med Pain* 20(2):85-94, 2001.

Reves J, Fragen RJ, Vinik HR et al: Midazolam: pharmacology and uses, *Anesthesiology* 62:310-324, 1985.

Sebel P, Larson J: Propofol: a new intravenous anesthetic, *Anesthesiology* 71:260-277, 1989.

Shepherd M: Multidisciplinary approach to developing guidelines for use of anesthetic agents in an intensive care unit, *Anesthesia Today* 6(1):15-18, 1995.

Short T, Chui P: Propofol and midazolam act synergistically in combination, *Br J Anaesth* 67:539-545, 1991.

Shorten G, Browne J, Carr D, Puig M et al: *Postoperative pain management: an evidence-based guide to practice,* Philadelphia, 2006, Saunders.

Spiess B: Two new pharmacological agents for the 1990s: flumazenil and propofol, *J Post Anesth Nurs* 5(3):186-189, 1990.

Spindler J, Mehlisch D, Brown C: Intramuscular ketorolac and morphine in the treatment of moderate to severe pain after major surgery, *Pharmacotherapy* 10:51S-58S, 1990.

Stoelting R: *Pharmacology and physiology in anesthetic practice,* ed 3, Philadelphia, 1999, Lippincott-Raven.

Stoelting R, Miller R: *Basics of anesthesia,* ed 4, New York, 2000, Churchill Livingstone.

Stone D: *Perioperative care: anesthesia, medicine, and surgery,* St Louis, 1998, Mosby.

Stoelting R: *Pharmacology and physiology in anesthetic practice,* ed 3, Philadelphia, 1999, Lippincott-Raven.

Stoelting R, Miller R: *Basics of anesthesia,* ed 5, Philadelphia, 2007, Churchill Livingstone.

White P: *Perioperative drug manual,* ed 2, Philadelphia, 2005, Saunders.

Vogelsang J, Hayes S: Butorphanol tartrate (Stadol): a review, *J Post Anesth Nurs* 6(2):129-135, 1991.

White P: *What's new in intravenous anesthesia,* 1990 International Anesthesia Research Society Review Course Lectures, Cleveland, 1990, IARS.

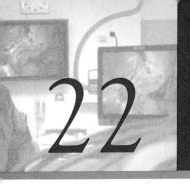

# 22

# OPIOID INTRAVENOUS ANESTHETICS

*Cecil B. Drain, PhD, RN, CRNA, FAAN, FASAHP*

Opioid intravenous anesthetics constitute a major portion of the clinical anesthesia process. These drugs enhance the effectiveness of the inhalation anesthetics. More specifically, the opioids meet much of the analgesic portion of the anesthesia process. Also, addition of the opioids to the drugs used for general anesthesia can reduce the concentration of the inhalation anesthetic; as a result, a safer anesthetic can be administered to the patient. Because opioids are used to manage acute and chronic pain and are administered for general inhalation anesthesia and sedation and pain relief during regional anesthesia, the implications for the postanesthesia nursing care of the surgical patient are profound.

The immediate postanesthesia phase is when the patient is most vulnerable to complications (see Chapter 29). Many drugs that have residual anesthetic effects well into the postanesthesia period are now used in modern anesthesia care. These agents include the potent inhaled agents, muscle relaxants, benzodiazepines, and opioids. Respiratory depression is the most common adverse event in the postanesthesia care unit (PACU); hence, the use and understanding of the various opioid agents optimize patient outcomes. Also, the reduction of pain in the PACU is one of the primary focuses of care in the perianesthesia phase. In addition to assessing pain, the perianesthesia nurse must take into the evaluation of pain the preoperative, intraoperative, and postanesthesia phase of the surgical patient. Because all pain-reducing drugs must be taken into account during the pain assessment in the PACU, the mixed action or agonist-antagonist combination drugs are presented in this chapter. To "balance out" all the different drugs given to the patient with the intended drug to be administered in the PACU is a difficult task. With a detailed description of the major opioids used in the the perianesthesia period provided, the PACU nurse will be able to make excellent informed decisions in regard to the anticipated outcome of the patient of pain reduction and comfort.

## DEFINITIONS

**Agonist:** A drug with a specific cellular or receptor affinity that produces a predictable response.

**Antagonist:** A drug that exerts an opposite action to that of another or competes for the same receptor site or sites.

**Breakthrough Pain:** A transient increase in the intensity of pain from a baseline pain level that is no greater than moderate.

**Dysphoria:** A disorder of affect that is characterized by depression and anguish.

**Endogenous:** Originating inside the body.

**Endorphins:** These opioid peptides are produced in the body and are composed of many amino acid (protein) substances that attach to opioid receptors in the central nervous system and the peripheral nervous system for reduction of pain.

**Exognenous:** Originating outside the body.

**Fixed Chest Syndrome:** Rigidity of the diaphragmatic and intercostal muscles.

**Micrograms (µg):** Also referred to as mcg; 1 µg is equal to 0.001 mcg.

**Mydriasis:** Dilation of the pupil of the eye.

**Opiate Receptor:** Receptors that are transmembrane proteins that bind to endogenous opioid neuropeptides and exogenous morphine and similar compounds. They are designated mu, kappa, and delta subtypes of the opiate receptor (Table 22-1).

**Opioid:** A drug that contains opium or a derivative of opium along with semisynthetic or synthetic drugs that have opium-like properties.

**Piloerection:** Erection of the hairs of the skin.

**Spasmolytic:** Stoppage of muscle group contractions.

## THE CONCEPT OF OPIOIDS AND OPIOID RECEPTORS

Opioids are the substances, either natural or synthetic, that are administered into the body (exogenous) and bind to specific receptors to produce a morphine-like or opioid agonist effect. The

## Table 22-1  Characteristics of Various Opioid Receptors

| Effects | MU RECEPTOR | | Kappa Receptor | Delta Receptor |
| --- | --- | --- | --- | --- |
| | Mu-1 | Mu-2 | | |
| Analgesia | Supraspinal | Spinal | Supraspinal, spinal | Supraspinal, spinal; modulates mu-receptor activity |
| Cardiovascular effects | Bradycardia | Bradycardia | | |
| Respiratory effects | | Depression | Possible depression | Depression |
| Central nervous system effects | Euphoria; sedation; prolactin release; hypothermia; catalepsy; indifference to environmental stimulus | Euphoria; dopamine turnover; possible growth hormone release | Sedation; dysphoria; psychotomimetic reactions (hallucinations, delirium) | |
| Pupil | Miosis | Miosis | Miosis | |
| Gastrointestinal effects | | Inhibition of peristalsis; nausea, vomiting | | |
| Genitourinary effects | Urinary retention | Urinary retention | Diuresis (inhibition of vasopressin release) | Urinary retention |
| Pruritus | | Yes | | Yes |
| Physical dependence | Low abuse potential | Yes | Low abuse potential | Yes |

Other opioid subtypes exist in animals, such as kappa-1, kappa-2, and kappa-3. Mu-1 and mu-2 agonists have not been developed for human use. From Nagelhout J, Zaglaniczy K: *Nurse anesthesia*, ed 3, St Louis, 2005, Saunders.

endogenous opioids are the endorphins. The endorphins, which are produced in the body, attach to the opioid receptors in the central nervous system (CNS) to activate the body's pain modulating system. The term opioid is used because of the multitude of synthetic drugs with morphine-like actions; with the advent of receptor physiology, opioid has replaced the term narcotic. Narcotic is derived from the Greek word for stupor and usually refers to both the production of the morphine-like effects and the physical dependence.

The naturally occurring alkaloids of opium are divided into two classes: phenanthrenes and benzylisoquinolines. The principal phenanthrene series of drugs includes morphine, codeine, and thebaine. Papaverine and noscapine, which lack opioid activity, represent the benzylisoquinoline alkaloids of opium.

The synthetic opioids have been produced with the modification of the chemical structure of the phenanthrene class of drugs. Drugs such as fentanyl (Sublimaze) and meperidine (Demerol) are examples of synthetic opioids.

The identification of specific opioid receptors has enhanced the understanding of the agonist and antagonist actions of this category of drugs. The opioid receptors are located in the CNS, principally in the brain stem and spinal cord. These receptors have been determined by the pharmacologic effect they produce when stimulated by a specific agonist along with how the effect is blocked by a specific antagonist. The three major categories of opioid receptors are the mu (μ), delta (δ), and kappa (κ).

The mu receptors are mainly responsible for the production of supraspinal analgesia effects with stimulation. These receptors are further divided into mu-1 and mu-2 types. Activation of the mu-1 receptors results in analgesia; when the mu-2 receptors are stimulated, hypoventilation, bradycardia, physical dependence, euphoria, and ileus can result. The mu receptors are activated by morphine, fentanyl, and meperidine. The drug that is specific to the mu-1 receptor is meptazinol, which is supraspinal in regard to analgesia; the mu-2 receptor analgesia occurs at the spinal level. Other characteristics of the mu-1 and mu-2 receptors are summarized in Table 22-1. Stimulation of the kappa receptors results in spinal analgesia, dysphoria, hallucinations, hypertonia, tachycardia, tachypnea, mydriasis, sedation, and miosis, with little effect on ventilation. The drugs that possess both opioid agonist and antagonist activities, such as nalbuphine (Nubain), have their principal action on the kappa opioid receptors. The delta opioid receptors, when stimulated, serve to modulate the activity of the mu receptors and cause depression and urinary retention. The drug naloxone (Narcan) attaches to all the opioid receptors and thus serves as an antagonist to all the opioid agonists (see Table 22-1).

### The Opioids

Opioids, or narcotics, are becoming quite popular in anesthesia practice. They are usually used in the nitrous-narcotic (balanced) techniques, which involve the use of a narcotic, nitrous oxide, and oxygen, with or without a muscle relaxant, and thiopental for induction.

The effects of narcotics generally last well into the PACU phase, and every perianesthesia nurse should have a good knowledge of the pharmacologic actions of each narcotic that is administered to the patient in the perioperative phase of the surgical experience.

The administration of opioids in the perioperative period is not without the concern of overdosage. The major signs of overdosage with opioids are miosis, hypoventilation, and coma. If the patient becomes severely hypoxemic, mydriasis can occur. Airway obstruction is a strong possibility because the skeletal muscles become flaccid. Also, hypotension and seizures may occur. The treatment for an opioid overdosage is mechanical ventilation and the slow titration of naloxone. Consideration must always be given to the fact that some patients who become overdosed with an opioid may indeed be already physically dependent. Naloxone can precipitate an acute withdrawal syndrome.

### Meperidine Hydrochloride

Meperidine (Demerol) was discovered in 1939 by Eisleb and Schauman. Because it is chemically similar to atropine, it was originally introduced as an antispasmodic agent and was not used as an opioid anesthetic agent until 1947. The main action of this drug is similar to morphine; it stimulates the subcortical mu receptors, which results in an analgesic effect. Meperidine is about 1/10 as potent as morphine and has a duration of action of about 2 to 4 hours. The onset of analgesia is prompt (10 minutes) after subcutaneous or intramuscular administration. All pain, especially visceral, gastrointestinal, and urinary tract, is satisfactorily relieved. This drug causes less biliary tract spasm than morphine; however, in comparison with codeine, meperidine causes greater biliary tract spasm. It produces some sleepiness but causes little euphoria or amnesia. Meperidine increases the sensitivity of the labyrinthine apparatus of the ear, which explains the dizziness, nausea, and vomiting that sometimes occur in ambulatory patients.

This narcotic may slow the rate of respiration, but the rate generally returns to normal within 15 minutes after intravenous injection. The tidal volume is not changed appreciably. In equivalent analgesic doses, meperidine depresses respiration to a greater extent than does morphine. Some authors have noted that meperidine may release histamine from the tissues. Occasionally, one may notice urticarial wheals that have formed over the veins where meperidine has been injected. The usual treatment is discontinuation of the use of meperidine and, if the reaction is severe, administration of diphenhydramine (Benadryl). Diphenhydramine further sedates the patient, however, and should be administered only if truly warranted.

Meperidine in therapeutic doses does not cause any significant untoward effects on the cardiovascular system. When this drug is administered intravenously, it usually causes a transient increase in heart rate. With intramuscular administration, no significant change in heart rate is observed. One of the major concerns with this drug is orthostatic hypotension, probably caused by meperidine's interference with the compensatory sympathetic nervous system reflex. Hence, after administration of meperidine, a patient should be repositioned slowly in a "staged" approach to avoid any possibility of hypotension.

Meperidine is generally metabolized in the liver; less than 5% is excreted unchanged by the kidneys. However, because of a toxic metabolite of meperidine, patients who are administered this drug may have seizures. Meperidine is partially metabolized to normeperidine and has some analgesic effects, but more importantly, it lowers the seizure threshold and can induce

CNS excitability. Meperidine probably should not be administered to elderly patients because renal dysfunction may occur.

Because of its spasmolytic effect, meperidine is the drug of choice for biliary duct, distal colon, and rectal surgery. It offers the advantages of little interference with the physiologic compensatory mechanisms, low toxicity, smooth and rapid recovery, prolonged postoperative analgesia, excellent cardiac stability in elderly patients and patients at poor risk, and ease of detoxification and excretion.

### Morphine

Morphine, one of the oldest known drugs, has only recently been used as an opioid intravenous anesthetic agent. Alkaloid morphine is from the phenanthrene class of opium. The exact mechanism of action of morphine is unknown. In humans, it produces analgesia, drowsiness, changes in mood, and mental clouding. The analgesic effect can become profound before the other effects are severe and can persist after many of the side effects have almost disappeared. With direct effect on the respiratory center, morphine depresses respiratory rate, tidal volume, and minute volume. Maximal respiratory depression occurs within 7 minutes after intravenous injection of the drug and 30 minutes after intramuscular administration. After therapeutic doses of morphine, the sensitivity of the respiratory center begins to return to normal in 2 or 3 hours, but the minute volume does not return to preinjection level until 4 or 5 hours have passed.

The greatest advantage of morphine is the remarkable cardiovascular stability that accompanies its use. It has no major effect on blood pressure, heart rate, or heart rhythm—even in toxic doses, when hypoxia is avoided. Morphine does, however, decrease the capacity of the cardiovascular system to adjust to gravitational shifts. This effect is important to remember because orthostatic hypotension and syncope may easily occur in a patient whose care necessitates a position change. This phenomenon is primarily the result of the peripheral vasodilator effect of morphine. Therefore, a position change for a patient who has received morphine should be accomplished slowly, with constant monitoring of the patient's vital signs.

Morphine may cause nausea and vomiting, especially in ambulatory patients, because of direct stimulation of the chemoreceptor trigger zone. The emetic effect of morphine can be counteracted with narcotic antagonists and phenothiazine derivatives such as prochlorperazine (Compazine), dexmedetomidine (Precedex), or the 5-HT$_3$ receptor antagonist ondansetron (Zofran). Histamine release has been noted with morphine, and morphine also causes profound constriction of the pupils, stimulation of the visceral smooth muscles, and spasm of the sphincter of Oddi.

Morphine is detoxified by conjugation with glucuronic acid. Ninety percent is excreted by the kidneys, and 7% to 10% is excreted in the feces via the bile.

Morphine is used in the balanced, or nitrous-narcotic, technique with nitrous oxide, oxygen, and a muscle relaxant. This technique is useful for cardiovascular surgery and other types of surgery in which cardiovascular stability is necessary. The patient may arrive in the PACU still narcotized from morphine with an endotracheal tube in place. Mechanical ventilation for 24 to 48 hours is usually warranted. Morphine may or may not be supplemented during the time of ventilation. This type of recovery procedure facilitates a pain free state and maximum ventilation of the patient during the critical phase of recovery. Morphine can also be used to provide basal narcosis when regional anesthesia is used.

In the PACU, morphine is an excellent drug for the control of postoperative pain. When given intravenously, this drug has a peak analgesic effect in about 20 minutes, with a duration of about 2 hours. With intramuscular administration, the onset of action is about 15 minutes, with a peak effect attained in about 45 to 90 minutes and a duration of action of about 4 hours.

### Methadone

Although methadone was introduced in the late 1930s in Germany and in the 1940s in the United States, it has returned to clinical use in the PACU for pain relief. The drug was originally introduced to help treat chronic pain, opioid abstinence syndromes, and heroin addiction.

Methadone undergoes slow metabolism and is high in lipid solubility, which makes it longer lasting that morphine-based drugs with a duration of action up to 24 hours that allows for less frequent dosing. It is a good drug for treatment of chronic pain, especially in patients who are thought to have a propensity for drug dependence. Methadone can be administered orally and intravenously; when administered intravenously at a dosage of 20 mg, methadone produces postoperative analgesia that lasts more than 24 hours.

This synthetic opioid agonist's actions resemble morphine; side effects include depression of ventilation, miosis, constipation, and biliary tract spasm. Clinically, the sedative and euphoric actions of methadone appear to be less than those produced by morphine.

## Hydromorphone

Hydromorphone (Dilaudid), which is a derivative of morphine, was developed in Germany in the 1920s and released to the mass market in the late 1920s. The drug has a renewed popularity for the PACU and can be administered intravenously, intramuscularly, rectally, or orally. The drug profile in regard to its analgesia and side effects is similar to morphine. Hydromorphone is recommended for patients in renal failure because of its virtual lack of active metabolites after its breakdown in the liver. It has a high solubility and a rapid onset of action and appears to have less troublesome side effects and dependence liability profile as compared with morphine. Because of its high lipid solubility, hydromorphone can be administered via epidural or spinal for a wide area of anesthesia as compared with duramophine.

Hydromorphone, like all opioids, is a CNS depressant and has actions and side effects similar to morphine. Its depressant effects can be enhanced with beta-blockers and alcohol. The duration of action of this drug is about 2 hours, with a peak action in about 30 minutes with intravenous administration.

## Fentanyl

Janssen and associates introduced a series of highly potent meperidine derivatives that were found to render the patient free of pain without affecting certain areas in the CNS. Fentanyl (Sublimaze) appeared to be of special interest. In regard to analgesic properties, fentanyl is approximately 80 to 125 times as potent as morphine and has a rapid onset of action of 5 to 6 minutes and a peak effect within 5 to 15 minutes. The analgesia lasts 20 to 40 minutes when administered intravenously. Via the intramuscular route, the onset of action is 7 to 15 minutes; the analgesia usually lasts 1 to 2 hours. When fentanyl is administered as a single bolus, 75% of the drug undergoes "first-pass" pulmonary uptake. That is, the lungs serve as a large storage site and this nonrespiratory function of the lung (see Chapter 12) limits the amount of fentanyl that actually reaches the systemic circulation. If the patient receives multiple doses of fentanyl via single injections or infusion, the first-pass pulmonary uptake mechanism becomes saturated and the patient has a prolonged emergence because of increased duration of the drug. Consequently, during the admission of the patient to the PACU, the postanesthesia nurse must determine the frequency and amount of intraoperative fentanyl administration. Patients who have received a significant amount of fentanyl via infusion or via titration should be continuously monitored for persistent or recurrent respiratory depression. Also, fentanyl has been implicated in what is called a delayed-onset respiratory depression. In some patients, a secondary peak of the drug concentration in the plasma occurs about 45 minutes after the apparent recovery from the drug. This syndrome may occur because some of the fentanyl can become sequestered in the gastric fluid and then can become recycled into the plasma in about 45 minutes. Hence, in the PACU, all patients who have received fentanyl should be continuously monitored for respiratory depression for at least 1 hour from the time of admission to the unit.

Fentanyl can be administered during surgery at three different dose ranges, depending on the type of surgery and the desired effect. For example, the low-dose range of 2 to 20 µg/kg attenuates moderately stressful stimuli. The moderate dose range is 20 to 50 µg/kg and strongly obtunds the stress response. The megadose range of as much as 150 µg/kg blocks the stress response and is particularly valuable when protection of the myocardium is critical.

Fentanyl shares with most other narcotics a profound respiratory depressant effect, even to the point of apnea. Rapid intravenous injection can provoke bronchial constriction and resistance to ventilation caused by rigidity of the diaphragmatic and intercostal muscles. This is commonly called the fixed chest syndrome, which can occur when any potent narcotic analgesic is administered too rapidly via the intravenous route. Should this syndrome occur, intravenous subclinical administration of succinylcholine (15 to 25 mg) relieves the rigidity of the chest wall muscles. Once succinylcholine is administered for this purpose, the perianesthesia nurse should be prepared for ventilation of the patient until the skeletal muscle relaxant properties of succinylcholine subside.

Fentanyl, unlike most narcotics, has little or no hypotensive effects and usually does not cause nausea and vomiting. Because of its vagotonic effect, it may cause bradycardia, which can be relieved with atropine or glycopyrrolate. Fentanyl can be reversed with the narcotic antagonist naloxone, which also reverses analgesia. Should fentanyl be reversed with naloxone in the PACU, the perianesthesia nurse should continue to monitor the patient for the possible return of respiratory depression because the

| Box 22-1 | Example of Conversion of Dosage Calculations from mg to mcg | |
|---|---|---|
| Milligrams | Micrograms | Milliliters of Fentanyl |
| 0.025 mg | 25 µg | 0.5 mL |
| 0.05 mg | 50 µg | 1.0 mL |
| 0.10 mg | 100 µg | 2.0 mL |
| 0.15 mg | 150 µg | 3.0 mL |
| 0.20 mg | 200 µg | 4.0 mL |
| 0.25 mg | 250 µg | 4.5 mL |
| 0.50 mg | 500 µg | 10.0 mL |
| 1.00 mg | 1000 µg | 20.0 mL |

duration of the respiratory depression produced by the fentanyl may be longer than the duration of action of naloxone.

Fentanyl can be used alone in a nitrous-narcotic technique (see Chapter 20). It also is used in the PACU in the form of a low-dose intravenous drip for pain relief; however, fentanyl is usually given slowly intravenously in the PACU for breakthrough pain (see Box 22-1 for helpful calculation of milligram to microgram dosage information).

## Sufentanil

Sufentanil is an analogue of fentanyl and is approximately five to seven times as potent as fentanyl. Anesthesia with sufentanil can be induced more rapidly, with basically the same technique as that used for fentanyl, without an increase in the incidence rate of chest wall rigidity. However, sufentanil can produce chest wall rigidity; so if it is administered in the PACU, equipment for administration of oxygen with positive pressure and the skeletal muscle relaxant succinylcholine should be on hand. The incidence rate of hypertension with sufentanil is lower than with comparable doses of fentanyl. Bradycardia is infrequently seen in patients who receive sufentanil, and when high-dose sufentanil is used in combination with nitrous oxide-oxygen, the mean arterial pressure and cardiac output may be decreased. The recovery time from sufentanil from the time of injection is about the same as with fentanyl because sufentanil is rapidly eliminated from tissue storage sites; consequently, the duration of action of sufentanil is about the same as with fentanyl. Also, initial study results indicate that the incidence rates of postoperative hypertension, the need for vasoactive agents, and the requirements for postoperative analgesics are generally reduced in patients who are administered moderate or high doses of sufentanil in comparison

with patients given inhalation agents. Of particular interest to the perianesthesia nurse is that sufentanil has an additive effect that is seen in patients who receive barbiturates, tranquilizers, other opioids, general anesthetics, or other CNS depressants. This effect is especially true of benzodiazepines because they can potentiate a profound hypotensive action. Hence, when sufentanil is combined with any of these drugs, particular attention should be paid to any signs of decreased respiratory drive, increased airway resistance, or hypotension. Immediate countermeasures include maintenance of a patent airway with proper positioning of the patient, placement of an oral airway or endotracheal tube, and administration of oxygen. If indicated, naloxone should be used as a specific antidote for management of the respiratory depression. The duration of respiratory depression after overdosage with sufentanil may be longer than the duration of action of the naloxone. Consequently, the patient should be constantly observed for the recurrence of respiratory depression, even after the initial successful treatment with naloxone. Hypotension can be treated with reversal with naloxone; however, fluids and vasopressors may be indicated (see Chapter 11).

## Alfentanil

Alfentanil is another analogue of fentanyl that is about 1/10 as potent and has about one third the duration of action of fentanyl. The onset of action of this drug occurs in about 1 or 2 minutes, and the duration of action is 20 to 30 minutes. Alfentanil appears to have significant advantages over currently available opioid anesthetics. For example, it has no cumulative drug effects, and once the infusion of alfentanil is terminated, the emergence time is quite predictable. Alfentanil, like fentanyl, produces minimal hemodynamic effects and offers a high therapeutic index. In fact, the therapeutic index for alfentanil is higher than those of fentanyl and other opioids. A therapeutic index is the ratio of the lethal dose to the effective dose; the higher the therapeutic index, the farther the lethal dose from the dose used for the desired effect. More specifically, the therapeutic index of fentanyl is 270, which means that it is about four times safer than morphine. Alfentanil's therapeutic index is about 2.5 times more favorable than that of fentanyl.

Alfentanil, in addition to its place in the operating room, may also have important uses in the PACU. Its rapid onset and brief duration of action make it advantageous for the immediate pain relief needs of PACU patients.

As previously stated, the drug has about one third the potency of fentanyl, but its onset of action is at least three times faster; its duration is one third that of fentanyl, and it has a high therapeutic index, which makes alfentanil well suited for pain relief in the immediate postoperative period. The drug produces few cardiovascular effects and thus should be of great value in the prevention of dangerous reflexes, such as tachycardia during intubation. Clinical observation indicates that the recovery time for this drug is extremely rapid. Hence, patients who receive this drug during surgery most likely have pain early in the immediate postoperative period and the appropriate analgesic should be administered.

### Remifentanil

Remifentanil is a selective mu opioid agonist that has an analgesic potency about equal to fentanyl and 20 times as potent as alfentanil. This drug has some excellent pharmacologic properties in that it is brief in action, titratable, and noncumulative; it lacks histamine release; and it has a rapid recovery after the discontinuation of the drug. The onset of this drug is within 1 minute. When the drug is discontinued, it is metabolized quickly; its effects disappear within 4 minutes. The remifentanil anesthetic technique is excellent for suppression of the stress response and allows for excellent depression of neurologic responses. In regard to the immediate postanesthesia period, remifentanil is better than most intravenous opioid drugs in regard to residual effects because it has a rapid recovery and less risk of postoperative respiratory depression.

This drug should probably not be used in the PACU; however, if the drug is administered in the PACU, it should be administered *only* by an anesthesia clinician who is experienced in the administration of the drug. Some of the adverse effects of the drug may accompany its administration.

Remifentanil is given via intravenous infusion with an infusion pump and should never be administered via intravenous bolus. The drug can produce the fixed chest syndrome and can also cause nausea and vomiting, respiratory depression, and mild-to-moderate depression of the heart rate and blood pressure.

## PARTIAL AGONIST-ANTAGONIST DRUGS

### Pentazocine

Pentazocine(Fortral, Talwin), an opioid agonist and antagonist analgesic, was first synthesized in 1959. The drug has significant activity and a low addiction potential. It is approximately one third as potent as morphine when given intramuscularly. Its advantage over morphine is that it can be given orally. Pentazocine can be used before and after surgery for the relief of pain from abdominal, cardiac, genitourinary, orthopedic, neurologic, and gynecologic surgery. The observed side effects of this drug include sedation, dizziness, nausea, and vomiting, but these occur infrequently.

Studies of the relative potency of this drug indicate that 30 mg of pentazocine is analgesically equivalent to 10 mg of morphine and 75 mg of meperidine. Pentazocine has been established to relieve severe pain and is approximately two to four times less potent than morphine when administered parenterally.

Pentazocine can be used in the nitrous-narcotic technique. The respiratory depression produced by pentazocine is potentiated when general anesthetics are used concomitantly. Pentazocine produces an increase in systolic blood pressure and does not appear to have depressant effects on cardiac output. The drug should be used with caution in patients with renal or hepatic impairment. Pentazocine depresses the respiratory system in a manner comparable with morphine in equivalent analgesic doses. Tolerance to the analgesic effect of the drug does not appear to develop as it does with other narcotics. Because pentazocine is a narcotic antagonist at the mu receptors, administration of this drug to a patient who depends on opiates may induce abrupt withdrawal symptoms.

The onset of analgesic activity of pentazocine is approximately 2 or 3 minutes when it is given intravenously and 15 to 20 minutes when given intramuscularly. The duration of action is about 3 hours. When given orally, the drug is about one third as potent as when it is given intramuscularly.

### Butorphanol

Butorphanol is a synthetic analgesic that is chemically related to the nalorphine-cyclazocine series with both narcotic and antagonist properties. More specifically, it serves as an agonist at the kappa and sigma opioid receptors. In regard to its analgesic potency, it is about 5 times more potent than morphine, 30 times more potent than meperidine, and 20 times more potent than pentazocine. Butorphanol can produce sedation, nausea, and respiratory depression. The respiratory depression is plateau-like in that 2 mg of butorphanol depresses respiration to a degree equal to 10 mg of morphine. The magnitude of respiratory depression with butorphanol is not appreciably increased at doses of

**Table 22-2    Comparison of Five Analgesics that Use Morphine as Drug with Primary Opioid Effects**

|  | Morphine | Meperidine | Pentazocine | Butorphanol | Nalbuphine |
|---|---|---|---|---|---|
| Indication | Moderate to severe pain | Moderate to severe pain | Moderate to severe pain | Moderate to severe pain | Moderate to severe pain |
| Recommended IM dose | 10 mg | 25-50 mg | 30 mg | 2 mg | 10 mg |
| Recommended IV dose | 4-10 mg | 100 mg | 30 mg | 1 mg | 10 mg |
| Time for onset of analgesia | Rapid IV 30 min IM | Rapid IV 30 min IM | Rapid IV 20 min IM | Rapid IV 30 min IM | Rapid IV 15 min IM |
| Duration of analgesia | 4 h | 2-4 h | 3-4 h | 3-4 h | 3-6 h |
| Respiratory depression | High | High | Occurs, but less than with morphine | Occurs, but less than with morphine | Occurs, but less than with morphine |
| Cardiovascular effect | Decreases cardiac workload | Decreases cardiac workload | Increases cardiac workload | Increases cardiac workload | Good cardiac stability |
| Abuse syndrome | High | High | Occurs; induces withdrawal syndrome | Occurs; induces withdrawal syndrome | Occurs; induces withdrawal syndrome |

*IM*, Intramuscular; *IV*, intravenous.

4 mg. The duration of the respiratory depression is dose-related and is reversible with naloxone. Intravenous administration of butorphanol can produce increased pulmonary artery pressure, pulmonary wedge pressure, left-ventricular end-diastolic pressure, systemic arterial pressure, and pulmonary vascular resistance. Consequently, this drug increases the workload of the heart, especially in the pulmonary circuit. Because of its antagonist properties, butorphanol is not recommended for patients who are physically dependent on narcotics because butorphanol can precipitate withdrawal symptoms in those patients. See Table 22-2 for an overview of the clinical pharmacology of butorphanol.

## Nalbuphine

Nalbuphine (Nubain) is a potent analgesic with narcotic agonist and antagonist actions. It is chemically related to oxymorphone and naloxone. This drug is an antagonist at the mu receptors, a partial agonist at the kappa receptors, and an agonist at the sigma receptors. Nalbuphine is as potent as morphine and about three times as potent as pentazocine on a milligram basis. At a dose of 10 mg/kg, nalbuphine causes the same degree of respiratory depression as does 10 mg of morphine. At higher doses, nalbuphine exhibits the same plateau effect as butorphanol

(i.e., respiratory depression is not increased appreciably with higher doses). The respiratory depression produced by nalbuphine can be reversed with naloxone. Nalbuphine does not appear to increase the workload of the heart or to decrease cardiovascular stability. This drug has a lower abuse potential than does morphine; however, if it is given to a patient who is physically dependent on narcotics, withdrawal symptoms may appear. Signs of withdrawal include abdominal cramps, nausea and vomiting, lacrimation, rhinorrhea, anxiety, restlessness, elevation of temperature, and piloerection. If these symptoms appear after the injection of nalbuphine, the administration of small amounts of morphine can relieve the objective effects of the syndrome. See Table 22-2 for an overview of the clinical pharmacology of nalbuphine.

## The Narcotic Antagonists

Narcotic antagonists are used to reverse narcotic-induced respiratory depression. An opioid antagonist, such as naloxone (Narcan), is a drug that completely antagonizes the effect of a narcotic. For completeness, older drugs such as nalorphine (Nalline) and levallorphan (Lorfan) best typify the agonist-antagonists. These drugs partially reverse the effects of narcotics but also produce autonomic, endocrine, analgesic, and respiratory depressant effects similar to those of morphine. Because the newer narcotic antagonists have pure opioid antagonist activity, the manufacture of the drugs nalorphine and levallorphan has ceased.

**Naloxone.** Naloxone (Narcan), a pure antagonist, reverses the depressant effects of narcotics. More specifically, this drug antagonizes the opioid effects at the mu, kappa, and sigma receptors. This drug also reverses the analgesic effect of the narcotic, which is important in assessment of the patient's respiratory effort. Naloxone should be titrated according to the patient's response. Usually, 0.1 to 0.2 mg given slowly intravenously should be adequate for reversal. The onset of action of naloxone is 1 or 2 minutes; if after 3 to 5 minutes inadequate reversal has been achieved, naloxone administration may be repeated until reversal is complete. If the patient shows no sign of reversal, assessment of other pharmacologic agents administered is indicated. Drugs such as halothane, barbiturates, and muscle relaxants are not reversed with naloxone.

The duration of action of naloxone is 1 to 4 hours, depending on the route and amount of drug used. If long-acting narcotics were used, the patient must be monitored for respiratory embarrassment after the administration of naloxone because the depressant activity of the narcotic may return. If this phenomenon occurs, supplemental doses of naloxone can be used. The intramuscular route of administration has been shown to produce a longer lasting effect.

An excessive dosage of naloxone may increase blood pressure, a finding that may be seen as a response to pain. Too rapid reversal may induce nausea, vomiting, diaphoresis, and tachycardia. During the reversal procedure, the vital signs should be monitored; naloxone should be used with caution in patients with cardiac irritability.

Naloxone does not produce respiratory depression as do other narcotic antagonists. It also does not produce any significant side effects or pupillary constriction. Naloxone reverses natural or synthetic narcotics, propoxyphene (Darvon), and the narcotic-antagonist analgesic pentazocine. Because reversal may precipitate an acute withdrawal syndrome, naloxone should be administered with great caution in patients who are physically dependent on opioids.

**Nalmefene.** Nalmefene is similar in chemical structure to naloxone and is considered a long-acting opioid antagonist. It has a rather rapid onset of about 2 to 5 minutes, with a duration of action of about 8 hours. Nalmefene, when given at the usual dose range, produces the same clinical effects as naloxone.

In the PACU, the dosage of this drug for reversal of respiratory depression is 0.1 to 0.5 µg/kg slowly titrated intravenously at 2-minute to 5-minute intervals. This drug should be titrated slowly with observation for a return of respiratory effort. Once the patient has a return of the appropriate rate and volume of breathing, titration should be stopped and a constant vigilance of the rate and volume of respiration should be continued throughout the PACU stay. This drug should not be administered in a dose of more than 1.6 µg because this does not elicit additional effects. As with naloxone, nalmefene should not be administered to a patient with opioid dependency. Both drugs should *always* be titrated slowly to all patients in case a patient is opioid dependent. If the PACU nurse is titrating these drugs and signs of acute opioid withdrawl are seen, titration should stop immediately.

**Naltrexone.** Naltrexone is a pure mu and kappa, and to a lesser extent delta, opioid receptor antagonist; therefore, its actions are similar to naloxone. This drug can produce sustained opioid antagonist activity for as long as 24 hours, with a peak action in 8 to 12 hours. This drug can *only* be administered orally and is used in opioid detoxification because it can facilitate withdrawal; once the patient has undergone complete detoxification, naltrexone can prevent relapses to opioids by blocking the euphoric effects of the opioid. Also, note that naltrexone is used to treat alcohol dependence; therefore, the same can be said in regard to titrating the drug slowly because it can also cause acute alcohol withdrawl.

## SELECTED METHODS OF OPIOID ADMINISTRATION

### Intrathecal and Epidural Routes of Administration

For management of acute and chronic pain, the opioids can be administered via the subarachnoid or epidural space. The technique is called the neuraxial administration of opioids. This concept of pain relief is based on the fact that opioid receptors exist in the substantia gelatinosa on the dorsal horn of the spinal cord. More specifically, mu, kappa, and delta opioid receptors are located in the substantia gelatinosa. The pain relieved with the administration of neuraxial opioids is usually of the visceral as opposed to the somatic type. When the opioid is administered via the epidural space, it crosses the epidural space to the opioid receptors in the spinal cord. Consequently, the dosage of the opioid, when administered into the epidural space, is usually 10 times the dosage of the opioid if it were administered via the subarachnoid space.

When 0.1 to 0.2 mg of preservative-free morphine (Duramorph) is administered into the subarachnoid space (intrathecal), the maximum concentration is reached in about 5 to 10 minutes, with a duration of about 80 to 200 minutes. When 5 mg of morphine is administered into the epidural space in the lumbar region, analgesia can last for as long as 24 hours. The patient should obtain pain relief in about 30 to 60 minutes after injection. If appropriate pain relief is not achieved, incremental doses of 1 to 2 mg can be administered. The maximum dose in a 24-hour period is 10 mg.

After spinal surgery, epidural morphine administered with the continuous epidural technique has both advantages and disadvantages. Its advantage is a profound degree of pain relief, especially for the first 12 to 18 postoperative hours. However, disadvantages are related to displacement of the epidural catheter and the length of action of the epidural morphine. If the epidural catheter becomes displaced and the morphine has been injected, only partial pain relief ensues. Because of the possibility of profound respiratory depression, opioids must be administered cautiously. In fact, a nonopioid drug such as ketorolac may be especially useful in this circumstance. Depending on the anticipated amount and length of pain, a patient-controlled analgesia (PCA) device can be started on the patient for an immediate result of pain resolution. Also, the postanesthesia nurse can have a profound impact on reduction of the pain threshold with repositioning and reassuring the patient. The new technology of apnea monitors can be quite useful in detection of hypoventilation or apnea that can be created by the opioid in this technique. Hence, the use of the apnea monitor on patients who are receiving epidural morphine certainly aids the postanesthesia nurse in monitoring for respiratory dysfunction.

Other opioids that can be administered epidurally are fentanyl and sufentanil. These drugs offer some advantages over morphine; they are more suited for continuous infusion techniques because of their rapid onset and short duration of action. Also, because they have such a rapid clearance from the cerebrospinal fluid, less chance exists for these drugs to spread toward the head (rostral spread). Rostral spread, which is associated more with morphine, has been shown to produce side effects such as nausea, pruritus, and the previously discussed delayed respiratory depression syndrome. Naloxone reverses this side effect; however, the analgesic effect also is reversed. In this instance, nalbuphine administration should be considered to reverse the respiratory depression and preserve some of the analgesia.

## Patient-controlled Analgesia

For the reduction of pain, the intramuscular injection of opioids and nonopioids has long been the standard route of administration used by nursing personnel. This method of administration has the advantage of simplicity and no requirement for specialized equipment. Its disadvantages include variable uptake, pain on injection, and patient dissatisfaction with the level of pain relief. Patient dissatisfaction is based on the cyclic effect of pain. If a level of analgesia were produced, the adverse effects of pain could be controlled. Intravenous administration offers some advantages over the intramuscular approach. The administration of an opioid via the intravenous route offers the patient an immediate reduction in pain. However, this reduction is only temporary because no appropriate blood level of the opioid has been established.

For an appropriate level of analgesia, a loading dose, followed by titration to effect, based on the pharmacokinetics of the opioid drug is used during surgery. The maintenance of an appropriate blood level of the opioid to achieve and maintain a level of analgesia is the goal of this technique. The blood level of the drug is called the minimum effective analgesic concentration (MEAC). Research has shown that the MEAC varies among individuals. Through the use of technology, the principles of this intraoperative technique have been continued into the immediate postoperative period. Intravenous PCA is the method of choice for those patients who need continued analgesia. The peaks and valleys of analgesia can be avoided without the patient becoming totally dependent on the nurse's response for pain relief. PCA allows the patient more control of the situation by allowing the patient to seek out a particular level of analgesia—the MEAC.

In the PACU, the patient is administered a loading dose of the intravenous opioid to achieve the MEAC and then a PCA infusion pump is set up for the patient. The PCA pump is programmed for the administration of a particular opioid based on the patient's analgesic needs and the pharmacokinetics of the drug to be administered. The parameters to be programmed are the bolus dose, the lockout interval, and the low-dose continuous basal infusion rate. Consequently, with a "push of a button" on the PCA pump, the patient can attain immediate analgesia and receive the benefits of controlled pain relief with low-dose continuous infusion of the opioid.

**Table 22-3    Protocol for Opioid Administration in Intravenous PCA**

| Drug | LOADING DOSE | | INTERVAL DOSE | |
|------|--------------|--|---------------|--|
| | Adult | By Weight | Adult | By Weight |
| Morphine | 0.5-4 mg every 10 min (total, 6-16 mg) | 0.05 mg/kg (total, 0.05-0.2 mg/kg) | 0.5-2 mg | 10-20 µg/kg |
| Meperidine (Demerol) | 12.5-25 mg every 10 min (total, 50-125 mg) | 0.5-1.5 mg/kg | 5-10 mg | 0.1-0.2 mg/kg |
| Fentanyl (Sublimaze) | 25-50 µg every 5 min (total, 50-300 µg) | 0.05-2.0 µg/kg (total, 0.5-4 µg/kg) | 10-30 µg | 0.25-0.5 µg/kg |

PCA, Patient-controlled analgesia. Basal rate or interval dose rate is optional because demand-only mode of PCA is often prescribed. Lockout intervals range generally between 6 and 12 minutes. Adapted from Bailey P: Respiratory effects of postoperative opioid analgesia, *Semin Anesth* 15(4):343-352, 1996.

The amount of the self-dose bolus should be low to avoid an acute increase in blood levels of the drug above the MEAC because, along with the concern about overdosage, blood levels above the MEAC have no analgesic value. The lockout interval, or delay, is the setting used to block the use of the self-dose bolus button for a period of time. During this time, the PCA pump does not deliver the drug, even when the patient pushes the button. The lockout interval is usually short, so the patient can self administer small incremental doses to maintain the MEAC; yet the interval should be long enough to prevent overdosage. The basal infusion rate is usually set at a rate necessary to provide analgesia when the patient is resting. See Table 22-3 for a suggested protocol for drug administration in PCA.

**Patient-controlled Epidural Analgesia**
The concept of PCA has been adapted to epidural analgesia. In this instance, the PCA infusion pump can be attached to the epidural catheter. The opioid drugs that can be used in this technique are fentanyl and sufentanil. They can be used with great success for analgesia after cesarean section. The basal infusion rate keeps the patient analgesic and comfortable. The patient can self administer a bolus of the opioid if the analgesia provided with the basal infusion rate is not sufficient. Also, the bolus opioid facilitates additional analgesia needed for turning and early ambulation. A suggested protocol for both fentanyl and sufentanil is provided in Tables 22-4 and 22-5. Because of the possibility of rostral spread (see Chapter 25), an apnea monitor is

suggested to be used on patients who are receiving patient-controlled epidural analgesia.

**Monitoring the Patient Receiving Opioids in the PACU**
In addition to routine monitoring for the patient receiving opioids in the PACU, the respiratory rate (RR) should be monitored for not only the rate but also the trend. For example, if the RR decreases from 18 to 16 to 12 in a 45-minute interval, strong suspicion exists that excessive opioid effect has occurred and the modified stir-up regime should be instituted.

Along with monitoring of respiratory rate and depth, peripheral pulse oximetry and, if necessary, detection of expired carbon dioxide or arterial blood gas monitoring can be used. The nervous system clinical indicators of significant opioid action should also be monitored and include observation for excess sedation, lethargy, apathy, dysphoria, nausea, vomiting, pruritus (especially facial), miosis, and cough suppression.

If the patient is determined to have opioid-induced respiratory depression, prophylactic supplemental oxygen should be administered and the modified stir-up regime should be instituted. If the patient is difficult to arouse, the airway should be supported and manually assisted ventilation with bag and mask may be needed. Should the patient have excessive secretions or vomitus, a person skilled in airway management should be summoned because tracheal intubation may be necessary. Pharmacologic treatment should include the use of naloxone. For the adult, treatment should start with lower doses

| Table 22-4 | Protocol For Administration of Fentanyl* via PCEA System for Patients After Cesarean Section | | |
|---|---|---|---|
| | PACU | Surgical Unit | For Pain |
| Bolus | 100 μg | — | 50-100 μg |
| Dose | 40 μg | 40 μg | 50-60 μg |
| Lockout | 10 min | 10 min | 10 min |
| Basal rate | 60 μg/h | 60 μg/h | 60-80 μg/h |
| Limit | 260 μg/h | 260 μg/h | 310-380 μg/h |

*Mix fentanyl in 20-μg/mL solution.
PCEA, Patient-controlled epidural analgesia. Adapted from Grass J, Harris A: Postcesarean section analgesia, *Wellcome Trends Anesthesiol* 9(6):3-8, 1991.

| Table 22-5 | Protocol for Administration of Sufentanil via PCEA System for Patients After Cesarean Section | | |
|---|---|---|---|
| | PACU | Surgical Unit | For Pain |
| Bolus | 30 μg | — | 20 μg |
| Dose | 8 μg | 4 μg | 8 μg |
| Lockout | 10 min | 10 min | 10 min |
| Basal rate | 6 μg/h | 6 μg/h | 6 μg/h |
| Limit | 46 μg/h | 26 μg/h | 26 μg/h |

PCEA, Patient-controlled epidural analgesia. Adapted from Grass J, Harris A: Postcesarean section analgesia, *Wellcome Trends Anesthesiol* 9(6):3-8, 1991.

such as 0.1 mg and titrate to effect to lessen the adverse cardiovascular effects that can occur when the opioid is completely reversed with high-dose naloxone.

## OPIATE DETOXIFICATION IN THE PACU

With the advent of more addiction to heroin, many methods of detoxification have been developed. The most common methods of opioid detoxification are methadone withdrawal, clonidine withdrawal, clonidine/naltrexone withdrawal, and anesthesia-assisted rapid opiate detoxification (AAROD).

The technique of AAROD is in its experimental stages but has advantages over the other methods of detoxification in that it is rapid and less costly than the other forms of treatment. In this method, the patient is admitted to the psychiatric unit of the hospital to ensure nothing per mouth status and a premedication is usually administered. The patient is usually administered multiple preprocedural oral medications, including clonidine (Catapres) to suppress the withdrawal symptoms, ondansetron (Zofran) to prevent nausea and vomiting, and metoclopramide (Reglan) to decrease gastric acidity. The patient is admitted to the PACU the next morning, and the procedure is initiated. Monitoring of this patient usually includes a continuous cardiac monitor, pulse oximeter, and a noninvasive blood pressure monitor. Oxygen is usually administered per nasal cannula, and emergency resuscitation equipment, including intubation equipment and cardiac arrest cart, is immediately available. Before the initiation of the procedure, midazolam and ondansetron may be given; and depending on the patient, droperidol (Inapsine) in small doses may be given as opposed to midazolam and ondansetron. Then, light sedation is produced with a propofol infusion, and the patient is dosed with intravenous naloxone. The patient has withdrawal signs and symptoms that usually include mydriasis, piloerection, and a mild increase in heart rate and blood pressure. After about 45 minutes, the propofol is discontinued and routine postanesthesia nursing care is provided. Emotional support and reassurance certainly are important to ensure an appropriate outcome. Once the patient's condition is stabilized, a report should be given to the receiving nurse on the psychiatric unit, and the patient is discharged from the PACU and transported to the psychiatric unit.

## SUMMARY

An excellent working knowledge of the pharmacology of opioids is critical in administration of perianesthesia care for the surgical patient. Opioids possess excellent qualities for pain relief; however, with incorrect administration or the absence of appropriate monitoring, drastic negative outcomes can occur. With the advent of newer opioids such as remifentanil, working with the anesthesia care team is important for prevention of adverse outcomes.

The pure opioid agonists were presented as were the mixed action agonist-antagonists. Also, appropriate reversal drugs were presented with the methods of administration of these drugs in the PACU.

## BIBLIOGRAPHY

Aitkenhead A, Smith G, Rowbotham D: *Textbook of anaesthesia*, ed 5, Philadelphia, 2007, Churchill Livingstone.

Alspach J: *Core curriculum for critical care nursing*, ed 6, Philadelphia, 2005, Saunders.

Atlee J: *Complications in anesthesia*, ed 2, Philadelphia, 2007, Saunders.

Bailey P: Respiratory effects of postoperative opioid analgesia, *Semin Anesth* 15(4):343-352, 1996.

Barash P, Cullen B, Stoelting R: *Clinical anesthesia*, ed 5, Philadelphia, 2005, Lippincott Williams & Wilkins.

Benumof J, Saidman L: *Anesthesia & perioperative complications*, ed 2, St Louis, 1999, Mosby.

Brunton L, Lazo J, Parker K: *Goodman and Gilman's the pharmacological basis of therapeutics*, ed 11, New York, 2005, McGraw-Hill Professional.

Cote C, Todres I, Goudsouzian N, et al: *A practice of anesthesia for infants and children*, ed 3, Philadelphia, 2001, Saunders.

Drake R, Vogl W, Mitchell A: *Gray's anatomy for students*, Philadelphia, 2005, Churchill Livingstone.

Estafanous F, Barash P, Reves J, editors: *Cardiac anesthesia: principles and clinical practice*, ed 2, Philadelphia, 2001, Lippincott Williams & Wilkins.

Evers A, Maze M: *Anesthetic pharmacology: physiologic principles and clinical practice*, Philadelphia, 2004, Churchill Livingstone.

Fisher L: *Benumof's anesthesia and uncommon diseases*, ed 5, Philadelphia, 2007, Saunders.

Gallager C, Issenberg B: *Simulation in anesthesia*, Philadelphia, 2007, Saunders.

Ganong W: *Review of medical physiology*, ed 22, New York, 2005, McGraw-Hill Medical.

Guyton A, Hall J: *Textbook of medical physiology*, ed 11, Philadelphia, 2006, Saunders.

Kaplan J, Slinger P: *Thoracic anesthesia*, ed 3, New York, 2003, Churchill Livingstone.

Kier L, Dowd C: *The chemistry of drugs for nurse anesthetists*, Chicago, 2004, AANA Publishing, Inc.

Lake C, Hines R, Blitt C: *Clinical monitoring: practical applications for anesthesia and critical care*, Philadelphia, 2001, Saunders.

Longnecker D, Murphy F: *Dripps, Eckenhoff, Vandam introduction to anesthesia*, ed 9, Philadelphia, 1997, Saunders.

Longnecker D, Tinker J, Morgan G: *Principles and practice of anesthesiology*, ed 2, St Louis, 1998, Mosby.

Miller R, editor: *Anesthesia*, ed 6, Philadelphia, 2005, Churchill Livingstone.

Murray J, Nadel J: *Textbook of respiratory medicine*, ed 4, Philadelphia, 2005, Saunders.

Nagelhout J, Zaglaniczy K: *Nurse anesthesia*, ed 3, St Louis, 2005, Saunders.

Ogden S: *Calculation of drug dosages*, ed 7, St Louis, 2005, Mosby.

Prielipp R, Young C: Current drugs for sedation of critically ill patients, *Semin Anesthesia Perioperative Med Pain* 20(2):85-94, 2001.

Shorten G, Browne J, Carr D, et al: *Postoperative pain management: an evidence-based guide to practice*, Philadelphia, 2006, Saunders.

Spindler J, Mehlisch D, Brown C: Intramuscular ketorolac and morphine in the treatment of moderate to severe pain after major surgery, *Pharmacotherapy* 10:51S-58S, 1990.

Stoelting R: *Pharmacology and physiology in anesthetic practice*, ed 3, Philadelphia, 1999, Lippincott-Raven.

Stoelting R, Miller R: *Basics of anesthesia*, ed 5, Philadelphia, 2007, Churchill Livingstone.

Townsend C, Beauchamp R, Evers B, et al: *Sabiston textbook of surgery: the biological basis of modern surgical practice*, ed 17, Philadelphia, 2004, Saunders.

Vogelsang J, Hayes S: Butorphanol tartrate (Stadol): a review, *J Post Anesth Nurs* 6(2):129-135, 1991.

White P: *Perioperative drug manual*, ed 2, Philadelphia, 2005, Saunders.

Wilson L, KeMaria P, Kane H, et al: Anesthesia-assisted rapid opiate detoxification: a new procedure in the postanesthesia care unit, *J Perianesth Nurs* 14(4):207-216, 1999.

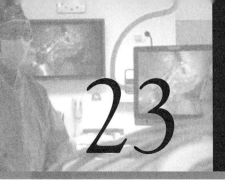

# 23

# NEUROMUSCULAR BLOCKING AGENTS

Cecil B. Drain, PhD, RN, CRNA, FAAN, FASAHP

Neuromuscular blocking drugs (NMBDs), or muscle relaxants, have been used in clinical anesthesia since the early 1940s. Significant advances have been made in understanding the physiology of neuromuscular transmission and the pharmacology of muscle relaxants and have contributed greatly to clinical anesthesia as it is now practiced. Muscle relaxants are not used exclusively in the field of anesthesia; in postanesthesia care units (PACUs), intensive care units (ICUs), and emergency department settings, these drugs may be needed to enhance patient care. Muscle relaxants are used: (1) for facilitaton of endotracheal intubation; (2) for procedures that necessitate muscle relaxation, such as intraperitoneal and thoracic surgery; (3) in ophthalmic surgery for relaxation of the extraocular muscles; (4) for termination of laryngospasm and elimination of chest wall rigidity, which may occur after rapid intravenous injection of a potent narcotic; and (5) for facilitation of mechanical ventilation with production of total paralysis of the respiratory muscles.

## DEFINITIONS

**Action Potential:** The passage of an electric impulse at any point on the nerve fiber where the inside becomes positive and the outside becomes negative; also referred to as action current.

**Anticholinesterase:** A drug that inhibits or inactivates the action of acetylcholinesterase.

**Antimuscarinic (Anticholinergic):** Drug that blocks the effects of acetylcholine receptors and results in the inhibition of the transmission of parasympathetic nerve impulses.

**Clinical Duration:** In reference to the use of neuromuscular blocking agents, the time from the administration of the drug to 25% recovery of the train-of-four twitch response.

**Defasciculating:** A result of the administration of a subclinical dose of a nondepolarizing skeletal muscle relaxant for prevention of the skeletal muscle twitches that occur after the

administration of the depolarizing skeletal muscle relaxant succinylcholine.

**Depolarizing Skeletal Muscle Relaxant:** A skeletal muscle relaxant that after administration produces skeletal muscle twitches by stimulating the nicotinic receptors on the neuromuscular end plate and remaining on the end plate for 3 to 5 minutes, which leads to muscle paralysis. Skeletal muscle function returns as the pseudocholinesterase metabolizes the succinylcholine, usually between 3 and 5 minutes.

**End Plate Potential (EPP):** One action potential at the myoneural junction.

**Excitation-Contraction (E-C) Coupling:** The entire process of muscle contraction, starting with the electric and then the chemical stimulus to the process of the release of calcium in the sarcoplasmic reticulum, which causes the muscle fibers (actin and myocin) to slide and thus contract.

**Extraocular Muscles:** The six sets of muscles that control the movement of the eyeball.

**Fasciculations:** Skeletal muscle twitches.

**Muscurinic:** Subset receptors of the parasympathetic nervous system.

**Myopathy:** An abnormal condition of skeletal muscle characterized by muscle weakness and wasting.

**Neurohumoral Transmission:** Combined electric and chemical transmission of an impulse.

**Nicotinic:** Subset of the parasympathic nervous system.

**Nondepolarizing Agents:** Drugs that cause paralysis of skeletal muscle by blocking neural muscular transmission at the myoneural junction.

**Onset time:** In reference to the use of neuromuscular blocking agents, the time from the administration of the drug to maximum effect.

**Pseudocholinesterase:** An enzyme that acts like cholinesterase and metabolizes acetylcholine.

**Recovery Index:** In reference to the use of neuromuscular blocking agents, the time from the train-of-four twitch index of 25% to 75% recovery of the twitch response.

**Total Duration of Action:** In reference to the use of neuromuscular blocking agents, the time from drug administration to 90% recovery of the train-of-four twitch response.

**Train-of-Four Ratio:** A term used in reference to neuromuscular blocking agents in which a comparison is made between the fourth twitch of the train-of-four with the first twitch; when the fourth twitch is 90% of the first twitch, recovery from the neuromuscular blocking agent is indicated.

## PHYSIOLOGY OF NEUROMUSCULAR TRANSMISSION

Because of the frequent and routine intraoperative and postoperative use of drugs that alter neuromuscular function, a review of the anatomy and physiology of the neuromuscular system is important, with emphasis on the chemical changes that occur at the receptor sites. Activation of skeletal muscle is both an electric and a biochemical event. The term conduction refers to the passage of an impulse along an axon to a muscle fiber. Transmission applies to passage of a neurotransmitter substance across a synaptic cleft (neuromuscular junction). The combined electric and chemical event is called neurohumoral transmission.

As the fine terminal branch of a motor neuron approaches the muscle fiber, it loses its myelin sheath and forms an expanded terminal that lies close to a specialized area of muscle membrane called the end plate (Fig. 23-1). Between the end of the muscle fiber and the end plate is the synaptic cleft, or neuromuscular junction. This space between the nerve and muscle fibers is about 20 nm wide. Acetylcholine is the biochemical neurotransmitter involved in the initiation of muscle contraction. Acetylcholine or cholinergic receptors are classified as nicotinic and muscarinic, respectively. The acetylcholine receptors are stimulated by acetylcholine. Anticholinesterase drugs such as neostigmine (Prostigmin), edrophonium chloride (Tensilon, Enlon) and pyridostigmine (Regonol) produce an increase in acetylcholine at the acetylcholine receptor. Therefore, the pharmacologic effects of the anticholinesterase drugs are on both the nicotinic and muscarinic receptors. The nicotinic receptors are further classified as either $N_1$ or $N_2$ receptors. The $N_1$ receptors are located at the presynaptic cleft and influence the release of acetylcholine. The $N_2$ receptors are situated on the postsynaptic cleft in the neuromuscular junction and, when occupied by acetylcholine, open their channels to allow the flow of ions down the cell membrane, thus

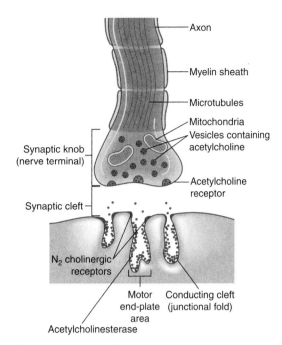

**Fig. 23-1** Myoneural junction at resting state.

resulting in the skeletal muscle contraction. The nondepolarizing neuromuscular blocking agents such as pancuronium (Pavulon) produce a block of the $N_2$ receptor and thus cause an inability of the channel to conduct ions, which results in skeletal muscle paralysis. Extrajunctional nicotinic receptors are located throughout the skeletal muscles. Their activity is normally suppressed by normal neural activity. However, when a patient has prolonged sepsis, inactivity, denervation, or burn trauma in the skeletal muscles, a proliferation of these extrajunctional nicotinic receptors results. Hence, these patients usually have an exaggerated hyperkalemic response when succinylcholine is administered.

The muscarinic receptors are also subdivided into $M_1$ and $M_2$ receptors. $M_1$ receptors are located in the autonomic ganglia and the central nervous system, and $M_2$ receptors are located in the heart and salivary glands. Atropine and glycopyrrolate (Robinul) block both the $M_1$ and the $M_2$ receptors.

Acetylcholine is formed in the body of the nerve cell and the cytoplasm of the nerve terminal and is stored in the small membrane-enclosed vesicles for subsequent release. A quantum is the amount of acetylcholine stored in each vesicle and represents about 10,000 molecules of acetylcholine. The presynaptic membrane contains discrete areas of specialization that are thought to be sites of release of the transmitter. These presynaptic active zones lie directly opposite the $N_2$ cholinergic receptors, which are located on the postsynaptic membrane. This alignment ensures that the acetylcholine diffuses directly to the $N_2$ receptors on the postsynaptic membrane quickly and in a high concentration. The $N_2$ receptor, which responds to the neurotransmitter acetylcholine, is a glycoprotein that is an integral part of the postsynaptic membrane of the neuromuscular junction (see Fig. 23-1). New evidence indicates that a positive feedback mechanism also exists at the neuromuscular junction. Acetylcholine has a presynaptic action; hence, acetylcholine receptors are located on the presynaptic membrane. This positive feedback mechanism enhances the mobilization and release of acetylcholine. Finally, the enzyme that hydrolyzes acetylcholine is acetylcholinesterase, which is located in the neuromuscular junction.

The initiation of skeletal muscle contraction occurs as a result of application of a threshold stimulus. An action potential that travels down the axon causes depolarization of the presynaptic membrane. As a result of this depolarization, the membrane permeability for calcium ions is increased and the calcium enters, or influxes, into the presynaptic membrane. Calcium acts to unite the vesicle to the presynaptic membrane and causes the rupture of that coalesced membrane, thus releasing acetylcholine into the fluid of the synaptic cleft (Fig. 23-2).

The acetylcholine molecules released from the nerve terminal into the synaptic cleft are subject to two main processes: (1) attachment to $N_2$ cholinergic receptors located on the postsynaptic membrane, which leads to an opening of calcium channels that results in the movement of sodium into the region and generates an end plate potential (EPP); and (2) attachment of acetylcholine to the presynaptic nicotinic receptor, which enhances the release of more acetylcholine. When enough EPPs are generated, an action potential is propagated and spreads throughout the muscle and causes a change in the ionic permeability of the muscle sarcolemma. This process results in the release of calcium from the sarcoplasmic reticulum with a resultant increase in free calcium concentration in the muscle fiber. The process of excitation-contraction (E-C) coupling then takes place within that skeletal muscle cell. The physiologic outcome of E-C coupling is the contraction of the skeletal muscle. The increased concentration of calcium in the muscle fiber leads to an interaction between troponin-tropomyosin and actin. This interaction causes the active sites on actin to be exposed and interact with

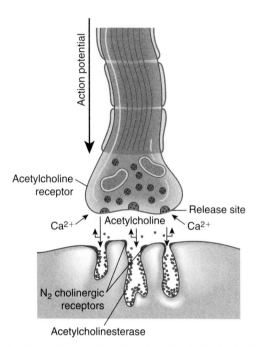

**Fig. 23-2**  Myoneural junction when threshold stimulus is applied.

myosin and slide together, thus resulting in muscle contraction. This sliding of actin and myosin is sometimes called the ratchet effect. The contraction of the muscle fibers is terminated when calcium is pumped back into the sarcoplasmic reticulum of the muscle fibers. The calcium is stored in the sarcoplasmic reticulum for use when another action potential is generated.

Regulation and control of skeletal muscle contraction are also based on the enzymatic breakdown of acetylcholine. As previously discussed, the stimulus must be strong enough to release enough acetylcholine to bind to the postsynaptic $N_2$ cholinergic receptor. This process of competition between the postsynaptic $N_2$ receptor and acetylcholinesterase allows for some degree of regulation of the excitation process and for the recovery of the muscle cell membrane. The molecules of acetylcholine either diffuse in a random fashion to the $N_2$ receptor or are destroyed by acetylcholinesterase. As the concentration gradient begins to decrease because of the destruction of acetylcholine by acetylcholinesterase, the $N_2$ receptor gives up its acetylcholine, which is then destroyed, and the skeletal muscle relaxes. A small portion of the acetylcholine can escape the acetylcholinesterase in the synaptic cleft and migrate into the extracellular fluid and from there into the plasma. Acetylcholine within the plasma is then destroyed by plasma acetylcholinesterase, or pseudocholinesterase, which is produced in the liver.

## PHARMACOLOGIC OVERVIEW OF THE SKELETAL MUSCLE RELAXANTS

With the anatomy and physiology of neuromuscular transmission as background, the principal pharmacologic actions of the nondepolarizing and depolarizing skeletal muscle relaxants are discussed. Table 23-1 presents a pharmacologic overview of the commonly used skeletal muscle relaxants.

The prototypical nondepolarizing skeletal muscle relaxants are pancuronium and vecuronium (Norcuron). Pancuronium is an inhibitor of acetylcholine, is chemically viewed as two acetylcholine-like fragments, and has a bulky inflexible nucleus. This drug attaches to the $N_2$ cholinergic receptors on the postsynaptic membrane and prevents depolarization. The skeletal muscle relaxant vecuronium has a chemical structure that is similar to a monoquaternary compound. The principal pharmacologic action

of this drug is to block the postsynaptic $N_2$ cholinergic receptor; in this way, it stops acetylcholine from binding to the receptor, which results in a competitive neuromuscular blockade. The nondepolarizing skeletal muscle relaxants also block the presynaptic cholinergic receptor and thus result in binding of the acetylcholine and thereby prevent activation of the positive feedback mechanism.

The pharmacologic actions of the nondepolarizing skeletal muscle relaxants can be reversed with anticholinesterase drugs such as neostigmine. In effect, these drugs increase the quantum of acetylcholine at the postsynaptic membrane by preventing destruction of the acetylcholine by acetylcholinesterase. This process promotes a more effective competition by the released acetylcholine with the nondepolarizing skeletal muscle relaxant that is occupying the $N_2$ receptor. Because of the increased availability and mobilization of the acetylcholine, the concentration gradients favor acetylcholine and remove the nondepolarizing agents from the $N_2$ receptor, with the

**Table 23-1  Pharmacologic Overview of the Commonly Used Neuromuscular Blocking Drugs**

| | Pancuronium (Pavulon) | Vecuronium Bromide (Norcuron) | Atracurium Besylate (Tracrium) | Cisatricurium Besylate (Nimbex) | Rocuronium Bromide (Zemuron) |
|---|---|---|---|---|---|
| Nondepolarizing | Yes | Yes | Yes | Yes | Yes |
| Depolarizing | No | No | No | No | No |
| Intubation dose (IV mg/kg) | 0.06-0.1 | 0.08-0.1 | 0.4-0.5 | 0.1-0.2 | 0.1 |
| Intubation time (injection to relaxation; min) | 4 | 2.5-3 | 2-2.5 | 2.8-3.4 | 1-2 |
| Muscle relaxation dose (IV mg/kg) | 0.04-0.08 | 0.05-0.06 | 0.2-0.5 | 2.5 | 0.6-1.0 |
| Recovery time (min) | 84-114 | 30-60 | 30-45 | 55-75 | 30-90 |
| Reversible? | Yes | Yes | Yes | Yes | Yes |
| Time to reversal (min; after initial dose) | 40-60 | 25-30 (for 0.1 mg/kg) 40-80 (for 0.2 mg/kg) | 20-35 | 10-15 | 5-10 |
| Cumulative effects? | Yes | Slight | No | No | No |
| Fasciculations and muscle soreness | No | No | No | No | No |
| Risk of histamine release | Slight to none | No | Minimal | No | No |
| Cardiovascular effects | Slight ↑ in pulse and ↑ in BP | None | Few | None | None |

*IV*, Intravenous; *BP*, blood pressure.

resultant return to normal contraction of the skeletal muscle.

The principal depolarizing skeletal muscle relaxant is succinylcholine (Anectine, Sucostrin). The molecular structure of this drug resembles two acetylcholine molecules back to back. Because of this structure, succinylcholine has the same effects as acetylcholine. Like acetylcholine, the succinylcholine molecule has a quaternary ammonium portion that is positively charged. This positively charged molecule is attracted by electrostatic action to the negatively charged $N_2$ receptor. Once the succinylcholine attaches to the receptor, a brief period of depolarization occurs that is manifested by transient muscular fasciculations. Succinylcholine also attaches to and activates the presynaptic acetylcholine receptor. This activation has an immediate effect of increased mobilization of acetylcholine in the motor nerve terminals, which explains why fasciculations are commonly observed after the administration of an intravenous bolus of succinylcholine. After the depolarization of the $N_2$ receptor takes place, succinylcholine promotes and maintains the receptor in a depolarized state and prevents repolarization. Succinylcholine has a brief duration of action because of its rapid hydrolysis of the succinylcholine by the enzyme pseudocholinesterase, which is contained in the liver and plasma. The actions of succinylcholine cannot be pharmacologically reversed.

## NONDEPOLARIZING NEUROMUSCULAR BLOCKING AGENTS

### Long-acting Nondepolarizing Skeletal Muscle Relaxants

*Pancuronium Bromide.* Pancuronium bromide (Pavulon) was introduced into clinical anesthesia in 1972. This drug has shown value (particularly in terms of its safety, cardiovascular stability, and skeletal muscle relaxant properties) and is receiving widespread clinical usage.

Chemically, pancuronium bromide is a biquaternary aminosteroid and is related to the androgens; however, it has no hormonal activities. Pancuronium is reversible with an anticholinesterase agent, such as neostigmine, that is administered in combination with an anticholinergic such as glycopyrrolate or atropine. This particular skeletal muscle relaxant has been shown clinically to be extremely difficult to reverse pharmacologically within the first 20 to 30 minutes after injection. In the PACU, if a skeletal muscle relaxant is needed for a short duration, another reversible skeletal muscle relaxant, such as vecuronium or atracurium, should be chosen. About 30 to 40 minutes

after injection, pancuronium is easily reversed with the combination of an anticholinesterase and anticholinergic drug preparation. Pancuronium is best suited for surgical procedures that last more than 1 hour. It is well suited for patients who need complete muscle relaxation with continuous mechanical ventilation. The dosage for adults is approximately 0.08 to 0.1 mg/kg of body weight. Relaxation lasts 60 to 85 minutes. If relaxation is necessary past this initial period, subsequent doses should be decreased to 0.02 to 0.04 mg/kg of body weight.

Pancuronium bromide does not produce ganglionic blockade, but it does block the $M_2$ cholinergic receptors in the heart. Consequently, when pancuronium bromide is administered, a slight 10% to 15% increase in heart rate is observed. Pancuronium activates the sympathetic nervous system by promoting the release of norepinephrine and blocking its uptake at the adrenergic nerve endings. Hence, after administration of this drug, a modest increase in mean arterial pressure and cardiac output is produced. Although isolated cases of histamine release have been reported, pancuronium can probably be used in patients who have a marginal allergy history. Pancuronium bromide is compatible with anesthetic agents used clinically and is safe for use in most patients when a nondepolarizing skeletal muscle relaxant is indicated. However, pancuronium bromide is not indicated when a nondepolarizing muscle relaxant is to be used with caution. In addition, pancuronium should not be used in patients who are undergoing chronic digitalis therapy because cardiac dysrhythmias have been reported. Finally, myocardial ischemia has been reported in patients with coronary artery disease when pancuronium is used. This ischemia is probably associated with the cardiac acceleration properties of the drug.

Pancuronium bromide should be avoided in patients with a history of myasthenia gravis. It is contraindicated in patients with true renal disease because a major portion of the drug is excreted unchanged in the urine. This agent is contraindicated in patients known to be hypersensitive to it or to the bromide ion.

### Intermediate-acting Nondepolarizing Skeletal Muscle Relaxants

*Vecuronium Bromide.* Vecuronium (Norcuron) is a nondepolarizing skeletal muscle relaxant with a more rapid onset of action and a shorter duration of action than pancuronium. Actually, vecuronium is pancuronium without the quaternary methyl group in the steroid nucleus. Because of this structural difference, vecuronium has no effect on heart rate, arterial pressure, autonomic ganglia, or the alpha and beta adrenal receptors. The potency of vecuronium is equal to or slightly greater than that of pancuronium. Vecuronium has little or no cumulative effect. Although a portion of vecuronium is metabolized, most of the drug is excreted unchanged in the urine and bile. However, the neuromuscular blockade produced by vecuronium is not prolonged by renal failure. The duration of neuromuscular blockade produced by vecuronium is increased in patients with impaired hepatic function. Of clinical interest is that vecuronium, like atracurium, is less influenced by general inhalation anesthetics than is pancuronium. The pharmacologic action of this drug is easily reversed with the combination of an anticholinesterase and an anticholinergic drug.

The onset of action of vecuronium is between 2.5 and 3 minutes, with the normal dosage of 0.08 mg/kg intravenously. Because of the rapid onset of action, vecuronium can be used for rapid-sequence intubation. In this instance, a doubling of the dosage of vecuronium to 0.2 mg/kg can be used to achieve intubation conditions within 45 seconds to 2 minutes. Another method for use of vecuronium for intubation is the priming technique. The object of this technique is administration of a small priming dose of vecuronium several minutes before the intubation dose is given to shorten the onset of neuromuscular blockade. The usual priming dose is 0.015 mg/kg; after 3 minutes, an intubation dose of 0.1 mg/kg is administered. The onset of neuromuscular blockade should be between 70 and 90 seconds. The main drawback of this technique is the potential development of symptoms of partial neuromuscular blockade. Sensations reported are heavy eyelids, blurred vision, and difficulty in swallowing. Therefore, if this technique is used in the PACU, the nurse should warn patients of the possible symptoms, and ventilatory support should always be available.

Because of concerns about the priming technique, the timing technique was developed. In the timing technique, which is used mainly in the operating room, the patient is given vecuronium before sodium pentothal. Consequently, the induction of anesthesia is specifically timed to the onset of clinical muscular weakness. In this technique, the patient is given intravenously 0.1 to 0.2 mg/kg of vecuronium; and at the onset of weakness, as determined with the peripheral nerve simulator, a 1.0-mg/kg to 2.5-mg/kg bolus dose of propofol is given. Intubating conditions occur within 1 minute.

Vecuronium is primarily used for intraoperative skeletal muscle relaxation and facilitation of mechanical ventilation in the critical care setting. Long-term infusions of this drug in the critical care situation may result in a prolonged recovery and an inability to pharmacologically reverse vecuronium because the metabolites are still in active form; if corticosteroid therapy is being used for patients with multiorgan failure, this prolonged effect can be exacerbated.

The dosage is 0.05 to 0.2 mg/kg for skeletal muscle paralysis, and the onset is 1 to 3 minutes, with a duration between 30 and 90 minutes. Prolonged skeletal muscle relaxing effects can be prolonged with patients with hepatic disease. No significant cardiac effects for this drug have been reported.

**Atracurium Besylate.** Atracurium (Tracrium) is a nondepolarizing skeletal muscle relaxant that offers an advantage over other skeletal muscle relaxants in that it does not depend on renal or hepatic mechanisms for its elimination. In fact, this quaternary ammonium compound breaks down in the absence of plasma enzymes through what is called Hofmann elimination and, to a lesser extent, through ester hydrolysis. Hofmann elimination is a nonbiologic method of degradation that occurs at a physiologic temperature and pH.

Atracurium is less potent than pancuronium and has a rapid onset of 1 to 3 minutes and a duration of action of about 30 to 45 minutes. For endotracheal intubation in the PACU setting, 0.3 to 0.5 mg/kg of atracurium should provide adequate skeletal muscle relaxation for intubation in about 2.5 minutes. For maintenance of mechanical ventilation in the PACU setting, an infusion rate of 10 μg/kg/min of atracurium may be used. Once the infusion has been discontinued, spontaneous ventilation by the patient occurs in about 30 minutes. The effects can be reversed with a combination of anticholinesterase and antimuscarinic in about 12 to 15 minutes after the discontinuation of the atracurium infusion.

Atracurium has many distinct advantages, such as its neuromuscular blockade not being prolonged by renal failure or impaired hepatic function. Also, it has little or no cumulative effect and is not influenced significantly by the specific general inhalation anesthetic dosage or concentration. Finally, this drug has little or no cardiovascular effect and is easily antagonized with the combination of an anticholinesterase and an anticholinergic.

**Cisatracurium Besylate.** Cisatracurium (Nimbex) is a stereoisomer of atracurium that is about three times as potent as atracurium with fewer side effects and is degraded by the same metabolic pathway as atracurium (i.e., the Hofmann elimination mechanism).

CONCEPTS IN ANESTHETIC AGENTS

The average adult intubation dose of cisatracurium is 0.2 mg/kg and has an onset of about 90 seconds, a peak in about 3 to 5 minutes, and a duration of action of about 40 to 50 minutes. A supplemental dose of 0.03 mg/kg provides an additional 20 minutes of skeletal muscle relaxation. For maintenance of a stable state of skeletal muscle relaxation in the PACU, cisatracurium can be administered via infusion at a rate of 1 to 2 µg/kg/min.

This drug has all the assets of atracurium plus a great advantage over atracurium of less histamine release. It does not have any particular effect on the cardiovascular system, and because it undergoes an organ-independent clearance, it can be used in patients with hepatic or renal failure without a noticeable change in duration of action. It is well suited for many patients who undergo intermediate to long surgical procedures.

### Short-acting Nondepolarizing Skeletal Muscle Relaxants

*Rocuronium Bromide.* Rocuronium (Zemuron) is a nondepolarizing skeletal muscle relaxant with a chemical structure related to vecuronium. It has a rapid onset (1 to 1.5 minutes) and a short duration of action of 30 to 120 minutes, depending on the total dose of the drug. The onset and duration of action are not altered in obese patients when the dose is based on the actual body weight. In patients who are more than 65 years of age, the duration of action is slightly prolonged. In pediatrics, the onset and duration is slightly faster.

Because rocuronium has such rapid effects and short duration of action, spontaneous recovery from neuromuscular blockade is possible. However, if a patient arrives to the PACU with spontaneous ventilation after rocuronium administration during surgery that was *not* reversed with anticholinesterase and anticholinergic, the patient still should be monitored in the PACU for neuromuscular function with the use of a peripheral nerve stimulator (PNS). In addition to use of the PNS, the patient should be evaluated for adequate clinical evidence of an adequate return of neuromuscular function with evaluation of the 5-second head lift, adequate phonation, ventilation, and upper airway maintenance.

Rocuronium can be used in patients with renal failure and has a low potential for histamine release. Although rare, its actions are prolonged in patients with cirrhosis of the liver. Also, rocuronium's muscle relaxant actions are potentiated by the inhalation anesthetics, which makes a prediction of a total recovery from neuromuscular blockade variable. Because rocuronium produces minimal cardiovascular effects,

it does not have significant histamine-releasing effects.

Rocuronium can be used as an agent of choice for nondepolarizing rapid sequence intubation in the PACU when appropriate intubation doses are used because it has such a fast onset and short duration of action and therefore is useful in intraoperative and postoperative periods. At a dose of 0.6 mg/kg to 1.0 mg/kg, rocuronium provides excellent intubating conditions in 60 to 90 seconds for both children and adults. Hence, before the intubation is attempted, the patient should undergo ventilation with 100% oxygen until appropriate paralysis of the skeletal muscle occurs to facilitate the intubation. The maintenance dose for rocuronium for adults is between 0.1 and 0.2 mg/kg and for children is 0.08 to 0.12 mg/kg intravenously. If rocuronium is to be used for continuous infusion, the initial rate is 0.01 to 0.012 mg/kg/min; at the desired level of neuromuscular blockade, the infusion of this drug can be individualized according to the patient's twitch response as monitored with the use of the PNS. The research indicates that infusion rates can range from 0.004 to 0.016 mg/kg/min. In assessment of the maintenance dosing of rocuronium, it should be administered at 25% of control T1, which is three twitches of the train-of-four. The infusion solutions for rocuronium can be prepared in solutions of 5% glucose and water or lactated Ringer's solution. Once the infusion is completed, the unused portions of the infusion solutions should be discarded.

### Reversal of Nondepolarizing Neuromuscular Blocking Agents

For restoration of neuromuscular transmission, the antagonist must displace the competitive neuromuscular blocking agent from the nicotinic receptor sites and open the way for depolarization of the postjunctional membrane. The antagonist is an antiacetylcholinesterase that blocks the enzymatic action of acetylcholinesterase located in the postsynaptic clefts so that acetylcholine is not hydrolyzed. The result is a buildup of acetylcholine at the end plate at the $N_2$ cholinergic receptor. The accumulated acetylcholine displaces the competitive neuromuscular blocking agent, which diffuses back into the plasma and thus reestablishes neuromuscular transmission.

Neostigmine and pyridostigmine are usually the anticholinesterase drugs of choice because of their long duration of action and reliability as compared with edrophonium chloride. However, research has shown that edrophonium chloride is an effective reversal agent of neuromuscular blockades produced by vecuronium and atracurium. Atropine or glycopyrrolate, both antimuscarinic (anticholinergic) drugs, can be administered immediately before or in conjunction with the anticholinesterase for minimization of the muscarinic effects of the anticholinesterase drug. The muscarinic effects include bradycardia, salivation, miosis, and hyperperistalsis. These effects are produced at lower concentrations of the anticholinesterase-type drug when administered (acetylcholine nicotinic effects are at the autonomic ganglia and the neuromuscular junction). Consequently, when an anticholinesterase drug is administered for reversal of the nondepolarizing neuromuscular blocking agent at the $N_2$ receptor, an antimuscarinic drug is also given for prevention of the adverse muscarinic cholinergic effects associated with the high dosage of anticholinesterase. Generally, 2.5 mg of neostigmine is the maximum dose necessary for reversal; however, the suggested limit is 5 mg. The method is administration of 0.4 mg atropine or 0.2 mg glycopyrrolate intravenously over a 1-minute period, observation for an increase in pulse rate, and then administration of 0.5 mg neostigmine intravenously and monitoring for the reversal. This procedure can be repeated until reversal has been achieved or until the limit of neostigmine that can be given is reached. If edrophonium chloride is indicated for reversal, the dosage is 0.5 mg/kg with 0.007 mg/kg of atropine.

Neostigmine should be administered cautiously. Cardiac monitoring is essential, especially in elderly or debilitated patients and in patients with cardiac disease. Atrioventricular dissociation and other dysrhythmias can be initiated by the anticholinesterases.

Pyridostigmine is an analogue of neostigmine. It facilitates the transmission of impulses across the myoneural junction by inhibiting the destruction of acetylcholine by acetylcholinesterase. Clinical data indicate a lower incidence rate of muscarinic side effects with this drug than with neostigmine. Like neostigmine, pyridostigmine should be administered with caution in patients with bronchial asthma or cardiac problems. Signs of overdosage are related to muscarinic and nicotinic receptor stimulation (Box 23-1). The muscarinic side effects are blocked with atropine or glycopyrrolate. Nicotinic responses can be blocked with drugs such as ganglionic or neuromuscular blocking agents. The recommended dosage for reversal is 0.15 mg/kg of intravenous pyridostigmine, in combination with 0.007 mg/kg of intravenous atropine. Full recovery occurs within 15 minutes in most patients; in other patients, 30 minutes or more may be necessary.

Another parasympatholytic agent, glycopyrrolate, has been substituted for atropine in the

---

### Box 23-1    Observable Responses to Stimulation of Receptors

**NICOTINIC**

Stimulation of autonomic ganglia: both sympathetic and parasympathetic

Stimulation of adrenal medulla, resulting in the release of both epinephrine and norepinephrine

Stimulation of skeletal muscles at the motor end plate

**MUSCARINIC**

Stimulation or inhibition of smooth muscle in various organs or tissues

Stimulation of exocrine glands (i.e., salivary and sweat glands)

Slowing of cardiac conduction

Decrease in myocardial contractile force

---

reversal technique. Its advantages over atropine are a longer duration of action and a lower incidence rate of arrhythmias; it causes small slow changes in the heart rate, and it does not cross the blood-brain barrier. The usual reversal dosage is 1 mg of neostigmine and 0.2 mg of glycopyrrolate in a 2-mL mixture. This dosage can be repeated if reversal is inadequate.

## DEPOLARIZING NEUROMUSCULAR BLOCKING AGENTS

### Succinylcholine

Succinylcholine (Anectine, Quelicin, Sucostrin) represents a valuable pharmacologic advance in modern anesthesia and in critical care, areas in which resuscitation is required. This agent is usually included as one of the drugs available for emergencies, especially with endotracheal intubation. Outside the operating room, succinylcholine is used for electroshock therapy, for relief of profound laryngospasm, for control of convulsions from tetanus, for management of ventilation of the flail chest, and during reduction of fractures or dislocations.

Although succinylcholine is widely used in the United States, it has side effects and complications that can be avoided with a basic understanding of the pharmacology of the drug.

Succinylcholine acts at the $N_2$ postsynaptic cholinergic receptor by causing a persistent depolarization of the end plate. It also acts on the presynaptic cholinergic receptor by causing an initial increase in acetylcholine at the motor end plate. This reaction is why patients who receive succinylcholine have fasciculations

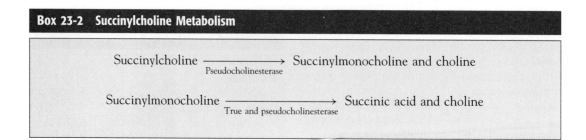

**Box 23-2   Succinylcholine Metabolism**

Succinylcholine $\xrightarrow[\text{Pseudocholinesterase}]{}$ Succinylmonocholine and choline

Succinylmonocholine $\xrightarrow[\text{True and pseudocholinesterase}]{}$ Succinic acid and choline

with initial administration. Succinylcholine is a synthetic quaternary ammonium compound with a chemical structure that closely resembles that of acetylcholine. The typical intravenous dose of succinylcholine to produce flaccid paralysis is 0.5 to 1.5 mg/kg; onset is 30 to 60 seconds with a duration of about 5 to 10 minutes. The drug is hydrolyzed rapidly by plasma pseudocholinesterase, an enzyme produced by the liver, to succinylmonocholine and choline. Succinylmonocholine is further hydrolyzed by pseudocholinesterase and true cholinesterase, which are found in the erythrocyte, to succinic acid and choline (see Box 23-2).

**Advantages and Uses.** Succinylcholine has certain advantages that, in most instances, justify its clinical use. Its rapid onset of action, coupled with its short duration of action, has made this drug valuable when: (1) rapid intubation is necessary; (2) laryngospasm is irreversible with positive pressure; (3) the skeletal muscles are rigid and prevent good ventilatory excursion; (4) procedures require a short duration of skeletal muscle relaxation, such as reduction of dislocations and fractures; and (5) electroconvulsive therapy is used to decrease the negative effects of seizures. Continued use over a 30-year period has shown succinylcholine to produce complications that can, in most instances, be prevented if the basic pharmacodynamics of the drug are understood.

In emergencies, succinylcholine remains the major muscle relaxant for facilitation of endotracheal intubation. Succinylcholine is contraindicated in children and adolescent patients except when used for emergency tracheal intubation or in instances in which immediate securing of the airway is necessary.

When this drug is used for a rapid-sequence intubation, the succinylcholine-induced fasciculations and the associated increase in gastric pressure should be reduced or eliminated with an intravenous injection of a small amount (3 mg per 70 kg of body weight) of vecuronium. This defasciculating dose of vecuronium should be administered about 1 or 2 minutes before the intravenous bolus injection of succinylcholine of 1.5 mg/kg.

**Untoward Reactions.** Because hydrolysis of succinylcholine depends on enzymatic activity, an understanding is important of the atypical responses that may occur. Pseudocholinesterase activity in the plasma may be increased or decreased. Cases with increased activity are congenital and occur rarely. Patients with atypical pseudocholinesterase are resistant to succinylcholine and do not relax well. The reductions in pseudocholinesterase activity may be acquired or congenital. Acquired deficiencies are more important to understand because they are more common. They occur with liver disease, severe anemia, malnutrition, prolonged pyrexia, pregnancy, and recent renal dialysis. Drugs such as quinidine and propranolol (Inderal) inhibit pseudocholinesterase, as do echothiophate iodide eye drops (Phospholine). Patients with low pseudocholinesterase activity have a prolonged response to these drugs.

Atypical pseudocholinesterase occurs alone in about one in 2800 people; this atypical form is inherited. Patients with genetically induced deficiencies of pseudocholinesterase have been seen to remain apneic for as long as 48 hours after a usual dose of succinylcholine. These patients need mechanical ventilation and constant nursing care. Patients with documented pseudocholinesterase deficiency should be advised to wear a Medic Alert bracelet. If anesthesia is necessary, these patients should be administered nondepolarizing skeletal muscle relaxants, such as pancuronium, vecuronium, and rocuronium, because these drugs can usually be reversed.

**Disadvantages and Side Effects.** Succinylcholine can be administered via single injection or continuous infusion. The single-injection method is used when neuromuscular relaxation is needed for a short time, such as facilitation of endotracheal intubation. The usual intubation dosage of succinylcholine is 1 mg/kg intravenously. During the first intravenous injection, cardiovascular status usually remains normal. If the injection must be repeated, the patient may have profound bradycardia and various arrhythmias. Therefore, monitoring of the patient's cardiovascular status with succinylcholine administration is important, especially if the dose is repeated.

Because children and adolescent patients are more likely than adults to have undiagnosed myopathies, a nondepolarizing skeletal muscle relaxant such as rocuronium (Zimuron) should be used for routine procedures in the PACU. More specifically, except when used for emergency tracheal intubation or in the instance in which immediate securing of the airway is necessary, succinylcholine is contraindicated in children and adolescent patients because a patient with a myopathy in this age group who is administered succinylcholine can have acute fulminating destruction of skeletal muscle (rhabdomyolysis) that results in hyperkalemia and cardiac arrest.

If succinylcholine must be administered to an adolescent or child, the patient must be monitored completely because the patient is especially prone to bradycardia, even on the initial injection of succinylcholine. This complication can be easily overcome with prior administration of glycopyrrolate or atropine sulfate, either alone or mixed with succinylcholine. This method appears to be the safest way of administration of intravenous succinylcholine in this age group.

A disadvantage of the single-injection method with succinylcholine is that it causes fasciculations of the muscles. These "mini" contractions are a result of the initial depolarization of the skeletal muscle from the positive feedback mechanism of initial stimulation of the presynaptic acetylcholine receptor. These contractions frequently lead to muscle pain, which is usually noted by the patient the day after surgery. This effect is particularly true in patients who are ambulatory soon after surgery. In ambulatory patients, muscle pains (myalgia) occur in 60% to 70% of cases. The incidence rate decreases to 10% in those patients confined to bed. Symptoms include pain in the neck, back, and abdomen; pain when blinking the eyes; pain when smiling; and generalized pain when ambulatory. These objective symptoms are usually noticed first by the nurse in the PACU. Skeletal muscle pain around the neck area is sometimes described to the perianesthesia nurse as a sore throat caused by the endotracheal tube; in fact, the pain is caused by the myalgia from the succinylcholine. The pain usually does not require analgesics and subsides in a day or two. The fasciculations can be prevented with administration of a nondepolarizing neuromuscular blocking drug at a pretreatment dose of between 5% and 10% of its normal intubation about 2 to 4 minutes before the injection of succinylcholine. If a pretreatment nondepolarizing drug was administered, the dose of succinylcholine should be increased by about 70%.

When succinylcholine is administered to patients in the presence of extensive burns, severe trauma, severe abdominal infections, tetanus, neuromuscular disease, or neurologic lesions such as paraplegia and quadriplegia, a release of potassium from the damaged muscle and nerve cells can result. The common denominator appears to be either massive tissue destruction or central nervous system injury with muscle wasting. This pathophysiologic process results when denervated muscle is stimulated by succinylcholine because of the extrajunctional nicotinic receptors proliferated during the skeletal muscle destruction. After activation of the nicotinic receptor by succinylcholine, response is enhanced in the ionic channels, with a resultant increase in the release of potassium into the circulation. Elevation of the serum potassium level, which can be as high as 10 to 15 mEq/L, has been reported. The result of this potassium elevation is cardiac dysrhythmias and cardiac arrest. The peak time for this reaction is 7 to 10 days after the injury. However, the critical period for these reactions is between posttraumatic days 1 and 180. Consequently, succinylcholine is contraindicated in patients who have injuries of major multiple traumas, extensive denervation of skeletal muscle, or upper motor neuron injury.

Succinylcholine has been implicated as one of the trigger agents of malignant hyperthermia (MH). Chapter 53 contains a complete description of the pathophysiology and treatment of MH.

In pediatric and adult patients anesthetized with halothane combined with succinylcholine as the muscle relaxant, an unusual incidence of plasma myoglobin has occurred. Myoglobin is an intracellular muscle protein and therefore should not be released into the plasma. If myoglobin is found in the plasma, it can only mean that the muscle membrane has been injured.

Succinylcholine can be administered in a drip infusion during a procedure that requires skeletal muscle relaxation for a longer period than a single injection can provide. It is usually administered in a 0.1% to 0.2% solution. If the infusion is administered for a prolonged period, the type of block can gradually change from a depolarizing block to a characteristic nondepolarizing block. The change is always from depolarization to nondepolarization, never in the reverse direction. This type of block is called a dual or phase II block. The exact time relationship and the mechanism of action are still uncertain. Treatment is via mechanical ventilation and careful monitoring of the patient until the dual block disappears.

Succinylcholine increases intraocular pressure by about 7.5 mm Hg in both children and adults, in part because of the contraction of the extraocular muscles. When administered before succinylcholine for prevention of contraction of the extraocular muscles, a nondepolarizing neuromuscular blocking drug does not completely extinguish the increase in intraocular pressure. Therefore, even if succinylcholine is used with an NMBD, it is contraindicated in patients in whom an increase in intraocular pressure would be detrimental.

## FACTORS THAT INFLUENCE THE NEUROMUSCULAR BLOCKING AGENTS

### Fluid Balance
Patients who are dehydrated are reported to be extremely sensitive to skeletal muscle relaxants. This finding is probably true because: (1) dehydration decreases neuromuscular excitability; (2) the contracted extracellular fluid compartment permits an increase in the plasma concentration of the relaxant and thus intensifies the relaxant action; and (3) renal function is slowed and the elimination time of the relaxant and its metabolites is prolonged.

### Sodium
A deficit of sodium may prolong the neuromuscular block. Experimental evidence indicates that a sodium deficiency itself may result in a partial neuromuscular block.

### Potassium
Potassium deficiency appears to increase the blocking action of pancuronium and other nondepolarizing neuromuscular blocking agents. On the other hand, depolarizing neuromuscular blocking agents are required in larger amounts when potassium deficiency exists. Depolarization is prevented to some extent because a potassium deficiency appears to stabilize the muscle end plate. Potassium depletion can occur from decreased intake or excessive loss, such as in chronic pyelonephritis, primary aldosteronism, chlorothiazide therapy, and chronic diarrhea.

### Magnesium
An increase in magnesium concentration causes a flaccid paralysis clinically similar to that caused by a nondepolarizing neuromuscular blocking agent. The principal action of magnesium is that it can enter the nerve terminal and replace or decrease the amount of calcium that enters, which stabilizes the postsynaptic membrane. Ultimately, depression of the release of acetylcholine occurs and reduces the EPP, which

causes a partial neuromuscular block. Consequently, magnesium enhances a neuromuscular block produced by a nondepolarizing agent and, to a lesser extent, potentiates the block produced by succinylcholine.

### Calcium
A deficiency in calcium prolongs the effects of nondepolarizing neuromuscular blocking agents by reducing the amount of acetylcholine released and by inhibiting neuromuscular transmission. The depolarizing neuromuscular blocking agents are also potentiated because a low calcium level aids depolarization. Conversely, the administration of calcium chloride solution in calcium deficiency states antagonizes the nondepolarizing effects of agents such as pancuronium. Calcium chloride has a pronounced antagonism to the respiratory depressant effects of succinylcholine.

### pH and Carbon Dioxide
The neuromuscular blocking effect of pancuronium is intensified in acidosis and in states of elevated carbon dioxide tension. With drugs such as rocuronium and succinylcholine, the neuromuscular blocking action is diminished. Alkalosis by itself decreases the effects of pancuronium. Hyperventilation has been thought to augment the abdominal muscle relaxation produced by pancuronium. One explanation of this phenomenon is that changes in pH or plasma concentrations of pancuronium reflect a change in binding to the receptor substance.

### Catecholamines
Epinephrine and ephedrine have a type of reversal effect on skeletal muscle. Clinically, an antagonism to pancuronium has been shown. This effect is caused by an increase in acetylcholine release, the inhibition of acetylcholinesterase, a decreased excitability of muscle fibers, and the release of potassium with administration of epinephrine and ephedrine.

### Mycins
Several antibiotics have a nondepolarizing neuromuscular blocking property because the aminoglycoside antibiotics potentiate the neuromuscular blockade by inhibiting the presynaptic release of acetylcholine. The resulting clinical difficulties are related to a combination of factors, including large doses of antibiotics, parenteral administration into body cavities that represent a large surface area for absorption, and concomitant use of a neuromuscular blocking agent. Neomycin and streptomycin have been most frequently implicated (Box 23-3).

**Box 23-3    Neuromuscular Blocking Properties of Various Antibiotics**

**ANTIBIOTICS THAT INCREASE THE ACTION OF THE NONDEPOLARIZING AGENTS**
Dihydrostreptomycin
Neomycin
Streptomycin
Kanamycin
Gentamicin
Polymyxin A
Polymyxin B
Lincomycin
Colistin
Tetracycline

**ANTIBIOTICS THAT INCREASE THE ACTION OF SUCCINYLCHOLINE**
Neomycin
Streptomycin
Kanamycin
Polymyxin B
Colistin

**ANTIBIOTICS THAT DO NOT EXERT ANY NEUROMUSCULAR BLOCKING ACTIVITY**
Penicillin
Chloramphenicol
Cephalosporins

**Cardiac Antidysrhythmic Drugs**
When administered intravenously, lidocaine potentiates a preexisting neuromuscular blockade that occurs because lidocaine stabilizes the postsynaptic membrane and depresses the skeletal muscle fibers. Quinidine interferes with the presynaptic release of acetylcholine at the neuromuscular junction. Consequently, it intensifies the neuromuscular blockade of both depolarizing and nondepolarizing skeletal muscle blocking agents. Finally, calcium channel blocking agents inhibit the calcium entry, with a resultant reduction in acetylcholine release followed by a reduction in neuromuscular function.

**Temperature**
Hypothermia antagonizes the action of pancuronium and potentiates the action of succinylcholine. During the recovery phase of an anesthetic, when a neuromuscular blocking agent has been administered, young infants should be specifically monitored for return of skeletal muscle tone. This rule is especially in effect when a nondepolarizing relaxant is administered to infants, who are prone to have

some hypothermia because of their immature heat-regulating systems.

**Inhalation Anesthetics**
The inhalation anesthetics produce a dose-dependent enhancement of the neuromuscular blockade of the nondepolarizing neuromuscular blocking agents. More specifically, this blockade is most pronounced when a patient has received isoflurane. Nitrous oxide only produces minimal potentiation of nondepolarizing neuromuscular blocking agents. This potentiation of the neuromuscular blockade by the inhalation anesthetics results from depression of the central nervous system and ultimately reduces skeletal muscle tone. Consequently, patients in the PACU who have received nondepolarizing neuromuscular blocking agents during surgery and have not completely emerged from the inhalation anesthetic should be closely monitored with a peripheral nerve stimulator for a reduction in skeletal muscle function. Also, an aggressive stir-up regimen should be instituted on these patients.

**ASSESSMENT OF NEUROMUSCULAR BLOCKADE**

In a study conducted in the 1940s, injection with d-tubocurarine (a nondepolarizing skeletal muscle relaxant) first caused motor weakness and then total muscle flaccidity. The small rapidly moving muscles, such as those of the fingers, toes, eyes, and ears, are involved before the long muscles of the limbs, neck, and trunk. The intercostal muscles and finally the diaphragm become paralyzed, and then respiration ceases.

The perianesthesia nurse should know the order of the return of muscle function after a patient has received a nondepolarizing muscle relaxant. The recovery of skeletal muscle function is usually in reverse order to that of paralysis; therefore, the diaphragm is ordinarily first to regain function. The order of appearance of paralysis after injection with a nondepolarizing neuromuscular blocking agent can be assessed electromyographically as follows:
1. Small-sized muscle groups: Oculomotor muscles, muscles of the eyelids; muscles of the mouth and face; small extensor muscles of the fingers, followed by the flexor muscles of the fingers.
2. Medium-sized muscle groups: Muscles of the tongue and pharynx; muscles of mastication; extensor muscles of the limb, followed by flexor muscles of the limbs.
3. Large-sized muscle groups: Neck muscles, shoulder muscles, abdominal muscles, dorsal muscle mass.

4. Special muscle groups: Intercostal muscles, larynx, and diaphragm.

The order of paralysis is essentially the same after injection with a depolarizing neuromuscular agent, except that the flexor muscles are paralyzed before the extensor muscles. Patients who arrive in the PACU must be evaluated for residual effects from a neuromuscular blocking agent that was administered during surgery. In most instances, the action of the nondepolarizing neuromuscular blocking agent is pharmacologically reversed at the end of the operation before the patient is admitted to the PACU; however, any patient who has received a neuromuscular blocking agent should be closely watched for signs of residual drug action. The goal of the assessment of the recovery from nondepolarizing neuromuscular blocking agents with the train-of-four is a ration of more than 75%. The residual actions of the depolarizing muscle relaxants are similar to those of the nondepolarizing muscle relaxants, and the same nonrespiratory parameters and respiratory variables can be used in evaluation of the neuromuscular blockade. The evoked (electric stimulation) responses differ between the depolarizing and nondepolarizing neuromuscular blocking agents.

The peripheral nerve stimulator (PNS; Fig. 23-3) can be used in the PACU for assessment of the type and degree of a neuromuscular blockade. This electric device can be used to stimulate the ulnar nerve at the wrist or elbow, and, on stimulation of the ulnar nerve, the nurse can observe the contraction of the fingers. Fig. 23-4 graphically shows the train-of-four test. The assessment of the depth of neuromuscular blockade with electric stimulation is useful when more than 70% of the $N_2$ receptors are blocked by a skeletal muscle relaxant. However, in most instances, if the patient has a normal tidal volume, vital capacity, and maximal inspiratory force and can lift the head for 5 seconds, the use of the PNS is not warranted. If identification of the type of neuromuscular blockade used (depolarizing or nondepolarizing) is needed, or if some of the aforementioned parameters are marginal, the train-of-four or sustained tetanus with the PNS can be used to provide the objective data for assessment.

Although the mechanisms that produce the nondepolarizing block differ from the depolarizing block, the diagnostic criteria with a PNS for assessment of a nondepolarizing and phase II dual block are basically the same. The hallmark of a nondepolarizing neuromuscular blockade is an inability to sustain contraction in response to a tetanic stimulus and posttetanic potentiation. A tetanic stimulus is the usual 50 Hz of current

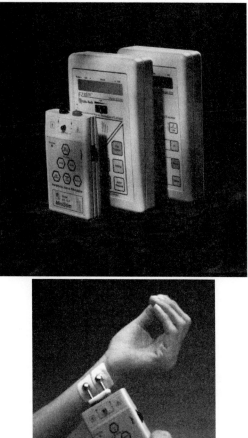

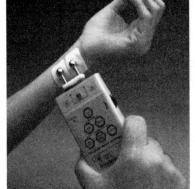

**Fig. 23-3**  Peripheral nerve stimulator. *(Courtesy Life-Tech, Inc, Stafford, Tex.)*

for 5 seconds (sustained tetanus) produced by a PNS. Posttetanic facilitation is a twitch after the response to tetanic stimuli higher than the twitch immediately before tetanus. If a patient has a partial nondepolarizing neuromuscular block, an unsustained contraction called fade is seen after the initial tetanic stimulus (Fig. 23-5). Fade is caused by the decreased mobilization of acetylcholine in the nerve terminal because the presynaptic acetylcholine receptor is blocked by the nondepolarizing muscle relaxant. The responses to electric stimulation result from the interaction of acetylcholine released and the number of $N_2$ cholinergic receptors occupied by the relaxant. In patients with a partial nondepolarizing neuromuscular block, the first three single electric stimuli are of enough intensity to produce a twitch, but the twitch produced is not of the same magnitude as a twitch

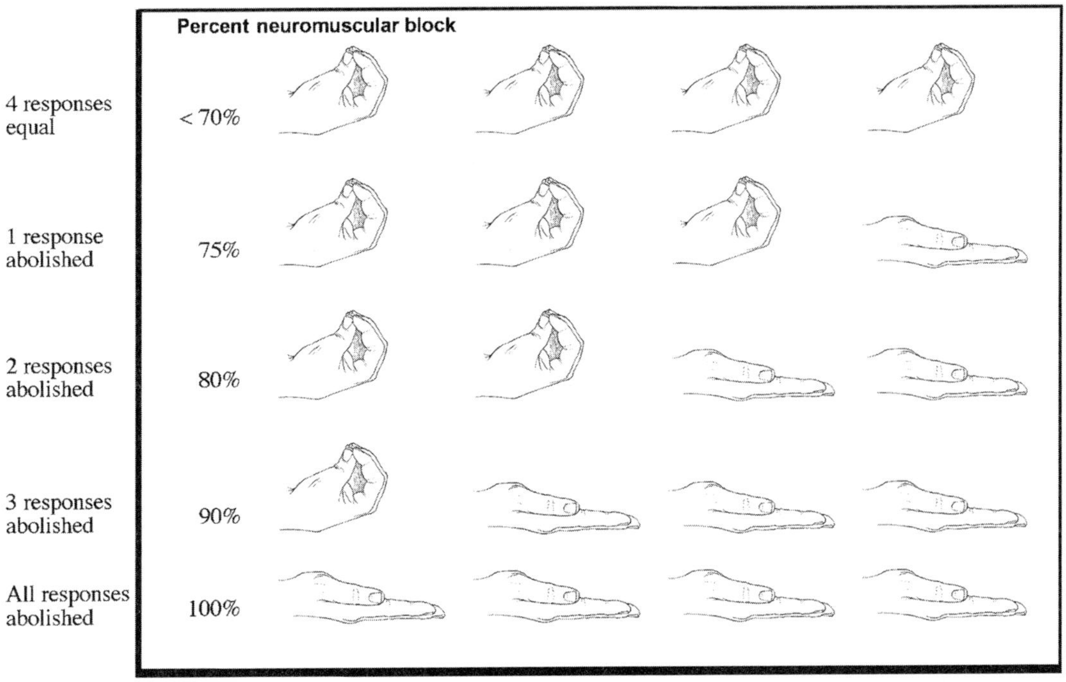

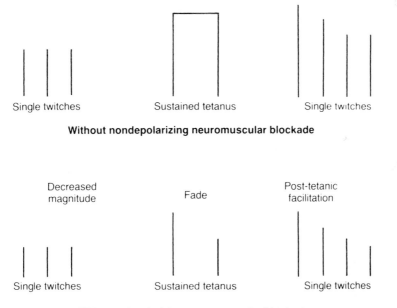

**Fig. 23-4** "Train-of-four" suppression. *(From Nagelhout J, Zaglaniczny K: Nurse anesthesia, ed 3, St Louis, 2005, Saunders.)*

**Fig. 23-5** Magnitude of posttetanic facilitation without and with nondepolarizing neuromuscular blockade. *(Adapted from Donati F: Monitoring neuromuscular blockade. In Saidman L, Smith NT, editors: Monitoring in anesthesia, ed 3, Woburn, Mass, 1993, Butterworth-Heinemann.)*

produced in a subject who has not received a nondepolarizing skeletal muscle relaxant (see Fig. 23-5). The three electric stimuli cause the normal quantum of acetylcholine to be released at the synaptic cleft; however, in this instance, the reduction in twitch magnitude is the result of the number of acetylcholine receptors being occupied by the nondepolarizing relaxant. Consequently, if the patient has had a complete nondepolarizing neuromuscular block in which all the $N_2$ cholinergic receptors were occupied, no twitch is elicited from the three electric stimuli.

In a healthy subject, when a tetanic stimulus is applied for 5 seconds, the quantum of acetylcholine that is released decreases during the stimulus period. Also, only a fraction of nicotinic cholinergic receptors are activated at any one time to trigger an action potential. The excess in nicotinic cholinergic receptors is the safety margin of neuromuscular transmission. Consequently, in the healthy subject who receives a tetanic stimulus, the magnitude of the twitch response is maintained because of the large nicotinic cholinergic receptor pool; however, if 75% of the nicotinic receptors are occupied by a nondepolarizing neuromuscular relaxant, for example, the twitch response is not maintained and fade (unsustained contraction) occurs because the usual margin of safety of excess acetylcholine receptors has been abolished. Between the termination of a tetanic stimulus and the first single-twitch stimulus, a buildup of acetylcholine occurs in the presynaptic knob. Thus, after sustained tetanus, when the first electric stimulus is administered, the height of the first twitch is greater than the pretetanic twitches. These large posttetanic twitches (posttetanic facilitation) return to the pretetanic height as the acetylcholine mobilization also returns to the pretetanic level. Finally, more than 70% of the nicotinic cholinergic receptors must be occupied before this tetanic stimulation test is sensitive enough for detection of neuromuscular blockade.

The major drawback to the delivery of a 50-Hz tetanic stimulus to an awakened patient in the PACU is pain and general discomfort. For the patient who is awake and reactive, the train-of-four stimulation is better for assessment of the degree of neuromuscular blockade caused by nondepolarizing skeletal muscle relaxants. In this test, the ulnar nerve is used, and four supramaximal electrical stimuli—2 Hz 0.05 seconds apart—are administered with a PNS. This test, which produces minimal discomfort to the awakened patient, is sensitive only when more than 70% of the nicotinic cholinergic receptors are occupied. The index of neuromuscular blockade in this test is the ratio of the fourth to the first twitch amplitude. More specifically, when the fourth response is abolished, a 75% block exists (Fig. 23-6). When the third and second responses to stimulation are abolished, the respective reductions in neuromuscular blockade are 80% and 90%. Finally, when all four twitch responses are absent, a 100%, or complete, block exists.

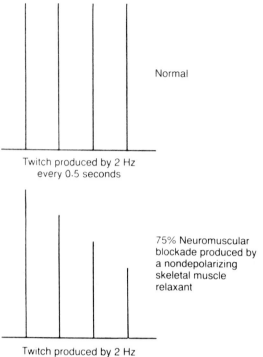

**Fig. 23-6**   Diagrammatic illustration of train-of-four in normal response and 75% neuromuscular blockade produced by nondepolarizing skeletal muscle relaxant.

The depolarizing neuromuscular blockade is characterized by an absence of posttetanic potentiation, a decreased response to a single impulse, a decreased amplitude (but sustained response to a tetanic stimulus), and, if present, a train-of-four ratio between the first and fourth stimulus that is greater than 70%. Refer to Table 23-2 for a complete overview of the commonly used monitoring tests and Table 23-3 for some key points related to the neuromuscular reversal.

## SPECIAL PROBLEMS IN THE PACU

A prolonged response to succinylcholine sometimes occurs because a patient does not possess the proper blood level of pseudocholinesterase. Other causes of a prolonged response include: (1) overdosage; (2) temperature changes; (3) acid-base imbalance; (4) carcinoma; (5) antitumor agents; (6) antibiotics; (7) myasthenia gravis; and (8) liver disease.

If a patient who arrives in the PACU is apneic, controlled respiration must be initiated and maintained as long as necessary. Careful monitoring of vital signs and evaluation of renal function are important. The

## Table 23-2  Neuromuscular Monitoring Methods

| Monitoring Test | Definition | Comments |
|---|---|---|
| Single twitch | Single supramaximal electric stimulus ranging from 0.1-1 Hz | Requires baseline before drug administration; generally used as qualitative rather than quantitative assessment |
| Train-of-four | Series of four twitches at 2 Hz every half-second for 2 s | Reflects blockade from 70% to 100%; useful during onset, maintenance, and emergence |
| Tetanus | Generally consists of rapid delivery of 30-Hz, 50-Hz, or 100-Hz stimulus for 5 s | Should be used sparingly for deep block assessment; painful |
| Posttetanic count | 50-Hz tetanus for 5 s, 3-s pause, then single twitches of 1 Hz | Used only when train-of-four or double-burst stimulation response is absent; count less than eight indicates deep block, and prolonged recovery is likely |
| Double-burst stimulation | Two short bursts of 50-Hz tetanus separated by 0.75 s | Similar to train-of-four; useful during onset, maintenance, and emergence; may be easier for detection of fade than with train of four; tactile evaluation |

From Nagelhout J, Zaglaniczny K: *Nurse anesthesia*, ed 3, St Louis, 2005, Saunders.

## Table 23-3  Key Points Related to Tests of Neuromuscular Transmission and Reversal

| Test | Acceptable Clinical Result to Suggest Normal Function | Approximate Percentage of Receptors Occupied When Response Returns to Normal Value | Comments, Advantages, and Disadvantages |
|---|---|---|---|
| Tidal volume | At least 5 mL/kg | 80 | Necessary, but insensitive as indicator of neuromuscular function |
| Single twitch strength | Qualitatively as strong as baseline | 75-80 | Uncomfortable; need to know twitch strength before relaxant administration; insensitive as indicator of recovery but useful as gauge of deep neuromuscular blockade |
| Train-of-four (TOF) | No palpable fade | 70-75 | Uncomfortable, but more sensitive as indicator of recovery than single twitch; used as gauge of depth of block with counting number of responses perceptible |
| Sustained tetanus at 50 Hz for 5 s | At lease 20 mL/kg | 70 | Very uncomfortable, but reliable indicator of adequate recovery |
| Vital capacity | At least 20 mL/kg | 70 | Requires patient cooperation, but is goal for achievement of full clinical recovery |

*CONCEPTS IN ANESTHETIC AGENTS*

*Continued*

| Table 23-3 | Key Points Related to Tests of Neuromuscular Transmission and Reversal—cont'd | | |
|---|---|---|---|
| Test | Acceptable Clinical Result to Suggest Normal Function | Approximate Percentage of Receptors Occupied When Response Returns to Normal Value | Comments, Advantages, and Disadvantages |
| Double-burst stimulation | No palpable fade | 60-70 | Uncomfortable, but more sensitive than TOF as indicator of peripheral function; no perceptible fade indicates TOF of at least recovery of 60% |
| Inspiratory force | At least −40 cm $H_2O$ | 50 | Difficult to perform with endotracheal intubation, but reliable gauge of normal diaphragmatic function |
| Head lift | Must be performed unaided with patient supine and sustained for 5 s | 50 | Requires patient cooperation, but remains standard test of normal clinical function |
| Hand grip | Sustained at level qualitatively similar to preinduction | 50 | Sustained stong grip, although also requires patient cooperation; is another good gauge of normal function |
| Sustained bite | Sustained jaw clench on tongue blade | 50 | Very reliable with patient cooperation; corresponds with TOF of 85% |

Modified with permission from Savarese JJ, Caldwell JE, Lien CA, et al: Pharmacology of muscle relaxants and their antagonists. In Miller RD, editor: *Anesthesia*, ed 5, Philadelphia, 2000, Churchill Livingstone; and from Nagelhout J, Zaglaniczny K: *Nurse anesthesia*, ed 3, St Louis, 2005, Saunders.

neuromuscular block can be identified with the PNS. If electric stimulation results in vigorous contractions, the apnea is unlikely to be the result of residual neuromuscular block. Consideration must then be given to other agents that may have caused the apneic state. The response of patients with neuromuscular disorders to muscle relaxants may include resistance, increased response, hyperkalemia, and even cardiac arrest. Table 23-4 is presented as a summary of the possible untoward responses in the clinical setting.

### Dual or Phase II Block

Various terms are used to describe the different types of blocks that succinylcholine is able to produce. The Phase I block is synonymous with the depolarizing block the drug ordinarily produces. It is characterized by a dose-dependent reduction in a single twitch without fade after a well-sustained tetanus and no posttetanic facilitation when the PNS is used.

Phase II block is also known as a dual block, desensitization, or open channel block. This block is caused by a conformational change in

the presynaptic and postsynaptic cholinergic receptors. This anatomic change results in desensitization to the stimulation of acetylcholine because of the prolonged depolarization at the motor end plate. The characteristics of this block as shown with the PNS are fade in response to tetanic stimuli, posttetanic potentiation, and antagonism with drugs such as neostigmine. The same clinical features are seen when vecuronium is used; however, this similarity does not mean that the two blocks are the same because good evidence suggests that the vecuronium and succinylcholine Phase II blocks differ in several respects. Some clinicians believe that the Phase II block produced by succinylcholine can be reversed with anticholinesterases, such as edrophonium, which has a shorter duration of action than neostigmine. Edrophonium is used in this situation because it either reverses or potentiates the block. If potentiation occurs, it is of a shorter duration than if neostigmine were used. Most experts believe that routine reversal to antagonize the dual block is unwarranted. Ventilation of the patient with a wait for return of the normal neuromuscular transmission

**Table 23-4  Summary of Response of Patients with Neuromuscular Disorders to Muscle Relaxants**

| Disorder | Pathophysiology | Response to Nondepolarizing Muscle Relaxant | Response to Depolarizing Muscle Relaxant |
|---|---|---|---|
| Hemiplegia | Sequelae of CVA; caused by upper motor neuron in cerebral motor cortex | Resistance | Hyperkalemia can occur as early as 1 wk and as late as 6 mo after stroke |
| Parkinson's disease | Extrapyramidal disorder | Normal | Hyperkalemia may occur |
| Multiple sclerosis | Demyelinating disorder of CNS | Normal | Hyperkalemia may occur |
| Diffuse intracranial lesions | No focal neurologic deficits or muscular denervation or paralysis (i.e., ruptured cerebral aneurysm) | Normal | Hyperkalemia and possible cardiac arrest |
| Tetanus | Acute infectious disease of CNS caused by endotoxin released by *Clostridium tetani* | Normal | Hyperkalemia and possible cardiac arrest |
| Paraplegia and quadriplegia | Traumatic or pathologic transection of spinal cord and interruption of pyramidal tracts | Increased response | Hyperkalemia as early as 3 wk and as late as 85 d after spinal cord injury |
| Amyotrophic lateral sclerosis (ALS) | Degenerative disease of motor ganglia in anterior horn of spinal cord and of spinal pyramidal tracts | Increased response | No reports of hyperkalemia in ALS; however, myotonia-like contracture may occur in patients with ALS; avoid succinylcholine in patients with significant muscular denervation |
| Muscular denervation | Result of traumatic peripheral nerve damage; muscles undergo atrophy | Normal response | Muscular contracture and hyperkalemia |
| Myasthenia gravis (MG) | Postsynaptic reduction in number of ACh receptors caused by autoimmune disease | Increased response and prolongation of effects | Resistance and early appearance of phase II (dual) block |
| Myasthenic syndrome | Differs clinically and electromyographically from MG; associated with small cell carcinoma of lung and results in presynaptic lesion at neuromuscular junction | Exaggerated response | Exaggerated response |
| Myotonias | Lesion in muscle fiber distal to neuromuscular junction; common symptom is delayed relaxation of skeletal muscles after voluntary contractions | Increased and prolonged; some report normal response | Unpredictable; many reports of increased rigidity |
| Muscular dystrophies (MD) | Disorder of muscle fiber proper that may be caused by neurogenic disorder | Normal to prolonged response; ocular MD has very high sensitivity to d-tubocurarine | Unpredictable; best to avoid use of succinylcholine |

CVA, Cerebrovascular accident; CNS, central nervous system; ACh, acetylcholine.

## Box 23-4   Summary of the Differentiating Characteristics of a Phase I and Phase II Block

**DEPOLARIZING (PHASE I BLOCK)**
Muscle fasciculation precedes the onset of neuromuscular blockade
Sustained response to titanic stimulation
Absence of posttetanic potentiation, stimulation, or facilitation
Lack of fade to train-of-four or double-burst stimulation
Block antagonized by prior administration of nondepolarizer as pretreatment (approximately 20% more succinylcholine necessary)
Block potentiated by anticholinesterase drugs

**NONDEPOLARIZING (PHASE II) BLOCK**
Absence of muscle fasciculation
Appearance of tetanic fade and posttetanic potentiation, stimulation, or facilitation
Train-of-four and double-burst fade
Reversal with anticholinesterase drugs
In rare cases, may be produced by an overdose and desensitization with succinylcholine at doses more than 6 mg/kg

From Nagelhout J, Zaglaniczny K: *Nurse anesthesia*, ed 3, St Louis, 2005, Saunders.

is more advisable. See Box 23-4 for a summary of the differentiating characteristics of a depolarizing (Phase I) block and a nondepolarizing (Phase II) block.

### Residual Paralysis
Residual paralysis is the reappearance after surgery of the pharmacologic actions of a nondepolarizing skeletal muscle relaxant that was administered during surgery. Other terms that are associated with this are compromised ventilation, partial reversal, or reduced train-of-four. This complication arises when renal insufficiency exists. The interesting facet of this complication is that even when a nondepolarizing skeletal muscle relaxant is reversed sufficiently at the end of the anesthetic, residual paralysis may still occur for as long as 8 hours. This reappearance may be partly caused by the fading of the effect of the neostigmine.

Symptoms of residual paralysis include clinical evidence showing a reduction of the return of neuromuscular function with evaluation of the 5-second head lift, adequate phonation, ventilation, and upper airway maintenance along with a poor twitch response with the PNS.

If symptoms appear, the required level of the reversal agent (neostigmine) must be maintained until that portion of the nondepolarizing skeletal muscle relaxant has been eliminated so that symptoms do not reappear. If residual paralysis occurs, the postoperative use of morphine and similar narcotics should be avoided because these agents enhance a residual neuromuscular block sufficiently to make it clinically

significant. Finally, because the patient becomes quite fearful, constant verbal reassurance by the PACU nurse helps in reduction of stress and anxiety.

### Bradycardia
Another problem that occurs in the PACU is the appearance of bradycardia when a patient has received an atropine-neostigmine combination at the end of the anesthetic. The bradycardia is usually the result of the longer duration of action of neostigmine in comparison with that of atropine. The treatment for this problem is glycopyrrolate. Glycopyrrolate should not be administered, however, until other causes of bradycardia are eliminated, such as pain, hypoventilation, and a full bladder.

## SUMMARY

The neuromuscular blocking agents used in today's perianesthesia practice produce excellent results with less disadvantages as compared with the drugs presented in the previous edition of this book. It is remarkable how the art and science of anesthesia has narrowed down the number of agents to be used in clinical practice to the most popular and those that possess excellent advantages over the neuromuscular agents used in the past. An overview of the process of excitation-contraction coupling was presented as were the current drugs in use. An in-depth approach was used in the discussion of the pharmacologic reversal of the nondepolarizing neuromuscular agents and in a discussion of the various methods of monitoring a patient who has received a skeletal muscle relaxant during surgery. Finally, an overview of the PACU nursing care was presented (an in-depth discussion on this topic can be found in Chapter 28).

Neuromuscular blocking agents are useful agents in the operating room for facilitation of the optimum surgical field for the physician to use life-saving skills effectively. In the PACU, neuromuscular blocking agents can be used for life-saving situations and facilitation of mechanical ventilation. In the PACU, these agents should only be administered by a practitioner skilled in airway management. Also, for those patients in the PACU who require mechanical ventilation and need neuromuscular blocking agents to enhance ventilatory care, the PACU nurse should be acutely aware that besides the skillful use of the neuromuscular blocking agent the patient also needs appropriate sedation and verbal support during that most fearful time of care.

## BIBLIOGRAPHY

Aitkenhead A, Smith G, Rowbotham D: *Textbook of anaesthesia*, ed 5, Philadelphia, 2007, Churchill Livingstone.

Alspach J: *Core curriculum for critical care nursing*, ed 6, Philadelphia, 2005, Saunders.

Atlee J: *Complications in anesthesia*, ed 2, Philadelphia, 2007, Saunders.

Barash P, Cullen B, Stoelting R: *Clinical anesthesia*, ed 5, Philadelphia, 2005, Lippincott Williams & Wilkins.

Benumof J, Saidman L: *Anesthesia & perioperative complications*, ed 2, St Louis, 1999, Mosby.

Bevan D, Smith C, Donati F: Postoperative neuromuscular blockade: a comparison between atracurium, vecuronium, and pancuronium, *Anesthesiology* 69(2):272–276, 1988.

Brown J, Foster S, Anderson C, et al: The literature and perspectives on muscle relaxants for rapid-sequence induction, *Nurse Anesth* 2(2):72–78, 1991.

Brunton L, Lazo J, Parker K: *Goodman and Gilman the pharmacological basis of therapeutics*, ed 11, New York, 2005, McGraw-Hill Professional.

Cote C, Todres I, Goudsouzian N, et al: *A practice of anesthesia for infants and children*, ed 3, Philadelphia, 2001, Saunders.

Drake R, Vogl W, Mitchell A: *Gray's anatomy for students*, Philadelphia, 2005, Churchill Livingstone.

Erkola O, Karhunen U, Sandelin-Hellqvist E: Spontaneous recovery of residual neuromuscular blockade after atracurium or vecuronium during isoflurane anaesthesia, *Acta Anaesthesiol Scand* 33:290–294, 1991.

Evers A, Maze M: Physiologic principles and clinical practice, *Anesthetic pharmacology*, Philadelphia, 2004, Churchill Livingstone.

Fisher L: *Benumof's anesthesia and uncommon diseases*, ed 5, Philadelphia, 2007, Saunders.

Ganong W: *Review of medical physiology*, ed 22, New York, 2005, McGraw-Hill Medical.

Goldhill D, Whitehead J, Emmott R, et al: Neuromuscular and clinical effects of mivacurium chloride in healthy adult patients during nitrous oxide-enflurane anaesthesia, *Br J Anaesth* 67(3):289–295, 1991.

Guyton A, Hall J: *Textbook of medical physiology*, ed 11, Philadelphia, 2006, Saunders.

Kier L, Dowd C: *The chemistry of drugs for nurse anesthetists*, Chicago, 2004, AANA Publishing, Inc.

Lake C, Hines R, Blitt C: *Clinical monitoring: practical applications for anesthesia and critical care*, Philadelphia, 2001, Saunders.

Longnecker D, Murphy F: *Dripps, Eckenhoff, Vandam introduction to anesthesia*, ed 9, Philadelphia, 1997, Saunders.

Longnecker D, Tinker J, Morgan G: *Principles and practice of anesthesiology*, ed 2, St Louis, 1998, Mosby.

Miller R, editor: *Anesthesia*, ed 6, Philadelphia, 2005, Churchill Livingstone.

Nagelhout J, Zaglaniczy K: *Nurse anesthesia*, ed 3, St Louis, 2005, Saunders.

Ogden S: *Calculation of drug dosages*, ed 7, St Louis, 2005, Mosby.

Ostheimer G: A comparison of glycopyrrolate and atropine during reversal of nondepolarizing neuromuscular block with neostigmine, *Anesth Analg* 56:182–186, 1977.

Shorten G, Browne J, Carr D, et al: *Postoperative pain management, an evidence-based guide to practice*, Philadelphia, 2006, Saunders.

Stoelting R: *Pharmacology and physiology in anesthetic practice*, ed 3, Philadelphia, 1999, Lippincott-Raven.

Stoelting R, Miller R: *Basics of anesthesia*, ed 5, Philadelphia, 2007, Churchill Livingstone.

White P: *Perioperative drug manual*, ed 2, Philadelphia, 2005, Saunders.

Wicks T: Mivacurium chloride, *Nurse Anesth* 3(4):173–182, 1992.

Zarr G: Pharmacology of neuromuscular blockade and antagonism. In Waugaman W, Foster S, Rigor B, editors: *Principles and practice of nurse anesthesia*, ed 3, Stamford, Conn, 1999, Appleton & Lange.

Zuurmond W, van Leeuwen L: Atracurium versus vecuronium: a comparison of recovery in outpatient arthroscopy, *Can J Anaesth* 35(2):139–142, 1988.

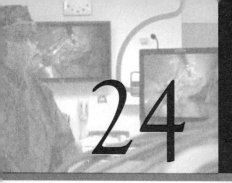

# 24

# LOCAL ANESTHETICS

*Thomas Corey Davis, CRNA, MSNA*

Local anesthetic agents are defined as pharmacologic agents capable of producing a loss of sensation in an area of the body. They were first used in 1884, when cocaine was used as a topical anesthetic agent by Freud and Köller, and in 1885, when Halsted used cocaine for prevention of nerve conduction in the lower extremities. The actual advent of the use of local anesthetics in anesthetic practice was not until 1943, when Lofgren synthesized procaine. Local anesthetics are used in all forms of regional anesthesia. The term *regional anesthesia* refers to the various anesthetic techniques that use local anesthetic agents to block nerve conduction in an extremity or a region of the body (see Chapter 25). The types of regional anesthesia are topical, infiltration, field block, and conduction. *Topical anesthesia* is produced when an anesthetic agent is applied to a surface, such as the skin, mucous membrane, urethra, nose, and pharynx. A topical anesthetic that can be used on the skin for analgesia during venipuncture is called *EMLA*. This eutectic mixture of local anesthetics is composed of lidocaine and prilocaine. *Infiltration anesthesia* is produced with injection of a local anesthetic into the tissue to be cut. *Field block anesthesia* is produced with injection of a local anesthetic agent into the surrounding tissues of an area containing the site of incision. *Conduction anesthesia* is produced with injection of a local anesthetic agent into a nerve that supplies a region of the body for elimination of sensation or motor control, or both. Epidural, subarachnoid, nerve, and nerve plexus blocks are *conduction blocks*.

The use of regional anesthesia has become popular in modern anesthesia practice because, when indicated, it offers many advantages over general inhalation anesthesia. For facilitation of optimal recovery of the surgical patient from this type of anesthetic, the postanesthesia care unit (PACU) nurse must first have a complete knowledge of the physiology of nerve conduction and the pharmacology of local anesthetic agents, including their mechanism of action, effects, and toxicity.

## PHYSIOLOGY OF NERVES, NERVE CONDUCTION, AND LOCAL ANESTHETICS

Nerves conduct impulses, or action potentials, that provide information to the central nervous system (CNS) about the type, degree, and magnitude of pain. As Wood and Wood describe, inside the nerve cell (including the axon) is cytoplasm that contains potassium ions that are positively charged and proteins that are negatively charged. The potassium ions can freely move in and out of the cytoplasm, whereas the proteins are not freely diffusible. The fluid outside the nerve cell and axon contains positively charged sodium ions and negatively charged chloride ions. These ions are freely diffusible into the cytoplasm. However, via a sodium pump, the sodium is quickly pushed out of the nerve cell. Outside the nerve cell, the concentration of the negatively charged chloride ion is large and the concentration of the positively charged potassium is low. Inside the nerve cell, this ratio is reversed: the concentration of potassium is high, and the concentration of the negatively charged chloride ions is low. The freely diffusible potassium ions are held inside the nerve cell by an excess of negatively charged ions. Because of the excess of negatively charged ions, an electric potential exists of about −70 to −90 mV (*resting potential*).

When the nerve impulse is conducted down the nerve fiber, the nerve membranes become permeable (because of depolarization) to the positively charged sodium ions. These sodium ions are conducted through pores, or sodium channels, in which a "gate" regulates their passage to the inside of the nerve cell. As the sodium ions reach the inside of the nerve cell, the electric potential changes to + 40 mV. This change from negative to positive of about 110 mV represents the movement of an action potential down a nerve fiber or, in neurophysiologic terms, propagation of an action potential. Once the sodium has reached a certain ionic concentration, the gate closes in the sodium channels. The membrane permeability to potassium increases, which allows potassium back into the cytoplasm, and sodium is pumped out of the nerve cell, which slowly returns the ionic potential to its resting level of –70 to –90 mV.

Local anesthetics are quite lipid soluble and, consequently, can diffuse through the cell membrane into the axoplasm. They ionize and occupy a receptor near the gate of the sodium channel. Thus, the local anesthetic prevents the opening of the gate, and sodium cannot enter the inside of the nerve, which results in a slowing of the rate of depolarization. Consequently, a nerve action potential cannot be reached, and the nerve's electric conduction system is blocked.

The afferent nerve fibers that conduct impulses to the spinal cord are classified as A, B, and C, on the basis of fiber diameter and conduction velocity. The A fibers are further divided into A-alpha, A-beta, A-gamma, and A-delta fibers. The large-diameter A fibers are myelinated and have the fastest conduction velocity. The A-alpha fibers have the largest diameter and the fastest conduction velocity. They provide innervation of motor function to the skeletal muscles. The moderately myelinated A-beta fibers are the next largest in diameter and speed, and they are responsible for touch and pressure. The sensation of proprioception and skeletal muscle tone are maintained by the A-gamma fibers, which are still smaller in diameter and slower than the preceding A-beta fibers. The A-delta fibers are lightly myelinated and are the smallest and slowest of the A fibers. They are responsible for conducting sensations of fast pain, touch, and temperature. The lightly myelinated B fibers are smaller than the A fibers and are the preganglionic autonomic fibers. The smallest fibers are the unmyelinated C fibers. They function as postganglionic sympathetic fibers and also conduct sensations such as slow pain and temperature.

Local anesthetics can penetrate and prevent nerve conduction in the smallest nerve fibers first and the large A-alpha fibers last. Consequently, during emergence from conduction anesthesia, a particular order of return is seen that is based solely on the reduced concentration gradient of the local anesthetic and the fiber size (Box 24-1). For example, after epidural and peripheral nerve or plexus blocks, the large A-alpha fibers return first and the patient has a return of motor function. The next fibers to return are the A-beta and A-gamma, and the patient has a return of proprioception, touch, and pressure. Finally, a return of pain and a loss of a sensation of warmth occurs as a result of low concentration of local anesthetic in the A-delta, B, and C fibers.

Pain, which is called *nociception*, is a protective mechanism that occurs when tissues are

---

**Box 24-1  Sequence of Nerve Blockade**

Motor paralysis
Loss of proprioception (awareness of body or extremity position)
Pressure sense abolished
Tactile sense lost
Slow and fast pain
Temperature discrimination lost
Sensation of warmth by patient
Block of cold temperature fibers
Vasomotor block dilation of skin vessels and increased cutaneous blood flow

---

damaged. The two major types of pain are fast and slow. *Fast pain* is a well-defined stabbing sensation that is rather short in duration. Causes of fast pain include surgical incision and pin pricks. Fast pain is conducted via the small afferent myelinated A-delta nerve fibers. *Slow pain* is not well defined and is characterized as a burning or aching sensation. In this type of pain, even after the pain stimulus is removed, the pain may continue. The efferent conducting nerves in this instance are the unmyelinated C fibers.

## THE LOCAL ANESTHETICS

The ideal local anesthetic should have the following properties: selectivity of action, low toxicity, complete reversibility, nonirritation, short latency, good penetrance, sufficient duration, solubility in saline and water, stability, and compatibility with vasoconstrictors. Not all local anesthetic agents possess all these attributes. As new agents are discovered, they are measured against these criteria.

In regard to analgesic activity, local anesthetic agents can be divided into three groups according to potency. Procaine and chloroprocaine are the least potent of the commonly used agents, whereas lidocaine, cocaine, mepivacaine, and prilocaine are compounds of intermediate potency; that is, they are twice as potent as procaine. Tetracaine, bupivacaine (and its isomers ropivacaine and chirocaine), and etidocaine are drugs of high potency that are approximately six to eight times more active than procaine.

The local anesthetic agents are grouped pharmacologically into two categories, on the basis of chemical structure: the amides and the esters (Table 24-1). The *amides* are metabolized in the liver, have no real history of documented allergic reactions, have good penetrance, and

## Table 24-1   Local Anesthetic Agents: Esters and Amides

| Agent | Use | Discussion |
|---|---|---|
| **ESTERS** | | |
| Cocaine | *Topical:* 4%-20% for use in nose and throat procedures; duration, 10-55 min; maximum dose, 3 mg/kg | Topical use only; vasoconstrictor; CNS stimulant in abuse |
| Procaine (Novocain) | *Topical:* 10%-20% required<br>*Infiltration:* 0.25%-0.5%<br>*Nerve block:* 1%-2%; duration, 20-30 min plain, 45 min with epinephrine; maximum dose, 10 mg/kg plain and 14 mg/kg with epinephrine | Low potency, rapid hydrolysis in plasma, mild acetylcholine inhibition, poor stability |
| Chloroprocaine (Nesacaine) | *Infiltration:* 10 mg/mL solution<br>*Peripheral nerve block:* 10 and 20 mg/mL solution<br>*Epidural block:* 20-30 mg/mL solution | Not topically active; more potent but shorter duration of action than procaine<br>Safest local anesthetic in regard to systemic toxicity<br>Onset of action is 6-12 min, and duration of anesthesia is 30-60 min<br>Total dose should not exceed 1 g with epinephrine and 800 mg without epinephrine; 12 times more potent than procaine |
| Tetracaine (Pontocaine) | *Topical:* 0.5%-1%; duration, 55 min<br>*Infiltration:* 0.1%-0.25%<br>*Nerve block:* 0.25%; duration, 3-4 h plain, 5-7 h with epinephrine; maximum dose, 1.5-2 mg/kg plain and 2-3 mg/kg with epinephrine | |
| **AMIDES** | | |
| Lidocaine (Xylocaine) | *Topical:* 2%-4%; onset, 2-4 min; maximum dose, 3 mg/kg<br>*Nerve block:* 1%-2%; maximum dose, 4-5 mg/kg plain or 7 mg/kg with epinephrine; duration, 1 h plain, 2 h with epinephrine; antiarrhythmic, 1 mg/kg bolus, then 1-2 mg/min intravenous drip | Rapid onset, intense analgesia, good penetrance, stable<br>As antiarrhythmic, it depresses automaticity of Purkinje fibers and decreases effective refractory period |
| Mepivacaine (Carbocaine) | *Infiltration:* 0.5%-1%<br>*Nerve block:* 1%-2%; maximum dose, 5-6 mg/kg plain, 7 mg/kg with epinephrine; duration, 1.5 h plain, 2 h with epinephrine | Derivative of lidocaine; less penetrance, slower metabolism; ineffective topically |
| Bupivacaine (Marcaine) | *Infiltration:* 0.1%-0.25%<br>*Nerve block:* 0.25%-0.5%; long-acting, up to 12 h | Less penetrance than other amides |
| Ropivacaine | *Epidural:* Labor: 0.1%-0.2% | Less motor block<br>Less cardiotoxicity than bupivacaine |
| Levobupivacaine | Similar to bupivacaine | Similar efficacy but enhanced safety profile compared with bupivacaine |

**Table 24-1  Local Anesthetic Agents: Esters and Amides—cont'd**

| Agent | Use | Discussion |
|---|---|---|
| Dibucaine (Nupercaine) | *Topical:* 2 mg/mL ointment, up to 15 mL <br> *Spinal:* 2.5-5 mg/mL | Mainly used as topical anesthesia; rarely used for spinal anesthesia because of high systemic toxicity |
| Etidocaine (Duranest) | *Infiltration:* 2.5-5 mg/mL solution <br> *Peripheral nerve block:* 5 and 10 mg/mL solution <br> *Epidural block:* 5 and 10 mg/mL solution | Greater potency and longer duration of action than lidocaine <br> Maximum dose of single injection should not exceed 400 mg in adult |

are stable. Drugs in this category are lidocaine, mepivacaine, prilocaine, etidocaine, and bupivacaine. The *esters*, except for cocaine, are hydrolyzed primarily in the plasma by plasma pseudocholinesterase and are metabolized more rapidly than the amides. Because the esters are metabolized to paraaminobenzoic acid (PABA), they are associated with an increased incidence rate of allergic reactions. In general, the esters have poor penetrance, rare allergic reactions, and fair to poor stability. Epinephrine is added to some local anesthetic agents because it is a vasoconstrictor and therefore prolongs the activity of the local agent and decreases its toxicity by slowing its uptake.

### The Short-Duration Local Anesthetics

**Procaine.** Procaine (Novocain) is one of the first ester local anesthetics; it was first synthesized by Einhorn in 1905. Because it ionizes so quickly, it has poor spreading and penetrating properties. Epinephrine is usually added to procaine to delay systemic absorption because it can produce vasodilatation. The use of procaine is usually for infiltration anesthesia in a 1% or 2% solution or spinal anesthesia in a 5% solution. Allergic reactions have been reported after repeated doses of procaine.

**Chloroprocaine.** Chloroprocaine (Nesacaine) is an analogue of procaine with low toxicity, a rapid onset of 10 minutes, and a short duration of action of about 45 minutes. Chloroprocaine can be used for most types of regional anesthesia. However, chloroprocaine with preservatives is rarely administered epidurally because of the risk of neurotoxicity from accidental injection into the subarachnoid space. Also, chloroprocaine is not used for spinal anesthesia because of the potential for neurotoxicity. Preservative-free chloroprocaine can still be used for epidural anesthesia without risk of neurotoxicity. The multiple-dose vial that contains chloroprocaine

with preservatives (sodium bisulfite and methylparaben) should be used only for infiltration anesthesia. Rapid inadvertent intrathecal injection of a low pH and bisulfite-containing solution can cause motor and sensory deficits.

### The Intermediate-Duration Local Anesthetics

**Cocaine.** Cocaine has three distinctive actions: (1) it can block nerve conduction; (2) it can produce euphoria and sympathetic and CNS stimulation; and (3) it is highly addictive. Cocaine is used primarily for topical anesthesia and probably should not be administered parenterally because it is addictive and has many toxic side effects when administered in any form other than topical. The major cardiovascular effect of cocaine is interference with the reuptake mechanism of catecholamines; consequently, cocaine can potentiate all vasopressors and cause cardiac dysrhythmias and seizures when administered in high doses.

**Lidocaine.** Lidocaine (Xylocaine) is one of the most widely used local anesthetics in the world. It can be used for topical, infiltration, field block, spinal, epidural, caudal, peripheral nerve and nerve plexus blocks, and intravenous regional (Bier) blocks. For topical anesthesia, a 4% solution is usually used; in this form, the onset of action is about 5 minutes and effects last for about 20 minutes. When lidocaine is administered for local infiltration in a 0.5% to 1% solution, the onset of anesthesia is from 2 to 5 minutes, with a duration of action of about 75 minutes. For brachial plexus (axillary) blocks, the drug has an onset of about 5 to 10 minutes and a duration of about 60 minutes without epinephrine and 120 minutes with epinephrine. A caudal block requires a 1% or 2% solution of lidocaine. The onset of anesthesia is between 5 and 15 minutes, with a duration of about 100 minutes with epinephrine and 60 minutes without epinephrine.

The safety of 5% lidocaine for spinal anesthesia has come into question. Case reports and other studies have implicated 5% lidocaine as the cause of neurologic symptoms after spinal anesthesia. To limit the potential for neurologic sequelae after spinal anesthesia with lidocaine, lidocaine is now recommended to be used in a 1.5% solution rather than the traditional 5% concentration. The onset of spinal anesthesia is between 5 and 10 minutes, and the duration is about 60 minutes without epinephrine and 90 minutes with epinephrine.

Lidocaine can be used as an antidysrhythmic at an intravenous dose of 1 mg/kg. Infusion rates for this drug range from 20 to 50 μg/kg/min. Lidocaine can be used for postoperative analgesia when it is administered in a slow continuous intravenous infusion. With this technique, the plasma level of lidocaine should be between 1 and 2 μg/mL. Lidocaine can also be used for prevention of increases in intracranial pressure and hypertension associated with endotracheal intubation; a bolus dose of 1.5 mg/kg of lidocaine given intravenously is helpful. The upper limits of safe dosage for this drug are between 200 and 400 mg without epinephrine and 500 mg with epinephrine. Toxic symptoms develop when the blood level of lidocaine increases about 5 μg/mL. Seizures and respiratory and cardiac depression have been reported when the blood level of lidocaine is higher than 8 μg/mL.

**Mepivacaine.** Mepivacaine (Carbocaine), an amide local anesthetic, is similar to lidocaine in its uses and onset of action; however, its duration of action is longer than that of lidocaine. Mepivacaine does not produce vasodilatation, and consequently, it is an attractive alternative to other local anesthetics that require epinephrine. The upper limits of safe dosage for the drug are 400 mg without epinephrine and 500 mg with epinephrine. At high doses, mepivacaine can depress both respiratory and cardiac functions.

**Prilocaine.** Prilocaine (Citanest)is similar to lidocaine in its uses and potency. However, it has a lower toxicity and shorter duration of action than lidocaine. Prilocaine is not as widely used as lidocaine because it can cause significant complications. One complication associated with prilocaine is methemoglobinemia, especially when the dosage exceeds 500 mg. The treatment for this problem is usually methylene blue given over 5 minutes intravenously at a dosage of 1 to 2 mg/kg.

## The Long-duration Local Anesthetics

**Bupivacaine.** Bupivacaine (Marcaine; Sensorcaine) is an amide local anesthetic that is about four times as potent as lidocaine. Like lidocaine, it is widely used in clinical practice. For infiltration anesthesia, it can be used in a 0.125% to 0.25% solution without epinephrine. For this type of anesthesia, bupivacaine has an onset of 5 to 15 minutes and a duration of about 200 minutes. The duration of action of bupivacaine can be doubled with the addition of epinephrine. For axillary block and other nerve block techniques, including epidural anesthesia, bupivacaine is administered in a 0.25% to 0.5% solution. In this instance, the onset of action is about 15 minutes and the duration is about 2 to 4 hours. For spinal anesthesia, 0.75% bupivacaine is in solution with dextrose. The dose range is between 5 and 20 mg, and the onset is between 8 and 15 minutes, with a duration of action between 2 and 4 hours. Bupivacaine is the drug of choice for lower extremity surgery when a tourniquet is used. Tourniquet pain is transmitted by the very small C fibers. Bupivacaine is able to better block the C fibers than is tetracaine.

A 0.75%, or 7.5 mg/mL, concentration of bupivacaine is not recommended for obstetric (except spinal) or intravenous regional anesthesia. The upper limits for safe dosage with this drug are 150 mg without epinephrine and 200 mg with epinephrine. In patients who receive diazepam (Valium), bupivacaine can be potentiated because diazepam increases the bioavailability of bupivacaine. If bupivacaine is accidentally administered intravenously, acute cardiovascular collapse can ensue.

**Ropivacaine.** Ropivacaine is a local anesthetic that resembles bupivacaine in potency and length of action. It may have certain advantages over bupivacaine when used in obstetrics because it produces less motor blockage while it keeps the patient in an analgesic condition. Ropivacaine can be used for epidural anesthesia because it produces a rapid onset of sensory loss and has a relatively long duration.

**Levobupivacaine.** Levobupivacaine (Chirocaine) is a newly released amide local anesthetic that contains only the pure S-enantiomer of bupivacaine. Studies indicate that levobupivacaine may be less toxic than bupivacaine at similar analgesic concentrations. Currently, however, levobupivacaine does not have widespread use.

**Etidocaine.** Etidocaine (Duranest) resembles lidocaine in time of onset; however, its duration of action is considerably longer than that of lidocaine. It is effective in infiltration, spinal, epidural, and caudal anesthesia, and it can cause a profound motor blockade and, consequently, should not be administered to obstetric patients. The safe dosage limit for etidocaine is 300 mg without epinephrine and 400 mg with epinephrine.

***Tetracaine.*** Tetracaine (Pontocaine) is an ester local anesthetic that resembles procaine and chloroprocaine. It is metabolized by plasma pseudocholinesterase at a slower rate than other ester local anesthetics. It is used predominately for spinal anesthesia in a 1% solution. The dosage range for spinal anesthesia is usually between 5 and 20 mg, with an onset of about 7 to 10 minutes and a duration of about 60 to 90 minutes. The addition of a vasoconstrictor increases the duration of the spinal block to about 120 to 180 minutes. Tetracaine can be potentiated by cimetidine (Tagamet). When the blood concentration of tetracaine exceeds 8 μg/mL, serious problems can occur, including seizures and severe depression of the respiratory and cardiovascular systems.

### Complications of Use of Local Anesthetics

***Allergic Reactions.*** Allergic reactions to local anesthetic drugs can be divided into four types: (1) contact dermatitis; (2) serum sickness, which includes fever, lymphadenopathy, and urticaria 2 to 12 days after injection; (3) anaphylactic reaction, characterized by dyspnea, cyanosis, and death; and (4) atopic response, which includes bronchospasm, urticaria, and angioneurotic edema.

When the allergy is evaluated, the first consideration is whether or not the reaction is caused by

added epinephrine. Symptoms such as tachycardia, palpitations, restlessness, and anxiety indicate epinephrine as the causative agent.

***Overdosage.*** Overdosage of local anesthetic agents can occur because of inadvertent intravenous injection of the local anesthetic, variation in patient response, or injection of the local anesthetic into a highly vascular area. Box 24-2 summarizes the signs of overdosage of the local anesthetic agents.

## SUMMARY

The treatment and nursing care of a patient who has had an overdosage of a local anesthetic agent begin with the administration of 100% oxygen. Oxygen should be administered to the patient at the first sign of local anesthetic toxicity and should be followed by preparation for the management of convulsions, hypotension, and respiratory depression. Diazepam should be administered for suppression of local anesthetic-induced seizures. Intubation and mechanical ventilation may be indicated. Vasopressors such as epinephrine may also be indicated.

### BIBLIOGRAPHY

Barash P, Cullen B, Stoelting R: *Clinical anesthesia*, ed 5, Philadelphia, 2006, Lippincott, Williams & Wilkins.

Cousins M, Bridenbaugh P: Neural blockade. In *Clinical anesthesia and management of pain*, ed 3, Philadelphia, 1998, Lippincott-Raven.

De Jong R: *Local anesthetics*, St Louis, 1994, Mosby.

Gilman A, Rall T, Nies A, et al: *Goodman and Gilman's the pharmacological basis of therapeutics*, ed 9, New York, 1996, McGraw-Hill Press.

Guyton A: *Textbook of medical physiology*, ed 8, Philadelphia, 1991, Saunders.

Macintyre P, Ready B: *Acute pain management: a practical guide*, ed 2, New York, 2001, Saunders.

Mcleod G, Burke D: Levobupivacaine, *Anaesthesia* 56:331-341, 2001.

Miller R, editor: *Anesthesia*, ed 5, Philadelphia, 2000, Churchill Livingstone.

Saleh K: Practical points in understanding local anesthetics, *J Post Anesth Nurs* 7(1):45-47, 1992.

Schneider M, Ettlin T, Kaufmann M, et al: Transient neurologic toxicity after hyperbaric subarachnoid anesthesia with 5% lidocaine, *Anesth Analg* 76(5):1154-1157, 1993.

Waugaman W, Foster S, Rigor B: *Principles and practice of nurse anesthesia*, ed 3, Norwalk, CT, 1999, Appleton & Lange.

Wood M, Wood A: *Drugs and anesthesia: pharmacology for the anesthesiologist*, ed 2, Baltimore, 1990, Williams & Wilkins.

---

**Box 24-2 Signs of Overdosage of Local Anesthetic Agents**

**CENTRAL NERVOUS SYSTEM**
**Stimulation of:**
*Cortex*: Excitement, disorientation, euphoria, dizziness, hallucinations, muscle twitching, numbness of fingers or lips, and convulsions
*Medulla*:
　*Cardiovascular center*: Hypertension, tachycardia
　*Respiratory center*: Increased respiratory rate and variations in rhythm
　*Vomiting center*: Nausea and vomiting

**Depression of:**
*Cortex*: Unconsciousness
*Medulla*:
　*Vasomotor center*: Hypotension
　*Respiratory center*: Apnea

**PERIPHERAL NERVOUS SYSTEM**
*Heart*: Bradycardia from direct depression
*Blood vessels*: Vasodilatation from direct action

CONCEPTS IN ANESTHETIC AGENTS

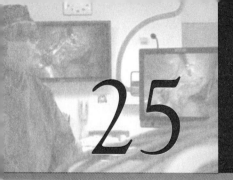

# 25

# REGIONAL ANESTHESIA

*Thomas Corey Davis, CRNA, MSNA*

Many surgical patients benefit greatly from the administration of regional anesthesia as opposed to general anesthesia. Regional anesthesia has the significant benefit of the ability for administration with medical conditions that require the patient to maintain many important physiologic functions during and after surgery. Consequently, the use of regional anesthesia has become popular in modern anesthesia practice because, when indicated, it offers many advantages over general inhalation anesthesia. For facilitation of optimal recovery of the surgical patient from this type of anesthetic, the perianesthesia nurse should have a strong knowledge base of all the particular regional anesthetic techniques used in today's art and science of anesthesia.

## DEFINITIONS

**Alpha-Adrenergic Vasopressors:** Drugs or substances used to cause peripheral vascular constriction that ultimately leads to increased blood pressure. Also referred to as alpha-adrenergic sympathomimetic drugs; agents that are in this classification include phenylephrine and norepinephrine. See Chapter 11 for a full description of the alpha-adrenergic system.
**Bradycardia:** Heart rate that is less than 60 bpm.
**Continuous (Serial) Epidural Technique (CSE):** Combined spinal-epidural technique is a combination spinal and epidural technique that is performed first with insertion of an epidural needle into the epidural space. A spinal needle is then passed through the epidural needle into the subarachnoid space, and spinal medication is injected. The spinal needle is then withdrawn, and a catheter is placed in the epidural space for future use.
**Dermatome Level:** That area of the skin that is supplied by a single spinal nerve.
**Epidural Block:** Produced by depositing an anesthetic agent in the epidural (peridural) space that results in a reduction in neuronal transmission of the exiting nerves from that area of deposition.
**High Spinal Block:** When the local anesthetic rises in the cerebrospinal fluid (CSF), the major nerves that exit the spinal cord can be effectively blocked.
**Hypotension:** Low blood pressure that is not adequate for normal perfusion and oxygenation of the tissues.
**Level of Anesthesia:** After a spinal or epidural anesthetic is administered, the level (or how high the numbness that was produced) is assessed with dermatones, which are determined by the area on the surface of the body that is innervated by afferent fibers from one spinal root. This assessment can be accomplished with a small pin, wet cotton ball, or alcohol sponge.
**Neuraxial Blocks:** The insertion of a needle and injection of a local anesthetic drug into a plane of the central nervous system or neuraxis that results in a motor, sensory, and sympathetic blockade. Spinal, epidural, and caudal blocks are examples of neuraxial blocks.
**Palsies:** A condition that is characterized by paralysis.
**Paralysis:** The loss of muscle function that includes the loss of sensation.
**Preemptive Analgesia:** Administration of a analgesic agent before surgery.
**Prophylactic:** Use of a drug or therapeutic agent for prevention of an untoward event. For example, administration of an antiemetic in its therapeutic range in an effort to prevent the untoward event of postoperative nausea and vomiting (PONV).
**Regional Anesthesia:** Refers to the various anesthetic techniques that use local anesthetic agents to block nerve conduction in an extremity or a region of the body.
**Spinal Headache:** Usually caused by a persistent leak of CSF through the needle hole in the dura mater; ranges from transient pain to quite severe.
**Tuffier's Line:** The imaginary line drawn between the iliac crests that aids the anesthesia practitioner in the identification of the L3-L4 interspace.

**Urinary Retention:** A condition in which the patient has an incomplete emptying of the bladder at the end of voiding.

## SPINAL AND EPIDURAL ANESTHESIA

### Anatomy of the Spine

The vertebral column comprises 33 vertebrae (7 cervical, 12 thoracic, 5 lumbar, 5 sacral, and 4 coccygeal). The ligaments of the vertebral column, which bind it together and protect the spinal cord, are the supraspinous ligament, intraspinous ligament, ligamentum flavum, posterior longitudinal ligament, and anterior longitudinal ligament (Fig. 25-1). When a midline spinal puncture is made, the needle traverses the first three ligaments.

The spinal cord, which is a continuation of the medulla oblongata, occupies the upper two thirds of the vertebral canal. It is approximately 18 inches long and ends at the lower border of L1. The lower portion of the spinal cord then becomes the filum terminale, which connects to the bone of the coccyx vertebra and holds the spinal cord in place. The spinal cord is encased by three membranes: the dura mater, the arachnoid, and the pia mater. The outermost membrane is the dura mater, which consists of two layers (periosteal and dural) and ends at S2. Between the dura and the ligamentum flavum is the epidural space, which is a potential space filled with loose fatty tissue and blood vessels. Local anesthetic solutions are introduced in this space when the epidural regional anesthetic technique is used. The arachnoid layer consists of a thin membranous sheath. The innermost layer is called the pia mater, and it is separated from the arachnoid layer by a subarachnoid space filled with cerebrospinal fluid (CSF).

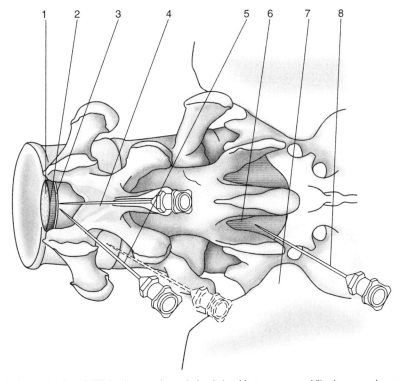

**Fig. 25-1** Dorsal view of fourth and fifth lumbar vertebrae, their relationship to sacrum and iliac bones, and most frequently used approaches for needle puncture in subarachnoid and lumbar peridural techniques. Numerals represent the following: (1), cauda equina; (2), dura mater; (3), ligamentum flavum at L3-L4 interspace; (4), midline approach for spinal and epidural techniques where needle is introduced between spines of L3 and L4 vertebrae, traversing supraspinous and interspinous ligaments before piercing ligamentum flavum; (5), paramedian approach at this level where needle puncture site is 1 to 2 cm lateral to above midline approach; if initial approach results in contacting lamina of vertebrae as shown in *dotted needle silhouette*, then needle is walked cephalad and medially until it slips off lamina and contacts ligamentum flavum as shown; (6), large interspace between S5 and L1, which is situated 2 cm medial and cephalad from; (7), posterior superior iliac spine; (8), needle can be introduced at this site in Taylor approach for either subarachnoid or epidural puncture. *(From Miller R: Anesthesia, ed 2, New York, 2000, Churchill Livingstone.)*

This space is where local anesthetic solutions are deposited when the spinal technique of producing regional anesthesia is used.

Thirty-one pairs of spinal nerves travel from the spinal column through the layers of the cord and exit at the intervertebral foramina. There are 8 cervical, 12 thoracic, 5 lumbar, 5 sacral, and 1 coccygeal pairs of spinal nerves. These nerves are blocked by the local anesthetic drug to produce anesthesia.

### Spinal Anesthetics

*Techniques of Administration.* Because a lumbar puncture may be performed in the postanesthesia unit (PACU), a brief description of the procedure of lumbar puncture is presented. Before the procedure is started, the perianesthesia nurse should ensure that the spinal (or epidural) procedure is not contraindicated. According to Barash, patient refusal is the only absolute contraindication to spinal anesthesia. Several preexisting conditions or treatments increase the risk-to-benefit ratio and must be carefully considered for each individual patient. These relative contraindications include uncorrected hypovolemia, infection at the planned site of injection, sepsis, anatomic abnormalities such as scoliosis, increased intracranial pressure, coagulopathy or thrombocytopenia, and a recent history of anticoagulation therapy.

Once the determination has been made that the spinal procedure is not contraindicated, the PACU nurse should obtain the patient's baseline vital signs. These include the blood pressure, pulse, respiratory rate, and oxygen saturation. The blood pressure cuff and pulse oximeter should remain in place throughout the procedure. Also, the nurse should describe the procedure to the patient and answer any questions the patient might have. Verbal contact with the patient throughout the procedure is important in reduction of fear and anxiety.

Proper positioning of the patient is of particular importance in the success of this procedure. The lateral decubitus position or sitting position can be used. For placement of the patient in the lateral decubitus position, the patient is turned on the side, the knees are bent and drawn up near the patient's chin, and the back is arched out toward the person who performs the lumbar puncture. A pillow may be placed under the patient's head to help align the spine and to add comfort during the procedure. The assistant should stand near the patient's stomach, securing the knees and providing for safety throughout the procedure. At this time, the patient's back should be inspected for signs of any dermatologic infectious process that may be present. If an infectious process near the lumbar puncture site is found, the procedure should be canceled. Once the patient is properly positioned, the person who performs the procedure should first wash his or her hands, then open the lumbar puncture tray so that the sterile components are available, and then, with sterile technique, don the sterile gloves. The drugs are then drawn into the syringes, and the needles and equipment are examined for any signs of damage. The back is then washed (prepped) with antiseptic solution, after which the sterile drapes are placed over the patient's back. Throughout the procedure, the PACU nurse should continue to explain each maneuver to the patient.

An imaginary line, called Tuffier's line, is then drawn between the iliac crests. This line crosses the spine between the third or fourth lumbar interspace. Because the spinal cord terminates at the L2 interspace, from L3 and below are used when the lumbar puncture is performed. Once the interspace has been identified, a local anesthetic (usually lidocaine) is deposited subcutaneously and into the supraspinous ligament with a 25-gauge needle. A needle introducer is then placed through the skin, the supraspinous ligament, and interspinous ligaments. The spinal needle is inserted through the introducer and is passed through the ligamentum flavum and the dura and enters the subarachnoid space. The stylet is removed, and CSF can be seen at the hub of the needle. Blood-tinged CSF or lack of free flow is a contraindication to the injection of the anesthetic solution. If the blood-tinged CSF becomes clear, the anesthetic solution can be administered. Before the syringe is connected to the hub of the needle, the patient should be secured and told not to move or cough by the PACU nurse. The patient should also be told that the legs will feel warm after the anesthetic solution is injected. The syringe is then secured to the hub of the needle, and after aspiration to ensure that CSF is still present, the anesthetic solution is injected. After the solution is injected, the syringe is aspirated for verification of the presence of CSF, confirming the introduction of the medications into the subarachnoid space. After confirmation, the syringe, needle, and introducer are removed simultaneously. Next, the patient is placed in the supine position by the PACU nurse and the person who performed the lumbar puncture. Before the patient is moved, the patient should be told not to try to move or cough because that increases the spread of the anesthetics.

Once the patient is supine, the blood pressure, pulse, respiratory rate, and oxygen saturation should be assessed at 1-minute intervals for the first 5 to 10 minutes and then every 5 minutes during the next half hour. If the oxygen saturation drops below 94% or the blood pressure decreases by 20% of the baseline reading, the anesthesia practitioner should be notified immediately.

If a local anesthetic was administered into the subarachnoid space, the dermatome level (Fig. 25-2) should be closely monitored with a supersaturated alcohol sponge or a pin. With either method, patients should be informed fully about the procedure to ascertain the dermatome level. In this procedure, the nurse touches the patient's shoulders with either the alcohol sponge or the pin. The patient is instructed to tell the nurse when the same sensation is felt. The nurse then touches the skin with the sponge or pin at about the sacral area and moves up slowly at intervals of about 1 inch, corresponding with the dermatomes. When the patient says the sensation is the same as the one felt on the shoulder, that dermatome is so noted (see Fig. 25-2) as the level of the anesthetic.

***Mechanism of Action.*** After the local anesthetic drug is injected into the subarachnoid space, a level of anesthesia is achieved that is dependent on the dosage of the agent used, the rate of injection, the specific gravity of the fluid injected, and the position of the patient after injection. The level of anesthesia is referred to as the dermatome level (see Fig. 25-2). A dermatome is that area of the skin that is supplied by a single spinal nerve. The face is supplied by the trigeminal nerve, and the remaining portions of the body's cutaneous areas are supplied in sequence by dermatomes C2 through S5. Some of the major topographic landmarks that can be depicted with a pinprick for detection of sensory loss are L1 to T12, the inguinal ligament and iliac crest; T10, the umbilicus; T6, the xiphoid; T4, the nipples; T1, the clavicle; and C7, the middle finger. The order of blockage of the various nerve modalities is shown in Table 24-1 in Chapter 24.

During the recovery from spinal anesthetic, the anesthesia works its way back from the extremities toward the site where the anesthetic was administered. Therefore, the areas near the site of injection are the last to recover.

***Complications.*** The complications of spinal anesthesia are high spinal block, hypotension, nausea and vomiting, backache, palsies and paralysis, urinary retention, postspinal headache, and meningitis.

**High Spinal Block.** When the local anesthetic rises in the CSF, the major nerves that exit the spinal cord can be effectively blocked. The effects of the spread of the anesthetic into the

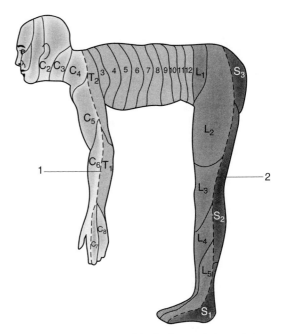

**Fig. 25-2** Dermatomes of body show orderly craniad to caudad sequence. By positioning the body as shown, complex arrangement of dermatomes on the limbs is more readily understood. On upper extremity, limb dermatomes are distributed symmetrically about axial line (1). Note that dermatomes C5 and C6 are distributed on preaxial border of limb and that postaxial dermatomes, C8, T1, and T2, are distributed on postaxial part of limb. C7, which is central dermatome of limb, is distributed more distally, that is, over middle finger. Orderly sequence on trunk from T3 to L1 is seen. Dermatome distribution of lower extremity is also arranged around axial line (2). Large areas of skin, that is, L2 and L3, have been borrowed from trunk to supplement true leg dermatomes of L4 through S3. Note that as in upper extremity, craniad dermatomes, L4 and L5, are distributed on preaxial border of limb and caudad dermatomes, S2 and S3, are distributed on postaxial border of limb. Central dermatome S1 is distributed over lateral aspect of plantar surface and lateral border of foot. *(Adapted from Foerster O: The dermatomes in man, Brain 56:1, 1933; by permission of Oxford University Press.)*

cervical region are usually short lived because dilution of the anesthetic produces a lower concentration of the drug. Some objective symptoms associated with a high spinal anesthetic are agitation, hypotension, nausea, diaphragmatic breathing (absence of intercostal muscle function), and an inability to speak in an audible fashion. The treatment of a high spinal block is initiated in the operating room and consists of efficient ventilation and oxygenation and the maintenance of the blood pressure with vasopressors. This block is a reversible complication; when the local anesthetic drug wears off, the patient recovers. PACU care consists of maintenance of the treatment initiated in the operating room. The patient may undergo intubation and possibly placement on a ventilator. As the local anesthetic agent wears off, the patient may not have maintenance of tidal volume because of partial paralysis of the respiratory muscles. Ventilation of the patient should be assisted until an adequate tidal volume can be spontaneously maintained. Placement of the patient in a head-up position in an effort to limit the spread of the anesthetic is inadvisable; the anesthetic is already "fixed" at a level in the CSF, and raising the head can reduce cerebral blood flow, resulting in medullary ischemia.

The PACU nurse should establish verbal contact with the patient to decrease the anxiety and apprehension felt because of partial sedation, difficulty in breathing, and inability to move about.

For enhancement of cardiac output, the patient's legs may be elevated to promote the return of venous blood from the lower extremities to the heart. If the vital signs still indicate neurogenic shock after this maneuver has been performed, vasopressor therapy usually is instituted. Vasopressors used to treat this complication are usually of the alpha-adrenergic variety because total spinal block produces a type of neurogenic shock. The alpha-adrenergic vasopressors produce peripheral vasoconstriction, which aids in returning the blood to the heart, thereby improving the cardiac output. Alpha-adrenergic vasopressors that may be used in this situation are phenylephrine (Neo-Synephrine) or norepinephrine (Levophed) and are discussed in Chapter 11.

Because of the height of the spinal block, the patient may also have some bradycardia, which can be treated with atropine or glycopyrrolate (Robinul). Nausea and vomiting may also occur. Suction should be available, and antiemetics may have to be administered to the patient.

**Hypotension.** Postoperative hypotension as a result of a sympathetic blockade from a spinal anesthetic leads to venous dilation, which results in a decreased venous return and a reduction in the cardiac output. This problem is most likely to occur during the first 30 minutes in the PACU. If the patient's condition is hypotensive, assessment for bleeding, which may be causing the hypotension, is important. If bleeding is not the cause, treatment should be instituted and the anesthesiologist or anesthetist should be notified. If bleeding is the cause, the attending physician should be notified. The first line of treatment is to ensure that hydration is adequate. Often, infusion of 500 mL of crystalloid along with elevation of the legs corrects the

postoperative spinal hypotension. If the hypotension continues, it can best be treated with vasopressors.

**Nausea and Vomiting.** Nausea and vomiting can be a result of hypotension, of hypertension from the vasopressors, of motion during change in position, or of apprehension. If hypotension or hypertension is present, the anesthetist should be notified. The PACU nurse must assess the cause of the nausea and vomiting. Blood pressure should be taken and oxygen administered to the patient. In the event of vomiting, the patient should be placed in a Trendelenburg position with the head to the side, and a clear airway should be established and maintained. The anesthetist should be summoned if the patient has nausea or vomiting (see Chapter 29).

**Palsies and Paralysis.** Palsies and paralysis usually occur after surgery in the peripheral nerves. Of the cranial nerves, the sixth cranial nerve is most often involved. In the PACU phase of the spinal anesthetic, the nurse should assess neurologic function of the extremities as the anesthetic wears off. If the patient has double vision or any other decrease in peripheral nerve function, the anesthetist and the surgeon should be notified.

**Urinary Retention.** Urinary retention is usually caused by trauma to the bladder during surgery or by a decrease in bladder tone from the anesthesia. The patient has severe pain and may have hypertension or bradycardia. If the condition is not diagnosed and corrected, the patient may become incoherent and thrash about in bed. The PACU nurse should assess the patient for a distended bladder or hypoxia because the symptoms are almost identical. If urinary retention is the problem, the patient should be encouraged to void. If the patient cannot void, the surgeon should be notified and an order for catheterization of the bladder obtained.

**Postspinal Headache.** The true postspinal headache is caused by a persistent leak of CSF through the needle hole in the dura mater. Postspinal headache is usually transient but annoying to the patient. The pain often becomes severe when the patient is upright and lessens with a supine position. The location of the pain is usually occipital or frontal. The patient may also have tinnitus and diplopia.

As a prophylactic measure, most patients who have received a spinal anesthetic are encouraged to remain in the supine position for at least 6 to 8 hours after surgery. Some research indicates that the supine-bedrest prophylaxis is unnecessary and of no value in prevention of postspinal headache. The advent of smaller-gauge needles has reduced the incidence rate of postspinal headache. Conservative treatment for this complication involves optimal hydration, analgesics, and reduction in environmental noise. However, if the postspinal headache becomes incapacitating or does not respond to conservative treatment within the first 2 days after the administration of the spinal anesthetic, an epidural blood patch procedure may be performed. This procedure involves administration of 10 to 20 mL of the patient's own blood into the epidural space at the site of the previous lumbar puncture. This procedure seals the hole in the dura mater; prompt pain relief usually follows.

### Epidural Anesthetics

*Mechanism of Action.* Epidural (peridural) block is produced by depositing an anesthetic agent in the epidural space. The location on the vertebral column or the segment where the epidural block is performed determines the type of epidural anesthesia the patient receives. Thoracic epidural block, lumbar epidural block, and caudal epidural block are the possible types of epidural anesthetic.

*Techniques of Administration.* Epidural block is usually performed in the same manner as the spinal block. The patient is placed into the sitting or lateral decubitus position, the back is prepped, and the needle is inserted into the epidural space. After the needle has been determined to be in the epidural space, a test dose of the anesthetic solution is injected. Blood pressure, pulse, respiratory rate, and oxygen saturation are then determined. If vital signs are unchanged, the remainder of the anesthetic is incrementally administered. The needle may be removed, or a catheter may be placed through the needle into the epidural space for the continuous (serial) epidural technique. Monitoring the patient after epidural block is similar to monitoring after the spinal technique.

The morphine epidural technique is becoming popular for reduction of postoperative pain. Epidural morphine may be administered during surgery or in the immediate postoperative period. The pharmacology of epidural morphine is discussed in detail in Chapters 22 and 31. The major risk with epidural morphine is respiratory depression. Epidural morphine can depress respiration with an onset of 2.5 to 16.5 hours or longer. Consequently, monitoring for respiratory depression requires close surveillance of the patient's respiratory rate and oxygen saturation. For enhancement of the monitoring parameters, an apnea monitor should be used as another alarm system to alert PACU personnel to the patient's respiratory depression. Fentanyl in a

continuous infusion or in a patient-controlled method is also used for postoperative pain management. Fentanyl may have a lower incidence rate of side effects such as pruritus and respiratory depression. This drug is discussed in Chapter 22.

The epidural block is the anesthetic technique of choice for cesarean section and is indicated in patients at high risk and in those with cardiac, pulmonary, and metabolic diseases. It is also well suited for patients who have had thoracic or upper abdominal surgical procedures. In this instance, the epidural is usually placed before surgery and the patient may receive both general and epidural anesthesia. This combination of two anesthesia techniques has been quite successful in reduction of postoperative pulmonary complications and enhancement of pain relief.

The epidural block is contraindicated in patients who refuse the block, in those undergoing anticoagulant therapy, when hemorrhage or shock is present, when the patient has had previous back surgery, and when local inflammation exists.

### Combined Spinal-epidural Technique

The combined spinal-epidural (CSE) technique is a combination spinal and epidural technique that is performed first with insertion of an epidural needle into the epidural space. A spinal needle is then passed through the epidural needle into the subarachnoid space, and spinal medication is injected. The spinal needle is then withdrawn, and a catheter is placed in the epidural space for future use. Because of the versatility of this combined technique, CSE is gaining in popularity. The CSE technique minimizes or eliminates some of the disadvantages of both spinal and epidural while maintaining the advantages. Specifically, CSE offers the rapid onset, profound analgesia, and reduced toxicity of spinal block combined with the potential for improving an inadequate block or lengthening the duration of anesthesia with epidural supplementation via epidural catheter. Preparation for anesthesia, side effects, precautions, contraindications, and postoperative care are essentially the same as for spinal and epidural block. The CSE technique is most commonly used in obstetrics and for orthopedic, general, urologic, and gynecologic surgery.

### PACU Care After Spinal, Epidural, or Combined Spinal-epidural Anesthesia

After the patient's arrival in the PACU, care must be exercised in moving the patient because the block's residual effects, such as lack of motor and sensory function, are still present. Care should be taken in positioning the patient because good body alignment is needed for reduction of muscle soreness or injury. The patient's joints should not be hyperextended, and the bedclothes should not press on the toes.

If a patient has any residual spinal anesthesia while in the PACU, care should be taken to avoid rapid position change, which causes severe decreases in blood pressure. The circulatory system cannot compensate adequately for rapid position change when anesthesia is present.

If intravenous sedation was given during the operation, respiratory function should be monitored closely with the use of a pulse oximeter. Oxygen should be administered to all patients with a block until the motor and sensory functions return adequately. The patient should be encouraged to cough and breathe deeply every 15 minutes to reduce the incidence of atelectasis.

The patient should be checked for any signs of bladder distention. Catheterization may be necessary, especially in patients who have had pelvic or perineal surgery.

## AXILLARY OR BRACHIAL PLEXUS BLOCK

Nerve blocks are used to produce anesthesia in specific areas of the body. They are usually used for orthopedic, obstetric, and vascular surgical procedures. They are relatively safe and usually have good patient acceptance.

The axillary or brachial plexus block is used to anesthetize the arm for surgery below the elbow. When this block is performed, either the axillary or the supraclavicular approach is used.

### PACU Care After Axillary or Brachial Plexus Block

The PACU care of the patient who has received an axillary block centers on patient education and observation for complications. The patient should be taught that motor function will be lost and that no attempts should be made to move the arm about. Injuries to the face and to the surgical site have been reported because of the patient's attempts to move the arm. With reduced motor control, the affected arm could flop onto the face or onto a side rail, resulting in injury.

If the supraclavicular approach was used, pneumothorax is a possible complication. The first sign is pain in the chest that is accentuated with deep breathing. Other signs of pneumothorax are increased resonance to percussion, absence of or decreased breath sounds, lag in expansion on the affected side in comparison with the unaffected side, and difficulty in "getting breath."

The PACU care involves administering oxygen and advising the anesthetist of the complication. Analgesics are usually administered, and after a chest radiograph is made, more definitive treatment may be instituted.

When the interscalene or supraclavicular approach is used in the brachial plexus block, Horner's syndrome can result. This syndrome occurs when the anesthetic solution spreads so that it involves the stellate ganglion. Symptoms of this syndrome, which appear on the side where the block is performed, are flushing of the face, constricted pupils, ptosis, and stuffiness of the nose. Horner's syndrome clears as the block wears off.

Another complication with the interscalene, infraclavicular, or supraclavicular approach is blockage of the phrenic nerve. This complication is related to the spread of anesthetic solution and is usually unilateral. Generally, no signs and symptoms occur, and the complication clears as the block dissipates itself.

Obliteration of the radial pulse is a possible complication of the axillary approach to the brachial plexus. It is caused by bleeding or the use of too large a volume of anesthetic solution. The radial pulse usually returns in 2 to 4 hours.

### The Brachial Plexus Indwelling Catheter

With the increasing use of ultrasound scan–guided approaches to the brachial plexus has come an increasing incidence rate of placement of a catheter into the brachial plexus. These catheters, much like the catheters placed for epidural anesthesia, eliminate the reliance on the single-shot approach to the brachial plexus by allowing the anesthetist to redose the anesthetic, or even provide a continuous infusion of local anesthetic. These catheters may be left in place for 4 to 7 days after the procedure to provide continued pain relief and even to induce vasodilation beneficial for limb replantation. Care of these patients follows the same guidelines as any other brachial plexus blocks, and care of the dressing and catheter site is the same as for an epidural catheter.

## INTRAVENOUS REGIONAL ANESTHESIA

The intravenous regional, or Bier, block was named for August K. Bier, who originated it in 1908. It is useful for emergency procedures on the forearm and hand, especially for a procedure such as Colles' fracture reduction, and is simple to administer. The Bier block involves starting an intravenous infusion in the hand, exsanguinating the arm with an Esmarch latex bandage, inflating a double pneumatic tourniquet above the elbow, and then removing the Esmarch bandage and injecting the local anesthetic agent (lidocaine) while the tourniquet remains inflated. At the end of the surgical procedure, the tourniquet is released and the analgesia ceases within 5 to 10 minutes. Usually, no sequelae occur from the anesthetic agent; by the time the venous blood from the limb has passed through the lungs and has mixed with the rest of the venous return, the systemic arterial blood levels are, because of the dilution effect, not clinically significant. Should the blood levels of the local anesthetic remain high, the patient will have cardiovascular depression, which is usually manifested by bradycardia. This cardiovascular depression is usually quite transient. If this situation arises, vigilant monitoring, coupled with appropriate interventions such as oxygen and glycopyrrolate (Robinul) or atropine, usually corrects the problem.

The intravenous regional technique can also be used for surgery on the lower leg and foot. Although it requires a larger tourniquet and more local anesthetic agent, it is an effective technique for this type of surgery.

### PACU Care After Intravenous Regional Anesthesia

When the patient arrives in the PACU, all analgesia provided by the local anesthetic agent used in the intravenous regional anesthesia has usually dissipated. Medication for the relief of pain can be given soon after the patient's arrival. The PACU nurse should assess the patient's level of sedation, including the amount of premedication and sedation during the surgical procedure, before administering the pain medication.

## SUMMARY

Regional anesthesia is a excellent adjunct anesthetic technique available to the anesthesia practitioner. It can be used as the anesthetic as opposed to a general inhalational anesthetic. Regional anesthetics can also be used as adjuncts to general anesthesia in an effort to reduce postoperative pain. This chapter introduced the basics of the subarachnoid and epidural regional anesthetics and the most popular peripheral nerve blocks used in the operating room and ambulatory surgery.

## BIBLIOGRAPHY

Barash P, Cullen B, Stoelting R: *Clinical anesthesia*, ed 5, Philadelphia, 2006, Lippincott, Williams, & Wilkins.

Cousins M, Bridenbaugh P: *Neural blockade in clinical anesthesia and management of pain*, ed 3, Philadelphia, 1998, Lippincott-Raven.

Cramer C: Postanesthetic management of regional anesthesia, *J Post Anesth Nurs* 1(4):243-256, 1986.

Gilman A, Rall T, Nies A, et al: *Goodman and Gilman's the pharmacological basis of therapeutics*, ed 9, New York, 1996, McGraw-Hill Press.

Kingsley C: Epidural analgesia: your role, *RN* 64(3):53-57, 2001.

Macintyre P, Ready B: *Acute pain management: a practical guide*, ed 2, New York, 2001, Saunders.

McCamant K: Peripheral nerve blocks: understanding the nurse's role, *J PeriAnesthesia Nurs* 21(1):16-23, 2006.

Miller R, editor: *Anesthesia*, ed 5, Philadelphia, 2000, Churchill Livingstone.

Rawal N, Van Zundert A, Holmstrom B, et al: Combined spinal-epidural technique, *Regional Anesthesia* 24(5):406-425, 1997.

Wood M, Wood A: *Drugs and anesthesia: pharmacology for the anesthesiologist*, ed 2, Baltimore, 1990, Williams & Wilkins.

CONCEPTS IN ANESTHETIC AGENTS

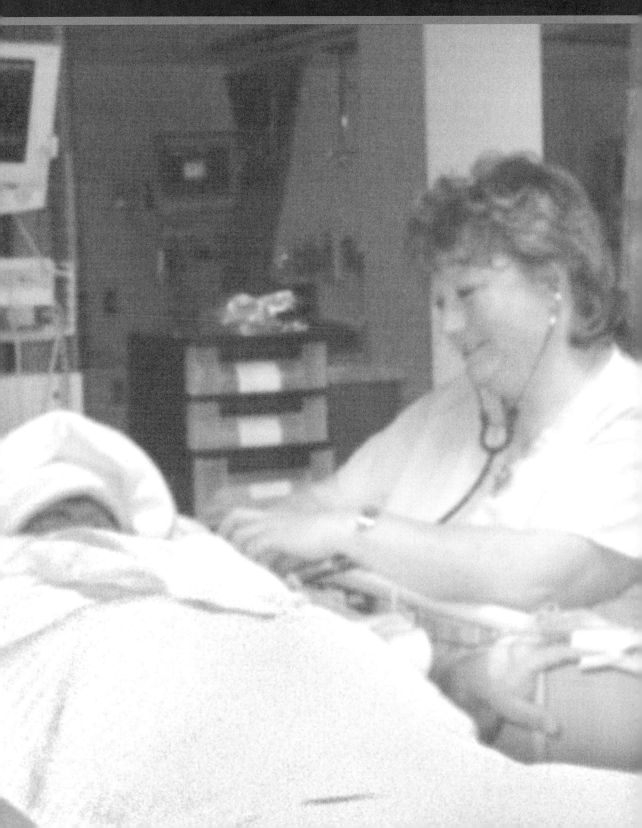

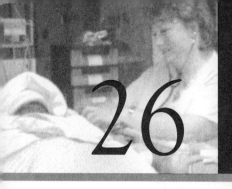

# 26

# TRANSITION FROM THE OPERATING ROOM TO THE PACU

*Kay Ball, RN, BSN, MSA, CNOR, FAAN*

The practice of nursing is directed toward the assessment, planning, implementation, and evaluation of the patient's care through a continuum of patient care services. Often the nurse is involved with the patient's transition from one level of care to another as the patient is transferred from one specialty area to another. This transition of care is common in the surgical environment as perioperative nurses and anesthesia providers transfer the patient's care to a perianesthesia nurse at the completion of an operative procedure or treatment. Clear communication among these professionals is critical and directly affects the patient's postoperative response and outcome.

Care of the surgical patient today is quite complex because advanced technology, minimally invasive techniques, and new anesthetic agents challenge perioperative nurses to communicate a comprehensive report when shifting the patient's care to the perianesthesia nurse. This chapter describes the importance of communication and what should be communicated when a patient is transitioned from the operating room to the postanesthesia care unit (PACU).

## PERIOPERATIVE NURSING

According to the Association of PeriOperative Registered Nurses (AORN), "the registered nurse specializing in perioperative nursing practice performs nursing activities in the preoperative, intraoperative, and postoperative phases of the patient's surgical experience."[1] Perioperative nursing services can be delivered in a variety of environments, from the preoperative area to the PACU. The model for competency for perioperative nurses is seen through perioperative assessment, diagnosis, outcome identification, planning, implementation, and evaluation. This "nursing process encompasses all significant actions taken by the nurse in providing care to all patients and forms the foundation of clinical decision making."[1] A perioperative nurse, therefore, has the requisite skills and knowledge to use the nursing process to design, coordinate, and

deliver care to patients to meet their specific needs when their protective reflexes or self-care abilities are potentially compromised because of an operative or invasive procedure.[1] The care of the surgical patient continues through the transportation to the PACU where this care is transferred to the perianesthesia nurse.

## PERIANESTHESIA NURSING

According to the American Society of Peri-Anesthesia Nurses, the Scope of PeriAnesthesia Nursing Practice involves the "assessment for, diagnosis of, intervention for, and evaluation of physical or psychosocial problems or risks for problems that may result from the administration of sedation/analgesia or anesthetic agents and techniques... [The practice] is systematic in nature and includes the nursing process, decision-making, analytical and scientific thinking, and inquiry... [Perianesthesia nursing's] unique knowledge base regarding sedation/analgesia and anesthetic agents and techniques, the physiological and psychological responses to them, and the vulnerability of the patient subjected to them is coupled with all the principles of age-specific medical-surgical and critical care nursing."[2] Perianesthesia nursing is multidimensional and encompasses patient care during the preanesthesia phase (patient assessment, preparation, and education) to postanesthesia phase I (transition from the immediate postanesthesia period to phase II), postanesthesia phase II (preparation of patient/family/significant other for care of the patient in the home or in an extended care environment), and postanesthesia phase III (ongoing care for those surgical patients who need extended observation or intervention after discharge from phase I or II).[2]

The perianesthesia nurse has a responsibility to the patient to provide quality care and safety. The Perianesthesia Standards for Ethical Practice state that the perianesthesia nurse "communicates pertinent information as the patient progresses through the continuum of perianesthesia care."[2] The nurse also has the professional responsibility to discuss "patient information with appropriate healthcare providers as needed to ensure optimum care."[2]

The American Society of PeriAnesthesia Nurses' (ASPAN) Resource 4 "Criteria for initial, ongoing, and discharge assessment and management" maintains that when the patient's care is transferred from the perioperative nurse to the perianesthesia nurse, the integration of the information about the patient should include[2]:

- Relevant preoperative status
- Anesthesia or sedation technique and agents
- Length of time anesthesia or sedation was administered; time reversal agents
- Pain and comfort management interventions and plan
- Medications administered
- Type of procedure
- Estimated fluid or blood loss and replacement
- Complications that occurred during anesthesia course; treatment initiated; response
- Emotional status on arrival to the operating or procedure room

The perioperative nurse or the anesthesia provider should remain in the PACU until the PACU nurse accepts the responsibility of the nursing care of the patient. Patient safety is compromised when a patient is transferred to the PACU and abandoned by the transporting surgical team members before the perianesthesia nurse is able to assume the responsibility for that patient's care.

## COMMUNICATION BETWEEN PERIOPERATIVE AND PERIANESTHESIA NURSES

However nurses describe their practices or roles (perioperative or perianesthesia), the basic foundation of nursing practice remains the same: high-quality care for the surgical patient. Therefore, nurses who provide care during surgical procedures that involve sedation, analgesia, or anesthetics must work closely with nurses who provide care after the procedure to foster continuity, quality services, and desired patient outcomes.

The perioperative nurse must establish a safe environment for the transportation of the surgical patient with use of transportation safety devices, plans for special patient needs during transfer (e.g., oxygen needs), and active participation in the safe transportation of the patient. An outcome that constantly should be addressed

is the "patient is free from signs and symptoms of injury related to transfer/transport."[1] The patient's individual needs are determined so that the patient can be transferred without injury and without alteration in the patient's condition, such as changes in temperature, respirations, tissue perfusion, discomfort, or pain.

The transportation and transference of care of the surgical patient involves planning, collaboration, and communication between the perioperative and perianesthesia registered nurses. Communication between perioperative and perianesthesia nurses is essential for patient safety and appropriate and consistent nursing care.[1] This communication can be in the form of verbal and written reports.

### Hand-off Communication

The Joint Commission's National Patient Safety Goals includes implementation of a standardized approach to hand-off communication.[3] This standardized approach to patient hand off must also include the opportunity to ask and respond to questions. Parameters for information to be shared depend on the situation. The interface between the preoperative nurse to OR nurse and the OR nurse to PACU nurse are crucial to continuity of care and safety for the patient. Standardizing a process where information about patient care is communicated in a consistent manner assures that the information about the patient will be accurate and pertinent.

### Written and Verbal Communication

Written documentation provides a basis for verbal reports and is usually in the form of standardized operative or anesthesia records. AORN's recommended practice for "Documentation of Perioperative Nursing Care" notes that the "patient's record should reflect the perioperative patient's plan of care, including assessment, diagnosis, outcome identification, planning, implementation, and evaluation."[1] Documentation should include information about the patient's status, assessment notes, plan of care, nursing interventions, and a continuous evaluation of nursing care and patient responses. The written patient operative record facilitates communication and provides continuity of care and also serves as a legal record of the care provided.

A verbal report is used for a "snapshot" or abbreviated synopsis of the patient status and care delivered. The perioperative nurse should give direct and concise information about the surgical patient in a consistent and organized manner. The perianesthesia nurse must listen to the report and ask questions when

NURSING CARE IN THE PACU

appropriate. Effective listening involves more effort than speaking because concentration is vital for processing of this critical information. Feedback by the perianesthesia nurse is often needed for clarification so that information is not misinterpreted.

For an examination of the issues of communication and documentation between the perioperative nurse and the perianesthesia nurse, the basic questions of why, when, where, who, how, and what must be explored.

WHY: Verbal reports highlight written documentation on the patient record. A written report records the details of the patient care, whereas a verbal report is a quick description or overview used when the patient's care is transferred to another nurse. This communication and documentation is vital so that continuity and safe patient care can be maintained.

WHEN: A formal written report begins with the admission of the patient for the surgical procedure and extends through discharge from the surgical arena. Written reports that document patient information before admission or after discharge may be added to the patient's chart. A verbal report from the perioperative nurse to the perianesthesia nurse begins with the call to the PACU to announce the completion of the surgical procedure and the request to transfer the patient to the PACU. At this time, any special needs must be communicated (i.e., ventilator needed). The verbal report continues when the patient is actually admitted to the PACU.

WHERE: Ideally the written patient record is kept with the patient during transfer from the operating room into the PACU. The verbal report is given when the patient's care is transferred from the perioperative nurse to the perianesthesia nurse in the PACU. Sometimes with a recovering patient from the obstetric unit, the postanesthesia care may be delivered in an area outside the normal postanesthesia care unit. Wherever the postanesthesia care is given, the standards of care (including communication) are no different than those used for nonobstetric surgical patients.[4]

WHO: Written patient reports are completed by the perioperative nurse, anesthesia provider, and the surgeon (or a designee). Usually the verbal report is given by the anesthesia provider and the perioperative registered nurse. In a few surgical environments, the perioperative nurse may phone the perianesthesia nurse to give a report while the anesthesia provider and an orderly (patient care assistant) transfer the patient to the PACU. Ideally the perioperative nurse and anesthesia provider should both accompany the patient to the PACU.

Sometimes the surgeon or the surgical assistant may also participate in the patient transportation and verbal report.

HOW: The written patient record is documented on a health care facility–approved standardized form. The verbal report is usually given in person from one professional to another, but verbal reports have also been given via telephone or computer, depending on the patient acuity and facility protocols.

WHAT IS REPORTED: The reporting of specific and appropriate information about the patient's surgical experience is critical. The perianesthesia nurse must receive the full details of the patient's condition, interventions, and plan of care so that continuity and safety can be maintained.

Care of certain patients, such as the patient recovering from cesarean section, can pose unique challenges. Documentation and verbal reports should alert the perianesthesia nurse to watch for signs and symptoms of adverse anesthetic effects, pulmonary problems, hemorrhage, infection, and other specific potential complications.[4] The care of a pregnant patient who is transferred from the operating room presents distinctive challenges because the status of the fetus must also be assessed, documented, and verbally reported.

The AORN Standards, Recommended Practices, and Guidelines are similar to the ASPAN recommendations previously noted; the AORN suggests that patient reporting should include but not be limited to:[1]

- Type of surgery; length of surgery; complications encountered
- Vital signs and airway patency (e.g., oxygen saturation)
- Level of consciousness
- Muscular strength (e.g., mobility limitations)
- Allergies
- Condition of operative site and dressing
- Location and patency of tubes or drains
- Medications given and response to those medications (e.g., anesthetic agents and technique, reversal agents)
- Intake and output (e.g., intravenous [IV], estimated blood loss)
- Tests ordered, with pertinent results, if available
- Pain level
- Nausea and vomiting
- Psychosocial status (e.g., substance abuse, physical or mental impairments, prostheses)
- Discharge orders

Surgical team members, including the anesthesia provider, perioperative nurse, and surgeon participate in giving the report during

## Box 26-1   Suggestions on Topics for Report from Each Professional

**ANESTHESIA PROVIDER MAY REPORT:**

Anesthesia Provider May Report:
Patient name, allergies, surgical procedures performed
Patient medical and surgical histories
Current medications
Anesthetic delivered
Medications administered
Regional anesthetic
Intraoperative course (anesthesia-related)
Lines, fluids, losses
Pain management
PACU orders
Questions and answers

**PERIOPERATIVE NURSE MAY REPORT:**

Identify patient
Preoperative diagnosis
Procedure performed
Drains, stomas
Surgical complications
Allergies and reactions
Medications, fluids, irrigations delivered by surgeon or RN
Positioning during surgery
Communication of other pertinent issues:
 Family or others
 Special devices
 Patient deficits
Questions and answers

Modified From: Sullivan EE: Handoff communication, J PeriAnesthesia Nurs 22:275–279, 2007.

transfer of the patient's care to the PACU nurse. Box 26-1 includes suggestions on what each professional should report.[5]

In the hustle and bustle of today's surgical environment, seemingly minor details that may have major effects on the patient's recovery can be disregarded or overlooked in the documentation and reporting during patient care transfer. For example, the perioperative nurse may not realize the importance of reporting the positioning used during a surgical procedure when transferring care to the PACU nurse. The following section explains why the documentation and reporting of patient positioning is so critical.

***Documentation and Reporting of Patient Positioning.*** Documentation and reporting of positioning used during a surgical procedure may seem trivial and insignificant and often may be overlooked by the surgical team members. However, patient injuries from prolonged or improper positioning during the surgical procedure have been assessed and documented by astute PACU nurses. AORN recommended practices note that perioperative documentation should include "patient positioning and/or repositioning devices and supports, including immobilization devices used during the surgical procedure."[1]

The impact of improper positioning may not be immediately recognized in the operating room; therefore, positioning must be documented and reported to allow the perianesthesia nurse to look for symptoms of potential problems. The results of improper positioning can be discovered during the assessment of various body systems, including the cardiac and vascular, skin, musculoskeletal, nervous, and respiratory systems. Positioning during a surgical procedure can influence breathing patterns, gas exchange, cardiac output, tactile sensory perception, mobility, and skin integrity. The perianesthesia nurse should assess the patient carefully with an understanding of the different systems that may be compromised from faulty positioning during surgery.

**Cardiovascular.** Cardiac output can indicate intraoperative positioning injuries and can easily be assessed with measurement of the patient's blood pressure. The following list provides some examples of how positioning in surgery can impact the patient's cardiovascular status after surgery:

- Hypotension or hypertension can be caused by the type of anesthesia administered but can be intensified by specific positioning during a surgical procedure.
- Regional or general anesthesia may cause peripheral blood vessels to dilate (from the relaxation of the muscle lining of the blood vessels) and may lead to venous pooling, a decrease in circulating blood volume, and a fall in blood pressure if the extremities are in a dependent position.
- Reverse Trendelenburg's, lithotomy, or jackknife positions can contribute to venous pooling because of the dependent position of the lower extremities.
- Pooling of the blood in the trunk may be caused from unusual pressure on the abdomen from the thighs during lithotomy position, which compresses the external iliac artery that distributes blood to the abdominal wall, external genitalia, and lower limbs.
- Lowered blood pressure may be the result of unusual pressure or tension on the major blood vessels (such as the inferior vena cava) from improper positioning or through the inappropriate positioning of deep retractors.

NURSING CARE IN THE PACU

- Hyperabduction of the arm (>90 degrees) can cause axillary and subclavian vessels to be stretched and compressed between the first rib and the clavicle, that can cause the radial pulse to be undetectable and could result in arterial thrombosis.

**Skin.** The skin is the largest organ of the body and the first line of defense against infection; therefore, the skin must be inspected thoroughly by the perianesthesia nurse for determination of whether any positioning injury has resulted.

The four potential positioning injuries that can cause skin problems are described in the following discussion.

*Pressure.* Pressure injuries are the most common skin injuries caused by inappropriate positioning. A lower pressure on the skin surface sustained for a prolonged time cannot be tolerated as easily as a greater pressure for a shorter time period. The PACU nurse should note the time surgery began to determine the possibility of the formation of pressure ulcers from lengthy surgical procedures.

If the patient's skin is thin, tissue can be easily compromised. With prolonged pressure, blood vessels may constrict and occlude and thus lead to possible ischemia, which is the first step in pressure ulcer formation. Years ago, researchers showed that pressures of more than 32 mm Hg cause arterioles to constrict and occlude, thus leading to decreased nourishment and oxygenation of the capillary beds. Ischemia and microscopic necrosis can then result and cause pressure ulcerations.[6] Injuries from prolonged pressure may not be evident for hours or even days and may even be missed by the perianesthesia nurse. Because a pressure ulcer starts at a bony prominence and extends to the skin, manifestation at the skin level takes time; therefore, a pressure ulcer may not be readily identified. Researchers have noted that one in every 12 patients who undergoes surgery for more than 3 hours can have at least one pressure ulcer develop within 4 days of surgery.[7]

Head injuries from pressure also may not be immediately evident in the PACU. With prolonged pressure on the scalp, localized postoperative alopecia may result. This condition may present with a reddened area or may not be evident until days or weeks after the surgery. Pain and swelling may occur where the pressure has been applied during surgery. Repositioning of the head every 30 minutes during a procedure and in the PACU can minimize this problem.

*Shearing.* Shearing injuries occur when the skin stays stationary while the underlying tissue moves during patient positioning. The moving of tissue layers on each other causes the tissue and vessels to be stretched and damaged. The perianesthesia nurse may note that the skin integrity has been broken, or a redness or discoloration may occur when shearing injuries are sustained.

*Friction.* Friction injuries occur when the skin is moved across a rough surface during positioning or when the skin is rubbed with operating room devices such as a safety strap or face mask. The perianesthesia nurse may note that the skin has become abraded during a potential friction injury that may lead to inflammation, infection, and pain. Friction injuries may involve deeper levels of skin and tissues, which may not be immediately evident during the PACU experience.

*Maceration.* Maceration injuries are caused by prolonged contact of the patient's skin with fluids (e.g., pooling of preparation solutions, incontinence, sweat, or irrigants) during a surgical procedure. This contact with fluids causes the skin to weaken and become more vulnerable to pressure, shearing, or friction injuries. The perianesthesia nurse should consider maceration injuries if the skin integrity has been compromised.

**Musculoskeletal System.** The structural framework of the body skeleton consists of more than 200 bones that provide support and allow movement to occur. Unusual pressure or overextension of a joint or extreme positioning coupled with anesthesia agents that lead to relaxation can cause musculoskeletal injuries. Stretching of a joint or ligament can lead to increased pressure on an area, thus compromising the bone by decreasing the blood supply. The perianesthesia nurse may notice discoloration or redness over a bony prominence or joint that could indicate an injury. Moreover, the patient's subjective symptoms of pain in a specific joint may suggest a musculoskeletal problem.

**Nervous System.** The two components of the nervous system are the central nervous system and the peripheral nervous system. The peripheral nervous system is more vulnerable to positioning injuries with pressure and stretching of structures that leads to pain. These injuries can be temporary or permanent and may result in a disability. Neural injuries from positioning usually are delayed in discovery in the PACU, which makes tracing the original injury back to the surgical experience more difficult.

The most frequently injured nerves from positioning problems are the following:
- Ulnar nerve, which extends from the upper arm to the lower arm. When the compression of the ulnar nerve is near the elbow, a clawing effect of the fingers may be present.

- Lower extremity nerves in the legs that may be injured by improper stirrup use or by improper use of positioning devices.
- Brachial plexus, which consists of a network of nerves from the clavicle down the upper arm. When the arm is overextended, a numbness or palsy of the hand, arm, or wrist may result.
- Lumbosacral nerves, which are located in the lower back region. When a patient is placed in the lithotomy position for a long procedure, the lumbosacral nerves can be stretched, thus leading to weakness of the quadriceps muscle or a sensory deficit in the anterior thigh area.

**Respiratory System.** If the lungs are not allowed to expand well because of positioning problems during a surgical procedure, the alveoli can begin to close, thus decreasing the exchange of respiratory gases. A pulse oximeter applied to the recovering patient in the PACU can be used to note any changes or respiratory problems that may have resulted from prolonged or improper positioning.

## SUMMARY

Thorough communication from the perioperative professionals to the perianesthesia nurse is imperative and directly impacts the outcomes in the care of the surgical patient. Whether written or verbal format is used, continuity of patient care and attention to the details of the surgical event and the patient's responses to the interventions are vital to ensure a smooth transition from the intraoperative surgical suite into the PACU. The perioperative nurse must be diligent in observing what details to document and verbalize, and the perianesthesia nurse must be unfailing in listening and observing patient details that could indicate untoward responses to the surgical event. Never should the importance of this critical part of communication within nursing be overlooked.

Florence Nightingale wrote in *Notes on Nursing* in 1860, "In dwelling upon the vital importance of sound observation, it must never be lost sight of what observation is for. It is not for the sake of piling up miscellaneous information or curious facts, but for the sake of saving life and increasing health and comfort."[8]

## REFERENCES

1. AORN: *Standards, recommended practices, and guidelines*, Denver, 2006, AORN.
2. ASPAN: *2006-2008 Standards of perianesthesia nursing practice*, Cherry Hill, NJ, 2006, ASPAN.
3. The Joint Commission: 2008 Hospital/critical access hospital national patient safety goals. Available at: http://www.jointcommission.org/PatientSafety/NationalPatientSafetyGoals/08_cah_npsgs.htm. Retrieved June 26, 2007.
4. Torgersen K: Communication to facilitate care of the obstetric surgical patient in a postanesthesia care setting, *J PeriAnesthesia Nurs* 20(3): 177-184, 2005.
5. Sullivan EE: Handoff communication, *J PeriAnesthesia Nurs* 22:275-279, 2007.
6. Kosiak M: Etiology and pathology of ischemic ulcers, *Physiol Med Rehabil* 40:60-69, 1959.
7. American Health Consultants: Are you overlooking your OR in the battle against pressure ulcers? Wound Care 3(6):61-63 1998.
8. Nightingale F: *Notes on nursing (an unabridged republication of the first American edition published by D. Appleton and Company in 1860)*, Toronto, 1969, Dover Publications.

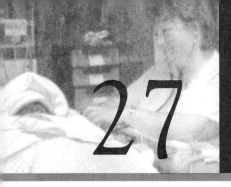

# 27

# ASSESSMENT AND MONITORING OF THE PERIANESTHESIA PATIENT

*Lois Schick, MBA, MNA, RN, CPAN, CAPA*

The primary purpose of the postanesthesia care unit (PACU) is the critical evaluation and stabilization of patients after procedures, with an emphasis on the anticipation and prevention of complications that result from anesthesia or the operative or interventional procedure. A knowledgeable skillful perianesthesia nurse must fully assess the condition of each patient not only at admission and at discharge but also at frequent intervals throughout the postanesthesia period. Assessment must be a continuous and complete process that leads to sound nursing judgment and the implementation of therapeutic care. Assessment includes the gathering of information from direct observation of the patient (the primary source), from the physician and other health care personnel, and from the medical record and the care plan. Traditionally, perianesthesia nurses have, with only limited information, performed the role of caring for the surgical and interventional patients in the vulnerable postanesthesia state. However, for assessment of the perianesthesia patient and plan and implementation of appropriate care, preoperative information must be available as a basis for comparison with postoperative data. The perianesthesia nurse has a professional obligation to consider the patient's history, clinical status, and psychosocial state. The necessary data may be gathered with chart review, personal preoperative visit, and consultation with other health care members who provide care to the patient. The collection of such information should be a coordinated effort with all involved members of the health care team. This chapter discusses the assessment of postprocedure patients and their common needs. Specific assessments related to patient age, the type of procedure, and problems that result from complicated diagnoses are dealt with in the following chapters. The assessment and management of postoperative pain is presented in Chapter 31.

## DEFINITIONS

**Alveolar Artery Carbon Dioxide Differences:** The end tidal carbon dioxide ($ETCO_2$) level is referred to as the alveolar-arterial $CO_2$ difference ($a\text{-}ADCO_2$).

**Alveolar Dead Space:** Alveoli that do not participate in gas exchange because of lack of blood flow.

**Anatomic Dead Space:** Areas of the tracheobronchial tree not involved in gas exchange.

**Capnography:** Measurement of $ETCO_2$ at the patient's airway that allows continuous assessment of the adequacy of alveolar ventilation.

**Dead Space Ventilation:** Includes anatomic, alveolar, and physiologic (total) dead space.

**End Tidal Carbon Dioxide ($ETCO_2$):** At the end of exhalation, the peak carbon dioxide occurs, which in the normal lung is the best approximation of alveolar carbon dioxide levels.

**Flow-Directed Pulmonary Artery Catheter (FDPAC):** Pulmonary artery thermodilution catheter used in hemodynamic monitoring.

**Hemodynamic Monitoring (Invasive Monitoring):** The monitoring of blood flow through the use of invasive catheters to provide pressure measurements in the systemic and pulmonary circulations, central veins, pulmonary capillary bed, and right and/or left atrium, as well as cardiac output.

**Hyperthermia:** A core temperature greater than 38° C (100.4° F).

**Hypothermia:** A core temperature less than 36° C (96.8° F).

**Left Atrial Pressure:** Measured with a catheter placed directly in the left atrium. Usually monitored only in open heart cases where direct access to the left atrium can be reached. In the absence of mitral valve disease or left atrial tumor, left atrial pressure reflects left ventricular end-diastolic pressure and left ventricle preload.

**Obstructive Sleep Apnea (OSA):** Repeated episodes of obstructive apnea during sleep together with daytime sleepiness, mood changes, and altered function.[1]

**Physiologic Dead Space:** The sum of anatomic and alveolar dead space.

**Pulmonary Artery Pressure:** Pressure in the pulmonary artery.

**Pulmonary Capillary Wedge Pressure (PCWP):** Also known as the pulmonary capillary occlusive pressure (PAOP); reflects the pressure in the left atrium.

**Pulmonary Vascular Resistance:** The resistance, impedance, or pressure the right ventricle must overcome to eject the blood into the pulmonary artery.

**Pulse Oximetry:** Pulse oximetry ($SpO_2$) is used for noninvasive measurement of arterial oxygen saturation ($SaO_2$) in the blood.

**Right Atrial Pressure:** Reflects venous return to the right side of the heart and right ventricular end diastolic pressure (preload).

**Systemic Vascular Resistance:** The resistance, impedance, or pressure the left ventricle must overcome to eject the blood from the left ventricle.

**Temporal Artery Temperatures:** Scanning of the forehead over the temporal artery with a noninvasive thermometer.

## PREOPERATIVE ASSESSMENTS

The preoperative evaluation of both the physical and the emotional status of the surgical patient is extremely important, and nursing brings a unique perspective to this assessment. The scope of perianesthesia nursing practice involves the assessment, diagnosis, intervention, and evaluation of physical or psychosocial problems or risks for problems that may result from the administration of sedation or analgesia or anesthetic agents and techniques.[2] Nurses in a number of subspecialties, including perianesthesia nurses, perioperative nurses, and general unit nurses, have advocated this assessment. A preoperative visit from each nurse who will care for the patient seems redundant and may be overwhelming for the patient. More appropriately, nurses should treat each other as colleagues who communicate needs for specific information, coordinate the collection of such information, and document data to be used for planning care. Multidisciplinary communications are instrumental in the education of all those who care for the patient and in the development of communication patterns.

Because many PACU departments now include preoperative holding areas, the perianesthesia nurse must participate in the patient's preoperative interview and assessment.

A complete preoperative nursing assessment should include relevant preoperative physical and psychosocial condition, spiritual and cultural status, medical history (including anesthesia history), length of fasting, understanding of the procedure and postprocedure course, and the need for follow-up services. The preoperative physical assessment should include documentation of temperature, pulse, blood pressure, respirations, oxygen saturation, height and weight, and a review of systems. Nursing diagnoses are established on the basis of analysis of data collected during the assessment phase, and an appropriate plan of care is generated.

## ADMISSION OBSERVATIONS

Physical assessment of the perianesthesia patient must begin immediately on admission to the PACU. The patient is accompanied from the procedure room to the PACU by the anesthesia provider or monitoring nurse, who reports to the receiving nurse on the patient's general condition, the procedure performed, and the type of anesthesia or sedation used. In addition, the nurse should be informed of any problems or complications encountered during the procedure and anesthesia or sedation (see Chapter 26). Because all anesthetics are depressants, postoperative assessment and care generally are the same, regardless of the specific agent used. For special precautions required for certain agents, review the chapters on anesthesia (see Chapters 19 through 25).

Rapid assessment of the life-sustaining cardiorespiratory system is of initial concern. The nurse ensures that the airway is patent and that respirations are free and easy; check and record the patient's blood pressure, pulse, rate of respiration, temperature, and oxygen saturation level; and quickly inspect all dressings and drains for gross bleeding. These baseline observations, which are made immediately on admission, should be reported to the anesthesia or sedation provider in attendance and recorded in the admission note.

Once these initial observations are made, systematic assessment of the patient's total condition is essential. This assessment may be made from head to toe or by systems, whichever the individual nurse prefers. These observations are essentially identical, and each system of the body has an integral function, making all observations interrelated.

## RESPIRATORY FUNCTION

Because the postanesthesia patient has had some interference with the respiratory system, maintenance of adequate gas exchange is a crucial aspect of care in the PACU. Any change in respiratory function must be detected early so that appropriate measures can be taken to ensure adequate oxygenation and ventilation. The most significant respiratory problems encountered in the immediate postoperative period include hypoventilation, airway obstruction, aspiration, and atelectasis.

Respiratory assessment is coupled with the related responses of the cardiovascular and neurologic systems for total evaluation of the adequacy of gas exchange and ventilatory efficiency. Respiratory function is evaluated with clinical assessment. Pulse oximetry is used for assessment of arterial oxygenation, and capnography is used in evaluation of the adequacy of alveolar ventilation. Arterial blood gas measurements may be a part of the respiratory assessment (see Chapters 12, 29, and 30).

### Clinical Assessment

*Inspection.* The resting respiratory rate of a normal adult is approximately 12 to 20 bpm. Infants and children have a higher respiratory rate and a lower tidal volume than adults (see Chapter 49). Respirations should be quiet and easy and have a regular rate and rhythm. The chest should move freely as a unit, and expansion should be equal bilaterally. Alterations in symmetry may be caused by many factors, including pain that may cause splinting at the incision site, consolidation, and pneumothorax. The nurse should note the character of the respirations; intercostal retractions, bulging, nasal flaring, or use of the accessory respiratory muscles are signs of respiratory distress. The depth of respiration is as important as the rate. Shallow respiration is the cardinal sign of continuing depression from anesthesia or preoperative medications, but it may be caused by many other factors, including incisional pain, obesity, tight binders, and dressings that restrict movements of the thoracic cage or abdomen. Shallow respirations and use of the neck and diaphragmatic muscles may also indicate reparalyzation from the use of skeletal muscle relaxants such as succinylcholine, atracurium, pancuronium, and vecuronium. The presence of chest movements alone does not provide evidence that adequate gas exchange is occurring.

Airway obstruction may be present when the normal duration of inspiration versus exhalation is altered. Restlessness, confusion or anxiety, and apprehension are the earliest signs of hypoxemia and $CO_2$ retention and should receive immediate attention for determination of cause. The patient's color is regularly evaluated. Although this assessment is difficult to make, the results provide important information about the respiratory function. Cyanosis is a late sign of severe tissue hypoxia, and if it appears, immediate and vigorous efforts must be instituted to determine and correct the cause of hypoxia. The noninvasive monitors that are increasingly used in the PACU provide an effective means of continuous and objective assessment of gas exchange; pulse oximeters are used in monitoring of hemoglobin oxygen saturation, and capnographs are used in evaluation of the adequacy of alveolar ventilation. A discussion of these monitors is forthcoming.

The presence of an artificial airway is noted; airways are used primarily for maintenance of a patent air passage so that respiratory exchange is not hampered. Four types of airways commonly used are: (1) the balloon-cuffed endotracheal tube (extends from the mouth through the glottis to a point above the bifurcation of the trachea); (2) the balloon-cuffed nasotracheal tube (extends from the nose to the trachea); (3) the oropharyngeal airway (extends from the mouth to the pharynx and prevents the tongue from falling back and obstructing the trachea); and (4) the nasopharyngeal airway (extends from the nose to the pharynx). The airway must be kept clear of secretions for adequate gas exchange to occur, and suctioning may be needed if gurgling develops. The airway should not be removed until the laryngeal and pharyngeal reflexes return; these reflexes enable the patient to control the tongue, to cough, and to swallow. If the patient "reacts on the airway" (attempts to eject it), gagging, which progresses to retching and vomiting, may occur. The airway should be removed as soon as clinically possible in this instance to avoid aspiration.

An endotracheal tube can be removed as soon as the patient's condition is adequately reversed, the patient can maintain an airway without the tube, and the danger of aspiration is over. Determination of this point may be difficult; the decision of when a patient needs an airway is usually much easier than the decision of when such an adjunct is not needed. If PACU policy permits removal of an airway, insertion of an airway should definitely be included and both procedures should be accompanied by appropriate education and skill training for the nurses who perform them.

*Palpation.* Palpation and inspection of the chest may be carried out simultaneously for validation of observations such as symmetry of expansion. Crepitation and fremitus may be heard and felt. The temperature, the level of moisture and general turgor of the skin, and the presence of any edema should be noted.

***Percussion.*** The normal sound over the lungs is resonance. Dullness heard where normally resonance should be heard indicates consolidation or filling of the alveolar or pleural spaces by fluid.

***Listening and Auscultation.*** First, the perianesthesia nurse should listen unaided to the patient's respirations. Normal respiration should be quiet; noisy breathing indicates a problem. Extraneous sounds always indicate some kind of obstruction; however, quiet breathing does not always indicate the absence of problems. An accumulation of mucus or other secretions evidenced by gurgling in any of the respiratory passages may cause airway obstruction and should be removed immediately. Purposeful coughing with good expiratory airflow is the most effective way of clearing secretions. If the patient is not yet reactive enough to do this alone, the secretions must be suctioned out orally and nasally. Nasotracheal suctioning may be useful to clear secretions and to stimulate cough, but the catheter is ineffective for reaching secretions distal to the carina. Obstruction may also occur from poor oropharyngeal muscle tone caused by the muscle-relaxant effect of general anesthesia plus the rolling back of the tongue. Patients with obstructive sleep apnea (OSA) are prone to airway obstruction and should not undergo extubation until they are fully awake. Tracheal extubation should be performed only when the patient is breathing spontaneously with adequate tidal volumes, oxygenation, and ventilation.[1,3] To relieve airway obstruction, use the jaw thrust maneuver by providing anterior pressure support on the angle of the jaw to open the air passages.

Crowing, a sudden violent contraction of the vocal cords, may indicate laryngospasm and result in complete or partial closure of the trachea. Other signs and symptoms of laryngospasm include wheezing, stridor, reduced compliance, cyanosis, and respiratory obstruction. If spasms continue and are not broken with jaw thrust and positive pressure, succinylcholine may be administered with subsequent positive pressure. As a last resort, an endotracheal tube may need to be inserted for maintenance of a patent airway. Total blockage of the airway caused by laryngospasm produces no sound because of the absence of moving air. Equipment and medications for management of a difficult airway should be readily available in the PACU.

Wheezing may indicate bronchospasm caused by a reflex reaction to an irritating mechanism. Bronchospasm occurs most often in patients with preexisting pulmonary disease, such as severe emphysema, reactive airway disease, pulmonary fibrosis, and radiation pneumonitis. Laryngeal edema after endotracheal intubation is not uncommon and can contribute significantly to airway obstruction. Acute changes in the patient's skin condition, cardiovascular status, and bronchospasm after regional anesthesia must alert the nurse to a possible rare allergic reaction.

The perianesthesia nurse should listen to the patient's chest with a stethoscope for quality and intensity of breath sounds. Any abnormality should be located and identified and then described in the patient's medical record. Total absence of breath sounds on one side may signal the presence of pneumothorax (collapsed lung), obstruction, or fluid or blood within the pleural space. Auscultation of breath sounds in the PACU is often difficult because the patient usually cannot sit up or respond to commands to breathe deeply with the mouth open. Positioning the patient on alternating sides during the stir-up regimen provides an opportunity for examination of the posterior lung field.

## Monitoring of Oxygenation with Pulse Oximetry

A pulse oximeter is used for noninvasive measurement of arterial oxygen saturation ($SaO_2$) in the blood ($SpO_2$ when measured with pulse oximetry) and is a valuable adjunct to the clinical assessment of oxygenation. Many clinical indicators, such as the patient's color and the characteristics of the respirations, are subjective, and the physical signs of cyanosis are not evident until hypoxia is severe. Pulse oximetry monitoring is objective and continuous and provides an early warning of developing hypoxemia, thus allowing intervention before signs of hypoxia appear. Consequently, pulse oximetry has been widely adopted in the PACU as a tool for both safety monitoring and patient management. As a confirmation of the importance of pulse oximetry, the American Society of PeriAnesthesia Nurses (ASPAN) Standards of Postanesthesia Nursing Practice[2] requires evaluation of all PACU patients with pulse oximetry at admission and discharge, and ASPAN recommends a pulse oximeter for every patient care unit in a phase I PACU.

A pulse oximeter consists of a microprocessor-based monitor and a sensor (Fig. 27-1). In addition to a $SpO_2$ display, most oximeters display the pulse rate and have an adjustable alarm system that sounds when values register outside a designated range. A variety of sensors is available, each intended for application to specific sites and for use on patients of various sizes (the manufacturer's instructions describe these

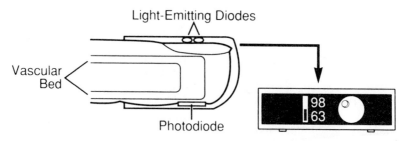

**Fig. 27-1**   Pulse oximeter uses two light-emitting diodes and photodiode to determine arterial hemoglobin saturation.

requirements). The sensor is applied to a site with a good arterial supply. The most common application site is a finger or toe (hand or foot in neonates); other sites include the nose, the forehead, the earlobe, or the temple. Both reusable sensors and disposable adhesive sensors are available, and disposable sensors allow for patient-dedicated monitoring when infection control concerns are present.

**Technology Overview.**   A pulse oximeter uses plethmysography for detection of the arterial pulse and spectrophotometry in determination of $SpO_2$. The pulse oximetry sensor incorporates a red and an infrared light-emitting diode (LED) as light sources and a photodiode as a light detector. In the most common type of sensor, a transmission sensor, the light sources and detector are positioned on opposite sides of an arterial bed, such as around the finger. In a reflectance oximetry sensor, they are positioned on the same surface, such as on the forehead.

With both transmission and reflectance sensors, red and infrared light passes into the tissue, and the detector measures the amount of light absorbed. Because oxyhemoglobin and deoxygenated hemoglobin differ in the absorption of red and infrared light, the detector can determine the percentage of oxyhemoglobin in the arterial pulse.

**Applications.**   Pulse oximetry is used in many clinical settings for safety monitoring and as a patient management tool. As a safety monitor, a pulse oximeter detects hypoxemia caused by unanticipated events such as severe atelectasis, bronchospasm, airway displacement, disconnections or kinks in the breathing circuit, and cardiac arrest. As a patient management tool, it is valuable in titrating oxygen therapy, weaning a patient from mechanical ventilation, and evaluating response to medications or other interventions that are intended for improvement of oxygenation.

In addition to these broad applications, certain uses of pulse oximetry are of particular value in the PACU. For example, patients after surgery can become significantly hypoxemic during transport to or from the PACU. Pulse oximetry during transport can be used to diagnose undetected hypoxemia and to identify a need for supplemental oxygen. Also, as indicated by the ASPAN standards, it is a valuable adjunct to clinical assessments in determination of readiness for PACU discharge. Some patients in PACU judged to be stable and ready for transfer on the basis of clinical evaluation alone have been found to be hypoxemic after evaluation with pulse oximetry.

**Interpretation of Pulse Oximetry Measurements.** Consideration of the mechanisms of oxygen transport is essential for adequate interpretation of $SPO_2^w$. Approximately 98% of the oxygen in blood is bound to hemoglobin; $SaO_2$ and $SpO_2$ reflect this blood oxygen. The remaining blood oxygen is dissolved in plasma; blood gas analysis measures the partial pressure exerted by this oxygen dissolved in plasma ($PaO_2 = 80 - 100$ mm Hg at sea level). The dissolved oxygen is used to meet immediate metabolic needs. The oxygen bound to hemoglobin serves as the reservoir that replenishes the pool of dissolved oxygen (see Chapter 12).

The rate at which oxygen binds to hemoglobin is primarily controlled by two factors: the $PaO_2$ and the affinity of hemoglobin for oxygen. This relationship between $SaO_2$ and $PaO_2$ is represented by the oxyhemoglobin dissociation curve. The curve is sigmoid in shape, and its position is affected by a number of physiologic variables that change the affinity of hemoglobin for oxygen (Fig. 27-2).

Many factors that shift the oxyhemoglobin dissociation curve are commonly seen in patients in the PACU. For example, a patient with hypothermia may have a left-shifted curve. In such a patient, a given $SpO_2$ as measured with pulse oximetry may correspond to a lower than normal $PaO_2$. Although oxygen saturation may be adequate, hemoglobin has a greater affinity for oxygen and is less willing to release oxygen to meet tissue needs. Warming the patient to a

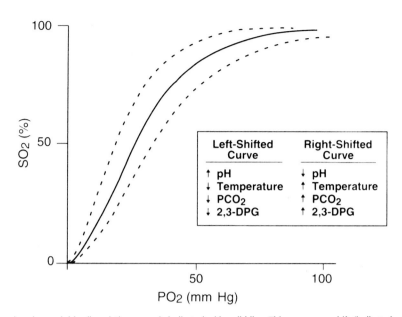

**Fig. 27-2**  Normal oxyhemoglobin dissociation curve is indicated with *solid line*. This curve may shift (indicated with *broken lines*) whenever pH, temperature, $PCO_2$, or 2,3-DPG values are increased or decreased. *$SO_2$,* Oxygen saturation; *$PO_2$,* partial pressure of oxygen; *$PCO_2$,* partial pressure of carbon dioxide; *2,3-DPG,* 2,3-diphosphoglycerate.

normothermic range facilitates oxygen unloading from the hemoglobin molecule and helps maintain adequate tissue oxygenation.

**Clinical Issues.** As with any technology, important clinical issues must be considered for appropriate use of pulse oximetry. As just discussed, shifts in the oxyhemoglobin dissociation curve that are caused by abnormal values of pH, temperature, partial pressure of carbon dioxide ($PCO_2$), and 2,3-diphosphoglycerate must be considered. Consideration of the patient's hemoglobin level is also important because a pulse oximeter cannot detect depletion in the total amount of hemoglobin. When pulse oximetry is used on a postoperative patient with a low hemoglobin level, a high $SpO_2$ value may not reflect adequate oxygenation. The amount of hemoglobin, although it is well saturated with oxygen, may be inadequate to meet tissue needs because fewer carriers are available to transport oxygen.

Adequate oxygenation is a factor of not only adequate oxygen saturation and hemoglobin values but also of adequate oxygen delivery (which necessitates appropriate cardiac output) and the ability of the tissues to effectively use oxygen. When oxygen demand exceeds oxygen supply, tissue hypoxia results. Pulse oximetry readings therefore should be assessed in conjunction with all other indices of oxygenation.

Dysfunctional hemoglobins, variants of the hemoglobin molecule that are unable to transport oxygen, present a similar problem. Despite the high $SpO_2$ level, hemoglobin may be insufficient to carry oxygen. Carboxyhemoglobin is hemoglobin that is bound with carbon monoxide and therefore is unavailable for carrying oxygen. Its effect must be considered in patients with burns or carbon monoxide poisoning and in those who smoke. In methemoglobinemia, the iron molecule on the hemoglobin is oxidized from the ferrous to the ferric state. This form of iron is unable to transport oxygen. Methemoglobinemia, although rare, may occur in patients who receive nitrate-based and other drugs and in those who are exposed to a variety of toxins. When dysfunctional hemoglobins are suspected, assessment of oxygenation with pulse oximetry must be supplemented with arterial blood gas saturations measured with a laboratory cooximeter for determination of whether dyshemoglobins are present and oxygenation is adequate.

Perfusion at the sensor application site must be sufficient for the pulse oximeter to detect pulsatile flow, which is an important consideration for some patients in the PACU, such as those treated with vasoconstrictors, those with marked hypothermia, and those with significantly reduced cardiac output. A well-perfused site should be selected for application of the sensor. If in doubt, the pulse and adjacent capillary refill can be checked.

If the monitor cannot track the pulse, the patient first is evaluated for adverse physiologic changes. Next, the perianesthesia nurse should ensure that blood flow is not restricted, such as by a flexed extremity, a blood pressure cuff, an arterial line, any restraints, or a sensor that is applied too tightly. Local perfusion to the sensor site can be improved by covering the site with a warm towel or with use of a forced air warming device. Certain sensors, such as nasal sensors, are designed for application to areas where perfusion is preserved even when peripheral perfusion is relatively poor. Finally, some pulse oximeters use an electrocardiographic (ECG) signal as an aid in identification of the pulse, thus enhancing the instrument's ability to detect a weak pulse.

The patient movement seen in the PACU can produce false signals that interfere with the pulse oximeter's ability to identify the true pulse, thus leading to unreliable $SpO_2$ and pulse rate readings. The sensor should be properly and securely applied; a sensor that is loosely attached or incorrectly positioned can magnify the effect of motion. If the problem persists, consideration should be given to moving the sensor to a less active site. Also, pulse oximeters that use the ECG signal as an aid in identification of the pulse can have an enhanced ability to distinguish between the true pulse and artifacts produced by motion. The result is more reliable $SpO_2$ readings.

Normally, venous blood is nonpulsatile and is not detected with a pulse oximeter. In the presence of venous pulsations, the $SpO_2$ value provided by the pulse oximeter may be a composite of both arterial and venous saturations. Venous pulsations may occur in patients with severe right-sided heart failure or other pathophysiologic states that create venous congestion and in patients receiving high levels of positive end-expiratory pressure. They may also occur when the sensor is placed distal to a blood pressure cuff or occlusive dressing and when additional tape is wrapped tightly around the sensor. When venous pulsations are present, the perianesthesia nurse should take care in interpreting the $SpO_2$ readings and, if possible, attempt to eliminate the cause.

Because pulse oximeters are optical measuring devices, the perianesthesia nurse must be aware of additional factors that can influence the reliability of $SpO_2$ readings. To ensure good light reception, the sensor's light sources and detector must always be positioned according to the manufacturer's specifications. In the presence of bright lights, such as infrared warming devices, fluorescent lights, direct sunlight, and surgical lights, the sensor must be covered with an opaque material to prevent incorrect $SpO_2$ readings. Also, agents that significantly change the optical-absorbing properties of blood, such as

recently administered intravascular dyes, can interfere with reliable $SpO_2$ measurements. The use of pulse oximetry with certain nail polishes, especially those that are blue, green, and reddish-brown in color, may result in inaccurate readings. If nail polish in these shades cannot be removed, the sensor should be applied to an alternate unpolished site.

### Monitoring of Ventilation with Capnography

Monitoring of $ETCO_2$ in respiratory gases provides an early warning of physiologic and mechanical events that interfere with normal ventilation. Capnography, which measures $ETCO_2$ at the patient's airway, is increasingly used in the PACU. It allows continuous assessment of the adequacy of alveolar ventilation, the function of the cardiopulmonary system, ventilator function, and the integrity of the airway and the breathing circuit. Consequently, it enables early detection of many potentially catastrophic events, including the onset of malignant hyperthermia, esophageal intubation, hypoventilation, partial or complete airway obstruction, breathing circuit leaks or disconnects, a large pulmonary embolus, and cardiac arrest.

Two variants of the instrument are available. A capnometer provides numeric measurement of exhaled $CO_2$ levels. A capnograph provides the same numeric information, and it also displays a $CO_2$ waveform. Both types of instruments usually incorporate an adjustable alarm system and often have trending and printing capabilities. The following discussion focuses on the use of capnographs because they allow more complete and effective patient assessment than do capnometers. As discussed subsequently, changes in the shape of the $CO_2$ waveform can provide crucial diagnostic information about ventilation, similar to the way in which the waveform provided with an ECG can provide crucial diagnostic information about the heart.

***Technology Overview.*** For measurement of exhaled $CO_2$, the most common type of capnograph passes infrared light at a wavelength that is absorbed by $CO_2$ through a sample of the patient's respiratory gas. The amount of light that is absorbed by the patient's gas reflects the amount of $CO_2$ in the sample.

Capnographs differ in the manner in which they obtain respiratory gas samples for analysis. Sidestream (or diverting) capnographs transport the sample through narrow-gauge tubing to a measuring chamber. Mainstream (or nondiverting) capnographs position a flow-through measurement chamber directly on the patient's airway.

Special adapters are available to allow sidestream capnographs to be used on patients who are not intubated. The sample adapter should be placed as close to the patient's endotracheal tube or airway as possible.

Sidestream capnographs incorporate moisture-control features that are designed to minimize clogging of the sample tube, protect the measurement chamber from moisture-induced damage, and minimize the risk of cross contamination. The design of these moisture-control systems significantly impacts a monitor's ease of use. Most rely on water traps, which must be emptied routinely. A new technology uses a special system of filters and tubing to dehumidify the sample and thus eliminate the need for water traps.

Capnographs also differ in calibration requirements. Many require removal of the patient from the respiratory circuit and adjustment of the instrument with special mixtures of calibration gases. Advanced capnographic technology includes automatic calibration and does not require any user calibration skills or time.

**The Normal Capnogram.** For effective use of capnography, an understanding is important of the components of the normal $CO_2$ waveform (capnogram), a square wave pattern with a plateau (Fig. 27-3). Early in exhalation, air from the anatomic dead space, which is virtually $CO_2$ free, is measured with the instrument. As exhalation continues, alveolar gas reaches the sampling site, and the $CO_2$ level increases rapidly. The $CO_2$ concentration continues to increase throughout exhalation and reaches the alveolar plateau because alveolar gas dominates the sample. At the end of exhalation, the peak (end tidal) $CO_2$ ($ETCO_2$) occurs, which in the normal lung is the best approximation of alveolar $CO_2$ levels. The $CO_2$ concentration then drops rapidly as the next inhalation of $CO_2$-free gas begins.

**End Tidal Versus Arterial Carbon Dioxide.** In normal conditions, when ventilation and perfusion are well matched, $ETCO_2$ closely approximates arterial $CO_2$ ($PaCO_2$). The difference between the $PaCO_2$ and the $ETCO_2$ level is referred to as the alveolar-arterial $CO_2$ difference (a-$ADCO_2$). $ETCO_2$ is usually as much as 5 mm Hg lower than $PaCO_2$. When the two measurements differ significantly, an anomaly in the patient's physiology, the breathing circuit, or the capnograph is usually present. Significant divergence between $ETCO_2$ and $PaCO_2$ is often attributable to increased alveolar dead space. $CO_2$-free gas from nonperfused alveoli mixes with gas from perfused regions, thus decreasing the $ETCO_2$ measurement. Clinical conditions that cause increased dead space, such as pulmonary hypoperfusion, cardiac arrest, and embolic conditions (e.g., air, fat thrombus, and amniotic fluid), can increase the alveolar-arterial $CO_2$ difference (a-$ADCO_2$). Changes in the a-$ADCO_2$ can be used in assessment of the efficacy of the treatment; as the patient's dead space improves, the partial pressure of the alveolar carbon dioxide less the partial pressure of arterial carbon dioxide ($PACO_2 - PaCO_2$) narrows. Increases in dead space ventilation lower $ETCO_2$ and therefore increase the $PaCO_2 - ETCO_2$ gradient. Widened $PaCO_2 - ETCO_2$ examples include embolic phenomena, hypoperfusion, and chronic obstructive pulmonary disease (COPD). Alternatively, a significant $PACO_2 - PaCO_2$ value can indicate incomplete alveolar emptying (such as with reactive airway disease), a leak in the gas-sampling system that allows loss of respiratory gas, and contamination of respiratory gas with fresh gas.[4]

**Interpretation of Changes in the Capnogram.** An abnormal capnogram provides an initial warning of many events that warrant immediate intervention. Abnormalities may be seen on a breath-by-breath basis or when the $CO_2$ trend is examined. For this reason, visualization is preferable of both the real-time waveform and the $CO_2$ trend on the monitor display. Examples follow for a look at changes produced by significant events that commonly occur in the PACU.

A sudden decrease in $ETCO_2$ to a near-zero level indicates that the monitor is no longer detecting $CO_2$ in exhaled gases (Fig. 27-4). Immediate action is crucial for detection and correction of the cause of this loss of ventilation. Possible causes include a completely blocked endotracheal tube, esophageal intubation, a disconnection in the breathing circuit, and inadvertent extubation. The latter three possibilities are particularly likely if the decrease in $ETCO_2$ coincides with movement of the patient's head. First, after elimination of possible clinical causes for this decrease in $ETCO_2$, a clogged sampling tube or instrument malfunction is investigated as the cause of the problem.

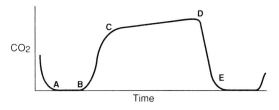

**Fig. 27-3** Normal capnogram. *AB,* Beginning exhalation, dead space; *BC,* initial alveolar emptying; *CD,* end-alveolar emptying; *D,* end tidal $CO_2$; *E,* inspiration ($CO_2$–free gas).

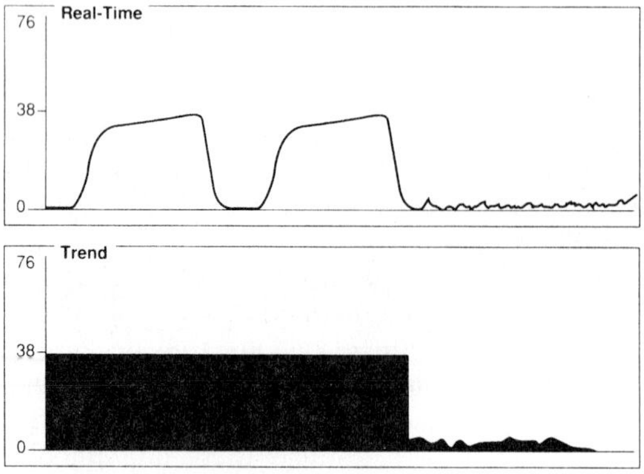

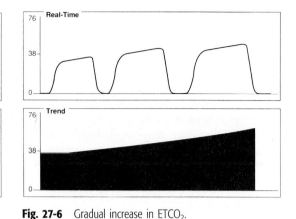

**Fig. 27-4**  Sudden decrease in $ETCO_2$ to near-zero level.

**Fig. 27-6**  Gradual increase in $ETCO_2$.

An exponential decrease in $ETCO_2$ over a small number of breaths usually signals a life-threatening cardiopulmonary event that has dramatically increased dead space ventilation (Fig. 27-5). Sudden hypotension, pulmonary embolism, and circulatory arrest with continued ventilation must be considered.

A gradual increase in the $ETCO_2$ level while the capnogram retains its normal shape usually indicates that ventilation is inadequate to eliminate the $CO_2$ that is produced (Fig. 27-6). This situation can be the result of a small ventilator leak or a partial airway obstruction that reduces minute ventilation. It can also reflect increased $CO_2$ production associated with increased body temperature, the onset of sepsis, or shivering. Of particular importance, a large increase in $ETCO_2$ can be one of the earliest signs of malignant hyperthermia, which may not begin until after emergence from anesthesia.

A gradual decrease in the $ETCO_2$ level commonly occurs in the patient who is anesthetized, narcotized, hyperventilated, or hypothermic (Fig. 27-7).

Assessment of the capnogram can reveal information about the quality of alveolar emptying. For example, the patient with bronchospasm is unable to completely empty the alveoli, and the resulting capnogram does not have an alveolar plateau (Fig. 27-8). The $ETCO_2$ reported by the capnograph in this instance is not a good estimate of alveolar $CO_2$. Effective administration of bronchodilator therapy commonly improves alveolar emptying and results in a more normal capnogram.

**Clinical Issues.** In addition to the diagnostic usefulness of changes in the capnogram, some specific applications of capnography are particularly valuable in the PACU. Of primary importance is its ability to provide early warning of hypoventilation that, in the PACU, may be the result of anesthesia, sedation, analgesia, or pain. A falling $ETCO_2$ value may indicate pulmonary hypoperfusion from blood loss or hypotension. During rewarming, $ETCO_2$ values are likely to increase as metabolic activity increases.

Capnography can signal when shivering produces an unacceptable increase in oxygen

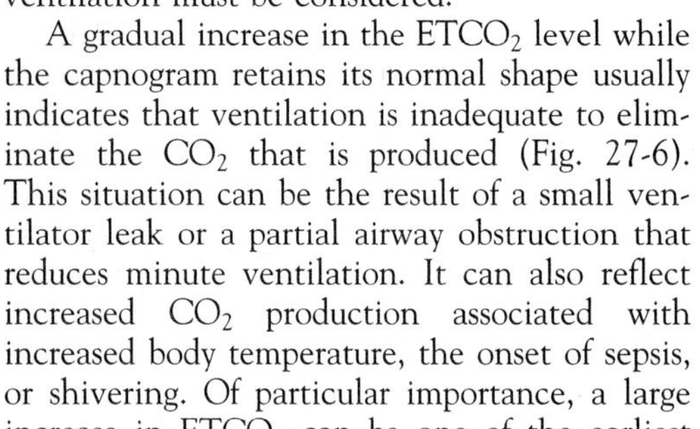

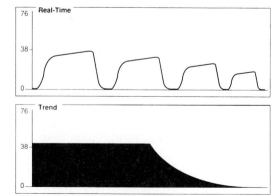

**Fig. 27-5**  Exponential decrease in $ETCO_2$.

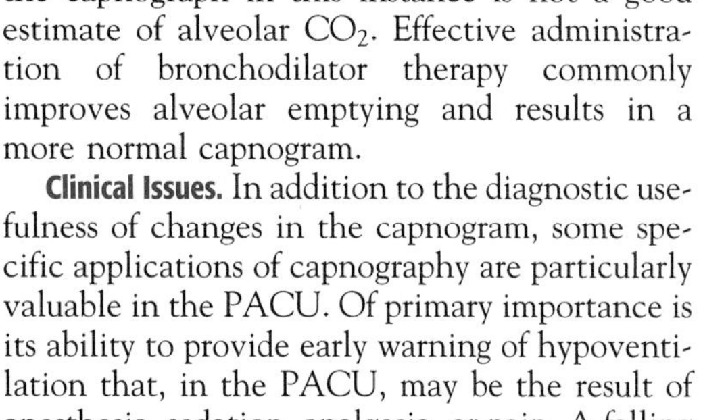

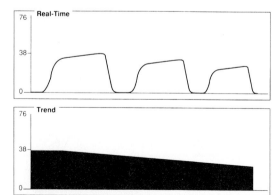

**Fig. 27-7**  Gradual decrease in $ETCO_2$.

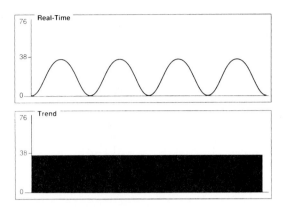

**Fig. 27-8** Incomplete alveolar emptying.

consumption and metabolic rate. During ventilator weaning, capnography is valuable in assessment of the adequacy of ventilation. Recent studies have shown the value of capnography in monitoring the course and efficacy of CPR. $ETCO_2$ measurements, which decrease during cardiac arrest, typically reach about 50% of normal levels during effective CPR. When spontaneous circulation is restored, $ETCO_2$ values increase dramatically. The presence and persistence of normal $ETCO_2$ values are also useful determinants in confirmation of tracheal intubation because $CO_2$ is not normally found in the esophagus. However, capnography cannot be substituted for chest auscultation and radiograph in elimination of the possibility of bronchial intubation.

## CARDIOVASCULAR FUNCTION AND PERFUSION

The three basic components of the circulatory system that must be evaluated are: (1) the heart as a pump; (2) the blood; and (3) the arteriovenous system. The maintenance of good tissue perfusion depends on a satisfactory cardiac output. Therefore, most assessment is aimed at evaluation of cardiac output.

### Clinical Assessment
Observe the overall condition of the patient, especially skin color and turgor. Peripheral cyanosis, edema, dilatation of the neck veins, shortness of breath, and many other findings may be indicative of cardiovascular problems. In addition to checking all operative sites for blood loss, note the amount of blood lost during surgery and the patient's most recent hemoglobin level.

### Blood Pressure Monitoring
Arterial blood pressure must be assessed in the preoperative physical assessment, on admission

to and discharge from the PACU, and at frequent regular intervals during the PACU stay. Arterial blood pressure is the pressure of blood in the arteries and arterioles. It is a pulsatile pressure because of the cardiac cycle, and systolic (peak) and diastolic (trough) numbers are reported in millimeters of mercury. Arterial blood pressure is regulated by the vasomotor tone of the arteries and arterioles, the amount of blood entering the arteries per systole, and blood volume. The pressure is currently measured either noninvasively (indirectly) or invasively (directly). Noninvasive methods include manual cuff measurement with either an aneroid sphygmomanometer or automatic measurement with an electronic blood pressure monitor. Invasive measurement may be accomplished via an arterial line connected to a transducer. A clear understanding of proper technique is essential to ensure accurate and reliable readings with all the blood pressure measurement methods.

### Noninvasive Measurement
**Manual Method.** An aneroid sphygmomanometer with inflatable cuff and stethoscope is needed for the standard auscultatory blood pressure measurement technique. Use of the correct cuff size is essential. The width of the inflatable bladder that is encased inside the cuff should be 40% to 50% of upper arm circumference. A bladder that is too wide underestimates blood pressure, whereas a bladder that is too narrow overestimates blood pressure. The length of the bladder should be at least 80% of the arm circumference.

The cuff is placed on the extremity, with the inflatable bladder positioned directly over the artery at the level of the heart. The brachial artery is the site most commonly used for blood pressure measurement. If the upper extremities are unavailable for cuff placement because of operative issues or other problems, the lower extremities may be used. The bladder of the cuff should be centered over the posterior surface of the lower third of the thigh, and pressure may be auscultated over the popliteal artery or at the ankle over the posterior tibial artery (just posterior to the medial malleolus). Systolic pressure in the legs is usually 20 to 30 mm Hg higher than in the brachial artery.

The cuff is inflated, and when cuff pressure exceeds the arterial pressure, arterial blood flow ceases and the pulse is no longer palpated. As pressure is released with turning the valve of the inflation bulb, blood flow resumes and audible (Korotkoff's) sounds are noted with the stethoscope. These sounds change in quality and intensity throughout further cuff deflation and generally disappear. Systolic pressure is noted as the first audible sound in the cuff-deflating process.[5] The diastolic pressure is marked by the disappearance of sounds in the adult patient and the muffling of sounds in the pediatric patient.

A common cause of error in blood pressure measurement is an auscultatory gap that may be present, especially in patients with hypertension. This gap is a silent interval between the systolic and diastolic pressures. During this gap, the pulse is palpable. Therefore, to avoid mistakenly low systolic readings, the cuff should be inflated until the pulse is obliterated. Blood pressure readings should be recorded completely, including the systolic pressure, the points at which the sounds become muffled and cease, and, if present, the range of the auscultatory gap.

Auscultatory blood pressure measurements may be completed quickly and easily in many circumstances. The accuracy and reliability of the readings may be affected by low flow states (including decreased cardiac output and vasoconstriction) or decreased sound transmission caused by factors related to the patient (edema and obesity) or the environment (noise). Cuff size and placement, user error, and improperly calibrated manometers may also contribute to unreliable readings. Because measurements are intermittent and must be initiated by the user, blood pressure changes may go unnoticed in the postoperative patient with labile hemodynamics or sudden blood loss. The use of automatic blood pressure monitors that can be set to measure blood pressure at regular frequent intervals can minimize some of this risk.

**Automatic Method.** Automatic blood pressure monitoring with electronic devices has become increasingly prevalent in the PACU. The devices are commonly used for frequent blood pressure measurements over relatively brief periods, when the need for arterial sampling is minimal to absent, and when the risks of arterial lines cannot be justified.

One of the most commonly used automatic noninvasive blood pressure methods is based on oscillometric technology. The cuff is chosen and applied according to conventional technique. Oscillations of the arterial wall are occluded as the cuff is inflated and are detected during cuff deflation. Systolic pressure is indicated at the onset of oscillations. As cuff pressure decreases, oscillations increase in amplitude and peak at the mean arterial pressure. The point at which oscillations disappear is the diastolic pressure (Fig. 27-9). All three pressures are normally reported on oscillometric monitoring devices.

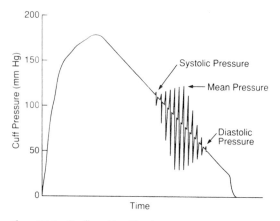

**Fig. 27-9** Oscillometric blood pressure measurement. Systolic pressure is indicated at onset of oscillations. Mean arterial pressure occurs when oscillations peak in amplitude. Point at which oscillations disappear is diastolic pressure.

Automatic noninvasive blood pressure monitors may be set to cycle at various measurement periods. The instruments alarm when systolic and diastolic pressures register outside of a preset range. Equipment should be calibrated on a regular basis, and preventive maintenance should include assessment for leaks. The use of automatic devices may be limited in patients with low-flow states or high peripheral vascular resistance and in those who are severely obese or edematous. These devices provide only intermittent measurements and are less desirable for assessment of the patient who is labile.

Newer advances in noninvasive blood pressure technology, currently available for intraoperative monitoring of the patient who is anesthetized, include continuous monitoring capabilities that ensure detection in sudden blood pressure variations. The only other reliable method of continuous blood pressure monitoring currently available is invasive arterial blood pressure technology.

***Invasive Measurement.*** Invasive arterial pressure measurements are most commonly obtained via cannulation of the radial artery but may also be obtained at other arterial sites. A continuous flush solution is connected to the intraarterial catheter and is slowly infused into the arterial vessel under pressure. The pressure within the artery is transmitted through the column of fluid via noncompliant pressure tubing to the transducer. The transducer then converts this pressure to an electric signal that can be converted to millimeters of mercury and displayed on the monitor. A corresponding arterial waveform, or pressure pulse, is also displayed on the monitor.

Arterial blood pressure measurements are continuous and are indicated for patients at high risk hemodynamically. Changes in patient pressures can be observed on an ongoing basis. This technology may also be chosen for patients in whom indirect measurements fail because of diminished or absent Korotkoff's sounds (as in patients who are obese or edematous) and for those with high peripheral vascular resistance. The direct arterial access is also beneficial if the patient needs frequent blood samples for laboratory analysis.

To ensure more reliable arterial blood pressure readings, the clinician should balance and calibrate the system according to the manufacturer's specifications. The transducer must always be balanced and positioned at the fourth intercostal level at the midaxillary line, known as the phlebostatic axis. Aseptic technique must always be used during placement and maintenance of the arterial line and transducer.

Damping of the arterial waveform with subsequent unreliable readings may occur for a variety of reasons, including clotting and kinking of the arterial catheter, positioning of the catheter against the arterial wall, and the presence of air bubbles within the arterial line system. Loose connections, calibration error, and equipment failure may also contribute to unreliable readings.

An Allen's test should be performed before radial artery cannulation for minimization of the risk of hand ischemia (see Chapter 11). If arterial lines are discontinued in the PACU, constant pressure should be applied to the site for 5 to 10 minutes or until bleeding has ceased. A pressure dressing should be applied, and the site should be checked frequently for any bleeding and radial pulse palpation.

Complications and risks of invasive arterial blood pressure monitoring include infection, thrombosis, emboli, tissue ischemia, hemorrhage, and vessel perforation. Arterial blood pressure monitoring is generally contraindicated in patients with septicemia, coagulopathies, irradiated arterial sites, anatomic anomalies, inadequate collateral blood flow, or thrombosis. No intravenous (IV) solution or medications should be administered through the arterial pressure monitoring system at any time. If the catheter patency is in question, blood and fluid are aspirated from the blood drawing port or stopcock and the system is flushed with the fast flush device, not a syringe.[6]

**Clinical Issues.** For assessment of significance, blood pressure readings in the postoperative period must be compared with preoperative baseline measurements. A low postoperative blood pressure may be the result of a number of factors, including the effects of muscle relaxants, spinal anesthesia, preoperative medication, changes in the patient's position, blood loss, poor lung ventilation, and peripheral pooling of blood. The administration of oxygen to help eliminate anesthetic gases and to assist the patient in awakening causes an increase in blood pressure. Deep breathing, leg exercises, verbal stimulation, and conversation can be instituted to raise the blood pressure. A low fluid volume may be augmented by increasing the rate of intravenous fluids, which helps maintain the arterial pressure. Any method designed to raise the pressure must be instituted with consideration for the patient's overall condition.

An increase in blood pressure after surgery is not uncommon because of the effects of anesthesia, respiratory insufficiency, or decreased respiratory rate and depth that cause $CO_2$ retention. The surgical procedure, with the accompanying discomfort, also causes increased blood pressure. Emergence delirium, with its excitement, struggling, and pain, may also be a causative factor in a transient increase in blood pressure. Obviously, determination of the cause is important before treatment is instituted. In patients with uncontrolled hypertension, continuous intravenous antihypertensive medications may be necessary. However, diagnosis of the cause of the hypertension is extremely important so that effective therapy may be administered rapidly.

### Pulse Pressure Monitoring

Pulse pressure is an important determinant in the evaluation of perfusion. Because of the pulsatile nature of the heart, blood enters the arteries intermittently, causing pressure increases and decreases. The difference between the systolic and diastolic pressures equals the pulse pressure. The pulse pressure is affected by two major factors: the stroke volume output of the heart and the compliance (total distensibility) of the arterial tree. The pulse pressure is determined approximately by the ratio of stroke output to compliance: therefore, any condition that affects either of these factors also affects the pulse pressure.

For accurate evaluation of the patient's cardiovascular status, all signs and symptoms must be evaluated individually and within the body system as a whole. For example, cool extremities, decreased urine output, and narrowed pulse pressure may be indicative of decreased cardiac output, even in the presence of normal blood pressure.

***Pulses.*** The rate and character of all pulses should be assessed bilaterally. The pulses should

NURSING CARE IN THE PACU

be examined simultaneously for determination of equality at time of arrival. Peripheral arterial occlusion is not uncommon; if it is suspected, a Doppler instrument can be of great value in detection of the presence or absence of blood flow. Occlusion is an emergency and must be reported to the surgeon at once. Irregularities in pulse are most commonly caused by premature beats, generally premature ventricular contractions (PVCs) or premature atrial contractions (PACs). These irregular rhythms should be thoroughly investigated before therapy is initiated.

## ELECTROCARDIOGRAPHIC MONITORING

The perianesthesia nurse must have a basic understanding of cardiac monitoring and should be able to interpret the basic cardiac rhythms and dysrhythmias and correlate them with expected cardiac output and its effects on the patient's condition. According to the most recent ASPAN standards, ECG monitoring should be performed for each patient in a phase I PACU and an ECG monitor should be readily available for patients in phase II units.[1] Dysrhythmias of any type may occur at any time and in any patient during the postoperative period; therefore, accurate ECG monitoring and interpretation are mandatory skills for the perianesthesia nurse. This section is designed to provide an introduction to specific problems of cardiac monitoring in the PACU.

Any type of cardiac dysrhythmia may be seen in the PACU. The causes of specific dysrhythmias must be carefully differentiated before any treatment is instituted. Some commonly encountered problems are reviewed here, but the list is by no means complete.

All abnormal rhythms should be documented with a rhythm strip and recorded in the patient's progress record. Any questionable rhythms should be documented with a complete 12-lead ECG.

Electric monitoring of the patient's heart is only one assessment parameter and must be interpreted in conjunction with other salient parameters before therapy is initiated. Cardiac monitors generally depict only a single lead. They do not detect all rhythm disturbances and alterations, and a 12-lead ECG is essential for accurate definition of a conduction problem.

### Lead Placement

The skin where the electrode will be placed should be clean, dry, and smooth. Excessive hair is removed; moisture or skin oils are removed with alcohol or acetone, and the skin is mildly abraded to obtain good adherence of the electrode.

Site selection on the chest is based on a triangular arrangement of positive, negative, and ground electrodes. Placement of electrodes directly over the diaphragm, areas of auscultation, heavy bones, or large muscles is avoided. Adequate space for application of defibrillator paddles is allowed in the event that defibrillation should become necessary. Fig. 27-10 depicts the most commonly used electrode leads. The modified lead II is the most commonly used in the PACU because it is the most versatile; it is useful in assessment of P waves, P-R intervals, and atrial dysrhythmias. The modified chest lead I is useful for assessment of bundle branch block and differentiation between ventricular dysrhythmias and aberrations. This lead is useful when the patient is known to have preexisting cardiac disease. The Lewis lead is useful when P waves are difficult to distinguish with other leads.

### Sinus Dysrhythmias

**Sinus Bradycardia.** Fig. 27-11 shows a slow heart rate, less than 60 bpm. Sinus bradycardia is a rhythm with impulses that originate at the sinus node at a rate of less than 60 bpm. Its rhythm may be irregular because of

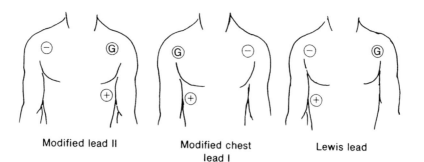

Modified lead II          Modified chest          Lewis lead
                          lead I

**Fig. 27-10**   Basic electrode placement.

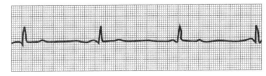

**Fig. 27-11** Sinus bradycardia (lead III).

accompanying sinus dysrhythmias. All other complex features are normal.

Sinus bradycardia is commonly encountered in the PACU because of the depressant effects of anesthesia. It may occur normally during sleep, and young healthy adults, especially those who are normally physically active, often have bradycardia. Usually no treatment is necessary except continuation of the stir-up regimen. Excessive parasympathetic stimulation from pain may cause bradycardia, in which case appropriate analgesics should be administered and other pain-relieving measures initiated. If the patient shows symptoms of low cardiac output, the physician should be notified and treatment instituted with atropine to block vagal effects or epinephrine and dopamine to stimulate the cardiac pacemaker. If temporary pacing wires are available, either atrial or ventricular pacing can be attempted. Bradycardia in conjunction with hypotension is considered an ominous sign for a pediatric trauma patient in shock because the major component of cardiac output in small children is the heart rate.[7]

***Sinus Tachycardia.*** Fig. 27-12 shows a fast heart rate, more than 100 bpm. The rhythm may be slightly irregular; all other complex features are normal.

Sinus tachycardia results from any stress and may be encountered in the PACU because of numerous causes, particularly factors relating to an increase in sympathetic tone, including the stress of surgery, anoxia, fever, overhydration, hypovolemia, pain, anxiety, or apprehension, or any combination of these factors. Tachycardia is an important postoperative sign and should be fully evaluated before treatment is instituted. Increasing tachycardia is an early sign of shock and must be thoroughly investigated. Treatment must be specific and based on removal of the underlying cause (see Chapter 54). The patient should be assessed carefully for the ability to tolerate the rapid rate. The deleterious effects of

tachycardias are generally related to diminished stroke volume and cardiac output. In general, the patient with previously normal cardiac function can tolerate tachycardias as high as 160 bpm without manifestation of symptoms. Poor tolerance with a resultant decrease in cardiac output occurs when the diastolic interval, and thus the ventricular filling time, is significantly compromised. Interventions for the compromised condition include beta-adrenergic blockers such as metoprolol and atenolol or calcium channel blockers such as verapamil.

***Sinus Arrest (Atrial Standstill).*** Sinus arrest is failure of the sinoatrial (SA) node to discharge, with the resulting loss of atrial contraction. The rate remains within normal ranges. The rhythm is regular except when the SA node fails to discharge. P waves and QRS complexes are normal when the SA node is firing and absent when it fails to discharge.

Common causes of sinus arrest in the PACU are the depressant effects of anesthesia or analgesics and electrolyte disturbances. Treatment is aimed at elimination of depressant drugs from the body and correction of electrolyte imbalances. This dysrhythmia must be brought to the attention of the physician immediately because persistent sinus arrest constitutes an emergency and CPR must be initiated.

### Supraventricular Dysrhythmias

Supraventricular dysrhythmias consist of supraventricular extrasystole (PAC), atrial tachycardia, atrial flutter, and atrial fibrillation. Supraventricular dysrhythmias occur in about 10% to 40% of patients after coronary artery bypass graft surgery. These rhythms should be documented with a 12-lead ECG. Their cause has been related to a number of possible factors, such as an inflammatory reaction to surgical trauma, insufficient "protection" of the atria during surgery, atrioventricular (AV) node ischemia, and sudden withdrawal of beta blockers. A correlation exists between persistent atrial activity during cardioplegia and postoperative supraventricular dysrhythmias.

***Premature Atrial Contraction.*** Premature atrial contraction, or atrial premature beat, occurs earlier than expected as a result of an irritable focus in the atrium (Fig. 27-13). Cardiac rate and rhythm are normal except for the prematurity. The P wave configuration of the premature beat usually differs from that of the normal beat. The PAC is followed by a pause that is not fully compensatory. This dysrhythmia results from anxiety and is commonly encountered in the PACU. No treatment is necessary unless the PACs become frequent or the patient

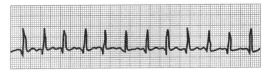

**Fig. 27-12** Sinus tachycardia (lead I).

NURSING CARE IN THE PACU

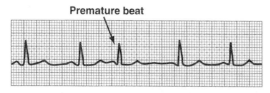

**Fig. 27-13**   Atrial premature beat (lead I).

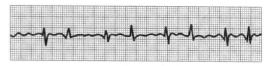

**Fig. 27-15**   Atrial flutter: 2:1 and 3:1 rhythm (lead I).

becomes symptomatic. Pharmacologic therapy may become necessary with agents such as digitalis, beta blockers, or verapamil if hemodynamic function is impaired.

*Atrial Tachycardia.* Atrial tachycardia is a rhythm disturbance that is a rapid regular supraventricular heart rate that results from an irritable focus of five or more PACs in succession (Fig. 27-14). The rate is 150 to 200 bpm with a regular rhythm.

This rhythm should be documented with a full 12-lead ECG. The physician should be notified for institution of therapy. Maneuvers that enhance vagal tone such as the Valsalva's maneuver and carotid sinus massage may be successful in termination of this dysrhythmia. Antiarrhythmic agents such as digitalis, quinidine, and verapamil may cause atrial tachycardia to revert to normal sinus rhythm. Adenosine can be used to stop atrial tachycardia, and quinidine or procainamide can be used to establish normal sinus rhythm. If these measures are unsuccessful, synchronized cardioversion is necessary.

*Atrial Flutter.* Atrial flutter consists of rapid supraventricular contractions that result from an ectopic focus with varying degrees of ventricular blocking (Fig. 27-15). Its cause is the same as that of PAC and atrial tachycardia. The rhythm is usually regular; the atrial rate is 250 to 350 bpm. Treatment is the same as for atrial tachycardia.

*Atrial Fibrillation.* In atrial fibrillation, one or more irritable atrial foci discharge at an extremely rapid rate that lacks coordinated activity (Fig. 27-16). Atrial fibrillation occurs commonly in patients with atrial enlargement from mitral valve disease or from long-standing coronary artery disease and is often preceded by PAC, tachycardia, or flutter. Clinically, the patient has an irregular heartbeat, pulse rate, and usually, a noticeable pulse deficit. Cardiac

output decreases in varying degrees. Normally, atrial filling and contraction account for 30% of ventricular filling. Without this atrial filling, or "atrial kick," of volume into the ventricle, stroke volumes and thus cardiac outputs are diminished. Treatment involves digitalis, quinidine, verapamil, atrial pacing, ablation, or cardioversion.

### Ventricular Dysrhythmias

Myocardial ischemia and perioperative myocardial infarction remain the two major causes of ventricular dysrhythmias; however, bradycardia, hypokalemia, hypoxemia, acidosis, and hypothermia are also potential causes.

*Premature Ventricular Contraction.* Premature ventricular contraction is a rhythm disturbance that involves an earlier-than-expected ventricular contraction from an irritable focus in the ventricle (Fig. 27-17). The rhythm is regular except for the premature beat, and the rate is normal.

The P wave is absent from the premature beat. A wide bizarre notched QRS complex that may be of greater-than-normal amplitude is present. A widened T wave of greater-than-normal amplitude is present after the premature beat and is of opposite deflection to that of the QRS complex.

The PVC is followed by a pause that is fully compensatory (i.e., the time of the PVC plus the pause time equals the time of two normal beats). PVCs are commonly encountered in the PACU and can occur in any patient. Occasional PVCs occur normally and need no treatment. Multiple PVCs may indicate inadequate oxygenation; when they occur, the patient's respiratory status should be thoroughly assessed. Other causative factors of PVCs include electrolyte disturbances, acid-base imbalance, drug toxicity, and hypoxemia of the myocardium.

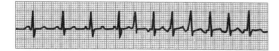

**Fig. 27-14**   Atrial paroxysmal tachycardia: onset in middle of record (lead I).

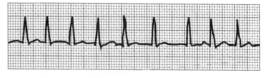

**Fig. 27-16**   Atrial fibrillation (lead I).

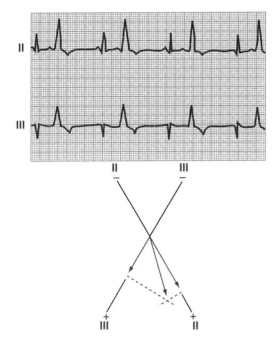

**Fig. 27-17** Premature ventricular contractions (leads II and III). (*From Guyton A, Hall J:* Textbook of medical physiology, *ed 10, Philadelphia, 2000, Saunders.*)

Treatment of PVCs is based on the underlying cause and obliteration of the irritable focus. Occasional isolated PVCs need not be treated. PVCs occur more frequently than five per minute, if a successive run of two or more occurs, if they are multifocal, or if they occur during the vulnerable period on the ECG complex, they must be treated because they are the precursors of the more lethal ventricular dysrhythmias.

Ventricular dysrhythmias present in the setting of bradycardia should be treated with atropine or with overdrive pacing for elimination of ventricular escape rhythms. Otherwise, lidocaine should be the first drug of choice for treatment of ventricular dysrhythmias.

**Ventricular Tachycardia.** Three or more consecutive PVCs constitute ventricular tachycardia (Fig. 27-18). The rhythm is fairly regular, and P waves are not seen. Occasionally, patients may have ventricular tachycardia and be asymptomatic, but usually they have anxiety,

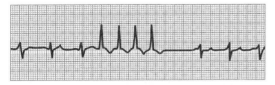

**Fig. 27-18** Ventricular paroxysmal tachycardia (lead III).

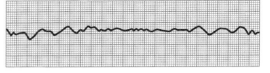

**Fig. 27-19** Ventricular fibrillation (lead II).

palpitations, fluttering, pounding in the chest, dizziness, faintness, and precordial pain. If ventricular tachycardia is prolonged, cyanosis, mental confusion, convulsions, and unconsciousness develop as a result of decreased blood and oxygen supply to the brain.

The causative factors of ventricular tachycardia are essentially the same as those for PVCs. Most commonly, ventricular tachycardia in the PACU is the result of hypoxia, drug toxicity, or underlying heart disease.

Ventricular tachycardia must be treated immediately. If the patient initially tolerates the dysrhythmia, treatment should be instituted with lidocaine. If the patient has cardiac decompensation and circulatory insufficiency, cardioversion with direct-current (DC) electric countershock should be immediately instituted. Immediate notification of the physician is essential.

**Ventricular Fibrillation.** A rapid irregular quivering of the ventricles that is uncoordinated and incapable of pumping blood characterizes ventricular fibrillation (Fig. 27-19). This rhythm disturbance is the major death-producing cardiac dysrhythmia. The immediate initial treatment is external DC countershock (Fig. 27-20). Ventricular fibrillation may occur spontaneously without any forewarning, or it may be preceded by evidence of ventricular irritability. Patients in whom ventricular fibrillation is likely to develop include those with underlying heart disease, those with ventricular irritability in the operating room during surgery, and those with symptoms of shock. All of these patients should be monitored continuously throughout the recovery period.

If ventricular fibrillation is not immediately terminated with countershock, CPR is instituted without delay. The anesthesiologist should be summoned immediately and a cardiac code initiated (see Chapter 57).

## HEMODYNAMIC MONITORING

Although more prominent in cardiac surgery, additional hemodynamic monitoring is commonly used with patients of higher acuity who receive care in many PACUs. Hemodynamic monitoring can be accomplished via the following invasive lines: a flow-directed pulmonary

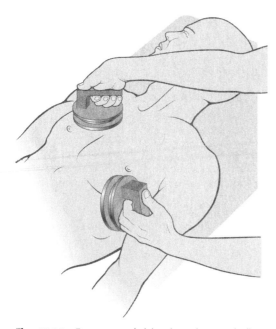

**Fig. 27-20** Emergency administration of external direct-current countershock. (*From Stoelting RK, Miller RD:* Basics of anesthesia, *ed 5, Philadelphia, 2007, Churchill Livingstone.*)

artery catheter, a central venous pressure catheter, a left-atrial or right-atrial catheter, a pulmonary artery thermistor catheter, or a peripheral arterial catheter (A-line). The parameters obtained from these various lines, the catheter insertion sites, and the placement and monitoring methods are presented in Table 27-1 and depicted in Fig. 27-21. Problems associated with maintenance of these lines are summarized in Table 27-2.

### Right-atrial Pressure

The normal right-atrial pressure ranges from 0 to 7 mm Hg. Pressures that exceed that level can be the result of fluid overload, right-ventricular failure, tricuspid valve abnormalities, pulmonary hypertension, constrictive pericarditis, or cardiac tamponade. Values in the lower range are usually indicative of hypovolemia.

### Pulmonary Artery Pressure

Pulmonary artery systolic pressures normally range from 15 to 25 mm Hg, whereas a normal pulmonary artery diastolic pressure is 8 to 10 mm Hg. Hypovolemia contributes to low pressure readings. Increased volume loads that can develop with an atrial or ventricular septal defect or left-ventricular failure can create elevations in pressure. In addition, obstructions to forward flow that can be caused by mitral stenosis or pulmonary hypertension can lead to an elevation in pulmonary artery pressures.

### Pulmonary Capillary Wedge Pressure

Normal pulmonary capillary wedge pressure (PCWP) recordings are between 6 and 12 mm Hg. Values in this range can be caused by an increased volume load, as is seen in left-ventricular failure, or they can be created by an obstruction to forward flow. Such obstructions may be caused by mitral stenosis or regurgitation or by a pulmonary embolism. Lower values may result from hypovolemia or indicate an obstruction to left-ventricular filling, which could occur with a pulmonary embolism, pulmonary stenosis, or right-ventricular failure.

### Left-atrial Pressure

Normal left-atrial pressures range from 4 to 12 mm Hg. As is seen with the PCWP, elevations in left-atrial pressure are associated with volume overloads or obstructions to forward flow, the latter of which may consist of left-ventricular failure states, mitral or aortic valve dysfunctions, or constrictive pericarditis. Lower recordings are generally a consequence of hypovolemia from inadequate volume or are related to an obstruction to forward flow. Such an obstruction may be a pulmonary embolism or pulmonic valve stenosis, or it may result from right-ventricular failure.

### Mean Arterial Pressure

Normal mean arterial pressures generally range between 80 and 120 mm Hg. In a postoperative cardiac surgical case, pressures lower than 60 mm Hg are generally avoided because coronary artery filling may be limited or impeded when parameters reach this level and may contribute to an ischemic or infarction state. Conversely, pressures higher than 120 mm Hg are avoided because they place too much stress on newly created suture lines that could readily rupture with sustained pressures.

### Cardiac Output and Cardiac Index

Cardiac output is the amount of blood ejected by the ventricle in 1 minute. Normal cardiac output is 4 to 8 L/min; it is calculated with the following formula:

$$SV \times HR \times CO$$

in which *SV* is stroke volume, *HR* is heart rate, and *CO* is cardiac output.

Cardiac index is calculated with the following formula:

$$CO/BSA = CI$$

in which *BSA* is body surface area in square meters and *CI* is cardiac index. Normal CI ranges from 2.5 to 4 Lmin/m$^2$. Because CI takes body size into

**Table 27-1  Methods for Invasive Monitoring of Hemodynamic Parameters**

| Parameters | Catheter Placement | Insertion Sites | Monitoring Method | Special Considerations |
|---|---|---|---|---|
| RAP | Proximal port of FDPAC lies in right atrium | Brachial<br>Jugular<br>Subclavian | Water manometer | Intermittent readings at lowest fluctuation* |
|  | Distal end of RAC or CVP lies in right atrium | Direct insertion through right atrial wall[†] | Transducer[‡] | Intermittent or continuous readings on mean[§] |
| PAP | Distal end of FDPAC lies in right or left branch of pulmonary artery | Brachial<br>Jugular<br>Subclavian | Transducer | Readings on systole and diastole |
|  | Distal end of PATC lies in main pulmonary artery | Direct insertion through pulmonary artery wall[†] |  |  |
| PCWP | Inflation of balloon on tip of FDPAC allows it to float into wedged position in smaller branch of pulmonary artery | Brachial<br>Jugular<br>Subclavian | Transducer | Intermittent readings on mean[§] |
| LAP | Distal end of LAC lies in left atrium | Direct insertion through left atrial wall[†] | Water manometer | Intermittent reading recorded at lowest fluctuation* |
| MAP | Distal end of catheter lies in peripheral artery | Radial<br>Brachial<br>Femoral | Anaeroid manometer | Midpoint of needle fluctuation |
|  |  |  | Transducer | Continuous readings on mean[§] |

*RAP*, Right-atrial pressure; *PAP*, pulmonary artery pressure; *RAC*, right-atrial catheter; *LAC*, left-atrial catheter; *CVP*, central venous pressure; *PATC*, pulmonary artery thermistor catheter. *FDPAC*, flow-directed pulmonary artery catheter.

*Fluctuation indicates patent catheter and good position in thorax.

[†]Direct insertion is achieved during open chest procedure via median sternotomy incision. Exit site is via stab wound at distal portion of median sternotomy. Catheter is attached to skin with suture. Removal is achieved with removal of suture and application of gentle traction to catheter to free it from chamber wall. Catheter is sutured to chamber wall with absorbable suture so that it releases easily. Chest tubes remain in place until such lines are removed because of possibility of bleeding.

[‡]To convert mm Hg to cm H$_2$O, multiply mm Hg reading times 1.36.

[§]Biphasic waves are measured on mean.

Adapted from Dennison R: *Pass CCRN*, ed 3, St Louis, 2007, Mosby; Smartt S: Hemodynamic monitoring. In DeFazio-Quinn D, Schick L, editors: *PeriAnesthesia Nursing core curriculum: preoperative Phase I and Phase II PACU nursing*, St Louis, 2004, Mosby.

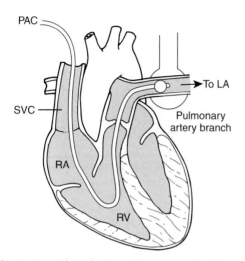

PAC

To LA

SVC

Pulmonary
artery branch

RA

RV

**Fig. 27-21** Schematic view of anatomy of pulmonary catheterization. (*From Papadakos P, Szalados J:* Critical care: the requisites in anesthesiology, *Philadelphia, Mosby.*)

consideration, it is a better indicator of the patient's perfusion status.[1,6,8,9]

### Systemic Vascular Resistance
Systemic vascular resistance (SVR) is the resistance the left ventricle must work against to eject its volume of blood. Normal SVR is 900 to 1300 dynes/s/cm$^{-5}$. An elevated SVR can create enough resistance to left-ventricular ejection that cardiac output and cardiac index decrease, which leads to a state of hypoperfusion or shock. Infusion of vasodilators and afterload-reducing agents can counteract this elevation. SVR is calculated with the following formula:

$$SVR = (MAP - CVP) \times 80/CO$$

in which *MAP* is mean arterial pressure and *CVP* is central venous pressure.[1,6,8,9]

### Pulmonary Vascular Resistance
Pulmonary vascular resistance (PVR) is the resistance the right ventricle must work against to eject blood into the pulmonary bed. Normal PVR is 80 to 240 dynes/s/cm$^{-5}$. An elevated PVR can create enough resistance to right-ventricular ejection that right-sided failure or infarction can develop. Infusion of vasodilators or pulmonary artery dilators such as aminophylline can counteract these elevations. PVR is calculated with the following formula:

$$PVR = [PAM - (PCWP \, or \, LAP)] \times 80/CO$$

in which *PAM* is pulmonary artery mean pressure and *LAP* is left-atrial pressure.[1,6,8,9]

## CENTRAL NERVOUS SYSTEM FUNCTION

All anesthetics affect the central nervous system (CNS), and one can assume for the present—even though we do not know exactly how narcosis occurs—that anesthetics are general nonselective depressants. The complexity of the CNS, coupled with our incomplete knowledge of how it functions, makes it a most difficult system to evaluate.

Assessment of the CNS in the PACU generally involves only gross evaluation of behavior, level of consciousness, intellectual performance, and emotional status. A more detailed assessment of CNS function is necessary for patients who have undergone CNS surgery; that discussion occurs in Chapters 10 and 38.

### Emergence from Anesthesia
Patients arrive in the PACU at all levels of consciousness, from fully awake to completely anesthetized. With modern anesthesia techniques, however, most patients respond appropriately by the time they are established in the PACU and become oriented quickly when the stir-up regimen is begun (see Chapter 28). With the use of fluorinated and opioid anesthetics, emergence is generally quiet and uneventful. Occasionally, a patient becomes agitated and thrashes about; this situation seems to occur more often in adolescents and young adults than in patients of other age groups. Emergence delirium also tends to occur more frequently in patients who have undergone intraabdominal and intrathoracic procedures (see Emergence Excitement in Chapter 29).

The perianesthesia nurse can facilitate patient orientation by telling the patient where he or she is, that the surgery is over, and what time it is as a part of the stir-up regimen. Reorientation occurs in reverse order from anesthesia: the patient first becomes oriented to person, then place, then time. This order, of course, may not hold true for the patient who was somewhat confused or disoriented before surgery, which emphasizes the importance of recording accurate information about the mental status of the patient before anesthesia.

Alterations in cerebral function are often the first signs of impaired oxygen delivery to the tissues. Therefore, an orderly and periodic assessment of mental function is necessary for detection of early evidence of abnormal cerebral function. Restlessness, agitation, and disorientation in the PACU may be ascribed to a number of other causes and are often difficult to evaluate. The use of continuous pulse oximetry can assist the perianesthesia nurse in

*Text continued on p. 383.*

**Table 27-2 Potential Problems Associated with Invasive Hemodynamic Monitoring**

| Potential Problems | Etiology | Precautions/Treatment |
|---|---|---|
| **ALTERATIONS IN PRESSURE WAVE CONFIGURATIONS** | | |
| Dampened tracings | **Technical** | |
| | Air in system | Check system for bubbles; flush bubbles out of system. |
| | Disconnection in system | Inspect and tighten all connections. |
| | Blood on transducer head | Flush until transducer dome clears of blood; change dome if necessary. |
| | Kinked catheter | Remove dressing to ascertain whether catheter is kinked externally. |
| | Catheter tip against wall | Turn patient's head or reposition extremity in which that catheter is inserted; watch for improvement in tracing. Gently aspirate catheter from various angles to determine at which angle best flow is achieved; tape and redress catheter at angle at which best flow is achieved. Gently flush catheter in attempt to push tip away from vessel wall. NEVER flush catheter in which clot is suspected. |
| | **Physiologic** | |
| | Clot on catheter tip | Attempt to aspirate blood from catheter. If possible, keep aspirating until clot is retrieved or blood no longer seems thickened. Flush system until line is cleared and readable tracing reappears. If blood cannot be aspirated, notify physician. |
| | With FDPAC, this may also indicate catheter has advanced forward and is in wedged position* | Ensure balloon is deflated. Recheck system and line. If no improvement, obtain chest radiograph and notify physician. |
| Abrupt exaggeration of pressure tracings | **Technical** | |
| | Loss of calibration of level of transducer | Recalibrate and relevel transducer. |
| | **Physiologic** | |
| | Slippage of catheter out of chamber or vessel | Avoid traction on intravascular lines; tape catheter to skin or secure with suture. |
| | FDPAC slipping from pulmonary artery to right ventricle; characterized by systolic pressure that | Inflate balloon in attempt to let catheter float back into pulmonary artery. If catheter does not migrate back |

*Continued*

**Table 27-2  Potential Problems Associated with Invasive Hemodynamic Monitoring—cont'd**

| Potential Problems | Etiology | Precautions/Treatment |
| --- | --- | --- |
| | remains same while diastolic pressure falls into range of right-ventricular end-diastolic pressure RAC, PAC, or PATC has slipped out of vessel wall into thoracic cavity | into pulmonary artery, obtain chest radiograph and notify physician. Attempt to aspirate to see whether catheter is still in vessel. If blood returns, flush system and attempt to obtain readable pressure tracings. If no blood return is achieved, notify physician and remove catheter, per protocol. |
| **ALTERATIONS IN VASCULAR INTEGRITY** | | |
| Venous and arterial spasms | Irritation to vessels during prolonged insertion attempts | Apply local anesthetic to catheter surface or administer anesthetic via intravenous route. Use guidewire to facilitate insertion. Cool catheter to make it less flexible and easier to insert. |
| Thrombophlebitis | Irritation to vessels from prolonged insertion attempts or from constant motion of catheter against vessel | See Venous and Arterial Spasms, discussed previously. Secure catheter in place with either tape or suture. Avoid prolonged infusions of chemically irritating medications. Maintain adequate dilutions. Observe for signs and symptoms of phlebitis, and notify physician for possible withdrawal of catheter. Distal placement of stopcocks, connecting catheters, and tubing permits atraumatic blood sampling and flushing. |
| Embolization | Clot embolization from thrombophlebitis or from clot on catheter tip<br>Pulmonary embolism with infarct from FDPAC<br><br>Cerebral embolization from LAC catheter<br><br>Peripheral embolization with extremity ischemia from peripheral arterial lines | Always aspirate catheter first if clot is suspected. NEVER FLUSH.<br>Observe for changes in chest radiograph that indicate pulmonary embolization.<br>Observe for neurologic changes that may indicate embolization from LAC.<br>Observe for ischemic changes of extremity in which catheter is located. |

| Complication | Cause | Nursing Intervention |
| --- | --- | --- |
| Air embolization | Loose connections | Secure and tighten all connections. Vigilantly observe LAC catheter because even minute amounts of air in this system can lead to serious neurologic complications. |
| | Rupture of balloon on FDPAC caused by overinflation or normal use because latex layer on balloon absorbs lipoproteins from blood and slowly loses elasticity, thus increasing its incidence rate of rupture | Inflate balloon slowly, and do not overinflate. Limit inflations. Allow balloon to empty air passively back into syringe. Avoid aspirating air back because this weakens integrity of balloon. Aspirate only if air fails to return passively. If air does not return and rupture is questioned, sterile saline solution can be injected into balloon and attempts made to aspirate it back. Failure to aspirate fluid back indicates leak; physician should be notified. |
| Vessel erosion or hemorrhage Bleeding from insertion site: Rupture of branch of pulmonary artery | Inadequate hemostasis after insertion Overinflation of balloon in normal-sized vessel | Apply firm pressure for 15 to 20 minutes. Do not attempt to inflate balloon if tracing already appears wedged. Inject only prescribed amount of air into balloon. |
| | Normal inflation of balloon in too-small vessel | Inject air slowly, and stop injecting if resistance is felt. Inject only amount of air necessary to obtain wedge tracing. |
| | Repeated normal inflations in brittle or susceptible vessel | Limit wedge intervals in patients at high risk, such as patients with pulmonary hypertension or long-standing mitral valve disease. |
| Atrial dysrhythmias | Irritation of right atrium from RAC or during insertion of FDPAC | Withdraw CVP catheter to level of superior vena cava, and obtain readings from that area. Continue with insertion of FDPAC because dysrhythmias are usually self limiting and stop once catheter tip exits right atrium. |
| Ventricular dysrhythmias | Irritation of right ventricle from tip of FDPAC during insertion procedure or from catheter tip slipping out of pulmonary artery and back into right ventricle | Continue with insertion of FDPAC because dysrhythmias are usually self limiting and stop once catheter passes into pulmonary artery. If catheter tip falls back into right ventricle from pulmonary artery, inflate balloon because this cushions tip of catheter and may alleviate dysrhythmias. Administer lidocaine if ventricular dysrhythmias continue. Notify physician, |

*Continued*

NURSING CARE IN THE PACU

## Table 27-2  Potential Problems Associated with Invasive Hemodynamic Monitoring—cont'd

| Potential Problems | Etiology | Precautions/Treatment |
|---|---|---|
| | | obtain chest radiograph, and manipulate catheter, per hospital policy. |
| **INFECTIONS** | | |
| Local infection | Faulty aseptic techniques during insertion or during subsequent dressing changes | Maintain sterility during insertion. Change dressings with sterile technique and tubings, per hospital policy. |
| Systemic infection | Faulty aseptic technique during insertion | Avoid spasms during insertion. Avoid development of thrombophlebitis along vessel. Change indwelling catheters and insertion sites every 48 to 72 hours, which may be impossible in patients with difficult vascular access sites. In these situations, rethreading new catheter over guidewire at previous insertion site can be done every 48 to 72 hours. However, once site is questionable or patient has symptoms of sepsis develop, such as elevated temperatures and white blood cell count, new line at new site is necessary. |
| Endocarditis | Extension of local insertion site<br>Infection along catheter and into circulation | Culture per hospital policy. Observe for development of new murmurs. |

*RAC*, Right-atrial catheter; *PATC*, pulmonary artery thermistor catheter; *LAC*, left-atrial catheter. *FDPAC*, flow-directed pulmonary artery catheter.
*Note: Wedging of catheter in postoperative patient may be common occurrence for two reasons: (1) catheter may have advanced forward during operative procedure when chest was open and lungs were not fully inflated because less resistance to forward advancement was found; and (2) as hypothermia is reversed and patient and catheter rewarm, its increased flexibility may allow it to float forward.
Adapted from Cole D, Schlunt M: *Adult perioperative anesthesia:the requisites in anesthesiology,* Philadelphia, 2004, Mosby; Dennison R: *Pass CCRN,* ed 3, St Louis, 2007, Mosby.

determination of whether symptoms may be related to hypoxemia.

## THERMAL BALANCE

The measurement of the patient's body temperature in the PACU is particularly important. The most recent ASPAN standards state that, at minimum, the preoperative assessment, initial postoperative physical assessment, and discharge evaluation of the patient in phases I and II PACUs should include documentation of temperature.[1] Normal body temperature may vary from 36° C to 38° C (96.8° F to 100.4° F). In the healthy adult, body temperature remains fairly constant because of the balance between heat production and heat loss. Alterations in body temperature occur often in the postoperative patient. Factors that affect the body temperature in the PACU patient are listed in Box 27-1.

Premedications, anesthesia, and the stress of surgery all interact in a complex fashion to disrupt normal thermoregulation. Both hypothermia (temperature less than 36° C) and hyperthermia (temperature more than 38° C) are associated with physiologic alterations that may interfere with recovery (Box 27-2).

Patients at the age extremes and those with extreme debilitation are at even greater risk for postoperative development of temperature abnormalities.

The accuracy of axillary, rectal, or oral measurement is often debated. Core temperature (approximate value of temperature of blood perfusing the major metabolically active organs) is only estimated with oral and rectal temperature readings. Invasive techniques that use the thermistor on a pulmonary artery catheter, the tympanic membrane, or the bladder as a site for monitoring temperature are more accurate. Unless necessary during surgery or because of a specific problem, these temperature-monitoring methods are seldom used in the PACU.

| Box 27-1 | Factors That Influence Body Temperature of the PACU Patient |
|---|---|

Anesthesia
Preoperative medications
Age of patient
Site and temperature of intravenous fluids
Vasoconstriction (from blood loss or anesthetic agent)
Vasodilation (from regional anesthesia or use of inhalational agent)
Body surface exposure
Temperature of irrigations
Temperature of ambient air

Shell (skin) temperature may be measured at the axilla or forehead with conventional thermometers or liquid crystal temperature strips. Shell temperature does not accurately reflect core temperature, although it may at least indicate gross trends.

Infrared tympanic membrane thermometry is often used in the PACU. The method is noninvasive and nontraumatic and may be used with patients of all sizes. With placement over the outer third of the auditory canal, the sensor on this otoscope-like thermometer gathers emitted infrared energy from the ear and translates this energy into a temperature reading within seconds. The infrared tympanic thermometer has been found to accurately track core temperature as measured with the thermistor tip of a pulmonary artery catheter.

The newer temporal scanner thermometer is a fast accurate noninvasive method of temperature measurement with gently scanning of the forehead over the temporal artery. Investigators in studies at Boston Children's Hospital and Harvard Medical School determined that temporal temperatures are as accurate as tympanic or rectal temperatures in children.[10,11] However, at the present time there is a lack of evidence to support accuracy for core temperature measurements in adults.[12] Some

| Box 27-2 | **Physiologic Alterations Associated with Hypothermia and Hyperthermia** |
|---|---|

| HYPOTHERMIA | HYPERTHERMIA |
|---|---|
| Bluish tint to skin (cyanosis) | Pale skin (mottled) |
| Increased metabolic rate with shivering, then decreased metabolic rate | Increased metabolic rate |
| Decreased oxygen consumption | Increased oxygen consumption |
| Decreased muscle tone | Decreased muscle tone |
| Decreased heart rate | Increased heart rate (rapid and bounding) |
| Dysrhythmias | Dysrhythmias |
| Decreased level of consciousness | Alterations in CNS (patient may be agitated) |

considerations include measurement of only the side of the head that is exposed. Any covering (hair, hat, etc.) prevents the heat from dissipating and causes the reading to be falsely high, which also applies with one side of the head in a pillow. Sliding the thermometer in a reasonably straight line across the forehead, midway between the eyebrows and the upper hairline, and not down the side of the face is the correct technique in taking the temperature. Midway on the forehead area, the temporal artery is less than 2 mm below the skin surface, but down the side of the face, it is much deeper; therefore, measurements are less accurate.

Management of the patient with hypothermia is directed toward the restoration of normothermia and the avoidance of shivering. Warm blankets may be placed over the patient as specific hospital protocol allows. Forced air warming systems provide a safe and effective means of gradually rewarming the patient. Hypothermia and hyperthermia are discussed in greater detail in Chapters 45 and 53.

## FLUID AND ELECTROLYTE BALANCE

Evaluation of a patient's fluid and electrolyte status involves total body assessment. Imbalances readily occur in the postoperative patient for a number of reasons, including the restriction of food and fluids before surgery, fluid loss during surgery, and stress (Table 27-3). The normal body response to stress of surgery is renal retention of water and sodium. In addition, patients often have abnormal avenues of postoperative fluid loss.

### Fluid Intake

Each patient must be evaluated for determination of baseline requirements and the fluid needed to replace abnormal losses. The healthy adult who is deprived of oral intake needs 2000 to 2200 mL of water per day to make up for urinary output and insensible loss.

*Intravenous Fluids.* Most patients admitted to the PACU from the operating room are receiving intravenous fluids. The anesthesia care provider must have an open intravenous line for the administration of necessary medications and replacement fluids during surgery, and an open line is needed after surgery for supply of necessary fluids, electrolytes, and medications. Because all efforts to substitute for normal oral intake of electrolytes and adequate volumes of fluid are at best temporary and inadequate, the first objective is to return the patient to adequate oral intake as soon as possible. Until this objective can be attained, an intravenous line must be maintained. The nurse should be aware of the type and amount of any fluid administered and any medications that may have been added to it.

The intravenous site should be checked to ensure that the needle or cannula is still in the vein and that no extravasation has occurred. Watch for kinks or disconnected tubing, and ensure that the rate of infusion is accurate. The intravenous site should be positioned comfortably; a board may be helpful in maintenance of the intravenous site if the patient should become restless.

Pediatric patients may need a protective device over the site or soft protective devices to prevent dislodging of the needle or cannula.

| Table 27-3 Common Clinical States that Affect Fluid and Electrolyte Balance in the PACU | |
|---|---|
| Clinical State | Effect on Fluid and Electrolyte Balance |
| Pain | Heightened response to stress |
| Anesthesia | Water and sodium retention |
| Fear | |
| Trauma | |
| Acute renal failure | Impaired acid-base regulatory mechanism |
| Blood loss | Impaired fluid circulation |
| Immobilization | |
| "–ostomies" | Excessive loss of fluid via abnormal routes |
| Nasogastric suction | Potassium and sodium deficit |
| Bleeding | |
| Vomiting | |
| Thyroidectomy | Calcium deficit |
| Treatment of acidosis | |
| Excessive administration of citrated blood | |

A simple paper cup device can be helpful in prevention of dislodgement of the intravenous line from the scalp veins of small infants. Snip the bottom out of the cup; thread the cup over the tubing; place the large opening over the intravenous site; and secure the cup to the baby's head with tape crisscrossed over the entire cup. In addition to providing protection for the intravenous site, this method allows the nurse to check the insertion site frequently.

After ensuring that the intravenous fluids are infusing correctly, check to see what fluids, if any, are to follow or if the infusion is to be discontinued. If the patient is receiving total parenteral nutrition and intralipids, only feeding solutions should go through this line; another intravenous pathway must be secured for other uses. Multilumen catheters allow for the administration of multiple fluids and medications and can be connected to a transducer to provide continuous hemodynamic monitoring, if indicated.

The flow of intravenous fluids in the patient receiving hyperalimentation, the patient who is fluid-restricted, the infant and small child, and the patient who is receiving intravenous analgesia or vasopressors should always be regulated with electronic fluid administration devices.

### Oral Fluids

Oral intake must be prohibited after anesthesia until the laryngeal and pharyngeal reflexes are fully regained, as evidenced by the patient's ability to gag and swallow effectively. If the patient is permitted oral intake, starting with small amounts of ice chips is best because these are less likely to cause nausea and vomiting. Some PACUs use isotonic ice chips that are made from a balanced electrolyte solution, such as Lytren, Pedialyte, and Ricelyte. If ice chips are well tolerated, the patient can progressively increase oral intake to include water and other clear liquids. Kool-Aid and fruit-flavored popsicles are well tolerated and accepted by both children and adults. In addition, carbonated beverages may be soothing to a patient who feels slightly nauseated. The management of postoperative nausea and vomiting is discussed in Chapters 16 and 29.

### Fluid Output

Normal output in the average adult results from obligatory urinary output and insensible avenues of loss, including evaporation of water from the skin and exhalation during respiration. The amount of urine necessary for the normal renal system to excrete waste products of a day's metabolism is approximately 600 mL. Optimally, 30 mL/h or more of urine should be obtained from an adult who is catheterized to ensure proper hydration and kidney function. Urinary output should be closely monitored in the recovery phase; measurement of urinary output and urine specific gravity yields important clues to the overall status of the patient and may alert the nurse to overhydration or dehydration or the development of shock.

A lower than normal urinary output can be expected in the postoperative patient as a result of the body's normal reaction to stress; however, an unduly small volume of urine (less than 500 mL in 24 hours) may indicate the presence of renal insufficiency, and the physician should be notified.

If a urinary catheter is in place, a more accurate observation of hourly output is available. If urine volume is low and specific gravity remains fixed at a low level, renal insufficiency is indicated. A small urine volume plus a high specific gravity indicates dehydration. In addition to the volume and specific gravity of urinary output noted, the urine should be examined for the presence of pus, blood, or casts.

The perianesthesia nurse must evaluate abnormal and normal avenues of output. Abnormal ways include external losses from vomiting, nasogastric tubes, T-tubes, and fistula or wound drainage and temporary functional losses from fluid shifting within the body, such as hemorrhage into soft tissues and the edema of surgical wounds.

The surgical site should be noted on admission to the PACU, and the dressing should be checked for drainage. The perianesthesia nurse must be aware of the presence of any drains and the expected amount of drainage. Drainage tubes should be checked to ensure patency, and the amount, color, and odor of any drainage should be observed and documented. All tubes should be secure and either clamped shut or connected to drainage apparatus as ordered by the physician. A summary of imbalances that may occur with abnormal avenues of output is presented in Table 27-4. Any deviations from the normally expected drainage in a specific route should be reported promptly to the surgeon.

Obviously, the accurate measurement and recording of all intake and output is vital to the assessment of each patient's fluid and electrolyte status. A running total kept on the postanesthesea flow sheet or online documentation system is essential for quick assessment of fluid status. In addition to observation and assessment of avenues of intake and output, the perianesthesia nurse should be alert to symptoms of fluid and electrolyte imbalance, which are summarized in Table 27-5.

NURSING CARE IN THE PACU

**Table 27-4   Imbalances that May Occur with Abnormal Avenues of Output**

| Fluid | pH | Content (mEq/L) | Likely Imbalances with Significant Losses |
|---|---|---|---|
| Gastric juice (fasting) (nasogastric suction) | 1-3 | $Na^+$ (60) $K^{++}$ (10) $Cl^-$ (85) $HCO^{-3}$ (0-15) | Metabolic alkalosis Potassium deficit Sodium deficit Fluid volume deficit |
| Small intestine (suction) jejunum | 7-8 | $Na^+$ (111) $K^+$ (4.6) $Cl^-$ (104) $HCO^{-3}$ (31) | Metabolic acidosis Potassium deficit Sodium deficit |
| Ileum | | $Na^+$ (117) $K^+$ (5.0) $Cl^-$ (105) | Fluid volume deficit |
| New ileostomy | | $Na^+$ (129) $K^+$ (11) $Cl^-$ (116) | Potassium deficit Sodium deficit Fluid volume deficit Metabolic acidosis |
| Biliary tract fistula | 7.8 | $Na^+$ (148) $K^+$ (5.0) $Cl^-$ (101) $HCO^{-3}$ (40) | Metabolic acidosis Sodium deficit Fluid volume deficit |
| Pancreatic fistula | 8.0-8.3 | $Na^+$ (141) $K^+$ (4.6) $Cl^-$ (76) $HCO^{-3}$ (121) | Metabolic acidosis Sodium deficit Fluid volume deficit |

Adapted from Bland J: *Clinical metabolism of body water and electrolytes*, Philadelphia, 1963, Saunders; and Guyton A, Hall J. *Textbook of medical physiology*, ed 11, Philadelphia, 2006, Saunders.

## PSYCHOSOCIAL ASSESSMENT

Assessment of the patient's psychologic and emotional well being is an important component of perianesthesia nursing. As with any other assessment, this assessment must be made in the context of the whole patient. Illness, hospitalization, surgery, and pain all take on a variety of values, depending on the person. The meaning of the surgery to the person must be explored before surgery and will probably have been obtained by other health care providers; this information should be communicated to the perianesthesia nurse who will care for the patient. Likewise, the perianesthesia nurse must ensure that additional assessment information and psychosocial care in the PACU are shared with those who care for the patient after discharge from the unit.

Almost all surgical patients have a degree of anxiety about anesthesia and the surgical procedure and a fear of postoperative pain. The physical signs and symptoms of anxiety are the same as those produced by any stressor. Reactions are mediated by the sympathetic nervous system and are listed in Box 27-3.

Symptoms of anxiety must be carefully differentiated from those of other causes. Differentiation is particularly difficult while the effects of anesthesia are still present. A quiet calm environment is important to the postanesthesia recovery of the surgical patient. A calm confident nurse can do much to allay anxiety for the postoperative patient through both verbal reassurance and touch. Hearing is the first sense to return after anesthesia. Yelling at patients is not necessary; they may not respond even if they can hear. In fact, yelling at patients may increase anxiety early in the PACU period because the patients may believe they are not recovering as quickly as they should.

Attention to comfort, including minimal environmental noise and stimuli, and the reassuring presence of the nurse are calming. Once the patient has fully regained consciousness, simply talking may help allay anxiety. Simple factual statements repeated often are best. At this point,

| Table 27-5 | Signs and Symptoms of Acute Fluid and Electrolyte Imbalance |
|---|---|
| **Imbalance** | **Symptoms and Findings** |
| Hyperosmolarity<br>   Water excess<br>   Sodium deficit | Polyuria (if kidneys are healthy), twitching, hyperirritability, disorientation, nausea, vomiting, weakness, serum Na $\uparrow$ 120 mEq/L |
| Isotonic disturbances<br>   Dehydration<br>   Circulatory collapse<br>   Volume excess | Weakness, nausea, vomiting, oliguria, postural drop in systolic BP, elevated hematocrit, normal serum $Na^+$<br>Shock<br>Dyspnea, cough, sweating, edema |
| Hydrogen ion imbalances<br>   Metabolic acidosis<br>   Metabolic alkalosis<br>   Respiratory acidosis ($CO_2$ retention) | Apathy, disorientation, increased rate and depth of respiration $\rightarrow$ Kussmaul's respiration, symptoms of $K^+$ excess, ABG pH $\downarrow$ 7.35, $HCO^{-3}$ $\downarrow$ 25, acid urine with pH $\downarrow$ 6.0<br>Increased irritability, disorientation, shallow slow respirations, periods of apnea, irregular pulse, muscle twitch, ABG pH $\uparrow$ 7.45, $HCO^{-3}$ $\uparrow$ 29, alkaline urine with pH $\uparrow$ 7.0<br>Increased rate and depth of breathing, tachycardia and other dysrhythmias, drowsiness, ABG pH $\downarrow$ 7.4, $PCO_2$ $\uparrow$ 40, $HCO^{-3}$ 25-35 |
| Potassium imbalances<br>   Deficit (hypokalemia)<br>   Excess (hyperkalemia) | Weakness, mental confusion, shallow respirations, hypotension, dysrhythmias, serum $K^+$ $\downarrow$ 3.5 (measurement of extracellular $K^+$ and only gives vague reflection of intracellular balance)<br>Four common causes of hypokalemia: Reduced intake; GI losses; excessive renal loss of $K^+$ $K^+$ shifts from extracellular to intracellular<br>Intestinal colic, oliguria, bradycardia, cardiac arrest, serum $K^+$ $\uparrow$ 5 mEq/L |
| Calcium imbalances<br>   Deficit (hypocalcemia)<br>   Excess (hypercalcemia) | Tingling of fingers, laryngospasm, facial spasms, painful muscle spasms, positive Trousseau's sign, positive Chvostek's sign, convulsions, palpitations, cardiac dysrhythmias, serum $Ca^{++}$ $\downarrow$ 4.5 mEq/L<br>Not usually seen in PACU; usually caused by pathology involving parathyroid glands |

*BP*, Blood pressure; *ABG*, arterial blood gas; *GI*, gastrointestinal.

the nurse may be able to explore the cause of the distress with the patient.

For the patient in acute distress from anxiety, a mild tranquilizer, such as diazepam (Valium), midazolam (Versed), or lorazepam (Ativan), may be indicated; however, these benzodiazepines should be used judiciously. One advantage of their use is that they potentiate opioids and often allow a reduction of the analgesic dosage necessary to control pain. Because apnea is a common side effect when benzodiazepines are given to patients receiving opioids, continuous respiratory monitoring with pulse oximetry and capnography is indicated.

Attention to the psychosocial ramifications of specific surgical interventions is provided in each of the following chapters on postanesthesia care. These comments are incorporated into the overall text whenever deemed appropriate. For further discussion of the relationship between pain and anxiety, see Chapter 31.

| Box 27-3    **Signs and Symptoms of Anxiety** |
|---|
| Tachycardia<br>Increased blood pressure<br>Pale cool skin<br>Increased respiratory rate<br>Hyperventilation<br>Increased muscle tone<br>Restlessness or agitation<br>Dilated pupils |

## SUMMARY

Obviously, the perianesthesia nurse must be an expert in assessment. The perianesthesia nurse must not only understand the normal physiologic functioning of the human body but also be able to differentiate and evaluate the variety of pathologic symptoms that may arise in the postprocedure patient. The perianesthesia nurse must be aware of the interrelationships between mind and body and must be sensitive to the psychosocial factors that influence the patient's reactions. Knowledgeable assessment of the postprocedure patient is essential for the provision of safe and effective medical treatment and nursing care.

## REFERENCES

1. Cole D, Schlunt M: *Adult perioperative anesthesia: the requisites in anesthesiology*, Philadelphia, 2004, Mosby.
2. American Society of PeriAnesthesia Nurses: *2006-2008 Standards of perianesthesia nursing practice*, Cherry Hill, NJ, 2006, ASPAN.
3. Atlee J: *Complications in anesthesia*, ed 2, Philadelphia, 2007, Saunders.
4. Miller R: *Miller's anesthesia*, ed 6, New York, 2005, Churchill Livingstone.
5. Stoelting R, Miller R: *Basics of anesthesia*, ed 5, Philadelphia, 2007, Churchill Livingstone.
6. Urden L, Stacy K, Lough M: *Priorities in critical care nursing*, ed 4, St Louis, 2004, Mosby.
7. Litman RS: *Pediatric anesthesia: the requisites in anesthesiology*, Philadelphia, 2004, Mosby.
8. Morton P, Fontaine D, Hudak C, et al: *Critical care nursing: a holistic approach*, ed 8, Philadelphia, 2004, Lippincott Williams & Wilkins.
9. Lessig ML: The cardiovascular system. In Alspach JG, editor: *Core curriculum for critical care nursing*, ed 6, St Louis, 2006, Saunders.
10. Siberry GK, Diener-West M, Schappell E, et al: Comparison of temple temperatures with rectal temperatures in children under two years of age, *Clin Pediatr (Phila)* 41(6):405–414, 2002.
11. Greenes DS, Fleisher GR: Accuracy of a noninvasive temporal artery thermometer for use in infants, *Arch Pediatr Adolesc Med* 155(3):376–381, 2001.
12. Hooper VD, Andrews JO: Accuracy of noninvasive core temperature measurement in acutely ill adults: the state of the science, *Biol Res Nurs* 8(1):24–34, 2006.

## BIBLIOGRAPHY

Alspach J: *Core curriculum for critical care nursing*, ed 6, Philadelphia, 2006, Saunders.
Arbour R: Impact of bispectral index monitoring on sedation and outcomes in critically ill adults: a case series, *Crit Care Nurs Clin North Am* 18:227–241, 2006.
Barash P, Cullen B, Stoetling R: *Clinical anesthesia*, ed 5, Philadelphia, 2005, Lippincott Williams & Wilkins.
Bickley L, Hoekelman R: *Bates' guide to physical examination and history taking*, ed 9, Philadelphia, 2005, Lippincott Williams & Wilkins.
Black J, Hokanson-Hawks J: *Medical-surgical nursing: clinical management for positive outcomes*, ed 7, St Louis, 2005, Saunders.
Brunton L, Lazo J, Parker K: *Goodman and Gilman's the pharmacological basis of therapeutics*, ed 11, New York, 2005, McGraw-Hill Professional.
Burden N, Defazio D, Quinn D, et al: *Ambulatory surgical nursing*, ed 2, Philadelphia, 2000, Saunders.
Cote C, Todres I, Goudsouzian N, et al: *A practice of anesthesia for infants and children*, ed 3, Philadelphia, 2001, Saunders.
DeFazio-Quinn D, Schick L: *PeriAnesthesia nursing core curriculum: preoperative phase I and phase II PACU nursing*, St Louis, 2004, Mosby.
Dennison R: *Pass CCRN*, ed 3, St Louis, 2007, Mosby.
Drew B, Funk M: Practice standards for ECG monitoring in hospital settings: executive summary and guide for implementation, *Crit Care Nurs Clin North Am* 18:157–168, 2006.
Estafanous F, Barash P, Reves J: *Cardiac anesthesia*, ed 2, Philadelphia, 2001, Lippincott Williams & Wilkins.
Fleisher L: *Evidence-based practice of anesthesiology*, Philadelphia, 2004, Saunders.
Ganong W: *Review of medical physiology*, ed 22, New York, 2005, McGraw-Hill Medical.
Guyton A, Hall J: *Textbook of medical physiology*, ed 11, Philadelphia, 2006, Saunders.
Hickey J: *The clinical practice of neurological and neurosurgical nursing*, ed 5, Philadelphia, 2002, Lippincott Williams & Wilkins.
Hill K, Klein D: Transcutaneous carbon dioxide monitoring, *Crit Care Nurs Clin North Am* 18:211–215, 2006.
Katzung BG: *Basic and clinical pharmacology*, ed 10, Los Altos, CA, 2006, Appleton & Lange.
Lake CL, Hines RL, Blitt CD: *Clinical monitoring: practical applications for anesthesia and critical care*, St Louis, 2001, Mosby.
McCance K, Huether S: *Pathophysiology: the biologic basis for disease in adults and children*, ed 5, St Louis, 2006, Mosby.
Murray J, Nadel J: *Textbook of respiratory medicine*, ed 4, Philadelphia, 2005, Saunders.
Nagelhout J, Zaglaniczny K: *Nurse anesthesia*, ed 3, Philadelphia, 2005, Saunders.
Rathmell J, Neal J, Viscomi C: *Regional anesthesia: the requisites in anesthesiology*, Philadelphia, 2004, Saunders.
Schumacker L, Chernecky C: *Critical care & emergency nursing*, St Louis, 2005, Saunders.

Springhouse: *Critical care nursing made incredibly easy*, Ambler, PA, 2003, Lippincott Williams & Wilkins.

Springhouse: *IV therapy made incredibly easy*, Springhouse, PA, 2005, Lippincott Williams & Wilkins.

Swearingen P: *Manual of medical-surgical nursing care*, ed 6, St Louis, 2006, Mosby.

Wadland D: Prevention, recognition, and management of nursing complications in the intraoperative and postoperative surgical patient, *Nurs Clin North Am* 41:151–171, 2006.

Zwerneman K: End-tidal carbon dioxide monitoring: a VITAL sign worth watching, *Crit Care Nurs Clin North Am* 18:217–225, 2006.

NURSING CARE IN THE PACU

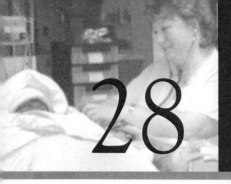

# 28

# PATIENT EDUCATION AND CARE OF THE PERIANESTHESIA PATIENT

*Denise O'Brien, MSN, APRN,BC, CPAN, CAPA, FAAN*

Patients primarily arrive for operative and interventional procedures on the day of the procedure, unlike many years ago, when most patients spent days in the hospital before procedures. This transition necessitated a change in preparation of patients and families for procedures and in focused interest on patient education processes and products. This chapter discusses effective patient education, which supports improved patient outcomes. Nursing care of postanesthesia patients who are emerging from anesthesia is also reviewed in this chapter. Postanesthesia care includes the stir-up regimen, intravenous therapy, maintenance of respiratory function, patient transfers, and general comfort measures.

## DEFINITIONS

**Affective Learning:** Relates to attitude and includes the ability to receive, respond, value, and organize a personal value system and internalize the value system.

**Cognitive Learning:** The human processing of information; application of knowledge.

**Continuous Positive Pressure Airway (CPAP):** Delivers air into the patient's airway and creates enough pressure to keep the airway open during inhalation.

**Intermittent Mandatory Ventilation (IMV):** Allows patients to breathe on their own as often and as deeply as they like and ensures that a set tidal volume is delivered at a predetermined back-up rate.

**Patient Education:** Useful information that helps patients and their families or companions become more informed about the medical and nursing care they receive before, during, and after surgical and diagnostic procedures.

**Positive End Expiratory Pressure (PEEP):** A technique that can be used to help prevent collapse of the alveoli during the expiratory phase of ventilation, to increase the lung's functional residual capacity (FRC), and to reduce the amount of physiologic shunting.

**Stir-up Regimen:** Consists of five major activities as the patient is recovering from anesthesia: deep-breathing exercises, coughing, positioning, mobilization, and pain management.

**Sustained Maximal Inspiratory (SMI) Maneuver:** The patient inhales as close to total lung capacity as possible and, at the peak of inspiration, holds that volume of air in the lungs for 3 to 5 seconds before exhaling.

**Synchronous Intermittent Mandatory Ventilation (SIMV):** Allows the patient to control the inspiratory time and the size of the spontaneous tidal volumes.

## PATIENT EDUCATION CONCEPTS AND PERIANESTHESIA CARE

Patient preparation for surgical and interventional procedures includes not only preanesthesia assessment and appropriate testing but also education individualized for the patient and the family or companion. The goals of patient education are to increase the patient's sense of self worth, decrease anxiety, and reduce facility and provider liability by ensuring the patient and family or companion receive information in a form that they can comprehend and use to enhance the operative experience. Ideally, the patient and family or companion has an opportunity to review the educational content and ask questions of the health care provider before the day of surgery.

The purpose of preoperative education is to empower patients, give them greater decision-making authority related to their care, and enable them to better manage their health. The patient benefits from learning before the surgery with decreased preoperative fear and anxiety, postoperative complications, recovery time, and postoperative pain. Education also increases patient compliance with instructions and improves coping mechanisms for the patient and preparation. Preoperative education is for the patient and the family or companion and is a professional responsibility of the professional registered nurse.

Before providing education for patients, perianesthesia nurses complete a self assessment that reflects on strengths and weaknesses such as knowledge base, understanding of the information to teach, and whether they like or dislike teaching. Consideration should be given to personal biases: does the nurse react negatively to patients with a history of alcohol use or who are obese? Does the nurse dislike children or the elderly? Do the religious or ethnic preferences of the nurse conflict with the patient population served? Sensitivity to diversity and cultural awareness of patients improve the professional registered nurse's ability to provide appropriate education for the patients and families or companions. The nurse may need to work on improving knowledge and teaching skills while preventing biases from affecting the duty to provide patient education.

### The Learning Environment and Learning Needs

If possible, education should take place in an environment that is conducive to learning. Unfortunately, the nurse is often challenged by noise, lack of privacy, and limited space. A quiet private space should help reduce the patient's anxiety and facilitate learning. An area that is family oriented and lacks physical barriers is best, especially when the population consists of children or elderly patients.

Methods for identification of learning needs of both the patient and the family or companions include asking open-ended questions, directly observing the patient and family, and hearing the verbal cues that indicate learning and knowledge. Nonverbal cues are also observed and noted. The patient's and family's or companion's current knowledge level can be identified through questionnaires, telephone conversations, observation, or interview. Rather than focusing on what the nurse wants to tell the patient and family or companion, the nurse should determine what the patient and family or companion want and need to know and teach them accordingly.

### Learner Characteristics

Patient demographic information includes age; primary language; reading level; sensory limitations; physical condition; developmental level; mental, emotional, or educational limitations; and motivation and attitude. Identification of how the patient prefers to learn is also essential in individualization of learning materials for the patient. For the pediatric patient,

developmental stage is evaluated. Age-related challenges need to be considered with the elderly patient.

### Types of Learners

The adult learner is internally motivated, self directed, and self governed; uses experience as a resource; may have difficulty accepting new concepts; and has a problem-centered orientation to learning. The child learner does not assume responsibility for learning, is totally dependent on adults, relies on a transmittal method of learning, is open to new concepts, and is subject centered.

When the child is the patient, the parents often begin education at home, depending on the age of the child and the preparation needed. Therefore, parent preparation is essential and requires knowledge of adult learning characteristics by the nurse. Typically, the younger the child, the closer to the day of the procedure the education occurs. Parents' and caregivers' understanding of the child's behavior and developmental stage should guide the nurse in choice of appropriate teaching tools and techniques. Even with preparation, separation anxiety for both child and parent occurs and may be especially difficult for the 1-year-old to 5-year-old child. See also Chapter 49 for specific information about caring for the pediatric patient.

The older adult may have had less formal education, and comprehension may be limited. However, the learning challenges of elderly patients may be related to sensory deficiencies that can interfere with the ability to learn and not educational level or intellect. Chapter 50 reviews the care of the geriatric patient and the specific challenges of this population.

### Influences on Learning

Physiologic, emotional, cultural, and environmental barriers can hinder the learning process for all ages and developmental levels. Language barriers can decrease the patient's ability to understand instructions and limit compliance with instructions because of lack of comprehension. Inadequate or poor teaching can also be a barrier to the learning process, and the professional registered nurse works on improving knowledge and skills of teaching and learning for the patient populations encountered. Another consideration is evaluation of the learner's present knowledge, previous experience, prior education, perceptions and expectations, and potential misinformation. The patient's health beliefs, attitudes, level of stress, coping skills, anxiety, and social support also influence learning.

Retention of information is dependent on how the information is presented. The reading of an educational pamphlet is less effective than hearing the same information while reading the material and talking about it. Content that is visually appealing, perhaps with photographs or diagrams, may also help the learner retain the information. Demonstration and return demonstration with the learner talking through the process is probably the most effective way to help the learner retain new information.

## Teaching Characteristics and Planning

The professional registered nurse needs to have knowledge of teaching-learning principles, to recognize that anxiety and pain impede learning, and to value reinforcement of learning. Common language, not medical terminology, should be used. Knowledge of the teaching tools available and the content to teach is essential for successful patient education.

Content knowledge guides the development of an individualized teaching plan for the patient and family or companion. The plan is based on assessment of learning needs. As part of the plan, one should consider developing a verbal or written contract with the patient or family or companion that helps meet the purpose of empowering the individual patient in the health care environment.

Learning goals focus on the domains of learning. Cognitive learning involves knowledge. Intellectual abilities such as the recall of facts and understanding of concepts, the application and analysis of learned ideas, and synthesis and evaluation fall in the cognitive domain. The affective learning domain relates to attitude and includes the ability to receive, respond, value, and organize a personal value system and internalize the value system. Skills are in the psychomotor domain. This domain includes imitation, manipulation, development of precision, skill integration, and expertise.

## Content of Teaching Plan

The teaching plan includes generic content, with general information about preoperative preparation, day of surgery activities, and postoperative issues. The environment is described as is the usual sequence of events. Individualized content is also integrated into the teaching plan to meet needs identified by the nurse's assessment of learning, review of the patient's history, and information requested by the patient or family.

Preoperative teaching content describes the procedure on the day of surgery, including expected behaviors to prepare the patient, possible alterations in comfort after the procedure, and strategies for pain reduction. Recommendations for fasting from solids and liquids are reviewed, as are medications to be held or taken on the day of surgery. Patients should be instructed to leave valuables and jewelry at home. Bathing or showering with an antibacterial cleanser may help reduce the risk of surgical infection; patients should be reminded to do this the evening before and the morning of the procedure if possible. For patients undergoing outpatient or ambulatory procedures, the requirement for a responsible adult companion and, if needed, a ride home at discharge should be reinforced. Facility policies vary regarding transportation requirements (e.g., whether the companion must stay in the facility during the procedure or if the companion may be called to pick up the patient). The professional registered nurse is responsible for knowing the facility policies; awareness of resources such as risk management or legal counsel is beneficial should questions arise regarding patient transportation or responsible adult companion issues.

Discussion related to possible alterations in comfort helps prepare the patient for what to expect after surgery. Common concerns include pain, sore throat, and nausea and vomiting. The patient's past experience may influence expectations. Descriptions of strategies for pain reduction, including request of pain medication and use of positioning, ice, or other techniques, may ease the patient's concerns about pain and discomfort. Postoperative nausea and vomiting may be minimized or controlled with medications, aromatherapy, hydration, and slow movements. Additional information on pain management can be found in Chapter 31; nausea and vomiting are discussed in Chapter 29.

A demonstration of equipment that the patient will see or hear during or after the procedure may ease fears of the unknown or unusual sounds and sights, especially for children.

The surgeon may discuss procedure-specific educational information for the patient. Brochures, booklets, videos, or group classes can be used. The anesthesia care provider may offer educational material for the planned anesthesia on the basis of the type of procedure and the patient's needs for the nurse to review or may provide the education personally.

Finally, postoperative behaviors are reviewed to complete the patient's preparation for surgery. The content includes passive exercises to reduce the risk of venous thromboembolism; safe ambulation; effective deep breathing and coughing to reduce the risk of respiratory complications;

dressing, drain, or cast care; diet and fluid needs or restrictions; signs and symptoms that indicate complications; follow-up care; and emergency contact information for use after leaving the facility.

## Teaching Strategies

The nurse's primary objectives when teaching are establishment of rapport to reduce anxiety and fear; assessment of patient and family knowledge and expectations for learning; and assessment of patient and family learning style to enhance the learning process. These objectives can apply to teaching before the day of surgery in a structured setting, patient education that occurs at the bedside while the patient is in the postanesthesia care unit (PACU), or teaching during preparation for discharge. The level of detail provided should be based on these assessments, with the education tailored specifically to the patient and family or companion. Teaching should be directed to the patient, but the family decision-maker or primary caregiver should also be considered as important to educational success. Ample opportunity for the patient and family to voice concerns and ask questions should be provided. If language is a barrier, interpreter services can assist in the teaching process. Short simple explanations are best, with the importance of the instructions and expected benefits of compliance with the instructions stressed. Jargon should be avoided and all terms clarified. Teachable moments should be used to advantage: those times when the patient and family are most likely to accept new information (e.g, symptoms are present).

Incorporation of more than one teaching method may enhance learning and reinforce teaching. A variety of teaching methods should be used, including written material and demonstration of skills. Formal education may occur in a classroom setting and involve lecture, group discussion, or audiovisual materials. Written material should be readable at a grade 5 or 6 level. Other options include play therapy, tours of the facility, films or videos, web-based learning activities, or games.

For children, factors that affect the choice of teaching method include the child's age and developmental level, the family's available resources, and the cognitive ability of the child and parent. The facility tour can be effective for 4-year-olds to 12-year-olds and may be combined with puppets or models. Play therapy provides an opportunity for the 3-year-old to 7-year-old child to draw, act out, or describe events. Puppets or dolls may be used. Films or videos can be viewed in multiple places and are most effective if the

patient is the same age, race, and gender as the children shown in the video. This method is most effective in the 7-year-old to 12-year-old age group but requires quiet time for viewing. Models allow visualization and manipulation of equipment such as breathing masks, circuits, splints, intravenous (IV) tubing, and anatomic parts. Although models are most effective with the 3-year-olds to 6-year-olds, they can be used with all ages.

Written material may include a description of events to be expected on the day of surgery and should be easy to understand. This material can be taken home for referral throughout the preparation period and after the procedure. Instead of text, picture or coloring books may be helpful to 4-year-olds to 8-year-olds or to patients with low literacy or language barriers. An advantage of preprinted instructions is the standardized information. Any written material needs to be legible with larger print size for the visually impaired and elderly. Use of internationally recognized symbols is also helpful.

## Patient Education on the Day of Surgery

The patient's greatest need on the day of surgery is psychosocial. Less emphasis should be placed on information and skills, and more on reassurance and support. Any information given is limited to the essential information for safe transitioning of the patient to the operative suite. The family or companion may have additional informational needs and also need support during this time.

## Discharge Instructions

Ideally, the patient and family or companion have had an opportunity to review any discharge instructions before the day of surgery to help prepare the home with any needed supplies or alterations (e.g., removal of rugs that increase fall risk, sleeping area moved closer to the bathroom) for minimization of safety concerns or enhancement of care. Discharge instructions are reviewed with the patient and family or companion before the patient is discharged. Included in the instructions are recommended diet; medications (new prescriptions, resumption of regular medications); pain management (when to take medications, when to call if pain not relieved); bowel habit (increase in dietary fiber and fluids, use of stool softener); wound, dressing, or drain care (when to change, supplies needed, when to call physician); follow-up plan and visit; resumption of activities of daily living and return to work; and emergency instructions (who to call, where to go).

### Documentation

Patient education completed by the nurse is documented as a record of education provided to the patient. Forms vary by institution and may be paper or electronic. Standardized care plans include documentation of individualized education. Checklists or flow sheets may be used. Whatever the form, teaching should be documented to support the work of the nurse and record what the patient was told and the response to the educational information. This documentation protects the patient, the nurse, and the facility should concerns arise over educational content and patient preparation. Additional information on documentation can be found in Chapter 7.

## CARE OF THE PERIANESTHESIA PATIENT

### The Stir-up Regimen

The stir-up regimen is an important aspect of postanesthesia nursing care, especially for the patient who has received general anesthesia. Patients transition to an awake state more quickly than in the past or even arrive in the PACU awake and alert; however, prevention of complications remains important and elements of the stir-up regimen can help minimize complications. Like most other PACU activities, the basics of the stir-up regimen are aimed at prevention of complications, primarily atelectasis and venous stasis. Five major activities constitute the stir-up regimen: deep-breathing exercises, coughing, positioning, mobilization, and pain management.

*Deep-breathing Exercises.* The primary factor that contributes to postoperative pulmonary complications is decreased lung volumes. The major factor that contributes to low lung volumes in the PACU patient is a shallow monotonous sighless breathing pattern caused by general anesthesia, pain, and opioids. Full inflation of the lungs prevents small areas of patchy atelectasis from developing and assists in the elimination of inhalation anesthetics, thus hastening the awakening process. Intravenous anesthesia differs from inhalation anesthesia in that, once injection has occurred, little can be done to expedite removal of the drug; however, the prevention of atelectasis with deep breathing remains just as important. The patient should be stimulated to take three or four deep breaths every 5 to 10 minutes. Full expansion is important but may be impeded by a number of factors. Every effort must be made to enhance the patient's ability to expand the lungs. Patients who are emerging from anesthesia may have difficulty participating in the

activity because of reduced levels of consciousness and awareness.

The sustained maximal inspiratory (SMI) maneuver is a method for enhancement of lung volumes after surgery. The SMI maneuver consists of the patient inhaling as close to total lung capacity as possible and, at the peak of inspiration, holding that volume of air in the lungs for 3 to 5 seconds before exhaling. Ideally, the patient has received instruction and coaching in the postoperative use of this maneuver. The patient may use an incentive spirometer that provides visual or auditory feedback and observation of inspiratory volume.

Incentive spirometry is used to prevent or assist reversal of atelectasis, promote normal lung expansion, and improve oxygenation. Instruction and practice before surgery provide patients the opportunity to master the device and establish a baseline for before anesthetic and surgical interventions. Devices currently available include disposable flow-oriented and volume-oriented incentive spirometers that are inexpensive and can be used by the patient at home. Incentive spirometry may have greater use after the immediate postanesthesia period because patients are more awake and capable of manipulating the devices than they are in the PACU.

*Coughing.* The patient must be instructed to cough in addition to the SMI maneuvers. The best way to clear the air passages of obstructive secretions is a purposeful cough. Cough effectiveness depends on the inspired tidal volume and the velocity of expired air flow. For the patient who is recovering from anesthesia, the cascade cough is the most effective cough maneuver. The patient should be taught to take a rapid deep inspiration to increase the volume of air in the lungs, which in turn dilates the airways, thus allowing air to pass beyond the retained secretions. On exhalation, the patient should perform multiple coughs at subsequently lower lung volumes. With each cough during exhalation, the length of the airways that undergo dynamic compression increases and cough effectiveness is enhanced.

Coughing is most effective when the patient is sitting. Splinting of incisions and adequate analgesia facilitate a good cough. If the patient is unable to sit upright, the side-lying position with hips and knees flexed or a semi-Fowler's position with head and arms supported with pillows and with knees flexed decreases abdominal tension and allows maximal movement of the diaphragm, thereby improving the effectiveness of the cough.

Preoperative teaching of postoperative breathing exercises and coughs and their importance is effective and should be included in the preoperative regimen whenever possible. Patients scheduled for surgery may attend formal teaching sessions before surgery or may receive instructions for coughing, deep breathing, and incentive spirometry through educational booklets, video programs, and visits to preoperative testing departments.

*Positioning.* When possible, patients in the PACU should be maintained in a semiprone or side-lying position. The semiprone position promotes maintenance of a patent airway, prevents aspiration of vomitus into the trachea, and permits optimal ventilation of the lower lung lobes. Frequent repositioning of patients (at least every hour) is essential for prevention of atelectasis and peripheral stasis. The patient's position should be changed from side to side. Care must be taken to ensure that all drainage tubes and intravenous catheters remain in place and patent and that no tension on any of these lines is created. As soon as they are able, patients should be encouraged to turn and change positions alone.

*Mobilization.* For prevention of venous stasis, patients are encouraged to move the legs and arms rhythmically. Patients should flex and extend the extremities. Mobilization and flexion of the muscles aid venous return, automatically cause deep breathing, and improve cardiac function.

*Pain Management.* Achievement of the stir-up regimen's first four activities is difficult if adequate pain relief is not provided. Opioids depress the cough reflex and ciliary action and may lower alveolar ventilation with direct depression of the respiratory center. If breathing is painful and splinting occurs or if the patient refuses to cough or move because of pain, respiratory or embolic complications may occur. Pain management is discussed in detail in Chapter 31.

*Modifications of the Stir-up Regimen.* Modifications of the stir-up regimen may be needed depending on the type of anesthesia used and the operative procedure performed. Ketamine may cause emergence excitement during the initial recovery period. When ketamine is used, a rigorous stir-up regimen is eliminated from routine PACU care and verbal and tactile stimulation of the patient is minimized as much as possible. Cough must be eliminated after eye surgery and other delicate plastic surgery procedures. Stimulation of the patient with increased or potentially increased intracranial pressure must be undertaken carefully to avoid dangerous and potentially life-threatening

pressure changes. If any doubt exists regarding purposeful coughing after a procedure, check with the surgeon for specific instructions.

Positioning is probably the activity most often modified in the stir-up regimen. Positioning of the patient and modifications of the stir-up regimen after specific surgical procedures and anesthetics are discussed in related chapters.

## Intravenous Therapy

Postoperative parenteral fluid requirements vary with the patient's preoperative status and with the surgical procedure. For a discussion of fluid and electrolyte imbalance, see Chapter 14.

## Maintenance of Respiratory Function

*Oxygen Therapy.* The optimization of the oxygen-carrying capacity of arterial blood is the goal of oxygen therapy. All anesthetized patients have had some interference with respiratory processes, so most experts suggest routine oxygen administration to all patients after anesthesia. However, oxygen is a drug and should be treated as such, with full prescription information provided by the anesthesia care provider. This information may be contained in standard orders that are individualized for each patient. Low-flow oxygen administration assists the patient in maintenance of adequate oxygenation of all tissues. Optimal arterial oxygen tension should be between 70 and 100 mm Hg. Patients with chronic lung disease may have maintenance with low-flow oxygen administration, which keeps the oxygen tension in the range of 50 to 70 mm Hg. Pulmonary processes should be monitored carefully in the PACU. Pulse oximetry monitoring of all patients who have received an anesthetic is recommended in the initial postanesthesia period.

Pulse oximetry, a noninvasive technique, is used to measure arterial oxygen saturation of functional hemoglobin. In the postanesthesia setting, continuous monitoring of a patient's oxygen saturation assists in manipulation of the fraction of delivered oxygen ($F_DO_2$) levels and in identification of episodes of desaturation and hypoxemia. Normal pulse oximetry values are 97% to 100%. Oxygen saturation as measured with pulse oximetry ($SpO_2$) values of 95% or greater are acceptable. Preanesthetic baseline $SpO_2$ values should be noted; patient levels may normally fall below the normal range in room air. Attempts to maintain higher oxygen saturation levels than the baseline level may result in prolonged oxygen therapy and PACU stays.

NURSING CARE IN THE PACU

Sensor site selection and application, ambient light, motion, electric interference, and impaired blood flow (low perfusion states, excessive edema) may influence $SpO_2$ levels. Temperature, pH, partial pressure of carbon dioxide ($PaCO_2$), hemodynamic status, and anemia affect accurate measurement. These factors alter the oxyhemoglobin dissociation curve and oxygen delivery. In addition, dysfunctional hemoglobins (carboxyhemoglobin, a byproduct of smoking and smoke; methemoglobin, formed from drugs such as lidocaine and nitroglycerin) may result in false elevation of oximetry values. Newer oximeters that measure eight wavelengths, rather than the two-wavelength pulse oximetry that has been in use, are now available and measure these dyshemoglobins.

Nurses may need to draw arterial blood gases to aid in the assessment of a patient's status. For discussion of arterial blood gases and the method for measurement, see Chapter 12.

Perianesthesia nurses should be aware of complications that can occur with oxygen therapy.

Oxygen-induced hypoventilation, atelectasis, substernal chest pain, and toxicity may occur when high concentrations are administered over prolonged periods (fraction of inspired oxygen concentration [$FiO_2$] > 0.5 for more than 24 hours). Clinical detection of decreased oxygen saturation levels is difficult without pulse oximetry or arterial blood gas sampling.

***Methods of Administration.*** Routine oxygen administration in the PACU can be accomplished with nasal cannula (prongs) or face masks. Table 28-1 lists commonly used oxygen delivery methods. Nasal cannulas are advantageous for routine short-term oxygen administration in the PACU. The cannula is made of plastic tubing with two soft plastic tips that insert into the nostrils about 1.5 cm. The prongs deliver 100% oxygen and thus yield a final inspired oxygen concentration of 30% to 40% when a 4 L/min to 6 L/min flow is used. The prongs are easily inserted, comfortable, inexpensive, and disposable. Simple clear plastic disposable face masks may be used for

| Table 28-1 | **Methods of Oxygen Administration** | | |
|---|---|---|---|
| Method | $FiO_2$ | Flow (L/min) | Comments |
| **LOW-FLOW METHOD** | | | |
| Nasal cannula (prongs) | 0.24-0.4 | 5-6 | Comfortable to wear; patient can breathe orally or nasally and still raise $FiO_2$; humidification unnecessary |
| Simple face mask | 0.4-0.6 | 10 | Adjustable to fit face; may be hot for patients Poorly tolerated; potential for skin irritation from tight fit and oxygen contact |
| Face tent | 0.3-0.55 | 4-10 | Less confining; useful when extra humidity is needed |
| Partial rebreathing mask | 0.35-0.6 | 6-10 | Mask with attached reservoir bag; no valves on mask (exhalation ports open) |
| **HIGH-FLOW METHOD** | | | |
| Nonrebreathing mask | 0.4-1 | 6-15 | Mask with reservoir bag; one-way valves on mask; side ports of mask; one-way valve between mask and bag for inhalation |
| Venturi mask | 0.24-0.55 | 2-14 | Believed accurate delivery of desired $FiO_2$; may be less if patient is hyperpneic or unable to keep mask in position on face |
| T-piece or Brigg's | 0.21-1 | 2-10 | Used with endotracheal or tracheostomy tube; provides accurate delivery of desired $FiO_2$ and humidification; most often used in weaning patients from ventilator assistance before endotracheal tube removal |
| Mechanical ventilator | 0.21-1 | Direct from supply | Pressure, volume, flow, and oxygen percentage all adjustable |

*$FiO_2$,* Fraction of inspired oxygen concentration.

oxygen administration in the PACU. They are also easy to apply and comfortable. The oxygen concentration inspired depends on the mask fit and the patient's inspiratory flow rate; however, an oxygen flow rate of 10 L/min yields an $FiO_2$ of up to 60%. A higher flow rate keeps the patient from rebreathing exhaled carbon dioxide ($CO_2$). Face masks in the PACU must be clear to provide adequate observation of the patient's nose and mouth. The mask should be removed intermittently to dry the face.

*Humidity.* Surgery and anesthesia often interrupt the normal functioning of the nose in heating and humidification of inspired air. When oxygen is administered via nasal cannula at flow rates of less than 4 L/min or via Venturi mask, humidification is generally unnecessary because adequate amounts of humidified room air are inspired. At higher flow rates, humidification or nebulization may be needed in the PACU.

Humidifiers convert water from the liquid to the gaseous state, whereas nebulizers produce tiny water particles. Humidifiers are used to add water vapor to the airway; a nebulizer can provide both water vapor and particulate water or medication or saline aerosols to the airway. Aerosol therapy can be used to administer antibiotics, bronchodilators, and corticosteroids. Care when filling humidifiers, avoidance of contamination of the water in the humidifier, and proper disposal of humidifiers after use avoid the spread of infectious agents.

*Mechanical Ventilation.* Rarely, some patients who are recovering from anesthesia may need some form of mechanical ventilation in the PACU. Various techniques such as positive end-expiratory pressure (PEEP), continuous positive airway pressure (CPAP), and intermittent mandatory ventilation (IMV) are used for improvement of the respiratory status of the patient. Table 28-2 gives the terminology of the common ventilatory modes.

**Positive End-Expiratory Pressure.** Positive end-expiratory pressure is a technique that can be used to help prevent collapse of the alveoli during the expiratory phase of ventilation, to increase the lung's functional residual capacity (FRC), and to reduce the amount of physiologic shunting. PEEP also increases the $PaO_2$, which usually enables the $FiO_2$ to be reduced, thus lessening the chances of oxygen toxicity. In patients with preexisting obstructive lung disease, PEEP should be used cautiously because it may overexpand relatively normal alveoli. When it is used in such circumstances, the dead space increases and occasionally causes a decrease in the $PaO_2$ and an increase in the $PaCO_2$.

When a patient is placed on PEEP therapy, hemodynamic status should be monitored because this ventilatory technique decreases venous return and may cause a decrease in cardiac output, especially in the patient with hypovolemia. In some instances, the reduced cardiac output can cause a decrease in systolic blood pressure. Other parameters to be monitored are vital signs, skin perfusion, and urine output.

**Continuous Positive Airway Pressure.** Continuous positive airway pressure helps keep the lungs expanded. The patient breathes out against increased pressure as high as 10 to 20 cm $H_2O$, but the mechanics of ventilation do not change. The lung performs at a larger, more inflated volume, thereby increasing the FRC and decreasing the tendency to atelectasis. CPAP is a technique that can be used for weaning a patient from a ventilator. When CPAP is used, the patient should be monitored

| Table 28-2 **Terminology: Common Ventilatory Modes** | |
|---|---|
| Abbreviation | Term |
| **MECHANICAL VENTILATION WITH POSITIVE AIRWAY PRESSURE** | |
| A/C | Assist–control ventilation |
| CMV | Continuous mandatory ventilation |
| IMV | Intermittent mandatory ventilation |
| SIMV | Synchronized intermittent mandatory ventilation |
| PSV | Pressure support ventilation |
| PEEP | Positive end-expiratory pressure |
| APRV | Airway pressure-release ventilation |
| **SPONTANEOUS BREATHING (SB) WITH POSITIVE AIRWAY PRESSURE** | |
| CPAP | Continuous positive airway pressure |
| BiPAP | Bilevel positive airway pressure |

for tachypnea, tachycardia, increases in blood pressure, dysrhythmias, or generalized distress, which should be reported to the physician, if detected.

**Bilevel Positive Airway Pressure.** Bilevel positive airway pressure (BiPAP) is another form of non-invasive positive-pressure ventilation that provides continuous high-flow positive airway pressure that cycles between a high positive pressure and a lower positive pressure. Gas exchange improves with BiPAP because of an increase in alveolar ventilation. Monitoring is similar to that for CPAP.

**Synchronous Intermittent Mandatory Ventilation.** Synchronous intermittent mandatory ventilation allows the patient to control the inspiratory time and the size of the spontaneous tidal volumes depending on patient effort and muscle strength, lung compliance, airway resistance, and whether or not pressure support is present to increase spontaneous tidal volume delivery. The patient receives three different types of breath: controlled (mandatory) breath, assisted (synchronized) breaths, and spontaneous breaths. SIMV can be combined with pressure support ventilation (PSV) to provide both a back-up support ventilation strategy and may also be implemented as SIMV (pressure mode).

**Intermittent Mandatory Ventilation.** Intermittent mandatory ventilation was originally devised for facilitation of the weaning process from mechanical ventilation. It is currently used when a patient is first given mechanical ventilation. This technique allows patients to breathe on their own as often and as deeply as they like; it also ensures that every minute a set tidal volume is delivered at a predetermined back-up rate. IMV allows gradual progression from complete ventilatory support with the ventilator to spontaneous provision of ventilation by the patient.

**Nursing Responsibilities.** All PACU nurses must be familiar with the specific types and modes of operation of ventilators used in the area (Fig. 28-1; see Table 28-2). However, some nursing responsibilities remain the same regardless of mechanical ventilator. The following list discusses these responsibilities.

1. Ascertain that the patient is ventilated with frequent observation of the chest for bilateral synchronous and equal expansion and by listening for bilaterally present and equal breath sounds.
2. Check the airway frequently for complete patency. See that the patient ventilator system is free of significant leaks by listening for air gurgling in the upper airway

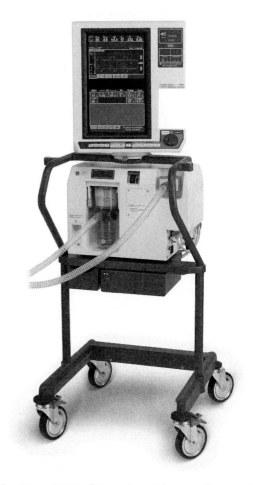

**Fig. 28-1**  840 Ventilator system. Volume ventilator used either to assist or to control patient's respirations. *(Reprinted by permission of Nellcor Puritan Bennett, Inc, Pleasanton, Calif.)*

during ventilation and by comparing the exhaled volume with the tidal volume set on the ventilator.
3. Ensure that the cuff is never overinflated. Inflate the cuff until no leak is identified on tidal ventilation and a small barely audible leak occurs on sigh volume.
4. Empty the ventilatory hoses frequently of excess water from condensation.
5. Ensure that proper humidification is delivered to the patient by noting the presence of water droplets in the ventilator hoses.
6. Check the humidifier and fill frequently to ensure proper humidification.
7. Ensure that the temperature gauge is between 32.2° C and 36.6° C, and that the ventilator hoses and humidifier are warm to the touch and never cold or hot.
8. Position the patient's endotracheal or tracheostomy tube so there is never any pull.

9. Perform the tracheostomy wound care as needed during the postanesthesia phase.

10. Ascertain frequently that all alarms on the ventilator are on, set appropriately, and functioning properly.

The observations and checks of mechanical devices often seem simple and routine but are an important part of nursing the patient who requires mechanical ventilation. Ideally, all these checks, along with measured parameters of the patient's respiratory status, should be recorded either on a flow sheet attached to the patient's bed or to the ventilator or electronically as defined by the facility. Frequently, respiratory therapists maintain and manage the ventilator in the PACU. The respiratory therapist is available to assist the nurse caring for the patient on the ventilator and to complete the appropriate documentation of ventilator and patient status.

***Suctioning.*** When large amounts of secretions accumulate that cannot be handled effectively with coughing, suctioning must be instituted to assist the patient in clearing air passages.

**Oral and Nasal Suctioning.** Suctioning the nose and mouth is simple and safe. This procedure is commonly used to assist patients in elimination of secretions when they have not yet regained full consciousness and cannot spit out secretions. The catheter used should be soft and pliable. The technique should be clean but need not be strictly sterile. A Yankauer or tonsil suction tip may be used to remove oral secretions from the mouth and over the tongue; however, care must be used to avoid breaking or chipping the teeth.

**Tracheal Suctioning.** Tracheal suctioning may be performed through the mouth or nose, via endotracheal tube, or through a tracheostomy tube (Fig. 28-2). Tracheal suctioning must be accomplished atraumatically with aseptic technique. A selection of sterile suctioning catheters in a variety of sizes should be kept at the bedside of every patient in the PACU along with sterile gloves and sterile water or normal saline solution. The catheter chosen for suctioning should not have an external diameter that exceeds by one third the internal diameter of the tube to be suctioned. Most commonly, a 14F or 16F size is used for adult patients. The catheter must not completely occlude the trachea or endotracheal tube.

The procedure should be explained to the patient even if the patient appears unconscious. Explanation of the procedure alleviates fear and also helps gain cooperation from the patient.

Before suctioning the patient, ensure proper ventilation. In most patients, suctioning lowers

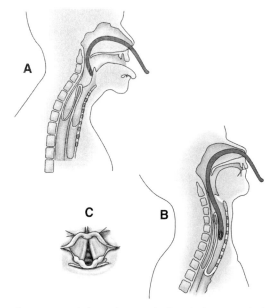

**Fig. 28-2** Technique of nasotracheal suctioning. **A,** Optimal position of head to direct catheter tip anteriorly into trachea. Neck is flexed, and head is extended. Tongue is protruded (and held in place with 4 × 4 gauze). **B,** After catheter has been advanced into trachea, tongue is released and patient's head may be more comfortably positioned. **C,** View of vocal cords from above. Cords are most widely separated during inspiration. *(Redrawn from Sanderson RG, editor: The cardiac patient, Philadelphia, 1972, Saunders.)*

the arterial pressure of oxygen 30 to 35 mm Hg. Because suctioning removes oxygen, which may in turn initiate cardiac dysrhythmias, the nurse should assess the total physiologic condition of the patient before beginning the procedure. Is the patient restless, agitated, or disoriented? Although these conditions can be caused by other factors, they often indicate inadequate oxygenation. Conscious patients can be asked to take four or five deep breaths. The patient who cannot cooperate must undergo preoxygenation with a bag-valve-mask (B-V-M) unit or anesthesia bag. A B-V-M device delivers variable oxygen concentrations ($FiO_2$ between 30% to 95%) and volumes. Flow rates should be at least 10 to 15 L/min for higher $FiO_2$. Higher volumes can be obtained with use of two hands to compress the bag. If the patient has an endotracheal airway in place and is on a ventilator, several sigh volumes can be delivered at 1.0 $FiO_2$ before suctioning.

For suctioning of the patient with no airway adjunct, the nurse should instruct the patient to stick out the tongue and then should grasp the tongue with a gauze pad and apply gentle traction to make the glottis open and move in line with the trachea. The nurse then lubricates the catheter tip with a small amount of water-soluble jelly and gently inserts the catheter into the nostril. A slight curvature in the tubing may facilitate intubation of the larynx. The catheter is advanced until intubation of the trachea is accomplished. The nurse listens through the catheter or feels for air movement against the cheek through the proximal end of the catheter. An increasing intensity of breath sounds or more air against the cheek indicates nearness to the larynx. If the breath sounds decrease or the patient begins to gag, the catheter is in the hypopharynx and the nurse needs to draw back and advance again. A sudden cough indicates the presence of the catheter in the larynx; the nurse should advance quickly with the next breath.

Once the catheter is positioned in the trachea, intermittent suction is applied with alternate occluding and opening of the vent of the Y-connector with the thumb and withdrawal of the catheter in a spiral motion. If an airway adjunct is present, suctioning may be accomplished through it.

Suction should never be applied until the catheter is in the trachea and never for longer than 15 seconds. One useful trick is for the nurse to hold his or her breath while suctioning the patient as a reminder of the time limits. The patient is monitored carefully during all suctioning procedures. Any form of suctioning can lead to dysrhythmias, and prolonged suctioning may produce hypoxia, asphyxia, and cardiac arrest. Suctioning removes oxygen and secretions; therefore, the patient should undergo oxygenation before and after the procedure.

Suctioning is not without risk of complication, nor should it be done routinely. Risks include bradycardia and vagal responses. Appropriate indications for suctioning are the presence of bronchial secretions, identified visually or with auscultation or, in the patient with mechanical ventilation, with rising airway pressures from retained secretions. Hypoxemia is the most common complication that can lead to atelectasis and dysrhythmias. Other complications include mucosal trauma, infection, paroxysmal coughing, and increased systemic and intracranial pressures.

Tracheostomy care is discussed in Chapter 32.

### General Comfort and Safety Measures

General comfort and safety measures are important parts of postanesthesia care. For safety, at least two nurses (one of whom is a registered nurse) should always be present in the same room whenever patients in PACU phase I level of care are recovering. An unconscious patient should never be left alone, and side rails should be raised on the bed or stretcher whenever direct patient care is not being provided. The wheels of the bed or stretcher should be locked to prevent sliding when care is rendered.

General physical measures such as cleanliness should not be overlooked in the PACU. Comfort measures, important to the total well being of the patient, are often forgotten in the hustle of caring for postanesthesia patients. As soon as the patient is settled into the unit and assessment has been accomplished, all excess skin preparations and electrodes should be removed; in addition to provision of comfort, the washing off of excess skin preparations gives the nurse an excellent opportunity to further assess the patient's general condition. This time is also good for changing the patient's position, assisting with range-of-motion exercises, and encouraging deep breathing. Frequent position changes help prevent atelectasis, promote circulation, and prevent pressure from developing on the skin surfaces.

Mouth care with moistened toothettes or swabs may be comforting to the patient who has not only had nothing by mouth but also has been medicated with an anticholinergic to reduce secretions. When patients are fully conscious and laryngeal reflexes have returned, they can rinse the mouth with water. Ice chips and small sips of water or juice may be offered to the patient who can tolerate fluids. A petrolatum-based ointment should be applied to the lips after mouth care to prevent drying and consequent cracking.

Patients often are cold when they return from the operating suite. This condition is caused in part by the effects of anesthesia and the cool atmosphere of the operating suite and the PACU. These reasons must be explained to the patient. Active warming measures, such as a convective warming device or intravenous fluid warmer, should be instituted on arrival to the PACU if the patient is hypothermic. Devices should be used according to the manufacturers' recommendations to avoid patient injury.

The patient who is normothermic may shiver or feel cold; warm blankets may provide psychologic comfort, and active warming interventions may be needed to reduce or eliminate shaking. Blankets of any type should not, however, obscure the intravenous lines, arterial lines, or other monitoring apparatuses from the direct view of the attending nurse. The patient's temperature must be monitored closely to avoid overheating. Shivering may be treated with low doses of meperidine, 12.5 to 25 mg intravenously, which attenuates the shivering response. Hypothermia is discussed in Chapter 53.

In addition to physical comfort measures, remember to provide psychologic comfort. Reorientation, especially to time and place, is important to the postanesthesia patient, as is constant reassurance that the surgery is completed and that all went well. The nurse's presence at the bedside or gentle touch may also be comforting to the patient.

### Transfer of the Patient from the PACU

When the patient has recovered from the effects of anesthesia, vital signs are stabilized; if no surgical complications have arisen, the patient is ready for transfer to the nursing unit or discharge area. The patient's postanesthesia recovery score, if a scoring system is used, should meet preestablished minimums, unless criteria for exception are noted. The patient should have regained a satisfactory level of consciousness to the point of being oriented and able to call for assistance, if necessary, and should be clean, dry, and dressed in appropriate hospital garb. All dressings should be dry and intact, and all drainage receptacles should be emptied. A licensed practitioner should see the patient before discharge, or the name of the responsible physician should be documented in the patient's record. The PACU nurse should discharge the patient when the patient meets medically approved discharge criteria.

No patient should be discharged immediately after receiving an initial dose of an opioid medication. Discharge should be delayed for assessment of pain relief and adverse side effects of the medication. Pain assessment and management should be documented in the patient's record for ongoing evaluation of pain intensity and treatment effectiveness.

A summarizing PACU discharge note should be written on the patient's progress record or entered into the electronic health record to indicate condition and time of transfer. The nurse should alert the receiving unit that the patient is being transferred and request the preparation of any specialized equipment for care and the assignment of a receiving nurse.

Patients may be transferred on a stretcher or bed as required by condition and operative procedure. The patient should be adequately covered with bed linens, including a warmed blanket if hallways are kept cool. The side rails of the stretcher should be locked in place. Ideally, two persons should be used to wheel the stretcher to the receiving unit. Transport personnel vary by institution, and decisions regarding who transports

may vary based on the patient's condition, staffing, and unit needs. The American Society of PeriAnesthesia Nurses (ASPAN) 2006-2008 Standards of Perianesthesia Nursing Practice, Resource 10, address required elements for the safe transfer of care. The handoff between providers should allow communication of patient status and care needs; the opportunity to ask questions of the transferring caregiver is required. The form of that transfer varies by facility policy and practice but must minimize patient risk.

A receiving nurse should meet the patient on arrival to the unit and direct the transfer to the patient's room. The patient is transferred to the bed along with all apparatuses. Safety precautions must be strictly followed. At least two people should always transfer the patient. A third person may be necessary to assist with the patient transfer if extra equipment or multiple drainage tubes are present. Use of transfer devices such as slider boards, roller tubes, or mechanical lifts facilitates the transfer and minimizes risk of injury for both the patient and the nursing staff. Both the bed and the stretcher should be stabilized by locking the wheels when transferring the patient from one to the other. The nurse should ensure that all drainage tubes and catheters are safely transferred, that no kinking occurs, and that they do not become tangled underneath the patient. All drainage receptacles should remain below the level of the patient. Intravenous tubing and solution must be carefully transferred from the portable stand attached to the stretcher to the bedside stand or holder. Drainage tubes should be connected to suction or gravity drainage as indicated, and their proper functioning checked. The patient's call light should be positioned within the patient's reach along with any other items that may be needed. The intravenous infusion rate should be assessed and adjusted as necessary. Side rails on the bed should be raised.

The report may be written, telephoned, faxed, printed from the electronic health record, or reviewed online before or at the time of transfer. It may be given in person to the receiving nurse. The PACU nurse should give a complete report to the receiving nurse, including pertinent facts about the following: patient demographic information; pertinent health history; the operative procedure performed; the type of anesthesia or sedation used and any reversal agents given; the patient's general condition and postanesthesia course; incision; any drains placed and the dressing; any drainage tubes or catheters; intake and output, including intravenous fluids given, estimated blood loss, and time of void or catheterization; any medications given in the PACU, especially analgesics; and the patient's response and level of comfort. As appropriate, orders are reviewed with the receiving nurse, the location of sensory aids and valuables is discussed, and social support availability is reviewed.

## SUMMARY

This chapter discussed patient education concepts including learner characteristics and teaching strategies. Nursing care of postanesthesia patients who are emerging from anesthesia is also reviewed in this chapter. Postanesthesia care discussed included the stir-up regimen, intravenous therapy, maintenance of cardiopulmonary function, and general comfort measures.

## BIBLIOGRAPHY

American Association of Critical-Care Nurses: *AACN procedure manual for critical care*, ed 5, Philadelphia, 2005, Saunders.

American Society of PeriAnesthesia Nurses: Clinical guideline for the prevention of unplanned perioperative hypothermia, *J Perianesth Nurs* 16(5):305–314, 2001.

American Society of PeriAnesthesia Nurses: *Standards of perianesthesia nursing practice 2006-2008*, Cherry Hill, NJ, 2006, American Society of PeriAnesthesia Nurses.

Black JM, Hawks JH: *Medical-surgical nursing: clinical management for positive outcomes*, ed 7, St Louis, 2005, Saunders.

Dark PM: Patient and family education. In Quinn DMD, Schick l, editors: *PeriAnesthesia nursing core curriculum*, St Louis, 2004, Saunders.

Finucane BT, Santora AH: *Principles of airway management*, ed 3, New York, 2003, Springer-Verlag.

Greensmith JE, Aker JG: Ventilatory management in the postanesthesia care unit, *J Perianesth Nurs* 13(6):370–381, 1998.

Hodgkinson B, Evans D, O'Neill S: *Knowledge retention from pre-operative patient information*, 2000 Report No. 6, 2000, The Joanna Briggs Institute for Evidence Based Nursing and Midwifery. Available at: http://www.joannabriggs.edu.au/pdf/BPISEng_4_6.pdf. Retrieved July 2, 2007.

Johansson K, Salantera S, Heiffinen K: Surgical patient education: assessing the interventions and exploring the outcomes from experimental and quasiexperimental studies from 1990 to 2003, *Clin Effectiveness Nurs* 8(2):81–92, 2004.

Longnecker DE, Murphy FL: *Dripps, Eckenhoff, Vandam introduction to anesthesia*, ed 9, Philadelphia, 1997, Saunders.

Marley RA: Postoperative oxygen therapy, *J Perianesth Nurs* 13(6):394–412, 1998.

Pasquina P, Tramer MR, Granier JM: Respiratory physiotherapy to prevent pulmonary complications after abdominal surgery: a systematic review, *Chest* 130(6):1887–1899, 2006.

Sjoling M, Nordahl G, Olofsson N: The impact of preoperative information on state anxiety, postoperative pain and satisfaction with pain management, *Patient Educ Counseling* 51:169–176, 2003.

Stoller JK, Kester L: Respiratory care protocols in postanesthesia care, *J Perianesth Nurs* 13(6):349–358, 1998.

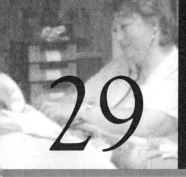

# 29

# POSTANESTHESIA CARE COMPLICATIONS

*Denise O'Brien, MSN, APRN,BC, CPAN, CAPA, FAAN*

Complications can occur during any phase of the patient's perianesthesia experience. From allergic reactions to preoperative medications in the holding area to postanesthesia airway obstruction, situations occur that require the perianesthesia nurse's vigilance, prompt action, and appropriate treatment. The postanesthesia period is a precarious time for the patient; prevention of complications is an essential role for the perianesthesia nurse. The perianesthesia nurse, whether in an inpatient or outpatient setting, must be prepared to respond to rapidly evolving potentially life-threatening situations. Complications that more commonly occur in the postanesthesia setting are addressed in this chapter, including respiratory and cardiovascular complications, thermoregulation, and anesthesia complications.

## DEFINITIONS

**Acute Myocardial Infarction:** Occurs when an area of heart muscle dies or is permanently damaged because of an inadequate supply of oxygen to that area.

**Anaphylactic Reactions:** Anaphylaxis is a severe whole-body allergic reaction that occurs rapidly and causes a life-threatening response that involves the whole body.

**Aspiration:** The inhalation of either oropharyngeal or gastric contents into the lungs.

**Awareness During Anesthesia:** Occurs when a person is aware of some portion of the procedure (sometimes even pain) during general anesthesia; can cause long-term psychologic effects and symptoms of posttraumatic stress.

**Bradycardia:** A heart rate of less than 60 bpm (adult) with a regular rhythm and P waves present; is seldom symptomatic in a healthy patient until the rate drops to less than 50 bpm.

**Bronchospasm:** Narrowing of the bronchi and bronchioles from smooth muscle contraction.

**Delayed Emergence (Awakening):** Patient emergence from anesthesia is delayed; failure to emerge can be classified as the result of drug effects, metabolic disorders, or neurologic disorders.

**Dilutional Hyponatremia:** Absorption of irrigating solutions through open blood vessels or perforation of the uterine or bladder wall that leads to circulatory overload from water intoxication.

**Emergence Excitement:** A condition characterized by restlessness, disorientation, crying, moaning, irrational talking, and inappropriate behavior.

**Hemolytic Reactions:** An ABO-incompatible blood reaction that precipitates a hemolytic reaction that results in agglutination, or clumping, of red blood cells (RBCs), which blocks the patient's capillaries and thus obstructs the flow of blood and oxygen to vital organs.

**Hemorrhage:** Bleeding after operative procedures.

**Hypertension:** A blood pressure increased 20% to 30% above the baseline blood pressure.

**Hyperthermia:** A core temperature of more than 38° C.

**Hypotension:** A blood pressure that is less than 20% to 30% of the baseline blood pressure.

**Hypothermia:** A core temperature of less than 36° C.

**Hypoventilation:** A decrease in respiratory rate that leads to an increase in partial pressure of carbon dioxide $PaCO_2$.

**Hypoxemia:** A $PaO_2$ of less than 60 mm Hg.

**Laryngospasm:** An involuntary partial or complete closure of the vocal cords, caused by secretions, or stimulation or irritation of the laryngeal reflexes during emergence.

**Malignant Hyperthermia (MH):** A hypermetabolic state of genetic origin (autosomal dominant inheritance) that can be triggered by succinylcholine or the volatile anesthetics.

**Noncardiogenic Pulmonary Edema:** Respiratory disorder that most commonly occurs after an obstructive event that results in pulmonary capillary leakage and pulmonary edema.

**Nonhemolytic Febrile Reactions:** Most often caused by sensitivity to leukocytes and platelets and seen most often in patients who have received multiple transfusions.

**Perforated Viscous:** Internal organs perforated during the operative procedure.

**Pneumothorax** An accumulation of air or gas in the pleural space.

**Postdischarge Nausea and Vomiting (PDNV):** Nausea or vomiting that occurs after discharge from the health care facility after ambulatory surgery.

**Postdural Puncture Headache:** A headache that typically presents 24 to 48 hours after lumbar puncture from a spinal needle placement or inadvertent dural puncture during an epidural placement.

**Postoperative Nausea and Vomiting (PONV):** Nausea or vomiting that occurs within the first 24 hours after inpatient surgery.

**Pseuodocholinesterase Deficiency:** Also referred to as plasmacholinesterase deficiency; an uncommon genetic disorder that renders the patient with an inability to hydrolyze the ester bonds in succinylcholine, resulting in prolonged skeletal muscle paralysis that can last 8 hours or more.

**Pulmonary Edema:** Increase in lung fluid as a result of leakage from pulmonary capillaries into the interstitium and alveoli of the lung; leads to impaired gas exchange and may cause respiratory failure.

**Pulmonary Embolism:** A sudden blockage of an artery in the lungs by fat, air, clumped tumor cells, or a blood clot; usually a blood clot that traveled to the lung from the leg.

**Spinal Epidural Hematoma:** A hematoma after spinal procedures or surgery; blood accumulates between the spinal dura and bone compressing nerves; without prompt treatment, it can cause permanent neurologic deficits.

**Tachycardia:** A heart rate greater than 100 bpm (adult) with a regular rhythm and P waves present.

**Transfusion-Related Acute Lung Injury (TRALI):** Rare but devastating complication of blood component therapy; findings are similar to adult respiratory distress syndrome and consist of hypotension, fever, dyspnea, and tachycardia.

## RESPIRATORY COMPLICATIONS

Airway management and respiratory care are first in the mind of the perianesthesia nurse when patients arrive in the postanesthesia care unit (PACU). Avoidance of postoperative pulmonary complications, including atelectasis, pneumonia, respiratory failure, and exacerbation, helps reduce patient morbidity and mortality rates. The perianesthesia nurse works to prevent these serious

longer term complications by maintaining and improving the patient's respiratory function in the immediate postanesthesia period of care. Some patients are at greater risk for development of these complications. Primarily these risk factors are patient-related or procedure-related. Box 29-1 lists the most common risk factors supported by evidence.

### Airway Obstruction

One of the most commonly occurring complications in the postanesthesia care setting is airway obstruction. Airway obstruction can be upper or lower in origin, from the simple problem of the tongue falling back and obstructing the upper airway to complete laryngospasm with no air movement.

Upper airway obstruction may be caused by tongue relaxation, which is most common, and is seen in the patient who has not fully recovered from anesthesia, who has received opioid or sedative drugs, or who has residual neuromuscular blocking agents on board. Other causes include swelling or edema of the airway, airway injury, or bleeding (hemorrhage). Treatment includes

---

**Box 29-1   Risk Factors for Postoperative Pulmonary Complications**

**PATIENT-RELATED RISK FACTORS**
Advanced age
ASA class greater than or equal to II
CHF
Functional dependence
Chronic obstructive pulmonary disease (COPD)
Weight loss
Impaired sensorium
Cigarette use
Alcohol use
Abnormal findings on chest examination

**PROCEDURE-RELATED RISK FACTORS**
Aortic aneurysm repair
Thoracic surgery
Abdominal surgery
Upper abdominal surgery
Neurosurgery
Prolonged surgery
Head and neck surgery
Emergency surgery
Vascular surgery
General anesthesia

Data from Smetana GW, Lawrence VA, Cornell JE: Preoperative pulmonary risk stratification for noncardiothoracic surgery: systematic review for the American College of Physicians, *Ann Intern Med* 144:581-595, 2006.

verbal or tactile stimulation of the patient, airway repositioning with chin lift or jaw thrust, placement of an oral or nasopharyngeal airway adjunct, and application of positive pressure with a bag-valve-mask device. If the patient's airway cannot be maintained with these methods, oral or nasal placement of an endotracheal tube may be necessary or emergency cricothyroidotomy or tracheostomy performed. Positioning the patient in the "recovery" position, side-lying with head down to facilitate drainage, may also help to maintain a patent airway in the patient at risk for soft tissue obstruction or significant oral drainage that interferes with the airway.

## Laryngospasm

Laryngospasm is an involuntary partial or complete closure of the vocal cords, caused by secretions, or stimulation or irritation of the laryngeal reflexes during emergence. Wheezing, reduced compliance, stridor (partial), paradoxic chest or abdominal movements, and absence of ventilation (complete) are signs and symptoms of laryngospasm. Ventilation is decreased or absent, and oxygenation of the patient is difficult as carbon dioxide release increases. Treatment includes airway maneuvers (chin lift/jaw thrust), elevation of the head of bed to maximize respiratory excursion, and application of bag-valve-mask for continuous positive pressure with oxygen. Secretions need to be carefully removed with suction. The patient may need reintubation to secure the airway. Medications may include succinylcholine or other neuromuscular blocking agents and lidocaine. Once the patient has received a neuromuscular blocking agent, the patient may need sedation to reduce anxiety related to apnea, muscle relaxation, and awareness.

## Subglottic Edema

For the pediatric patient, obstruction may be caused by subglottic edema, usually observed in children aged 1 to 4 years. Traumatic intubation, tight fit of the endotracheal tube, coughing with the tube in place, position change with the tube inserted, surgery of the head or neck, and procedures that last more than 1 hour may result in subglottic edema. Crowing respirations, stridor, and rocking chest wall respiratory attempts may signal subglottic edema. Postoperative supplemental humidified oxygen may diminish airway swelling. Initial treatment includes humidified oxygen and nebulized mist treatment with racemic epinephrine. Further treatment may include inhalation of a helium/oxygen mixture, administration of dexamethasone, and calming with analgesics and parental or caregiver

presence. Ambulatory surgery patients with subglottic edema who are treated with racemic epinephrine may be considered for overnight admission because of the risk of rebound edema. Extended observation for up to 8 hours may be sufficient if the parents are comfortable and emergency resources are readily available.

## Bronchospasm

Narrowing of the bronchi and bronchioles from smooth muscle contraction results in bronchospasm. Bronchospasm may be the result of preexisting asthma; allergy or anaphylaxis; histamine release; mucous plugging; aspiration; pulmonary edema; wheezing with acute heart failure, but without any other acute pulmonary pathology (cardiogenic asthma); or foreign body aspiration. Signs and symptoms include cough, expiratory wheezing, dyspnea, use of accessory muscles, and tachypnea. Treatment of the patient includes removal of the identified cause, oxygen administration, inhaled bronchodilators, and epinephrine. Depending on cause, an antihistamine or dexamethasone may be appropriate. Secretions should be suctioned. If the condition results from foreign body aspiration, such as a tooth, emergent bronchoscopy is needed. Ventilatory support may be necessary, and the patient may need reintubation for maintenance of oxygenation and ventilation.

## Aspiration

Identified as a high-risk low-frequency occurrence, aspiration may be observed in the postanesthesia setting. The patient with a full stomach or nasal or oropharyngeal airway in place and returning gag reflexes may become nauseated and vomit. In a nonresponsive state and supine position, the patient is at greater risk for aspiration. Types of aspirates include large particle, clear acidic or nonacidic fluid, foodstuff or small particle, and contaminated material. Also, foreign bodies such as teeth or blood may be aspirated. Symptoms include unexplained tachypnea and tachycardia, cough, bronchospasm, hypoxemia, atelectasis, interstitial edema, hemorrhage, and acute respiratory distress syndrome (ARDS). The aspiration can trigger laryngospasm, infection, and pulmonary edema. Prevention of aspiration is preferred. Patients at risk should be identified before surgery and premedicated. Patients at risk are patients with emergent procedures, known full stomachs, or history of gastroesophageal reflux disease; those older than age 65 years; and laboring women. Medications include histamine blockers, nonparticulate antacids, and anticholinergic agents. During surgery, rapid sequence induction and nasogastric tube placement may help minimize the risk of aspiration. After surgery, maintenance of the endotracheal tube until airway reflexes have returned and positioning of the patient with the head to the side or in a left lateral decubitus position may aid in decreasing the risk of aspiration. Should aspiration occur, one should correct hypoxemia and maintain hemodynamic stability. The patient may need reintubation and suctioning and mechanical ventilation. Arterial blood gases assist in planning respiratory management of the patient. Chest x-ray is obtained, but findings may be inconclusive initially; radiographic findings may lag behind clinical signs by 24 hours after the suspected aspiration event. Prophylactic antibiotics or steroids are not recommended. Tracheal secretions should be cultured; if results are positive, antibiotics can be prescribed.

### Hypoventilation

Hypoventilation may be the result of residual anesthetic agents; opioids; neuromuscular blocking agents; inadequate reversal of opioids, sedatives, or neuromuscular blocking agents; thoracic or abdominal incisions and procedures; or neuromuscular diseases.

Signs and symptoms include decreased respiratory rate, shallow respirations, increased end-tidal carbon dioxide ($ETCO_2$), and increased $PaCO_2$ (>45 mm Hg [hypercarbia]). Treatment includes identification and management of the cause of the hypoventilation, supplemental oxygen administration, verbal and tactile stimulation, deep breathing exercises, repositioning, and cautious use of analgesics or sedatives. Oxygen saturation monitoring is necessary, and capnographic monitoring may be appropriate for patients at risk.

### Hypoxemia

Hypoxemia in the postanesthesia patient is not as common since the advent of noninvasive oxygen saturation monitoring with pulse oximetry. Hypoxemia may be the result of low inspired concentration of oxygen, hypoventilation, ventilation/perfusion inequality, increased intrapulmonary right to left shunt, or pneumothorax. It may also be caused by diffuse airway collapse, pulmonary edema, and pulmonary embolism. Treatment includes identification and correction of the cause, stimulation of the patient, supplemental oxygen administration, and continuous positive airway pressure (CPAP), which may be used in the spontaneously breathing patient. Patients who cannot maintain oxygen levels may need tracheal intubation and mechanical ventilation and positive end-expiratory pressure support.

### Pneumothorax

Pneumothorax, an accumulation of air or gas in the pleural space, may occur during the perianesthesia period. It may be the result of percutaneous internal jugular and subclavian vein cannulation, hemodynamic monitoring line placement, certain upper extremity blocks (supraclavicular and infraclavicular approaches to the brachial plexus), or operative procedures of the chest. The patient may have sharp ipsilateral chest pain and dyspnea. Assessment findings include decreased breath sounds and hyperresonance on the affected side of the chest. Treatment includes supplemental oxygen administration and ordering of a chest x-ray. If the chest x-ray results indicates a less than 20% pneumothorax, the treating physician may want to observe the patient for a period of time until the pneumothorax either resolves or increases. If the pneumothorax is greater than 20% or the patient has cardiovascular compromise, a chest tube is placed immediately.

### Pulmonary Edema

Fluid overload, congestive heart failure (CHF), or acute pulmonary injury can result in pulmonary edema. Signs and symptoms include hypoxemia, rales, and decreased pulmonary compliance. Pulmonary infiltrates are seen on chest x-ray results.

Identification and treatment of the cause of the pulmonary edema is the first step in treatment. In addition, diuretics and fluid restriction to decrease afterload and supplemental oxygen administration may be ordered. Patients with an inability to maintain oxygenation or adequate ventilation may undergo intubation and mechanical ventilation and PEEP.

### Noncardiogenic Pulmonary Edema

Noncardiogenic pulmonary edema may be the result of upper airway obstruction, laryngospasm, bolus dosing with naloxone, incomplete reversal of neuromuscular blockade, or a significant period of hypoxia. When the cause is obstructive in origin, two types of postobstructive pulmonary edema (POPE) have been identified: type I and type II. Both are present with acute respiratory distress. Type I usually occurs within 60 minutes of a precipitating event, but onset can be delayed up to 6 hours. Type I POPE may follow postextubation laryngospasm, epiglottitis, croup, choking or foreign body, strangulation, hanging, endotracheal tube obstruction, laryngeal tumor, goiter, mononucleosis, postoperative vocal cord paralysis, migration of Foley catheter balloon used for tamponade epistaxis, near drowning, and intraoperative direct suctioning of an endotracheal tube adapter. Type II POPE develops soon after relief of chronic upper airway obstruction, such as after tonsillectomy or adenoidectomy, removal of upper airway tumor, choanal stenosis, and hypertrophic redundant uvula.

Signs and symptoms include hypoxemia, cough, failure to maintain oxygen saturation levels, tachypnea, and frothy sputum. Treatment includes supplemental oxygen administration and maintenance of a patent upper airway. CPAP may be used. Patients with an inability to maintain a patent airway may need intubation and mechanical ventilation with PEEP. For patients with significant compromise, hemodynamic support and continued observation in an intensive care unit may be needed. Patients with noncardiogenic pulmonary edema typically recover rapidly after the intense initial phase and leave the critical care unit within approximately 24 to 36 hours and without permanent sequela from the event.

### Pulmonary Embolism

Patients predisposed to development of pulmonary emboli include patients who are obese or immobile, who are undergoing pelvic or long bone procedures, and who have a history of congestive heart failure or malignant disease. Signs and symptoms may include tachypnea, pleuritic chest pain, hemoptysis, breathlessness, and a sense of impending doom. Treatment is supportive for correction of hypoxemia and hemodynamic instability. Intravenous heparin and morphine sulfate may be given to help stabilize the pulmonary capillary membrane. Prevention of deep vein thrombosis and subsequent pulmonary emboli development includes subcutaneous unfractionated heparin, low–molecular weight heparins, or intermittent/sequential compression devices.

## CARDIOVASCULAR COMPLICATIONS

Cardiovascular complications that occur in the PACU range from relatively benign ectopic beats to hemodynamic collapse from an acute myocardial infarction. The perianesthesia nurse monitors the patient continuously in phase I, observing rate and rhythm and blood pressure and noting any signs or symptoms of hemodynamic compromise. The following section briefly discusses the more common cardiovascular complications seen in the perianesthesia setting.

Major cardiovascular perioperative risks are identified as myocardial infarction, heart failure, and death. Clinical predictors of increased perioperative cardiovascular risk

are divided into major, intermediate, and minor predictors. These predictors are listed in Box 29-2.

### Dysrhythmias

Dysrhythmias may occur as the result of hypoxia, hypercarbia, electrolyte abnormalities, acid-base alterations, myocardial ischemia, drug effects, pain, hypovolemia, bladder distention, and hypothermia. Occasional ectopic beats may be seen in healthy patients. Significant dysrhythmias necessitate immediate identification and treatment; these include premature ventricular contractions (more than five per minute, coupled [more than two together], or multifocal), ventricular tachycardia, ventricular fibrillation, asystole, heart block, pulseless electric activity, and new onset atrial fibrillation. Treatment includes identification and treatment of the cause, supplemental oxygen administration,

---

**Box 29-2  Clinical Predictors of Increased Cardiovascular Risk**

**MAJOR**
Unstable coronary syndromes: acute or recent myocardial infarction (MI) with evidence of important ischemic risk, unstable or severe angina
Decompensated heart failure
Significant dysrhythmias: atrioventricular block, symptomatic ventricular dysrhythmias, supraventricular dysrhythmias with uncontrolled ventricular rate
Severe valvular disease

**INTERMEDIATE**
Mild angina pectoris
Previous myocardial infarction with history or pathologic Q waves
Compensated or prior heart failure
Type I diabetes mellitus
Renal insufficiency

**MINOR**
Advanced age
Abnormal ECG
Rhythm other than sinus
Low functional capacity
History of stroke
Uncontrolled systemic hypertension

Data from Eagle KA, Berger PB, Calkins H, et al: ACC/AHA guideline update for perioperative cardiovascular evaluation for noncardiac surgery: executive summary, *Anesth Analg* 94:1052-1056, 2002.

ventilatory and hemodynamic support, and pharmacologic therapy. Advanced cardiac life support (ACLS) or pediatric advanced life support (PALS) protocols are initiated when appropriate.

## Bradycardia

Sinus bradycardia may occur as the result of vagal responses, hypoxia, drug effects, increased intracranial pressure (ICP), or distended bladder. Treatment is dependent on the cause and may include anticholinergic agents (e.g., atropine), supplemental oxygen administration, and stimulation. If the condition is the result of elevated ICP, hyperventilation and pharmacologic therapy may be indicated.

## Tachycardia

Sinus tachycardia is the most commonly occurring postanesthesia dysrhythmia. Causes include hypoxia, hypercarbia, hypovolemia, sepsis, hyperthermia, heart failure, pain, drugs, and psychologic stress. Treatment includes administration of supplemental oxygen, ventilation support, and evaluation of fluid and cardiac status. If the condition results from pain, medication with analgesics is the treatment. Sedatives may be needed if the condition is from anxiety or stress. If the patient is hyperthermic, the patient's temperature is lowered with recommended cooling devices.

## Hypotension

Hypotension is defined as blood pressure that is less than 20% to 30% of the baseline blood pressure. Causes range from use of an inappropriately sized cuff, to hypovolemia, myocardial dysfunction, and a decrease in systemic vascular resistance (Fig. 29-1). Management and treatment of hypotension in the PACU includes use of a cuff of the appropriate size, administration of supplemental oxygen, initiation of fluid resuscitation, stoppage of drug infusions if causative, and

elevation of the legs. Inotropic agents or vasopressor or vasoconstrictive agents may be ordered.

## Hypertension

Hypertension is defined as blood pressure increased 20% to 30% above the baseline blood pressure. Too small or narrow of a cuff can result in abnormally elevated blood pressures. Pain, stress, hypoxemia, hypercarbia, fluid overload, delirium, drugs, bladder, bowel or stomach distention, or hypothermia can cause hypertension. Many of the patients in PACU in whom hypertension develops have preexisting hypertension. The elevation in blood pressure is usually benign and short lived; however, the hypertension can precipitate myocardial ischemia in the patient with coronary artery disease (CAD) as a result of stimulation of the sympathetic nervous system. Treatment for hypertension includes use of an appropriately sized cuff and identification and management of the underlying cause first. This condition may necessitate ventilatory support and oxygen administration, analgesics or sedatives, bladder decompression, and antihypertensive agents.

Patients who have had a cervical or thoracic (above T6) spinal cord injury are at risk for development of autonomic dysreflexia, which is a massive uninhibited sympathetic cardiovascular response to noxious stimuli (e.g., bowel or bladder overdistention) characterized by paroxysmal hypertension, pounding headache, facial flushing, sweating, temporal/neck vessel engorgement, nasal congestion, blurred vision, chill bumps, chills, nausea, and occasional bradycardia. Treatment includes elimination of the precipitating stimuli if known and elevation of the head of bed. Pharmacologic treatment may be needed to reduce the blood pressure if the blood pressure remains elevated after these measures.

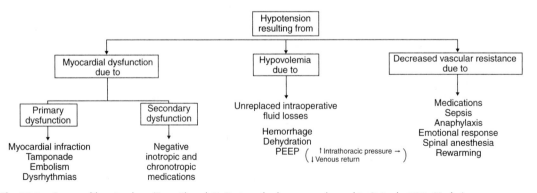

**Fig. 29-1**    Causes of hypotension. *(From Litwack K: Postanesthesia care nursing, ed 2, St Louis, 1995, Mosby.)*

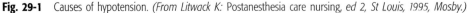

## Acute Myocardial Infarction

The patient with a history of preexisting CAD, diabetes, and significant dysrhythmias is at risk for perioperative cardiac events (see Box 29-2). The pathology of perioperative myocardial infarction is shown in Fig. 29-2.

When a patient has chest pain in the PACU, the cause needs to be evaluated, with the first consideration for the source as cardiac in origin (Box 29-3). The signs and symptoms of myocardial infarction include chest pain, tachypnea, tachycardia or other dysrhythmias, hypotension or hypertension, pallor, diaphoresis, cool extremities, nausea, vomiting, and generalized weakness. New Q waves or increasing prominence of existing ones, ST segment elevations, and T wave inversions may be seen on electrocardiographic (ECG) results. Initial treatment is aimed at relief of chest pain, reduction of cardiac workload, stabilization of cardiac rhythm, limiting of infarct size, prevention of further damage, and detection and treatment of complications. The first response is to order a 12-lead ECG; initiate supplemental oxygen; administer morphine, nitrates, and antiplatelet/anticoagulant agents; and continuously monitor the ECG. Laboratory blood studies are obtained, including troponin-I,

troponin-T, MB fraction of creatine kinase (CK-MB), and CK-MB isoforms. The patient is evaluated and transferred to a critical care unit for continued monitoring and possible interventional procedures and management.

## THERMOREGULATION

For a more detailed discussion of thermoregulation, see Chapter 53.

### Hypothermia

Hypothermia is defined as a core temperature of less than 36° C. Signs and symptoms of hypothermia include shivering, restlessness, discomfort, and cold pale cyanotic extremities and distal appendages from peripheral vasoconstriction. This state may lead to delayed drug clearance, myocardial ischemia, unexplained hypertension, and residual paralysis from

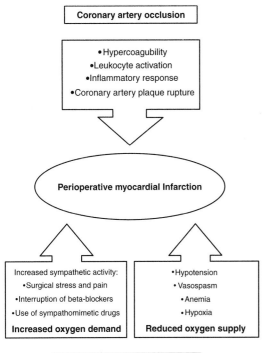

**Fig. 29-2** Pathology of perioperative myocardial infarction. *(From Kertai MD, Klein J, Bax JJ, et al: Predicting perioperative cardiac risk, Progress Cardiovasc Dis 47[4]:240-257, 2005.)*

**Box 29-3 Differential Diagnosis of Chest Pain**

**CARDIOVASCULAR ORIGIN**
Angina
Acute myocardial infarction
Aortic dissection
Mitral valve prolapse
Pericarditis
Postpericardiotomy syndrome

**GASTROINTESTINAL ORIGIN**
Reflux esophagitis
Esophageal spasm
Peptic ulcer disease
Pancreatitis

**PULMONARY ORIGIN**
Pleuritic chest pain
Pleural effusion
Pneumothorax
Pneumonia
Pulmonary embolism
Pulmonary hypertension

**MUSCULOSKELETAL ORIGIN**
Costochondritis
Rib fracture

**MISCELLANEOUS ORIGIN**
Herpes zoster
Anxiety disorder

From Litwack K: *Postanesthesia care nursing,* ed 2, St. Louis, 1995, Mosby.

neuromuscular blocking agents. The American Society of PeriAnesthesia Nurses Clinical Guideline for The Prevention of Unplanned Perioperative Hypothermia offers the perianesthesia nurse guidance for assessment and management of the patient who is hypothermic during the perianesthesia period. Recommendations for treatment of the patient include active rewarming, supplemental oxygen administration, and ventilatory support if necessary.

## Hyperthermia

Hyperthermia is defined as a core temperature of more than 38° C. Temperature elevations may be the result of blood transfusion reactions, warm environment, drug-induced fever, use of anticholinergics, overcorrected hypothermia, endocrine disorder, hypothalamic injury, or malignant hyperthermia (MH). Signs and symptoms include fever, tachycardia, and warm flushed skin and other sign and symptoms depending on the cause of the hyperthermia (shaking, chills or rigors, agitation). The cause should be identified and corrected when possible. Cooling blankets or pads may be used; antipyretic agent may be given.

## Malignant Hyperthermia

Malignant hyperthermia is a drug-induced hypermetabolic state of genetic origin (autosomal dominant inheritance) that can be triggered by succinylcholine or the volatile anesthetics. It may occur on induction, during emergence, or up to 24 hours after anesthesia. The exact incidence rate is unknown but is thought to be approximately 1:15,000 in children and less common in adults after age 30 years. Patients with central core disease and other muscle diseases may be at added risk for development of MH.

The signs and symptoms of MH include the earliest sign of an unanticipated doubling or tripling of end-tidal $CO_2$ in the anesthetized patient. This sign may be followed by unexpected tachycardia, tachypnea, and jaw muscle rigidity. Respiratory acidosis and, after severe temperature increase, metabolic acidosis is present. Body rigidity is a specific sign of MH syndrome. Fever, when it develops, is a late sign of MH; the temperature may rise at a rate of 1° C every 3 to 5 minutes. The urine may become dark and cola colored from the breakdown of myoglobin.

Early recognition of MH is essential; additional help needs to be summoned. If it occurs in the operating suite, discontinue all anesthetics, hyperventilate the patient with 100% oxygen with a new circuit, and end the operative

procedure as soon as safely possible. Dantrolene sodium (Dantrium should be available in sufficient quantities [36 vials recommended in all locations where volatile anesthetics or succinylcholine are administered]) as should diluent. Dosing begins at 2.5 mg/kg of dantrolene sodium, up to 10 mg/kg. Laboratory blood studies including coagulation profile, creatine, electrolytes, arterial blood gas, and CK should be obtained. Acidosis not reversed with dantrolene sodium can be treated with sodium bicarbonate. The patient's temperature should be monitored and cooling measures initiated if the temperature is more than 38.5° C. Dysrhythmias may be treated with standard antiarrhythmics, but calcium channel blockers should be avoided. Elevated potassium levels are treated with intravenous (IV) insulin, glucose, and calcium. Hydration and diuretics ensure urine output of at least 2 mL/kg/h.

Once the MH crisis is treated and the patient's condition is stabilized, the patient should be transferred to a critical care unit for continued monitoring, including temperature, for at least 24 hours because recrudescence can occur and does in about 25% of MH cases.

Patients who have had a MH episode during a previous surgery or have a family history of MH are treated as MH susceptible; triggering agents are avoided. Dantrolene sodium prophylaxis is not recommended for these patients. The patient who undergoes an uneventful anesthetic and is scheduled as an outpatient may be discharged home on the day of surgery; this patient should be monitored in the phase I PACU for a minimum of 1 hour and in the phase II PACU for an additional 1.5 hours.

Diagnosis of MH susceptibility involves a skeletal muscle biopsy from the thigh. Only eight medical centers in the United States and Canada perform the test on fresh muscle. Genetic testing is available, but not all the genes responsible for MH have been identified, so risk may still exist for the patient whose test results are negative and who has unidentified genes.

When an MH crisis occurs, consultation is available from the MH Hotline at 1-800-MH-HYPER (1-800-644-9737) in the United States or 1-315-464-7079 outside of the United States. Additional information and resources can be found at www.mhaus.org.

## ANESTHESIA-RELATED COMPLICATIONS

### Awareness Under Anesthesia

One to two per thousand patients at low risk has an ability to recall some aspect of the surgical experience. The impact of awareness with anesthesia varies from pleasant recall to terror that leads to posttraumatic stress disorder. Difficulty in diagnosis of awareness adds to the challenge of this event. Patient recall can include events such as conversations, pain, or anxiety related to perception of an inability to breathe. Risk factors include a history of drug or alcohol abuse, extreme anxiety, or a previous episode of awareness. Patients undergoing cardiac, major trauma, and obstetric procedures are at greatest risk of awareness. Patients who are defined as sicker by the American Society of Anesthesiologists (ASA) status appear to be at higher risk for awareness under anesthesia. They may receive lower doses of anesthetic agents to minimize physiologic impact of the agents, thus resulting in "lighter" anesthesia and greater potential for awareness, or other factors may be the cause.

These events may be caused by delivery of inadequate hypnotic agent, an unreliable technique for delivery of hypnotic agents, unappreciated increased anesthetic requirements (history of drug tolerance), equipment malfunction, or lack of vigilance. Classically, autonomic nervous system responses have been used as a measure of the state of consciousness; these can be inaccurate. Mean arterial blood pressure may be a good correlation to consciousness, but heart rate is not. Movement may be an attempt by the patient to communicate or a reflexive spinal response; regardless of whether movement is caused by an attempt to communicate or spinal reflexes, it indicates inadequate anesthesia. Treatment should not be with muscle relaxants alone; additional sedatives or hypnotics are needed. Use of brain function monitors was recommended by The Joint Commission in a Sentinel Event Alert, published in October 2004. These devices may help prevent and detect awareness in patients at high risk, although concerns exist over accuracy and artifacts and cost of these monitors.

When patients arrive in the postanesthesia care unit, nurses tell the patients that surgery is over, they are in the PACU or wake-up room, they are doing well, and the nurses are going to take care of them while they are awakening. This reassurance can minimize fears of waking up while still in the operating suite. Frequent reminders to the patients of status and safety help reduce anxiety related to awareness or awakening. If a patient indicates recall of events from the operating suite, the perianesthesia nurse should contact the anesthesia care provider to come to the bedside and interview the patient. Telling the patient an event did not occur or was a

---

**Box 29-4    The Original Brice Questionnaire**

1. What was the last thing you remember before you went to sleep for your operation?
2. What was the first thing you remember after your operation?
3. Can you remember anything in between those two periods?
4. Did you dream during your operation?
5. What was the worst thing about your operation?

From Brice DD, Hetherington RR, Utting JE: A simple study of awareness and dreaming during anesthesia, *Br J Anaesth* 42:535-542, 1970.

---

dream is inappropriate. If an awareness event is suspected, the nurse should sympathize and apologize to the patient, explain and answer questions as appropriate, and notify the anesthesia care provider, surgeon, and risk management department.

Through staff education, use of monitoring devices, awareness of patients at risk, and establishment of procedures to provide postoperative counseling, awareness events may be avoided. Anesthesia care providers, when interviewing patients after procedures, may use a structured interview tool, such as the Brice questionnaire (Box 29-4). This interview may dispel concerns and identify awareness events with greater frequency.

## Emergence Excitement

Most patients emerge from general anesthesia in a calm tranquil manner. Some patients, however, emerge in a state of "excitement," a condition characterized by restlessness, disorientation, crying, moaning, irrational talking, and inappropriate behavior. In the extreme form of excitement, which is also called emergence delirium (Fig. 29-3) or agitation, the patient screams, shouts, and wildly thrashes. Postoperative delirium or emergence excitement is defined as responsive or unresponsive agitation.

The incidence rate of emergence excitement is higher among children, the elderly, and those with a history of drug dependency or psychiatric disorders. Medications administered before or during surgery, including ketamine, droperidol, opioids, benzodiazepines, large doses of metoclopramide, and atropine or scopolamine, may precipitate delirium. Patients who are emotional or anxious before induction of anesthesia or who awaken restrained are at increased risk of emergence excitement or delirium.

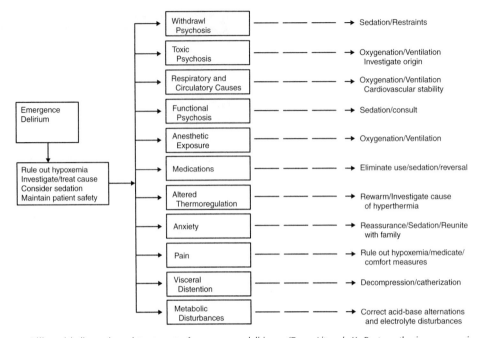

**Fig. 29-3** Differential diagnosis and treatment of emergence delirium. *(From Litwack K:* Postanesthesia care nursing, *ed 2, St Louis, 1995, Mosby.)*

The PACU nurse should assess the patient's status if emergence excitement is encountered. The patient's cardiopulmonary function, airway patency, and oxygen saturation should be checked first because restlessness and agitation are well-known manifestations of hypoxemia. Other causes include bladder distention, cramped or sore muscles and joints from prolonged abnormal positioning on the operating table, the presence of pain, incomplete reversal of neuromuscular blockade, withdrawal from alcohol and other drugs, central anticholinergic syndrome, acid-base disturbances, and electrolyte abnormalities.

The restless patient needs constant careful observation. Gentle physical restraint may be necessary for prevention of injury. Several nurses or attendants may be needed to provide safety for the patient, and for the caregivers too. Treatment is symptomatic. If hypoxia, pain, and full bladder are ruled out, a change in position may have a quieting effect. Physostigmine may be used to reverse central anticholinergic drug effects. Anxiolytics, such as midazolam, usually calm the patient. If sedative treatment is instituted, the patient should be monitored for respiratory depression. Nurses should be alert to increased agitation after benzodiazepine administration. These agents may contribute to restlessness rather than decreasing it; a paradoxical reaction to benzodiazepines.

Anticholinergic syndrome (ACS), or central anticholinergic syndrome, is rare but occurs most frequently with atropine and scopolamine. Other agents that cause ACS are glycopyrrolate, antihistamines, and antipsychotics. This syndrome or response to anticholinergic agents may present as emergence excitement in the PACU. It is produced by the inhibition of cholinergic neurotransmission at muscarinic receptor sites. It can manifest before surgery or in the PACU when patients are given atropine or have applied transdermal scopolamine patches. Signs and symptoms include sinus tachycardia, agitation, flushing, dry skin and mucous membranes, mydriasis with loss of accommodation, altered mental status, fever, decreased bowel sounds, functional ileus, urinary retention, hypertension, tremulousness, and myoclonic jerking. Patients with central ACS may have ataxia, disorientation, short-term memory loss, confusion, hallucinations (visual, auditory), psychosis, agitated delirium, seizures (rare), coma, respiratory failure, and cardiovascular collapse. Supportive care, removal of scopolamine patches, and administration of intravenous physostigmine constitute initial treatment of ACS.

Physostigmine is a reversible acetylcholinesterase inhibitor that directly antagonizes the central nervous system (CNS) manifestations of anticholinergic toxicity. Increased acetylcholine allows for stimulation at muscarinic and nicotinic receptors. The drug crosses the blood-brain barrier and reverses the central effects of coma, seizures, severe dyskinesias, hallucinations, agitation, and respiratory depression.

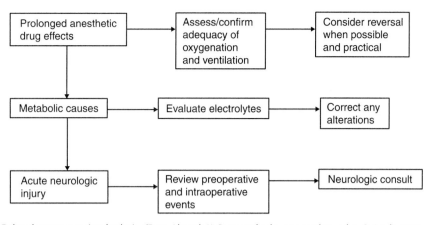

**Fig. 29-4** Delayed emergence (awakening). *(From Litwack K:* Postanesthesia care nursing, *ed 2, St Louis, 1995, Mosby.)*

Adverse effects include vomiting, diarrhea, abdominal cramps, diaphoresis, and rare brady-asystole in the presence of prolonged PR or QRS intervals on the ECG.

### Delayed Emergence (Awakening)
Occasionally patients awaken from anesthesia more slowly than expected. Causes include prolonged action of anesthetic and other drugs; metabolic problems such as hypoglycemia, hypocalcemia, hyponatremia, and hypermagnesemia; hypovolemia; hypothermia; and neurologic injury. Respiratory inadequacy with resultant hypercarbia and hypoxemia may result from opioids, sedatives, other anesthetic agents and adjuncts, or neurologic causes. The most common cause of delayed awakening is prolonged drug effects (Fig. 29-4).

Treatment consists of thorough assessment and identification of the cause or causes of the delayed arousal. Oxygenation and ventilation along with adequate cardiac output must be maintained. Residual anesthetic agents may be treated with maintenance of ventilation. Residual opioids, sedatives, neuromuscular blocking agents, and anticholinergics may be reversed with the appropriate antagonists. Metabolic disturbances should be corrected. If hypothermia is the suspected cause, warming measures are instituted with appropriate temperature monitoring. Neurologic evaluation may be needed if other causes of delayed arousal have been excluded.

### Nausea and Vomiting
One of the most perplexing problems for the perianesthesia nurse is postoperative nausea and vomiting (PONV). The incidence rate of nausea and vomiting has remained between 20% and 30% of all patients undergoing anesthesia and rises up to 80% in patients at high risk. PONV contributes to postoperative complications, increases the costs of care, and delays patient recovery and return to work. PONV is a major source of patient discomfort and fear.

*Mechanism of Action.* The vomiting (emetic) center is located in the medulla near the dorsal nucleus of the vagus nerve (Fig. 29-5). It can be excited by reflex impulses that arise in the pharynx, stomach, or other portions of the gastrointestinal tract. Foreign materials, such as blood and mucus or irritant gases in the stomach or other portions of the gastrointestinal tract, can produce nausea and subsequent vomiting. The vomiting center can be excited by impulses received from cerebral centers because the vomiting center is located very close to the fourth cerebral ventricle (see Chapter 10) and receives impulses from the chemoreceptor trigger zone (CTZ), cerebral cortex, and vestibular center. Of these physiologic centers, the CTZ has the greatest impact on the vomiting center. In fact, the CTZ, when stimulated by the appropriate stimuli, can initiate vomiting independent of the vomiting center. The CTZ is rich in the receptors serotonin, dopamine, histamine, and opioids and is not protected by the blood-brain barrier. This lack of protection allows the CTZ to be directly stimulated by chemical stimuli from the systemic circulation or the cerebral spinal fluid (CSF).

Drugs such as anesthetic agents and opioids sensitize the vestibular apparatus, the organ of balance. This sensitization explains why two of the principal causative factors of nausea and vomiting are rough handling of the patient during transportation and regular changes of position in the immediate recovery period.

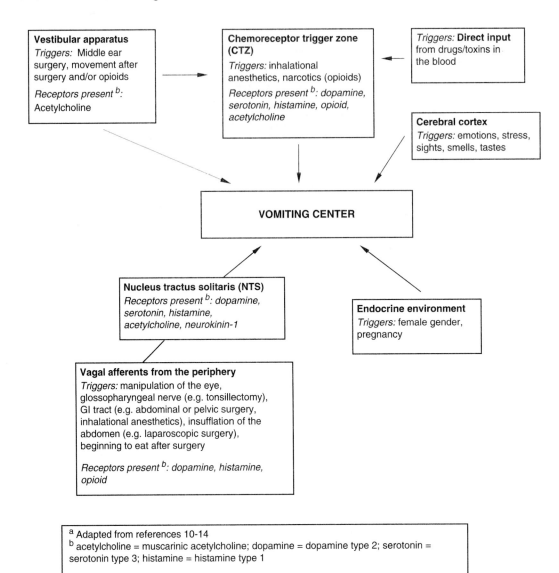

**Fig. 29-5** Mechanisms and neurotransmitter systems of PONV.

The vomiting center and the CTZ can be excited by chemical materials carried in the blood. Drugs such as morphine and meperidine directly excite the vomiting center, which is designated as central vomiting. The vomiting center can be excited by interference with its blood supply. Severe cerebral anoxia and increased intracranial pressure are such examples. Finally, the vomiting center can be excited by dehydration and electrolyte imbalance.

***Incidence of Postoperative Nausea and Vomiting.*** Primary risk factors for postoperative nausea and vomiting fall into three categories: patient-specific, anesthetic-related, and surgery-related. Patient-specific risk factors include female gender, nonsmoking status, history of

PONV, and history of motion sickness. Use of volatile anesthetics, nitrous oxide, and postoperative opioids are the anesthetic-related factors. Duration of surgery and anesthesia and the type of surgery are the surgery-related factors.

Simplified risk factor assessment tools are used to identify patients at greatest risk for development of PONV. Risk can be predicted depending on the number of factors that are present. The factors in these tools include female gender, nonsmoker, history of PONV or motion sickness, postoperative opioid use, or duration of surgery greater than 60 minutes.

The presence of each additional factor predicts increased risk of development of PONV and guides antiemetic prophylaxis for the prevention of PONV. Patients with zero to one

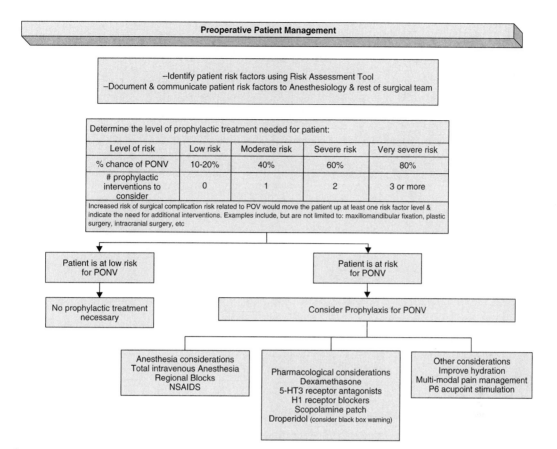

**Fig. 29-6**   Preoperative patient management. *(From American Society of PeriAnesthesia Nurses,* J PeriAnesth Nurs 2006; 21:230-250.)

factor have a low level risk of PONV; those with two are at moderate risk, with an approximately 40% chance of PONV. With three or more factors, patients have a 60% chance of development of PONV. Very severe risk, a more than 80% risk of PONV, can be found in patients with four to five risk factors. See Fig. 29-6 for recommendations for preoperative antiemetic prophylaxis from the American Society of PeriAnesthesia Nurses (ASPAN) Evidence-Based Clinical Practice Guideline for the Prevention and/or Management of PONV/PDNV.

### Care of the Patient with Nausea and Vomiting.
In most cases, vomiting is preceded by nausea. Nausea is a feeling of impending vomiting. Several signs accompany the feelings of nausea. The patient usually has excessive salivation, dilated pupils, tachypnea, swallowing, pallor, sweating, and tachycardia. If the patient's nausea worsens, retching usually occurs and the tachycardia may change to bradycardia. If patients have nausea, they should be encouraged to deep breathe. A cool washcloth placed on the patient's forehead and words of encouragement sometimes help ease the nausea. The nurse remains with the patient because the patient may begin vomiting at a moment's notice and the danger of aspiration of vomitus and obstructed airway is always present.

***Pharmacologic Interventions.*** If the previous intervention does not relieve the nausea and vomiting, a pharmacologic intervention is needed (Table 29-1; Fig. 29-7). As previously discussed, the following receptors are in the CTZ: serotonin ($5\text{-}HT_3$), dopamine ($D_2$), histamine, and muscarinic. Drugs that block serotonin ($5\text{-}HT_3$) receptors are ondansetron (Zofran), dolasetron (Anzemet), or granisetron (Kytril), and the drugs that block the dopamine ($D_2$) receptors are droperidol (Inapsine), prochlorperazine (Compazine), or metoclopramide (Reglan). For the histamine receptors, promethazine (Phenergan) or diphenhydramine (Benadryl) can be given. For the muscarinic receptors, atropine, glycopyrrolate (Robinul), or scopolamine patches may be used. Dexamethasone (Decadron) is often administered in combination with a serotonin ($5\text{-}HT_3$)–blocking drug and dopamine ($D_2$)–blocking agent. Another neurotransmitter of interest is substance P, which belongs to the

**Table 29-1  Pharmacologic Interventions**

| Drug (Trade Name; Receptor Site Affinity*) | Dose* | Duration of Action* | Adverse Effects* | Comments and Recommendations for Use |
|---|---|---|---|---|
| Droperidol (Inapsine; *Dopamine*) | *Adult:* 0.625-1.25 mg IV<br>*Pediatric:* 20-50 mcg/kg IV | 12-24 h | Sedation, hypotension (especially in patients with hypovolemia), EPS | Higher doses and doses that are repeated too soon can cause sedation, EPS, and QT prolongation (US FDA black box warning; ECG monitoring)<br><br>Effective first line agent |
| Prochlorperazine (Compazine; *Dopamine*) | *Adult:* 5-10 mg IM or IV; 25 mg PR<br>*Pediatric†:* 0.13 mg/kg IM; 0.1 mg/kg po; 2.5 mg PR | 2-6 h (12 h when given PR) | Sedation, hypotension (especially in patients with hypovolemia), EPS | |
| Promethazine (Phenergan; *Dopamine, Histamine, Acetylcholine*) | *Adult:* 6.25-25 mg IM, IV, or PR<br>*Pediatric (>2 y of age):* 0.25-0.5 mg/kg IV, IM, or PR‡ | 4 h | Sedation, hypotension (especially in patients with hypovolemia), EPS | Good for patients with motion sickness or undergoing surgery affecting vestibular apparatus |
| Diphenhydramine (*Benadryl*; *Histamine, Acetylcholine*) | *Adult:* 12.5-50 mg IM or IV<br>*Pediatric:* 1 mg/kg IV or PO (maximum, 25 mg for <6 y old) | 4-6 h | Sedation, dry mouth, blurred vision, urinary retention | Good for patients with motion sickness or undergoing surgery affecting vestibular apparatus |
| Dimenhydrinate (*Dramamine*; *Histamine, Acetylcholine*) | *Adult:* 50-100 mg IV or IM<br>*Pediatric:* 1.25 mg/kg IV or IM§ | 6-8 h | Sedation, dry mouth, blurred vision, urinary retention | Good for patients with motion sickness or undergoing surgery affecting vestibular apparatus |
| Metoclopramide (Reglan; *Dopamine*) | *Adult:* 10-20 mg IV<br>*Pediatric:* 0.15-0.25 mg/kg | 6-8 h | Sedation, hypotension, EPS | Increases gastric motility; good if nausea or vomiting is from gastric stasis; reduce dose to 5 mg in renal impairment; consider diphenhydramine to prevent EPS in children |
| Ondansetron (Zofran; *Serotonin*) | *Adult:* 4 mg IV<br>*Pediatric:* 0.05-0.1 mg/kg | Up to 24 h | Headache, lightheadedness | Much more effective for vomiting than nausea; 2 mg |

| Drug (Trade; Mechanism) | Dose | Duration | Side effects | Comments |
|---|---|---|---|---|
| | | | | may be sufficient to treat PONV in PACU |
| Dolasetron (Anzemet; *Serotonin*) | *Adult:* 12.5 mg IV / *Pediatric:* 0.35 mg/kg | Up to 24 h | Headache, lightheadedness | Much more effective for vomiting than nausea |
| Granisetron (Kytril; *Serotonin*) | *Adult:* 1 mg IV over 30 s / *Pediatric:* N/A | Up to 24 h | Headache, lightheadedness | Much more effective for vomiting than nausea |
| Scopolamine (Transderm Scop; *Acetylcholine*) | *Adult:* 1.5 mg transdermal patch / *Pediatric:* N/A | 72 h ‖ | Sedation, dry mouth, visual disturbances, dysphoria, confusion, disorientation, hallucinations | Good for patients with motion sickness or undergoing surgery affecting vestibular apparatus; apply 4 h before exposure |
| Dexamethasone (Decadron; *None; works by another mechanism*) | *Adult:* 4-8 mg IV / *Pediatric:* 0.5-1 mg/kg | Up to 24 h | Watch blood sugar in patients with diabetes; watch for fluid retention, especially in cardiac patients | Generally well tolerated in healthy patients; may take time (hours) to work |
| Propofol (Diprivan; *None*) | *Adult:* 10-20 mg IV / *Pediatric:* N/A | < 10 min | Sedation | Very short acting (off-label use) |
| Aprepitant (Emend) | *Adult:* 40 mg po 1-3 h before anesthesia | Up to 24 h | Generally well tolerated | Oral prophylaxis only; caution with patients on warfarin; may reduce effectiveness of oral contraceptives |

*Adapted from references 14, 39 and 40.

14. Kovac AL: Prevention and treatment of postoperative nausea and vomiting. Drugs 59:213-243, 2000.

39. Tramer MR: A rational approach to the control of postoperative nausea and vomiting: Evidence from systematic reviews. Part I. Efficacy and harm of antiemetic interventions, and methodological issues. Acta Anaesthesiol Scand 45:4-13, 2001.

40. Taketomo CK, Hodding JH, Kraus DM: Pediatric Dosage Handbook (ed 6). Hudson, OH, LexiComp, 1999-2000.

Unless otherwise indicated, pediatric doses should not exceed the adult dose for each antiemetic agent.

†Children more than 10 kg or 2 years of age only. Change from IM to oral as soon as possible. With administration PR, dosing interval varies from 8 to 24 hours depending on child's weight.

‡Maximum of 12.5 mg in children less than 12 years of age.

§Children more than 2 years of age only; do not exceed 75 mg/dose or 300 mg/d.

‖Remove after 24 hours when used to prevent or treat PONV. Instruct patient to wash site where patch was and hands thoroughly.

EPS, Extrapyramidal symptoms, such as motor restlessness or acute dystonia; FDA, Food and Drug Administration; PR, per rectum; po, orally; N/A, not applicable.

Modified from Golembiewski JA, O'Brien D: A systematic approach to the management of postoperative nausea and vomiting, J Perianesth Nurs 17(6):364-376, 2002.

NURSING CARE IN THE PACU

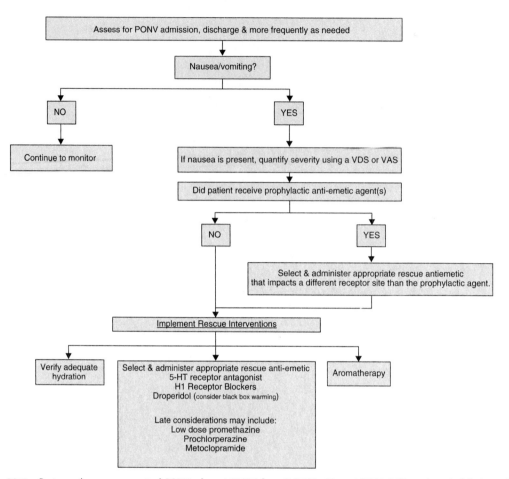

**Fig. 29-7** Postoperative management of PONV: phase I PACU/phase II PACU. *(From ASPAN: Evidence-based clinical practice guideline for the prevention and/or management of PONV/PDNV, J PeriAnesthesia Nurs 21(4):230-250, 2006.)*

tachykinin family of neurotransmitters, known as neurokinins. Substance P has the greatest affinity for neurokinin 1 (NK-1) receptors, which are found centrally in the brainstem vomiting center and peripherally in the gastrointestinal tract. Currently, the only available medication that targets these NK-1 receptors is aprepitant (Emend), available orally for prophylaxis of PONV.

**Nonpharmacologic Interventions.** In addition to pharmacologic interventions to manage nausea and vomiting, nonpharmacologic interventions are useful adjuncts. Adequate hydration with intravenous fluids and modified fasting protocols can help to minimize PONV. Aromatherapy (e.g., isopropyl alcohol, peppermint oil) is equal in benefit and risk and easy for the nurse to perform or administer. P6 acupoint stimulation with acupuncture or acupressure techniques has been shown to be effective and is recommended for use.

**Airway Management.** Perianesthesia care of the patient who is vomiting focuses on airway management. The patient should be placed in a head-down position so that the vomitus drains away from the lungs. Oral suctioning should be instituted if the patient is not completely able to control the airway. Oxygen should be administered when any question of compromise of the respiratory status arises. Rapid assessment of the patient's respiratory status should be made during and after the vomiting episode. This assessment is done with bilateral auscultation of the chest for adventitious sounds. Any possible aspiration of vomitus should be reported immediately to the physician. If the airway becomes obstructed, place the patient in a head-down position, turn the head to one side, and try to remove foreign material with suctioning or with the finger. While performing this maneuver, the nurse should send another person for an anesthesia care provider.

**Postdischarge Nausea and Vomiting.** After discharge, up to 30% to 50% of patients undergoing outpatient surgery have postdischarge nausea

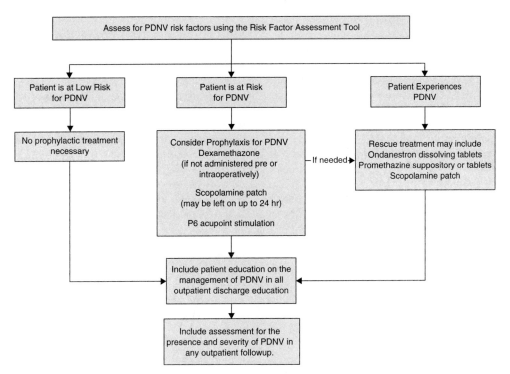

**Fig. 29-8** Management of PDNV. *(From ASPAN: Evidence-based clinical practice guideline for the prevention and/or management of PONV/PDNV, J PeriAnesthesia Nurs 21(4):230-250, 2006.)*

and vomiting (PDNV). PDNV affects the quality of recovery, increases the potential for patient morbidity and hospitalization of patients at high risk, and decreases patient satisfaction. PDNV is defined as nausea and vomiting that occurs up to 24 hours after the patient is discharged from the facility. See Fig. 29-8 for rescue and treatment recommendations. More research is needed to establish the scope of the PDNV problem and the effectiveness of these recommendations.

## OTHER COMPLICATIONS

### Spinal Epidural Hematoma
Particular attention should be paid to patients who have undergone spinals or epidurals who are seen in the PACU with severe back pain and symptoms of cord compression. The severe pain is a cardinal symptom of an emergent situation: spinal epidural hematoma. Typically, a rapid onset of sensory and motor deficits progresses to paralysis if not identified and promptly treated. Rapid action is needed to prevent permanent neurologic sequela.

Patients at greatest risk for development of this serious complication are female and older, who may have had a traumatic needle or catheter placement, and those with indwelling epidural catheters. Also at risk are patients who received low–molecular weight heparin therapy near the time of the epidural placement. In addition, concomitant dosing with anticoagulants or antiplatelet agents contributes to risk.

If the patient has severe back pain during recovery and has had an epidural or spinal, the nurse should immediately notify the anesthesia care provider to evaluate the patient. Definitive diagnosis of an epidural hematoma is with magnetic resonance imaging. Once the condition is determined to be a hematoma, emergency laminectomy and hematoma evacuation needs to occur quickly, ideally within 6 to 8 hours, to minimize the risk of permanent neurologic damage from the cord compression.

### Pseudocholinesterase Deficiency
Pseudocholinesterase (also referred to as plasma-cholinesterase) deficiency is an uncommon genetic disorder that creates unusual sensitivity to succinylcholine and ester local anesthetic agents. The typical response to succinylcholine is skeletal muscle paralysis that lasts approximately 5 to 10 minutes. The patient with abnormal or deficient pseudocholinesterase may remain apneic and paralyzed for up to 8 hours or more. The deficiency renders the patient with an inability to hydrolyze the ester bonds in succinylcholine, which leads to the prolonged skeletal muscle paralysis.

Questioning the patient regarding a blood relative's history of any anesthetic events may help to identify the patient at risk. The deficiency in pseudocholinesterase may also be acquired as the result of liver disease, malignant disease, pregnancy, collagen vascular disease, malnutrition, hypothyroidism, chronic infections (tuberculosis), extensive burn injuries, organophosphate pesticide poisoning, or uremia. Neonates and elderly patients are at risk. Other causes of lower pseudocholinesterase activity include plasmapheresis and medications such as anticholinesterase inhibitors, contraceptives, echothiophate eye drops, esmolol, glucocorticoids, metoclopramide, monoamine oxidase inhibitors, and pancuronium.

Care is supportive, with mechanical ventilation until the patient regains spontaneous respiratory effort because succinylcholine is not reversible. After recovery, the patient should be counseled to carry identification that indicates pseudocholinesterase deficiency and to alert blood relatives that they may also have this genetic variant.

Testing for pseudocholinesterase deficiency can be accomplished with dibucaine, an amide local anesthetic agent, combined with the patient's blood, which reflects the ability of pseudocholinesterase to metabolize succinylcholine. This test does not measure levels of the enzyme in the plasma. Also available is a simplified screening test of pseudocholinesterase enzyme activity that can be performed with specialized test paper (the Acholest Test Paper).

### Postdural Puncture Headache

Postdural puncture headache typically presents 24 to 48 hours after lumbar puncture from spinal needle placement or inadvertent dural puncture during epidural placement. Patients may either contact the facility with severe headache relieved by lying down or respond on follow-up by the perianesthesia nurse that they have a severe headache. The headache is caused by leakage of cerebrospinal fluid. The incidence rate of postdural puncture headache is greater in younger patients and women, especially during pregnancy.

Treatment is initially conservative; recommendations include mild analgesics, bed rest, caffeinated beverages, and increased fluid intake. Caffeine may also be given intravenously. If the symptoms continue, definitive treatment is an epidural blood patch, where fresh autologous blood is injected into the epidural space until the headache resolves or fullness or pain is felt. Epidural blood patches are effective in greater than 95% of symptomatic patients.

## PROCEDURE-RELATED COMPLICATIONS

### Perforated Viscous

Internal organs may be perforated during the operative procedure. Commonly caused by various types of endoscopic procedures (e.g., laparoscopy, gastroscopy), perforations can present as pain out of proportion to the procedure; a distended firm abdomen; hypotension, or bleeding. The esophagus, stomach, bladder, uterus, or bowel may be damaged and not noticed until after the patient arrives in the PACU and becomes symptomatic. The nurse should call the surgeon immediately, provide hemodynamic support as ordered (fluid resuscitation, blood component therapy, vasoactive medications, positioning, additional line placement), and analgesia or sedation if appropriate. The nurse may need to prepare for emergent transfer to the operative suite for repair of the perforation.

### Hemorrhage

Bleeding after operative procedures should be minimal. Dressings remain dry with minimal bloody drainage. However, hemorrhage can and does occur in the PACU and requires the attentive nurse to respond promptly to avert potential serious events. Any operative site may bleed if hemostasis is inadequate. Some sites may be more prone to bleeding, such as the tonsillar beds, nasopharynx resulting in epistaxis, the cervix after conization, and the uterus after dilatation and curettage vaginal/cervical. Signs and symptoms of overt or hidden hemorrhage include bright red bleeding; saturation of more than one pad per hour after uterine, cervical, or vaginal procedures; hypotension; tachycardia; restlessness; hematoma formation; and pain. Initial treatment for minor bleeding may be the application of ice or reinforcement of dressings or binders. More severe bleeding requires immediate action by the nurse. Pressure is applied depending on the location of the bleeding, the surgeon is called, fluid resuscitation is initiated, and preparations are made to return the patient to the operative suite for ligation of bleeders, hematoma evacuation, or other necessary surgical interventions to stop the bleeding.

### Dilutional Hyponatremia

Referred to as TURP syndrome when primarily seen in men undergoing prostate resections, dilutional hyponatremia can also occur in women undergoing hysteroscopic procedures. The usual cause is absorption of irrigating solutions through open blood vessels or perforation of the uterine or bladder wall that leads to circulatory overload from water intoxication. Signs and symptoms include hyponatremia, hypertension, bradycardia, agitation, nausea, CNS aberrations, muscle twitching, visual disturbances, excessive sedation, obtundation, increased ICP, seizures, coma, cardiovascular compromise including hemodynamic instability, pulmonary edema, and cardiovascular collapse. Patients may behave in a confused manner, have difficulty seeing, or be difficult to arouse. Treatment includes diuresis with loop diuretics and intravenous normal saline solution administration. If the serum $Na^+$ level is less than 120 mEq/L, 3% to 5% saline solution should be given and hemodynamic support provided. Visual disturbances generally resolve with prompt treatment. Permanent blindness can occur if the severe hyponatremia is left untreated.

## OTHER EMERGENCIES

### Allergic Reactions or Anaphylaxis

Although allergic reactions to anesthetics are rare, they can occur. Patients also react to antibiotics, latex products, analgesics, and other agents while in the perianesthesia setting. The target organs in an allergic response are the cutaneous, gastrointestinal, respiratory, and cardiovascular.

Cutaneous responses include erythema, flushing, and pruritus, especially of the palms, soles, and groin. Nausea, cramping, abdominal pain, vomiting, and diarrhea are the gastrointestinal responses. The respiratory responses involve laryngeal edema with hoarseness, dysphonia or a "lump in throat," chest tightness, shortness of breath, coughing, and wheezing. Cardiovascular responses may be most significant with hypotension, tachycardia, lightheadedness, faintness, syncope, myocardial infarction, dysrhythmias, and cardiovascular collapse experiences. Other symptoms may include nasal, ocular, and palatal pruritus; sneezing; diaphoresis; disorientation; or incontinence.

The nurse should respond immediately when a patient exhibits signs and symptoms of an allergic or potential anaphylactic reaction. The nurse should stop the administration of drugs, attempt to reduce the absorption of the offending agent, maintain the airway, and administer 100% oxygen. Intubation may need to be considered particularly if significant respiratory distress or laryngeal swelling is present. Fluid bolus for volume expansion is initiated. Epinephrine should be administered: start with 0.1 mL/kg of 1:1000 subcutaneously (SC) or intramuscularly

(IM) or 0.1 mL/kg of 1:10,000 IV (maximal dose, 5 mL) and titrate to effect on the basis of physician orders. Secondary treatment includes antihistamines, glucocorticoids, continuous catecholamine infusion, and sodium bicarbonate if acid-base status indicates the need. With supportive care, and especially if the patient is not intubated and symptoms continue, continually reevaluate the airway to ensure adequate oxygenation and ventilation.

### Transfusion Reactions

The exact incidence rate of transfusion reactions is unknown. Reports of the incidence rate vary from 0.2% to 10%, and some reactions are undoubtedly unrecognized and unreported.

Nurses in the PACU must be especially adept at assessment of the patient receiving blood because many of the signs and symptoms of an adverse reaction to blood may be difficult to separate from those caused by other variables, such as the patient's illness, surgery, or medications (including anesthesia). In addition, the patient who is not fully conscious may not report symptoms. Blood transfusion reactions or complications may be either immediate or delayed. Immediate reactions include hemolytic, nonhemolytic febrile, and anaphylactic reactions. Other reactions include transmission of infectious disease (acquired disease), graft-versus-host disease, and transfusion-related acute lung injury.

***Hemolytic Reactions.*** Fifty to 75 mL of ABO-incompatible blood can precipitate a hemolytic reaction that results in agglutination, or clumping, of RBCs, which blocks the patient's capillaries, thus obstructing the flow of blood and oxygen to vital organs. In time, hemolysis of the RBCs occurs, thus releasing free hemoglobin into the plasma. Free hemoglobin may plug the renal tubules and disrupt the work of the nephrons and result in renal failure. Improper storage, overheating, or freezing of blood may also cause hemolysis of the cells and release of free hemoglobin.

The clinical signs of the hemolytic reaction occur quickly and include sudden hypotension; tachycardia; chest tightness; abdominal, leg, and back pain; dyspnea; and sensorium changes, most often restlessness and apprehension. Headache may be one of the awakened patient's first symptoms. Pain may occur along the vein path. Fever and chills develop later, along with hemoglobinuria, which leads to oliguria. The patient may also have nausea and flushing of the skin. Many of these symptoms may be significantly masked by the influence of anesthesia. Bleeding from the wound strongly suggests that the patient has received incompatible blood; it is also a poor prognostic sign.

**Nonhemolytic Febrile Reactions.** Febrile reactions are most often caused by sensitivity to leukocytes and platelets and are seen most often in patients who have received multiple transfusions. The thought now is that these reactions stem from the formation of cytokines during blood storage. A febrile reaction may also be attributed to bacterial contamination. The symptoms do not occur as rapidly as in hemolytic reactions. In febrile or bacterial contamination reactions, the patient may have headache and chills, followed by a rapid rise in temperature. Backache, nausea, vomiting, diarrhea, and abdominal pain follow. Hypotension and tachycardia develop quickly. Pyrogenic reactions caused by the polysaccharide products of bacterial metabolism are manifested by the same symptoms, except that blood pressure does not drop and the temperature usually returns to normal within 12 hours. Patients at risk for febrile responses may be premedicated with acetaminophen and diphenhydramine to minimize the discomfort associated with this reaction.

**Anaphylactic Reactions.** Anaphylactic reactions occur in about 1 in 20,000 of all transfusions and are most often seen in patients who have a history of allergy. The reactions are more frequently seen in transfusions of large plasma amounts, as found in whole blood, pooled platelets, and fresh frozen plasma. Symptoms, which may occur after transfusion of as little as 10 mL of blood, include chills, abdominal cramps, dyspnea, vomiting, and diarrhea. Minor allergic reactions are associated with urticaria. Wheezing, laryngeal edema, and hypotension are associated with more severe reactions.

**Transfusion-related Acute Lung Injury.** Patients who receive blood products, particularly plasma-containing products, may be at risk for transfusion-related acute lung injury (TRALI), a serious pulmonary syndrome that can lead to death if not recognized and treated appropriately. The syndrome may be confused with non-cardiogenic pulmonary edema, which can be a symptom of TRALI. Symptoms typically begin 1 to 2 hours after transfusion and are fully manifested within 1 to 6 hours. Any transfusions should be stopped immediately. The condition is poorly understood and underdiagnosed. Patients may have dyspnea, hypoxemia, fever, and hypotension. Care is supportive; the condition may be mild to fatal, with a mortality rate of approximately 10%. Most cases resolve within 72 hours.

**Treatment of Immediate Reactions.** At the first sign of a reaction, the transfusion must be stopped and the physician notified. The donor blood is replaced with a new infusion set and normal saline solution. Recheck the patient's identity and blood label information match. The donor blood unit and administration set, along with a sample of the recipient's blood (drawn atraumatically from a site other than the intravenous catheter where the blood was administered), should be sent to the blood bank for transfusion reaction investigation. Urine output must be monitored carefully. Ideally, a Foley catheter should be inserted and hourly output recorded. Vital signs must be monitored and the patient treated according to symptoms. Blood transfusion with properly matched blood may be needed to correct blood volume deficits and control shock. Vasopressors may be necessary to control blood pressure but must be used with caution because they may contribute to renal damage, especially if blood volume has not been restored. Oxygen and epinephrine may be used to treat dyspnea and wheezing. Steroids and broad-spectrum antibiotics may be necessary to treat reactions caused by bacterial contamination. Antihistamines and antipyretics are given to the patient with an allergic reaction. Diuretic therapy (e.g., furosemide) and the infusion of 0.9% sodium chloride or 5% dextrose in 0.45% sodium chloride may be prescribed to maintain hydration and urine flow of more than 100 mL/h.

### Delayed Reactions

Delayed reactions include the transmission of disease (hepatitis, cytomegalovirus, HIV, human T-cell lymphotropic virus–I/II), graft-versus-host disease, circulatory overload, citrate intoxication, cardiac dysrhythmias, and bleeding caused by depleted coagulation factors. Delayed hemolytic reactions commonly occur 4 to 8 days after blood transfusion but may develop up to 1 month later. Symptoms are generally mild and can include a mild elevation in serum bilirubin or fever.

Circulatory overload results when fluid is infused into the circulatory system either too rapidly or in too great a quantity. Elderly patients and those with minimal cardiac reserve are particularly susceptible. The use of packed RBCs in these patients should be considered carefully. Symptoms of circulatory overload include cough, dyspnea, edema, tachycardia, hemoptysis, and frothy pink-tinged sputum. If the patient is conscious, the patient may have a pounding headache, a feeling of constriction around the chest, back pain, and chills. If these symptoms develop, the transfusion should be stopped and the physician notified.

When large amounts of banked blood are transfused, citrate intoxication may occur. If the blood is infused rapidly, the liver cannot metabolize the citrate ions, which combine with the calcium in the blood and cause calcium deficit symptoms such as tingling of the fingers, muscular cramps, and nervousness. If the calcium deficit is not corrected, cardiac dysrhythmias, including ventricular fibrillation, may occur. Treatment consists of slow intravenous administration of calcium gluconate, 1 g for every 1000 mL of blood the patient received. If calcium gluconate is unavailable, calcium chloride may be used, but this is more irritating to the veins.

The rapid infusion of cold blood may result in cardiac dysrhythmias or cardiac arrest. Blood should be warmed to room temperature or passed through a warming infuser, with care taken not to overheat it, which would cause hemolysis of the RBCs.

In cases of massive blood replacement, bleeding from dilution of coagulation factors and platelets can occur. If massive transfusions are necessary, several fresh blood infusions (<4 hours old) are suggested to be used along with banked blood.

Blood must be properly stored and refrigerated at 5° C, except for platelets. In most instances, blood should be stored in the blood bank until needed. If blood is to be kept in the PACU, proper storage requirements must be met. When units of blood prepared for a given recipient are not used, they should be promptly returned to the blood bank.

Following blood bank protocols for acquiring blood specimens, proper handling and storage of the blood products, checking patient identification with blood products before transfusion, and managing transfusion reactions are necessary for safe blood product administration.

## SUMMARY

The perianesthesia nurse in the postanesthesia care unit monitors the patient, vigilant and mindful of the potential for complications and adverse events. Proactive and responsive, the nurse reacts with sound clinical judgment to intervene quickly and assertively for the patient. Some complications are minor and transitory and easily resolved; others are life threatening and require skillful intervention by the nurse and the anesthesia care team to save the patient's life or avoid permanent injury. All perianesthesia nurses, regardless of the facility size or location, need competence in management of potential postanesthesia complications.

## BIBLIOGRAPHY

Ali SZ, Taguchi A, Roesenberg H: Malignant Hyperthermia, *Best Practice Res Clin Anaesthesiol* 17(4):519–533, 2003.

American Association of Critical-Care Nurses: *AACN procedure manual for critical care*, ed 5, Philadelphia, 2005, Saunders.

American Association of Nurse Anesthetists: *Considerations for policy development: unintended intraoperative awareness*, available at http://www.aana.com/news.aspx?ucNavMenu_TSMenuTargetID=62&ucNavMenu_TSMenuTargetType=4&ucNavMenu_TSMenuID=6&id=712, accessed March 15, 2007.

American Society of Anesthesiologists TAsk Force on INtraoperative Awareness: Practice advisory for intraoperative awareness and brain function monitoring, *Anesthesiology* 104:847-864, 2006.

American Society of PeriAnesthesia Nurses: Clinical guideline for the prevention of unplanned perioperative hypothermia, *J PeriAnesth Nurs* 16(5): 305-314, 2001.

American Society of PeriAnesthesia Nurses: *Standards of perianesthesia nursing practice 2006-2008*, Cherry Hill, NJ, 2006, American Society of PeriAnesthesia Nurses.

ASPAN: Evidence-based clinical practice guideline for the prevention and/or management of PONV/PDNV, *J PeriAnesthesia Nurs* 21(4):230-250, 2006.

Brice DD, Hetherington RR, Utting JE: A simple study of awareness and dreaming during anaesthesia, *Br J Anaesth* 42:535–542, 1970.

Bruns JJ Jr: *Anticholinergic toxicity*, available at http://www.emedicine.com/EMERG/topic36.htm, accessed March 9, 2007.

Bycroft J, Shergill IS, Choong EAL, et al: Autonomic dysreflexia: a medical emergency, *Postgrad Med J* 81:232–235, 2005.

Couture DJ, Maye JP, O'Brien D, et al: Therapeutic modalities for the prophylactic management of postoperative nausea and vomiting, *J PeriAnesth Nurs* 21(6):398–403, 2006.

Cullen DJ, Bogdanov E, Htlut N: Spinal epidural hematoma occurrence in the absence of known risk factors: a case series, *J Clin Anes* 16(5):376–381, 2004.

Eagle KA, Berger PB, Calkins H, et al: ACC/AHA guideline update for perioperative cardiovascular evaluation for noncardiac surgery: executive summary, *Anesth Analg* 94:1052–1064, 2002.

Finucane BT, Santora AH: *Principles of airway management*, ed 3, New York, 2003, Springer-Verlag.

Golembiewski JA, O'Brien D: A systematic approach to the management of postoperative nausea and vomiting, *J Perianesth Nurs* 17(6):364–376, 2002.

Joint Commission: Preventing, and managing the impact of anesthesia awareness, *Sentinel Event*

Alert 32: 2004. Accessed July 3, 2007, online at http://www.jointcommission.org/SentinelEvents/SentinelEventAlert/sea_32.htm

Kardon E. *Transfusion reactions*, available at http://www.emedicine.com/emerg/topic603.htm, accessed March 9, 2007.

Kertai MD, Klein J, Bax JJ, et al: Predicting perioperative cardiac risk, *Progress Cardiovasc Dis* 47(4):240–257, 2005.

Lepouse C, Lautner CA, Liu L, et al: Emergence delirium in adults in the post-anaesthesia care unit, *Br J Anaesth* 96(6):747–753, 2006.

Litwack K: *Post anesthesia care nursing*, ed 2, St. Louis, 1995, Mosby.

Mamaril ME, Windle PE, Burkard JF: Prevention and management of postoperative nausea and vomiting: a look at complementary techniques, *J PeriAnesth Nurs* 21(6):404–410, 2006.

Mathews DM, Brauer SD: Awareness during anesthesia, *Audio-Digest Anesthesiol* 48(19), 2006.

Murphy MJ, Hooper VD, Sullivan E, et al: Identification of risk factors for postoperative nausea and vomiting in the perianesthesia adult patient, *J PeriAnesth Nurs* 21(6):377–384, 2006.

Odom-Forren J, Fetzer SJ, Moser DK: Evidence-based intervention for post discharge nausea and vomiting: a review of the literature, *J PeriAnesth Nurs* 21(6):411–430, 2006.

Osborne GA, Bacon AK, Runciman WB, et al: Crisis management during anaesthesia: awareness and anaesthesia, *Qual Saf Health Care* 14(3):e16, 2005.

Siegmeth R, Bergman I, Absalom AR: Does depth of anaesthesia monitoring reduce the incidence of awareness? *Royal College Anaesthetists Bull* 29:1463–1467, 2005.

Smetana GW, Lawrence VA, Cornell JE: Preoperative pulmonary risk stratification for non-cardiothoracic surgery: systematic review for the American College of Physicians, *Ann Intern Med* 144:581–595, 2006.

Vlajkovic GP, Sindjelic RP: Emergence delirium in children: many questions, few answers, *Anesth Analg* 104(1):84–91, 2007.

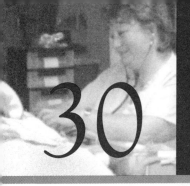

# 30

# ASSESSMENT AND MANAGEMENT OF THE AIRWAY

*Suzanne M. Wright, MSNA, CRNA*

Airway management is a fundamental skill essential to all personnel in perianesthesia nursing. Airway assessment and airway management are crucial in the provision of safe and effective care to patients after surgery. As these vulnerable patients enter the postanesthesia care unit (PACU), they are extremely susceptible to many events that can compromise ventilation and adequate oxygenation of vital body tissues. Of particular concern are the residual effects of many potent potentially life-threatening medications given by anesthesia personnel during the intraoperative period. These medications include, but are not limited to, narcotics, sedatives, hypnotics, inhalational gases, neuromuscular blockers, insulin, intravenous fluids, and blood products. In addition, predisposing factors have the potential to affect the patency of the postsurgical airway. These factors include histories of obstructive sleep apnea, snoring, smoking, asthma and ear, nose, throat (ENT), and neck surgery. Anticipation and early recognition of respiratory distress coupled with adequate airway assessment and management skills are paramount in assuring the best possible surgical outcome.

## DEFINITIONS

**Airway Obstruction:** A mechanical impediment to the delivery of air to the lungs or to the absorption of oxygen in the lungs.

**Auscultate:** To listen, most commonly with a stethoscope, for sounds within the body to aid in assessment of the frequency, intensity, duration, and quality of sounds.

**Blind Nasotracheal Intubation:** Nasotracheal intubation performed without the use of a laryngoscope.

**Cricothyrotomy:** A puncture through the cricothyroid membrane with a large bore cricothyrotomy catheter or large bore intravenous catheter for immediate access to the airway.

**Extubate:** The removal of an endotracheal or nasotracheal tube from the trachea.

**Laryngoscopy:** Use of a laryngoscope to view the anatomy of the larynx.

**Laryngospasm:** A involuntary, spasmodic closure of the vocal cords of the larynx.

**Nasopharyngeal Airway:** A device, usually a flexible tube, placed through the nares to create an air passage between the nose and the nasopharynx.

**Nasotracheal Intubation:** Insertion of a breathing tube through the nose into the trachea for facilitation of a patent airway.

**Oropharyngeal Airway:** A device placed in the oropharynx to conduct air or gases into the trachea; commonly referred to as an oral airway.

**Oropharynx:** One of three anatomic components of the pharynx; extends behind the mouth from the soft palate to directly above the hyoid bone. The oropharynx contains the palatine and lingual tonsils and lies between the nasopharynx and the laryngopharynx.

**Orotracheal Intubation:** The insertion of a breathing tube through the mouth into the trachea for facilitation of a patent airway.

**Sellick Maneuver:** Also referred to as cricoid pressure; the application of external pressure to the cricoid bone before and during laryngoscopy in an effort to compress the esophagus, preventing regurgitation through the esophagus during intubation of the trachea.

**Tracheostomy:** An opening through the neck into the trachea that provides a conduit for the placement of an indwelling tube to establish a patent airway.

## AIRWAY MANAGEMENT

Patients present to the PACU still experiencing the depressant effects of anesthesia. They may be obtunded, which renders them with the inability to maintain their own airway. Loss of important airway reflexes soon leads to airway obstruction. In some instances, the obtunded patient's tongue and epiglottis fall back on the posterior pharyngeal wall, further occluding the airway. Indications of airway obstruction include increased respiratory effort, retraction of the muscles of

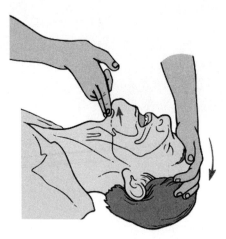

**Fig. 30-1**   Opening of airway with head-chin-lift manuever. *(From Lewis S, Heitkemper M, Dirksen S, et al: Medical-surgical nursing: assessment and management of clinical problems, ed 7, St Louis, 2007, Mosby.)*

| Box 30-1   Requirements for Bag-Valve-Mask Unit |
| --- |
| • Self-refilling but without sponge rubber inside (because of the difficulty in cleaning and disinfecting and in eliminating ethylene oxide and because of fragmentation)<br>• Nonjam valve system at 15-L/min oxygen inlet flow<br>• Transparent plastic face mask with an air-filled or contoured resilient cuff<br>• Standard 15-mm/22-mm fittings<br>• No pop-off valve, except in pediatric models<br>• System for delivery of high concentrations of oxygen through an ancillary oxygen outlet at the back of the bag or via an oxygen reservoir<br>• True nonrebreathing valve<br>• Oropharyngeal airway<br>• Satisfactory practice on mannequins<br>• Availability in adult and pediatric sizes |

respiration, a rocking chest motion, abnormal or absent breath sounds, cyanosis, and signs associated with hypoxemia and hypercarbia. On recognition of an airway obstruction, the nurse should place the patient supine, position a pillow beneath the head, tilt the head backward, and hyperextend the neck, unless contraindicated. The nurse should then lift the angle of the lower jaw upward with moderate pressure (Fig. 30-1). Often, this maneuver is all that is necessary for spontaneous respiratory effort to be effective. If the airway obstruction does not clear, the oral cavity should be inspected for foreign material and the oral pharynx suctioned if necessary. If large particles are present, the nurse should turn the patient's head to the side and remove the particles manually.

If spontaneous respiratory effort is absent, positive pressure breathing must be initiated. A bag-valve-mask unit that is connected to an oxygen source should be used. The requirements for a bag-valve-mask unit are addressed in Box 30-1. For optimal airway management, the perianesthesia nurse should be positioned behind the patient's head. The mask should be securely placed over the patient's mouth and nose with the neck hyperextended. The lower jaw should be lifted at its angle with the other fingers of the hand holding the mask. The thumb of that hand should be placed at the top of the mask. Moderate downward pressure provides compression over the bridge of the nose and reduces air leaks (Fig. 30-2).

After the mask is properly placed, ventilation of the patient should be attempted. While the perianesthesia nurse is ventilating the patient, an assistant should auscultate the chest and

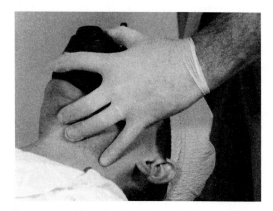

**Fig. 30-2**   Holding of mask with one hand. *(From Miller R: Miller's anesthesia, ed 6, St Louis, 2005, Churchill Livingstone.)*

assess the quality of breath sounds. If an assistant is unavailable, the perianesthesia nurse should check to see whether the chest rises with inspiration and falls with expiration. This observation is merely a crude estimate of ventilation. If breath sounds are not audible during auscultation, or if the crude estimate of ventilation is inconclusive, an appropriately sized oropharyngeal airway should be inserted (Fig. 30-3). The oral airway is noxious to awake or lightly sedated patients and should be used with extreme caution in this population. The untoward consequences associated with inappropriate use of the oral airway include bradycardia, retching, vomiting, and laryngospasm.

The oropharyngeal airway relieves an airway obstruction by providing a mechanical conduit

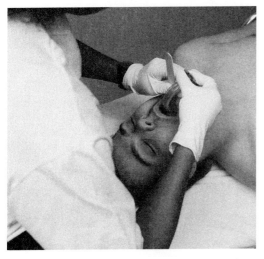

**Fig. 30-3** Insertion of oral airway. Airway is inserted with use of tongue blade to displace tongue forward. *(From Sanders, M: Mosby's paramedic textbook, ed 3, St Louis, 2007, Mosby.)*

for air to pass between the base of the tongue and the posterior oropharynx. For placement of an oropharyngeal airway, the perianesthesia nurse should first open the patient's mouth with the right hand and place a tongue blade toward the posterior aspect of the tongue with the left hand. Slight pressure should then be applied to draw the tongue forward. With the oropharyngeal airway held in the right hand, the nurse should slip the airway in over the tongue blade into the oropharynx. The airway should not be twisted or forced into place, and placement should be accomplished quickly with careful avoidance of trauma to the soft tissue and teeth.

In comparison with the oropharyngeal airway, the nasopharyngeal airway is less stimulating to the irritant receptors in the upper airway, especially in awake or lightly sedated patients. The nasopharyngeal airway should be lubricated with a local anesthetic water-soluble lubricant, such as 1% lidocaine gel or ointment, and gently passed with the right hand through the nostril along the curvature of the nasopharynx into the oropharynx. The nasopharyngeal airway should never be forced. If resistance is encountered on placement, the other nostril should be considered unless otherwise indicated. When positioned properly, the nasopharyngeal airway should rest between the base of the tongue and the posterior pharyngeal wall. This airway should not be used in a patient with a nasal-septal deformity, a leakage of cerebrospinal fluid from the nose, or a coagulation disorder.

Once the oropharyngeal or the nasopharyngeal airway has been placed properly, ventilation

should be attempted. Assessment of ventilatory effort should be continuous. With insertion of the oropharyngeal airway, the airway obstruction often clears. In this instance, the patient should be given a breath via the bag-valve-mask unit to assist with the spontaneous ventilatory effort and to help with removal of accumulated carbon dioxide. If apnea persists, positive-pressure breathing should be initiated via bag-valve-mask with large tidal volumes (10 to 12 mL/kg) at a rate of 14 to 16 breaths per minute. For prevention of oxygen delivery into the stomach, pressure on the bag-valve-mask device should not exceed 30 cm $H_2O$.

## INTUBATION OF THE TRACHEA

Intubation of the trachea is a proficiency reserved for nursing personnel who are specifically trained to perform this maneuver. The perianesthesia nurse should be familiar with intubation technique and capable, according to local hospital policy, of performing it quickly and efficiently should it be necessary. Airway management skills, such as endotracheal intubation, can be developed in the operating room setting under the mentorship of a certified registered nurse anesthetist (CRNA) or a physician anesthesiologist. With the same mentor, the perianesthesia nurse should continue to practice the intubation skills on a monthly basis in the operating room. In an airway emergency, the perianesthesia nurse should intubate the trachea if ventilation of the patient is unsuccessful. Endotracheal intubation indicates the placement of an endotracheal tube directly into the trachea. When the endotracheal tube is placed through the mouth, the method is called orotracheal intubation. When the endotracheal tube is placed through the nose, the method is called nasotracheal intubation. Other indications for endotracheal intubation in the PACU include the inability of the patient to protect the airway, prolonged mechanical ventilation, and cardiac and respiratory arrest.

The perianesthesia nurse should be familiar with the technique of endotracheal intubation and be capable of performing it quickly and efficiently, with recognition that the conditions in which intubation is performed in the PACU are less than ideal. The patient's position in the bed, excess upper airway secretions, and intact airway reflexes contribute to the degree of difficulty in performance of this maneuver in the PACU.

### Equipment for Endotracheal Intubation
Adult and pediatric intubation equipment should be kept in the PACU at all times. This equipment should be inspected daily and after

each use for proper functioning. For a list of the suggested items to be kept in the PACU, see Box 30-2. Table 30-1 shows the recommended sizes for endotracheal tubes. Because of their importance, the laryngoscope and endotracheal tubes are discussed in detail.

*Laryngoscope.* The laryngoscope is used for visualization of the larynx and the anatomic structures in close proximity to the larynx (Fig. 30-4). The laryngoscope has two main parts: the handle and the blade. The handle holds the laryngoscope and houses batteries that provide electricity for the light on the side of the blade. The blade consists of three sections: the spatula, the flange, and the tip. The spatula can be straight or curved; it is the long main shaft of the blade. It compresses and moves the soft tissue of the lower jaw for facilitation of direct vision of the larynx. The flange, which is on the side of the spatula, deflects tissue that may obstruct the direct vision of the larynx. The tip, at the distal end of the spatula, is either curved or straight and serves to elevate

| Box 30-2 | Suggested Equipment for PACU Pediatric and Adult Airway Management Carts |
| --- | --- |

**PEDIATRIC ENDOTRACHEAL EQUIPMENT**
Small laryngoscope handle
No. 2 Macintosh curved blade
No. 1 Miller straight blade
Pediatric oral airways
Assorted pediatric masks
Child's anatomic masks
Randell-Baker-Soucek masks
Assorted tracheal tubes
Reverse-angle endotracheal tubes
Cole tubes
Reinforced latex tube with stylet
Plastic thin-walled tube

**PEDIATRIC LMA EQUIPMENT**
LMA-Classic: sizes 1, 1½, 2, 2½, and 3
LMA-Unique: sizes 3 and 4
20-mL Syringes for inflation of LMA
Pediatric oral airways

**ADULT ENDOTRACHEAL EQUIPMENT**
Laryngoscope handle
Laryngoscope blades
Nos. 2 and 4 Miller
No. 3 Macintosh
Stylet
Sterile gauze with topical water-soluble anesthetic lubricant
Sizes 6-mm through 9-mm cuffed tracheal tubes
10-mL Syringe for inflation of the cuff
Small hemostat
Tongue blades for airway insertion
Assorted-sized oropharyngeal airways

**ADULT LMA EQUIPMENT**
LMA-Classic: sizes 3, 4, 5, and 6
LMA-Unique: sizes 3, 4, and 5
60-mL Syringes for inflation of LMA

| Table 30-1 | Recommended Sizes For Endotracheal Tubes | |
| --- | --- | --- |
| Age/Gender | | Internal Diameter (mm) |
| **PEDIATRIC** | | |
| Premature | | 2.0 |
| Newborn | | 2.5 |
| 6 months | | 3.5 |
| 1 year | | 4.0 |
| 2 years | | 5.0 |
| 4 years | | 5.5 |
| 6 years | | 6.0 |
| 8 years | | 6.5 |
| 10 years | | 6.5-7.0 |
| 12 years | | 7.0-7.5 |
| 14 years | | 7.5-8.0 |
| **ADULT** | | |
| Female | | 8.0-8.5 |
| Male | | 9.0-9.5 |

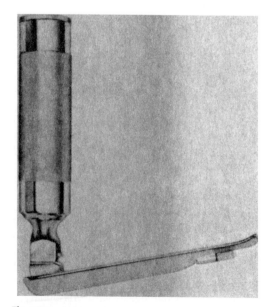

**Fig. 30-4** Laryngoscope.

the epiglottis, either directly or indirectly. The blade is attached to the handle at a connection called the hook-on fitting. The perianesthesia nurse is strongly encouraged to practice connecting the blade to the handle before using the laryngoscope in an emergency.

The Macintosh and Miller blades are the most popular types of laryngoscope blades in clinical use. The Macintosh is a curved blade with the flange on the left side for aid in moving the tongue, which enhances visual exposure of the larynx. The Macintosh blade (Fig. 30-5) comes in four sizes: No. 1 for the infant, No. 2 for the child, No. 3 for the medium adult, and No. 4 for the large adult. For most adults, the No. 3

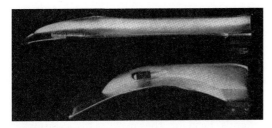

**Fig. 30-5** Most frequently used laryngoscope blades: Miller (top) and Macintosh (bottom). *(From Miller R, editor:* Anesthesia, *New York, 1981, Churchill Livingstone.)*

medium adult is the blade of choice. The Miller blade (see Fig. 30-5) has a straight spatula with a slightly curved tip. This blade has five sizes: No. 0 for the premature infant, No. 1 for the infant, No. 2 for the child, No. 3 for the medium adult, and No. 4 for the large adult. The Miller Nos. 0 and 1 are the blades of choice for premature and full-term infants, whose anatomic structures are more receptive to the use of a straight blade. Many anesthesia practitioners use the No. 2 Miller for intubation of adults. The perianesthesia nurse is encouraged to use both the straight and the curved blades while learning the technique. In most instances, the curved blade is easier to use than the straight blade; however, the exposure of the vocal cords is not as good as with the straight blade.

***Endotracheal Tube.*** The endotracheal tube is also called the tracheal tube, intratracheal tube, or catheter (Fig. 30-6). It is usually made from natural or synthetic rubber or plastic. The proximal, or machine, end protrudes from the patient's mouth and receives the adaptor. The distal, or patient end, has a slanted portion called the bevel. Endotracheal tubes are numbered according to the internal diameter in millimeters. Endotracheal tubes are available in many variations; some with inflatable cuffs and some without. Uncuffed endotracheal tubes are

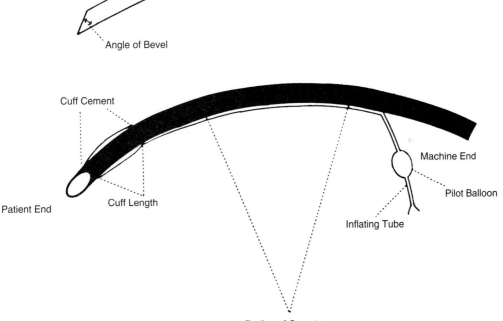

Angle of Bevel

Cuff Cement

Machine End

Pilot Balloon

Patient End

Cuff Length

Inflating Tube

Radius of Curvature

**Fig. 30-6** Curved tracheal tube. *(From Dorsch J, Dorsch S:* Understanding anesthesia equipment, *Baltimore, 1975, Williams & Wilkins.)*

usually seen in the pediatric population. Near the distal end of the endotracheal tube is the inflatable cuff. Leading away from the cuff is a long thin inflating tube with a pilot balloon at its proximal end. The pressure within the pilot balloon indicates whether the cuff is inflated. Above the pilot balloon is a one-way valve to which the inflation syringe is attached.

The cuff is an inflatable sleeve that provides a leak-resistant fit between the tube and the trachea when inflated. It also prevents aspiration and allows positive-pressure ventilation of the lungs. The cuff is permanently attached to the endotracheal tube at the distal end. High-volume or low-volume cuffs are available. The high-volume cuff is also referred to as a low-pressure cuff. The low-volume cuff is also referred to a high-pressure cuff. The arterial pressure in the tracheal wall is about 30 torr, and the venous pressure in that area is about 20 torr. Most clinicians agree that a low-pressure (high-volume) thin-walled cuff should be inflated to a pressure of about 17 to 23 torr. Local tracheal damage is associated with high cuff pressures, especially after long periods of intubation. Excessive cuff pressure is the primary factor that leads to ulceration, necrosis, and tracheal stenosis. These complications occur because high cuff pressure reduces the blood supply to the tracheal mucosa. For long-term ventilation, the cuff should be long, with a large residual volume (low-pressure).

In an emergency, the perianesthesia nurse should choose a cuffed endotracheal tube that is one size smaller than the size normally recommended for the patient. In making this choice, many clinicians look at the little finger of the patient; a smaller than normal little finger indicates that the patient has an opening at the vocal cords that is smaller than normal. Also, a stylet made of malleable metal or plastic should be inserted inside the endotracheal tube to improve its curvature and maintain its shape on insertion. A stylet should never be used with nasotracheal intubation. Before the stylet is placed inside the tracheal tube, it must be covered with a water-soluble lubricant to ease its withdrawal from the tube after placement. The end of the stylet should be about 3 cm from the distal end of the tracheal tube and should not protrude beyond the bevel because damage to the vocal cords can occur.

### Oral Endotracheal Intubation

Before oral endotracheal intubation is attempted, additional equipment should be immediately available and ready for use. Such equipment includes a tonsil suction connected to a working suction device, McGill forceps, 1-inch tape, a 10-mL empty syringe, and an anesthesia bag system or bag-valve unit. Also, throughout the procedure, the patient's oxygen saturation should be monitored continuously with a pulse oximeter.

The essential steps in the technique of oral endotracheal intubation are proper positioning of the patient, proper positioning of the patient's head, insertion of the laryngoscope blade, lifting of the epiglottis, visualization of the vocal cords, placement of the endotracheal tube, and assessment of the patient for correct tube placement. The methods for accomplishing these steps are discussed in the following sections.

***Positioning the Patient.*** Position the patient so that the head is near the top of the bed. Raise the entire bed so that the patient's face is approximately at the level of the standing perianesthesia nurse's xiphoid process.

***Positioning the Head.*** Place a firm 4-inch pillow or blanket under the head. Flex the patient's head at the neck. This position is called the sniffing position (Fig. 30-7). Extend the patient's head unless contraindicated.

***Insertion of the Laryngoscope Blade.*** With the fingers of the right hand, open the jaw, ensuring that the lips are not entangled in the teeth. With the laryngoscope in the left hand, insert the blade between the upper and lower teeth at the right side of the patient's mouth. Advance the blade slowly inward, past the tonsillar pillars and toward the midline of the oral cavity. Sweep the tongue toward the left side of the mouth. The key to successful intubation is moving the tongue to the left, out of the visual path to the vocal cords. At this point, the right hand can be placed under the patient's occiput to lift the head. The epiglottis should now be visualized. It is a red leaf-shaped structure that appears behind the tip of the blade as the laryngoscope is advanced down the oral cavity.

***Raising the Epiglottis and Visualizing the Vocal Cords.*** With the epiglottis in direct vision, slip the straight blade just beneath the tip of the epiglottis, gently lift the blade forward and upward at a 45-degree angle, and hold the wrist rigid (Fig. 30-8). If a curved blade is used, slip the tip of the blade between the epiglottis and the base of the tongue (see Fig. 30-8). With the left hand, lift forward and upward on the handle at a 45-degree angle. The epiglottis folds onto the blade, and the vocal cords should then be visible.

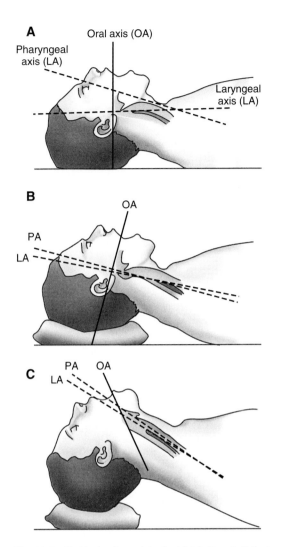

**Fig. 30-7** Positioning for endotracheal intubation. **A,** Patient is in supine position, with alignment of oral, pharyngeal, and laryngeal axes. **B,** Placement of pad or ring under patient's occiput (sniffing position) aligns pharyngeal and laryngeal axes. **C,** Extension of patient's head at atlanto-occipital joint now aligns all three axes, which provides shortest distance and most nearly straight line from mouth to larynx. *(Redrawn from Miller R, editor:* Anesthesia, *ed 5, New York, 2000, Churchill Livingstone.)*

Regardless of whether a curved or straight blade is used, the handle should not be used as a lever nor should the upper teeth be used as a fulcrum because the tip of the blade will push the larynx up and out of sight and the teeth can become chipped or broken.

At this point, if the vocal cords cannot be visualized, an assistant should apply gentle external downward pressure on the larynx (the Sellick maneuver). The vocal cords should come into view. If the blade is inserted too deeply, it enters the esophagus. At this point, withdraw the blade, ventilate the patient with 100% oxygen, and attempt the procedure again. During ventilation of the patient, review what went wrong and design an alternative strategy to facilitate successful intubation of the trachea.

***Placing the Endotracheal Tube.*** When the vocal cords are visualized, an assistant should place the endotracheal tube, with a stylet properly inserted to maintain a curve and the cuff deflated, in the laryngoscopist's right hand. The laryngoscopist should never lose sight of the cords once they are visualized. Pass the endotracheal tube with the right hand along the right side of the tongue and blade and through the vocal cords until the cuff disappears beyond the vocal cords or until the tip of the endotracheal tube protrudes 2 or 3 cm into the trachea.

***Assessing the Patient.*** Once the endotracheal tube is placed, correct placement must be verified. Remove the blade with the left hand while holding onto the endotracheal tube with the right hand. Place the laryngoscope on the patient's bed or on a table, and slowly remove the stylet without dislodging the tracheal tube. The cuff can be inflated at this time. With a 10-mL syringe full of air, inject a volume of air (about 4 to 6 mL) into the pilot balloon until leakage around the cuff is minimal or stops. A cuff leak is assessed with placement of the bell of the stethoscope over the larynx. The end of the endotracheal tube should be connected to a bag-valve unit or an anesthesia bag system and ventilated while an assistant auscultates the chest for breath sounds. Breath sounds should be assessed in all four quadrants, and the stomach should also be auscultated. If no breath sounds are audible or if a gurgling sound is heard over the stomach, deflate the cuff, remove the endotracheal tube, and ventilate the patient by mask, with 100% oxygen. These signs indicate an esophageal intubation. While ventilating the patient, consider why the attempt was unsuccessful, review the procedure, and reintubate the patient. If breath sounds are audible on only the right side of the chest, a right endobronchial intubation is indicated. If this condition occurs, withdraw the tube at 1-cm intervals and auscultate until breath sounds are bilateral. Confirmation of endotracheal intubation is also verified with bilateral and symmetric chest rise and the presence of expiratory carbon dioxide. Expiratory carbon dioxide can be measured with spectroscopy or disposable carbon dioxide detectors used specifically for this purpose. Once correct endotracheal tube placement and cuff pressure are confirmed, insert an oral airway and secure the tube with adhesive tape.

NURSING CARE IN THE PACU

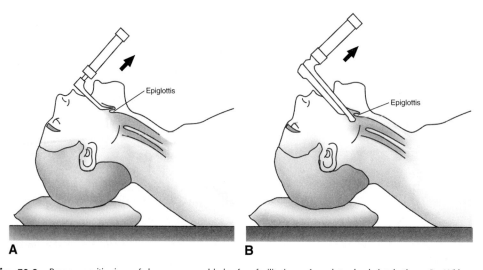

**Fig. 30-8** Proper positioning of laryngoscope blade for facilitation of endotracheal intubation. **A,** With curved blade (e.g., Macintosh), tip is placed into space between base of tongue and pharyngeal surface of epiglottis, which is called vallecula. **B,** With straight blade (e.g., Miller), tip is placed on laryngeal surface of epiglottis. Regardless of type of blade used, once blade is in position, forward and upward movements on handle (arrows) exert pressure on long axis of blade, which serves to elevate epiglottis and expose vocal cords. *(Redrawn from Miller R, editor:* Anesthesia, *ed 5, New York, 2000, Churchill Livingstone.)*

Documentation of the procedure should include the number of attempts, the degree of visualization of the vocal cords, whether the intubation was traumatic or atraumatic, the quality of breath sounds, the amount of air injected into the cuff, the cuff pressure, the endotracheal tube size, and the laryngoscope blade type and size.

***Ventilating the Patient.*** The adult patient should be ventilated approximately 14 to 18 times a minute at a tidal volume of 8 to 10 mL/kg. Infants should be ventilated at approximately 26 to 30 times a minute at a volume large enough to raise the chest on inspiration. However, when time permits, a tidal volume of 7 mL/kg should be used. Children should be ventilated at a rate of 18 to 24 bpm. The tidal volume to be delivered can be determined in the same manner for infants.

### Nasotracheal Intubation

When the endotracheal tube is inserted through the nose, the method is called nasotracheal intubation. When nasotracheal intubation is done without the use of a laryngoscope, the method is called a blind nasotracheal intubation. Direct-vision intubation is the insertion of an endotracheal tube with the aid of a laryngoscope. With the direct-vision method for performance of a nasotracheal intubation, the perianesthesia nurse may use Magill forceps (Fig. 30-9). A description of the nasal intubation technique can be found in many anesthesia textbooks.

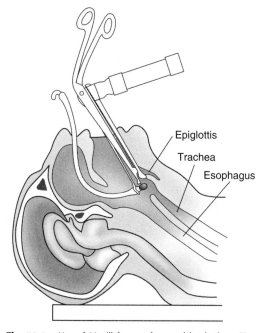

**Fig. 30-9** Use of Magill forceps for nasal intubation. *(From Collins VJ:* Principles of anesthesiology, *ed 2, Philadelphia, 1976, Lea & Febiger.)*

Intubation has many advantages. It provides a route for mechanical ventilation, reduces the amount of anatomic dead space, and protects the patient from aspiration of blood, mucus, or foreign material into the tracheobronchial tree. It also relieves upper airway obstruction and provides an access route for removal of excess secretions in the airways.

The disadvantage of intubation is that it can produce trauma to the teeth, lips, soft palate, epiglottis, vocal cords, and other tissues in that region.

## Emergency Airway Management

At times, the perianesthesia nurse is called on to care for a patient with a documented or undocumented difficult airway. A difficult airway implies an inability to ventilate or intubate in optimal conditions by an airway expert. The perianesthesia nurse must be familiar with methods to manage this life-threatening event. The American Society of Anesthesiologist's (ASA) Difficult Airway Algorithm is a helpful tool and can be easily referenced. A copy of this algorithm, or one like it, should be available in the postanesthesia care unit at all times.

Cricothyrotomy is a puncture through the cricothyroid membrane with a large bore cricothyrotomy catheter or large bore intravenous catheter. The perianesthesia nurse should become familiar with locating the cricothyroid membrane, which falls midline between the thyroid cartilage and the cricoid cartilage on the anterior portion of the neck around the level of the sixth cervical vertebra. Before ventilating through this *temporary* airway, the nurse should confirm correct placement into the trachea, which is evidenced by the aspiration of air through the catheter into an attached syringe. A jet ventilator, which delivers oxygen at a very high pressure, is ideal for ventilating through this type of airway because the resistance is difficult to overcome. Witnessing the egress of air after each inspiration with the jet ventilator is crucial to avoid excessive accumulation of pressure in the lungs. Cricothyrotomy is a last attempt at securing an airway. It is instituted only after all other viable options to securing the airway have been exhausted. For this procedure to be successful, the nurse must know where the requisite supplies are located and how the equipment functions. Cricothyrotomy is merely a bridge until a more definitive airway, such as a surgical cricothyrotomy or tracheostomy, can be performed.

## Perianesthesia Care of the Intubated Patient

Nursing care of the intubated patient involves: (1) frequent auscultation of the chest for bilateral breath sounds to ensure correct placement of the endotracheal tube; (2) frequent suctioning of the oral cavity and, if clinically necessary, suctioning inside the endotracheal tube to remove secretions; and (3) maintenance of communication to reduce anxiety. The perianesthesia nurse must reassure the patient of continuous observation and monitoring. In addition, the nurse should provide the patient with a means of communication. Also, delivery of at least five maximal ventilations of 100% oxygen before endotracheal suctioning is performed is important.

## Extubation of the Patient

With determination that the patient can be safely extubated, the perianesthesia nurse should first ensure that all intubation, suction, and ventilation equipment is functioning properly and is at the patient's bedside. The entire procedure should be explained to the patient. Depending on the amount and location of secretions, the trachea and the nasopharynx should be suctioned. All secretions must be aspirated from the upper airway to reduce the incidence of coughing and laryngospasm. Next, the patient should be ventilated with 100% oxygen for at least 2 minutes. A syringe is then placed into the side valve of the pilot balloon and the endotracheal tube cuff is deflated. The patient should be asked to take a deep breath, and at the end of inspiration, the tube should be gently removed. If the patient is completely awake and responding, the oral airway should also be removed. Oxygen (100%) should be administered via mask, and the patient assessed for dyspnea, stridor, and airway obstruction. Oxygenation should be assessed continually by the pulse oximeter and the clinical picture.

## Adverse Sequelae after Tracheal Intubation

*Hoarseness and Sore Throat.* On emergence from anesthesia, some patients who have been intubated during surgery have a sore throat. Although the incidence of a sore throat after intubation is low, it is a significant discomfort to the patient. The incidence of sore throat increases dramatically when the patient's head is turned frequently or is placed in an abnormal position during surgery.

Assessment of the patient with a sore throat should include visual assessment of the oropharynx and auscultation of the chest. Abnormal findings should be reported to the anesthesia provider. Counseling the patient is probably the most important nursing intervention. The nurse should review the anesthesia record to determine whether the patient was intubated and whether the procedure was traumatic (such as multiple attempts and difficult intubation). A sore throat can result from a traumatic intubation.

Interventions consist of communicating to the patient that an endotracheal tube was placed in the throat during surgery to help with breathing and that throat discomfort may persist for 1 to 3 days. When the patient understands the reason for the discomfort and learns that it is not life-threatening, the perception of the discomfort often becomes less severe. If treatment is necessary, medications such as dexamethasone may be given to reduce the inflammation. Also, an ice bag or ice chips may be given to the patient to relieve symptoms.

**Laryngospasm.** Partial or complete closure of the vocal cords can occur because of increased secretions or as a reflex caused by stimulation of the irritant receptors. Assessment reveals reduced or no breath sounds. If partial laryngospasm is present, the patient makes crowing sounds, especially on inspiration. Interventions include the administration of 100% oxygen under positive pressure with a bag-valve-mask unit. If the patient cannot be ventilated, intravenous administration of succinylcholine and reintubation are mandated (see Chapter 23).

**Aspiration of Gastrointestinal Contents.** Aspiration of gastrointestinal contents is a complication that may be seen in weak and debilitated patients, those with neurologic disease, or those with an intestinal obstruction. See Chapter 16 for a complete discussion of this syndrome.

**Laryngeal Mask Airway.** The laryngeal mask airway (LMA) was developed in the 1980s by a British anesthesiologist, Dr Archie Brain. The product first became available in the United States in 1992. During the last 15 years, modifications have been made to the design of the original LMA, known as the LMA-Classic, that have resulted in numerous LMA products that are useful for a variety of patient airway needs.

**Laryngeal Mask Airway–Classic.** The LMA-Classic was designed to provide an alternative method of airway management that is intermediate in invasiveness between the face mask and the endotracheal tube (ETT; Fig. 30-10). The reusable latex-free device consists of three basic components. The first component is the

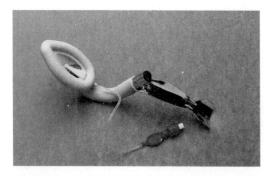

**Fig. 30-10**  LMA-Classic. *(Used with permission of The Laryngeal Mask Company Limited, United Kingdom.)*

soft inflatable cuff that, when inserted correctly, conforms to the hypopharynx with its opening facing the patient's laryngeal opening. At the proximal end, on the inside of the cuff, is a set of aperture bars located at the junction of the cuff and airway tube. The aperture bars allow passage of air into the cuff yet prevent airway anatomy, such as the epiglottis, from entering the tube and blocking the airway passage. The cuff is connected to the second component, an airway tube, which is a large bore tube with a 15-mm standard connector on the end. The tube acts as a gas conduit for ventilation, and if needed, an endotracheal tube can be passed through the LMA through the vocal cords for intubation. The size of the ETT able to pass through the LMA depends on the size of the LMA inserted. Lastly, a long thin inflation tube is attached to a pilot balloon that permits inflation and deflation of the LMA cuff.

The LMA-Classic is used for a variety of patient circumstances during general anesthesia and is commonly used for patients with spontaneous breathing during the anesthetic. The LMA is often well tolerated in the patient who is lightly anesthetized and semiconscious. The LMA is available in eight sizes and can be used in patients ranging in size from neonates to more than 100 kg. More importantly, the LMA has been used routinely in management of difficult and emergent airway situations. The device has proven successful in providing a bridge or temporary airway in patients in whom a permanent airway has not been obtained. Recently, the LMA has been included in two nationally recognized association protocols: the ASA Difficult Airway Algorithm and the American Heart Association Guidelines for 2000 for Cardiopulmonary Resuscitation and Emergency Cardiovascular Care for Advanced Cardiac Life Support (ACLS).

Insertion of the LMA is simple, and most providers find the learning curve to be gentle. After the cuff is deflated so that it is flat and free of wrinkles, the anterior portion of the cuff is lubricated with a water-soluble product. The patient then is placed in the preferred position, the sniffing position, although a neutral position can be used in patients with actual or suspected cervical spine injury. The provider places the dominant index finger at the junction between the cuff and the airway tube while ensuring the solid black line on the tube faces the patient's upper lip. The cuff is placed against the patient's hard palate and is moved back and forth against the palate to effectively lubricate the airway and prevent the cuff from folding over on insertion. Without forcing, the

LMA is advanced as far down into the pharynx as possible. The nondominant hand holds the tube, and the dominant finger is withdrawn from the LMA device. Without the nurse holding onto the device, the LMA is inflated following the recommended maximum cuff inflation volumes. Correct placement of the LMA may be observed during inflation; a slight and upward movement of the LMA in the airway and notable swelling in the neck may occur after cuff inflation. Insertion of an oral airway next to the LMA tube may be necessary for prevention of occlusion of the airway tube as the patient regains consciousness. Auscultation of bilateral breath sounds and the presence of end-tidal carbon dioxide confirm placement of the LMA device.

**Other Laryngeal Mask Airway Products.** Additional LMA products are available for management of the patient's airway. The LMA-Unique is the disposable version of the LMA-Classic. This product is often found in prehospital settings and in code carts and other airway management carts. The LMA-Flexible is a wire-reinforced device used primarily for procedures that involve the head or neck area. The flexible airway tube permits the airway product to be positioned away from the surgical field while an adequate seal is maintained. The LMA-Fastrach is designed to facilitate endotracheal intubation (Fig. 30-11). The reusable device differs from the classic LMA design primarily in its rigid anatomically curved airway tube that is connected to a metal handle.

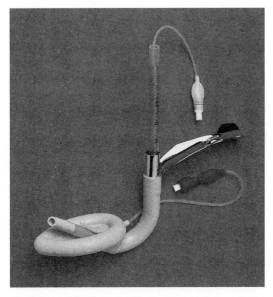

**Fig. 30-11** LMA-Fastrach. *Used with permission of The Laryngeal Mask Company Limited, United Kingdom.*

The handle is used to facilitate one-handed insertion and removal and to adjust the LMA cuff's position and the glottic alignment of the ETT. The aperture bars of the classic LMA have been replaced in the Fastrach with an epiglottic elevating bar. The elevating bar is designed to lift the epiglottis as the ETT passes through the LMA device, which may decrease the risk of arytenoid trauma or esophageal placement.

The newest LMA product, introduced in 2000, is the LMA-ProSeal. The LMA-ProSeal is designed specifically for separation of the alimentary and respiratory tracts with improvement of the laryngeal seal. The newly improved seal offers a higher airway seal pressure during positive pressure ventilation and may be used in the patient who is either spontaneously breathing or paralyzed. A built-in bite block provides protection from occlusion by the patient, and a removable introducer allows insertion of the product without the need to place fingers directly in the patient's mouth. Another unique feature of this product is the ability to blindly pass a gastric tube through the device, which allows for stomach decompression and drainage.

The following guidelines are for the perianesthesia nurse caring for patients in the PACU who have or have had an LMA inserted for surgery. If an LMA is present in the patient in the PACU, a few important points should be remembered. The LMA is designed to be removed in either an awake patient or a deeply anesthetized patient. Removal of the LMA while the patient is awake is the most common and preferred technique, especially in adult patients. Most patients are able to open their mouths on command for removal of the LMA. Because cuff deflation before the return of effective swallowing and coughing reflexes may allow secretions in the upper airway to enter the larynx and cause laryngospasm, the LMA cuff should not be deflated until the LMA is being removed. Also, the bite block or oral airway should not be removed before removing the LMA device. This precaution prevents occlusion of the airway from the patient biting down on the LMA tube. For patients who still have an LMA present in the PACU, manual support of the airway is not necessary. In fact, lifting of the jaw may actually displace the LMA cuff and cause laryngospasm or malposition.

Although LMA products may differ regarding indications for use in patient airway management, important similarities for product usage exist. The LMA products are contraindicated in patients at risk for aspiration and regurgitation because the devices do not protect the airway from gastric secretions.

The LMA products are also contraindicated in patients with upper airway pathology or obstruction. LMA devices are advantageous for use in patients who are professional speakers who need a general anesthetic. Because LMA devices do not come in contact with the vocal cords, voice changes caused by vocal cord trauma are less likely. The devices are especially useful in patients who have a difficult mask airway because of distorted facial anatomy or the presence of a beard. LMA products have gained acceptance in many areas of health care. The ease of insertion combined with a variety of different products has allowed health care professionals to offer a greater degree of airway management and safety for surgical patients.

## SUMMARY

The perianesthesia nurse is in a good position to respond to airway problems that may arise in the PACU. Patients who enter this environment are vulnerable to airway compromise because of medical history and the residual effects of anesthesia and surgery. Knowledge of airway management techniques coupled with early recognition of difficulties are key in optimization of patient outcomes in the perioperative setting.

## BIBLIOGRAPHY

Aitkenhead A, Smith G, Rowbotham D: Textbook of anaesthesia, ed 5, Philadelphia, 2007, Churchill Livingstone.

Alspach J: Core curriculum for critical care nursing, ed 6, Philadelphia, 2005, Saunders.

Atlee J: Complications in anesthesia, ed 2, Philadelphia, 2007, Saunders.

Austin R: Respiratory problems in emergence from anesthesia, Int Anesthesiol Clin 29(2):25–36, 1991.

Barash P, Cullen B, Stoelting R: Clinical anesthesia, ed 5, Philadelphia, 2001, Lippincott Williams & Wilkins.

Bickley L: Bates' guide to physical examination and history taking, ed 9, Philadelphia, 2005, Lippincott Williams & Wilkins.

Bowdle T, Horita A, Kharasch E: Pharmacologic basis of anesthesiology: basic science and practical applications, Philadelphia, 1994, Saunders.

Brimacombe JR, Brain AIJ: The laryngeal mask airway: a review and practical guide, Philadelphia, 1997, Saunders.

Brunton L, Lazo J, Parker K: Goodman and Gilman's the pharmacological basis of therapeutics, ed 11, New York, 2005, McGraw-Hill Professional.

Butterworth J, Marlow G: Atlas of procedures in anesthesia and critical care, Philadelphia, 1992, Saunders.

Class P: Nursing considerations for airway management in the PACU, Curr Rev Post Anesth Care Nurses 14(1):3–7, 1992.

DeFazio-Quinn D, Schick L: Perianesthesia nursing core curriculum, Philadelphia, 2004, Saunders.

Dolenska S: Basic science for anaesthetists, London, 2006, Cambridge University Press.

Fisher L: Benumof's anesthesia and uncommon diseases, ed 5, Philadelphia, 2007, Saunders.

Gallager C, Issenberg B: Simulation in anesthesia, Philadelphia, 2007, Saunders.

Ganong W: Review of medical physiology, ed 22, New York, 2005, McGraw-Hill Medical.

Guyton A, Hall J: Textbook of medical physiology, ed 11, Philadelphia, 2006, Saunders.

Hagberg C: Benumof's airway management, ed 2, St Louis, 2007, Mosby.

King T, Adams A: Failed tracheal intubation, Br J Anaesth 65:400–414, 1990.

Lake C, Hines R, Blitt C: Clinical monitoring: practical applications for anesthesia and critical care, St Louis, 2001, Mosby.

Longnecker D, Murphy F: Dripps/Eckenhoff/Vandam introduction to anesthesia, ed 9, Philadelphia, 1997, Saunders.

Longnecker D, Tinker J, Morgan G: Principles and practice of anesthesiology, ed 2, St Louis, 1998, Mosby.

Martin J, Warner M: Positioning in anesthesia and surgery, ed 3, St Louis, 1997, Mosby.

McIntosh L: Essentials of nurse anesthesia, New York, 1997, McGraw-Hill.

Miller R, editor: Miller's anesthesia, ed 6, Philadelphia, 2005, Churchill Livingstone.

Motoyama E, Davis P: Smith's anesthesia for infants and children, ed 7, St Louis, 2006, Mosby.

Nagelhout J, Zaglaniczny K: Nurse anesthesia, ed 3, St Louis, 2005, Saunders.

Pesola G, Kvetan V: Ventilatory and pulmonary problem management, Anesthesiol Clin North Am 8(2):287–309, 1990.

Stoelting R, Miller R: Basics of anesthesia, ed 5, New York, 2007, Churchill Livingstone.

Stoelting R, Miller S: Pharmacology and physiology in anesthetic practice, ed 4, Philadelphia, 2005, Lippincott Williams and Wilkins.

Stone D, editor: Perioperative care: anesthesia, medicine, and surgery, St Louis, 1998, Mosby.

Whitten C: Anyone can intubate, ed 2, San Diego, 1990, Medical Arts Publications.

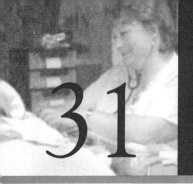

# 31

# PAIN MANAGEMENT IN THE PACU

Michael J. Boss, MD
Philip H. Ewing, MD
Stephen P. Long, MD

Pain is a response to a noxious stimulus and has evolved over many years as a defensive mechanism designed to protect the human body. It is defined as an unpleasant sensation and emotional experience that is associated with a damaging or noxious stimulus. Although minor injuries and sore muscles are consequences of everyday activities, pain in an operative setting should never be viewed as an acceptable consequence by either the clinician or the patient. Pain has no beneficial value in the postoperative setting; the undertreatment of pain can result in negative physiologic, psychologic, and economic effects. Increasingly, poorly managed pain has become a legal issue as patients have sought legal advice after inadequately treated pain in the hospital setting.

As science and practice continue to mature, the responsibility for the management of pain in surgical patients is shared among all caregivers from the time of admission to the time of discharge. However, the role of the postanesthesia care unit (PACU) nurse does not diminish with this team-oriented approach. Effective interventions begin both before surgery and from the moment the patient arrives in the PACU from the operating room. In spite of the many advances in pain control options and in the PACU care approach, the overall challenge of pain management remains unchanged: to provide analgesia in the narrow window that lies between sedation and the numerous undesirable states of pain. To aid the perianesthesia nurse in accomplishing this goal, the American Society of PeriAnesthesia Nurses (ASPAN) has developed a position statement regarding the optimal management of pain (Appendix A).

## UNDERSTANDING PAIN: A BASIC FUND OF KNOWLEDGE

The perianesthesia nurse should have a solid understanding of anesthesia, analgesia, stress and inflammatory responses to surgery, and hemodynamics. For effective pain treatment, the perianesthesia nurse also needs a working knowledge of the concepts of pain management to augment knowledge of the treatment of postoperative pain. A strong foundation in the understanding of pain management should begin with understanding the different mechanisms and manifestations of pain and with the requirements for the production of pain.

The three commonly reported types of pain are visceral, nociceptive or somatic, and neuropathic pain. Visceral pain is poorly localized and often referred to as a distant pain. This pain is produced by activation of nociceptors in any of the visceral tissues. Good examples of visceral pain are the right upper quadrant abdominal and shoulder pain with cholecystitis, the crushing pain of angina pectoris, and the back and epigastric pain with pancreatic carcinoma. Nociceptive pain, also known as somatic pain, is well localized, referred to as familiar in quality, and often associated with inflammation. Somatic pain is produced by the activation of nociceptors in the somatic tissues. Examples of nociceptive pain are those of surgical pain and bone metastasis. The final type of pain is neuropathic pain. This type of pain can be regarded as the most complicated in regard to its multiple mechanisms and manifestations. Neuropathic pain is most often localized within the distribution of a central nervous system or peripheral nerve tract. Its quality is often referred to as unfamiliar and can be described as burning, lancinating, or squeezing in quality. Neuropathic pain is often intermittent and can be experienced as areas of sensory loss or numbness. Multiple mechanisms exist for the creation of neuropathic pain, including compression of peripheral nerves, inflammatory changes in a sensory ganglion, demyelination in sensory tracts, ectopic discharges, and the loss of small and large sensory fibers. Some familiar examples

437

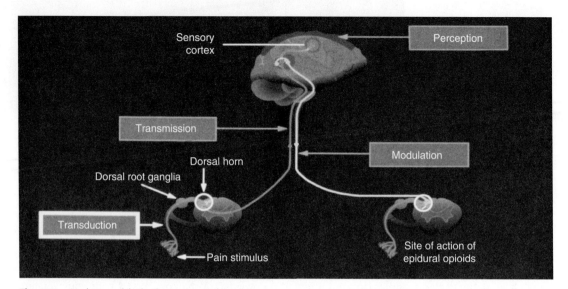

**Fig. 31-1** Modern model of pain: sensory pathway.

of neuropathic pain are carpal tunnel syndrome, herpes zoster, multiple sclerosis, trigeminal neuralgia, and diabetic neuropathy. These three types of pain all share one thing in common: the requirements for their production.

The modern model of pain identifies the following four requirements for the production of pain: transduction, transmission, modulation, and perception (Fig. 31-1).

Transduction occurs when mediators such as substance P, serotonin, histamine, and bradykinin are released at the site of tissue injury. These mediators stimulate peripheral sensory afferent nerves that extend to the dorsal horn of the spinal cord. Transmission of this stimulus occurs when ascending nerves running from the dorsal horn of the spinal cord to the brain are stimulated by the peripheral sensory afferents. Descending pathways to the dorsal horn modulate the activity of the peripheral nerves with the release of enkephalins and endorphins. Perception of pain occurs at the level of the brain and reflects modulation of the transduction of the pain stimulus, ranging from amplification to suppression.

Pain is not only an unpleasant experience, but it can also cause undesirable physiologic (Box 31-1) and psychologic (Box 31-2) consequences.

Effective pain management in any setting, before surgery through postoperative recovery, requires thorough evaluation of the patient's condition, determination of the severity of the pain, a search for the cause of the pain, and linking of the pathogenesis of that pain with an appropriate targeted treatment approach. In many cases, the preoperative evaluation of pain includes recognition of the likely possibility

---

**Box 31-1  The Physiologic Consequences of Pain**

Increased metabolic rate
Increased blood clotting
Water retention
Tissue breakdown
Impaired immune function
Autonomic hyperactivity
Pulmonary dysfunction
Delayed return of bowel function
Development of chronic pain syndromes

---

**Box 31-2  The Psychologic Consequences of Pain**

Negative emotions
Anxiety
Depression
Sleep deprivation
Suffering

---

of postoperative pain, and with the anesthesiologist, preemptive provision of the proper treatment modality for lessening this pain.

A systematic approach to assessment of a patient's pain is strongly recommended. The goal of this assessment is an attempt to quantify the intensity of the patient's pain and determine its cause. The evaluation of any patient with pain should begin with a data-gathering phase in which a careful pain-related history is

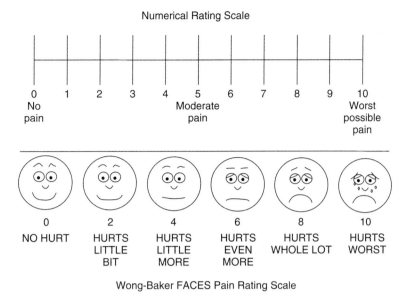

**Fig. 31-2** Pain rating scales. Numeric rating scale or visual analog scale is useful for evaluation of adult pain status. Wong-Baker FACES pain rating scale is useful in rating of pain in pediatric population. *(From Hockenberry M, Wilson D:* Wong's nursing care of infants and children, *ed 8, St Louis, 2007, Mosby.)*

essential. This evaluation should elicit information concerning medical history including coexisting diseases and other symptomatology, any relevant existing laboratory data, and a thorough behavioral and social history, including the use of preoperative analgesics (both duration of use and quantity). The behavioral and social history should begin to define the patient's level of functioning and the extent to which the pain has interfered with or interrupted the patient's ability to perform activities of daily living. In addition, this detailed history should provide some insight into whether preexisting psychosocial impairment may influence the pain symptom or affect the patient's perception of pain.

In pain management, one should evaluate additional issues such as personality, coping and pain beliefs, health care utilization, medication use, and any previous adverse effects from drug therapy the patient may have had. Furthermore, if the patient is a potential candidate for opioid medications, an inquiry about the patient's history of drug use (prescription, over-the-counter, and illicit), chronic pain, psychiatric disorders, and substance abuse may assist the perianesthesia nurse and ultimately the medical team in determining the patient's suitability for opioid analgesics. This information may also facilitate determination of the intensity of supervision that may be needed should an opioid medication be deemed appropriate. If a history of long-term opioid use is elicited from the patient, consideration of possible patient

tolerance to or addiction to opioids becomes important. Tolerance is defined as a phenomenon in which exposure to a drug results in a reduction in the effect or in the need for a higher dose of medication to maintain the desired effect, whereas addiction is defined as the compulsive use of a substance that results in physical, psychologic, or social harm to the user with continued use despite the harm inflicted.

An important aspect of the evaluation of pain is the assessment of pain severity. Numerous scales and tools have been developed to assist in the assessment of pain severity. Frequently used scales include the Visual Analog Scale (VAS), the Verbal Rating Scale (VRS), the Numeric Pain Intensity Scale, the Simple Descriptive Pain Intensity Scale, and the Wong-Baker FACES Pain Rating Scale (Fig. 31-2). In general, these scales ask patients to rank pain as mild, moderate, or severe on a scale of 1 to 10, with 1 indicating mild pain and 10 indicating severe unbearable pain. The FACES Pain Rating Scale incorporates "happy" or "sad" faces and a numeric scale from 0 to 10 to aid the patient in describing pain. The FACES Pain Rating Scale is particularly useful in the pediatric population and in the illiterate or mentally challenged populations. Another particularly useful scale for the preverbal or nonverbal child is the FLACC (Face, Legs, Activity, Cry, Consolability) scale. This scale evaluates the aforementioned areas each on a scale of 0 to 2, which provides a total pain rating of 0 to 10. Preoperative education of the patient regarding the use of these scales is paramount to provision of the most accurate representation of pain. Pain intensity has an impact not only on the pharmacologic agent selected but also on the dose and route of administration and the titration rate.

In addition to pain intensity, assessment is important of the quality of the pain, its distribution, and its relationship to time or other events. These descriptors are helpful in determination of the cause of the pain and selection of appropriate therapy. An attempt to get as detailed a description as possible of the patient's pain experience assists in clarification of the mechanism of pain and in identification of the possible etiology. An example of the importance of the previously listed descriptors is in the evaluation of the temporal aspects of pain: that is, whether the pain occurs on a more or less continuous basis or is interrupted by discrete episodes of breakthrough pain, a common scenario during the postoperative period. In the latter case with breakthrough pain, one manages the breakthrough pain and contemplates a dosing adjustment of the maintenance analgesic or administers supplemental "rescue doses" of the medications to manage the breakthrough episodes.

An essential part of any evaluation is a careful physical examination and assessment of the patient's functional capacity, including any impairments or physical symptoms other than pain that may be attributed to the pain syndrome. Such information is obviously critical in determination of the efficacy of whatever treatment method is selected. Among the issues that should be investigated are questioning the patient regarding ability to get dressed and perform activities of daily living, such as walking and climbing stairs, and specific estimates of "up time." In addition, inquiries about the patient's quality of sleep and nutritional issues, such as appetite and weight gain or loss, are important. This additional evaluation of the patient's function establishes a baseline that can ultimately be used to gauge the effectiveness of pain management and overall progress throughout the recovery period.

## PAIN MANAGEMENT

After patient assessment, an appropriate strategy for the management of preoperative and postoperative pain must be developed. Studies have increasingly suggested that procedure-specific management of postoperative pain provides far superior analgesia and patient comfort than previous methods used to choose appropriate analgesics. Preoperative pain management becomes important not only for patient comfort but also for the management of postoperative pain. A direct correlation has been shown between the severity of preoperative pain and the severity of postoperative pain and opioid requirements. Investigators have also found a direct link between the severity of preoperative and postoperative pain levels and the development of chronic or neuropathic pain. The pain management strategy may include nonopioid medications, short or long half-life opioids either orally or parentally, patient-controlled analgesia (PCA), epidural or intrathecal analgesia, epidural PCA, regional anesthesia, skin infiltration of local anesthetic via elastomeric pump, iontophoresis, or a combination of any of these methods. The method of pain control chosen depends on several factors including the anticipated mechanisms of pain production (somatic, visceral, or neuropathic), severity of the pain, type of surgery performed, history of opioid use, previous successful methods of pain management in the operative setting, and patient preference. Some patients may not need aggressive preoperative intervention because the particular procedures may not induce enough pain to warrant such measures. Those patients who have neuropathic pain may need medications outside of the scope of opioid medications. These may include anticonvulsant medications, tricyclic antidepressants, or $\alpha$-2 agonists, to name a few. Each viable option should be explained to the patient, with a description of possible risks, benefits, and alternative options. Once the patient has made a decision regarding treatment of the anticipated postoperative pain, consent should be obtained by appropriate personnel and the chosen plan implemented.

The intraoperative management of pain is critical to the patient's overall perception of pain. Although the perianesthesia nurse usually does not have contact with the patient in the intraoperative setting, an understanding is still important of the multiple methods of pain management that may occur before patient arrival in the PACU. Both inhalation and intravenous anesthetics provide poor analgesia; therefore, opioid analgesics are administered to better decrease intraoperative pain. Anesthesia alone allows the transmission and transduction of pain to occur in the absence of perception and perhaps modulation. Opioid analgesics are administered intravenously to decrease transmission and downregulate the activity of ascending and descending neuronal pathways. Local anesthetics are often used to dampen the transduction of nociceptive signals that are produced at the site of the surgical incision or, in laparoscopic surgeries, the sites of trocar insertion. For many operative cases, an appropriately placed epidural or a regional block placed before surgery provides superior analgesia and anesthesia when compared with other methods. Also, skin infiltration pumps such as the OnQ series of elastomeric pumps, which infuse a steady dose of local anesthetic, may be inserted in the operating room.

The immediate postoperative setting is perhaps the most difficult and challenging arena for pain management. During this period, pain may be produced by many different mechanisms, both surgical and nonsurgical in nature. The PACU nurse is faced with many challenges during the postoperative period and must effectively address the components of the stress response after surgery, the psychological duress associated with emergence from anesthesia and the many other side effects associated with anesthesia, and other bothersome concomitants of surgical procedures such as catheters, restraints, and drains. To lessen environmental stressors, the PACU should be a soothing location for the patient to recover. Every attempt should be made to minimize unpleasant environmental stimuli, such as bright lights, loud noises, or extremes of temperature. To ensure optimal pain control in the PACU, the verbal report from the anesthesiologist to the PACU nurse immediately on arrival of the patient must include information about the type of anesthesia used and the type, administration time, and amount of analgesics used in the operating room. Determination of the type of incision used during the surgery is also critical because incisions of the upper abdomen, chest, back, anorectal region, joints, and vertical abdominal incisions are noted to be the most painful and may necessitate increased doses of pain medication.

Objective assessment, including careful monitoring of vital signs and a focused physical examination, should begin as soon as the patient arrives in the PACU from the operating room. The patient is sometimes transported to the PACU with monitoring systems in place. If not, these monitors are connected immediately on arrival to the PACU. Parameters such as blood pressure, respiratory rate, and heart rate are routinely recorded and are all excellent indicators of a patient's level of pain. Physiologic changes related to activation of the sympathetic nervous system as a result of pain include hypertension, tachycardia, tachypnea, pallor, dilated

pupils, and increased muscle tone. Nausea, vomiting, bradycardia, and hypotension are all parasympathetically mediated changes caused by pain in the visceral organs. Patients who are in pain have also been suggested to have irregular respiratory patterns with short or nonexistent pauses between breaths, a trait that may be used to monitor analgesic effectiveness. The elevation or depression of blood pressure, heart rate, and respiratory rate may also occur because of underlying pathologic processes such as primary hypertension, myocardial infarction, and various respiratory diseases, to name a few. Collection of subjective data from the patient, as the patient's level of sedation permits, is also equally important. Sedated patients are not able to fully and accurately verbalize the level of discomfort. Stoic patients may not voice any symptoms in spite of intense pain, whereas some patient groups may have an exceedingly poor tolerance for pain and act out, cry, moan, or exhibit other unusual behaviors despite the nurse's perception that adequate analgesia has been provided. The basic questions to be asked of the patient focus on the onset of pain and its location, intensity, quality, timing, and modifying factors (what improves or worsens the pain). The onset of pain after surgery most often indicates the decreasing effect of analgesia and anesthesia but may also indicate discomfort caused by poor positioning both in the operating room and in the PACU. An unexpected new onset of pain such as chest pain or lower extremity tenderness should alert the PACU nurse to a more serious pathologic problem, including myocardial infarction, pulmonary embolus, or deep venous thrombosis, especially when the pain occurs at a site distant to the surgical incision. The location of pain in patients after surgery is most often noted to come from the site of surgical incision, pressure points, venous or arterial access sites, and surgical drain sites. Referred pain may also occur in laparoscopic abdominal procedures (cholecystectomy, hernia repair, etc.) where right shoulder pain is caused by irritation of the right hemidiaphragm from the use of pneumoperitoneum. The intensity of pain should be quantified with one of the many available pain scales discussed previously, with the appropriate scale chosen on the basis of the patient's ability to comprehend the scale and respond effectively. Again, the Visual Analog Scale (VAS), the Verbal Rating Scale (VRS), the Numeric Pain Intensity Scale, or the Simple Descriptive Pain Intensity Scale suffice for most patient populations. However, the FACES Pain Rating Scale or the FLACC scale may be more appropriate for use with children who have difficulty verbally expressing pain. With pain scales, having the patient identify the worst imaginable pain is often helpful. This mark can help serve as an anchor for the scale that may be used to better understand the context of the patient's pain and as an aid in evaluation of the success of any therapeutic interventions. The quality of pain often helps better identify its source. Recall the three different mechanisms of pain production: visceral, nociceptive, and neuropathic pain. Identification of which mechanisms are functioning helps to identify different types of pain, such as incisional, nociceptive pain, dull aching visceral right upper quadrant and shoulder pain associated with cholecystectomy, or burning, neuropathic pain associated with nerve injury. The timing and modifying factors of pain are often used to identify additional components, such as positioning and activity level, which may affect the overall pain experience.

The evaluation of a patient's psychologic state should be of high priority during both the preoperative and postoperative periods. A patient may display excitement, irritability, depression, unusual quietness, withdrawal, or behavioral reverses. One must exercise caution in identification of pain as the source of these psychologic alterations because some patients display these changes when placed into an anxiety-provoking situation such as surgery. Others may simply have these traits at baseline, as seen with a previously diagnosed psychologic problem. To aid in the differentiation between causes of anxiety in operative patients, Drain and Cain have recommended differentiation between state and trait anxiety. They define state anxiety as that which is related to the fright, uncertainty, and helplessness that patients have as a result of the process of surgery. On the other hand, trait anxiety describes the feelings that a patient has without the stress factors of surgery.

Withdrawal syndromes in patients with tolerance who have been taking either prescribed or illicit opioids or benzodiazepines or other drugs are an important aspect of perianesthesia nursing assessment that often goes unrecognized. Identification of these syndromes can help clarify the clinical picture and prevent potentially life-threatening complications, such as the delirium tremens. The opiate withdrawal syndrome includes anxiety, agitation, rhinorrhea, hypotension, myoclonic twitches, sweating, pupillary dilation, piloerection, nausea, and vomiting. This syndrome shares many symptoms with those that may indicate postoperative pain. However, rhinorrhea and marked piloerection

may be subtle indicators that the patient is experiencing withdrawal and not just pain. The alcohol withdrawal syndrome includes headaches, malaise, and agitation that may progress to seizures, autonomic instability, and delirium with auditory and tactile hallucinations. The generalized seizures that accompany frank delirium tremens can be lethal. Treatment of these conditions is beyond the scope of this chapter and requires additional physician input, diagnosis, and treatment options.

## IMPLEMENTATION OF PAIN MEDICATIONS

After the assessment of the patient, a plan should be devised for the implementation of pain medications. Three particular types of medications are particularly important in the PACU setting: antiinflammatories, opioids, and local anesthetics. The route of administration for each of these drug classes depends on the particular medication but may include oral, parenteral, intramuscular, epidural, intrathecal, transdermal, skin infiltration, or rectal.

### Nonsteroidal Antiinflammatory Drugs

Nonsteroidal antiinflammatory drugs (NSAIDs) are often a first line choice of pain management, especially after minor surgeries or in conjunction with opioids. Several varieties of NSAIDs exist, most notably cyclooxygenase (COX)–1 inhibitors, which actually inhibit COX-1 and COX-2, such as ibuprofen or ketoralac and COX-2 inhibitors such as celecoxib (Celebrex). NSAIDs function by reducing the effects of inflammatory mediators produced via the arachidonic acid cascade (Fig. 31-3).

Cyclooxygenase-1 inhibitors inhibit COX-1, which is responsible for the normal physiologic production of prostaglandins, powerful inflammatory mediators. With this inhibition, COX-1 inhibitors also inhibit the production of prostaglandins in the stomach, thus decreasing the mucous lining that predisposes the operative patient to nausea and gastrointestinal bleeding. COX-1 inhibitors also inhibit platelet aggregation. Therefore, administration of oral COX-1 inhibitors on an empty stomach should be avoided, especially for patients with a history of gastrointestinal bleeding or with bleeding diatheses. The advent of the first injectable COX-1 inhibitor, ketorolac tromethamine, revolutionized perioperative analgesia. This inhibitor has been shown to be equianalgesic to opioids and can actually replace opioid analgesia in some surgical procedures. Ketorolac has been shown to be an effective intraoperative and postoperative analgesic in many patients. Studies

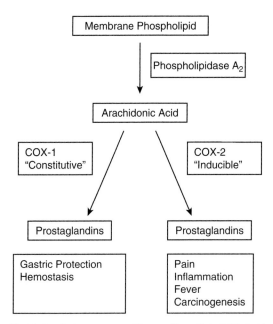

**Fig. 31-3** Cyclooxygenase pathways. *(From Gajraj NM, Joshi GP: Role of cyclooxygenase-2 inhibitors in postoperative pain management,* Anesthesiol Clin North Am *23:49-72, 2005.)*

have also shown that ketorolac reduces intraoperative and postoperative analgesic requirements. COX-2 inhibitors avoid many of these adverse affects by targeting inflammatory mediators only at the site of tissue injury or inflammation. Therefore, COX-2 inhibitors avoid the adverse gastrointestinal effects seen with use of COX-1 inhibitors. Also, platelet aggregation is not inhibited by COX-2 inhibitors. Several COX-2 injectable agents are currently being explored for the marketplace. One major benefit of NSAID use after surgery is the opioid-sparing effect produced by the drug class. The use of NSAIDs has been shown to decrease the use of opioids after surgery, which in turn decreases the severity and frequency of opioid-induced side effects simply as a result of the decreased use. Another benefit of NSAID use is the decrease in inflammation produced with surgical procedures. NSAIDs should be used cautiously in patients with decreased renal function because they have been known to cause electrolyte abnormalities and acute renal failure, although these adverse effects are rare. Unfortunately, in 2004, the safety of some of the COX-2 inhibitors came into question as studies showed an increase in cardiovascular risk to patients. As a result, some COX-2 inhibitors were withdrawn from the market.

## Oral, Intramuscular, and Intravenous Opioids

Although NSAIDs are suitable for postoperative pain management, most patients need a more potent analgesic, such as an opioid, or a multimodal treatment approach after surgical procedures. Multiple routes of administration exist for opioid analgesics, all with specific indications and contraindications. Oral analgesia is typically avoided after major surgeries in which general analgesia was used, and a postoperative ileus is expected, especially after abdominal surgery. Oral analgesia may, however, be appropriate in ambulatory surgery settings depending on the nature of the procedure performed. In terms of particular opioid agents, μ-agonists are the first-line agents historically used for analgesia. The μ-agonists reduce the release of excitatory neurotransmitters by the primary afferent neuron at its synapse in the spinal cord, affecting both transmission and modulation. Several oral opioid preparations are currently in use. Codeine, a weak opioid agonist, is often combined with acetaminophen (Tylenol #3) and is available in tablet or liquid form and in a parenteral form (seldom used). Propoxyphene (Darvocet, Wygesic) is also a weak opioid combined with acetaminophen. Oxycodone (Percocet, Tylox, Roxicet, Roxicodone, OxyContin) is usually combined with either aspirin or acetaminophen but can be administered alone and is available in tablet form or as a liquid when administered alone. OxyContin is a controlled-release form of oxycodone. Hydrocodone (Vicodin, Vicoprofen, Lortab, Lorcet) is combined with either acetaminophen, aspirin, or ibuprofen and is available in either tablet or liquid form. Morphine, the gold standard of opioid therapy, is a potent opioid agonist that can be administered orally or rectally but is most often given parenterally. Sustained-release forms of morphine (MS Contin, Oramorph, Kadian, Avinza) are also available. Hydromorphone (Dilaudid), a strong opioid agonist that is seven to eight times more potent than morphine, is available in oral, rectal, or parenteral forms. One major benefit of hydromorphone is that it does not have active metabolites, which makes it ideal for patients with renal failure. Levorphanol (Levo-Dromeran), available in oral and parenteral preparations, is a strong opioid agonist with a longer duration of action than that of morphine because of an extended half-life. Methadone (Dolophine) is a strong opioid agonist with the longest duration of action of the previously mentioned opioids. Methadone takes several days of administration to reach a steady state and is available in oral, rectal, and parenteral formulations. Because of its long half-life, methadone is not an easily administered postoperative medication. Meperidine (Demerol) has a potency and duration of action less than those of morphine and thus requires more frequent dosing; it is available in oral and parenteral forms. It can also be used for the prevention and treatment of postoperative shivering and rigors. Meperidine has fallen out of favor with many organizations because of its limited analgesic effectiveness and its problematic side effect profile. These side effects include the potential for the induction of seizures as a result of the epileptogenic metabolite normeperidine. For this reason, meperidine should not be administered for more than 48 hours or in doses greater than 600 mg in 24 hours. Meperidine also exhibits strong anticholinergic effects. Elderly patients in particular may have anticholinergic side effects of meperidine that can cause long-lasting sedation, which is particularly problematic in the patient with Alzheimer's. Many researchers also believe that meperidine is the drug of choice in patients with biliary or pancreatic disease because of its alleged decreased spasmogenic effect on smooth muscle, specifically the sphincter of Oddi and the sphincter mechanism of the common bile duct. Most of these claims are based on data that have not been borne out in the clinical setting. On the contrary, meperidine does cause spasmogenic effects on smooth muscle and, when given in an equianalgesic dose, causes smooth muscle spasm analogous to that of other opioids. An area in which meperidine has been found to be useful is that of postoperative shivering. Studies suggest that both meperidine and clonidine, an $\alpha$-2 agonist, are useful in providing prophylactic cessation of postoperative shivering and cessation of established postoperative shivering.

Intramuscular injection of opioids is an ineffective method of administration because the delivery and absorption of the particular medication used is inconsistent among patients. The results incurred consist of unpredictable peak concentration and varying analgesic effect. Another downside to the intramuscular injection of opioids is the resulting injection site pain after injection. In the past, the intramuscular injection of meperidine was considered the standard of care. However, for the reasons listed previously, this method is rarely, if ever, used.

Intravenous analgesics are most often the preferred method of analgesic administration after surgery because they provide rapid titratable pain relief while bypassing the need to use the gastrointestinal tract. Intravenous access also allows patients to titrate their own pain medication via a PCA pump when the level of pain indicates its use. Also, PCA pumps require that the patient be coherent enough to press the dose button and thus administer medication. If the patient is sedated or cannot understand the proper use of the PCA, then bolus dosing of intravenous opioids is more practical. Bolus doses of opioid medications afford the PACU nurse the ability to titrate analgesic levels and therefore effectively meet the patient's unique pain control requirements. The most commonly used opioids for parenteral administration are morphine, hydromorphone (Dilaudid), and fentanyl (Sublimaze) all of which can be administered in bolus doses or given via a PCA pump. General guidelines for PCA dosing can be found in Table 31-1.

Several questions must be considered in deciding which opiate and which route of administration are most appropriate for the treatment of postoperative pain. Is the opiate in use the most suitable one for the type of pain being treated? In the treatment of acute pain, multiple doses of a short-acting opiate are appropriate, whereas if an element of chronic pain is also present, a longer acting sustained-release preparation may be more appropriate. The combination of assessment, including the use of pain scales and physical examination, should provide the PACU nurse with enough information to determine whether the current opioid dose is sufficient to provide adequate pain relief or whether the dose is supratherapeutic and causes undesirable side effects. As stated previously, certain routes of opioid

| Table 31-1    General Guidelines for PCA Dosing | | | |
|---|---|---|---|
| Opioid | Bolus (PCA) Dose | Lockout (min) | Infusion Rate* |
| Morphine | 1-3 mg | 10-20 | 0-1 mg/h |
| Hydromorphone (Dilaudid) | 0.1-0.3 mg | 10-20 | 0-0.5 mg/h |
| Fentanyl (Sublimaze) | 15-25 µg | 10-20 | 0-50 µg/h |

*Continuous infusion rates are not recommended for most patients.
Adapted from Morgan EG, Maged MS, Murray MJ: *Clinical anesthesiology*, New York, 2006, Lange Medical Books/McGraw-Hill Medical.

administration are more appropriate depending on the particular surgical procedure performed. Oral preparations may be appropriate in the ambulatory setting, whereas parenteral or epidural administration is more appropriate for major procedures and for procedures that require an increased amount of pain control. The PACU nurse must also be aware of dose timing and the duration of action of the opioid in use to provide a steady state of pain relief. If any of the previously mentioned areas are not met satisfactorily, or if undesirable side effects are present, a change to a different opioid preparation should be considered. Recommended starting doses are listed in Table 31-2. An equianalgesic dosing table can be helpful in provision of adequate pain relief with a change to an opioid of increased or decreased potency or with a change to a different route (Table 31-3).

Rapp and Gordon provide two simple equations for the adjustment to an alternate route of administration or a different opioid.

*Switching routes of administration:*
Chart dose of oral opioid (mg)
   = Current or desired (×) 24-h dose of oral opioid (mg)

Chart dose of parenteral opioid (mg)
   Current or desired (×) 24-h dose of parenteral opioid (mg)

*Switching opioids:*
Chart dose of current opioid
   = 24-h dose of current opioid

Chart dose of desired opioid 24-h dose of desired opioid

Keep in mind that the equianalgesic dosing table is provided for general dosing estimates. Many other considerations must be taken into account with dosing of opioids, such as coexisting diseases, a patient's current level of pain and sedation, previous tolerance to opioids, chronic pain, and cross tolerance. Cross tolerance, or a patient's tolerance to analgesia and side effects of a particular opioid, may not be complete with a change to a different opioid. Therefore, recommendations are that with a change to a new opioid, the starting dose be decreased by 50% to 75% of the equianalgesic dose.

### Epidural and Intrathecal Opioids

The development of epidural and intrathecal delivery of analgesics and anesthetics in the early 1980s revolutionized the way in which postoperative pain is managed. Not only do the epidural and intrathecal delivery of analgesics and anesthetics provide preemptive analgesia and anesthesia, they also provide more consistent stable levels of both with the use of smaller amounts of medications. Of particular interest with this delivery method is the ability for smaller amounts of opioid to provide significantly longer duration of analgesia because of the placement of the opioid in close proximity to the site of action, the $\mu$-receptors of the spinal cord.

Epidural administration of opioid agents represents a nearly direct delivery system of analgesics to the substantia gelatinosa in the dorsal horn. This specific area of administration provides an optimal ratio of analgesic effect to safety of delivery. Opioids or local anesthetics are generally administered via a catheter placed in the epidural space either before the start of surgery or at the conclusion of the procedure before emergence from general anesthesia. Normally, but not always, the epidural catheter is used as an anesthetic adjunct during the surgical procedure and is continued after surgery as the primary method of analgesic and anesthetic delivery. With the combination of a dilute concentration of local anesthetic agent, such as 0.0625% bupivacaine (blocking the sensory/sympathetic, A-delta, and C-polymodal fibers), with an opioid agent, sensory blockade is achieved without major motor blockade, which allows optimal pain management without an affect on a patient's ability to ambulate during recovery. When combination therapy is used, better analgesia is achieved with fewer side effects primarily because the use of single agents is lessened. With use of epidurally administered opioids, the amount of opioid agent that is normally administered via the intravenous (IV) or intramuscular (IM) routes is reduced by 10 fold. So, a patient may need 100 mg of IV morphine over a 24-hour period, but that same patient would need only 10 mg of epidurally administered morphine. The addition of a local anesthetic may reduce the opioid requirement to an even greater extent.

Epidural medications can be delivered in several fashions, including "single shot" one time doses, intermittent bolus doses, continuous infusion of medications, or epidural PCA. In best case scenarios, with morphine as the agent for single shot delivery, analgesia lasts approximately 12 hours in the epidural space. With delivery via the intrathecal space, medication is deposited even closer to the $\mu$-receptors within the dorsal horn of the spinal cord. Analgesia with morphine administered intrathecally may last up to 24 hours. An additional alternative for single dose opioids is the use of the drug DepoDur. DepoDur is a long-acting preparation of morphine.

## Table 31-2   Recommended Starting Doses

| | Adults (>50 kg body weight) | | Children or Adults (<50 kg body weight) | |
|---|---|---|---|---|
| | PO | Parenteral | PO | Parenteral |
| **OPIOID AGONISTS** | | | | |
| Morphine | 30 mg q 3-4 h | 10 mg q 3-4 h | 0.3 mg/kg q 3-4 h | 0.1 mg/kg q 3-4 h |
| Hydromorphone (Dilaudid) | 6 mg q 3-4 h | 1.5 mg q 3-4 h | 0.06 mg/kg q 3-4 h | 0.015 mg/kg q 3-4 h |
| Oxymorphone (Numorphone) | Not available | 1 mg q 2-3 h | Not recommended | Not recommended |
| Oxycodone (Roxicodone, Roxicet, Percocet) | 10 mg q 3-4 h | Not available | 0.2 mg/kg q 3-4 h [4] | Not available |
| Codeine | 60 mg q 3-4 h | 60 mg q 2h (IM/IV/SQ) | 1 mg/kg 3-4 h [4] | Not recommended |
| Hydrocodone (Vicodin, Vicoprofen, Lortab, Lorcet) | 10 mg q 3-4 h | Not available | 0.2 mg/kg q 3-4 h [4] | Not available |
| Meperidine (Demerol) | Not recommended | 100 mg q 3 h | Not recommended | 0.75 mg/kg q 2-3 h |
| Levorphanol (Levo-Dromeran) | 4 mg q 6-8 h | 2 mg q 6-8 h | 0.04 mg/kg q 6-8 h | 0.02 mg/kg q 6-8 h |
| Methadone (Dolophine) | 20 mg q 6-8 h | 10 mg q 6-8 h | 0.2 mg/kg q 3-4 h [4] | 0.1 mg/kg q 6-8 h |
| **OPIOID AGONIST-ANTAGONISTS AND PARTIAL AGONISTS** | | | | |
| Buprenorphine (Buprenex) | Not available | 0.4 mg q 6-8 h | Not available | 0.0004 mg/kg q 6-8 h |
| Butorphanol (Stadol) | Not available | 2 mg q 3-4 h | Not available | Not recommended |
| Nalbuphine (Nubain) | Not available | 10 mg q 3-4 h | Not available | 0.1 mg/kg q 3-4 h |
| Pentazocine (Talwin) | 50 mg q 4-6 h | Not recommended | Not recommended | Not recommended |

PO, Oral; q, every; SQ, subcutaneously.
Adapted from National Library of Medicine: Dosing data for opioid analgesics: health services/technology assessment text: AHCPR archived clinical practice guidelines, available at http://www.ncbi.nlm.nih.gov/books/bv.fcgi?rid=hstat6.table.9290, accessed February 25, 2007.

## Table 31-3 Equianalgesic Table

| Drug | Parenteral (mg) | PO (mg) | Parenteral:PO Ratio | Duration of Action (h) | Comments |
|---|---|---|---|---|---|
| Morphine | 10 | 30 | 1:3 | 3-4 | |
| Hydromorphone (Dilaudid) | 1.5 | 7.5 | 1:5 | 3-4 | |
| Oxymorphone (Numorphone) | 1 | 10 | 1:10 | 3-4 | |
| Oxycodone (Roxicodone, Roxicet, Percocet) | N/A in United States | 20-30 | – | 3-4 | Available alone or combined with aspirin or acetaminophen |
| Codeine | 130 | 200 | 1:1.5 | 3-4 | Increased side effects with doses >1.5 mg/kg |
| Hydrocodone (Vicodin, Vicoprofen, Lortab, Lorcet) | – | 30 | – | 3-4 | Combined with aspirin, acetaminophen, or ibuprofen |
| Propoxyphene (Wygesic, Darvocet) | – | 100 | – | 4-6 | |
| Meperidine (Demerol) | 75 | 300 | 1:4 | 3-4 | Toxic metabolite normeperidine may cause CNS excitability and convulsions; dose no more than 48 h or 600 mg/24 h |
| Levorphanol (Levo-Dromeran) | 2 | 4 | 1:2 | 4-8 | |
| Methadone (Dolophine) | 10 | 3-5 | – | 4-12 | |
| Fentanyl (Sublimaze; Duragesic) | 0.1 | – | – | 1-3 | Continual infusion produces lipid accumulation and prolonged terminal excretion |

PO, Oral; N/A, not available.
Adapted from Rapp CJ, Gordon DB: Understanding equianalgesic dosing. *Orthopaedic Nursing* 19(3):65-70, May/June, 2000.

NURSING CARE IN THE PACU

The medication consists of morphine suspended within a delivery system of microscopic liposomal chambers (DepoFoam). After injection, the liposomal chambers slowly degrade, providing a sustained release of epidural morphine that can provide analgesia for up to 48 hours. Although more effective than IV or IM bolus doses, epidural bolus doses are not as effective at maintaining consistent levels of analgesia as is the continuous delivery of epidural medication or that of epidural PCA. Epidural PCA is a commonly applied delivery method used for patients undergoing major extremity, abdominal, vascular, or cardiothoracic surgery. Epidural PCA uses the same principles as IV PCA, with less nursing time, less total drug needed, increased patient sense of control, and fewer side effects. However, epidural PCA provides more profound analgesia and even fewer side effects as shown in comparative studies of epidural PCA versus IV PCA. Common dosing guidelines for epidural opioids and epidural PCA can be found in Table 31-4.

In comparison with epidural opioids, the side effects of intrathecally administered opioids may be more intense and severe, especially pruritus, nausea, urinary retention, and respiratory depression. In both epidural and intrathecal delivery of opioids, one must be extraordinarily judicious in providing supplemental opioid analgesia for breakthrough pain via the oral or IV route because dangerous side effects can occur. Vigilant monitoring becomes a requirement in these circumstances, and postoperative oxygen saturation, level of sedation, arousability, pupil size and reactivity, and respiratory rate must be monitored frequently. The benefits of the superb analgesia provided with the epidural administration of opioids along with the concomitant reduction in both morbidity and mortality rates far outweigh the reported but infrequent risks. Although the extent of these benefits remains unclear in some cases, the overall findings promote more extensive use of neuraxial blockade.

Morphine and fentanyl are the medications most often used for epidural delivery of opioids. The choice of drug depends on the type of analgesia needed. Morphine is less lipophilic (more hydrophilic) than fentanyl and therefore spreads easily throughout the epidural space, providing for more diffuse spinal mediated analgesia. Morphine can be delivered in the lumbar space and can provide analgesia to surgical dermatomes far from the site of injection. Fentanyl, which is more lipophilic, has a limited distribution in the epidural space and offers an analgesic effect in a classic dermatomal distribution. Intrathecal dosing allows even more direct delivery of the opioid to the site of action in the spinal cord. Reduction of the intrathecal doses of morphine and fentanyl by a factor of 10 is necessary in comparison with epidurally administered opioids. A lesser amount is needed because the opioids do not need to cross the dura to reach the target. Some authors support the use of hydromorphone for epidural and intrathecal analgesia, although at this point, hydromorphone is not US Food and Drug Administration (FDA)–approved for either method of delivery. However, because hydromorphone has properties somewhere between those of morphine and fentanyl, it may provide analgesia with less rostral spread and central nervous system (CNS) depression as seen with morphine and with less systemic uptake as seen with fentanyl. Often, patients with chronic pain may become tolerant to opioids. This scenario requires continuous dosage increases of opioid medication to reach an acceptable level of analgesia. Unfortunately, these dosage increases are often met with intolerable side effects. When this situation occurs, as it sometimes does with patients with chronic or neuropathic pain, exploration of the use of additional nonopioid medications may be necessary for epidural or intrathecal administration. Clonidine has been shown to be effective in this situation when combined with morphine and administered intrathecally. Investigators have shown that this

| Table 31-4 | | **General Guidelines for Epidural Opioid Dosing** | | | | | | | |

| Opioid | Relative Lipid Solubility | Dose | Onset (min) | Peak (min) | Duration (h) | Infusion Rate | PCA Dose | PCA Lockout (min) |
|---|---|---|---|---|---|---|---|---|
| Morphine | 1 | 2-5 mg | 15-30 | 60-90 | 4-24 | 0.3-0.9 mg/h | 0.2-0.3 mg | 30 |
| Fentanyl (Sublimaze) | 600 | 50-100 μcg | 5-10 | 10-20 | 1-3 | 25-50 μg/h | 20-30 μg | 15 |

Adapted from Morgan EG, Maged MS, Murray MJ: *Clinical anesthesiology*, New York, 2006, Lange Medical Books/McGraw-Hill Medical.

morphine/clonidine mixture can remain stable for long periods of time, which allows for increased ease of use in implantable infusion systems.

Although most researchers agree that epidural opioid administration is far superior to and provides better pain management than parenterally administered opioids, several limitations do exist. Gaps in effective analgesia can occur because of improper catheter placement, kinks in the catheter, medication leaks, inadvertent removal of the catheter, and pump malfunctions. Other problems include hypotension and an interference with mobility depending on the dose and type of local anesthetic used. Particular care must be used with administration of epidural medications to a patient with hypotension because the medications may increase the severity of the hypotension. Epidurals also pose a risk to patients undergoing anticoagulation therapy because epidural and intrathecal instrumentation may cause spinal hematoma. A complete list of recommendations for the use of neuraxial anesthesia in the patient with anticoagulation therapy can be found in Appendix B at the end of this chapter.

### Transdermal, Transmucosal, and Iontophoretic Opioids

Several additional routes of administration are currently used for opioid medications, particularly fentanyl. These routes include transdermal fentanyl patches (Duragesic), oral transmucosal fentanyl lozenges (Actiq), the fentanyl buccal tablet (Fentora), and the fentanyl iontophoretic transdermal system (IONSYS). The transdermal patches, buccal tablets, and lozenges are recommended for the treatment of chronic pain, such as cancer pain. The transdermal patches have the advantage of easy dosing, with one patch lasting for 3 days. Unfortunately, after application, the system takes a total of 12 hours to reach full analgesic effect. Similarly, the pharmacologic effect of the patch remains for up to 12 hours after removal. Therefore, patients with respiratory depression from supratherapeutic opioid dosing may need repeated doses of opiate antagonists as the drug, which is readily absorbed by fat, becomes available for systemic absorption. Oral transmucosal fentanyl lozenges and buccal tablets are absorbed quickly through the buccal mucosa and thereby avoid first pass metabolism, which increases the medication's bioavailabilty. The lozenges and buccal tablets provide analgesia quickly and have a short duration of action that lasts approximately 15 minutes. Transdermal patches, buccal tablets, and oral transmucosal lozenges are not indicated for the treatment of acute postoperative pain and should not be used as such. Transdermal patches are prescribed for

the treatment of chronic pain, including cancer pain. Oral transmucosal lozenges and buccal tablets are only indicated for the treatment of breakthrough cancer pain in patients currently undergoing long-term treatment with opioids or in patients who already have a tolerance to opioids. The fentanyl iontophoretic transdermal system, which was just recently approved by the FDA in May 2006 for use in treatment of acute postoperative pain, works with a mild electric field for quick transport of fentanyl across the skin on patient demand. The use of this system requires that the patient undergo titration to a satisfactory level of analgesia before initiation. The iontophoretic transdermal system is currently indicated for short-term postoperative management of acute pain during hospitalization and is not approved for home use. This system allows for the delivery of a controlled dose of fentanyl without the use of needles or the restriction of IV lines.

### Opioid Side Effects

Opioid medications provide patients with much needed pain relief during the postoperative period, but they are not without adverse side effects. One of the most common side effects is decreased gastrointestinal motility. Opioids cause the inhibition of motor activity in the intestines, increase gastric emptying time, and increase the intestinal transit time and therefore lead to constipation. These gastrointestinal side effects can be compounded by postoperative ileus, particularly after abdominal surgery or after the bowel has been handled. For this reason, when patients are treated with opioid medications, they should also be placed on a sufficient bowel regimen to help prevent constipation (Table 31-5).

Opioids may also cause nausea and vomiting through action on the chemoreceptor trigger zone. Nausea and vomiting may also occur as a side effect from anesthesia, decreased intestinal motility, and constipation. Promethazine (Phenergan) and ondansetron (Zofran) are two effective antiemetics that may be used for treatment of nausea and vomiting, along with constipation if present. Promethazine increases somnolence in most patients and should be avoided in situations where respiratory depression is of concern. Pruritus caused by opioids can often be treated with an antihistamine or with a switch to a different opioid. Urinary retention can be seen after the epidural or intrathecal administration of opioids. Foley or straight catheterization is usually necessary in this situation for prevention of painful urinary retention and bladder distention. Hypotension

| Table 31-5    **Prevention and Treatment of Opioid-Induced Constipation** | | |
|---|---|---|
| | | **If Not Effective...** |
| **Prevention** | **Increase Dose** | **Or Add** |
| Docusate Sodium 100 mg PO BID | 200 mg PO TID | Milk of magnesia |
| + | 34.4 mg PO TID | Mineral oil |
| Sennosides 17.2 mg PO BID | | |
| Add Bisacodyl 10 mg PO HS PRN | | Lactulose |
| If no bowel movement in 24 h | | Citrate of magnesium |
| Repeat in AM if still no bowel movement | | Phosphosoda |

PO, Oral; *BID*, twice a day; *TID*, three times a day; *HS*, at bedtime; *PRN*, as necessary.
Adapted from Payne R, Levy MH, Long SP, et al: *Advances in the use of opioids in pain management: monograph*, presented at the Eighth World Congress on Pain, Vancouver, British Columbia, 1996, Annenberg Center for Health Sciences at Eisenhower.

is sometimes noted, especially with spinal analgesia. Therefore, the PACU nurse must be vigilant in regard to vital signs before the administration of opioids. Perhaps the most feared side effect of opioid medications is the ability to cause profound respiratory depression, including a decrease in respiratory rate, decreased minute and tidal volume, and hypoxia. In this situation, an opioid antagonist such as naloxone (Narcan) should be used or ventilatory assistance provided to return the patient to a normal respiratory status. Naloxone should be administered intravenously at a starting dose of 0.01 mg for treatment of moderate respiratory depression. The dose can then be doubled every 2 minutes until a sufficient respiratory status has been reached. If a patient has severe respiratory depression, then naloxone should be given at doses of 0.1 to 0.4 mg. The half-life of naloxone is much shorter than that of many opioid agonists; therefore, repeated dosing of the antagonist may be needed for maintenance of adequate respiration while the opioid is metabolized. In cases of severe opioid overdose, once respiratory status has been stabilized, a naloxone infusion may be started at up to 5 μg/kg to continue reversal of respiratory depression while maintaining appropriate analgesia. Naloxone may also be used to alleviate opioid side effects such as severe pruritus with spinal analgesia.

Benzodiazepines, such as lorazepam and midazolam, are frequently used to treat anxiety both before and after surgery. They are also used for the induction of anesthesia, the maintenance of sedation, the treatment of alcohol withdrawal, and the interruption of seizure activity. Benzodiazepines also have the ability to cause respiratory depression, especially when given with opioid medications. Respiratory depression caused by benzodiazepines can be reversed with the benzodiazepine antagonist flumazenil. A starting dose of 0.2 mg intravenously over 15 seconds is recommended. An additional dose of 0.2 mg may be given after 45 seconds and repeated at 60-second intervals to a total dose of 1 mg until a satisfactory level of respiratory function and consciousness has been reached. If respiratory depression recurs, an additional 1 mg may be given every 20 minutes at 0.5 mg/min. Flumazenil should be given per recommendations because precipitous administration can induce seizure activity.

### Local and Regional Anesthesia

The use of both local and regional anesthesia (see Chapters 24 and 25) can be widely observed in the operative patient population. The medications used in this particular type of anesthesia play a critical role in the prevention and suppression of pain during the preoperative, intraoperative, and postoperative periods. Local anesthetics, such as those listed in Table 31-6, provide anesthesia to the particular areas of medication infiltration by stabilizing cell membranes and thus preventing excitation of nerves that detect painful stimuli. Local anesthetics are classified in two different groups: those local anesthetics that are amides and those that are esters. Ester-based local anesthetics, although still useful in some situations, have fallen out of favor because of toxicity and adverse allergic reactions that can be caused by one of the metabolites.

One of the simplest preoperative applications of local anesthetics is use before the insertion of an intravenous catheter. An eutectic mixture of local anesthetics, more commonly known as EMLA, can be applied topically to intact skin before the insertion of IV catheters or the initiation of minor

| Table 31-6 Local Anesthetic Agents | | | | | |
|---|---|---|---|---|---|
| Agent | Drug Class | Concentration (%) | Onset | Duration | Maximal Dose (mg/kg) |
| Lidocaine (Xylocaine) | Amide | 1 | Rapid | 30-60 min | 4 |
| Mepivicaine (Carbocaine) | Amide | 1 | Moderate | 45-90 min | 4 |
| Bupivicaine (Marcaine) | Amide | 0.25 | Slow | 2-4 h | 3 |
| Procaine (Novocain) | Ester | 1-2 | Slow | 15-60 min | 7 |
| Tetracaine (Pontocaine) | Ester | 0.25 | Slow | 2-3 h | 1.5 |
| Chloroprocaine (Nesacaine) | Ester | 2 | Slow | 30 min | 6-7 |

Note: Duration is increased in agents combined with epinephrine.
Adapted from Salam GA: Regional anesthesia for office procedures: part I, head and neck surgeries, *Am Fam Physician* 69(3):585-590, 2004.

surgical procedures. This method of local anesthesia is particularly useful in the pediatric population because needles are not necessary. A small amount of 1% lidocaine may also be infiltrated under the skin before IV insertion to aid in elimination of the most painful aspect of IV insertion, the actual skin puncture. Local anesthetic use for IV insertion can greatly improve patient comfort especially in patients who have an aversion to needles or in those with difficult intravenous access. Local anesthetics are also useful for local infiltration of surgical wounds and for field blocks. Field blocks are commonly used to anesthetize nerves that supply sensation to small surgical fields. This technique involves injection of local anesthetic around the margins of the surgical field and lasts for a greater amount of time than local infiltration of anesthetic. Investigators have shown, for instance, that the addition of an ilioinguinal field block to local infiltration of anesthetic can greatly reduce intraoperative pain during inguinal hernia repair. This type of regional anesthesia also allows the procedure to be performed without the use of general anesthesia techniques. Local anesthetics can also be injected intraarticularly after procedures such as arthroscopic knee surgery. This use of local anesthesia has been shown by investigators to significantly reduce pain and convalescence after diagnostic knee arthroscopy. Furthermore, the addition of methylprednisolone, a potent injectable steroid, to this local anesthetic/opioid combination has been shown to reduce pain, swelling, convalescence, and the need for additional analgesics even further.

Although local infiltration of anesthetic provides excellent anesthesia for small surgical sites, sometimes larger areas need to be anesthetized. Infiltration of enough anesthetic to anesthetize large areas, such as an entire leg or arm, is impractical and unsafe because of the amount of anesthetic necessary. Regional anesthesia avoids these potential complications by allowing the placement of local anesthetic in the extraneuronal or paraneuronal spaces. Once this placement has been achieved, anesthesia is provided distal to the injection site in the distribution of the nerve near which the anesthetic has been placed. This type of anesthesia is particularly useful in orthopedic procedures or any procedure that involves the extremities. Regional anesthesia may also be used for intercostal blocks before a thoracotomy incision or for intrapleural analgesia before upper abdominal procedures or in the event of a fractured rib. Administration of local anesthetic can be given as a one time injection, or a catheter may be inserted and left in place to provide extended anesthesia. These catheters may be connected to automated pumps, similar to those used for epidural infusions, or they may be connected to an elastomeric pump system.

The elastomeric pump system is a newer technology that is quickly gaining popularity. It can provide local anesthesia via skin infiltration systems such as the OnQ PainBuster or may be used to provide regional anesthesia using the OnQ C-Bloc system. These systems are comprised of elastomeric pumps that administer a set dose of local anesthetic to the skin surrounding a surgical site or to a regional nerve block site via an imbedded catheter. Several key points and suggestions for patient monitoring regarding the OnQ elastomeric pump systems can be seen in Boxes 31-3 and 31-4, respectively.

Regional anesthesia possesses several benefits; the current literature suggests that it enables improved return of gastrointestinal functioning, decreased incidence of deep venous thrombus formation, and improved pulmonary function

---

**Box 31-3    OnQ PainBuster and C-Bloc Systems: Key Points**

*Dressing:* Ensure that dressing over catheter site remains secure. Do not remove dressing; this may dislodge the catheter.

*Filter:* Do not tape over inline filter.

*Tubing Clamp:* Ensure that clamp is open. Check for tubing kinks. If tubing appears crimped, massage area to facilitate flow.

*Flow Restrictor:* Located at end of pump tubing. Placement is important for accurate flow rates.

*ON-Q C-Bloc and PainBuster:* Flow restrictor should be in contact with patient's skin. Tape if necessary.

*ON-Q C-Bloc with On-Demand:* Restrictor is inside bolus device. Skin contact is not necessary. Bolus device should be worn outside of patient's clothing.

*ON-Q C-Bloc with Select-A-Flow:* Rate is controlled by the controller. Skin contact is not necessary. Variable rate controller should be worn outside the patient's clothing.

- Flow restrictor should not be in contact with cold therapy pads. Contact with cold therapy decreases flow rate.
- Do not squeeze pump. Pump provides the force needed to deliver the medication.
- Patient discharge: If patient is discharged home with C-bloc, provide patient with patient guidelines.

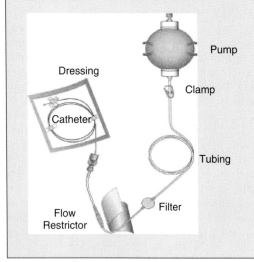

Adapted from I-Flow Corporation: Nursing guidelines: OnQ C-Bloc: OnQ C-Bloc continuous infusion system, 2006, available at http://www.iflo.com/pdf/products/1303734a.pdf, accessed February 9, 2007.

---

**Box 31-4    OnQ PainBuster and C-Bloc Systems: Patient Monitoring**

Assess patient's pain and administer postoperative pain medication as ordered.

Routinely evaluate catheter site and dressing.

Do not attempt to remove occlusive dressing; this may dislodge catheter.

Confirm catheter placement.

Diminished pain relief or presence of signs or symptoms of local anesthetic toxicity may indicate catheter migration.

If any of the following symptoms are assessed, close the tubing clamp and notify the physician immediately:

    Increase in pain
    Redness, swelling, pain, or discharge at the catheter site
    Dizziness or light headedness
    Blurred vision
    Ringing or buzzing in ears
    Metal taste in mouth
    Numbness or tingling around the mouth, fingers, or toes
    Nausea or vomiting
    Drowsiness
    Confusion

*Patient precautions:*

Patient may have loss of motor control or feeling at and around the affected limb. Ensure appropriate measures are followed to avoid patient injury. Patient should be instructed not to drive or operate heavy machinery.

Adapted from I-Flow Corporation: Nursing guidelines: OnQ C-Bloc: OnQ C-Bloc continuous infusion system, 2006, available at http://www.iflo.com/pdf/products/1303734a.pdf, accessed February 9, 2007.

---

after surgery. However, as with any anesthetic methods, several risks and shortcomings also are seen to regional anesthesia. The method of placement of an appropriate peripheral nerve blockade requires time and does not always provide complete anesthesia to the target area. Intraneuronal injection of an anesthetic can cause nerve damage in several different ways, including neurotoxicity, mechanical trauma, and ischemia. Nerves are often found in neurovascular bundles; therefore, vascular puncture during placement of a peripheral nerve block is always a possibility and may cause a hematoma, resulting in neural ischemia. Side effects can also occur with local anesthetic medications. With correct administration, large doses of anesthetic are needed to precipitate known side effects. However, inadvertent intravascular administration can quickly elicit the following side effects: tinnitus; a metallic taste in the mouth; perioral and glossal numbness; lightheadedness; and rarely, a loss of consciousness, coma, or seizures. Intravascular anesthetics may also cause a loss of vasomotor tone, decreased cardiac conduction, or decreased ventricular contractility. Regional anesthesia should not be attempted on patients with a known allergy to a specific anesthetic agent, an infection at the intended injection site, or a coagulopathy or with certain anticoagulants or thrombolytics (Appendix B).

## SUMMARY

The role of the perianesthesia nurse has changed as the understanding of pain has improved. Aggressive interventions that are available today allow for optimal pain control and rapid recovery. The key to understanding these interventions lies in the physiologic basis of pain, analgesic and anesthetic pharmacology, and the methods used to deliver analgesics and anesthetics. A working clinical and basic science knowledge of these topics is essential to the mastery of pain management in the postoperative setting. Implementation of basic pain management principles coupled with newer state-of-the-art and standard-of-care techniques can reduce postoperative morbidity and mortality rates. In the practical sense, aggressive postoperative analgesia by a caring staff creates a hospital stay that is not only safer but more cost effective and pleasant for all of those involved.

## BIBLIOGRAPHY

Abram S: Preemptive analgesia, *Semin Anesth* 16(4):263-270, 1997.

Allen H: Difficult cases in postoperative pain management, *Semin Anesth* 16(4):271-279, 1997.

Anderson FH, Nielsen K, Kehlet H: Combined ilioinguinal blockade and local infiltration anesthesia for groin hernia repair: a double blind randomized study, *Br J Anaesth* 94(4):520-523, 2005.

Atsberger DB, Shrewsbury P: Postoperative pain management: the PACU nurse's challenge, *J Post Anesth Nurs* 3(6):399-403, 1988.

Bates JJ, Foss JF, Murphy DB: Are peripheral opioid antagonists the solution to opioid side effects, *Anesth Analg* 98:116-122, 2004.

Berry PH, Dahl JL: Making pain assessment and management a healthcare priority through the new JCAHO pain standards, *J Pharmaceutic Care Pain Symptom Control* 8(2):5-20, 2000.

Drain CB, Cain RS: The nursing implications of postoperative pain, *Military Med* 146:127-130, 1981.

Edwards WT, Breed RJ: The treatment of acute postoperative pain in the postanesthesia care unit, *Anesthesiol Clin North Am* 8(2):235-265, 1990.

Eisenach JC: Treating and preventing chronic pain: a view from the spinal cord: Bonica Lecture, ASRA Annual Meeting 2005, *Reg Anesth Pain Med* 31(2):146-151, 2006.

Gajraj NM, Joshi GP: Role of cyclooxygenase-2 inhibitors in postoperative pain management, *Anesthesiol Clin North Am* 23:49-72, 2005.

Gray A, Kehlet H, Bonnet F, et al: Predicting postoperative analgesia outcomes: NNT league tables or procedure-specific evidence? *Br J Anaesth* 94(6):710-714, 2005.

Hildebrand KR, Elsberry DD, Hassenbusch SJ: Stability and compatibility of morphine clonidine admixtures in an implantable infusion system, *J Pain Symptom Manage* 25(5):464-471, 2003.

Horlocker TT, Wedel DJ, Benzon H, et al: Regional anesthesia in the anticoagulated patient: defining the risks (the second ASRA consensus conference on neuraxial anesthesia and anticoagulation), *Reg Anesth Pain Med* 28(3):172-197, 2003.

I-Flow Corporation: *Nursing guidelines: OnQ C-Bloc: OnQ C-Bloc continuous infusion system*, 2006, available at http://www.iflo.com/pdf/products/1303734a.pdf, accessed February 9, 2007.

Kehlet H: Labat Lecture 2005: Surgical stress and postoperative outcome: from here to where, *Reg Anesth Pain Med* 31(1):47-52, 2006.

Kehlet H: Procedure-specific postoperative pain management, *Anesthesiology Clin North Am* 23:203-210, 2005.

Kranke P, Eberhart LH, Roewer N, et al: Single-dose parenteral pharmacological interventions for the prevention of postoperative shivering: a quantitative systematic review of randomized controlled trials, *Anesth Analg* 99:718-727, 2004.

Latta KS, Ginsberg B, Barkin RL: Meperidine: a critical review, *Am J Ther* 9:53-68, 2002.

Long SP: The management of post-operative pain and the rationale for pre-emptive anesthesia, *J Back Musculoskeletal Rehabil* 9:279-297, 1997.

Morgan EG, Maged MS, Murray MJ: *Clinical anesthesiology*, New York, 2006, Lange Medical Books/McGraw-Hill Medical.

National Library of Medicine: *Dosing data for opioid analgesics: Health services/technology assessment text: AHCPR archived clinical practice guidelines*, available at http://www.ncbi.nlm.nih.gov/books/bv.fcgi?rid=hstat6.table. 9290, accessed February 25, 2007.

Payne R, Levy MH, Long SP, et al: *Advances in the use of opioids in pain management: monograph, presented at the Eighth World Congress on Pain*, Vancouver,

British Columbia, 1996, Annenberg Center for Health Sciences at Eisenhower.

Pereira J, Lawlor P, Vigano A, et al: Equianalgesic dose ratios for opioids: A critical review and proposals for long-term dosing, *J Pain Symptom Manage* 22(2):672-687, 2001.

Perkins FM, Kehlet H: Chronic pain as an outcome of surgery, *Anesthesiology* 93:1123-1133, 2000.

Rapp CJ, Gordon DB: Understanding equianalgesic dosing, *Orthop Nurs* 19(3):65-70, 2000.

Rathmell JP, Wu CL, Sinatra RS, et al: Acute post-surgical pain management: a critical appraisal of current practice, *Reg Anesth Pain Med* 31(4):1-42, 2006.

Rasmussen S, Lorentzen JS, Larsen AS, et al: Combined intraarticular glucocorticoid, bupivicaine, and morphine reduce pain and convalescence after diagnostic knee arthroscopy, *Acta Orthop Scand* 73(2):175-178, 2002.

American Society of Regional Anesthesia: *Recommendations: neuraxial anesthesia and anticoagulation* by American Society of Regional Anesthesia, 2003, available at http://www.anesth.utmb.edu/ASRA.htm, accessed January 23, 2007.

Rizzotti L, Roussakis G, Tringa E, et al: Continuous wound instillation of local anesthetic via pump infuser after major abdominal surgery: a prospective comparative study, *Reg Anesth Pain Med* 31(5):25, 2006.

Rocca GD, Chiarandini P, Peitropaoli P: Analgesia in PACU: nonsteroidal antiinflammatory drugs, *Curr Drug Targets* 6(7):781-787, 2005.

Rodgers A, Walker N, Schug S, et al: Reduction of post-operative mortality and morbidity with epidural or spinal anaesthesia: Results from overview of randomized trials, *Br Med J* 321:1-12, 2000.

Salam GA: Regional anesthesia for office procedures: part I, head and neck surgeries, *Am Fam Physician* 69(3):585-590, 2004.

Sinatra RS, Levin S, Ocampo CA: Neuroaxial hydromorphone for control of postsurgical, obstetric, and chronic pain, *Semin Anesth* 19(2):108-131, 2000.

Sites BD, Brull R: Ultrasound guidance in peripheral regional anesthesia: philosophy, evidence-based medicine, and techniques, *Curr Opin Anaesthesiol* 19:630-639, 2006.

U.S. Department of Health and Human Services, Agency for Health Care Policy and Research: *Clinical practice guideline for acute pain management: operative or medical procedures and trauma,* AHCPR publication number 92-0032, Rockville, MD, 1992, U.S. Department of Health and Human Services.

Vaglienti CS, Grinberg M: Emerging liability for the undertreatment of pain, *J Nurs Law* 9(3):7-17, 2004.

Van Poznak A: The role of respiratory patterns in the treatment of pain and anxiety, *J Post Anesth Nurs* 3(3):189-191, 1987.

Viscusi ER: Emerging techniques in the management of acute pain: epidural analgesia, *Anesth Analg* 101:S23-S29, 2005.

Weir MR: Renal effects of nonselective NSAIDs and coxibs, *Cleve Clin J Med* 69(S1):53-58, 2002.

Wetchler BV: Managing pain in the postanesthesia care unit, *J Post Anesth Nurs* 1(1):52-56, 1986.

Wu CL, Fleisher LA: Outcomes research in regional anesthesia and analgesia, *Anesth Analg* 91:1232-1242, 2000.

Zuckerman LA, Ferrante FM: Nonopioid and opioid analgesics. In Ashburn MA, and Rice LJ: *The management of pain*, Philadelphia, 1998, Churchill Livingstone.

# APPENDIX A

## ASPAN POSITION STATEMENT ON PAIN MANAGEMENT

ASPAN has the responsibility of defining the practice of perianesthesia nursing. An integral part of this responsibility involves identifying the educational requirements and competencies essential to perianesthesia nursing practice and the educational needs of the patients and family regarding pain assessment and management.

ASPAN sets forth this position statement to promote the optimal level of practice and to present a consistent standard of care that documents sound clinical judgment in the management of postoperative pain.

### BACKGROUND

ASPAN has defined a standard for pain management (Standard XI) with the intent of providing guidelines that represent what is believed to be an optimal level of practice. To assist members in achieving this standard, ASPAN published pain management competency material in the Competency Based Orientation and Credentialing Program. In response to continued concerns from perianesthesia nurses, ASPAN's Standards and Guidelines Committee conducted a review of literature to identify current issues related to pain assessment and management. The following issues were identified:

1. As many as 50% of postoperative patients in both hospitals and outpatient surgical centers are undermedicated and have unrelieved pain.[1-4]
2. The practice of undermedicating for pain occurs regardless of the patient's age.[5,6]
3. Frequently the patient's self report of pain is not taken into consideration in the dosage of medication given for pain relief.[7,8]
4. Inadequate pain management affects postoperative recovery and behaviors associated with that recovery.[5,6,9]
5. A prevalent cause of ineffective pain management is the professional's lack of knowledge related to pain physiology, medications, and protocols.[4,10]
6. An overriding concern still exists that the use of opioids in the treatment of acute postoperative pain control contributes to psychologic dependence.[11]
7. Patient and family education that addresses postsurgical pain management remains inconsistent.[12]
8. Pain management should begin before surgery with patient and family education that addresses the use of a pain scale and methods of postoperative pain control.
9. The Agency for Health Care Policy and Research (AHCPR) suggests that practitioners are too rigid in the management of acute postoperative pain and should set goals to reduce its incidence rate and severity. Guidelines have been published by this agency for acute pain management.[13]

## POSITION

Therefore, the position of ASPAN is that a collaborative plan should be developed between the anesthesia department and the perianesthesia nurses to address pain management within the perianesthesia setting. The following points of action should be addressed:

1. The goal should be relief of as much pain as possible to allow for activity, relaxation, prevention of complications, and promotion of optimal health and heating.
2. Areas of education in pain management for health care professionals should include the following:
   a. Physiology of pain management.
   b. Assessment techniques.
   c. Methods of intervention (pharmacologic and nonpharmacologic).
   d. Management of side effects and complications related to each intervention.
   e. Evaluation of successful management.
   f. Ethical considerations.
   g. Age and cultural considerations.
   h. Patient and family education issues.
3. Whenever possible, the patient's plan of care for pain management should begin during the preoperative interview.
4. The patient's self report of pain is the best measurement tool to use in assessment of pain.
5. The use of reliable and valid pain scales should be a standard part of the pain assessment.
6. Measurement of outcomes should reflect timely appropriate interventions and achievement of desired effects.

## EXPECTED OUTCOMES

Perianesthesia nurses need to familiarize themselves with this position statement and inform and educate peers, nurse managers, hospital administrators, and physicians.

Anesthesiologists and perianesthesia nurses need to collaborate in the development of a multidisciplinary plan of care (protocol, critical pathway, care map, etc.) to provide safe, appropriate, and effective pain management.

ASPAN, as the voice of perianesthesia nursing practice, must externalize this information by sharing this position statement with regulatory agencies and professional organizations that interface with perianesthesia nursing areas.

## APPROVAL OF STATEMENT

This statement was recommended by a vote of the ASPAN Board of Directors on April 16, 1999, and approved by a vote of the ASPAN Representative Assembly on April 18, 1999, in Honolulu, Hawaii.

## REFERENCES

1. Anonymous: Most patients face pain, often unrelieved, after surgery, *Am J Nurs* 96:68, 1996.
2. Campese C: Development and implementation of a pain management program, *AORN J* 64:931-940, 1996.
3. Bormarm D, Hansen K: Improving pain management through staff education, *Nurs Manage* 28:55-57, 1997.

4. Thornborough J: Developing a pain management protocol in the PACU, *Today Surg Nurse* 20:23-27, 1998.
5. Fortin J, Schwartz-Barcott D, Rossi S: The postoperative pain experience: a description based on the McGill Pain Questionnaire, *Clin Nurs Res* 1:292-304, 1992.
6. Pasero C, McCaffrey M: Managing postoperative pain in the elderly, *Am J Nurs* 96:38-46, 1996.
7. Reid D, Evans M, Topiko J, et al: Postoperative pain, *Can Nurse* 88:55, 1992.
8. Malek C, Olivieri R: Pain management: documenting the decision making process, *Nurse Case Manage* 1:64-76, 1996.
9. Getker Black S, Hart F, Hoffman J, et al: Preoperative self-efficacy and postoperative behaviors, *Appli Nurs Res* 5:134-139, 1992.
10. Carr E: Overcoming barriers of effective pain control, *Professional Nurse* 12:412-416, 1997.
11. Aiher J, Coghlan A, Martin K, et al: Children win with improved pain management, *Can Nurse* 88:19-21, 1992.
12. Jones S, Villalobos J: Incorporating clinical research findings into practice, *J Nurs Staff Develop* 12:46, 1996.
13. Agency for Health Care Policy and Research: *Acute pain management in infants, children, and adolescents: operative and medical procedures*, Rockville, MD, 1992, Department of Health and Human Services.

## BIBLIOGRAPHY

ANA: *Code for nurses with interpretive statements*, Washington, DC, 1995, American Nurses Association.

Anonymous: Surgical patient's no. 1 fear: pain, *Today Surgl Nurse* 18:7, 1996.

ASPAN: *Competency based orientation and credentialing program*, Cherry Hill, NJ, 1997, American Society of PeriAnesthesia Nurses.

Bishop A, Scudder J: *Nursing ethics: therapeutic caring presence*, Boston, 1996, Jones and Bartlett Publishers.

Heiser R, Chiles K, Fudge M, et al: The use of music during the immediate postoperative recovery period, *AORN J* 65:777-778, 781-785, 1997.

Miaskowski C, Jacox A, Hester N: Interdisciplinary guidelines for the management of acute pain: implications for quality improvement, *J Nurs Care Qual (Educ)* 7:1-6, 1992.

Schwartz-Barcott C, Fortin J, Kim-Hesook S: Client-nurse interaction: testing for its impact in preoperative instruction, *Int J Nurs Studies* 31:23-35, 1994.

Wong: *Pain assessment in children and infants*, video presentation. From the American Society of PeriAnesthesia Nurses, 10 Melrose Ave, Ste 110, Cherry Hill, NJ 080037-3696; (phone) 877-737-9696 (toll-free); (fax) 7 856-616-9601.

# APPENDIX B

## RECOMMENDATIONS: NEURAXIAL ANESTHESIA AND ANTICOAGULATION

### UNFRACTIONATED HEPARIN

1. A delay of the first dose of such heparin is prudent after the block to minimize the chances of bleeding.
2. Continuous SC heparin therapy for more than 4 days can cause thrombocytopenia, so a platelet count should be done before the neuraxial block is placed.
3. Neuraxial techniques and intraoperative anticoagulation:
   - Avoid the technique if the patient is on other anticoagulant therapy.
   - Administer heparin 1 hour after the needle placement.
   - Remove the epidural catheter 1 hour before the next dose of heparin.
   - Wait 2 to 4 hours before removing the epidural catheter if heparin is already given.
   - Stop systemic heparinization, wait 2 to 4 hours, and evaluate coagulation status before removing the epidural catheter.
   - Do neurologic checks:
     Limit the dose of local anesthetics.
     Use epidural narcotics for pain control.
   - Difficult placement or blood in the needle may increase the risk, but the case does not have to be cancelled; no supporting data exist. Be advised to use clinical judgment.

### LOW–MOLECULAR WEIGHT HEPARIN (LMWH)

#### Preoperative LMWH
Administration requires coordination and communication.

Monitoring of anti-Xa level is **not recommended.**

- Single injection spinal anesthetic is the safest technique but must be done 10 to 12 hours after the LMWH dose.
  For patients receiving:
  Enoxaparin 1 mg/kg × 12 h
  Enoxaparin 1.5 mg/kg × 24 h
  Dalteparin 120 U/kg × 12 h
  Dalteparin 200 U/kg × 24 h
  Tinzaparin 175 U/kg × 24 h
- Delay neuraxial block for 24 hours.

### Postoperative LMWH
If LMWH is to be started after surgery:
*LMWH twice a day:*
- Single injection spinal and catheter techniques are okay.
- The first dose of LMWH should be given 24 hours after surgery.
- Remove the catheter before starting LMWH; wait 2 hours and then start LMWH.
- If the dose is already given, then wait 10 to 12 hours to remove the catheter; wait 2 hours and then give the next dose of LMWH.
*LMWH once a day:*
- The first dose should be given 6 to 8 hours after surgery.
- The second dose should be given 24 hours after the first dose.
- Remove the indwelling catheter only after 10 to 12 hours after the last dose of LMWH. Wait 2 hours after removing the catheter to administer the next dose of LMWH.

Concurrent use of medications like oral anticoagulants, LMWH, or antiplatelet drugs with heparin may increase the risk of bleeding.

### ORAL ANTICOAGULANTS

- For chronic oral anticoagulation, stop 4 to 5 days before the procedure. Measure PT/INR and perform neuraxial block if the PT/INR are within normal limits.
- After surgery, if anticoagulation therapy is continued, monitor PT/INR daily (for the 5-mg dose of warfarin); higher doses may require more frequent monitoring.
- The neuraxial catheter should be removed when the INR is less than 1.5.

- Neurologic checks should be made for 24 hours, or longer if the INR is more than 1.5.
- An INR of more than 3.0 should alert the physician to decrease the dose of warfarin and delay removal of the catheters.

### ANTIPLATELET MEDICATIONS

- No single test is available to define platelet activity.
- Spinal and epidurals can be safely done in the presence of NSAIDS.
- If used with ticlopidine, clopidogrel, or platelet GP IIb/IIIa, beware of the potential for spinal hematoma.
- Discontinue ticlopidine 14 days before the neuraxial block.
- Discontinue clopidogrel 7 days before the neuraxial block.
- Discontinue eptifibatide 8 hours before the neuraxial block.
- Discontinue abciximab 48 hours before the neuraxial block.

Duration action for platelet GP/IIIa inhibitors ranges from 8 hours for eptifibatide to 48 hours for abciximab.

### NEW ANTICOAGULANTS

#### Fondaparinux
- Actual risk is unknown; it has sustained antithrombotic effect and irreversibility, so avoidance of neuraxial block is best.

### HERBAL THERAPY

- No significant risk is known at the present time.
- No accepted test exists for homeostasis.
- No specific concerns exist for the timing of the neuraxial blocks.

From American Society of Regional Anesthesia: Recommendations: neuraxial anesthesia and anticoagulation by American Society of Regional Anesthesia, 2003, available at http://www.anesth.utmb.edu/ASRA.htm, accessed January 23, 2007.

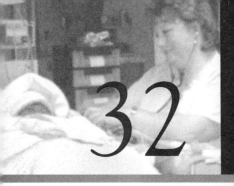

# 32

# CARE OF THE EAR, NOSE, THROAT, NECK, AND MAXILLOFACIAL SURGICAL PATIENT

*Cecil B. Drain, PhD, RN, CRNA, FAAN, FASAHP*

The patient with ear, nose, and throat (ENT) dysfunction presents many challenges to the perianesthesia nurse. These patients often have a difficult airway for management (see Chapter 30), which in itself can be most challenging. These patients also often have abnormal or dysfunctional anatomy that presents major concerns and requires enhanced awareness of the "normal" anatomy of the structures associated with ENT surgical procedures. Also, the patient emerging from maxillofacial surgery, which usually consists of dental or plastic surgery, needs close monitoring of airway patency and clearance along with management of the pain associated with those surgical procedures in a way that does not depress respiratory status. The perianesthesia nurse who manages these types of surgical procedures needs a strong knowledge of airway anatomy and physiology and excellent skills in the management of a difficult airway. Finally, the perianesthesia nurse must also manage the behavioral component of patients who undergo ENT or maxillofacial surgery. These patients have all kinds of emotions: from fright because of wiring of the jaw to fear because of the tight bandaging and pain. Because patients who undergo ENT and maxillofacial surgery present a great challenge to the perianesthesia nurse, a complete review of this category of surgical patients is presented. The reader is encouraged to read as follow-up Chapters 12 and 30, which present more information on the respiratory system and airway management.

## DEFINITIONS

**Ankyloglossia (Tongue Tied):** A short lingual frenulum that may cause difficulty with suckling in the infant and subsequent speech impairment. It is treated surgically with clipping of the frenulum.

**Cochlear Implant:** A prosthesis with an internal electrode is surgically implanted into the cochlea so that an external microphone later can be applied for stimulation of the eighth cranial nerve and provision of sound for a deaf person.

**Electrocautery Unit:** Application of a snare heated with electricity for the purpose of cauterization of small vessels to bleeding or for cutting tissue, without blood loss.

**Endoscopy:** Nasal surgery performed with direct vision with endoscopic equipment.

**Ethmoidectomy:** Removal of ethmoid bone.

**Fenestration:** Reconstruction of the outer and middle parts of the ear by means of a new drum or skin flap; creation of a new window into the internal ear mechanism with a newly established drum or skin flap.

**Glossectomy:** Removal of the tongue.

**Intranasal Antrostomy (Antral Window):** Creation of an opening in the lateral wall of the nose under the middle turbinate and the removal of the anterior end of the inferior turbinate.

**Labyrinthectomy:** Opening of the labyrinth to destroy the inner ear in an attempt to relieve medically uncontrollable symptoms of unilateral Meniere's syndrome.

**Laryngectomy:** Removal of the larynx; total laryngectomy is the complete removal of the cartilaginous larynx, the hyoid bone, and the strap muscles connected to the larynx and the possible removal of the preepiglottic space along with the lesion.

**Laryngofissure:** Opening of the larynx for exploratory, excisional, or reconstructive procedures.

**Laryngoscopy:** Direct examination of the interior of the larynx with a laryngoscope.

**Mastoidectomy:** Removal of mastoid air cells and of the tympanic membrane. Radical mastoidectomy also involves removal of the malleus, incus, chorda tympani, and mucoperiosteal lining.

**Myringotomy:** Incision of the tympanic membrane with direct vision and insertion of tubes for facilitation of drainage.

**Ossiculoplasty:** Reconstruction of the ossicular chain.

**Paletouvuloplasty:** The reconstruction of the posterior section of the palate and the uvula.

**Radical Antrostomy (Caldwell-Luc Operation):** Use of an incision into the canine fossa of the upper jaw and exposure of the antrum for removal of bony diseased portions of the antral wall and contents of the sinus; establishment of drainage by means of a counteropening into the nose through the inferior meatus for establishment of a large opening in the nasoantral wall of the inferior meatus, which ensures adequate gravity drainage and aeration and permits removal of all diseased tissue in the sinus with direct vision.

**Semi-Fowler's Position:** The patient is in a inclined position, with the upper half of the body raised with elevation of the head of the bed by about 30 degrees.

**Sensorineural Hearing Loss:** The sound is conducted normally through the external and middle ear, but a defect in the inner ear or auditory nerve results in a loss or deficit in hearing.

**Serosanguineous:** A discharge from the body that is composed of serum and blood.

**Stapedectomy:** Removal of the stapes, followed by the placement of a prosthesis.

**Stents** A rod for supporting tubular structures.

**Submucosal Resection:** Removal of either cartilaginous or osseous portions of the septum that lie between the flaps of the mucous membrane and the perichondrium for establishment of an adequate partition between the left and right nasal cavities, thereby providing a clear airway for both the internal and the external cavities and the parts of the nose.

**Tonsillectomy and Adenoidectomy (T&A):** Surgical removal of the tonsils and adenoids.

**Tracheostomy:** Opening of the trachea and insertion of a cannula through a midline incision in the neck below the cricoid cartilage.

**Tympanoplasty (Myringoplasty):** Reconstruction of the tympanic membrane.

## SURGERY ON THE EAR

Otologic surgery has been revolutionized by antibiotics, the operating microscope, new and more delicate instruments, and an increased understanding of the anatomic structures involved (Figs. 32-1 and 32-2). New methods have been devised for the surgical treatment of hearing loss with correction of conduction apparatus abnormalities, and selected patients can now be surgically relieved of the disabling symptoms of sensorineural hearing loss.

Most otologic procedures are now performed in the day surgery arena. The immediate postanesthesia care for patients who have undergone surgery on the ear is generally the same, regardless of the procedure. Immediate postoperative complications are rare. Occasionally, excessive bleeding may occur, especially if a large blood vessel has been entered during the operation. If bleeding has occurred, the incident should be reported to the postanesthesia care unit (PACU) nurse who provides care for the patient

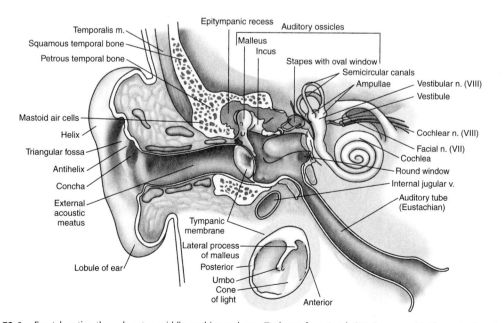

**Fig. 32-1** Frontal section through outer, middle, and internal ear. (*Redrawn from Jacob SW, Francone CA:* Elements of anatomy and physiology, *ed 2, Philadelphia, 1989, Saunders.*)

NURSING CARE IN THE PACU

on admission. Immediate postanesthesia assessment should follow the same format as for any patient who undergoes general anesthesia. In addition, postanesthesia assessment should include testing for function of the facial nerve.

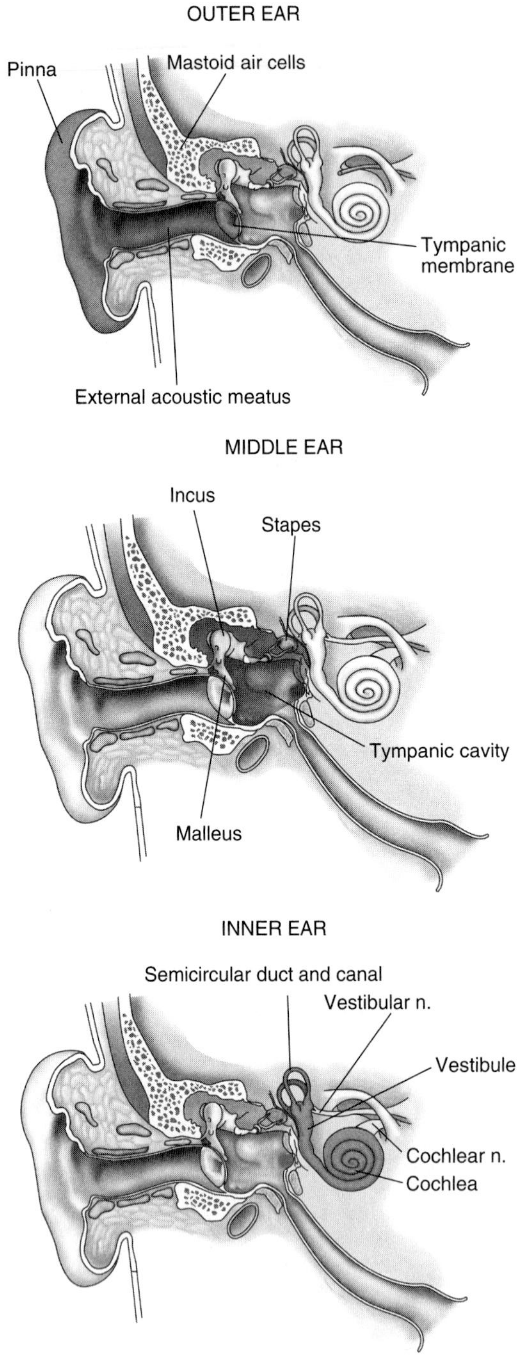

**OUTER EAR**

**MIDDLE EAR**

**INNER EAR**

**Fig. 32-2** Three divisions of ear. (Redrawn from Jacob SW, Francone CA: Elements of anatomy and physiology, ed 2, Philadelphia, 1989, Saunders.)

The patient should be instructed to frown, smile, wrinkle the forehead, close the eyes, bare the teeth, and pucker the lips. An inability to perform these actions indicates injury to the facial nerve and should be appropriately indicated in the patient's medical record and reported to the surgeon.

If surgery has been performed near the brain (inner ear), check for clear fluid in the ear or on the dressings that may indicate cerebrospinal fluid leakage. Aseptic technique for all dressings and protection from infection are especially important elements in the care of the patient who has undergone surgery on the ears because infection can easily be transmitted to the meninges and the brain. The outer ear is highly vascular and susceptible to circulatory damage and excoriation. The outer ear may even become necrotic if circulation is impaired by excessive pressure from or malpositioning of a dressing. Assessment of the dressing should therefore include proper positioning.

Positioning of the postanesthesia patient who has undergone ear surgery should be indicated by the surgeon. If position is unimportant, the patient should be allowed to assume a position of comfort, usually with the head of the bed elevated to facilitate drainage. This position also decreases the need to move the head to see. Generally, lying on the unoperated side is most comfortable for the patient.

Nausea, vertigo, and nystagmus commonly occur in patients after ear surgery. The patient may minimize discomfort by remaining in the position ordered, moving slowly, and avoiding quick jerky movements. The patient should be advised to take slow deep breaths through the mouth to minimize nausea. Antiemetic drugs and sedatives such as low-dose droperidol (Inapsine) or a 5-HT$_3$ antagonist such as ondansetron (Zofran) may be ordered for prevention or treatment of nausea and vertigo. The nurse should avoid jarring the bed. When approaching the patient, the nurse should place a hand on top of the patient's head as a reminder not to turn suddenly when the nurse speaks. Sudden turns should be avoided, and movement should be slow in patient transport. Particular attention must be paid to maintaining the integrity of the airway should nausea and vomiting occur.

### Special Considerations

*Myringotomy.* Myringotomy is the most common procedure performed on infants and small children. Special pediatric considerations must be given in the immediate postanesthesia phase to airway management, safety, parental involvement, and outpatient teaching. The patient should be positioned to promote drainage from the ear. A small piece of sterile cotton may be placed loosely in the external ear to absorb the drainage that commonly occurs. The cotton should be changed often to avoid contamination.

***Mastoidectomy.*** A firm bulky dressing is placed over the ear and held in place with a circular head bandage after mastoidectomy. This dressing may be reinforced, if necessary, but should be changed only by the physician. Minimal serosanguineous drainage may be expected, but bright bloody drainage should be reported to the surgeon.

The patient should be placed in a position of comfort, usually on the unoperated side. Grafts are often taken from the arm or leg for radical mastoidectomy, and the donor sites should be assessed for drainage and treated according to local policy. Dizziness and vertigo are common after mastoidectomy and may be treated with the previously mentioned measures.

***Tympanoplasty.*** Patients are usually positioned on the unoperated side after tympanoplasty. Care must be taken to keep bandages and grafts in place. Patients should be instructed not to blow the nose or cough and to avoid sneezing to prevent disruption of the grafts.

***Fenestration.*** Fenestration is not commonly performed; however, it may occasionally be the procedure of choice for patients who have lost effective hearing in both ears. Fenestration is a major surgical procedure and is usually performed with general anesthesia. Nausea, vertigo, and pain on moving the jaws can be expected after fenestration. The patient is usually placed on the operated side to keep drainage from the operative site from entering the ear. The patient may be allowed to change position from the operated side to the back for nursing care and comfort.

***Stapedectomy.*** Patients who have undergone stapedectomy are usually admitted to the PACU with ear packing in place; this packing should not be disturbed (Fig. 32-3). Occasionally, patients have vertigo after surgery. Patients should be advised to avoid blowing the nose, coughing, and sneezing.

***Cochlear Implant.*** Patients who have undergone a cochlear implant need the same postanesthesia care as any other patient for ear surgery. Verification of the integrity of the facial nerve is important. These patients do not have hearing immediately after surgery and need emotional support and a means of communication.

## SURGERY ON THE NOSE AND SINUSES

Nasal and sinus surgery may be accomplished with local or general anesthesia. The disposition of the patient is determined by the nature and type of surgery and anesthesia and by the perianesthesia course related to complications and sedation required in the PACU. Overnight observation of the patient in an inpatient setting may be necessary before discharge from the hospital. The anatomy of the nasal cavity is shown in Fig. 32-4.

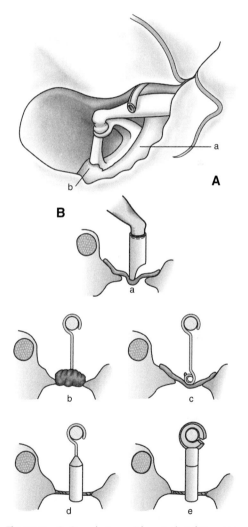

**Fig. 32-3** **A**, Stapedectomy. Adequate footplate exposure is achieved when facial canal (*a*) and pyramidal process (*b*) are seen. **B**, Stapedectomy prostheses: (*a*) vein/polyethylene strut (Shea); (*b*) wire/fat (Schuknecht); (*c*) wire on compressed Gelfoam (House); (*d*) wire/Teflon piston; (*e*) Teflon piston (Shea). *(From Paparella MM, Shumrick DA: Otolaryngology, vol 2, Philadelphia, 1973, Saunders.)*

NURSING CARE IN THE PACU

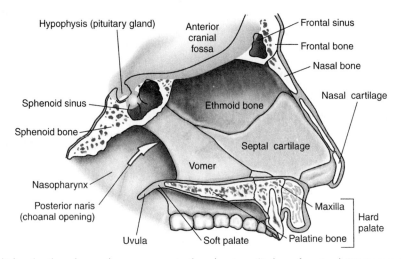

**Fig. 32-4** Sagittal section through nose shows components of nasal septum. *(Redrawn from Jacob SW, Francone CA:* Elements of anatomy and physiology, *ed 2, Philadelphia, 1989, Saunders.)*

### Nasal Surgery

Conscious patients admitted to the PACU after nasal surgery should be placed in a semi-Fowler's position to promote drainage, reduce local edema, minimize discomfort, and facilitate respiration. Some postoperative serosanguineous drainage is expected; however, the nurse should observe closely for gross bleeding. The patient is usually admitted with one or both nostrils packed and a mustache dressing in place to catch any drainage from the packing. The position of the nasal packs and the amount of drainage should be checked frequently. The mustache dressing may be changed as necessary; two or three changes within a 4-hour period are not unusual. Another method commonly used to facilitate postoperative drainage is the insertion of nasal stents. This approach affords more comfort and permits nasal breathing.

The back of the patient's throat should be checked frequently for blood. Frequent belching (from the accumulation of blood in the stomach) and frequent swallowing and the classic signs of hemorrhage, such as tachycardia, are additional signs of unusual bleeding. The patient should be instructed not to blow the nose and not to swallow secretions but rather to spit them into a basin. An ample supply of disposable tissues along with an emesis basin should be placed within easy reach of the patient.

Airway obstruction or laryngeal spasm may occur if a postnasal pack accidentally slips out of place. A flashlight, scissors, and a hemostat for emergency removal of nasal packing and emergency airway equipment must be kept readily available at the patient's bedside.

Fluids are withheld until bleeding is controlled, vomiting and nausea have subsided, and independent airway management has been established. Occasionally, an antiemetic may be ordered to alleviate nausea and vomiting.

Mouth breathing, bleeding, and postnasal drainage create a dryness and an offensive taste and odor in the patient's mouth, so once the gag reflex has returned, oral hygiene is a priority. Lemon-glycerine swabs or mouthwash may be used for mouth care and to make the patient more comfortable. A petrolatum-based ointment may be applied to the lips to prevent drying and cracking.

Ice packs across the nose may be ordered to minimize pain, edema, discoloration, and bleeding. These ice packs should be small and lightweight.

Oxygen should be delivered via cool mist mask through a face tent because dry mucus membranes often produce coughing, dyspnea, and decreased respiratory exchange. Ice chips may be a comfort measure if intake is warranted.

### Sinus Surgery

After surgery on the sinuses, the patient is usually admitted to the PACU with packing in place. Reports of feelings of numbness in the upper lip and teeth are not unusual. After general anesthesia, the patient should be positioned well on one side to prevent aspiration of drainage. The conscious patient should be placed in a semi-Fowler's position, with the head elevated 45 degrees to promote drainage and minimize edema. The same general care, including oral hygiene and instructions to the patient not to blow the nose, should be followed as for the patient with nasal surgery.

## SURGERY ON THE TONGUE

The tongue occupies a large portion of the floor of the mouth. Surgery on the tongue generally involves excision of benign or malignant lesions, correction of congenital anomalies, or repair of traumatic lacerations. Lesions may be excised without associated neck dissection; however, when the lesion is malignant, surgical treatment usually involves a combined operation that may include radical neck dissection and resection of both the mandible and the tongue.

Local anesthesia is used for minor surgical procedures, such as incision and longitudinal closure of the frenulum in ankyloglossia. Local infiltration is also used for repair of lacerations caused by trauma. More extensive surgical procedures on the tongue require endotracheal anesthesia.

After surgery, the patient must be placed in a side-lying position with the head slightly dependent to allow for the drainage of secretions out of the mouth. When protective reflexes have returned, the patient should be placed in a sitting position to promote venous and lymphatic drainage.

Maintenance of the airway is the most crucial nursing concern. Suctioning equipment with soft-tipped catheters must be immediately available at the bedside. The patient should be instructed to allow saliva to run out of the mouth. A wick of gauze may be placed in the patient's mouth to assist in the elimination of secretions. Swelling of the tongue may occur and obstruct the airway; therefore, an intubation tray should be readily available.

Because of the vascular nature of the tongue and oral cavity, postoperative bleeding may be a problem. If excessive bleeding occurs, local pressure should be applied until the surgeon can be notified and repair effected in the operating room.

## THROAT SURGERY

Surgery on the throat and neck is generally accomplished with general anesthesia. Aside from routine care and assessment, specific post-anesthesia care for the patient who has undergone surgery on the throat involves: (1) close observation for bleeding from the surgical site; (2) maintenance of a patent airway; (3) prevention of aspiration of secretions; and (4) awareness of possible cerebral neurologic complications that may develop.

The most common procedures are tonsillectomy, either alone or in combination with adenoidectomy, and tracheostomy.

### Tonsillectomy and Adenoidectomy

Most patients who undergo tonsillectomy (Fig. 32-5) and adenoidectomy (T&A) are children and young adults. However, the number of the young children for T&A continues to be reduced each year as a result of excellent antibiotic treatment. Adult patients who have undergone T&A with local anesthesia or are admitted to the PACU fully conscious may be positioned on their backs with the head elevated 45 degrees. Patients who return after general anesthesia and who are unconscious or semi-conscious must be placed in the tonsillar position—well over on the side with the face partially down. The Trendelenburg's position may be used to facilitate drainage. The patient's airway and chest expansion must be in full view of the nurse to ensure maximum respiratory integrity at all times. In this position, secretions are easily drained from the mouth. An oral airway should be left in place until the swallowing reflex has returned and the patient can handle secretions. The patient should be advised to spit out secretions as much as possible and to try not to cough, clear the throat, blow the nose, or talk excessively. An ice collar may be applied to minimize pain and postoperative bleeding. The administration of cool humidified air to the patient after T&A provides comfort, helps minimize swelling, and supplies oxygen.

The most common complication of T&A is postoperative bleeding, for both children and adults. Frequent swallowing, clearing of the throat, and vomiting of dark blood are indications of possible bleeding. The nurse should frequently check the back of the throat with a flashlight for trickling blood. If any of the cardinal symptoms of hemorrhage occur, such as decreased blood pressure, tachycardia, pallor, and restlessness, the surgeon should be notified. Because the surgeon may want to treat a bleeding episode in the PACU, a tonsil tray should be available (Box 32-1). An electrocautery unit and appropriate illumination with a headlight should also be available, along with suction equipment. Postoperative bleeding after T&A can often be controlled with the application of vasoconstrictors via nasal packing with pressure. If significant bleeding occurs, however, the patient may have to return to the operating room for suturing or cauterizing of blood vessels.

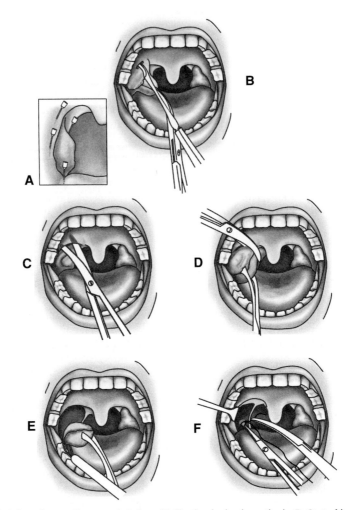

**Fig. 32-5** Method of dissection tonsillectomy. **A,** Points of infiltration for local anesthesia. **B,** Start of incision with tonsil knife at attachment of anterior pillar to tonsil superiorly. **C,** Separation with scissor dissection of superior pole of tonsil. **D,** Continuation of dissection of tonsil from its attachment to pillars and bed of tonsillar fossa. **E,** Separation of tonsil with snare at lower pole, including plica triangularis. **F,** Hemostasis. *(From Boies LR, Hilger JA, Priest RE:* Fundamentals of otolaryngology: a textbook of ear, nose, and throat diseases, *ed 4, Philadelphia, 1964, Saunders.)*

With the advent of laser dissection of tonsils and adenoids, swelling of the tissue in the hypopharyngeal area is increased. Close observation and measures to alleviate swelling are crucial. The advantage of laser dissection is that the potential for bleeding is significantly decreased.

Once the patient is conscious and the reflexes have returned, ice chips and fluids may be offered. Large swallows of lukewarm fluids seem to cause the least discomfort to these patients. Sucking may precipitate bleeding, so a straw should not be offered to the patient. Oral hygiene, including alkaline mouthwash, may provide comfort. Petrolatum ointment should be applied to the lips to prevent drying and cracking.

Patients who have undergone T&A are especially prone to laryngospasms and must be observed closely for patency of the airway. Airway obstruction may be created by swelling of the palate or nasopharynx, swelling in the retropharyngeal space, or swelling of the tongue and nose. If laryngospasm does occur, positive pressure via Ambu bag and 100% fraction of inspired oxygen ($FiO_2$) is administered. If this method is not effective in breaking the spasm, reintubation and administration of succinylcholine and narcotics as prescribed may be necessary.

### Laryngoscopy

Laryngoscopy may be accomplished with local or general anesthesia. If the patient's gag and cough reflexes have been obliterated, the patient should not be given anything orally until these reflexes have fully returned. The conscious

| Box 32-1 **Contents of Tonsil Tray** |
| --- |
| Tongue depressors |
| Hurd retractor (1) |
| Mouth gags (2) |
| Allis clamp (1) |
| Tonsil hemostats (2) |
| Short sponge forceps (1) |
| Pair of scissors (1) |
| Sterile towels |
| Epinephrine hydrochloride (Adrenalin) 1:1000 |
| Set of tonsil suture needles (1) |
| Needle holder (1) |
| Glass medicine cup (1) |
| Sterile basin (1) |
| Cotton balls |
| Tonsil tampons |
| Soft rubber catheter (1) |
| Petrolatum |

| Box 32-2 **Contents of Tracheostomy Tray** |
| --- |
| Adson or Poole suction (without guard; 1) |
| No. 3 knife handle with no. 15 blade (1) |
| No. 11 blade (1) |
| Metzenbaum scissors (1) |
| One-point sharp scissors (1) |
| Curved tenotomy scissors (1) |
| Collier needle holder (1) |
| Six-inch needle holder (1) |
| Adson forceps (2) |
| Tissue forceps (1) |
| Dressing forceps (1) |
| Curved mosquito forceps (4) |
| Straight mosquito forceps (2) |
| Allis clamps (2) |
| Small towel clips (4) |
| Sponge stick (or forceps; 1) |
| Probe (1) |
| Grooved director (1) |
| Goiter right-angle retractor (1) |
| Tracheostomy hook (1) |
| Vein retractors (2) |
| Army-Navy retractors (2) |
| Tonsil suction with tip screwed on (1) |
| Ten-mL, 3-ring syringe (1) |
| Needle, 25-gauge, 5/8-inch (1) |
| Prep cup (1) |
| Medicine glass (1) |
| Tracheostomy tubes, sizes 00-8 (1 each) |
| Hand towels (4) |
| Trousseau tracheal dilator (1) |

patient may be placed in a semi-Fowler's position on either side. If unconscious, the patient should be placed in the side-lying position to avoid aspiration. Cool mist, sips of water, and intravenous narcotics may help relieve the coughing that often occurs.

These patients are especially susceptible to the development of laryngospasm, and the most important observations in the patient after laryngoscopy are aimed at ascertaining the patency of the airway. Laryngeal stridor, dyspnea, decreased oxygen saturation, or shortness of breath should alert the nurse to respiratory impairment, and the anesthesiologist should be notified. Equipment for endotracheal intubation and emergency tracheostomy should be immediately available at the bedside should laryngeal edema or laryngospasm develop (Box 32-2).

A certain amount of throat discomfort can be expected and may be relieved with the use of an ice collar. The administration of high-humidity oxygen via face tent or mask decreases throat irritation. After the cough and gag reflexes have returned, the patient may be allowed sips of warm normal saline solution, which is soothing to irritated tissues. If severe pain occurs in either the throat or the chest, the physician should be notified. The nurse should watch for signs of hemorrhage, including coughing or regurgitation of blood, apprehension, and the classic signs of tachycardia and lowered blood pressure.

In patients who have undergone laryngoscopy (with biopsy) or removal of polyps, vocal rest is important. Coughing should be avoided if possible, and paper and pencil or a "Magic Slate" should be made available so the patient can communicate without talking. If intractable coughing does occur, the anesthesiologist may need to be consulted for further measures of control, including pharmacotherapeutics such as codeine and lidocaine to suppress the cough reflex.

Because laser surgery is so frequent in ENT surgery and the technology has improved to a significant degree, Chapter 47 is devoted to the care of the patient after laser and laparoscopic surgery. Patients for ENT surgery, especially involving the upper airway, may undergo laser surgery because lasers enable a precise excision of tissue without significant edema and bleeding. Lasers emit one wavelength, whereas light emits multiple wavelengths. Lasers with shorter wavelengths allow for less absorption by water and therefore less tissue penetration. Patients who are received in the PACU after laser surgery may still have the endotracheal tube in place. Although the "perfect" endotracheal tube for laser surgery has not been developed, Table 32-1 describes the advantages and disadvantages of the laser-resistent tracheal tubes. A debate between cuffed and uncuffed tracheal tubes continues. However, from a perianesthesia point of view, when a laser case arrives in the PACU, the nurse must inquire whether the tube is cuffed or uncuffed. If the tracheal tube is cuffed, the cuff was probably inflated with a methylene blue-tinged normal saline solution. This solution is used because it absorbs and disperses heat and also does not act as a reservoir of combustion-supporting gas. Extubation should be handled as described in this chapter and in Chapter 30. Also, Chapter 47 provides an excellent description of the use of lasers during surgery.

### Tracheostomy

A tracheostomy, an incision into the trachea and the insertion of a cannula, may be done as either an emergency or an elective procedure (Fig. 32-6). Ideally, a tracheostomy is performed in the operating suite with controlled conditions. Tracheostomies are performed to improve the airway and to provide access for suctioning of secretions from the trachea and bronchi. The PACU nurse should know what condition necessitated the tracheostomy.

The PACU personnel should anticipate the arrival of a patient with a tracheostomy and have the necessary items at the bedside (Box 32-3).

A variety of tracheostomy tubes are available, and the nurse should be familiar with those used in the particular institution. Several common types are shown in Fig. 32-7.

Immediate postanesthesia care of the patient with a new tracheostomy includes a complete assessment of the patient's general condition

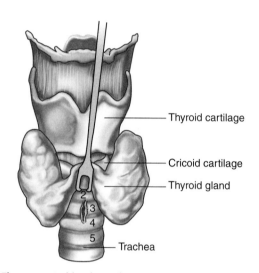

**Fig. 32-6**   Incision for tracheostomy. *(Redrawn from Jacob SW, Francone CA:* Elements of anatomy and physiology, *ed 2, Philadelphia, 1989, Saunders.)*

| Table 32-1 | Advantages and Disadvantages of Commonly Available Laser-Resistant Tracheal Tubes | |
|---|---|---|
| Tube Type | Advantages | Disadvantages |
| Metal | Atraumatic external surface<br>Double cuff maintains seal even if punctured with laser<br>Kink resistant | Thick-walled nonflammable cuff reflects laser and transfers heat |
| Polyvinyl chloride (PVC) | Inexpensive<br>Nonreflective<br>Maintains shape well<br>Double cuff maintains seal after proximal cuff puncture | Burns vigorously and yields pulmonary toxin (hydrogen chloride)<br>Cuffed version contains flammable material |
| Red rubber | Wrapping protects flammable material but dries tube<br>Maintains structure<br>Nonreflective | Red rubber itself is highly flammable<br>Tubes are thick walled |
| Silicone rubber | Wrapping protects flammable material<br>Methylene blue aids in detection of cuff perforation<br>Nonreflective | Contains flammable material<br>Turns to toxic ash<br>Single cuff is vulnerable to laser damage |

From Nagelhout J, Zaglaniczny K: *Nurse anesthesia*, ed 3, St Louis, 2005, Saunders.

and detailed attention to respiratory status and tracheostomy wound care. Because of the many nursing needs and the necessity of intensive ongoing respiratory assessment, the patient with a new tracheostomy needs constant attendance.

Assessment of respiratory function should include all parameters mentioned in previous chapters. The nurse should auscultate the patient's chest frequently for normal bilateral breath sounds and report any adventitious

sounds or indications of pulmonary congestion. Pulse oximetry should be used to assist in assessment.

### Suctioning and Tracheostomy Care.

Patency of the newly created airway is vital, and frequent suctioning is necessary because of increased secretions from the tracheobronchial tree caused by trauma. Suctioning of the tracheostomy must be sterile and atraumatic; a sterile disposable catheter and glove should be used for each procedure. A suction catheter in a plastic sleeve provides a means of suctioning without the use of gloves and is most convenient for use in the PACU. Catheters should be smooth and small enough to pass easily into the lumen of the tracheostomy tube without obstructing it.

As with any suctioning technique, the patient should undergo hyperventilation with increased $FiO_2$ both before and after the procedure. For suctioning, insert the catheter 6 to 8 inches into the tracheostomy tube. Do not apply suction during insertion. Apply suction intermittently by occluding the air valve with the thumb and at the same time slowly withdrawing the catheter in a twisting motion. Suctioning should not continue for longer than 5 seconds. Time should be allotted between each suctioning for adequate oxygenation of the patient. Suctioning often stimulates forceful coughing, which is effective in bringing up secretions, so the nurse should be prepared to wipe expelled

---

### Box 32-3 Bedside Equipment Needed for a Patient With Tracheostomy

Suction equipment
Respirator
Ambu or anesthesia bag
Extra sterile tracheostomy tray, including tracheostomy tubes of proper size, sterile forceps, tracheal hook, and Trousseau tracheal dilator (see Box 32-2)
Sterile gauze squares
Sterile scissors
Tracheostomy ties
Cleaning solutions for the tracheostomy tube and the incision
Syringe
Hemostat (for inflation of the tracheostomy tube cuff)

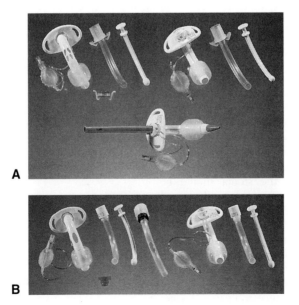

**Fig. 32-7 A,** Shiley Tracheosoft XLT tracheostomy tubes (Nellcor Puritan Bennett Inc, Pleasanton, Calif). **B,** Shiley fenestrated low-pressure cuffed tracheostomy tube, showing: (*a*) outer cannula with fenestration above cuff; (*b*) decannulation cannula used to plug tracheostomy tube. *(Reprinted with permission of Nellcor Puritan Bennett Inc, Pleasanton, Calif.)*

secretions away from the tracheostomy tube orifice with plain gauze squares. For determination of the effectiveness of the suctioning, the chest should be auscultated immediately afterward.

If deep suctioning is indicated, a coudé-tip catheter should be used. Insert the catheter with the tip pointing in the direction of the main stem bronchus to be suctioned. Recent evidence indicates that positioning the patient's head to the left or the right has little effect, if any, on which bronchus is entered.

If the patient's secretions are exceptionally thick, the physician may order instillation of 3 to 5 mL of sterile normal saline solution into the tracheostomy tube to help loosen secretions and promote coughing. Although this procedure is common, whether it is actually effective is questionable; and if the normal saline solution is not immediately removed with suctioning, it may produce the effects of any inhaled fluid and act as a contaminant. More effective measures to ensure liquefaction of secretions include providing inspired air that is well humidified and ensuring that the patient is well hydrated.

Immediate postanesthesia care of the patient with a new tracheostomy also includes care and cleaning of the tracheostomy tube, which may be necessary as often as every hour. A variety of methods may be used to clean the inner cannula of the tracheostomy tube, including normal saline solution and hydrogen peroxide or 2% sodium bicarbonate solution. A small test tube brush or pipe cleaners may be used to scrub off sticky crusts of mucus. Regardless of the method, the procedure must be sterile, and no supplies should be used that may leave on the cannula any lint or other debris that may be inhaled by the patient.

Wound drainage from the tracheostomy is generally minimal; however, soiling of the tracheostomy dressing occurs from secretions and sweating. The dressings should be changed as often as necessary, and the skin should be kept clean and dry to prevent maceration and infection. The skin around the stoma should be cleansed with hydrogen peroxide and normal saline solution and dried with sterile gauze pads, and an antibiotic ointment such as bacitracin should be applied. The tracheostomy dressing should be plain gauze with the edges bound and should have no cotton filling or loose strings. Special tracheostomy "pants" that fit over the tracheostomy tube and have all edges sewn make the best dressing. Sterile gauze may be cut halfway to the center and fitted over the tube (Fig. 32-8); however, this approach has the disadvantage of cut edges that may fray and

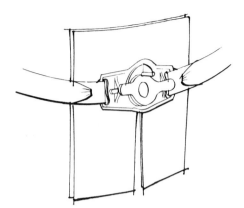

**Fig. 32-8**   Gauze square cut to use as tracheostomy dressing. *(From Sutton AL: Bedside nursing techniques in medicine and surgery, ed 2, Philadelphia, 1969, Saunders.)*

allow bits of gauze to enter the wound or the trachea.

Fabric tapes or ties or Velcro devices are used to secure the tracheostomy tube in place. These should be checked frequently to ensure the proper tension. If they are too tight, they are uncomfortable for the patient and may compress the external jugular veins. If they are too loose, the cannula slides up and down in the trachea or is even expelled. When the tapes are tied so that one finger can easily slip underneath, the tension is right.

**Complications.**   When complications of a tracheostomy occur, PACU nurses should be especially astute in observing for signs of danger. The most common complication is respiratory obstruction caused by external pressure, foreign bodies, tracheal edema, or excessive secretions. If suctioning does not relieve airway obstruction, the tracheostomy tube may be removed immediately, the tracheal stoma held open with a tracheal dilator and hook or forceps (Fig. 32-9), and the surgeon or anesthesiologist summoned.

Occasionally, a tube is coughed out either because the ties are not sufficiently tight or

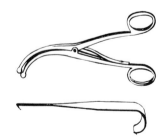

**Fig. 32-9**   Tracheal dilator and hook. *(Adapted from Sutton AL: Bedside nursing techniques in medicine and surgery, ed 2, Philadelphia, 1969, Saunders.)*

because the tube is too short. If a tube is accidentally expelled, it must be reinserted by persons qualified to do so. In some institutions, nurses practice changing tracheostomy tubes under the supervision of physicians so that if accidental expulsion should occur in the PACU, the nurse is skilled in replacement. If the tube cannot be inserted easily, the stoma should be held open and the surgeon called. Misplacement or displacement of the tube is a common complication and must be corrected immediately (Fig. 32-10).

Obstruction below the tracheostomy tube may create respiratory insufficiency. Respiratory adventitious sounds, unequal lung expansion, and marked respiratory efforts, including supraclavicular, intercostal, and substernal retractions, should alert the nurse to this problem, and the physician should be notified.

Some bloody secretions from the tracheal stoma may be expected in the immediate postoperative period, but frank bleeding is abnormal and the surgeon should be notified. Sometimes,

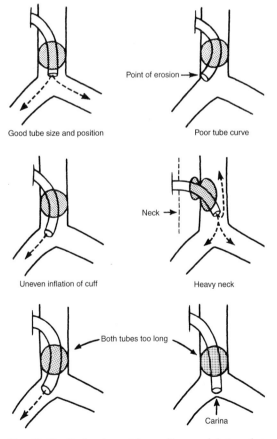

Good tube size and position

Point of erosion →

Poor tube curve

Uneven inflation of cuff

Neck →

Heavy neck

Both tubes too long

Carina

**Fig. 32-10** Tracheostomy tube positions and factors that affect them. *(From Murphy ER: Intensive nursing care in a respiratory unit,* Nurs Clin North Am *3:433, 1968.)*

bleeding from a thyroid vein or other neck vessel next to the tube occurs, and blood, which runs down into the trachea, is sprayed about with every cough. This situation is usually not serious and can often be controlled with local packing with petrolatum gauze. Occasionally, however, serious bleeding does occur and the patient must be taken back to the operating room, where the wound is reopened and the bleeding vessel ligated.

Subcutaneous emphysema may occur as a complication of tracheostomy if the wound is sutured too tightly about the tracheostomy tube, thus allowing air to enter the subcutaneous tissues, or it may result from an overly large incision or a partially obstructed tube. Although subcutaneous emphysema is annoying, it is usually not serious and generally clears after several days. If the nurse notices a crackling sensation under the skin of the neck, chest, or face of the patient, it should be reported to the surgeon because removal of a suture or two may readily correct this problem.

The complications of tracheostomy in infants and children are almost always more serious because the relative size of the airway is smaller and tolerance for any obstruction is lessened.

Emotional support of the patient with a new tracheostomy is important and begins immediately on the patient regaining consciousness. Although the patient may have been well prepared with regard to the loss of ability to speak, awakening in that state is still a traumatic event. A pad and pencil should be readily available to allow the patient to communicate.

### Laryngectomy

Partial laryngectomy (Table 32-2) is the surgical treatment of choice for patients with a limited malignant process of the vocal cords. It is commonly performed through a laryngofissure, and tracheostomy is usually performed concomitantly to ensure a good airway during the immediate postoperative period. Postanesthesia nursing care is essentially the same as that for a patient after tracheostomy.

Postoperative subcutaneous emphysema is not uncommon and should be reported to the surgeon. Patients after laryngectomy have trouble swallowing and need frequent suctioning and reassurance.

Supraglottic laryngectomy is performed for carcinoma of the epiglottis and adjacent structures above the level of the true vocal cords. A tracheostomy is mandatory for these patients; they also have a great deal of difficulty swallowing and need close observation and assistance with elimination of saliva and other secretions.

NURSING CARE IN THE PACU

| Table 32-2 Laryngectomy | | |
| --- | --- | --- |
| Structures Removed | Structures Remaining | Postoperative Conditions |
| **TOTAL LARYNGECTOMY** | | |
| Hyoid bone | Tongue | Loss of voice; breathing through tracheostomy; no problem swallowing |
| Entire larynx (epiglottis, false cords, true cords) | Pharyngeal walls | |
| Cricoid cartilage | Lower trachea | |
| Two or three rings of trachea | | |
| **SUPRAGLOTTIC OR HORIZONTAL LARYNGECTOMY** | | |
| Hyoid bone | True vocal cords | Normal voice; occasional aspiration may occur, especially with liquids; normal airway |
| Epiglottis | Cricoid cartilage | |
| False vocal cords | Trachea | |
| **VERTICAL (OR HEMI-) LARYNGECTOMY** | | |
| One true vocal cord | Epiglottis | Hoarse but serviceable voice; normal airway; no problem swallowing |
| False cord | One false cord | |
| Arytenoid | One true vocal cord | |
| One half thyroid cartilage | Cricoid | |
| **LARYNGOFISSURE AND PARTIAL LARYNGECTOMY** | | |
| One vocal cord | All other structures | Hoarse but serviceable voice; occasionally almost normal voice; no airway problem; no swallowing problem |
| **ENDOSCOPIC REMOVAL OF EARLY CARCINOMA** | | |
| Part of one vocal cord | All other structures | Possibility of normal voice; no other problems |

Total laryngectomy is reserved for patients with advanced carcinoma of the true cords (Fig. 32-11). Tracheostomy is always performed. Some means of communication should be established before surgery for postoperative use.

The primary nursing concern after laryngectomy is maintenance of an adequate airway. Tracheostomy care, as previously discussed, should be deftly carried out and the air well humidified. In the immediate postanesthesia period, patients need frequent suctioning, not only of the tracheostomy but also of the nose and mouth, because they cannot blow the nose and may have difficulty spitting. Frequent mouth care provides additional comfort, and a petrolatum ointment should be applied to the lips to prevent drying and cracking.

After surgery, the patient should be positioned on the side until full consciousness is regained. When conscious, the patient may be positioned in a low semi-Fowler's position with the head elevated about 30 degrees. This position promotes drainage, minimizes edema, prevents uncomfortable pressure on suture lines, and facilitates respirations.

Dressings should be checked frequently for excessive drainage and reinforced or changed as necessary. Sometimes, drainage catheters are placed under the wound flaps for removal of fluid from the potential dead space left after removal of the larynx and related structures. Drainage catheters must be connected to a constant vacuum source at 40 to 60 mm Hg, and free drainage must be maintained within the system, which may be accomplished with a Hemovac drainage device (Fig. 32-12). Excessive bloody drainage should be reported to the surgeon. The most common site of hemorrhage is the base of the tongue.

Patients after laryngectomy are frequently apprehensive on awakening and should have someone in close attendance at all times. Although patients may be prepared for the postoperative loss of the voice, the first experiences

Before laryngectomy

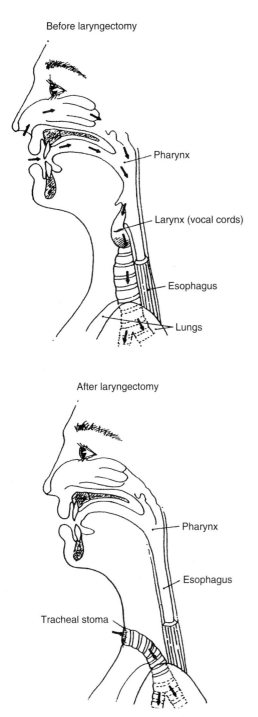

After laryngectomy

**Fig. 32-11** Total laryngectomy. *(From Keith RL: Looking forward . . . a guidebook for the laryngectomy, ed 3, Rochester, MN, 1995, Mayo Foundation. With permission of Mayo Foundation for Medical Education and Research.)*

of being voiceless and unable to call for help are always extremely frightening. A bell to ring or other noisemaker is more reassuring in this instance than the routine pencil-and-paper communication system.

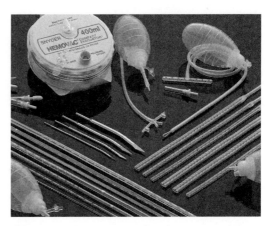

**Fig. 32-12** Silicone evacuator (Snyder Hemovac drainage) device is closed suction apparatus and blood receptacle for facial and neck surgery. *(Courtesy of Zimmer Inc., Warsaw, Ind.)*

## RADICAL NECK SURGERY

The radical neck procedure itself is relatively simple; it involves removal of all the subcutaneous fat, lymphatic channels, and some of the superficial muscles within a prescribed area of the neck (Fig. 32-13). Generally, the procedure involves the removal of the sternocleidomastoid muscle, omohyoid muscle, internal and external jugular veins, and all lymphatic tissue on one side of the neck. The purposeful resection of the XIth cranial (spinal accessory) nerve causes atrophy of the large trapezius muscle. In the modified neck dissection, the accessory nerve and the internal jugular vein are spared.

Postanesthesia nursing care of the patient after radical neck surgery is somewhat less demanding than that after laryngectomy because these patients do not have a tracheostomy and can talk and eat normally. The patient should be placed in a low semi-Fowler's position with the head elevated 30 to 45 degrees to improve venous return. Pillows must be used cautiously when patients are positioned to avoid restriction of venous return or compression of the bases of pedicle flaps. Venous congestion, when present, gives the patient's face a purplish hue. This hue can be differentiated from cyanosis caused by inadequate ventilation with observation of the color of the extremities to confirm good circulation and close monitoring of oxygen saturation. Postoperative pain is usually minimal after radical neck dissection and can be managed with the usual analgesics.

Dressings are minimal. Skin flaps are secured over drainage tubes, which should be connected to constant suction at 40 to 60 mm Hg. The

NURSING CARE IN THE PACU

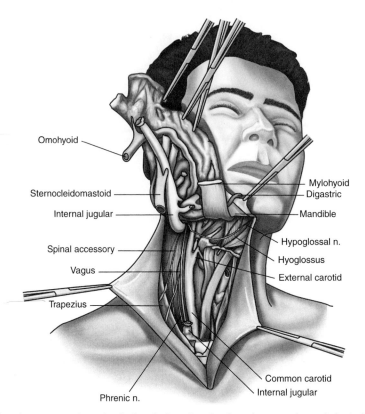

**Fig. 32-13** Drawing shows extent of usual radical neck dissection. Specimen is retracted superiorly. As is shown, resection of posterior belly of digastric muscle permits high ligation of internal jugular vein and also facilitates dissection around hypoglossal nerve. (*Redrawn from Converse JM: Reconstructive plastic surgery, vol 3, Philadelphia, 1964, Saunders.*)

suction catheters constantly working under the skin flaps suck them firmly against the neck. Approximately 70 to 120 mL of serosanguineous drainage can be expected the day of operation. This amount drastically decreases the second day and becomes minimal (less than 30 mL) the third day. If the dressing soaks through with blood, the surgeon should be notified immediately.

Edema of the recurrent laryngeal nerve and of the nerves to the pharynx may cause difficulty in swallowing and in expectorating secretions; therefore, frequent gentle suctioning of oral secretions may be needed. Extreme care must be taken to avoid any trauma to the internal suture lines. A gauze wick placed in the corner of the patient's mouth can alleviate the annoyance of constant dribbling of mucus and saliva. Mouth care is important for the comfort of this patient and can be accomplished with any of the conventional methods.

**Complications**

Edema of the lower part of the face on the same side as the surgery is to be expected. Lower facial paralysis may occur because of

injury of the facial nerve during dissection. The most common complication after radical neck dissection is hemorrhage, which is most often the result of inadequate hemostasis in the immediate postoperative period. The most serious complication is rupture of the carotid artery ("carotid blowout"). This event is uncommon and occurs almost exclusively when radical neck dissection is combined with total laryngectomy. It is more likely to occur in a patient who before surgery has had a course of radiation therapy or who has a fistula that bathes the carotid artery in secretions. If the danger of a blowout of the carotid artery is present, all personnel should be aware of it and know what to do if it occurs.

If a carotid blowout occurs, digital pressure with gauze pads, bath towels, or anything available should be applied immediately and help summoned. Intravenous fluids must be started immediately if they are not already infusing. Fluids should be administered at an increased rate to replace loss and combat shock. The nurse should inflate the cuff on the tracheostomy tube and perform tracheal suctioning to prevent aspiration of blood. Most importantly, a patent airway needs to be maintained and oxygen administered. Patients on carotid precautions—that is, those who may have this complication—should be typed and cross-matched for whole blood, and appropriate emergency equipment, including gauze pads, vascular clips, and suture ties, should be immediately available at the bedside.

### Reconstruction Surgery in Head and Neck Cancer

A large variety of reconstructive procedures may be used to reestablish both contour and function after the removal of large areas of the head and neck for malignant disease. Skin grafts have largely been replaced with skin flaps or muscle-skin combined flaps that can cover extensive areas both inside and outside the neck. These flaps provide a lining of the throat or mouth and can also replace excised skin on the external surfaces. The commonly used flaps are the pectoralis major muscle-skin unit and the deltopectoral flap, both from the anterior chest area. In rare instances, a free flap may be used. This flap is usually a muscle-skin flap that is moved a long distance from one area of the body to another. For this procedure to be successful, this type of flap requires the microsurgical repair of its tiny artery and vein with an artery and vein in its new location. In general, these reconstructive flaps must be free of any pressure or dressings. A light coat of antibacterial ointment is usually applied along the suture lines, and the area is frequently observed for color, warmth, and bleeding. Because these flaps depend on a single small artery and vein, any kinking or external pressure may result in the death of the flap.

## MAXILLOFACIAL SURGERY

The care of patients with extensive maxillofacial surgery follows the principles outlined earlier for tracheostomy care and care after laryngectomy or radical neck dissection. The care of these patients is extremely demanding, and attention to detail is the basis for the prevention of complications.

Maxillofacial surgery may be needed to correct trauma and fractures or congenital skeletal deformities. After this type of surgery, the patient is in intermaxillary fixation (IMF) with the jaws wired shut. Care revolves around protection of the airway and includes wire cutters at the bedside. Maxillofacial surgery is lengthy, and the anesthesia time can exceed 3 hours. Hence, the patient usually arrives in the PACU in a rather sleepy condition and has a slow emergence from the anesthesia; yet in most cases, the patient is able to respond to stimuli and verbal commands.

Some additional emergency equipment is needed at the bedside of patients who are admitted with IMF, including wire cutters, a suture set, additional nasal airways, small suction catheters, and gauze pads. On admission of the patient, the surgeon should review placement of the IMF wires with the nurse. A line drawing of these wires that indicates which to cut in case of extreme emergency (e.g., cardiac or respiratory arrest) should be posted at the head of the bed.

Preoperative preparation of the patient who is undergoing IMF is particularly important and should include instructions on how to clear secretions or remove vomitus while remaining in IMF. The patient should also be taught how to use the suction catheter. These instructions have to be repeated frequently in the PACU as the patient recovers. Having the jaws wired closed is a frightening experience for any patient, no matter how well prepared that patient is. Blood, emesis, lingual and pharyngeal edema, hematoma formation, or laryngospasm may further compromise the oral airway, which is already obstructed as much as 90% by fixation of the jaws. Reassurance is provided with proximity to the patient, ensuring a means to attract attention, and explaining fully all treatments and procedures.

The patient arrives in the PACU with a nasotracheal tube in place. Extubation should not be considered until the patient is fully awake and reflexes have returned sufficiently to allow handling of secretions. A soft nasal airway may be inserted after extubation to assist in maintenance of a patent airway.

The patients should be observed closely for bleeding. Some oozing of blood is normal, but excessive amounts should be reported to the surgeon. Frequent gentle suctioning with a small catheter assists in keeping the airway clear by removing blood and saliva. The patient may be more comfortable doing this independently when able. A suction catheter in hand for use as necessary is reassuring to these patients.

Vomiting and subsequent aspiration is a significant risk for this patient. A nasogastric tube is frequently used to reduce the likelihood of nausea and vomiting. The nurse should ensure that it is correctly positioned and patent. Antiemetics should be administered as necessary, and pain should be treated promptly to prevent the development of nausea and vomiting.

NURSING CARE IN THE PACU

Despite all efforts at prevention, vomiting may occur. If still drowsy, the patient should be turned immediately to the lateral or semi-prone position and the emesis suctioned out via the nose or mouth. If the patient is awake, the nurse should help the patient sit up, lean over, and allow emesis to flow out of the mouth and nose. The cheeks are retracted by holding them out with the fingers. Most importantly, instructions and reassurances need to be repeated quietly but confidently to keep the patient calm. Rarely is cutting the wires necessary, but if any question exists, an anesthesia practitioner should be notified immediately; with a team approach, airway management and resolution of the postoperative nausea and vomiting (PONV) should be initiated.

The patient should be positioned with the head of the bed elevated 30 degrees to assist in maintaining the airway with control of edema. Ice packs are usually ordered after surgery to assist in control of edema and to promote comfort. A surgical glove partially filled with cracked ice can be used, or ice collars can be molded to the jaws, chin, or nose. Iced saline solution gauze pads may be applied to the eyes.

Petrolatum ointment or other emollient cream should be applied to the lips and corners of the mouth to relieve tenderness and prevent drying and cracking. Dental wax can be molded and applied to protruding wires, which are quite irritating to the oral mucosa.

When the patient is fully awake and protective reflexes have sufficiently returned, rinsing the mouth with warm saline solution provides additional comfort. The patient may then also have small sips of liquids.

## SUMMARY

Perianesthesia care of the patient after ENT and maxillofacial surgery requires basic knowledge of the pathophysiology of the face and neck. Advanced airway management skills are important in rendering nursing care to these patients. Also, the perianesthesia nurse must use enhanced behavioral techniques to aid the patient through the initial fear and anxiety generated by the many appliances and devices that can be placed about the oral airway. Patients who undergo maxillofacial surgery may have serious complications from the possibility of the jaw being wired or rubber bands placed to stabilize the jaw. Therefore, complications such as delayed emergence from lengthy surgery and anesthesia time, possible airway obstruction from bleeding, edema,

and the possibility of postoperative nausea and vomiting all become quite serious.

## BIBLIOGRAPHY

Aitkenhead A, Smith G, Rowbotham D: *Textbook of anaesthesia*, ed 5, 2007, Churchill Livingstone, London, 2007.

Alspach J: *Core curriculum for critical care nursing*, ed 6, Philadelphia, 2005, Saunders.

Arnet G, Basehore LM: Dentofacial reconstruction, *Am J Nurs* 84(12):1488-1490, 1984.

Atlee J: *Complications in anesthesia*, ed 2, Philadelphia, 2007, Saunders.

Balkany TJ: The Cochlear implant, *Otolaryngol Clin North Am* 19:217-449, 1986.

Ball KA: *Lasers: the perioperative challenge*, St Louis, 1990, Mosby.

Barash P, Cullen B, Stoelting R: *Clinical anesthesia*, ed 5, Philadelphia, 2005, Lippincott Williams & Wilkins.

Benumof J, Saidman L: *Anesthesia & perioperative complications*, ed 2, St Louis, 1999, Mosby.

Bickley L, Szilagy P: *Bates' guide to physical examination and history taking*, ed 9, Philadelphia, 2005, Lippincott Williams & Wilkins.

Brunton L, Lazo J, Parker K: *Goodman and Gilman's the pharmacological basis of therapeutics*, ed 11, New York, 2005, McGraw-Hill Professional.

Cote C, Todres I, Goudsouzian N, et al: *A practice of anesthesia for infants and children*, ed 3, Philadelphia, 2001, Saunders.

Darvich-Kodjouri C: Nursing care of the patient with a new tracheostomy, *Curr Rev Recov Room Nurses* 3(7):18-23, 1985.

DeFazio-Quinn D, Schick L: *PeriAnesthesia nursing core curriculum*, Philadelphia, 2004, Saunders.

Drake R, Vogl W, Mitchell A: *Gray's anatomy for students*, Philadelphia, 2005, Churchill Livingstone.

Estafanous F, Barash P, Reves J, editors: *Cardiac anesthesia: principles and clinical practice*, ed 2, Philadelphia, 2001, Lippincott Williams & Wilkins.

Evers A, Maze M: *Anesthetic pharmacology: physiologic principles and clinical practice*, Philademphia, 2004, Churchill Livingstone.

Fisher L: *Benumof's anesthesia and uncommon diseases*, ed 5, Philadelphia, 2007, Saunders.

Frost CM, Frost DE: Nursing care of patients in intermaxillary fixation, *Heart Lung* 12(5):524-528, 1983.

Gallager C, Issenberg B: *Simulation in anesthesia*, Philadelphia, 2007, Saunders.

Ganong W: *Review of medical physiology*, ed 22, New York, 2005, McGraw-Hill Medical.

Gotta A: Airway management for maxillofacial trauma, *Curr Rev Post Anesth Nurses* 10(5):34-39, 1988.

Guyton A, Hall J: *Textbook of medical physiology*, ed 11, Philadelphia, 2006, Saunders.

Kaplan J, Slinger P: *Thoracic anesthesia*, ed 3, New York, 2003, Churchill Livingstone.

Kier L, Dowd C: *The chemistry of drugs for nurse anesthetists*, Chicago, 2004, AANA Publishing, Inc.

Lake C, Hines R, Blitt C: *Clinical monitoring: practical applications for anesthesia and critical care*, Philadelphia, 2001, Saunders.

Litwack K, Zeplin K: Practical points in the management of laryngospasm, *J Post Anesth Nurs* 4(1):36-39, 1989.

Longnecker D, Murphy F: *Dripps, Eckenhoff, Vandam introduction to anesthesia*, Philadelphia, 1997, Saunders.

Longnecker D, Tinker J, Morgan G: *Principles and practice of anesthesiology*, ed 2, St Louis, 1998, Mosby.

Lyons RJ, Coren DA: The head and neck patient, *AORN J* 40(5):751-760, 1984.

Mapp C: Trach care: are you aware of all the dangers, *Nursing* 18(7):34-43, 1988.

Miller R, editor: *Anesthesia*, ed 6, Philadelphia, 2005, Churchill Livingstone.

Murray J, Nadel J: *Textbook of respiratory medicine*, ed 4, Philadelphia, 2005, Saunders.

Nagelhout J, Zaglaniczy K: *Nurse anesthesia*, ed 3, St Louis, 2005, Saunders.

Ogden S: *Calculation of drug dosages*, ed 7, St Louis, 2005, Mosby.

Patton C: The critical airway, *Curr Rev Post Anesth Nurses* 13(5):35-39, 1991.

Rook JL, Rook M: Head and neck cancer, *J Post Anesth Nurs* 4(6):263-277, 1989.

Shorten G, Browne J, Carr D, et al: *Postoperative pain management: an evidence-based guide to practice*, Philadelphia, 2006, Saunders.

Smalley PJ: Lasers in otolaryngology, *Nurs Clin North Am* 25(3):645-655, 1990.

Stoelting R: *Pharmacology and physiology in anesthetic practice*, ed 3, Philadelphia, 1999, Lippincott-Raven.

Stoelting R, Miller R: *Basics of anesthesia*, ed 5, Philadelphia, 2007, Churchill Livingstone.

Thompson J, McFarland G, Kirsch J, et al: *Mosby's clinical nursing*, ed 5, St Louis, 2002, Mosby.

Townsend C, Beauchamp R, Evers B, et al: *Sabiston textbook of surgery: the biological basis of modern surgical practice*, ed 17, Philadelphia, 2004, Saunders.

White P: *Perioperative drug manual*, ed 2, Philadelphia, 2005, Saunders.

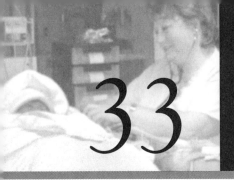

# 33

# CARE OF THE OPHTHALMIC SURGICAL PATIENT

*Carole Muto, RN, BSN, CPAN*

The care for patients undergoing eye surgery presents unique rewards and challenges in the perianesthesia setting. Often, the postanesthesia care unit (PACU) nurse shares in the joy and excitement as a patient experiences dramatically improved vision minutes after cataract surgery. Conversely, the same nurse may care for a toddler with weeping parents after the distressing loss of the child's eye from retinoblastoma. The primary goals of the plan of care after eye surgery are safe and successful postanesthetic recovery and comfort in keeping with ASPAN guidelines, but the special cognitive and advocacy needs of these patients should be identified first in the preoperative holding area. These needs are met through education and discharge planning that begins in the preanesthesia phase and continues to the phase II or ambulatory surgery setting.[1]

Ophthalmologic advances have proceeded at an incredible pace during the past few decades.[2] Ophthalmic surgery is performed safely on fragile premature infants and neonates and on the elderly. The special concerns that apply to specific age groups must be considered. In the care of infants and children, a thorough understanding of normal growth and development is essential. The perianesthesia nurse who works with the pediatric population should be certified in pediatric advanced life support (PALS) and advanced cardiac life support (ACLS). Elderly patients for ophthalmic surgery may have complex medical histories, sensory deficits, and senile dementia. Diabetes mellitus, a leading cause of blindness in adults between the ages of 21 and 60 years, leads to eye surgery for many in this age group.[3] Meticulous attention to details of the patient's ocular and medical history and type and course of anesthesia is vital to optimal perianesthesia care.

Most eye surgical procedures today are performed as same-day or ambulatory outpatient surgery. Cataract surgery has few restrictions and is often performed with topical anesthesia and almost exclusively on an outpatient basis.

Many patients, including those who have had an eye removed, may be discharged home the same day of general anesthesia. Discharge criteria are in keeping with other nonophthalmic types of surgery. In all cases, postoperative care instructions should be discussed both before and after surgery with the patient and a significant other. Instructions should also be written, preferably in large type, so that they may be reviewed as necessary after discharge. Special postoperative instructions that pertain to patients for ophthalmic surgery may include self administration of eye drops, proper application of the protective eye shield, face-down or other positioning techniques after retina surgery, and emphasis on stringent handwashing for prevention of infection. For enucleated cases with hydroxyapatite orbital implant, multidisciplinary involvement may include referral to an ocularist. Care of the patient who undergoes day surgery is outlined in Chapter 46.

Ophthalmic surgical procedures for which patients may be admitted to the hospital for inpatient care include repair of ruptured globe caused by trauma, which requires intravenous antibiotics; application of radioactive plaque for eye tumors; glaucoma surgery that requires postoperative measurement of intraocular pressure, especially if the patient is monocular; and enucleation in children.

## DEFINITIONS

**Anterior Segment:** The intraocular segment of the eyeball occupied by the aqueous fluid that lies in front of and is separated from the vitreous-filled posterior segment by the lens and zonule of Zinn (also called ocular zonule); it is subdivided by the iris into anterior and posterior chambers.

**Blepharophimosis:** Horizontal narrowing of the palpebral fissures (eye slits).

**Blepharoplasty:** Surgical repair of the eyelid. Often performed for ptosis or blepharophimosis of the eyelid (Fig. 33-1).

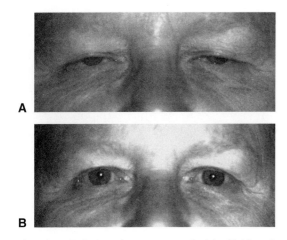

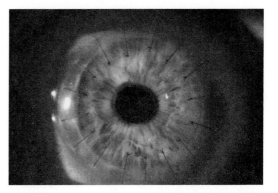

**Fig. 33-1** **A,** Preoperative appearance of adult with bilateral ptosis. **B,** Postoperative appearance after bilateral ptosis repair. *(Courtesy of Dr. Robert B. Penne, Wills Eye Hospital, Philadelphia.)*

**Fig. 33-3** Traditional corneal grafts with use of penetrating keratoplasty require variety of suturing techniques. Evolving DLEK procedure negates use of sutures and may decrease risk of infection, ulceration, and perforation of cornea. *(Courtesy of Dr. Christopher J. Rapuano, Thomas Jefferson University Hospital, Philadelphia.)*

**Cataract:** Opacity of the lens. Surgical treatment consists of removal of the lens.

**Chalazion:** A chronic granulomatous inflammation of one or more of the meibomian glands in the tarsal plate of the eyelid. Surgical treatment consists of incision and curettage.

**Choroid:** The vascular layer of the eye that lies between the retina and the sclera.

**Choroidal Melanoma:** The most common primary intraocular tumor in adults (Fig. 33-2).

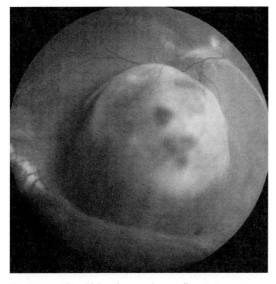

**Fig. 33-2** Choroidal melanoma is a malignant tumor composed of melanocytes: pigment that contains and produces cells normally present in choroid. Initially appearing as small freckle, it can grow and spread to other organs of body. *(Courtesy of Dr. C.L. Shields, Thomas Jefferson University Hospital, Philadelphia.)*

**Ciliary Body:** The part of the eye that contains the ciliary muscle and ciliary processes.

**Ciliary Muscle:** A smooth muscle that affects zonules, enabling changes in lens shape for light focusing.

**Ciliary Process:** Any of the radiating pigmented ridges on the inner surface of the ciliary body that, with the folds in the furrows between them, constitute the anterior portion of the ciliary body.

**Dacryocystitis:** Infection of the lacrimal sac.

**Dacryocystorhinostomy:** Creation of a new pathway from the lacrimal sac to the nasal cavity.

**Deep Lamellar Endothelial Keratoplasty (DLEK):** A new method of corneal transplant that uses a small incision that leaves the surface of the recipient cornea untouched (Fig. 33-3).

**Dermatochalasis:** Relaxation of the skin of the eyelid because of atrophy. Surgical treatment is blepharoplasty.

**Ectropion:** Eversion of the margin of the eyelid. Surgical treatment is shortening of the lower lid in a horizontal direction (Fig. 33-4).

**Entropion:** Inversion of the margin of the eyelid; this condition usually affects the lower lid but may affect the upper lid. Surgical treatment involves either removing a base triangle of skin, muscle, and tarsus and suturing the edges together to evert the lid margin or exposing the orbicular muscle, dividing it, and suturing it to the lower border of the tarsus (Fig. 33-5).

**Enucleation:** Removal of the entire eyeball after the eye muscles and optic nerve have been severed.

**Epiphora:** Excess tearing; epiphora may be caused by a blocked lacrimal drainage system.

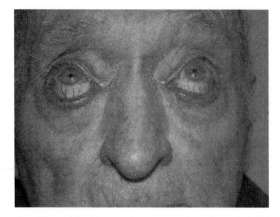

**Fig. 33-4** Bilateral ectropions; outward turning of eyelid margins. *(Courtesy of Dr. Edward H. Bedrossian, Jr, Thomas Jefferson University Hospital, Philadelphia.)*

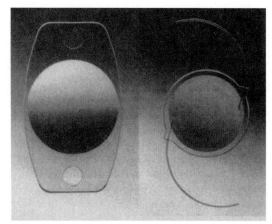

**Fig. 33-6** Examples of intraocular lens implants used today. *(Courtesy of Wills Eye Hospital, Philadelphia.)*

Surgical treatment for epiphora and dacryocystitis caused by blockage is probing of the lacrimal duct.

**Evisceration of the Eye:** Removal of the contents of the eye, with the sclera left intact and the muscles attached to the sclera.

**Exenteration of the Eye:** Radical removal of all orbital contents, usually for unresectable malignant tumors of the eyelids, conjunctiva, intraocular structures, and orbit. In many cases, an eyelid-sparing technique may be used to expedite healing.[4]

**Glaucoma:** A disease of the eye characterized by increased intraocular pressure. Surgical treatment is aimed at establishment of an evacuation route for outflow of aqueous fluid.

**Goniotomy:** Surgery for congenital glaucoma in which the trabecular meshwork is incised.

**Hydroxyapatite Implant:** An orbital implant made of natural material derived from ocean coral that resembles human bone in chemical and porous structure. After enucleation, the eye muscles can be attached directly to this implant, thus allowing it to move within the orbit just like the natural eye.

**Intraocular Lens (IOL) Implant:** Synthetic lens used to replace the crystalline lens after cataract extraction surgery. The latest versions include a soft foldable multifocal lens that can fit through 1.4-mm or smaller incisions, which allows for faster healing and significantly improved vision (Fig. 33-6).

**Keratoplasty:** Transplantation of a portion of the entire thickness of the cornea (Fig. 33-7).

**Lacrimal Punctum:** The opening of either the upper or the lower lacrimal duct at the inner canthus of the eye.

**LASIK (Laser-Assisted in Situ Keratomileusis):** A corneal procedure in which the excimer laser is used to reshape the cornea and thus correct farsightedness (hyperopia), nearsightedness (myopia), and astigmatism.

**Miosis:** Contraction of the pupil; the opposite of mydriasis.

**Mydriasis:** Dilation of the pupils induced by eyedrops; the opposite of miosis.

**Oculocardiac Reflex (OCR):** A decrease in pulse rate associated with traction on extraocular muscles or compression of the eyeball; especially sensitive in children; may produce bradycardia, junctional rhythm, and asystole.

**Phacoemulsification:** The procedure of fragmentation of the lens with ultrasound vibrations combined with aspiration for cataract surgery (Fig. 33-8).

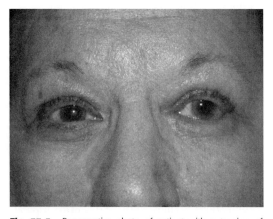

**Fig. 33-5** Preoperative photo of patient with entropion of left lower lid. Entropion is inward rotation of eyelid margin. *(Courtesy of Dr. Edward H. Bedrossian, Jr., Thomas Jefferson University Hospital, Philadelphia.)*

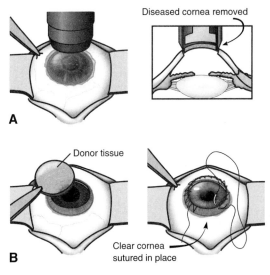

**Fig. 33-7** Corneal transplant surgery. **A,** Diseased cornea is removed. **B,** Donor corneal tissue is placed in opening and is sewn in place with fine suture. *(Courtesy of the Department of Medical Illustration and Audio Visual Education, Baylor College of Medicine, Houston.)*

**Plaque:** A radioactive device (that usually contains iodine 125) that is surgically applied to the sclera over an intraocular neoplasm. It is used to treat retinoblastoma and choroidal melanoma.

**Presbyopia:** A condition in which the lens of the eye loses its ability to focus. The condition is associated with aging and is progressive. People with presbyopia have difficulty seeing objects up close.

**Proliferative Diabetic Retinopathy:** The latter stages of diabetic retinopathy in which new abnormal blood vessels grow on the surface of the retina, which leads to vitreous hemorrhage and detachment of the retina.

**Proptosis:** Protrusion of the eyeball.

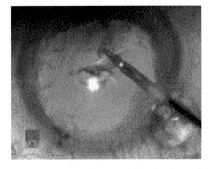

**Fig. 33-8** Microincision phacoemulsification is a technologic advance that allows surgeon to operate through wounds nearly half the size of usual phacoemulsification. *(From Alio J, Rodriguez-Prats JL, Ramzy GA: Outcomes of microincision cataract surgery versus coaxial phacoemulsification, Ophthalmology 112(11):1999, 2005.)*

**Pterygium:** A fleshy triangular growth that extends from the conjunctiva and encroaches on the cornea. Surgical treatment is excision.

**Ptosis:** Drooping of the upper eyelid. Surgical treatment involves either elevating the lid with a sling or shortening the levator muscle of the lid (levator resection).

**Retinoblastoma:** Malignant retinal tumor of infancy.

**Retinopexy:** Surgical correction of retinal detachment (Fig. 33-9) with sealing of the hole. Sealing is accomplished by causing scar formation with heat, electric current, or cryotherapy.

**Scleral Buckle:** Surgical correction of a retinal detachment with compression of the sclera to rejoin the underlying retinal pigment epithelium to the detached sensory retina; used in conjunction with retinopexy.

**Strabismus:** Condition in which the eyes are not simultaneously directed toward the same object. Esotropia is inward deviation of the eyes; exotropia is outward deviation. Surgical treatment involves changing the relative strength of individual muscles either with resection (the shortening of a muscle with removal of part of the tendon) or with recession (the surgical transfer of a muscle insertion backward from the original attachment on the eye).

**Tonometer:** A hand-held noncontact instrument used for measurement of intraocular pressure in postoperative eyes.

**Topical Anesthesia:** The topical application of local anesthetic that dispenses with akinetic anesthesia with use of regional blocks. Topical anesthesia avoids anesthesia-related complications (e.g., retrobulbar hemorrhage, globe perforation).

**Trabecular Meshwork:** A group of tiny canals through which most of the fluid in the eye drains.

**Trabeculectomy:** Creation of a drainage channel from the anterior chamber to the subconjunctival space; used for treatment of intractable glaucoma.

**Vitrectomy:** Surgical removal of the vitreous gel from the eye, usually to clear blood or opacified vitreous fluid that blocks sight or to sever vitreous traction bands that pull on the retina and detach it. The clouded gel is replaced with specialized gas or silicone oil (Fig. 33-10).

**Vitreous Fluid:** A clear jelly-like substance that fills the posterior chamber of the eyeball.

**Vitreous Hemorrhage:** Bleeding into the vitreous fluid as a result of the vitreous pulling away from and tearing the retina.

**Zonule of Zinn:** A ring of fibrous strands that connects the ciliary body with the crystalline lens of the eye.

NURSING CARE IN THE PACU

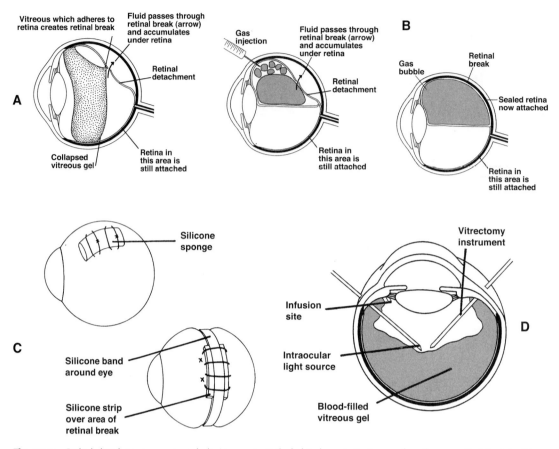

**Fig. 33-9** Retinal detachment surgery and vitrectomy. **A,** Retinal detachment; **B,** Pneumatic retinopexy; **C,** Scleral buckling; **D,** Vitrectomy. *(Courtesy of Wills Eye Hospital, Philadelphia.)*

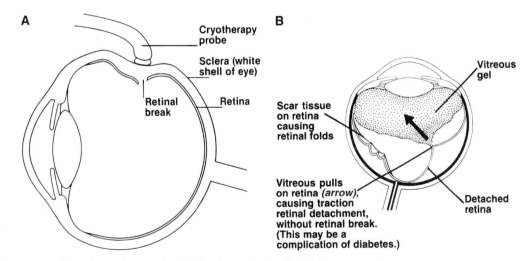

**Fig. 33-10** **A,** Cryotherapy is process in which freezing probe is applied briefly to outside of eyewall to promote sealing of retinal hole. **B,** Traction retinal detachment for which patient may undergo vitrectomy. *(Courtesy of Wills Eye Hospital, Philadelphia.)*

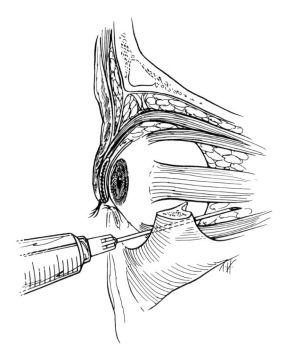

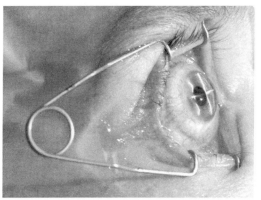

**Fig. 33-12** Speculum used for LASIK procedure separates eyelids widely. *(In McLeod SD, McDonnell, PJ: Refractive surgery, Ophthalmol Clin North Am 14(2):288, 2001. Copyright 2001. Ray Swords Photography [swordsra@mindspring.com].)*

**Fig. 33-11** Retrobulbar anesthesia. Injection with 31-mm 26-gauge needle carried out with eye in primary position. Injection begins at inferotemporal orbital margin, and needle is aimed at lower edge of superior orbital fissure. *(From Spaeth GL: Ophthalmic surgery: principles and practice, ed 3, Philadelphia, 2003, Saunders.)*

## ANESTHESIA

Many anesthetic methods and agents are available in ophthalmology surgery. The type of anesthesia used is based on factors such as the type of ocular surgery to be performed, the patient's medical status, and the patient's pain and anxiety level.[5] Ophthalmic procedures are most often performed with monitored anesthesia care (MAC) with the administration of intravenous sedation in conjunction with local anesthesia. Local anesthetic agents can be administered topically or intraocularly or via block injection. Midazolam, fentanyl, and propofol are administered in the preoperative area before the block injection. Commonly used local anesthetics for eye surgery are bupivicaine, mepivacaine, lidocaine, and procaine. The type of block (retrobulbar, peribulbar, parabulbar, subconjunctival, lid, or facial) also depends on the type of surgery. Risks of local anesthesia are injection into the optic nerve, globe perforation, or retrobulbar hemorrhage with peribulbar and retrobulbar blocks (Fig. 33-11). The perianesthesia nurse should be alert to the potential for these complications, although they are rare. Facial drooping on the side of the operated eye after a facial nerve block is sometimes present on the patient's arrival to the PACU. Usually this condition resolves as the anesthetic wears off.

Topical anesthesia is used more often in less invasive, relatively atraumatic, and short duration procedures. Patients should understand the sensations that may be experienced during surgery, and they should be able to tolerate the lid speculum (Fig 33-12). Monocular patients are well suited for topical anesthesia because of the unique need for quick recovery of vision from the operated eye. Tetracaine (0.5%) and proparacaine (0.5%) are generally used. Injection agents, such as bupivacaine (0.75%), mepivicaine (4%), and lidocaine (1.0% to 4.0%), may also be used topically. Benefits of topical anesthesia include avoidance of the risks associated with general, retrobulbar, and peribulbar anesthesia. Patients have better visual acuity immediately after surgery and less pain.[7] Another advantage of topical anesthesia is that anticoagulant or antiplatelet therapy does not need to be interrupted. In some practice settings, eye procedures of short duration, such as nasolacrimal duct probing, may be performed on children with topical 5% cocaine placed on the lacrimal punctum with a cotton-tipped applicator.[6] A disadvantage to topical anesthesia may be the patient's awareness during surgery, the feeling of the speculum, the microscopic light, and the potential sensation of pain. In the preoperative setting, the perianesthesia nurse should report to the surgeon if the patient is apprehensive or confused or has language problems; in these cases, topical anesthesia may not be the best technique.[6]

Infants, children, uncooperative or particularly anxious patients, and mentally challenged persons usually need general anesthesia. General anesthesia is also indicated when a local anesthetic might exacerbate an eye problem; when surgery is to be performed on a lacerated cornea, ruptured globe, for optic nerve decompression; or when the surgery planned is extensive, as in enucleation or evisceration. The goals of general anesthesia for ophthalmic surgery include a smooth induction with stable intraocular pressure, avoidance or treatment of severe oculocardiac (OCR) reflexes, maintenance of a motionless field, a smooth emergence, and avoidance of postoperative nausea and vomiting (PONV).[7] The patient for ophthalmic surgery who undergoes general anesthesia is assessed and receives care as described in Chapters 27 and 28. The special precaution for these patients is modifications in care that must be made to prevent stress on the eyes and surrounding musculature. Intraocular pressure may be increased significantly during emergence from general anesthesia. Coughing, straining, bucking, breath-holding, obstructed airway, or Valsalva's maneuvers can elevate the intraocular pressure as much as 30 to 40 mm Hg.[7] The perianesthesia nurse must respond immediately, with collaboration with anesthesiology, to treat emergence delirium and help to ensure an optimal surgical outcome.[7]

## PERIANESTHESIA CARE

### Preoperative period
Patients are generally more apprehensive about procedures performed on the eyes than about procedures performed on other parts of the body.[7] In many cases, patients may be facing repeat eye surgery for conditions such as recurrent retinal detachment after failed scleral buckle, failed corneal graft, retained lens fragments, retinal detachment, or IOL dislocation subsequent to cataract extraction.[8] Patients awaiting enucleation may worry about how the loss of an eye will affect appearance and lifestyle.[9] Parents of premature infants scheduled for eye surgery may have fears regarding the possibility of poor functional vision outcomes for their child.[10] In the busy perianesthesia setting, the nurse must maximize opportunities for promotion of an environment in which the patients and parents express feelings and concerns. Interventions include active listening, validation of the patient's fears, and reassurance to the patient that anxiety and fear are normal and expected responses to upcoming eye surgery.[9]

In keeping with universal protocol mandates, the perianesthesia nurse participates in the preoperative verification process by properly identifying the patient's name and birthdate, asking the patient to state and point to the eye that is to be operated on, and documenting when the ophthalmologist initials the skin over the brow of that eye.[11] The nurse assigned to the anesthesia holding room may also be asked to administer eye drops to dilate the pupils and block accommodation for surgery. Eye drops commonly ordered are cyclopentolate hydrochloride (1%), phenylephrine (2.5%), and tropicamide (1%). Compression of the lacrimal punctum during and after administration of eye drops minimizes the potential of systemic reaction to the drops.[12]

### Postoperative Nursing Management
The patient is usually awake on arrival in the PACU. Immediate postoperative assessment of the cardiorespiratory system should proceed as described in Chapters 27 and 28. Vital signs are monitored, and the stir-up regimen is started. One challenge is to keep the patient's lungs clear without an increase in intraocular pressure. Deep rhythmic breaths at frequent intervals assist in the prevention of atelectasis. The nurse should coach the patient in deep inspirations and concentration on breathing to help avoid coughing. Sucking on ice chips or throat lozenges may soothe the throat and prevent coughing. Antitussives and opioids are generally not prescribed in the PACU, however, if coughing persists and cannot be controlled, the surgeon must be notified.

### Positioning
The nurse should begin to orient the patient as soon as the patient enters the PACU. To avoid any startle reflexes, a warning is of particular importance before moving or touching the ophthalmic patient. Every caution is observed when the patient is transferred from stretcher to bed to avoid bumping and jarring. Movement should be slow and smooth and kept to a minimum. The patient's head should be positioned comfortably so that straining of the neck does not occur.

Specific instructions on head positioning are provided by the surgeon and vary according to the type of eye surgery. For retinal reattachment surgery, a face-down position commonly is ordered to promote continuing reattachment. The patient assumes this position only when fully recovered from the anesthetic. The head of the stretcher generally is elevated at least 30 degrees for patients with oculoplastic, eye muscle, and enucleation surgeries. Care should be taken to prevent pressure on the operated eye.

**Table 33-1  Drugs Administered to Patients Undergoing Eye Surgery**

| Ophthalmic Indication | Drug | Mechanism of Action | Systemic Effect |
|---|---|---|---|
| Miosis | Acetylcholine | Cholinergic agonist | Bronchospasm, bradycardia, hypotension |
| Glaucoma (increased intraocular pressure) | Acetazolamide | Carbonic anhydrase inhibitor | Diuresis, hypokalemic metabolic acidosis |
| | Echothiophate | Irreversible cholinesterase inhibitor | Prolongation of succinylcholine's effects Reduction in plasma cholinesterase activity up to 3-7 wk after discontinuation |
| | Timolol | β-Adrenergic antagonist | Bradycardia, bronchospasm Atropine-resistant bradycardia, bronchospasm, exacerbation of congestive heart failure; possible exacerbation of myasthenia gravis |
| Mydriasis, ophthalmic capillary decongestion | Atropine | Anticholinergic | Central anticholinergic syndrome ("mad as a hatter," delirum, agitation; "hot as a hare," fever; "red as a beet," flushing; "dry as a bone," xerostomia, anhidrosis) Blurred vision (cycloplegia, photophobia) |
| | Cyclopentolate | Anticholinergic | Disorientation, psychosis, convulsions, dysarthria |
| | Epinephrine | α-Adrenergic agonist, β-Adrenergic agonist | Hypertension, tachycardia, cardiac dysrhythmias; epinephrine paradoxically leads to decreased intraocular pressure and can also be used for glaucoma |
| | Phenylephrine | α-Adrenergic agonist, β-Adrenergic agonist, direct-acting vasopressor | Hypertension (one drop, or 0.05 mL, of a 10% solution contains 5 mg of phenylephrine) |
| | Scopolamine | Anticholinergic | Central anticholinergic syndrome (see atropine) |

From Stoelting R, Miller R: *Basics of anesthesia*, ed 5, Philadelphia, Churchill Livingstone, 2007.

If the patient has had an operation on only one eye or has only one eye bandaged, determination of just how much sight exists in the unaffected eye is important. The assumption is not safe that the patient can see with the unoperated eye. The patient who cannot see out of the unaffected eye may agree to wear a patch on the unaffected eye, which serves to remind the nursing personnel that the patient is sightless and needs additional care. The nurse should explain all nursing actions and tell the patient exactly what is expected.

Special cardiorespiratory situations may arise related to the patient's eye condition or surgery (Table 33-1). Vasovagal syncope is not uncommon in the PACU after eye surgery. The patient becomes lightheaded, nauseated, and flushed; feels warm; and may even lose consciousness for several seconds. Immediate therapy includes intravenous fluids, oxygen, lowering the head of the stretcher, and raising the feet. If the patient has symptomatic bradycardia and hypotension that does not respond to these interventions, atropine, glycopyrrolate, or ephedrine may be ordered.

The use of intravenous mannitol for its ocular hypotensive effect during eye surgery increases the potential for congestive heart failure in elderly patients or in patients with poor cardiac output. The supine position for eye surgery tends to compound this potential because a nonupright position can cause abdominal organs to shift to the chest, preventing sufficient lung expansion.[8] Many patients with eye problems use ophthalmic medications that may interact with the medications used in anesthesia.[13] Patients with glaucoma who are treated with topical beta-blockers may have serious systemic effects from the eye drops, such as bradycardia, heart failure, hypotension, dysrhythmias, and myocardial infarction.[13] An understanding of these associated complications is necessary because these patients may need a medical doctor's evaluation and transfer to a tertiary facility for continued monitoring.

The OCR is a response to manipulation of eye muscles and tissue during surgery. Strabismus repair, retinal surgery, or direct pressure on the orbital contents can also trigger this reflex response. Bradycardia is the most common manifestation of OCR and may cause hypotension and dysrhythmias (junctional rhythm, ectopic atrial rhythm, atrioventricular rhythm, and ventricular bigeminy), which can continue into the postoperative period.[7,13]

Malignant hyperthermia (MH) may be more likely to develop in patients with strabismus because of the possibility of underlying myopathy.[13] The perianesthesia nurse should consider this increased risk for MH when caring for these patients before and after surgery because early recognition and efficient appropriate response are critical.

## Nausea and Vomiting

The increased incidence rate of PONV in patients for ophthalmologic surgery compared with many other types of surgery is well documented.[7,14,15] In particular, strabismus surgery is associated with PONV in more than 50% of pediatric patients.[7,13] PONV may lead to increased anxiety and bleeding in the PACU.[5] As a precaution, oral fluids and diet may be delayed for a brief period after general anesthesia. The anesthesia team often administers a prophylactic antiemetic regimen of ondansetron (Zofran), ranitidine (Zantac), metoclopromide (Reglan), or dexamethasone (Decadron), alone or in combination (see Chapter 29) The use of propofol infusion, with the anesthetic agent discontinued after induction, has also been shown to be effective in reduction of PONV in outpatient surgical settings.[7] In the PACU, patient movement should be minimized and hypotension avoided. If the patient has thirst, the mouth may be moistened with oral swabs dipped in ice water (with care taken to minimize stimulation of the oropharynx). Despite preventative measures, nausea and vomiting may still occur, and prompt recognition is important so treatment can begin without delay. Usual therapies are the administration of oxygen with nasal prongs or with the patient encouraged to breathe slowly and deeply to avoid retching, appropriate fluid volume replacement for treatment of hypovolemic hypotension, and antiemetics. Pediatric patients with nausea and vomiting in the PACU may receive ondansetron usually at a dose of 0.15 mg/kg intravenously.

The perianesthesia nurse must determine whether pain is contributing to nausea and vomiting. Although opioids can precipitate nausea, unrelieved eye pain and headache may actually require opioid administration to relieve nausea. Opioids can be especially effective if given in conjunction with antiemetics. Persistent nausea and vomiting accompanied by pain may indicate intraocular hemorrhage, which necessitates immediate intervention by the ophthalmologist.

## Pain Management

Many patients report no pain in the PACU after eye surgery. The patient is usually quite comfortable because of the residual effects of the local block, the intraoperative use of topical anesthesia, topical nonsteroidal antiinflamma-tory agents, and anticholinergics such as atro-pine and tropicamide, which paralyze the ciliary muscle. Ophthalmic ointments that con-tain antiinflammatory or antibiotic agents are often applied to the eye before patching. These ointments soothe the eye and promote comfort but may blur vision.

When localized pain in the eye does occur, it can be related to the use of surgical retractors (see Fig. 33-12), surgical wounds, and pressure dressings. Symptoms of itching, scratchy or grat-ing feelings, or a "pins and needles" sensation should be interpreted as pain and treated as such. Patients may also have headache, particu-larly after anterior segment surgery. Reassurance and acetaminophen are usually quite effective with these discomforts; however, codeine with acetaminophen (Tylenol #3) or oxycodone and acetaminophen (Percocet) may be prescribed by the surgeon if acetaminophen alone does not provide adequate pain relief.[5]

Injuries to the eyes and the surrounding tissue are quite common after blunt or penetrating facial trauma and often result in emergency eye surgery.[7] Pain from intraocular foreign bodies, eyelid lacerations, orbital fractures, and sharp injuries to the globe may be quite intense. The administration of opioids may be necessary to control pain. If fentanyl, morphine sulfate, or other opiates are necessary for pain relief, they should be used in conjunction with an anti-emetic to decrease the chance of nausea and vomiting. Eye pain in some adult patients for same-day surgery may be treated with intrave-nous or intramuscular ketorolac (Toradol). However, ketorolac is generally not used for patients with oculoplastic procedures or proce-dures in which bleeding may be a postoperative concern. Infants and children should be assessed for pain and medicated depending on age, surgi-cal procedure performed, and severity of pain.

Corneal abrasion is an ocular injury that can occur during the perioperative period, usually to the unoperated eye. The patient may report blurry vision, sensitivity to light, and tearing in the PACU. Pain during blinking occurs because of chafing of the eyelid against the corneal abrasion. Early detection and intervention by the PACU nurse may help to avoid corneal erosion. Gentle irrigation with ophthalmic eye wash often allevi-ates irritation from residual surgical preparation, but the ophthalmologist should be called to exam-ine the patient. Antibiotic ointment and patching may be ordered for more painful abrasions. Although corneal abrasions usually resolve quickly, careful attention by the perianesthesia nurse to prevent an occurrence is recommended.[16]

Moist, cold, or iced compresses are routinely ordered for patients who are recovering from oculoplastic procedures and eye muscle surgery. The compresses help prevent swelling and pro-mote comfort. Compresses should be lightweight and may be applied to the surgical eye in awake patients as early as possible for 15 to 20 min-utes.[5] The perianesthesia nurse should be alert to the possibility of OCR being elicited by pres-sure on the eye and should remove the com-presses at once if symptoms occur.

**Intraocular Pressure**

The potential for increased intraocular pressure is an important consideration in the care of patients after ophthalmic surgery.[17] As described previously, prompt management of pain, nausea, and vomiting is indispensable in promoting patient comfort and avoiding ocular injury. Other factors associated with increased intraocu-lar pressure that should be avoided are coughing, bucking, breath-holding, obstructive airway, or straining, as in Valsalva's maneuver.[7] The exer-tion of hard crying, often a problem with chil-dren and infants, should be minimized as much as possible. Some children respond well to being held by the nurse, or if feasible, a parent may be called to the PACU to hold the child. Because exertion against restraints increases intraocular pressure, patients should not be restrained. In both children and adults, benzodiazepines may be needed to ensure patient cooperation and a smooth recovery course.

Excessive lid swelling, periorbital swelling, or evidence of proptosis and abnormally severe symptoms of eye pain should be promptly reported to the patient's surgeon. Diffuse perior-bital pain may indicate acute glaucoma, a serious postoperative complication of eye surgery.[7] Acute glaucoma may occur after glaucoma surgery, cataract extraction, corneal transplanta-tion, and vitreoretinal surgery.[7,18] For significant pain that is not relieved with the prescribed analgesics, an ophthalmologist must be con-sulted immediately. In cases of suspected ocular hypertension, the ophthalmologist may measure the intraocular pressure in the PACU with a pneumatic tonometer (Fig. 33-13).

**Dressings**

Dressings are not always necessary, especially after relatively minor procedures, topical anesthesia, or plastic ophthalmic surgery. Often one or both of the eyes are bandaged with sterile eye patches. If bandages are present, they should not be disturbed. The patient must be prevented from disturbing the bandage or inadvertently rubbing the eyes. After enucleation, a firm

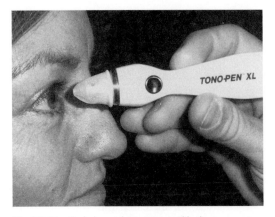

**Fig. 33-13**  Technique of tonometry with the pneumoton-ometer. *(Courtesy of Wills Eye Hospital, Philadelphia, 2002.)*

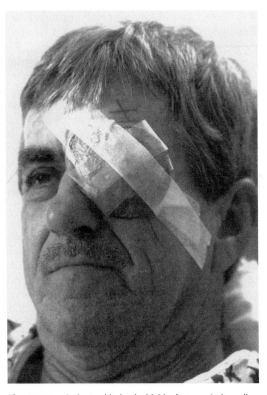

**Fig. 33-14**  Patient with lead shield after surgical applica-tion of iodine plaque. *(Courtesy of Wills Eye Hospital, Philadelphia.)*

pressure dressing is applied for 24 hours. An alternative to enucleation for treatment of ocular tumors is the use of iodine plaque irradia-tion. The iodine plaque is sutured over the base of the tumor with local anesthesia. The plaque remains in place for a calculated amount of time, depending on the strength of the iodine plaque and the size of the tumor. A lead shield is placed over the operative eye to protect the health care personnel and visitors from radiation exposure (Fig. 33-14).

Hemorrhage or excessive discharge is uncom-mon. A slight blood-tinged watery discharge from the eyes is not unusual and may be gently wiped from the face, with care taken not to apply pressure to the eye. Although infrequent, hem-orrhage may be a problem after enucleation, exenteration, or orbital surgery. If bleeding occurs in the PACU, the surgeon may be able to control it with pressure, but in some instances, the patient may need to return to the operating room.

Whenever both eyes are bandaged, extra care must be taken to orient the patient and to pro-vide reassurance. Eye shields made of clear plas-tic or perforated metal may be placed alone or over the dressing as an additional protection for the eye. Dressings should not be changed unless ordered by the surgeon, and if they are acciden-tally dislodged, they should be replaced and the physician notified. The tape used to hold eye patches or shields in place should not extend to the maxilla because movement of the jaw may cause disruption of the dressing. The perianesthesia nurse should reinforce the shield as necessary.

## Psychologic Aspects of Care

Perianesthesia care of patients after ophthalmic surgery requires not only keen physical assessment skills but also a serious sensitivity to the meaning of sight. A proactive creative approach to promoting comfort and preventing complications is essential.

The perianesthesia nurse must be prepared to provide significant support through both verbal communication and gentle touch. Unnecessary noise can be especially annoying to visually impaired patients and can heighten feelings of stress and pain. Promotion of a quiet peaceful PACU environment helps soothe patients who may be worried or nervous about the outcome regarding vision.

Some patients may leave the PACU fully recovered from the anesthetic and elated with the immediate result of improved vision. Blepharoplasty, one of the most common eye cosmetic surgeries, offers patients hope of a desired esthetic outcome. Even patients with the disfiguring effects of facial palsy can have excellent results from oculoplastic surgery to correct brow ptosis and paralytic ectropion.[5] Most patients, however, have some degree of emotional distress and may need a great deal of empathy and reassurance.[19] Eyes and the sense of sight are precious, and when sight is threatened by disease or surgery, individuals are understandably anxious and apprehensive. Injuries, particularly those produced by imbedded foreign bodies, may provoke even greater anxiety for the patient who goes to surgery with the prognosis for visual acuity completely unknown. Loss of an eye and vision from cancer may give rise to feelings of powerlessness, anger, and profound sadness.[9] The perianesthesia nurse must be armed with factual information from the surgeon about expectations for the patient so that reassurances are realistic.

## SUMMARY

As eye surgery continues to change from the traditional hospital PACU to more diverse practice settings, the perianesthesia nurse's role is expanding; advocacy and interpersonal understanding are as important as hemodynamic monitoring and pain management. PACU nurses who participate in evidence-based practice studies, which investigate critical events after eye surgery, may help to ensure that adequate staffing patterns are maintained.[20] A collaborative approach with other members of the perianesthesia and surgical teams and a holistic picture of patients' needs are crucial to avoiding complications and ensuring optimal outcomes for patients after ophthalmic surgery.

## REFERENCES

1. Niehbuhr BS, Muenzen P: A study of perianesthesia nursing practice: the foundation for newly revised CPAN and CAPA certification examinations, *J Perianesth Nurs* 16(3):163-173, 2001.
2. Singh RP, Lewis H: Innovations in eye surgery, *Clin Geriatric Med* 22(3):659-675, 2006.
3. Proliferative diabetic retinopathy, *Insight J Am Soc Ophthal Reg Nurses* 26(3):88-91, 2001.
4. Shields JA, Shields CL, Demirci H, et al: Experience with eyelid-sparing orbital exenteration: the 2000 Tullos O. Coston Lecture (electric version), *Am Soc Ophthal Plast Reconstr Surg* 17(5):355-361, 2001.
5. Della Rocca RC, Bedrossian EH Jr, Arthurs BP: *Ophthalmic plastic surgery: decision making and techniques,* New York, 2002, McGraw-Hill.
6. Livingston M: Cataract surgery with topical anesthesia-a mixed blessing, *J Cataract Refractive Surg* 29(11):2248, 2003.
7. Spaeth GL: *Ophthalmic surgery: principles and practice,* ed 3, Saunders, Philadelphia, 2003.
8. Arbisser LB, Charles S, Howcroft M, et al: Management of vitreous loss and dropped nucleus during cataract surgery, *Ophthal Clin North Am* 19(4):495-506, 2006.
9. Carpenito-Moyet LJ: *Nursing care plans & documentation: nursing diagnoses and collaborative problems,* ed 4, Philadelphia, 2004, Lippincott Williams & Wilkins.
10. Lakhanpal R, Sun RL, Albini TA, et al: Anatomic success rate after 3-port lens-sparing vitrectomy in stage 4a or 4b retinopathy of prematurity, *Ophthalmology* 112(9):1569-1573, 2005.
11. Dunn D: Surgical site verification: A through Z, *J PeriAnesthesia Nurs* 21(5):317-331, 2006.
12. Williams LS, Hopper PD: *Understanding medical surgical nursing,* ed 2, Philadelphia, 2003, F.A. Davis.
13. Stoelting R, Miller R: *Basics of anesthesia,* ed 5, Philadelphia, 2007, Churchill Livingstone.
14. Williams KS: Postoperative nausea and vomiting, *Surg Clin North Am* 85(6):1229-1241, 2005.
15. Gregory GA: *Pediatric anesthesia,* ed 4, New York, 2002, Churchill Livingstone.
16. Moos D, Lind D: Detection and treatment of perioperative corneal abrasions, *J PeriAnesthesia Nurs* 21(5):332-341, 2006.
17. Spaeth GL: The use of antimetabolites with trabeculectomy: a critical appraisal, *J Glaucoma* 10(3):145-150, 2001.
18. Anderson N, Fineman M, Brown G: Incidence of intraocular pressure spike and other adverse events after vitreoretinal surgery, *Am Acad Ophthalmol* 113(1):42-47, 2005.
19. Scott IU, Schein OD, Feuer WJ: Emotional distress in patients with retinal disease, *Am J Ophthalmol* 131(5):584-589, 2001.
20. Channel DA, Navarro VB, Nolan MT: An evidence-based practice study: critical events following eye surgery in one ophthalmicx PACU, *Insight J Am Soc Ophthal Reg Nurses* 27(4):92-94, 2002.

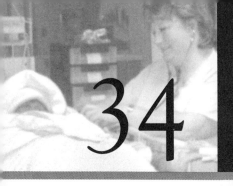

# 34

# CARE OF THE THORACIC SURGICAL PATIENT

*Jan Odom-Forren, RN, BSN, MS, CPAN, FAAN*

Thoracic surgery involves procedures in the structures within the chest cavity, including the lungs, heart, great vessels, and esophagus. In this chapter, discussion centers on procedures of the lungs and respiratory system. Specific postanesthesia care after cardiac surgery is discussed in Chapter 35, care after surgery of the great vessels is discussed in Chapter 36, and care after surgery of the esophagus is discussed in Chapter 40.

Lung surgery may be recommended for the diagnosis and treatment of:

- Persistent cough
- Hemoptysis
- Wheezing
- Obstruction
- Abnormal chest x-ray results
- Cancer
- Tumors (solitary pulmonary nodules)
- Small areas of long-term infection (highly localized tuberculosis or mycobacterium)
- Pockets of infection (abscess)
- Permanently enlarged (dilated) bronchus (bronchiectasis)
- Permanently enlarged (dilated) section of lung (lobar emphysema)
- Permanently collapsed lung tissue (atelectasis)
- Injuries with collapsed lung tissue (atelectasis, pneumothorax, hemothorax)
- Correction of congenital or acquired chest wall deformities

## DEFINITIONS

**Atelectasis:** Collapse of the alveoli, caused primarily by obstruction of lower airways. Most commonly, this obstruction is caused by accumulation of respiratory secretions, but it may also be caused by diminished lung volumes, tumors, prolonged bronchospasm, and foreign bodies.

**Bronchoscopy:** Direct visualization of the tracheobronchial tree with use of a lighted scope (Fig. 34-1). It is used for diagnostic and therapeutic interventions for visualization of structures of the tracheobronchial tree; removal of secretions, washings, mucus plugs, or foreign bodies; and performance of a tissue biopsy or application of medication. Bronchoscopy may be combined with laser (YAG) therapy for ablation of tracheal and bronchial obstructions. It may be performed in the operating room, special procedures unit, or at the patient's bedside, depending on the degree of urgency and the patient's status.

**Chest Tube:** Placement of a drainage tube into the intrapleural space to remove air, fluid, or blood with the goal of restoring normal negative pressure and to allow reexpansion of the lung. The tube is placed on the operative side after open chest procedures.

**Chest Wall Reconstruction:** Repair of chest wall defects caused by trauma or tumor, with use of muscle or omentum (underlying abdominal tissue). It provides for protection of underlying structures and organs and provides support for respiration.

**Decortication of the Lung:** Removal of fibrous deposits or restrictive membranes on the visceral or parietal pleura that interfere with ventilatory action. The goal is restoration of normal lung function.

**Hemothorax:** Accumulation of blood or serosanguineous fluid or both within the pleural cavity, compromising lung expansion.

**Lobectomy:** Removal of one or more lobes of the lung. Lobectomy is the preferred procedure when a cancerous lesion involves a single lobe of the lung. It is used primarily in the treatment of bronchial cancer and is also used in the treatment of bronchiectasis, emphysematous blebs, large benign tumors, fungal infections, and congenital anomalies.

**Mediastinoscopy:** Direct visualization of lymph nodes or tumors at the tracheobronchial junction, subcarina, or upper lobe bronchi via a lighted scope. This procedure is done by passing the mediastinoscope through a small incision at the suprasternal area and then down along the anterior course of the trachea. It is a diagnostic procedure for patients with identified changes on chest x-ray results.

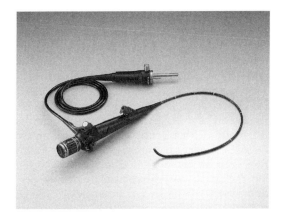

**Fig. 34-1** Flexible fiber-optic bronchoscope. *(Courtesy Olympus America., Inc, Melville, NY.)*

**Needle Biopsy:** Insertion of a needle with subsequent aspiration of lung tissue or fluid for diagnostic purposes. It is generally performed with local anesthesia via a percutaneous approach.

**Pneumonectomy:** Removal of an entire lung, most commonly for lung cancer when lobectomy cannot be performed for total removal of bronchial cancer.

**Pneumothorax:** Accumulation of air or gas within the pleural cavity, thus compromising lung expansion. Pneumothorax may occur as direct result of a thoracotomy incision or after chest wall trauma such as a stab wound.

**Segmentectomy (Segmental Resection):** Excision of individual bronchovascular segments of the lobe of the lung with ligation of segmental branches of the pulmonary artery and vein and division of the segmental bronchus. Segmentectomy conserves healthy tissue while allowing for removal of localized lesion.

**Sleeve Resection:** Surgical removal of part of the bronchi, with healthy tissue left for reanastomosis, thus preserving some tissue and lung function. Sleeve resection is used primarily for metastatic disease in either the right or left upper bronchus.

**Sternotomy:** Incision through the sternum.

**Thoracentesis:** Insertion of a needle through the chest wall into the pleural space to remove either air or fluid to relieve lung compression or for diagnostic purposes. Removed fluid is evaluated for chemical, bacteriologic, and cellular composition. This procedure may be performed at the bedside, generally with local anesthesia.

**Thoracoplasty/Thoracostomy:** Removal of ribs or portions of the ribs to reduce the size of the thoracic space and to collapse a diseased lung.

**Thoracoscopy:** The insertion of an endoscope, a narrow-diameter tube with a viewing mirror or camera attachment, through a small incision in the chest wall for examination of the lungs or other structures in the chest cavity, without a large incision. The procedure may be diagnostic or therapeutic.

**Thoracotomy:** Incision into the chest cavity that may be used as a diagnostic tool to diagnose or stage cancer. It provides a definitive diagnosis in more than 90% of cases. Closed thoracotomy is used to place chest tubes or catheters for drainage of air or fluid to restore normal negative pressure within pleural space. It also may be used to create a surgical access port for video-assisted lobectomy and other endoscopic procedures.

**Transplantation:** Removal of a diseased recipient lung with an immediate replacement of a cadaveric donor lung.

**Volume Reduction Surgery:** Incision and removal of those parts of the lung that are the most destroyed, most commonly from emphysema, to allow for full function of remaining lung structures.

**Wedge Resection:** Excision of a small wedge-shaped section from the peripheral portion of the lobe of a lung that is commonly used to remove cancerous growths in the outer section of the lung to spare lung tissue and function.

## ANESTHESIA

Invasive surgery that involves the chest cavity is generally performed with general anesthesia, although diagnostic procedures such as bronchoscopy, needle biopsy, and thoracentesis are commonly performed with local (topical) anesthesia, often with small titrated amounts of intravenous sedation. Epidural catheters may also be placed before surgery for use during surgery and for extended postoperative pain control after pneumonectomy or lobectomy. Because these procedures all involve the airway in addition to anesthesia, patients are given nothing by mouth status (NPO) before any procedure.

Topical anesthesia involves the instillation or spray of a local anesthetic, commonly 4% lidocaine hydrochloride (Xylocaine), onto the laryngeal and pharyngeal surfaces. Although uncommon, toxic reactions or bronchospasm can occur; therefore, emergency equipment should be readily available. Recovery of the patient after topical anesthesia requires airway assessment, ready availability of emergency resuscitation equipment, and the administration of humidified oxygen after the procedure. The patient must be given nothing by mouth until the pharyngeal and laryngeal reflexes have returned (2 to 4 hours). Patients should be advised to rest their voices after the procedure; in fact, the surgeon may prescribe a time interval for voice rest. Once the gag reflex has returned, throat lozenges and warm drinks may help to relieve the sore throat that inevitably follows bronchoscopy.

Epidural anesthesia involves placement of a catheter into the epidural space of the thoracic vertebrae with subsequent instillation of an infusion combination of an opioid and local anesthetic to achieve sensory blockade of pain without compromising motor function needed for coughing, deep breathing, and ambulating. The catheter may be left in place for up to 3 days after surgery for pain control and may be regulated solely by medical personnel or controlled by the patient. Epidural anesthesia is commonly used as an adjunct to general anesthesia.

General anesthesia involves the administration of some combination of inhalational anesthetics, intravenous anesthetics, benzodiazepines, opioids, muscle relaxants, and reversal agents and aims to render the patient amnestic and pain free. Somatic, autonomic, and endocrine reflexes are eliminated, and skeletal muscle relaxation is achieved. Because of the effects of general anesthesia on respiratory function and effort, in conjunction with a preexisting compromise in the respiratory system that necessitates surgery, nursing care must emphasize respiratory assessment, monitoring, and application of prompt intervention if evidence of compromise is noted after surgery.

## SURGICAL PROCEDURES

Surgical procedures can be diagnostic or therapeutic in nature. Diagnostic procedures can include bronchoscopy, mediastinoscopy, laryngoscopy, and thoracoscopy. Bronchoscopies are performed to visualize the airway or remove abnormal tissue, mucous plugs, or foreign bodies. They also aid in evaluation of lung lesions and staging of lung cancer. Complications can include airway obstruction, hypoxemia, pneumothorax, hemorrhage, or cardiovascular problems such as dysrhythmias or hypotension. Mediastinoscopy is performed for direct visualization of lymph nodes or tumors at the tracheobronchial junction, subcarina, or upper lobe bronchi via a lighted scope. Complications can include hemorrhage; venous air embolism; airway or esophageal injury, including subcutaneous emphysema; chest pain; or pneumothorax. Recurrent laryngeal nerve injury may occur, such as hoarseness or vocal cord paralysis. A laryngoscopy is performed to visualize or biopsy the oropharynx, laryngopharynx, larynx, or proximal trachea. Complications include trauma to the lips, mucous membranes, teeth, or eyes; rupture of the esophagus; hypoxemia; or laryngospasm.

Thoracoscopy is the insertion of an endoscope, a narrow-diameter tube with a viewing mirror or camera attachment, through a small incision in the chest wall for examination of the lungs or other structures in the chest cavity, without a large incision. Video-assisted thoracic surgery (VATS) is often performed with monitored anesthesia care and local anesthesia. VATS can be diagnostic or therapeutic and is used often for biopsy of mediastinal masses, to perform wedge resections, to obtain hemostasis, or to evacuate blood clots. A variety of procedures can be performed via thoracoscopy, from lung volume reduction to a biopsy and excision of mediastinal lesions. A significant advantage of thoracoscopy is that it is minimally invasive and results in less incisional pain. It can also decrease recovery time and length of hospital stay. In some facilities, patients come to the PACU with a small chest tube that is pulled if chest radiograph results are clear; the patient then is allowed to go home in a few hours.

Therapeutic thoracic surgeries may include pectus excavatum, chest wall reconstruction, wedge resection of a lung lesion, segmentectomy, lobectomy, or pneumonectomy. Excision of the right lung is less tolerated than removal of the left lung because of the larger vascular bed and breathing capacity. Other thoracic surgeries include lung volume reduction, for removal of emphysematous lung tissue, or lung transplant.

## PERIANESTHESIA NURSING CARE AFTER THORACIC PROCEDURES

Admission assessment in the PACU is the same as for any other surgical patient (see Chapters 27 and 28). Some specific issues for the patient after thoracic surgery are discussed.

### Positioning

Positioning after thoracic procedures varies; therefore, medical orders must be checked. The patient may be kept in a side-lying position until awake, and then the head of the bed is elevated 30 to 45 degrees to facilitate ventilation. This position allows the diaphragm to drop into normal position, thus enhancing lung expansion and, if present, facilitating chest tube drainage. After lobectomy, segmentectomy, and wedge resection, the patient can be turned freely from side to side to allow full expansion of lung tissue on both the operative and nonoperative side. After pneumonectomy, the patient may be placed on the back or on the operative side. The patient is *not* positioned side lying on the nonoperative side because the mediastinum is no longer confined by lung tissue and may move freely, thereby compressing the remaining lung or creating traction or torsion of the vena cava. In addition, if the bronchial stump ruptures and bleeds profusely, the unaffected lung is compressed by secretions from the pneumonectomy site.

Position changes are important after thoracic surgery. If the patient undergoes an outpatient procedure, such as bronchoscopy, position changes are made independently. If the patient has a chest tube in place, the perianesthesia nurse needs to assist with position changes to ensure system patency and patient comfort. Position changes also include early return to ambulation, with the goal of promoting patient comfort, drainage of secretions, and prevention of venous stasis and atelectasis.

### Respiratory Assessment and Care

On arrival, the patient is placed on oxygen via the delivery system required per the extent of the patient's surgery, preexisting medical conditions, and need for continued assistance. Continued assistance may include a nasal cannula after bronchoscopy, face mask or face tent, or mechanical ventilation. Delivered oxygen should be given with humidification to help thin tracheobronchial secretions and thus permit the ciliary mechanism and coughing to clear the airway.

The perianesthesia nurse should assess respiratory function on arrival, beginning with inspection of the patient's respiratory effort and ease of effort. Respiratory rate is noted; a rate of 10 to 20 breaths per minute is considered normal. A rate of greater than 20 is considered to be tachypnea and may be caused by pain, hypoxemia, hypoventilation, or secretions. The use of pulse oximetry helps in the quick assessment for hypoxemia. A rate of less than 10 is considered bradypnea, which may occur as a result of anesthetic and opioid administration. The patient should also be assessed for the quality of respirations. The patient may have a respiratory rate within normal limits but not deep enough to blow off the carbon dioxide of normal respirations. Some PACUs have the capability to monitor end tidal $CO_2$ with a capnograph. The nurse should auscultate the patient's lungs to assure that respirations are of good quality. Appropriate pain management can promote effective ventilation. The patient may also arrive in the PACU intubated with either a T-piece, if respiratory effort is sufficiently present but loss of airway patency is a concern, or mechanical ventilation, if airway and ventilation are concerns.

Breath sounds should be assessed for depth, clarity, and the presence of adventitious sounds, including crackles, rhonchi, or a pleural friction rub. The use of accessory muscles should be noted. Accessory muscle actions include nasal flaring, suprasternal retractions, diaphragmatic breathing, and intercostal retractions.

The regularity of breathing is assessed as regular, irregular, or ventilated. Ventilator settings are confirmed; if arterial blood gases are drawn, adjustments are made, if necessary, after assessment of results. Ongoing pulse oximetry monitoring is necessary for any patient who has undergone a thoracic surgical procedure.

If the patient is intubated, the intubation may be to protect the airway, to assist ventilation, or to provide a means for management of secretions through suctioning. Tracheal suctioning of the patient after thoracic surgery may be necessary to assist in removal of accumulated secretions.

### Respiratory Management

The modified stir-up regimen, including positioning, mobilization, sustained maximum inspiration (SMI), cascade coughing, and pain relief, is especially important for a patient recovering from a thoracic surgical procedure. Positioning and mobilization have already been discussed. The SMI and cascade coughing exercises are the easiest ways to maintain a patent airway after the patient is reactive to verbal commands. Preoperative teaching is extremely important; the patient who has been well educated and knows what is expected after surgery can cooperate by taking a deep breath, holding it for 3 seconds, and then exhaling (the SMI), and then taking a deep breath and coughing throughout exhalation (the cascade cough). Effective preoperative teaching enhances the effectiveness of the modified stir-up regimen even if the patient is not fully reactive.

Once the patient is fully conscious, rigorous SMIs and cascade coughing are continued every hour. This regimen is most effective with the patient sitting to allow full lung expansion. If the patient cannot sit, raise the head of the bed and have the patient bend the knees to relax the abdominal muscles. The patient is instructed to inspire deeply and hold the breath for 3 seconds to expand the lungs and relax the abdominal muscles so that the belly pouches out. Four to five SMIs are taken, and then the patient is instructed to perform the cascade cough to clear the tracheobronchial tree of accumulated secretions. After the patient performs about three cascade coughs, a "forceful" cough is then usually produced spontaneously, thus clearing the airways of secretions. Endotracheal secretions are usually excessive after thoracic surgery because of the tracheobronchial tree during the operation and intubation, decreased lung ventilation, and a decreased cough reflex. Pain or fear, or both, may interfere with the patient's ability to perform the SMI and cascade cough.

## Pain Management

Although pain after bronchoscopy is usually limited to a sore throat, the patient for thoracic surgery should be told before surgery to expect a fair amount of postoperative incisional pain. The patient should also be told that pain relief measures are available and may include epidural analgesia, patient-controlled analgesia, and nurse-administered opioids. Because acute pain after thoracic surgery has been linked to chronic thoracic pain months later, appropriate pain relief must occur. Severe pain during the first couple of days after surgery is predictive of postthoracotomy pain. Pain management via epidural catheter has been shown to provide more effective pain relief after thoracotomy. Of best benefit is epidural analgesia with an opioid and local anesthetic that has begun at least 30 minutes before induction of anesthesia. Pain medications should be given in adequate doses and in a timely manner because pain interferes with needed activities after surgery, including deep breathing, coughing, and progressive mobilization. Because opioids can diminish respiratory function, care must be taken in their administration, especially after general anesthesia. However, a patient whose pain is not adequately controlled is unable to deep breath effectively to maintain oxygenation and prevent atelectasis.

In addition to analgesics, pain relief measures can include use of a pillow to splint the incision while coughing. Because coughing is the most effective way to clear secretions, pain medication should be offered and given regularly.

## Fluid Management

Optimal hydration after thoracic surgery is important to prevent the increased viscosity of mucus to facilitate the removal of secretions. Oral fluids may be started as soon as the patient recovers from anesthesia and the danger of nausea and vomiting has passed. Intravenous fluids are also used after more extensive surgery to ensure hydration and to continue fluid replacement for losses in the operating room. Removal of large segments of lung or of a total lung (pneumonectomy) significantly reduces the size of the pulmonary circulation, thus predisposing the patient to the development of pulmonary edema if fluids are administered too rapidly or in too large a volume. The

surgeon writes postoperative fluid orders. Accurate intake and output records are particularly important.

## Chest Tube Management

Surgery on the structures of the chest that involves entry into the thoracic cavity results in air entry and the development of a pneumothorax (atmospheric pressure admitted into the pleural cavity and collapse of the lung). Placement of a pleural chest tube after open-chest procedures allows for drainage of air and blood, restoration of normal negative pressure, and reexpansion of the collapsed lung. Because blood is heavier than air, blood pools in the lower portion of the pleural space, whereas air accumulates in the upper portion. Therefore, two chest tubes usually are placed through the chest wall via a stab wound or incision. An upper or anterior chest tube is placed in the second intercostal space to allow for air removal. A lower or posterior chest tube is placed in the sixth to eighth intercostal space to allow for drainage from the pleural space (Fig. 34-2). The chest tubes are sutured in place with purse-string sutures and covered with a dressing. The chest tube insertion site should be palpated for the presence of crepitus (also known as subcutaneous emphysema) caused by air trapping in subcutaneous tissue. Crepitus feels like crunchy cereal under the skin. If noted, the surgeon should be notified for probable resecuring of the chest tube.

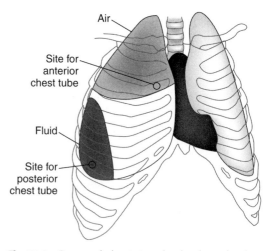

**Fig. 34-2**   Because air rises to top of cavity, chest tube placement for treatment of pneumothorax is at second intercostal space, close to sternum. Chest tube placement for fluid removal is generally at level of sixth to eighth lateral intercostal space because this is where fluid collects.

The chest tubes are connected to a drainage system that uses positive pressure, gravity, and suction to facilitate evacuation of air and fluid to reexpand the collapsed lung. The air trapped in the chest creates the positive pressure. Gravity assists primarily in fluid evacuation, and suction, when applied, facilitates removal of both air and fluid. Suction is generally established at 20 cm negative pressure, unless specifically ordered differently. Wall units have a manometer in place to allow for correct setting of suction pressure. Once the air and fluid are removed, the visceral and parietal pleura are brought back together again, and the pressure in the interpleural space becomes negative once again, thus reexpanding the lung.

In the past, drainage systems ranged from one-bottle to two-bottle to three-bottle systems, all with water seal to draw out air and fluid, thus allowing for reexpansion of the lung. These systems had to be set up by nursing personnel, which included gathering the required number of bottles, establishing a system for measurement, and maintaining sterility. Cumbersome in nature and subject to breakage, they have been replaced with disposable prefabricated chest drainage units such as the Pleur-Evac or Atrium systems (Fig. 34-3).

The principles of positive pressure, gravity, and suction still apply to these systems, yet they are simpler to use and transport and are associated with a lower rate of infection and system disruption. The pleural drainage system has three basic compartments, each with its own specific function. The first compartment, the collection chamber, receives air and fluid from the chest cavity. This compartment is vented to the second chamber, known as the water-seal chamber. This chamber acts as a one-way valve so that air can enter from, but not back into, the collection chamber. If bubbling is noted in this chamber, the lung has not reexpanded. The third chamber is the suction control chamber, which is used to apply controlled suction to the system to facilitate evacuation of air and fluid and to promote reexpansion of the lung. Some of these units have even been designed to allow for reinfusion of collected drained blood for autotransfusion.

Because the goal of chest tube placement is evaluation of air and fluid, the system must remain patent. The perianesthesia nurse must ensure patency of the chest tubes, drainage tubing, and the system through periodic regular assessments. A chest x-ray is often performed on admission to the PACU to ensure placement and lung function. Proper functioning of the system is evidenced by fluctuation or bubbling of the fluid in the water seal tubing in response to the patient's respiration. If no fluctuation is noted, the system should be evaluated for proper functioning. The tubing must not kink and should form a straight line from patient to collection unit to allow for unobstructed gravitational flow. "Milking" or "stripping" of the chest tube may dislodge clots of blood that block the tubing. This procedure should be done in the direction away from the patient, toward the drainage system, to prevent forcing clots back into the pleural space. If the system shows no fluctuation or bubbling with respiration and the tubing has been deemed clear, the physician should be notified, especially in the immediate postoperative period. In the latter

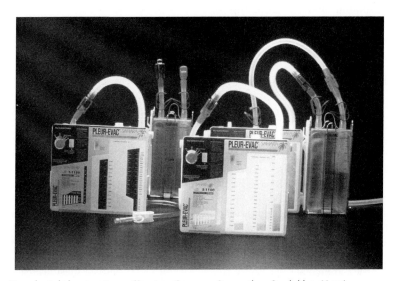

**Fig. 34-3** Pleur-Evac chest drainage systems. *(Courtesy Genzyme Corporation, Cambridge, Mass.)*

days of recovery, the absence of fluctuation or bubbling signals reexpansion of the lung, with further evidence provided by full return of breath sounds and chest x-ray results. However, in the PACU, failure of the system prevents lung reexpansion. Any acute respiratory difficulty or pain should be referred immediately to the surgeon.

## Complications

*Risks of General Anesthesia.* The risks of general anesthesia for any patient, regardless of the underlying medical condition and surgical procedure, include the potential for respiratory and cardiovascular compromise. In the presence of underlying pulmonary disease and surgery that involves the thoracic cavity, the potential for respiratory compromise, including hypoxemia, hypoventilation and atelectasis, increases greatly. The perianesthesia nurse should be prepared to evaluate for respiratory and ventilatory adequacy and to intervene with appropriate interventions if compromise is noted. This intervention may include the need to simply stimulate the patient to take deep breaths, to increase the concentration of oxygen delivered, or to anticipate and assist with reintubation if necessary.

*Wound Infection.* As with any surgical procedure, the risk of infection is possible. Prophylactic antibiotics may be given for major thoracic surgical procedures, including lobectomy and pneumonectomy, and are used if prolonged postoperative mechanical ventilation is anticipated.

*Bleeding.* After bronchoscopy, bleeding should be limited to no more than lightly pink-tinged or slightly blood-streaked sputum. Grossly bloody sputum and coughing up of frank blood should be reported to the surgeon and anesthesia provider immediately. After a more invasive procedure such as lobectomy or pneumonectomy, the surgical site must be inspected for bleeding and the chest tube for the presence of bloody drainage. If chest tube drainage seems excessive (greater than 100 mL/h) or does not decrease in volume over time or if fresh bleeding is noted, the physician should be notified to evaluate for hemorrhage. Even if drainage is excessive, the chest tube should never be clamped unless specifically ordered. Clamping of the chest tube may result in the development of a tension pneumothorax, which is considerably more dangerous than an open pneumothorax.

*Pneumonia.* Although pneumonia is unlikely to develop in the immediate postoperative period, diminished ventilatory effort and prolonged bedrest are strong predictors of pneumonia potential. The patient should be encouraged on arrival to the PACU to take deep breaths, to cascade cough, and, if ordered, to use the incentive spirometer to prevent atelectasis and pneumonia. The use of sterile technique when suctioning is essential.

*Worsening of Existing Heart Problems.* Underlying cardiac disease should be carefully evaluated and documented before surgery. In any patient with preexisting cardiac disease, close attention to continuous electrocardiographic (ECG) monitoring in the PACU is of vital importance because cardiac dysrhythmias commonly develop in these patients. These dysrhythmias may range from benign to life threatening. Sinus tachycardia and atrial fibrillation are the most commonly seen dysrhythmias in the early recovery phases.

## SUMMARY

Care of patients undergoing thoracic surgery or procedures of the lungs and respiratory system was discussed in this chapter. These procedures range from minimally invasive procedures to open thoracotomies. The procedures are performed on patients with underlying conditions such as emphysema or malignant disease that must be surgically treated. Care of these patients in the PACU involves respiratory function, observation for complications, and promotion of ventilation.

## BIBLIOGRAPHY

Atlee J: *Complications in anesthesia*, ed 2, Philadelphia, 2007, Saunders.

Barash PG, Cullen BF, Stoelting RK: *Clinical anesthesia*, ed 5, Philadelphia, 2005, Lippincott Williams & Wilkins.

Benumof J, Saidman L: *Anesthesia & perioperative complications*, ed 2, St Louis, 1999, Mosby.

Cafarelli JM: Respiratory anesthesia: thoracic surgery. In Nagelhout J, Zaglaniczny K, editors: *Nurse anesthesia*, ed 2, Philadelphia, 2001, Saunders.

Coughlin AM, Parchinsky C: Go with the flow of chest tube therapy, *Nursing* 36(3):L36-42, 2006.

Crum BG: Thoracic surgery. In Rothrock J, editor: *Alexander's care of the patient in surgery*, ed 13, St Louis, 2007, Mosby.

Fibla JJ, Molins L, Perez J, et al: Early removal of chest drainage and outpatient program after videothoracoscopic lung biopsy, *Eur J Cardiothor Surg* 28:604-606, 2005.

Fleisher LA: *Anesthesia and uncommon diseases*, ed 5, Philadelphia, 2006, Saunders.

Gotoda Y, Kambara N, Sakai T, et al: The morbidity, time course and predictive factors for persistent post-thoracotomy pain, *Eur J Pain* 5:89-96, 2001.

Longnecker D, Murphy F: *Dripps/Eckenhoff/Vandam introduction to anesthesia*, ed 9, Philadelphia, 1997, Saunders.

Marley RA: Respiratory surgery. In Quinn DM, L Schick, editors: *Perianesthesia nursing core curriculam, preoperative, Phase I and Phase II PACU nursing*, St Louis, 2004, Saunders.

Miller RD: *Anesthesia*, ed 6, New York, 2005, Churchill Livingstone.

Moon MR, Luchette FA, Gibson SW, et al: Prospective, randomized comparison of epidural versus parenteral opioid analgesia in thoracic trauma, *Ann Surg* 5:684-692, 1999.

Mason RJ, Broaddus VC, Murray JF, et al: *Textbook of respiratory medicine*, ed 4, Philadelphia, 2005, Saunders.

Senturk M, Ozcan PE, Talu GK, et al: The effects of three different analgesia techniques on long-term postthoracotomy pain, *Anesth Analg* 94:11-15, 2002.

Thys D: *Textbook of cardiothoracic anesthesiology*, New York, 2001, McGraw-Hill Professional.

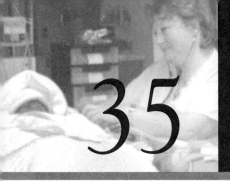

# 35

# CARE OF THE CARDIAC SURGICAL PATIENT

*Patricia C. Seifert, RN, MSN, CNOR, CRNFA, FAAN*

Traditionally, the beginning of cardiac surgery is associated with Rehn's suture repair of a right ventricular stab wound in 1896. Rehn's action showed that the heart could be manipulated and sutured without causing ventricular fibrillation (VF) and without entering the pleural cavity and creating a pneumothorax. With the introduction of positive-pressure endotracheal anesthesia, the dangers of a pneumothorax were obviated because clinicians could access the heart and enter the pleural cavities without causing the lungs to collapse. The introduction by Gibbon in 1953 of extracorporeal circulation (i.e., cardiopulmonary bypass) allowed surgeons to isolate the heart and lungs from the circulation without producing irreversible tissue anoxia. The development of electric defibrillation and induced chemical cardiac arrest made stopping and restarting the heart possible with consistent predictability. Myocardial protection techniques promoted by Buckberg greatly improved cardiac surgery outcomes by protecting and conserving the myocardial energy resources during the period of induced cardiac arrest when the cardiac repair was performed. Advances in diagnostic imaging and monitoring capabilities have allowed clinicians to visualize the heart, identify specific pathoanatomy, record the heart's electric activity, measure blood pressure and flow, and assess ventricular function. These imaging and monitoring improvements, along with the creation of mechanical and bioprosthetic materials, improved anesthetic agents, and other technologic advances, have made development of newer more effective procedures possible to revascularize the myocardium, repair valves, treat aneurysms, alter conduction disturbances, and assist and replace a failing heart.[1] Many of the improvements that affect the intraoperative care of patients for cardiac surgery also positively affect the preoperative and postoperative recovery periods, which commonly occur in a specialized cardiac surgical intensive care unit (CSICU).

Before surgery, documentation of the history and physical examination, surgical consents, the results of diagnostic and laboratory tests, and additional pertinent information are reviewed by the nurse. Among the significant factors are estimates of left ventricular (LV) function (e.g., ejection fraction), a history of medications that may affect perioperative bleeding (e.g., aspirin, clopidogrel bisulfate [Plavix]), oxygen-carrying capacity (e.g., hematocrit, hemoglobin), renal function (creatinine), pulmonary function (spirometry tests), cardiac anatomy (e.g., of the valves, coronary arteries), and the presence of concomitant carotid artery disease.

An increasing number of patients are admitted the morning of surgery, which shortens the period of time for teaching. Many institutions have preoperative laboratory testing and requests for packed red blood cells (RBCs) performed a few days before the scheduled surgery; patient teaching can be accomplished at this time. The postanesthesia care unit (PACU) nurse should be aware of the level of knowledge, understanding, and anxieties of both the patient and the family before surgery. When possible (and depending on the individual institution's policies and procedures), the PACU nurse may provide preoperative instruction for the patient and family or make an introductory visit before surgery. Teaching content for coronary or valve surgery (Table 35-1) can be initiated in the preoperative period and reinforced after surgery.

Discharge from the CSICU or open heart PACU to a step-down unit now commonly occurs within 1 day or sometimes hours. A reduction has also been seen in the overall length of stay (LOS) from a week (or more) to a few days. The movement toward rapid postoperative endotracheal extubation and shortened LOS has been spurred not just by costs but also by improved pain control that facilitates earlier extubation and by fundamental shifts in anesthetic management from a high-dose opioid technique to a more balanced approach with moderate-dose opioids, shorter acting muscle relaxants, and volatile anesthetics. The so-called fast track approach (i.e., extubation in 2 to 8 hours after surgery or in the operating

## Table 35-1 Patient Teaching for Coronary Artery Bypass Graft Surgery and Valve Surgery

| Topic | CABG Surgery | Valve Surgery |
|---|---|---|
| **PERIOPERATIVE POINTERS** | | |
| Medical diagnosis | Coronary artery occlusive disease | Valve regurgitation, stenosis, or mixed |
| Diagnostic tests | ECG, chest radiograph, nuclear imaging, cardiac catheterization | Same, plus echocardiogram |
| Routine preoperative tests | CMP, ECG, T&C, pulmonary function, PT, PTT, INR | Same |
| Incision site | Midsternal or anterior thoracotomy; multiple leg incisions for vein harvest, arm incision for radial artery harvest | Ministernotomy or full sternotomy |
| Resumption of eating | 2-3 d after removal of ET and NG tubes | Same |
| Pain control | IM, PO, PCA | Same |
| Estimated length of procedure | 4-6 h | Same |
| Estimated length of hospital stay | 5-7 d | 6-8 d |
| Long-term effects of surgery | Loss of saphenous vein, possible intermittent lower leg ischemia | Possible chronic anticoagulation therapy; differences between biologic and mechanical prostheses, valve repair |
| Drains or tubes | 2 d: mediastinal chest tube, pleural tube; 2-3 d: leg drains, urinary drainage catheter | 2 d: mediastinal and pleural tubes, urinary catheter |
| **POSTOPERATIVE POINTERS/HOME INSTRUCTIONS** | | |
| Food | Cardiac diet | Same |
| Wound care | Wounds covered if draining; redress after shower or bath; contact clinician if signs of infection | Same |
| Bathing | Daily | Same |
| Driving | 4-6 wk (automatic shift only) | Same |
| Sex | Restricted by limits of ability to bear weight on upper arms and chest | Same |
| Return to work | 8-12 wk | Same |
| Medications | Aspirin anticoagulant, cardiac drugs | Warfarin (Coumadin), cardiac drugs |
| Follow-up | 7-14 d | Same, plus laboratory tests for determination of bleeding times |
| Special restrictions | Upper body movement restricted for 6 wk for sternal healing | Same |
| Lifestyle changes | Reduction of coronary risk factors; rehabilitation | Risk factor reduction; rehabilitation |
| Worrisome but normal | Fatigue, swelling in leg; leg discomfort 4-6 wk; weakness, emotional let down | Fatigue; sound of mechanical valve; weakness; emotional let down |

From Seifert PC: *Cardiac surgery: perioperative patient care*, St Louis, 2002, Mosby.
*CMP*, comprehensive metabolic panel (includes glucose, blood urea nitrogen, sodium, potassium, chloride, creatinine, albumin, bilirubin, calcium, alkaline phosphatase, total protein); *T&C*, type and cross match (blood); *PT*, prothrombin time; *PTT*, partial thromboplastin time; *ET*, endotracheal; *NG*, nasogastric; *IM*, intramuscular; *PO*, by mouth (per ora); *PCA*, patient-controlled analgesia.

room)[2] is becoming a standard of care in a number of centers.[3] The longer LOS sometimes seen in the rapidly growing number of patients 80 years and older may be the result of comorbid conditions such as peripheral vascular disease, renal pathology, diabetes mellitus, hyperlipidemia, and hypertension, but advances in anesthetic techniques and myocardial protection during surgery have improved morbidity and mortality rates in elderly and younger patients.[4,5] This chapter is designed to familiarize the PACU nurse with the perioperative care for the adult cardiac patient. Understanding what the patient has experienced before and during surgery assists the nurse after surgery to tailor the care to the patient's needs and to strengthen the continuity of that care.

## DEFINITIONS

**Allograft (Homograft):** Tissue from another human. In cardiac surgery, allografts are commonly taken from cadaver aortic valves with a portion of the attached aorta (Fig. 35-1). The aortic allograft is obtained in a sterile manner; tested to rule out communicable disease, malignant disease, diabetes, and other pathologic conditions; treated with antibiotics; measured; placed in a sterile bag; and cryopreserved in a special freezer. When needed for surgery, the correct size of allograft is thawed and implanted. Allografts are advantageous because they do not require warfarin anticoagulation, are resistant to

infection, have excellent hemodynamics, and are useful in patients with small aortic roots because no sewing ring exists to decrease the size of the aortic valve orifice, unlike prosthetic biologic or mechanical valves. Disadvantages are less availability, technical difficulties of implantation, and some concern about potential graft failure, especially in patients with severe or poorly controlled hypertension.[5]

**Annuloplasty:** The surgical repair of a dilated valve annulus that causes valvular regurgitation. The valve leaflets may be normal, but they are unable to coapt and create a competent valve because the dilated annulus pulls the leaflet edges away from one another. The procedure commonly is performed on the mitral or tricuspid valve or both. A cloth-covered prosthetic annuloplasty ring (Fig. 35-2) in a size smaller than the dilated native annulus is sutured to the valve annulus (Fig. 35-3). When the stitches are tied, excess annular tissue is pulled up against the ring, thereby reducing the overall circumference of the valve orifice and allowing the valve leaflets to coapt properly. Annuloplasty rings have different configurations (e.g., circular, almond-shaped, C-shaped) and may be flexible, rigid, or semirigid. The surgeon's selection of the prosthesis is based on factors such as the underlying pathology, anatomy, annular dynamics, remodeling of the annular geometry, and preservation of valve function. Prosthetic valvular annuloplasty itself does not require postoperative long-term anticoagulation therapy.

During ring insertion for tricuspid annulus repair (Fig. 35-4), the surgeon is especially cautious when inserting stitches near the atrioventricular (AV) node and the bundle of His (in the area of the tricuspid septal leaflet) to avoid creating complete heart block or other injury to the conduction system.[6] A suture annuloplasty (i.e., without the insertion of a prosthetic ring) called the DeVega technique[7] can be used

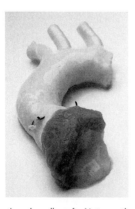

**Fig. 35-1** Aortic valve allograft. Note aortic arch branches (*top*), tissue from left ventricle (red-brown tissue in lower portion of graft), and attached anterior leaflet of mitral valve (white smooth tissue in lower right portion of graft). Depending on graft material required, surgeon trims excess or unneeded tissue. *(From Rothrock JC: Alexander's care of the patient in surgery, ed 13, St Louis, 2007, Mosby. Courtesy CryoLife, Inc., Marietta, GA.)*

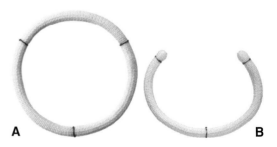

**A**          **B**

**Fig. 35-2** Annuloplasty rings. **A,** Duran ring. **B,** Colvin-Galloway (i.e., CG) ring. *(Courtesy of Medtronic Heart Valves, Minneapolis, MN.)*

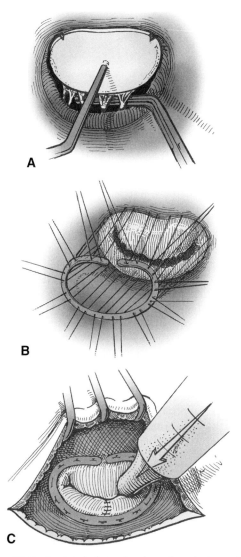

**A**

**B**

**C**

**Fig. 35-3** **A,** Annuloplasty ring bean-shaped sizer with handle used to measure annulus (note retraction of chordae tendineae to facilitate sizing). **B,** Stitches are inserted into annulus and into prosthetic ring. **C,** Sutures are tied and cut; bulb syringe squirts saline solution into orifice to determine whether repair has produced competent valve. Portion of excess posterior leaflet tissue has been resected. *(From Rothrock JC: Alexander's care of the patient in surgery, ed 13, St Louis, 2007, Mosby.)*

also for some tricuspid valve repairs (see also definition of valvuloplasty).

**Aortic Aneurysm:** A localized or diffuse dilation of the arterial wall. Weakening and degeneration of the medial layer of the aortic wall leads to progressive enlargement of all layers of the aorta. Surrounding tissue may be compressed by the enlarging vessel, and eventual rupture with exsanguination can occur without treatment. Thoracic aortic aneurysms may occur in

the ascending aorta, the aortic arch, or the descending aorta and may extend into the abdominal aorta and branch vessels. Surgical treatment consists of excision of the aneurysmal tissue with insertion of a prosthetic (e.g., Dacron) graft (Fig. 35-5). An endovascular stented graft made from expanded polytetrafluoroethylene (PTFE) is available for repair of descending (and abdominal) aortic aneurysms. The prosthesis is initially compressed, inserted percutaneously into the femoral artery, and guided to the desired position in the aorta where it is expanded.

**Aortic Dissection:** A unique condition that affects the aortic media in which repeated stress (often from hypertension) and a congenital predisposition produce a tear in the intimal layer. Blood enters the tear, creating a dissecting hematoma within the tunica media and forming a false lumen. As the false lumen enlarges, with more blood entering the tear, the true lumen compresses and eventually compresses branches of the aorta. The intimal tear usually forms in the ascending aorta, although it can originate in any portion of the thoracic aorta. Surgery (excision of the aorta that contains the tear and replacement with a graft) is indicated for ascending aortic and transverse aortic arch dissections. Uncomplicated descending thoracic aortic dissections are more commonly managed medically with antihypertensive medications and analgesics; surgery is indicated with impending rupture.[8]

**Aortic Insufficiency (AI):** Also called aortic regurgitation; a condition that occurs when the aortic valve leaflets do not close properly (or have tears) and the valve becomes incompetent, thereby allowing regurgitation of blood from the aorta back into the left ventricle (LV) during diastole (Fig. 35-6). AI can be the result of a primary valve disorder or aortic root disease. Valve disorders may be the result of congenital or rheumatic heart disease, infective endocarditis, torn leaflets (Fig. 35-7), or trauma; aortic root disease may include aneurysmal dilatation, aortic dissection, Marfan's syndrome, or some other condition that predisposes the root to dilatation (i.e., ectasia). Mild chronic AI can be tolerated by the LV for almost two decades with more forceful dilation and contraction to eject the additional regurgitant volume. Eventually the LV is stimulated to hypertrophy and decompensates if corrective therapy is not implemented. Symptoms include dyspnea from pulmonary edema and fatigue and other symptoms associated with LV failure. Sudden acute AI (e.g., from bacterial endocarditis that causes tearing of the leaflets or acute aortic dissection

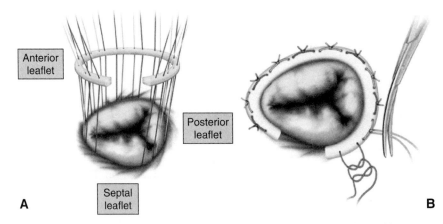

**Fig. 35-4    A,** Tricuspid valve repair is similar to mitral valve repair. Note that stitches are not inserted in area of atrioventricular conduction tissue (see text). **B,** Completion of tricuspid valve repair. *(Courtesy of Medtronic Heart Valves, Minneapolis, MN.)*

that dilates the aortic annulus) is poorly toler-ated because the normal-sized LV cannot accom-modate the sudden increased volume and the lowered diastolic pressure that results from a por-tion of the cardiac output (CO) being regurgi-tated into the LV impairs coronary filling. Emergency aortic valve replacement is indicated for acute AI.[9] Aortic valve replacement (see the definition of valve replacement) is generally indicated for AI; some reparative techniques are available for the aortic valve, but they tend to have less successful outcomes.

**Aortic Stenosis (AS):**  The development of stiff and fibrotic valve leaflets or a narrowing of the orifice of the aortic valve itself. Valvular AS is often characterized by a fusion of the commis-sures of the valve leaflets that leaves only a small opening. A calculated aortic valve orifice of less than 1 cm$^2$ is considered critical AS. Cardinal symptoms are syncope, angina pectoris, and dys-pnea; these symptoms are related respectively to insufficient cerebral and myocardial blood flow and impaired LV function. Sudden death may be the presenting symptom. AS can occur as a con-genital process, as in the bicuspid valve (a common congenital anomaly first diagnosed in adulthood; Fig. 35-8, A)[10]; as an acquired disease process related to a history of rheumatic heart disease (Fig. 35-8, B); or as calcific AS (Fig. 35-8, C). A form of subvalvular stenosis occurs when the intraventricular septum becomes hypertrophied and creates an obstruc-tion to left-ventricular outflow. This lesion is known as idiopathic hypertrophic subaortic ste-nosis (IHSS) or hypertrophic obstructive cardi-omyopathy; surgical treatment for subaortic stenosis with a hypertrophied septum involves excision of a portion of the hypertrophied septum; cardiomyopathy may require heart

transplantation. Supraaortic valvular stenosis occurs when the aorta above the valve is nar-rowed from a congenital anomaly. Repair involves opening of the affected portion of the aorta and insertion of a patch graft to enlarge the narrowed vessel.

The regurgitating blood in AI creates an increased volume load on the LV (Fig. 35-9), and AS represents an increased pressure load on the LV (increased afterload). The LV responds by developing left-ventricular hypertro-phy (LVH), which results in decreased LV com-pliance. The LV cavity becomes reduced (from the hypertrophying muscle invading the ventri-cular cavity). During cardiac catheterization for study of the valve, calculated pressure gradients between the LV and the aorta may exceed 50 mm Hg. As an example, the aortic pressure may be 100 mm Hg, but the LV pressure may be 150 mm Hg, which shows the work required by the LV to eject an adequate cardiac output. LV dila-tation and failure can develop when the myocar-dium is no longer capable of generating sufficient pressure to eject an adequate CO.

The atrial contribution to cardiac output becomes especially important to maintain an adequate preload and forward flow of blood and to contribute to a more forceful ventricular contraction. Loss of this atrial contribution, or kick, through the development of supraventricu-lar dysrhythmias (e.g., atrial fibrillation) can result in a marked decrease in cardiac output with resultant pulmonary edema.

**Aortocoronary Bypass Grafts:**  See myocardial revascularization.

**Atrial Septal Defect (ASD):**  An opening in the atrial septum (Fig. 35-10). ASDs are among the frequently seen congenital anomalies in adult-hood.[11] The most common form in the adult is

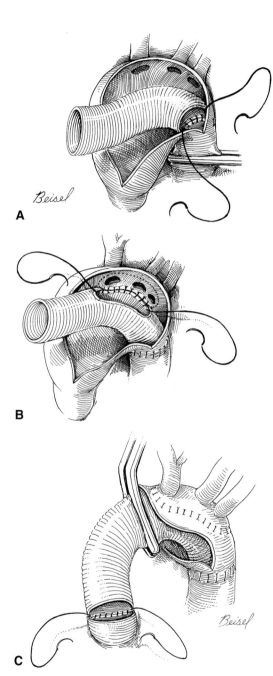

**Fig. 35-5** Resection of aneurysmal portion of ascending aorta and transverse arch and insertion of prosthetic patch. Circulatory arrest is instituted until arch vessels are repaired. **A,** Graft anastomosed to distal portion of aorta. **B,** Arch vessels are anastomosed as island to prosthetic graft. **C,** After arch vessels are connected, cross clamp is placed on graft, CPB is resumed, and proximal anastomosis is completed. *(In Seifert PC: Cardiac surgery, St Louis, 2002, Mosby. From Waldhausen JA, et al: Surgery of the chest, ed 6, St Louis, 1996, Mosby.)*

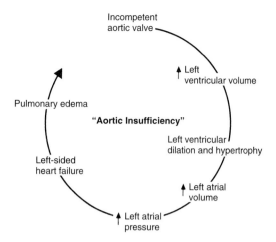

**Fig. 35-6** Pathophysiology of aortic insufficiency/regurgitation. *(In Seifert PC: Cardiac surgery, St Louis, 2002, Mosby. From Kinney MR, et al: Andreoli's comprehensive cardiac care, ed 8, St Louis, 1996, Mosby.)*

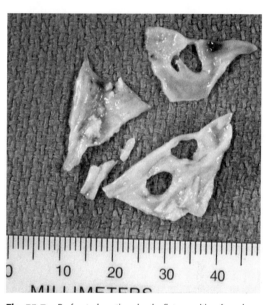

**Fig. 35-7** Perforated aortic valve leaflets resulting from bacterial endocarditis. Patient had aortic insufficiency. *(From Seifert PC: Cardiac surgery, St Louis, 2002, Mosby. Courtesy Edward A Lefrak, MD.)*

the ostium secundum defect, located in the mid-portion of the septum in the vicinity of the fossa ovalis (formerly the intrauterine shunt known as the foramen ovale). Depending on the size of the defect (commonly the size of a quarter coin), a shunting of blood from the left atrium to the right atrium, and subsequently increased pulmonary flow, is seen.

The sinus venosus defect is located near the entrance of the superior vena cava (SVC) in

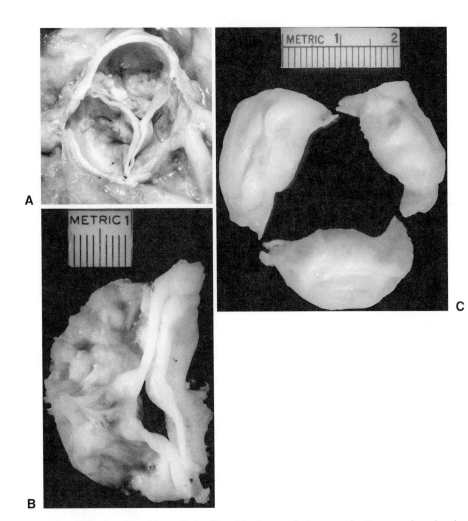

**Fig. 35-8   A,** Bicuspid aortic valve with calcified stiffened leaflets producing stenosis. Note greatly reduced orifice area. **B,** Rheumatic trileaflet (e.g., morphologically normal) aortic valve. Thickened, glistened, and smooth leaflets are typical of rheumatic changes. **C,** Calcific aortic stenosis of trileaflet aortic valve. *(From Seifert PC: Cardiac surgery, St Louis, 2002, Mosby. Courtesy William C Roberts, MD; Michael Spencer, photographer.)*

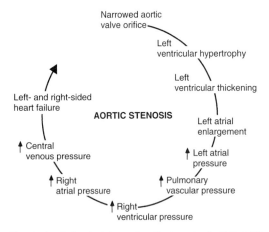

**Fig. 35-9**   Pathophysiology of aortic stenosis. *(In Seifert PC: Cardiac surgery, St Louis, 2002, Mosby. From Kinney MR, et al: Andreoli's comprehensive cardiac care, ed 8, St Louis, 1996, Mosby.)*

the high right atrium. Sinus venosus defects are associated with partial anomalous pulmonary venous return (commonly of the right superior pulmonary vein), whereby the anomalous pulmonary vein enters the right atrium (rather than the left atrium) and returns oxygenated blood from the lungs into the SVC or the upper right atrium. The amount of anomalous pulmonary venous return can be estimated with blood samples from the SVC, the high right atrium (RA), the mid RA, and the low RA during cardiac catheterization. In patients with anomalous pulmonary venous return, the SVC and high RA blood samples (compared with blood samples in the lower RA) show an increased oxygen saturation (step-up) in what normally should be desaturated venous blood returning to the right heart.

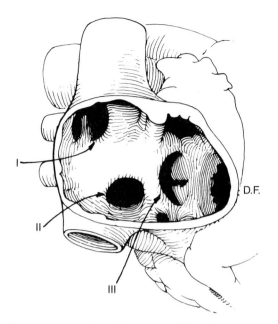

**Fig. 35-10** Location of three types of ASD. Sinus venosus defect (*I*) is shown with anomalous drainage of right upper pulmonary vein. Ostium secundum defect (*II*) is in midportion of septum in area of fossa ovalis. Ostium primum defect (*III*) is located in base of septum, with its inferior edge formed by continuity of tricuspid and mitral valves. Often a cleftlike anomaly is seen in anterior leaflet of mitral valve visible through defect. (*In Seifert PC: Cardiac surgery, St Louis, 2002, Mosby. From Bove EL: Congenital heart lesions. In Miller TA, editor: Physiologic basis of modern surgical care, St Louis, 1988, Mosby.*)

Closure of the secundum and sinus venosus septal defects is accomplished with suturing or patching the defect with a patch of pericardium or prosthetic material. During repair of a sinus venosus defect, the patch is placed in such a way that anomalous pulmonary venous drainage is diverted into the left atrium.

The ostium primum lesion is a defect that occurs low in the atrial septum and is more commonly seen initially in the pediatric population. This anomaly is an embryonic endocardial cushion defect that commonly involves the tricuspid and mitral valves and portions of the intraventricular septum. Repair is more complex than the secundum defect and involves valve repair and closure of the defect.

**Atrial Septal Defect:** See previous definition.

**Balloon Valvotomy/Valvuloplasty:** A catheter-based interventional (i.e., nonsurgical) procedure that consists of the percutaneous insertion of a balloon-tipped catheter (commonly inserted into the femoral artery or femoral vein) that is threaded through the aorta or inferior vena cava

(IVC) to the intended location to enlarge a (stenotic) valve opening. For aortic valvuloplasty, the balloon tip is positioned across the aortic valve and the balloon is inflated to dilate the aortic valve orifice. This technique is useful for children, young adults, and patients who are too elderly or medically compromised to withstand an operation. Balloon valvotomy for the mitral valve is performed with a catheter percutaneously inserted into a large vein and threaded to the RA where a septal puncture is made to allow access to the mitral valve. Occasionally, the catheter is threaded up the aorta and through the aortic valve into the LV and then placed across the mitral valve where the balloon is inflated. Complications of valvotomy include development of aortic or mitral regurgitation (depending on the affected valve), cardiac perforation, pulmonary edema, and cerebral embolus.[12]

**Bicuspid Aortic Valve:** See aortic stenosis.

**Cardiac Catheterization:** A technique in which a radiopaque plastic catheter is inserted into the left or right heart via a percutaneous puncture (or if necessary, a cutdown) into the femoral artery or vein (Judkins technique) or brachial artery or vein (Sones technique) to obtain pressure, volume, and oxygen saturation determinations from the intracardiac chambers and the great blood vessels (i.e., superior and inferior vena cava, pulmonary artery, and aorta). Cardiac catheterization is commonly performed for identification of areas affected by obstructive atherosclerotic coronary artery disease; selective coronary angiography with an injection of contrast medium into the right and left coronary ostia illustrates coronary anatomy, distal coronary perfusion, the location of atherosclerotic lesions, the status of coronary collateral circulation, and the percentage of narrowing of coronary arteries affected by coronary artery disease (CAD). Coronary angiography is also performed for assessment of the patency of previously inserted bypass grafts. Left ventriculography is accomplished with an injection into the LV chamber and filming of the movement of the dye. Cardiac output, ejection fraction values (normal value, 60% to 70%), wall motion (e.g., hypokinesia, dyskinesia/paradoxic motion), and valvular function (e.g., mitral regurgitation, prosthetic valve function) can be assessed during ventriculography. Generally, a right-heart catheterization yields data concerning the inferior and superior vena cava, the right atrium and ventricle, tricuspid and pulmonary valves, and the pulmonary artery. A left-heart catheterization yields information concerning the left atrium and ventricle, the proximal aorta, aortic and mitral valves, and the coronary arteries.[13] Aortography displays the size and function of the aorta and can be used to identify the location of the intimal tear in a dissection. Computed tomographic (CAT) scan and magnetic resonance arteriography have largely replaced aortography for imaging of aortic disease.

**Cardioplegia:** Literally, "paralysis of the heart"; pharmacologically induced cardiac arrest during surgery on the heart. The purposes of cardioplegia are protection of the myocardium against irreversible ischemic injury during the aortic cross-clamp period when the heart is arrested and conservation of energy resources that can be used after removal of the cross clamp. Effective intraoperative myocardial protection positively affects the patient's postoperative recovery.

The goal of myocardial protection is achieved with induced hypothermia and rapid diastolic arrest. Hypothermia reduces the metabolic rate (and therefore the energy demands) of the tissue being cooled. Rapid diastolic arrest conserves existing cellular energy resources (e.g., adenosine triphosphate [ATP]) by avoiding the energy-expensive state of ventricular fibrillation before the heart achieves an arrested state. Quick arrest of a beating heart (e.g., 10 to 20 seconds) enhances myocardial energy conservation. Potassium is the most commonly used arresting agent, but the solutions may also contain electrolytes, buffers to maintain appropriate pH, glucose, metabolic substrates, calcium antagonists, tromethamine, heparin, and antiarrhythmic agents; the carrying solution may be crystalloid or blood (preferable for its oxygen carrying capacity).[14]

Methods of infusion of cardioplegia include the antegrade and retrograde routes and the direct coronary ostial route of infusion. With the antegrade method, a needle catheter is inserted into the anterior aorta proximal to the aortic cross clamp (Fig. 35-11). The cardioplegia solution is infused with sufficient pressure to close the aortic valve; with the cross clamp applied distally and a competent aortic valve proximally, the only paths for the solution to travel are the right and left coronary ostia lying between the cross clamped aorta and the closed aortic valve. In patients with aortic valve insufficiency, cardioplegia flow into the coronary ostia is significantly reduced because the incompetent aortic valve provides a lower pressure pathway into the inner ventricular chamber, thereby distending the heart (and increasing myocardial wall tension). Retrograde delivery is indicated.

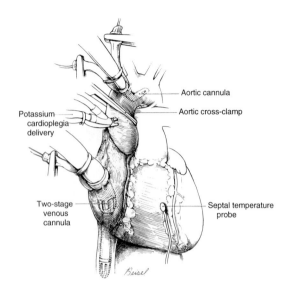

**Fig. 35-11** Antegrade cardioplegia infusion catheter is inserted proximal to aortic cross clamp and arterial infusion cannula. Two-stage (single) venous cannula drains sysemic venous return. Openings in distal end of cannula drain blood from lower body; openings in midportion of cannula (within right atrium) drain blood returning from upper body and coronary venous drainage exiting from coronary sinus. Septal temperature probe monitors myocardial septal temperature. *(From Rothrock JC: Alexander's care of the patient in surgery, ed 13, St Louis, 2007, Mosby.)*

With the retrograde route, a catheter is inserted through the right atrial wall and the catheter tip is inserted into the coronary sinus. Cardioplegia is infused and travels through coronary venous tissue to the capillary beds and then to the arterial system where it exits through the coronary ostia. With the cross clamp applied, the exiting blood places excess tension on the aorta, so a suction catheter is used to vent the effluent from the aorta. With both antegrade and retrograde cardioplegia, transmural delivery of the arresting solution can be achieved. In patients with coronary lesions, the antegrade route alone does not achieve transmural delivery. In some cases where the aorta has been opened (e.g., aortic valve replacement), retrograde cardioplegia may be sufficient. Occasionally, however, insertion of the retrograde catheter cannot be performed. In these cases, direct ostial infusion of the cardioplegia with hand-held cannulas may be used.

**Cardiopulmonary Bypass (CPB):** A temporary substitution for the heart and lungs with a mechanical device that drains systemic venous return (thereby decompressing the heart) into an oxygenator that removes excess carbon dioxide and adds oxygen (simulating the lungs) and pumps arterialized blood into the systemic circulation (simulating the heart). The development of CPB enabled surgeons to isolate the heart by cross clamping the aorta and to pharmacologically induce cardiac arrest to create a dry quiet operative field in which to perform the surgical repairs. During the period of cardiac arrest, the rest of the body can be adequately perfused via CPB (Fig. 35-12).

Systemic venous return flows by gravity drainage (the level of the patient needs to be above that of the bypass machine to facilitate drainage) into one or two large-bore (e.g., 32F to 36F) cannulas inserted into the right atrium. With the single two-stage cannula (see Fig. 35-11), openings in the distal tip drain blood returning from the inferior vena cava (IVC) and openings in the mid portion of the cannula drain venous blood from the superior vena cava (SVC) and the coronary circulation exiting from the coronary sinus. Some blood enters the RA and the pulmonary circulation. With double cannulation (Fig. 35-13), individual cannulas are inserted into the IVC and the SVC, thereby forcing all venous return into the cannulas. Generally the two-stage cannula is used for coronary artery bypass grafting and aortic valve surgery when total right side decompression is not generally needed and blood entering the right side of the heart does not obscure the surgical field; individual (double) venous cannulation may be used for procedures in the right side (e.g., tricuspid valve repair) to keep the right heart free of blood. Occasionally, two cannulas may be used when greater decompression of the RA is necessary (e.g., mitral valve surgery).

After the blood is oxygenated, it is pumped into the systemic circulation via an arterial cannula, commonly located in the aorta (Fig. 35-14). When aortic pathology (e.g., aortic aneurysm) prevents cannulation, the femoral artery may be cannulated (retrograde flow) for arterial return. The axillary artery may be needed when the aorta or both of the femoral arteries are unavailable.

In addition to the standard cannulation techniques for CPB, minimally invasive systems use endovascular catheters (Fig. 35-15). A venous catheter is inserted into the femoral vein, and the arterial cannula is placed into the femoral artery. The ipsilateral femoral artery is also used for insertion of a multilumen catheter; one lumen serves as an endovascular cross clamp that occludes the aorta with inflation of an intraaortic balloon at the tip of the catheter, and the other lumen can be used for infusion of antegrade cardioplegia. Pressure lines, venting catheters, and a coronary sinus retrograde cardioplegia catheter can be inserted via the jugular vein. This system does not require median sternotomy and is an important adjunct for minimally invasive surgery.

A number of risks are associated with the use of CPB (e.g., particulate or air embolus), and some form of checklist is often used before CPB is instituted (Box 35-1) and before the patient is weaned from CPB (Box 35-2). Such checklists help to enhance the safety of CPB. In addition, the clinical sequelae of CPB can affect all body systems; caregivers in the postoperative period should be aware of the effects that CPB may have (Table 35-2).

**Coarctation of the Aorta:** A narrowing of the thoracic aorta, usually in the area of the ligamentum arteriosum (formerly, the fetal patent ductus arteriosus [PDA], that shunts blood from the pulmonary artery to the aorta).[10] Of the two types of coarctation, preductal and postductal, the postductal type is more likely to be seen in the adult because the heart in utero has been stimulated to develop extensive collateral circulation in response to the increased afterload represented by the coarctation's position distal to the aortic exit of the PDA. (In preductal coarctations, the fetal heart is not stimulated to develop collaterals because blood flow from the heart to the aorta via the PDA is not restricted.) In the adult, a coarctation may be identified when preoperative bilateral arm blood pressure measurements are unequal. A common repair in the adult is accomplished with excising the coarctation and interposing a prosthetic graft.

**Commissurotomy:** The opening or separation of fused valvular commissures (in the adult, generally the mitral or pulmonary valve). Open commissurotomy is now commonly performed (versus closed commissurotomy). The procedure consists of exposing the affected valve (with the use of CPB and induced cardiac arrest) and sharply incising the fused commissures. The procedure is done on young adults with a history of rheumatic fever that leads to fusion of the leaflets. The leaflets tend to become progressively more fibrotic and stenotic. A commissurotomy performed at an earlier age can delay the inevitable future need for more extensive valve repair or replacement, which is a significant consideration because the patient can avoid the potential complication of prosthetic valve replacement. Balloon valvulotomy may be performed in some instances.

**Congenital Heart Disease:** Anomalies apparent at birth or later in life. In this section, some of the congenital anomalies that are seen in adulthood are discussed.[15]

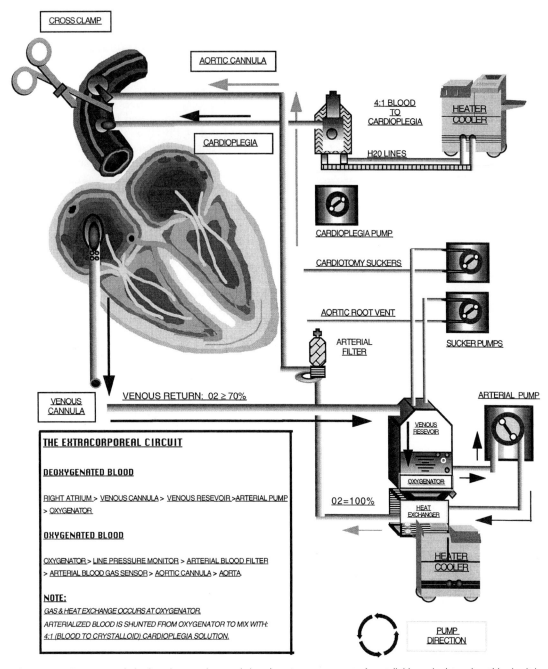

**Fig. 35-12**  Extracorporeal circuit and anatomic cannulation sites. Average amount of crystalloid required to prime this circuit is 2000 mL. Heparin, mannitol $NaHCO_3^-$, albumin, corticosteroids, and antifibrinolytics such as aminocaproic acid are also added, depending on institutional preferences. Most circuits incorporate inline arterial and venous blood as monitoring, line pressure manometers, anesthetic vaporizers, temperature monitoring systems, and numerous safety devices with computerized override mechanisms to be used in event of mechanical failure or operator error. *(From Nagelhout JJ, Zaglaniczny KL: Nurse anesthesia, ed 3, St Louis, 2005, Saunders.)*

**Dysrhythmia Surgery for Atrial Fibrillation (AF):** Surgery designed to block or redirect aberrant atrial fibrillatory impulses toward the atrioventricular (AV) node to achieve normal sinus rhythm. AF is associated with significant morbidity and mortality rates. In 1991, the Cox Maze procedure[16] showed excellent results in redirecting the impulses of AF with incisions made and then sutured closed. Electric impulses cannot cross sutured (or ablated) tissue. Because

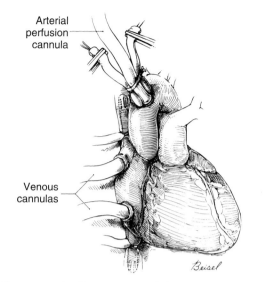

**Fig. 35-13** Double venous cannulation. One cannula is inserted into inferior vena cava (IVC), and the other into superior vena cava (SVC). Also shown is arterial infusion catheter. *(In Seifert PC: Cardiac surgery, St. Louis, 2002, Mosby. From Rothrock JC: Alexander's care of the patient in surgery, ed 13, St Louis, 2007, Mosby.)*

electric impulses can travel only through normal tissue, the surgeon locates the various incisions in such a way to create a pathway toward the AV node, thereby returning the heart to normal sinus rhythm.[16] More recent research has shown that the source of 90% of the aberrant impulses come from the area that surrounds the pulmonary veins.[17] Ablation of the targeted tissue (with cold energy, radiofrequency, or

other energy source) has been successful with a more than 90% success rate in achieving sinus rhythm.[18]

**Hypothermia:** Cooling of the patient during cardiac surgery. Hypothermia may be induced (elective) or inadvertent. Induced systemic hypothermia is achieved with a heat exchanger incorporated into the CPB circuit (see Fig. 35-12). For most cardiac procedures of less than 1 hour of induced cardiac arrest (e.g., coronary artery bypass grafting), the perfusionist cools the systemic circulation from a normal temperature of 37° C to approximately 30° C (86° F). The cardioplegia solution is cooled to a lower temperature (near freezing) for intracardiac cooling as a method of myocardial protection. For procedures with a longer cross-clamp time, the systemic temperature may be further reduced to protect the brain, kidneys, and other organs while the heart is arrested by reducing energy demands and limiting ischemic injury. Topical cooling of the heart with cold lavage or frozen "slush" placed on the heart and in the pericardial well helps to achieve transmural cooling.

Although induced hypothermia plays an important role in minimization of tissue ischemia during selected portions of cardiac procedures, inadvertent hypothermia has become an important consideration for cardiac patients because of associated risks for perioperative complications. Before surgery, shivering increases myocardial oxygen demands and further taxes hearts that have diminished myocardial energy supplies. During surgery, before and after CPB,

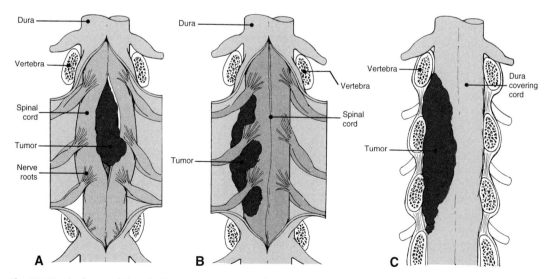

**Fig. 35-14** Aortic cannulation. **A,** Two concentric purse string sutures are placed in anterior aorta and tourniquets attached. **B,** Stab wound is made in aorta, and arterial cannula is inserted. **C,** Tourniquets are tightened and tied to arterial cannula. *(From Waldhausen JA, et al: Surgery of the chest, ed 6, St Louis, 1996, Mosby.)*

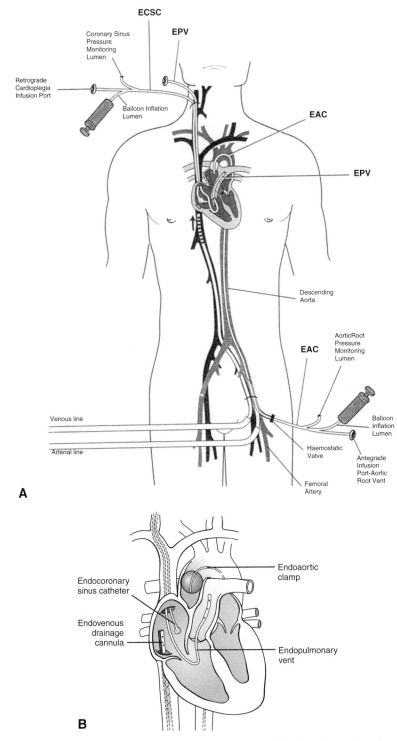

**Fig. 35-15**   Minimally invasive cardiopulmonary bypass technique. **A,** Positioning of endovascular catheters (see text). *EAC,* Endoaortic clamp; *ECSC,* endocoronary sinus catheter; *EPV,* cardiopulmonary vent. **B,** Correct positions of endocoronary sinus catheter, endoaortic clamp, endovenous drainage cannula, and endopulmonary vent for port-access cardiopulmonary bypass. (**A,** *From Toomasian M, et al: Extracorporeal circulation for port-access cardiac surgery,* Perfusion *12:83, 1997.* **B,** *From Kaplan J, editor:* Kaplan's cardiac anesthesia, *ed 5, Philadelphia, 2006, Saunders.)*

---

**Box 35-1    Checklist for Initiation of Pump**

Heparin administered

ACT checked and at least 350 to 400 seconds

Muscle relaxant adequate (or infusion turned on for maintenance)

Inotropic infusions turned off

Pupil symmetry assessed for later comparison (unilateral dilation may indicate unilateral carotid perfusion on cardiopulmonary bypass)

Pulmonary artery catheter (if used) pulled back 5 cm

Urinary output emptied before bypass (start anew with initiation of bypass)

Proper functioning of all monitors ensured

From Brouillette CV: Cardiac anesthesia. In Nagelhout JJ, Zaglaniczny KL, editors: *Nurse anesthesia*, ed 3, St Louis, 2005, Saunders.

---

**Box 35-2    Checklist for Weaning from the Pump**

Patient is warm (to at least 35°C)

Heart rhythm has returned

All monitors are functioning; electrocardiogram, pulmonary artery tracing, arterial line tracing, central venous pressure reflect heart filling

Heart rate is 70 to 100 beats per minute (< 60 bpm is reduced cardiac output; ≥ 120 bpm is detrimental to left ventricular filling)

Infusions are prepared as necessary

Lungs are inflated (but kept out of the surgeon's field)

Pressure becomes pulsatile as ventricles fill

Blood drawn for measurement of electrolytes, hematocrit, arterial blood gases, and activated clotting time

Surgeon clamps venous drain and removes cannula

Patient is off pump

From Brouillette CV: Cardiac anesthesia. In Nagelhout JJ, Zaglaniczny KL, editors: *Nurse anesthesia*, ed 3, St Louis, 2005, Saunders.

---

inadvertent cooling of the patient is associated with increased surgical bleeding and a diminished immune response. After surgery, hypothermia contributes to patient discomfort, impaired wound healing, prolonged bleeding, longer lengths of stay, and cardiac events such as ischemia and tachyarrhythmias.[19,20] Active measures, such as the application of warm blankets before surgery and the intraoperative (before and after

induced hypothermia), the postoperative use of forced warm air devices and intravenous fluid warmers, and an increased ambient room temperature, can help to maintain normothermia.

**Implantable Cardioverter-Defibrillator (ICD):** A device that provides a shock to the heart for tachycardia above a predetermined rate or ventricular fibrillation and also has the capability to provide bradycardia therapy. The device is usually inserted transvenously in the electrophysiology or cardiac catheterization laboratory. Patients with ICDs who undergo surgery have a magnet placed over the generator (usually in the right or left upper chest) to turn off the device and avoid frequent shocks during induced cardiac arrest. After surgery, the magnet is removed and the ICD is again activated.

**Minimally Invasive Cardiac Surgery:** Operations that use smaller incisions, endoscopic access, endovascular techniques, or off-pump (i.e., no CPB) procedures. Some controversy exists over the definition of "minimally invasive." Some clinicians define minimally invasive surgery as procedures that use smaller incisions; others consider the use of CPB as invasive and define minimally invasive surgery as that which does not use CPB.

The most common procedure in minimally invasive surgery (MIS) is the endoscopic video-assisted excision of saphenous vein coronary bypass grafts. In other cases, smaller sternal or thoracic chest incisions or ports may be used for target areas of the heart that can be accessed through these minimal incisions (e.g., certain coronary bypass operations for single vessel disease and some valve procedures; Fig. 35-16). With smaller incisions or port access, endovascular techniques to establish CPB may be used (see Fig. 35-15). MIS can speed patient recovery, allow the patient to return faster to normal activities, and reduce costs.

When the surgery requires a thorough assessment of, and complete access to, the heart (as with global CAD), a traditional sternotomy is usually used, although CPB may not be used. So-called "off-pump" procedures for myocardial revascularization (see subsequent definition) can be performed while the heart is beating with the use of special devices to isolate the section of the coronary artery to be grafted. For procedures that require entry into the chambers of the heart (e.g., valve replacement), CPB and cardioplegic arrest is necessary for perfusion of the body, avoidance of air emboli that originate from the open cardiac chamber, and myocardial preservation.

**Mitral Regurgitation (MR):** A condition that occurs when one or more components of the

## Table 35-2   Effects of Cardiopulmonary Bypass

| Effects | Contributing Factors |
| --- | --- |
| **CARDIOVASCULAR SYSTEM** | |
| Perioperative myocardial infarction | Inadequate myocardial protection and emboli |
| Low cardiac output syndrome after surgery | Preexisting heart disease, inadequate myocardial protection, alteration in colloidal osmotic pressure, left ventricular dysfunction, hypoperfusion injury, hypothermia, long pump run |
| Increased afterload | Catecholamine release |
| Hypertension | Elevated rennin, angiotensin, and aldosterone levels |
| Hypotension | Postoperative diuresis, sudden vasodilation (rewarming), third spacing |
| **PULMONARY SYSTEM** | |
| Respiratory insufficiency | Alterations in colloidal osmotic pressure, interstitial pulmonary edema, decreased perfusion, alterations in ventilatory patterns, decreased surfactant production, pulmonary microemboli |
| Atelectasis | Complement activation and inflammatory response, emboli, alveolar-capillary membrane damage |
| **NEUROLOGIC SYSTEM** | |
| Cerebrovascular accident | Cerebral emboli |
| Transient motor defects | Decreased cerebral blood flow |
| Cerebral hemorrhage | Systematic heparin administration |
| Neuropsychologic deficits | Microemboli, ischemia, altered perfusion flow of bypass |
| **GASTROINTESTINAL SYSTEM** | |
| Gastrointestinal bleeding | Hormonal stress and coagulation diatheses |
| Intestinal ischemia or infarction | Emboli and decreased perfusion |
| Acute pancreatitis | Pancreatic vasculature emboli |
| **RENAL SYSTEM** | |
| Acute renal failure | Decreased renal blood flow, microemboli, and myohemoglobin release |
| Hemoglobinuria | Red blood cell hemolysis |
| **FLUID AND ELECTROLYTE BALANCE** | |
| Interstitial edema, weight gain | Increased extravascular fluid and organ dysfunction, fluid shifts, decreased plasma protein concentration, increased capillary permeability |
| Intravascular hypovolemia | Decreased intravascular volume, bleeding, and interstitial edema |
| Hypokalemia | Dilution, polyuria, intracellular shifts of potassium ions |
| Hyperkalemia | Potassium cardioplegia and increased intracellular exchange of glucose and potassium, cellular destruction |
| Hyponatremia, hypocalcemia, and hypomagnesemia | Dilution, fluid shifts, diureses |
| **ENDOCRINE SYSTEM** | |
| Water and sodium retention | Increase in antidiuretic hormone |
| Hypothyroidism | Increased levels of thyroxine (T4) and decreased levels of triiodothyronine (T3) and thyroid-stimulating hormone |
| Hyperglycemia | Depressed insulin response, stimulation of glycogenesis |
| **IMMUNE SYSTEM** | |
| Infection | Exposure to multiple pathogens, decreased immunoglobin levels, and hypothermia |
| Postperfusion syndrome | Release of anaphylactic toxins, complement activation |
| **HEMATOLOGIC FACTORS** | |
| Bleeding | Blood cell hemolysis, heparin rebound, reduction in platelet count and coagulation factors, coagulopathy, systemic heparin administration, depressed liver function from hypothermia |

From Seifert PC: *Cardiac surgery: perioperative patient care*, St Louis, 2002, Mosby.

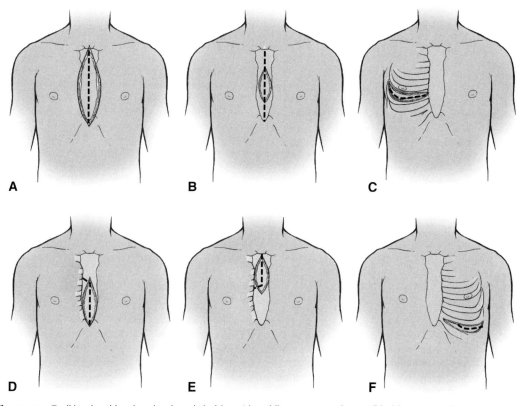

**Fig. 35-16** Traditional and less invasive thoracic incisions (*dotted lines* represent chest wall incisions). **A,** Traditional sternotomy. **B,** Full sternotomy with limited skin incision. **C,** Parasternal incision (infrequently used). **D** and **E,** Partial lower and upper sternotomy incisions used mainly for valve procedures. **F,** Right thoracotomy incision can be used for mitral valve procedures; left anterior thoracotomy (*not shown*) can be used for single coronary bypass graft to left anterior descending coronary artery. *(In Rothrock JC: Alexander's care of the patient in surgery, ed 13, St Louis, 2007, Mosby. From Braunwald E, Zipes DP, Libby P, editors: Heart disease, ed 6, Philadelphia, 2001, Saunders.)*

mitral valve apparatus prevents competent closure of the valve, with subsequent regurgitation of blood into the left atrium (Fig. 35-17). The causes of MR may be inflammatory, degenerative, infective, structural, or congenital. Components of the mitral valve apparatus include the valve leaflets, the annulus, chordae tendineae, papillary muscles, and the endoventricular wall (the tricuspid valve is similarly configured). The leaflets may not close properly because of leaflet tears, leaflet degeneration from fibroelastic changes (Fig. 35-18), or mitral valve prolapse (whereby the leaflets balloon into the left atrium). Annular dilation prevents the leaflets from approximating one another. Chordae tendineae may be ruptured or excessively elongated or shortened and fused from bacterial endocarditis, one or more papillary muscle heads may have ruptured as a result of ischemic heart disease, or the ventricular endocardium may be dilated. Annuloplasty and valvuloplasty (see subsequent definition) may be

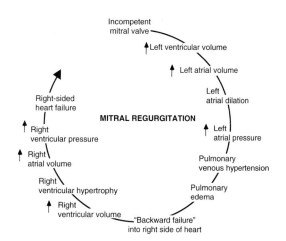

**Fig. 35-17** Pathophysiology of mitral regurgitation. *(In Seifert PC: Cardiac surgery, St Louis, 2002, Mosby. From Kinney MR, et al: Andreoli's comprehensive cardiac care, ed 8, St Louis, 1996, Mosby.)*

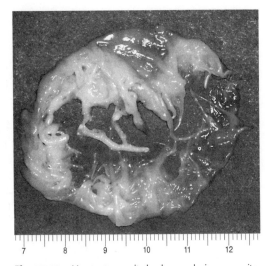

**Fig. 35-18**  Myxomatous mitral valve producing regurgitation. Thin elongated leaflets are rarely amenable to valve repair and usually require valve replacement. *(From Seifert PC: Cardiac surgery, St Louis, 2002, Mosby. Courtesy Edward A. Lefrak, MD.)*

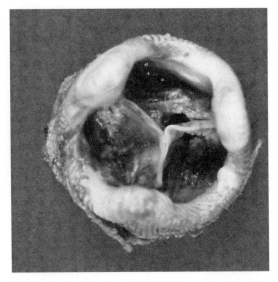

**Fig. 35-19**  Explanted porcine mitral valve prosthesis. Leaflets are torn and calcified. *(From Seifert PC: Cardiac surgery, St Louis, 2002, Mosby. Courtesy Edward A. Lefrak, MD.)*

performed on the affected component. When valvular deformation injury is severe, prosthetic replacement may be required. MR also may be related to fibrosis, calcification, or tears in a previously implanted valve prosthesis (Fig. 35-19). Chronic MR produces an enlarged atria where stasis of blood can lead to thrombus formation and subsequent thromboembolism (TE); the dilated atrium can also lead to conduction disturbances such as atrial fibrillation. Pulmonary overloading occurs and eventually can produce pulmonary hypertension; the subsequent increased pulmonary pressures may produce functional tricuspid valve regurgitation. Acute MR is poorly tolerated because the left atrium is unable to contain the sudden regurgitant volume overload and pulmonary overload ensues rapidly; emergency valve replacement or repair (if possible) is indicated.

**Mitral Stenosis (MS):**  A narrowing of the mitral valve orifice that creates an impedance to flow across the valve (Fig. 35-20). MS is the result of changes in one or more of the components of the mitral apparatus. The causes of MS may be inflammation, calcification, tumors (i.e., left atrial myxoma), and infection. Bacterial vegetations and the sequelae of rheumatic fever continue to be significant causes of MS. Fig. 35-21 illustrates the classic "fish mouth" appearance of a rheumatic mitral valve: smooth fibrotic thickened leaflets, commissural fusion, and shortened thickened chordae tendineae. Reparative surgical options for MS are more limited than those for MR because the deformities seen in

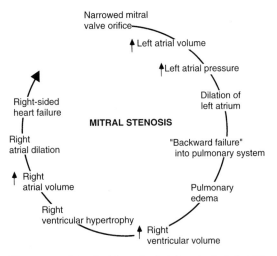

**Fig. 35-20**  Pathophysiology of mitral stenosis. *(In Seifert PC: Cardiac surgery, St Louis, 2002, Mosby. From Kinney MR, et al: Andreoli's comprehensive cardiac care, ed 8, St Louis, 1996, Mosby.)*

severe MS (such as thickened leaflets) are less amenable to repair. Techniques such as chordal splitting and debridement of valvular calcific nodules may be used, but valve replacement is often necessary. In the earlier stages of MS, mitral commissurotomy for fused commissures may provide acceptable postoperative valve function for years. Unlike AS, AI, or MR, stenosis of the mitral valve is the only lesion that does not place either a volume or a pressure load on the left ventricle. However, chronic MS

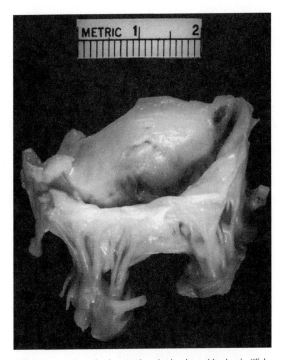

**Fig. 35-21** Stenotic rheumatic mitral valve with classic "fish mouth" appearance. Leaflets are smooth and thickened; chordae tendineae arising from papillary muscle tips are shortened and fused. *(From Seifert PC: Cardiac surgery, St Louis, 2002, Mosby. Courtesy William C Roberts, MD; Michael Spencer, photographer.)*

(like MR) produces an enlarged atria and stasis of blood (with the risk of TE) and frequently leads to atrial fibrillation. Functional tricuspid regurgitation may develop.

**Myocardial Protection Techniques:** Techniques or procedures designed to conserve myocardial energy resources and limit the amount of ischemic tissue injury that can occur. The use of cardioplegia and induced hypothermia (see previous definition) to arrest and preserve the heart form the foundation of myocardial protection. Additional myocardial protective measures may include minimization of the risk of an air embolus from ambient room air trapped inside the heart with insufflation of $CO_2$ gas through a catheter into the pericardial well. The $CO_2$ gas not only displaces ambient air but also dissolves approximately 25 times faster in the blood than room air and is less harmful to cardiac tissue.

The best way to achieve adequate myocardial energy conservation is to implement actions that consistently maximize myocardial energy supplies and minimize myocardial energy demands. Thus, surgeons and assistants, for example, use caution in touching the heart before bypass to lessen the risk of ventricular fibrillation;

anesthesia providers pharmacologically decrease cellular oxygen demand and increase cellular oxygen supply.

Other considerations in protecting the heart include minimization of cross-clamp time with availability of the appropriate supplies and equipment, a plan for surgery (this applies to surgeons, anesthesia providers, perfusionists, and nursing personnel), anticipation and ability to respond to potential risks and complications applicable to one's professional responsibilities and skills, implementation of safety procedures, and frequent and collaborative communication. Each member of the surgical team plays a critical role in achieving optimal outcomes because "time is muscle" in cardiac surgery and small delays can have a negative impact.

**Myocardial Revascularization:** Also called coronary artery bypass grafting (CABG). Surgical procedure performed for CAD in which conduits of the patient's own tissue (autograft), most commonly the internal mammary artery (IMA) or other arteries (e.g., radial artery, gastroepiploic artery) and the greater saphenous vein, are attached directly to the affected coronary artery at a site distal to the narrowed atherosclerotic lesion. Generally, coronary narrowing of 70% or greater in arteries of 1 mm or more is an indication for bypass grafting; narrowing of less than 70% may create competitive flow between the conduit and the native artery and reduce the amount of blood that perfuses the bypass graft (and the anastomosed coronary artery). Fig. 35-22 illustrates possible arterial and venous autologous conduits. Grafts from cadaver human saphenous vein, human and bovine umbilical vein, and synthetic grafts have been used when other conduits were unavailable. CABG does not cure CAD; its purpose is to increase blood flow to the myocardium beyond the obstructive lesions. CAD is a progressive disease, and retardation of the atherosclerotic process requires life style changes and pharmacologic support (e.g., statins). Gender-based differences in CABG outcomes are under scrutiny, and guidelines have been published to provide (Box 35-3) evidence for the selection of techniques.[21]

The left IMA is commonly used in bypass of the left anterior descending coronary artery. The IMA is dissected from its retrosternal bed to the required length (Fig. 35-23), leaving intact the proximal attachment to the left subclavian artery. Greater saphenous vein is commonly harvested with video-assisted endoscopic techniques (Fig. 35-24); because leg veins have valves that facilitate flow towards the right heart, reversal of the vein is necessary so that

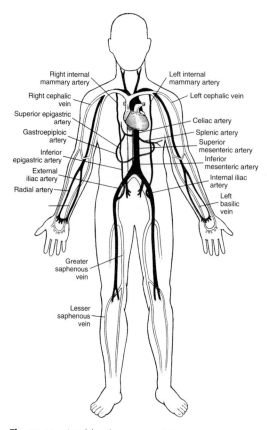

**Fig. 35-22** Arterial and venous conduits for coronary bypass surgery. *(From Seifert PC:* Cardiac surgery, *St Louis, 2002, Mosby.)*

flow as a bypass graft is not impeded. The distal anastomosis is created with attaching the end of the graft conduit to the side of the coronary artery. Veins grafts may be attached to the diagonal, obtuse marginal, posterior descending, or right coronary arteries, as indicated. Proximally, the IMA graft remains attached to the subclavian artery; for vein grafts, the proximal end of the vein is attached to an opening created in the side of the proximal aorta (Fig. 35-25).

Off-pump CABG has been facilitated with the use of stabilizing devices that isolate and reduce the motion of the portion of the artery to be anastomosed (Fig. 35-26, A). An attachment applies suction to the LV apex and allows the heart to be retracted for access to the lateral (i.e., obtuse marginal branches) and posterior (i.e., posterior descending or distal right coronary artery) portions of the heart (Fig. 35-26, B). Patient teaching considerations related to on pump/off pump surgery are listed in Table 35-3.

Another form of myocardial revascularization is repair of a left ventricular aneurysm. An LV aneurysm most often results from a large myocardial infarction or numerous smaller adjacent infarctions that cause a portion of the myocardial wall to become scarred, necrotic, thin, and weak. Scar tissue does not contract during systole but instead bulges outward (paradoxic motion/dyskinesia), which decreases the patient's cardiac output. Thrombus can form within the trabeculations of the LV, and pieces of thrombus can break off and embolize to the systemic circulation. In addition, the perimeter around the scarred fibrotic aneurysmal area can alter conduction pathways and create reentrant ventricular dysrhythmias. Surgical repair consists of excision of the aneurysmal tissue, removal of existing thrombus, and insertion of a patch into the LV in a manner that restores a more normal (i.e., elliptic) ventricular geometry. If the patient continues to have recurrent ventricular tachycardia (VT), electrophysiologic (EP) mapping and possible insertion of an ICD may be performed after surgery in the EP laboratory.

**Patent Ductus Arteriosus (PDA):** A duct between the pulmonary artery and the aorta. This structure, present in fetal life, usually closes within 1 or 2 weeks after birth (and becomes the ligamentum arteriosum). Failure to close can predispose the patient to the development of pulmonary hypertension, endocarditis, or cardiac failure. Closure can be surgically achieved with ligation of the ductus or with division of the ductus followed by oversewing of the ends.

**Percutaneous Transluminal Coronary Angioplasty (PTCA) with Stent Insertion:** A catheter-based interventional technique performed with fluoroscopy in the cardiac catheterization (see previous definition) laboratory for acute or chronically obstructed coronary arteries. A percutaneously inserted balloon catheter is threaded to the right or left coronary os, where the catheter is positioned across the coronary artery at the site of the narrowing. The balloon is inflated to compress the atherosclerotic lesion and enlarge the coronary lumen. Equalized pressure measurements above and below the lesion indicate a successful angioplasty. Because the restenosis rate for angioplasty at 6 months has been approximately 30%, insertion of a stent (bare metal or coated) is commonly performed in conjunction with the PTCA. Complications from the PTCA procedure include prolonged chest pain, myocardial infarction, coronary spasm, or coronary artery dissection (that often necessitates emergency CABG).

**Pericardiectomy, Pericardial Window:** Pericardiectomy is the partial excision of an

| Box 35-3    Guidelines for Female Patients Undergoing Coronary Artery Bypass Surgery |
|---|

In an effort to resolve the numerous inconsistencies that surround the issue of gender-based differences between the outcomes of women and men who undergo CABG, the Society of Thoracic Surgeons (STS) Workforce on Evidence-Based Surgery reviewed published information on this subject. The following guidelines focus specifically on perioperative management and are based on the evidence available to the authors of the Guidelines.

1. Use of the internal mammary artery (IMA)
   - The IMA is underused in women
   - Use of the IMA is associated with a significant reduction in mortality rate (compared with CABG with venous conduits alone)
   - At least one IMA is used to bypass stenotic coronary artery
2. Management of hyperglycemia
   - Diabetes is more common in women than in men who undergo CABG
   - The adverse effects of diabetes are more pronounced in women
   - Hyperglycemia produced an incremental risk in CABG
   - Blood glucose levels should be maintained at less than 150 mg/dL (range, 100-150 mg/dL)
3. Intraoperative management of anemia
   - Hematocrits of less than 22% are associated with operative mortality
   - Strategies to increase red blood cell concentration include hemoconcentration, ultrafiltration, minimization of pump prime volume, rapid autologous priming (see text)
   - Adequate hematocrit levels should be maintained at or greater than 22%
4. Use of off-pump CABG (OPCAB)
   - Improved outcomes after OPCAB versus on-pump CABG may be related to increased use of IMA with OPCAB
   - No major differences in outcomes are associated with valve surgery
   - With the absence of firm evidence that OPCAB is superior, the Guidelines suggest that the indications for OPCAB are the same for women as for men
5. Optimization of thyroxine treatment for women with hypothyroidism
   - Hypothyroidism is associated with impaired contractility and increased risk of myocardial infarction
   - A greater incidence rate is seen of women with hypothyroidism (compared with men) undergoing CABG
   - A euthyroid state should be maintained during surgery
6. Consideration of preoperative hormone replacement therapy (HRT)
   - HRT is not a significant predictor of mortality rate in multivariate analyses
   - HRT is associated with complications such as thromboembolism
   - HRT is not used for postmenopausal women undergoing CABG

From Rothrock JC: *Alexander's care of the patient in surgery,* ed 13, St Louis, 2007, Mosby.

adhered thickened fibrotic pericardium to relieve constriction of the heart and great blood vessels. In patients with chronic cardiac effusions, the creation of a pericardial window (excision of a portion of the pericardial/pleural wall) between the pericardial sac and the pleural space drains the fluid. In patients with chronic effusions, the window to the pleural space generally allows future fluid accumulation to be reabsorbed.

**Pulmonary Stenosis:** Fusion of the valve cusps at the commissures, which creates an obstruction to the right-ventricular outflow tract. Repair may be accomplished surgically via an open procedure with direct visualization; the fused commissures are sharply divided to improved leaflet motion. Balloon angioplasty in the cardiac catheterization laboratory also may be performed.

Another form of pulmonary stenosis occurs in the infundibular portion where fibromuscular obstruction occurs proximal to the valve, creating right ventricular outflow tract (RVOT) obstruction. Repair may involve opening of the RVOT and insertion of a patch to enlarge the outflow tract.

**Tetralogy of Fallot (TOF):** A congenital entity with four distinctive features: (1) a high ventricular septal defect (VSD); (2) pulmonary stenosis that affects the valve or the infundibular

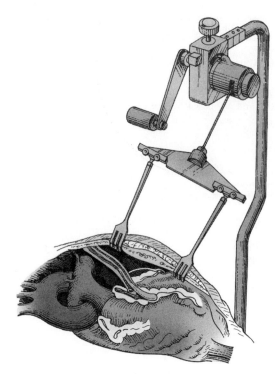

**Fig. 35-23**    Dissection of left internal mammary artery (LIMA) from retrosternal bed with use of special retractor that elevates sternal border. *(From Rothrock JC: Alexander's care of the patient in surgery, ed 13, St Louis, 2007, Mosby. Courtesy Rultract, Inc, Cleveland.)*

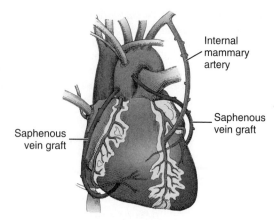

**Fig. 35-25**    Coronary artery bypass grafts with left internal mammary artery to left anterior descending coronary artery, and saphenous vein grafts to obtuse marginal and distal right coronary arteries. *(In Rothrock JC: Alexander's care of the patient in surgery, ed 13, St Louis, 2007, Mosby. From Zipes DP, et al: Braumwald's heart disease: a textbook of cardiovascular medicine, ed 7, Philadelphia, 2005, Saunders.)*

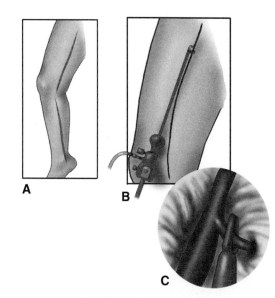

**Fig. 35-24**    Minimally invasive approach to saphenous vein harvesting. **A,** Traditional open incision. **B,** Insertion of endoscopic camera and dissector. **C,** Venous tributaries cut and clipped, cauterized, or ligated to prevent leaking of blood. *(In Rothrock JC: Alexander's care of the patient in surgery, ed 13, St Louis, 2007, Mosby. From Zipes DP, et al: Braumwald's heart disease: a textbook of cardiovascular medicine, ed 7, Philadelphia, 2005, Saunders.)*

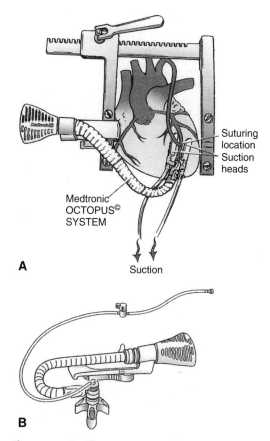

**Fig. 35-26**    **A,** Off pump retractor stabilizes site of coronary anastomosis. **B,** Suction device attached to left ventricular apex exposes apical and lateral coronary arteries for coronary bypass. *(Courtesy of Medtronic Heart Valves, Minneapolis, MN.)*

## Table 35-3 Patient Teaching Considerations for Minimally Invasive Surgery (On/Off Pump)

| | Beating Heart/Off-Pump | Arrested Heart |
|---|---|---|
| Definition | CABG without CPB or induced cardiac arrest; HR and contractile force may be pharmacologically reduced; stabilizer used at anastomotic site; apical retractor used to expose lateral and posterior coronary arteries | CABG with CPB and endovascular technique for CPB and induced cardiac arrest |
| Indications | Multiple-vessel disease, angioplasty contraindicated, medical problems, poor anatomy, accessible target arteries, previous CABG with blocked grafts | Multiple-vessel disease; angioplasty contraindicated, need to stop heart to enhance technical precision, accessible target arteries, mitral valve disease |
| Contraindications | Intramyocardial lesions, hemodynamic instability | High complex lesions, posterior targets |
| Incisions | Sternotomy or ministernotomy (cephalad or caudad); 1-3 small right or left rib or submammary incision | 1-4 small rib incisions, 1 or 2 groin inscisions |
| CPB | No, available on standby | Yes |
| Cardioplegia | No | Yes |
| Procedure time | 2 h or more | 2 h or more |
| Hospital LOS | 3-5 d (versus 4-6 d for sternotomy) | 3-5 d (versus 4-6 d for sternotomy) |
| Advantages | Avoids CPB, ischemic arrest, and hypothermia; may enable more complete revascularization with postoperative insertion of intracoronary stents into posterolateral coronary arteries in cardiac catheterization laboratory ("hybrid" procedure) | Allows repair of more complex lesions without technical challenge of moving heart; better ability to produce more complete revascularization |
| Potential complications and disadvantages | Learning curve technically more challenging; may cause VF; may have to revert to standard sternotomy with CPB and induced arrest | Learning curve technically more challenging; may have to revert to standard sternotomy; potential for endovascular injury to cannulated blood vessels |
| Discharge planning | Anticipated faster recovery of 1-2 wk (versus 4-12 wk for sternotomy), earlier ambulation, need to identify reportable signs and symptoms (angina, difficulty breathing, infection) | Anticipated faster recovery of 1-2 wk (versus 4-12 wk for sternotomy), earlier ambulation, need to identify reportable signs and symptoms (angina, difficulty breathing, infection) |

*HR,* Heart rate; *CABG,* coronary artery bypass grafting; *CPB,* cardiopulmonary bypass.
From Rothrock JC: *Alexander's care of the patient in surgery,* ed 13, St Louis, 2007, Mosby.

region; (3) overriding of the ventricular septal defect by the aorta; and (4) hypertrophy of the right ventricle. In the adult (and commonly in the child), correction includes closure of the VSD with a patch and enlargement of the pulmonary valve (or stenosed infundibular region) with dilators, via commissurotomy, valve replacement, infundibular resection, or insertion of an allograft, depending on the underlying pathology.

**Transplantation:** With the improvement in pharmacologic management and infection prophylaxis, cardiac transplantation 1-year survival rates are approaching 90%. Potential candidates are patients who are considered to be in the New York Heart Association's Functional Classification System's class IV (four classes are within class IV, which denotes the most compromised cardiac status) and who have less than a 10% chance of survival for 6 months. Contraindications for transplantation include significant pulmonary hypertension, the presence of systemic disease, a recent pulmonary infarction, or active systemic infection. Heart donors are persons with irreversible catastrophic brain injury who do not have atherosclerotic heart disease; age limitations have become less restrictive, and donors and recipients may be 60 years or older in certain cases.

Removal of the donor heart is accomplished with transection of the venae cavae, the pulmonary artery, the left atrium, and the aorta. The donor heart is placed in a sterile bag with cold preservation fluid and transported to the recipient's institution. The recipient is cannulated for CPB, and the heart is surgically removed after the donor heart has been judged acceptable and has arrived in the operating room. The pulmonary artery, the SVC and the IVC, the pulmonary veins, and the aorta are anastomosed. This technique has been modified from the traditional technique in which a right atrial anastomosis was performed. The newer technique reduces some of the dysrhythmias and tricuspid valve dysfunction associated with the previously created atrial connections. After surgery, except for the addition of infection and rejection monitoring, transplant patients receive the same care provided other cardiac surgery patients.

**Tricuspid Regurgitation:** A condition that occurs when the tricuspid valve does not totally close because the leaflets do not completely approximate in diastole (Fig. 35-27). This lesion may be the result of severe mitral stenosis that produces significant back pressure that affects the right side of the heart. It may develop also as a result of rheumatic changes, a right-ventricular infarction, or annular dilatation

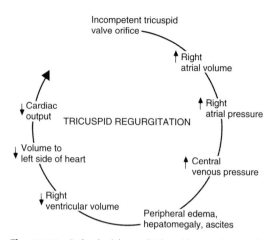

**Fig. 35-27** Pathophysiology of tricuspid regurgitation. *(In Seifert PC: Cardiac surgery, St Louis, 2002, Mosby. From Kinney MR, et al: Andreoli's comprehensive cardiac care, ed 8, St Louis, 1996, Mosby.)*

from right atrial remodeling that occurs with right-ventricular failure. Annuloplasty repair is generally performed (see Fig. 35-4).

**Tricuspid Stenosis:** A narrowing of the orifice of the tricuspid valve (Fig. 35-28). Although this condition occurs infrequently in the adult, it can occur as a result of rheumatic heart disease or bacterial endocarditis. Tricuspid valve replacement is performed if a repair to the native valve cannot be accomplished.

**Valve Replacement:** A surgical procedure in which the native valve is replaced with a mechanical (Fig. 35-29) or biologic (Fig. 35-30) prosthesis; allograft valve replacement also may be performed. The advantage of mechanical valves is their durability; the

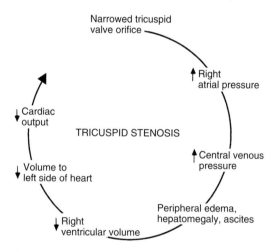

**Fig. 35-28** Pathophysiology of tricuspid stenosis. *(In Seifert PC: Cardiac surgery, St Louis, 2002, Mosby. From Kinney MR, et al: Andreoli's comprehensive cardiac care, ed 8, St Louis, 1996, Mosby.)*

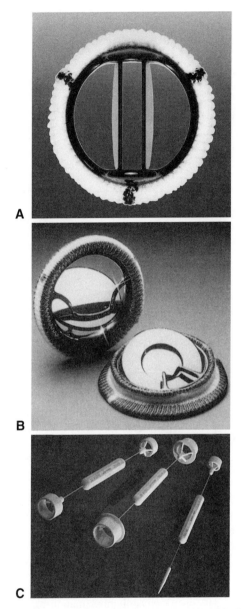

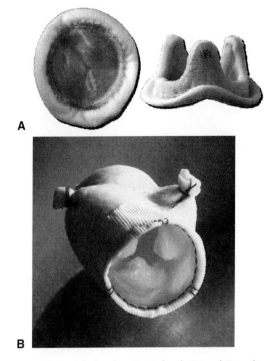

**Fig. 35-30** Biologic valves. **A,** Medtronic Hancock II porcine bioprosthesis. **B,** Stentless porcine aortic root bioprosthesis. Use of porcine stentless valves has reduced demand for cadaver allografts. These valves are especially useful in patients with small aortas. *(Courtesy of Medtronic Heart Valves, Minneapolis, MN.)*

**Fig. 35-29** Mechanical valves. **A,** St Jude Medical bileaflet tilting disk valve prosthesis. **B,** Medtronic-Hall tilting disk valve prosthesis. **C,** Double-ended obturators *(left and center)* for sizing patient's valve; probe *(right)* used to test prosthetic leaflet motion. Sizing obturators are specific to prosthesis. *(**A,** Courtesy St. Jude Medical Inc, St. Paul, MN. From Rothrock JC: Alexander's care of the patient in surgery, ed 13, St Louis, 2007, Mosby. **B** and **C,** Courtesy of Medtronic Heart Valves, Minneapolis, MN. From Rothrock JC: Alexander's care of the patient in surgery, ed 13, St Louis, 2007, Mosby.)*

disadvantage is that they require continuous anticoagulation therapy after surgery because mechanical prostheses are thrombogenic. The advantage of biologic prostheses is that they do not require continuous anticoagulation therapy (although in patients with preexisting conditions such as atrial fibrillation, chronic anticoagulation therapy does need to be continued); the disadvantage is that biologic valves are less durable than mechanical prostheses.

Valve replacement is performed more commonly on valves in the left side of the heart (i.e., aortic and mitral valves) because the higher pressures on the left side aggravate traumatic, infectious, or other preexisting injury to the valves and valve components. After the valve tissue is excised, the aortic or mitral valve annulus is sized with obturators specific to the prosthesis desired (Fig. 35-31), and the appropriate prosthesis is opened and inserted. Biologic valves are stored in glutaraldehyde; before implantation, the solution must be rinsed off the prosthesis in three baths of normal saline solution.

For aortic valve replacement (Fig. 35-32), the leaflets are excised, the annulus is sized, and the selected prosthesis is implanted. For mitral valve replacement (Fig. 35-33), the anterior leaflet is usually (but not always) excised, but often all or part of the posterior leaflet and its attached chordae are retained to preserve the LV geometry and enhance LV function. Although valve

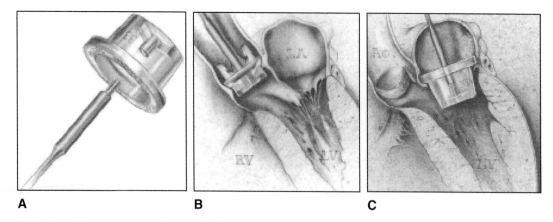

**Fig. 35-31**    Valve sizers in use. **A,** Obturator/sizer is screwed onto handle. **B,** Obturator used to size aortic annulus. **C,** Sizing mitral valve annulus. *(Courtesy of Medtronic Heart Valves, Minneapolis, MN.)*

replacement improves cardiac function with removal of the stresses associated with volume or pressure overloading, transient symptoms of ventricular failure may exist after mitral valve replacement for chronic MR because the LV no longer has the release valve represented by the incompetent valve. With the insertion of a competent mitral prosthetic valve, the LV must now develop sufficient pressure to push all of the left ventricular end-diastolic volume forward through the aortic valve; afterload reduction (e.g., with sodium nitroprusside) assists LV ejection.

After surgery, anticoagulation therapy is usually initiated 3 to 5 days after surgery, when the patient's intravascular lines and chest tubes are discontinued and immediate postoperative hemorrhage is no longer a concern. Oral coumadin therapy is then started and titrated appropriately to achieve an international normalized ratio (INR) of 2.5 to 3.5 times normal (target, 3.0 for mechanical valves).[22]

**Valvuloplasty:** The repair of one or more components of the right (tricuspid) or left (mitral) atrioventricular valve complex that consists of the valve annulus (see definition of annuloplasty), the valve leaflets, the chordae tendinae, the papillary muscles, and the endoventricular wall. When possible, repair, rather than replacement, of the native valve is preferable to avoid the potential complications associated with prosthetic valve replacement: thromboembolism, anticoagulation-related hemorrhage, prosthetic valve endocarditis, perivalvular leak, and prosthetic failure.[23] In addition to insertion of a prosthetic annuloplasty ring for annular dilation (see Figs. 35-1 and 35-2), excess portions of the posterior leaflet of the mitral valve can be excised and the remaining edges sewn together to promote leaflet coaptation and to reduce the

annular circumference. Torn leaflets can be repaired with a patch of pericardium. Ruptured chordae tendineae can be replaced with suture or reattached to the valve leaflet; shortened thickened chordae can be incised to increase length and improve flexibility; and excessively lengthened chordae may shortened with implantation of a portion of the chord into a papillary muscle head.

**Ventricular Assist Device (VAD):** Mechanical devices to support the LV (LVAD), the RV (RVAD), or both ventricles (BiVAD) now can be used long term as a bridge-to-transplant or an end-destination therapy, depending on the underlying pathology. VADs decrease the workload of the heart by diverting blood from the ventricle to an artificial pump that maintains systemic (LVAD) or pulmonary (RVAD) perfusion. Currently, patients can be ambulatory with implantable VADs powered by batteries, which has substantially improved the quality of life for many VAD patients. Placement of a transplant candidate on a VAD enhances anabolism, ambulation, and improved organ function. Improvements in VAD therapy have significantly reduced the incidence rate of infection and thromboembolism. In 2002, the U.S. Food and Drug Administration approved a vented electric LVAD for destination therapy/permanent replacement for the left ventricle.[24-26]

Short-term assist devices include the intraaortic balloon pump (IABP), a sausage-shaped balloon mounted on a catheter percutaneously inserted into the aorta distal to the left subclavian artery via the femoral artery. The balloon inflates during diastole, propelling blood proximally to the aortic root and into the coronary ostia to enhance coronary perfusion; distally, blood is propelled into the peripheral vascular bed to enhance organ blood flow. When the

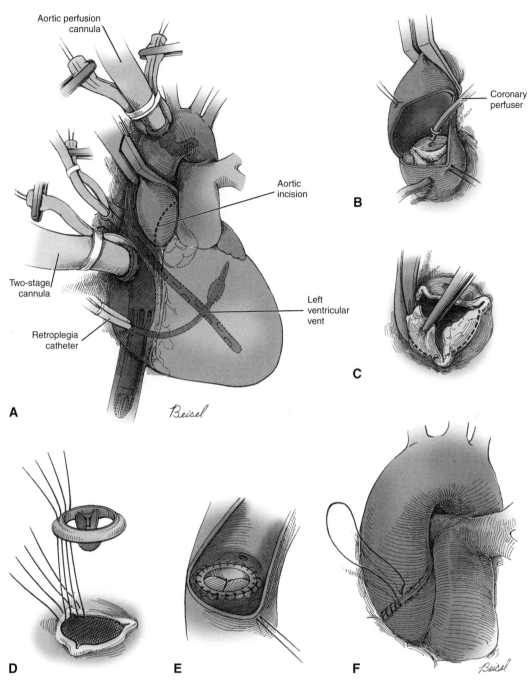

**Fig. 35-32** **A,** Aortic valve replacement. Cardiopulmonary bypass cannulation, retrograde cardioplegia, and left ventricular vent (inserted via right superior pulmonary vein) are shown. Note incision site on aorta (*dotted line*). **B,** If retrograde cardioplegia is not used, hand-held ostial catheters may be used for cardioplegia infusion. **C,** Valve leaflets are completely excised. **D,** Sutures are placed in aortic annulus and prosthetic sewing ring. **E,** Stitches are tied and cut. **F,** Aorta is closed. *(In Rothrock JC: Alexander's care of the patient in surgery, ed 13, St Louis, 2007, Mosby. From Doty DB: Cardiac surgery: operative techniques, St. Louis, 1997, Mosby.)*

balloon deflates during systole, LV afterload has been reduced by the movement of blood during balloon inflation. With the increase in coronary blood flow and the decrease in afterload, the total work of the heart is reduced, thereby providing an environment that supports the recovery of a failing myocardium and improves peripheral vascular perfusion.

**Ventricular Septal Defect (VSD):** Consists of a hole through the ventricular septum. Congenital

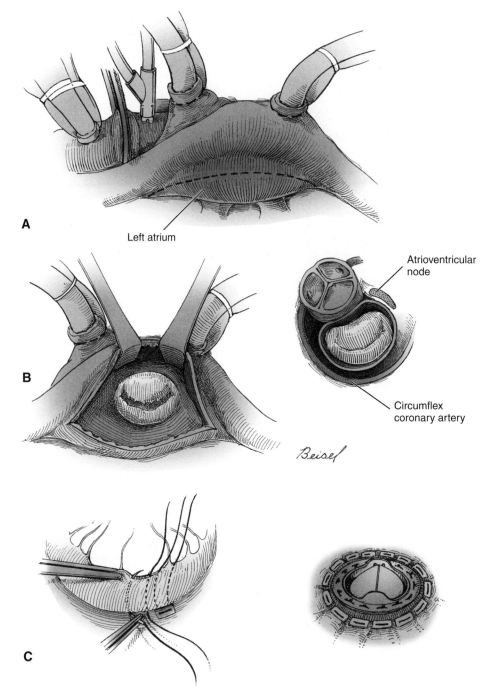

**Fig. 35-33**  Mitral valve replacement. **A,** Incision (*dotted*) line in left atrium, exposure of mitral valve, and illustration of relationship between mitral and aortic valves and atrioventricular node. Double venous cannulas shown for cardiopulmonary bypass; antegrade cardioplegia catheter inserted into aorta below the cross clamp and aortic cannula are shown. **B,** Sutures are placed in native valve annulus and then prosthetic. **C,** Completed valve replacement. *(In Rothrock JC: Alexander's care of the patient in surgery, ed 13, St Louis, 2007, Mosby. From Waldhausen JA, et al: Surgery of the chest, ed 6, St Louis, 1996, Mosby.)*

VSDs may be small enough to close spontaneously; VSDs that persist necessitate surgical closure before irreversible pulmonary hypertension develops.

Adult acquired VSDs usually develop suddenly after myocardial infarction (MI) of one or more coronary arteries perfusing the ventricular septum. These postinfarction VSDs create pulmonary overloading rapidly and require emergency surgery to close the defect (commonly with a prosthetic patch).

## INTRAOPERATIVE CONSIDERATIONS

Monitoring (Table 35-4) of the patient's electrocardiographic (ECG) and direct blood pressure (commonly via the radial artery in the nondominant wrist) results is initiated when the patient arrives in the preoperative area. Central lines are usually inserted after transport into the operating room (OR) but occasionally are inserted in another designated location, such as the holding area. Whether the patient first undergoes intubation before insertion of central lines (i.e., central venous pressure [CVP], pulmonary artery catheter) or after line insertion is at the discretion of the anesthesia provider; the sequence varies among institutions. Increasingly, a transesophageal echocardiographic (TEE) probe is inserted to illustrate cardiac function; use of TEE for valve surgery and for patients with compromised LV function is routine.

Anesthesia for cardiac surgery varies from hospital to hospital and also can vary with the type of cardiac repair. Ideally, anesthetic management includes drugs that have rapid onset and termination, minimize ischemia, and are nontoxic to myocardial and other tissue.[27] For example, in patients with significant pulmonary involvement, agents that increase pulmonary vascular resistance should be avoided. Hemodynamic effects of some anesthetic drugs are shown in Table 35-5.

After the patient has been anesthetized, positioned, and washed (prepped), the chest is opened. The most commonly used chest incision in cardiac surgery is the median sternotomy. However, ministernotomy, anterolateral or posterolateral thoracotomy incisions, or transverse sternotomy also may be used (see Fig. 35-16). The sternum is split with a saw from the sternal notch to the xiphoid process. After the sternum is opened, the exposed pericardial sac is incised anteriorly and the pericardial edges are tacked up along the chest wall incision to allow complete access to the entire pericardium without the necessity of entering the pleural cavities. For CABG procedures, once the sternum is opened, the surgeon dissects the required length of the mammary artery and the assistant harvests additional bypass conduits, such as the saphenous vein or the radial artery. After conduit harvesting is completed, or if another procedure is planned (e.g., valve repair), the surgeon proceeds to cannulate for CPB. The body is cooled to the desired temperature, and the heart is arrested with cardioplegia.

Coronary bypass surgery may be performed without the use of CPB, thereby avoiding the deleterious effects associated with extracorporeal circulation (see Table 35-2). However, in operations that necessitate entry into the heart (valve repair or replacement), CPB is required for perfusion of the body while the heart is arrested and opened. (During CABG, the procedure is performed on the epicardial coronary arteries that lie on the surface of the heart, not inside the heart; the heart can beat to perfuse the systemic, pulmonary, and coronary circulations.)

After the cardiac repair is completed, temporary pacing wires are attached to the right atrial and ventricular surface, brought out through the chest below the sternal incision, and connected to an external pacemaker generator. One or more chest tubes are placed anteriorly, laterally, or posteriorly in the pericardium to facilitate drainage. They exit via stab wounds below the sternal incision. If either of the pleurae were opened during the procedure, the tip of one of the pericardial chest tubes is inserted into the affected pleura. The pericardial sac is rarely closed so any remaining blood or fluid can drain freely into the chest tubes (avoiding the creation of cardiac tamponade). Occasionally, when a repeat operation is anticipated (e.g., after a biologic valve replacement in a young person), the upper (cephalid) portion of the pericardium may be closed so that less scar tissue forms over the cannulation sites for CPB (e.g., the aorta). The lower portion of the sac remains open to drain fluid. The sternum is closed with stainless steel wires, and the fascia, subcutaneous tissue, and skin are closed with suture. Before transfer from the OR to the postanesthesia care unit (or intensive care unit [ICU]), portable monitoring lines for heart rate and rhythm, arterial blood pressure, and oxygen saturation are connected for transport to the postoperative unit. Patients can have acute circulatory instability develop either because of the normal recovering physiologic state or inadvertent movement or displacement of the numerous invasive lines and tubes needed. A portable defibrillator is often placed on the transport bed for use if ventricular tachycardia or ventricular fibrillation develops during transport.

## POSTANESTHESIA CARE

All patients in the open heart PACU or CSICU need intensive continuous hemodynamic monitoring and rapid intervention to prevent

## Table 35-4 Physiologic Monitoring

| Monitoring Device | Location | Assesses/Measures |
|---|---|---|
| **CARDIOVASCULAR SYSTEM** | | |
| Electrocardiogram (ECG) | Electrodes placed on shoulders, hips, and left axillary line | Electrical activity of heart: lead II useful to monitor cardiac rhythm (good visualization of P wave and QRS) and myocardial ischemia (inferior surface); lead V5 useful to detect myocardial ischemia (anterior surface) |
| Intraarterial catheter | Radial artery (also femoral artery) aorta, bypass circuit; in children, may use superficial temporal or dorsalis pedis arteries; in neonates, may use umbilical artery | Direct arterial BP; blood gases; blood chemistries |
| Blood pressure cuff | Right or left arm | Indirect BP |
| CVP line | RA | RA pressure (CVP); RV filling pressure; RV preload |
| PA catheter (addition of fiberoptics provides additional information about mixed venous oxygen saturation [$SvO_2$]) | PA (proximal and distal) | PA pressures: systolic, diastolic, mean, wedge; pulmonary vascular resistance; LV filling pressure; LV preload; CO; assessment of stroke volume, stroke work, systemic vascular resistance; mixed venous saturation (continuous indirect assessment of CO and reflection of tissue oxygenation); RV function |
| LA catheter (when used) | LA | LA pressure (direct); LV filling pressure; LV preload |
| TEE | Esophagus | Valve function before and after repair; LV wall motion, failure; intracardiac air bubbles |
| Urinary drainage catheter | Urinary bladder | Urinary output, renal perfusion; indirect measure of CO |
| **RESPIRATORY SYSTEM** | | |
| Mass spectrometry | Anesthesia circuit | Inspired/expired $O_2$, $CO_2$, and anesthetic gases; used to avoid hypoxia, hypercarbia, anesthetic overdose |
| Pulse oximeter | Finger or toe cot; earlobe, nose | Oxygen saturation of arterial hemoglobin; tissue oxygenation |
| Capnography | Anesthesia circuit | End-tidal $CO_2$; used to detect integrity of anesthesia circuit; avoid disconnections of monitor, endotracheal tube; detect spontaneous ventilation, rebreathing, obstructive pulmonary disease |
| **CENTRAL NERVOUS SYSTEM** | | |
| Temperature | Esophagus, nasopharynx, urinary bladder, rectum, ventricular septum, bypass circuit, PA catheter | Core and peripheral temperature of heart, brain, and other organs |

**Table 35-4 Physiologic Monitoring—cont'd**

| Monitoring Device | Location | Assesses/Measures |
|---|---|---|
| Electroencephalogram | Scalp electrodes | Detect cerebral ischemia, embolus; indication of depth of anesthesia |
| **RENAL SYSTEM** | | |
| Urinary discharge catheter | Bladder | Urinary output; indirect measure of cardiac output |

From Seifert PC: *Cardiac surgery: perioperative patient care*, St Louis, 2002, Mosby.
BP, Blood pressure; RV, right ventricular; PA, pulmonary artery; LA, left atrial.

complications from the surgery and CPB. Patients are routinely monitored for dysrhythmias, pleural effusion, bleeding, and cardiovascular, neurologic, renal, pulmonary/respiratory, and temperature alterations. The nurse's role is critical to ensure that anticipated clinical changes (e.g., temperature, fluid shifts) do not progress to more serious complications that can jeopardize optimal patient outcomes. In addition, nurses in the postoperative unit and the step-down unit educate patients about the plan of care and involve patients and family members to implement the plan designed for patients and their families (Table 35-6).

On admission to the postoperative unit, the nurse immediately assesses the parameters currently monitored. If any of these parameters indicates circulatory or ventilatory dysfunction, immediate resuscitative measures are instituted. On entry to the postoperative unit, if circulatory and ventilatory statuses appear adequate, then admission routines are initiated. The respiratory

**Table 35-5 Hemodynamic Effects of Anesthetic Drugs**

| Drug | HEMODYNAMIC EFFECT | | | | | |
|---|---|---|---|---|---|---|
| | CI | BP | SVR | PLVED | HR | Contractility |
| Tubocurarine | ↓ | ↓ | ↓ | ↓ | ↑ | ↔ |
| Diazepam | ↓ | ↓ | ↓ | ↓ | ↔ | ↔ |
| Dimethyl tubocurarine | ↑ | ↔↑ | ↔↓ | ↔↓ | ↑ | ↔ |
| Droperidol | ↔↑ | ↓ | ↓ | ↓ | ↑ | ↔ |
| Enflurane | ↓ | ↓ | ↓ | ↔↓ | ↔↓ | ↓ |
| Fentanyl | ↔ | ↓ | ↓ | ↔ | ↔ | ↔ |
| Halothane | ↓ | ↓ | ↔↓ | ↔↑ | ↔↑↓ | ↓ |
| Innovar | ↔↑ | ↓ | ↓ | ↓ | ↔ | ↔ |
| Isoflurane | ↔ | ↓ | ↓ | ↔ | ↑ | ↓ |
| Ketamine | ↑ | ↑ | ↑ | ↑ | ↑ | — |
| Methoxyflurane | ↓ | ↓ | ↓ | ↔ | ↔ | ↓ |
| Midazolam | ↔ | ↔ | ↔↓ | ↓ | ↑ | ↔↓ |
| Morphine | ↔↑ | ↔↓ | ↓ | ↔↑ | ↓ | ↔ |
| Nitrous oxide | ↓ | ↔↓ | ↔↑ | ↑ | ↔↓ | ↓ |
| Pancuronium | ↑ | ↑ | ↔ | ↓ | ↑ | ? |
| Succinylcholine | ↓ | ↔↓ | ↓ | ↓ | ↑↓ | ? |
| Thiopental | ↔↓ | ↔ | ↑ | ↔ | ↑ | ↓ |
| Vecuronium | ↔ | ↔ | ↔ | ↔ | ↔ | ↔ |

From Rothrock JC: *Alexander's care of the patient in surgery*, ed 13, St Louis, 2007, Mosby. From Kouchoukos N, Blackstone EH, Doty DB, et al: *Kirklin/Barratt-Boyes cardiac surgery*, ed 3, vol I, Philadelphia, 2003, Churchill Livingstone.
↓, Decrease; ↑, increase; ↔, no change; CI, insufficient data; BP, blood pressure; SVR, systemic vascular resistance; PLVED, left-end distal pressure; HR, heart rate.

NURSING CARE IN THE PACU

## Table 35-6  Cardiac Surgery Plan of Care

| Therapies | Day Before Surgery | Day of Surgery/ Intensive Care Unit | Day 1 After Surgery | Day 2 After Surgery | Day 3 After Surgery | Day 4 After Surgery |
|---|---|---|---|---|---|---|
| Visits | • Surgeon<br>• Physician's assistant/nurse practitioner<br>• Anesthesiologist<br>• Mended Hearts<br>• Research nurse | • Surgeon<br>• Physician's assistant<br>• Anesthesiologist<br>• Mended Hearts | • Surgeon<br>• Physician's assistant/nurse practitioner<br>• Mended Hearts | • Surgeon<br>• Physician's assistant/nurse practitioner<br>• Mended Hearts | • Surgeon<br>• Physician's assistant/nurse practitioner<br>• Mended Hearts | • Surgeon<br>• Physician's assistant/nurse practitioner<br>• Mended Hearts |
| Lines and Tubes | | • Breathing tube<br>• Tube for stomach<br>• Catheter for urine<br>• Chest tubes<br>• IV lines<br>• Pacer wires<br>• Heart monitor<br>• Breathing tube removed<br>• Tube for stomach removed<br>• IV lines capped | • Breathing tube<br>• Tube for stomach<br>• Catheter for urine<br>• Chest tubes<br>• IV lines<br>• Pacer wires<br>• Heart monitor<br>• Breathing tube removed<br>• Tube for stomach removed<br>• Catheter for urine removed<br>• Chest tubes removed<br>• IV lines capped | • Chest tubes<br>• Heart monitor<br>• Pacer wires<br>• Capped IV | • Heart monitor<br>• Pacer wires<br>• Capped IV | • Heart monitor<br>• Pacer wires<br>• Capped IV |
| Treatments | • Exidine shower at bedtime or in the morning | | | • Remove chest tubes<br>• Remove bandages<br>• Wash incisions with Dial soap and water<br>• Remove pacer wires | | |

| | Column 1 | Column 2 | Column 3 | Column 4 | Column 5 | Column 6 |
|---|---|---|---|---|---|---|
| **Medications** | • Stop aspirin or non-steroidal anti-inflammatory drugs, e.g., ibuprofen, 5 days prior to surgery<br>• Sleeping pill available if needed | • IV fluids<br>• Pain medication if needed | • Ask for pain medication and sleeping pill if needed<br>• Valve patients begin Coumadin | • Ask for pain medication and sleeping pill | • Ask for pain medication and sleeping pill<br>• Ask for laxative if needed | • Ask for pain medication and sleeping pill<br>• Ask for laxative if needed |
| **Nutrition** | • Eat what you like for dinner, but nothing by mouth after midnight except medications | • Nothing by mouth<br>• Ice chips and sips of clear liquids if breathing tube out | • Sips of liquid after breathing tube out<br>• Solid foods when ready, then healthy heart diet | • Healthy heart diet | • Healthy heart diet | • Healthy heart diet |
| **Activity/Safety** | • Unrestricted activity | • Bed rest<br>• Wrists will be loosely restrained to protect breathing tube<br>• IS every hour while awake if breathing tube out<br>• Dangle legs on side of bed<br>• If breathing tube out and able to dangle legs, transfer to Step-Down Unit | • Sit on side of bed<br>• Up in chair 1 to 2 times<br>• Walk with assistance to bathroom<br>• Feed self<br>• Daily weight and measure urine<br>• IS every hour while awake<br>• Transfer to Step-Down Unit | • Up in chair<br>• Walk in hall 1 to 3 times, 100 to 200 ft.<br>• Daily weight and measure urine<br>• Feed self<br>• Bathe at sink with assistance<br>• IS every hour while awake | • Up in chair<br>• Walk in hall 3 to 4 times, 200 to 400 ft.<br>• Daily weight and measure urine<br>• Feed self<br>• Bowel movement<br>• Shower<br>• IS every hour while awake<br>• Late morning discharge | • Up in chair<br>• Walk in hall 3 to 4 times, 200 to 400 ft.<br>• Daily weight and measure urine<br>• Shower<br>• IS every hour while awake<br>• Morning discharge |

*Continued*

NURSING CARE IN THE PACU

**Table 35-6  Cardiac Surgery Plan of Care—cont'd**

| Therapies | Day Before Surgery | Day of Surgery/ Intensive Care Unit | Day 1 After Surgery | Day 2 After Surgery | Day 3 After Surgery | Day 4 After Surgery |
|---|---|---|---|---|---|---|
| Discharge Planning | • Complete home needs assessment | | • Discuss discharge, social and nutritional needs with nurse | • Discuss discharge, social and nutritional needs with nurse | • Driver designated and clothes for home at bedside | • Driver designated and clothes for home at bedside |
| Education | • Review this plan of care<br>• Review advance directives<br>• Breathing/coughing exercises and IS (Incentive Spirometer)<br>• Sternal precautions | • Family orientation to ICU<br>• Nurse will update your family<br>• Education reinforced as needed | • Read and review discharge instruction packet | • Review discharge instruction packet | • Review discharge packet<br>• Review "survival skills" and medications<br>• Receive prescriptions and appointment schedule | • Review discharge packet<br>• Review "survival skills" and medications<br>• Receive prescriptions and appointment schedule |

The plan, especially designed for patients and families, is used by patients to assist them in participating more fully in their own care. It is used as a guide and may be modified as patient situations warrant. (Permission to reproduce from Inova Heart and Vascular Institute, Inova Health System, Falls Church, VA).

therapist or anesthesia care provider usually attaches the patient to the ventilator, establishes the initial ventilator settings, and sets the alarms. Once the patient is attached to the ventilator, the nurse auscultates both lung fields and repeats the assessment often until discharge from the PACU.

Invasive monitoring lines are attached to transducers or manometers. Patency is ascertained, and values and wave tracings are continuously displayed and recorded. Commonly measured intravascular parameters include mean arterial, right atrial, mean pulmonary artery, pulmonary artery systolic, pulmonary artery diastolic, pulmonary capillary wedge, and left atrial pressures. In addition to these directly measured parameters, these values assist in calculation of indirect or derived hemodynamic parameters, such as cardiac output and cardiac index, systemic vascular resistance, and pulmonary vascular resistance. These parameters assist in assessment of both left-ventricular and right-ventricular status and are used in determination of pharmacologic, fluid, and mechanical therapies for the postoperative patient. Once these invasive lines are connected, the nurse reviews and assesses with the anesthesia provider the intravascular lines and solutions with regard to type, drugs infused, flow rates, patency, and expiration times. Intake and output recordings with running totals are made and documented hourly (or more often as clinically indicated). Volume administration and replacement treatments are largely determined by the individual patient's hemodynamic parameters, and responses can vary greatly from hour to hour.

Chest tube drainage systems inserted in the OR are connected to suction. Water-seal drainage or autotransfusion systems with 15 cm to 20 cm of negative suction are most commonly used. The amount and type of chest tube drainage are frequently assessed and recorded on an hourly basis. Drainage that exceeds 100 mL/h should be brought to the attention of the physician. Chest tubes are usually removed on the first or second postoperative day, as long as intracardiac lines have been removed, no evidence of fluid accumulation is present on chest radiograph results, and drainage has been less than 200 mL in the last 6 hours. Most patients have one or two mediastinal chest tubes that facilitate pericardial drainage after surgery. If the pleural spaces were opened during the procedure or the internal mammary arteries were dissected off the chest wall, or both, then pleural chest tubes are also present to facilitate drainage and to prevent a pneumothorax.

Arterial blood gas values are determined on admission and as needed thereafter. Patients remain intubated until the effects of anesthesia subside and hemodynamic stability is achieved and maintained. Controlled ventilation is used initially. As patients begin to generate their own respirations, they are switched to intermittent mandatory ventilation modes, in which they gradually increase their spontaneous respirations to maintain adequate minute ventilations. Once patients maintain an adequate respiratory rate, they are switched to continuous positive airway pressure (CPAP) systems. With CPAP, the patient determines the respiratory rate and the ventilator provides the positive pressure to the airway that the glottis normally provides when the patient is not intubated. The use of CPAP prevents microatelectasis and increases the functional residual capacity of the lung by increasing lung expansion. Once the patient maintains adequate arterial blood gas levels on CPAP, extubation usually follows quickly. After extubation, face masks or nasal cannulas are used to deliver supplemental oxygen.

A continuous ECG recording is established, alarm limits are set, and a strip recording is obtained. A 12-lead ECG is obtained as soon as possible and repeated as necessary. Cardiac rhythm is assessed frequently and documented at least every 2 hours. Lead selection varies, but modified chest lead one ($MCL_1$), in which the left-atrial and right-atrial leads are in their respective places and the third lead is placed on the fourth right intercostal space, is commonly used. Electrode placement with this lead does not interfere with defibrillation procedures or with mediastinal or chest tube dressing placement. The apical pulse is auscultated and validated with the ECG recording. Most patients have a temporary external pacer, and the nurse checks and records the type of pacer, the mode, the rate, and the milliamperage and determines whether the pacer is functioning adequately. If the patient is not being paced, then the nurse needs to ensure that the unused pacemaker wires are covered with gauze or electrical tape, placed in a plastic covering (a finger cot), and securely dressed and attached to the chest to protect the patient from electrical hazard. Usually, two ventricular and two atrial pacing wires are attached to the epicardium with a fine suture before the chest is closed. These wires then exit the chest via stab wounds on either side of the sternal incision. The atrial wires are usually on the right, and the ventricular wires on the left. They are most often left in place for a few days after surgery and may be used to assist in cardiac rate and rhythm control. Before the patient is discharged from the hospital, the wires are totally removed with gentle traction or they are clipped off at the skin level, with a portion left attached to the epicardium and residing in the subcutaneous tissues.

The patient's neurologic status is assessed on admission and every 30 to 60 minutes and thereafter until arousal from anesthesia. The Aldrete Postanesthesia Recovery Score can be used to assess for recovery from anesthesia. Once the patient has been aroused, neurologic assessments are decreased to every 2 hours.[28,29]

An admission temperature is obtained and active rewarming therapies are instituted. During this period, temperatures are recorded hourly; rewarming devices are discontinued when the patient's condition reaches normothermia. One temperature-related condition is hypothermia-related hypocarbia. The body temperature usually remains lower than normal during the early postoperative hours. Slowly, the body temperature returns to normal; occasionally, rebound hyperthermia occurs. However, as rewarming takes place, carbon dioxide is produced. Consequently, hypercarbia can develop, and ventilator settings should be adjusted to produce a minute volume necessary to facilitate normocarbia. In addition, if rebound hyperthermia occurs or if rewarming devices are not regulated and monitored appropriately, a hyperthermic overshoot may occur, which increases myocardial oxygen demand and consumption.[30]

An abdominal assessment is performed on admission and every 2 hours thereafter until bowel sounds return. A nasogastric tube (inserted in the OR) relieves gastric distention and facilitates removal of gastric contents. It is usually attached to low intermittent suction or gravity drainage and removed at the time of extubation. Analysis of pH and tests for the presence of occult blood may be performed on gastric secretions if they begin to resemble coffee grounds. Once the nasogastric tube is removed, the patient is given ice chips and resumes a clear liquid diet within the first 24 hours.

Urinary drainage from the catheter inserted in the OR should be recorded on admission to the PACU and then hourly. The appearance of the urine is also monitored closely. During the first few hours after surgery, massive diuresis of 2 to 3 L of pale dilute urine is usually common from diuretics that are generally administered during the discontinuation of CPB to facilitate the removal of fluid that has sequestered during surgery in the interstitial space. Once this initial diuresis resolves, urine color and consistency return to normal. Urinary output should be more than 0.5 mL/kg/h; a lower urine output is commonly the result of decreased renal perfusion.[30]

Peripheral pulses and skin color and temperature are assessed and recorded hourly. All incisions and intravascular and tube insertion sites are observed. The patient is placed in a semi-Fowler's position with the legs supported at the knees and the calves slightly elevated. This position facilitates venous return from the legs and limits swelling, particularly in patients with saphenous vein excision. Legs are wrapped from toes to hips with elastic leg wraps or anti-embolism stockings.

Cardiopulmonary bypass affects every body system, and a brief review of some of the effects on the patient seen in the postoperative period is useful to the nurse. For example, epinephrine and norepinephrine levels are markedly elevated during CPB. Hyperglycemia and impaired insulin responses are present and result in use of fat stores for energy until carbohydrate metabolism returns to normal levels. Secretion of antidiuretic hormone and aldosterone is also increased, stimulated by different mechanisms associated with the physiologic components of stress. Serum complement that is activated when blood contacts the inner surfaces of the bypass circuit cause an inflammatory response with a marked increase in total body water and interstitial edema. Postoperative fluid requirements are affected by rewarming because rewarming itself causes fluid shifts. This excess fluid usually redistributes itself by the second or third day after surgery and is excreted spontaneously or with diuretic therapy. CPB and hypothermia also alter coagulation factors, platelet formation, and the immune system.[20]

In addition, when exposed to the foreign surfaces of the CPB circuit, platelets clump together. A decrease in the number of functional platelets occurs along with a decrease in the aggregative and adhesive functions of remaining platelets. Release of vasoactive substances occurs as platelets are destroyed. In addition, exposure to the CPB circuit (and suctioning devices) causes a breakdown of plasma proteins, including gamma globulin, which in turn may cause fat microemboli release, microcoagulation, clotting factor consumption, and increased vascular permeability. The shear stresses caused by suction catheters and the tubing and connectors within the circuit also damage the formed elements of the blood (e.g., erythrocytes and leukocytes).

After admission routines, a written assessment is performed. The frequency of assessment and documentation of the hemodynamic parameters and routines is dictated by the patient's response to and recovery from surgery. Recovery time varies from patient to patient but generally occurs within 12 to 24 hours (except with impaired cardiac, pulmonary, renal, or other organ function). During that time, largely because of the techniques of CPB, hypothermia, anesthesia, and surgical manipulation of the myocardium, numerous expected postoperative physiologic alterations occur. With correct interventions, these physiologic responses are short lived and reversible. However, two problems do exist. First, although these alterations are reversible, if they are not identified early and quickly treated, they can lead to complications. Such is the case with uncontrolled hypertension that can develop into hemorrhage if fresh suture lines are disrupted. Second, these alterations often resemble complications and thus may be missed in the early stages. For example, the initial absence of a pedal pulse may be attributed to hypothermia and vasoconstriction only to be traced later to a vascular embolism. For these reasons, the PACU nurse must be knowledgeable about the causes, assessment factors, and interventions for both expected physiologic alterations and complications that can occur after cardiac surgery. In the following section, these alterations and potential complications are briefly reviewed.

## COMPLICATIONS

### Cardiovascular System

A number of predisposing factors are known to increase the incidence rates of postoperative complication and early mortality. These factors include preoperative cardiac conditions such as myocardial dysfunction, recent myocardial infarction, and previous CABG surgery or systemic conditions such as advanced age, obesity, diabetes mellitus, and chronic obstructive pulmonary disease. The surgical risks of CABG can be assessed before surgery, and complications can be anticipated with these preoperative risk factors taken into consideration.

Complications related to CABG and valvular surgery can generally be classified as either cardiac or noncardiac. Cardiac complications include myocardial infarction, congestive heart failure, tamponade, dysrhythmias, and postoperative hypertension. Each of these complications can contribute to decreased cardiac output.

Noncardiac complications include hemorrhage; wound dehiscence and infection; and neurologic, renal, pulmonary, and gastrointestinal problems. Each complication is addressed individually.

### Cardiac Complications of Coronary Artery Bypass Grafting and Valvular Surgery

*Myocardial Infarction.* Despite improved myocardial protection with induced hypothermia, cardioplegic arrest, and topical hypothermia during surgery, myocardial infarction (MI) still remains the most common and serious postoperative complication and the main cause of early death after surgery. Suboptimal myocardial protection may result from uneven distribution of cardioplegic solutions in the coronary arteries. Subendocardial ischemia may occur from a distended or hypertrophic left ventricle and incomplete revascularization. Sudden bypass graft closure (from thrombus) may be a contributing factor. The patient's own underlying heart disease may be too severe for reversal with attempted revascularization. Some patients with CAD are treated medically (i.e., pharmacologically, lifestyle changes) for prolonged periods; because CAD is a progressive disease, cardiac function can deteriorate significantly without catheter-based (PTCA with stent) or surgical (CABG) revascularization. In patients with valvular heart disease, the degree of ventricular dysfunction is difficult to gauge accurately because the heart is capable of performing work by relying on compensatory mechanisms and patients may not be symptomatic until serious myocardial injury has occurred.

Another contributing factor may be reperfusion injury from sudden reperfusion of an ischemic area causing necrosis as a result of a rapid influx of calcium ions, oxygen-free radicals, and other metabolic waste products into the ischemic myocardial cells. The appearance of new Q waves after surgery also has been shown to adversely affect early and late survival. Other predictors of perioperative MI include left main coronary artery stenosis, multivessel disease, minimal collateral circulation, and the duration of CPB.

*Congestive Heart Failure (Alterations in Myocardial Contractility).* Alteration in myocardial contractility with resultant low cardiac output and shock-like states also can develop after surgery and may be the result of a perioperative ischemia, MI, incomplete revascularization or repair, myocardial edema from surgical manipulation, metabolic disturbances, and depression from hypothermia and anesthesia. The patient clinically has a decrease in cardiac output (CO) and cardiac index (CI), hypotension, elevated systemic vascular resistance, elevated filling pressures, acidosis, tachycardia, and decreased urine output. If the condition occurs during surgery after the surgical repair and the discontinuation of CPB, an intraaortic balloon pump (IABP) may be inserted or CPB may be reinstituted for approximately 30 minutes to "rest" the heart, relieve myocardial ischemia, and improve ventricular contractility to a level that allows smooth weaning with low dosages of inotropic support. (CPB decompresses the heart and removes cardiac volume and pressure work.) If the heart cannot be weaned from CPB, even with IABP support, insertion of a ventricular device may be necessary to support one or more ventricles.

After surgery, treatment can include a combination of pharmacologic and mechanical circulatory support throughout the period of recuperation. Depending on the hemodynamic status of the patient, different combinations of inotropic and vasopressor agents are used as initial therapy, with the addition of mechanical support (i.e., IABP) if cardiac output remains low despite inotropic stimulation and optimal filling pressures, as indicated by a pulmonary capillary wedge pressure higher than 22 to 25 mm Hg.

***Cardiac Tamponade.*** Cardiac tamponade develops when the amount of blood or fluid accumulated in the pericardial cavity is sufficient to compress the heart. Cardiac compression produces ineffective filling and ejection of an adequate CO. Signs of tamponade consist of low CO and CI, hypotension, tachycardia, equalization of the right-atrial and left-atrial pressures, development of pulsus paradoxus, narrowed pulse pressure, muffled heart sounds, widening of the mediastinum on chest radiograph, and alteration in neurologic status. Observation of the quality of chest tube drainage is critical, especially in the first 6 hours when tamponade is more likely to occur. Generally, chest tube drainage in cardiac surgical patients is thin, red, or serosanguinous and nonclotted because blood is exposed to the mechanical effects of the contracting heart and the motion of the lungs. Blood in the pericardium that normally begins to clot is defibrinated by this mechanical trauma and becomes thin non-clotted chest tube drainage.[5] When clots begin to appear in the chest tubes, relatively fresh bleeding may be indicated. In this situation, the incidence rate of tamponade is higher because clot can occlude the chest tube lumen, preventing chest drainage. Sudden cessation of previously heavily clotted drainage should be promptly investigated for signs of tamponade. The specific cause can be either rapid active bleeding from a suture line or continuous slow oozing from a coagulopathy. Mediastinal exploration in the OR (or in the postoperative unit if the patient's condition is unstable) may be

necessary to control surgical bleeding; treatment for coagulopathy is determined with assessment of the underlying cause of the bleeding (e.g., insufficient number of functional platelets) and treatment of the specific problem.

***Dysrhythmias.*** Rhythm disturbances of the atria or ventricles are common after surgery and may be caused by ischemia, hypoxia, hypotension, or pharmacologic or metabolic factors. Inotropic drugs (with their contractile and chronotropic effects), acid-base imbalances, and electrolyte abnormalities can also cause dysrhythmias. The high incidence rate of dysrhythmias necessitates continuous monitoring for the first 48 hours in the critical unit and the step-down unit. Correction of electrolyte imbalances and hypoxia are basic requirements. Massive diuresis can precipitate hypokalemia, promoting the development of dysrhythmias; potassium replacement should be aggressive to maintain serum potassium concentrations at levels higher than 4 mEq/L. An intravenous infusion of magnesium may reduce premature atrial contractions and promote atrial contraction to enhance preload and CO.[30]

Premature ventricular contractions necessitate electrical (cardioversion) or pharmacologic (amiodarone, magnesium) intervention. If the ventricular rhythm deteriorates into ventricular tachycardia or fibrillation, cardiopulmonary resuscitation with defibrillation should be initiated promptly.

Atrial fibrillation (AF) is common after cardiac surgery, and procainamide and amiodarone may be infused to promote new onset AF conversion to sinus rhythm. For patients with persistent or permanent AF, the goal is rate control of the ventricular response to the atrial ectopic impulses. If cardioversion is considered, a TEE first should be performed for identification of the presence of left atrial thrombus (that could break off and embolize).[30] If thrombus is present, an increased risk for TE after cardioversion exists.

Patients with transient heart block (e.g., from edema of conduction tissue during valve surgery) can be paced sequentially (in patients with an intact atrioventricular node) with the temporary pacemaker wires until the edema resolves. For patients with bradycardia, temporary pacing at a rate of 90 bpm can be initiated to maintain an acceptable CO.

***Peripheral Vasoconstriction (Postoperative Hypertension).*** Factors that contribute to the development of peripheral vasoconstriction include the patient's own sympathetic drive triggered by anxiety, surgical manipulation of the heart and the great vessels with the attached pressor receptors, vasoactive drugs, and systemic hypothermia. Patients may appear pale, with cool extremities and temperature lower than 37° C (98.6° F). Patients may also display increased systemic vascular resistance, weak or impalpable pulses, tachycardia, and varying degrees of hypertension. Hypertension needs to be controlled so that the elevated pressure does not disrupt the surgical anastomoses. Increased systemic vascular resistance increases ventricular afterload and stresses the myocardium. Treatment approaches include active rewarming and administration of vasodilating agents (e.g., intravenous sodium nitroprusside, nitroglycerin, and phentolamine). These agents have relatively immediate effects and can be easily reversed once use is discontinued. Dosages should be titrated to achieve a mean arterial blood pressure of 70 to 80 mm Hg.[30]

### Noncardiac Complications of Coronary Artery Bypass Grafting and Valvular Surgery

*Hemorrhage.* Coagulation disorders and hemorrhage pose a potential threat to the cardiac surgical patient. Coagulation dysfunction is often the result of CPB,[5] from direct trauma to the blood components from solid synthetic surfaces and inline tubing connectors in the CPB circuit, inadequate surgical hemostasis, coagulation disorders, preoperative use of antiplatelets or anticoagulants, or insufficient heparin reversal with protamine sulfate. Preoperative evaluation can be used to detect some coagulation disturbances that can be treated before surgery (e.g., discontinuation of anticoagulant medications or switching from coumadin to heparin). Previous health problems such as uremia and hepatic disease also should be taken into account as possible causes of coagulation disturbances. Adequate heparin reversal with confirmation with a whole-blood activated coagulation time (ACT) or activated partial thromboplastin time (APTT) should be performed. Even if the results of these studies are normal, heparin may still be released from body stores (e.g., adipose tissue) and cause a heparin rebound phenomenon. Therefore, an initially normal ACT or APTT result does not guarantee that subsequent bleeding is unrelated to the effects of heparin. Another prophylactic measure for reduction of intraoperative and postoperative bleeding is use of antifibrinolytic drugs (e.g., aprotinin, epsilon-aminocaproic acid).[5] Aprotinin may be indicated for patients who are undergoing repeat or complicated cardiac procedures and for patients who have taken aspirin in the perioperative period.

Surgical hemostasis at the end of the surgical procedure can prevent most postoperative bleeding. Particular attention is paid to the internal mammary artery sites because of the extensive dissection from the chest wall, but all areas incised and sutured during operation are assessed for hemostasis. In patients undergoing reoperation, extensive adhesions and neorevascularization increase the risk of bleeding.

Mediastinal exploration is indicated when signs of cardiac tamponade develop with bleeding of more than 500 mL/h or less or more than 300 mL/h for 6 hours or longer. The decision to reoperate should be made before the patient's condition becomes hemodynamically unstable. On reexploration for bleeding, oozing from the mediastinal wound or active bleeding may be found. During exploration, clots and hematoma are removed, the heart and pericardium are explored, and active bleeders are controlled. The pericardium is irrigated, and the chest is closed. Occasionally, no discrete source of bleeding can be found, even after extensive scrutiny of the surgical site.

Bleeding from minimally invasive endoscopic sites (e.g., saphenous vein incision site) may not be noticeable until increased swelling from the leg is seen. The leg may need exploration to find and repair the bleeding site. With endovascular thoracic aneurysm repair (see Fig. 35-5, *D*), identification and confirmation of bleeding sites may require a CAT scan, with severe bleeding necessitating a return to the OR for an open exploration to control bleeding.

**Sternal Wound Dehiscence and Infection.** Superficial wound infection, sternal osteitis, and mediastinitis can occur after surgery, although superficial wound problems are the most common. Predisposing factors for impaired sternal healing include advanced age, obesity, diabetes mellitus, long-term steroid use, and chronic obstructive pulmonary disease. Postoperative bleeding that necessitates reexploration also contributes to sternal wound infection. Infection can occur at any time but is usually diagnosed 6 to 12 days after surgery. Treatment consists of intravenous antibiotics, opening of the wound, removal of clot, débridement, and irrigation. After the sternal wound has been debrided, primary closure may be performed. In more severe cases, sternal reconstruction (occasionally with muscle flaps)[31] may be needed and be performed about 1 or 2 weeks after débridement. Intravenous antibiotics are continued for at least 1 week after wound closure.

**Inadequate Volume Status.** Inadequate volume status can easily develop in postoperative patients. Hypovolemia can be induced by inadequate volume management during rewarming with rapid vasodilatation. Hypovolemia can also be associated with diuretic and vasodilator therapies, hemorrhage, coagulopathies, or inadequate reversal of systemic heparinization required for CPB.

Hypervolemia develops as interstitial fluid moves back into the intravascular space or if overaggressive volume replacement occurs. Assessment of these states requires extensive hemodynamic monitoring and understanding of the numerous processes involved. Signs and symptoms specific to hypovolemia or hypervolemia should be investigated. Interventions for hypovolemia initially consist of replacement with crystalloid fluids. Colloidal solutions may be more appropriate in patients with significant peripheral edema because colloidal solutions can pull fluid more aggressively into the vascular bed where excess fluid can be excreted through the kidneys. If persistent hemorrhage from coagulopathies exists, transfusion with fresh-frozen plasma, platelet concentrates, or other factors may be indicated. If hemorrhage is related to technical factors, reoperation is necessary and replacement solutions in the interim can consist of autotranfused blood, whole blood, or packed cells.

### Respiratory System
The effects of anesthesia, sedation, and the deflation of the lungs during CPB commonly create moderate episodes of impaired gas exchange with concurrent alterations in the arterial blood gas values. These episodes, largely atelectatic in nature, are usually self limiting or easily resolved with sustained maximal inspiration, chest physiotherapy, and administration of supplemental oxygen. If a hemothorax or a pneumothorax develops, more negative pressure may be added to the drainage systems or additional chest tubes may be inserted. A volume overload from overaggressive replacement or mobilization of fluid from the third spaces may exist and can hamper gas exchange; diuretic therapy is indicated.

### Nervous System
Temporary and permanent sensory, motor, perceptual, and cognitive deficits can occur during the perioperative period. Permanent deficits can usually be attributed to a low cerebral perfusion state from inadequate cardiac output or to an embolic phenomenon from intracardiac thrombi, calcified valve fragments, aortic plaque dislodgement and subsequent embolization from application of the aortic crossclamp, or air embolization from intracardiac chambers of invasive lines.[31] The magnitude of the deficit is determined by the degree of neurologic involvement. Deficits are usually identified early in the postoperative period when the effects of anesthesia have resolved. Some of these deficits may not be identified until after extubation. Transient deficits, lasting from hours to days, can range in degree from slowness to arousal to confusion and delirium. Deficits can be caused by microemboli from tissue debris, air bubbles, or platelet aggregation and are associated with CPB.

### Renal System
Prerenal and acute renal failure states can develop after cardiac surgery. Inadequate CO from myocardial depression or inadequate volume replacement can lead to prerenal oliguria. Blood urea nitrogen and serum sodium levels increase, and serum creatinine levels remain the same. Low sodium content is seen in the urine as the body attempts to save sodium and thus increase its intravascular volume. If these states continue for prolonged periods, acute renal failure can ensue. Treatment focuses on maintenance of adequate volume replacement and increase in CO, with an inotropic agent if necessary. In addition, renal emboli from intracardiac thrombi or hemolysis from blood transfusions or prolonged CPB runs (from trauma to the formed elements of the blood producing hematuria) can also lead to the development of acute renal failure. In acute renal failure, serum creatinine and urea levels elevate and remain in a 10:1 ratio, urine sodium levels increase, and the plasma urine osmolality ratio falls to 1:1. Transient hematuria is usually short lived and may resolve after infusion of an osmotic diuretic (e.g., mannitol).

### Gastrointestinal System
Gastrointestinal (GI) complications are similar to those for general surgery.[31] After extubation, the patient may remain on nothing by mouth (NPO) status for a few hours with a nasogastric tube to decompress the stomach. Small amounts of ice or water are then allowed. Gastric distention can occur if air enters the stomach and can cause cardiac problems and pulmonary complications. Rarely, mesenteric or splenic ischemia or infarction from intracardiac thrombi or air emboli may occur; surgical revascularization can be performed.

### Peripheral Vascular System
Vascular complications can include both venous and arterial thrombus formation and embolism development. Venous thrombus can develop as a result of blood stasis from immobilization and

inactivity in the immediate postoperative period. Arterial complications are largely associated with various intravascular devices such as intraarterial lines and (when present) intraaortic balloon catheters. Assessment of pulses should be ongoing, and a Doppler pencil may be used to confirm the patency of the radial artery after removal of the intraarterial pressure monitoring line. The status of lower extremity pulses, skin color and temperature, and motor activity should be monitored closely, particularly in the presence of an intraaortic balloon catheter and particularly during insertion and removal. Passive and active range-of-motion exercises and early ambulation are advocated and encouraged in these patients to prevent complications. Patients are instructed and assisted in performing active dorsiflexion and extension of the feet and ankles. These maneuvers facilitate venous return and decrease stasis.

## SUMMARY

This chapter was intended to familiarize the PACU nurse with the perioperative care for the adult cardiac patient. The cardiac surgery patient has complex needs and may have resulting complications. Knowledge of the patient's experiences before and during surgery assists the nurse afte surgery to tailor the care to the patient's needs and to strengthen the continuity of that care.

## REFERENCES

1. Westaby S: *Landmarks in cardiac surgery*, Oxford, 1997, Isis Medical Media.
2. Jiricka MK: Ask the experts, *Crit Care Nurse* 26(3):70-72, 2006.
3. Cheng DCH, Bainbridge D: Postoperative cardiac recovery. In Kaplan J, editor: *Kaplan's cardiac anesthesia*, ed 5, Philadelphia, 2006, Saunders.
4. Rosborough D: Cardiac surgery in elderly patients, *Crit Care Nurse* 26(5):24-31, 2006.
5. Kouchoukos NT, Blackstone EH, Doty DB, et al, editors: Aortic valve disease. *Kirklin/Baratt-Boyes cardiac surgery*, ed 3, vol I, Philadelphia, 2003, Churchill Livingstone.
6. Waldhausen JA, et al: *Surgery of the chest*, ed 6, St Louis, 1996, Mosby.
7. Rabago G, et al: The new DeVega technique in tricuspid annuloplasty, *J Thoracic Cardiovasc Surg* 21:231, 1980.
8. Pantin EJ, Cheung AT: Kaplan's cardiac anesthesia. In Kaplan JA editor: *Thoracic aorta*, ed 5, Philadelphia, 2006, Saunders.
9. Cook DJ, Housmans PR, Rehfeldt KH: Valvular heart disease: replacement and repair. In Kaplan JA editor: *Kaplan's cardiac anesthesia*, ed 5, Philadelphia, 2006, Saunders.
10. Aboulhosn J, Child JS: Left ventricular outflow obstruction, *Circulation* 114:2412-2422, 2006.
11. Webb G, Gatzoulis MA: Atrial septal defects in the adult: recent progress and overview, *Circulation* 114:1645-1653, 2006.
12. Rocchini AP: Interventional cardiology. In Mavroudis C, Backer CL, editors: *Pediatric cardiac surgery*, ed 3, St Louis, 2003, Mosby.
13. Kern MJ, editor: *The cardiac catheterization handbook*, Philadelphia, 2003, Mosby.
14. Guru V, Omura J, Alghamdi AA, et al: Is blood superior to crystalloid cardioplegia? A meta-analysis of randomized clinical trials, *Circulation* 114(suppl I):I331-I338, 2006.
15. Marelli AJ, Mackie AS, Ionescu-Ittu R, et al: Congenital heart disease in the general population: changing prevalence and age distribution, *Circulation* 115:163-172, 2007.
16. Cox JL, Schuessler RB, D'Agostino HJ Jr, et al: The surgical treatment of atrial fibrillation; development of a definitive surgical procedure, *J Thoracic Cardiovasc Surg* 101:569-583, 1991.
17. Haisaguerre M, Jais P, Shah DC, et al: Spontaneous initiation of atrial fibrillation by ectopic beats originating in the pulmonary veins, *N Engl J Med* 339:659-666, 1998.
18. Ad N: The cryosurgical Maze procedure, *Cardiothoracic Surg Network*, 2006, available at http://www.ctsnet.org/sections/clinicalresources/adultcardiac/expert_tech-5.html, accessed July 7, 2006.
19. Panagiotis K, Maria P, Argiri P, et al: Is postanesthesia care unit length of stay increased in hypothermic patients? *AORN J* 81(2):379-392, 2005.
20. Kurz A, Sessler DI, Lenhardt R: Perioperative normothermia to reduce the incidence of surgical wound infection and shorten hospitalization, *N Engl J Med* 334:1209-1215, 1996.
21. Edwards FH, Ferraris VA, Shahian DM, et al: Gender-specific practice guidelines for coronary artery bypass surgery: perioperative management, *Ann Thoracic Surg* 79:2189-2194, 2005.
22. Finklemeier BA: *Cardiothoracic surgical nursing*, ed 2, Philadelphia, 2000, Lippincott.
23. Seifert PC: Cardiac surgery. In Rothrock JC, editor: *Alexander's care of the patient in surgery*, ed 13, St Louis, 2007, Mosby.
24. Rose E, Moskowitz AJ, Packer M, et al: The REMATCH trial: rationale, design, and end points: randomized evaluation of mechanical assistance for the treatment of congestive heart failure, *Ann Thoracic Surg* 67(3):723-730, 1999.

NURSING CARE IN THE PACU

25. Rose E, Gelijns AC, Moskowitz AJ, et al: Long-term mechanical left ventricular assistance for end-stage heart failure, *N Engl J Med* 345:1435-1443, 2001.

26. Park SJ, Tector A, Piccioni W, et al: Left ventricular assist devices as destination therapy: a new look at survival, *J Thoracic Cardiovasc Surg* 129(1):9-17, 2005.

27. Brouillette CV: Cardiac anesthesia. In Nagelhout JJ, Zaglaniczny KL, editors: *Nurse anesthesia*, ed 3, St Louis, 2005, Saunders.

28. Odom J: Management and policies. In Drain C editor: *Perianesthesia nursing: a critical care approach*, ed 4, St Louis, 2003, Saunders.

29. Aldrete J, Kroulik D: A post anesthetic recovery score, *Anesthesia Analgesia* 49:924-933, 1970.

30. Munro N: Cardiac surgery. In Morton PG, Fontaine DK, Hudak CM, et al editors: *Critical care nursing: a holistic approach*, ed 8, Philadelphia, 2005, Lippincott Williams.

31. Seifert PC: *Cardiac surgery*, St Louis, 2002, Mosby.

## BIBLIOGRAPHY

Adams DH, Filsoufi F, Antman EM: Medical management of the patient undergoing cardiac surgery. In Zipes DP, Libby P, Bonow RO, et al editors: *Braunwald's heart disease*, ed 7, Philadelphia, 2005, Saunders.

Andrew MJ, Baker RA, Kneebone AC, et al: Mood state as a predictor of neuropsychological deficits following cardiac surgery, *J Psychosom Res* 48(6):537-546, 2000.

Buckberg GD: Overview: procedure versus protection: an impossible separation, *Semin Thoracic Cardiovasc Surg* 13(1):29-32, 2001.

Cameron A, Davis KB, Green G, et al: Coronary bypass surgery with internal-thoracic-artery grafts: effects on survival over a 15-year period, *N Engl J Med* 334(4):216-219, 1996.

Carpino PA, Khabbaz KR, Bojar RM, et al: Clinical benefits of endoscopic vein harvesting in patients with risk factors for saphenectomy wound infections undergoing coronary artery bypass grafting, *J Thoracic Cardiovasc Surg* 119:69-76, 2000.

Care after coronary-artery bypass surgery, *N Engl J Med* 384(15):1456-1463, 2003.

Carvalho G, Moore A, Qizilbash B, et al: Maintenance of normoglycemia during cardiac-surgery, *Anesthesia Analgesia* 99(2):319-324, 2004.

Conway DG, House J, Bandt K, et al: The elderly: health status benefits and recovery of function one year after coronary artery bypass surgery, *J Am Coll Cardiol* 42(8):1421-1426, 2003.

DiMattio MJK, Tulman L: A longitudinal study of functional status and correlates following coronary artery bypass graft surgery in women, *Nurs Res* 52(2):98-107, 2003.

Douville EC, Asaph JW, Dworkin RJ, et al: Sternal preservation: a better way to treat most sternal wound complications after cardiac surgery, *Ann Thoracic Surg* 78(5):1659-1664, 2004.

Eagle KA, et al: ACC/AHA guideline update for coronary artery bypass graft surgery, *Circulation* 110(9):1168-1176, 2004.

Edmunds LH: Cardiopulmonary bypass after 50 years, *N Engl J Med* 351(16):1603-1606, 2004.

Fransen EJ, Diris JH, Maessen JG, et al: Evaluation of "new" cardiac marker for ruling out myocardial infarction after coronary artery bypass grafting, *Chest* 122(4):1316-1321, 2002.

Furnary AP, Zerr KJ, Grunkemeier GL, et al: A continuous insulin infusion reduces the incidence of deep sternal wound infection in diabetic patients after cardiac surgical procedures, *Ann Thoracic Surg* 67:352-360, 1999.

Garrett K, Lauer K, Christopher BA: The effects of obesity on the cardiopulmonary system: implications for critical care nursing, *Prog Cardiovasc Nurs* 19(4):155-161, 2004.

Hessel EA: Abdominal organ injury after cardiac surgery, *Semin Cardiothor Vasc Anes* 8(3):243-263, 2004.

Kern LS: Postoperative atrial fibrillation: new directions in prevention and treatment, *J Cardiovasc Nurs* 15(2):103-115, 2004.

King KB, Rowe MA, Zerwic JJ: Concerns and risk factor modification in women during the year after coronary artery surgery, *Nurs Res* 49(3):167-172, 2000.

King KM: Gender and short term recovery from cardiac surgery, *Nurs Res* 49(1):29-36, 2000.

Knotzer H, Dunser MW, Mayr AJ, et al: Post bypass arrhythmias: pathophysiology, prevention, and therapy, *Curr Opin Crit Care* 10(5):330-335, 2004.

Leung JM, Bellows WH, Schiller NB: Impairment of left atrial function predicts postoperative atrial fibrillation after coronary artery bypass graft surgery, *Eur Heart J* 25(20):1836-1844, 2004.

Lorenz RA, Lorenz RM, Codd JE: Perioperative blood glucose control during adult coronary artery bypass surgery, *AORN J* 81(1):126-150, 2005.

Lu CY, Grayson AD, Jha P, et al: Risk factors for sternal wound infection and mid-term survival following coronary artery bypass surgery, *Eur J Cardiothoracic Surg* 23:943-949, 2003.

Lutarewych M, Morgan SP, Hall MM: Improving outcomes of coronary artery bypass graft infections with multiple interventions: putting science and data to the test, *Infect Control Hosp Epidemiol* 25(6):517-519, 2004.

Maglish Ehrman BL, Moore HA: Blood conservation strategies in cardiovascular surgery, *Dim Crit Care Nurs* 23(6):244-252, 2004.

Mason VF, Miller KH: Optimizing outcomes: nurses caring for patients after cardiac surgery can promote early transfers, *AJN* 101(Suppl):13–15, 2001.

Milgrom LB, Brooks JA, Qi R, et al: Pain levels experienced with activities after cardiac surgery, *Am J Crit Care* 13(2):116-125, 2004.

Miller KH, Grindel CG: Comparison of symptoms of younger and older patients undergoing coronary artery bypass surgery, *Clin Nurs Res* 13(3):179-193, 2004.

Mooss AN, Wurdeman RL, Sugimoto JT, et al: Amiodarone versus sotalol for the treatment of atrial fibrillation after open heart surgery: the reduction in postoperative cardiovascular arrhythmic events (REDUCE) trial, *Am Heart J* 148:641-648, 2004.

Paparella D, Brister SJ, Buchanan MR: Coagulation disorders of cardiopulmonary bypass: a review, *Intens Care Med* 30:1873-1881, 2004.

Rantanen A, Kaunonen M, Astedt-Kurki P: Coronary artery bypass grafting: social support for patients and their significant others, *J Clin Nurs* 13(2):158-166, 2004.

Salamon T, Michler RE, Knott KM, et al: Off-pump coronary artery bypass grafting does not decrease the incidence of atrial fibrillation, *Ann Thor Surg* 75:505-507, 2003.

Sharma M, Berriel-Cass D, Baran J: Sternal surgical-site infections following coronary artery bypass graft: prevalence, microbiology, and complications during a 42-month period, *Infect Control Hosp Epidemiol* 25:468-471, 2004.

Simani-Oren L: The ten commandments of caring for patients after open heart surgery, *Home Healthcare Nurse* 21(8):551-556, 2003.

Suma H, Isomura T, Horii T, et al: Late angiographic result of using the right gastroepiploic artery as a graft, *J Thoracic Cardiovasc Surg* 120:496, 2000.

Theobald K, McMurray A: Coronary artery bypass graft surgery: discharge planning for successful recovery, *J Advanced Nursing* 47(5):483-491, 2004.

Timothy PR, Rodeman BJ: Temporary pacemakers in critically ill patients: assessment and management strategies, *AACN Clin Issues Adv Pract Acute Crit Care* 15(3):305-325, 2004.

Tranmer JE, Parry MJE: Enhancing postoperative recovery of cardiac surgery patients: a randomized clinical trial of an advanced practice nursing intervention, *West J Nurs Res* 26(5):515-532, 2004.

Vaccarino V, Lin ZQ, Kasl SV, et al: Gender differences in recovery after coronary artery bypass surgery, *JACC* 41(2):307-314, 2003.

Vallerand AH, Hasenau SM, Templin T: Barriers to pain management by home care nurses, *Home Healthcare Nurse* 22(12):831-838, 2004.

Villareal RP, Hariharan R, Liu BC, et al: Postoperative atrial fibrillation and mortality after coronary artery bypass surgery, *JACC* 43(5):742-748, 2004.

Watt-Watson J, Stevens B, Katz J, et al: Impact of preoperative education on pain outcomes after coronary artery bypass graft surgery, *Pain* 109:73-85, 2004.

Wilson JA, Clark JJ: Obesity impediment to wound healing, *Crit Care Nurs Q* 26(2):119-132, 2003.

Wynne R: Postoperative pulmonary dysfunction in adults after cardiac surgery with cardiopulmonary bypass: clinical significance and implications for practice, *Am J Crit Care* 13(5):384-393, 2004.

Yorke J, Wallis M, McLean B: Patients' perceptions of pain management after cardiac surgery in an Australian critical care unit, *Heart Lung* 33(1):33-41, 2004.

NURSING CARE IN THE PACU

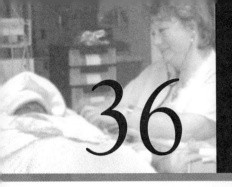

# 36

## CARE OF THE VASCULAR SURGICAL PATIENT

*Melody S. Heffline, MSN, RN, APRN,BC, ACNP*

Integrity and patency of the vascular system, which includes arteries, veins, capillaries, and lymphatic vessels, are essential to the life of human tissues. Before the 1950s, a limited number of surgical procedures was available for treatment of impaired blood flow through the vascular system. Loss of limb or life as a result of impaired blood flow was common, and vascular surgical procedures were experimental. Vascular surgery advancements occurred as a result of the development of diagnostic tools, such as arteriography, and improvements in medications, such as antibiotics and anticoagulants. The development and refinement of surgical instruments and techniques also contributed to the growth of vascular surgery as a specialty.

During the past two decades, a rapid growth has been seen in the technology and instrumentation available for the vascular surgeon. The development of improved instrumentation, suture materials, synthetic graft materials, and improved monitoring techniques has also contributed to the advancement of vascular surgery. Minimally invasive techniques available include placement of endografts, percutaneous transluminal angioplasty (PTA) with or without stenting, atherectomy, cryoplasty, and fibrinolytic therapy. Although many of these procedures can be performed percutaneously, these techniques require sedation and close observation after the procedures.

## DEFINITIONS

**Aneurysm:** A localized abnormal dilation, distention, or sac in an artery.

**Angiography (Arteriography):** The injection of radiopaque dye into the arteries followed by rapid sequential radiographs of the vascular tree for determination of abnormalities.

**Atherectomy:** Procedure performed with a special catheter that contains a special shaver device at the distal tip. The rotating blade shaves the plaque from the inner lining and removes it from the vessel through a suction device.

**Bypass:** Performed to reroute blood flow around an area of stenosis in a blood vessel.

**Cryoplasty:** A technique that uses cooling and balloon angioplasty to open occluded vessels.

**Embolectomy:** Extraction of an embolus from an artery.

**Embolus:** Fragments of thrombus, atherosclerotic debris, or other material that migrate through a vessel.

**Endarterectomy:** Surgical removal of atheromatous plaque from an occluded vessel.

**Endograft:** Device designed to exclude an area of a blood vessel and provide a new conduit through which blood flows. It may be delivered percutaneously (puncture site only) or through small incisions made at the insertion site. It is primarily used to exclude aneurysmal vessels.

**Fibrinolytic (Thrombolytic) Therapy:** Technique that uses clot-dissolving agents to dissolve clot material in a blood vessel.

**Ischemia:** Lack of adequate blood flow to an area to meet the needs of the tissues.

**Ligation:** Transection and tying off of a blood vessel.

**Stent:** Device made of metal or other material used to maintain patency of a blood vessel after angioplasty. The device may be balloon expandable or self expanding.

**Sympathectomy:** Interruption of the sympathetic nerve chain performed to produce vasodilation of blood vessels distal to the surgical site. Cervical, thoracic, and lumbar sympathectomy may be performed.

**Thrombectomy:** Surgical removal of a thrombus.

**Thrombus:** Stationary blood clot or atheromatous plaque that totally occludes a blood vessel.

**Transluminal Angioplasty:** The use of a special catheter with a balloon at the distal tip that is passed through the vessel to the area of stenosis and inflated to compress the stenosis and widen the vessel lumen. The balloon is deflated before removal of the catheter from the vessel. This procedure may be done percutaneously (with only a puncture site) or open (through an incision in the vessel) and may be done in conjunction with a stent, atherectomy, or cryoplasty.

## TREATMENT OF VASCULAR DISEASE

### General Considerations

Peripheral arterial disease (PAD) is among the most common causes of disability and death in the Western world. The arterial system is a complex organ with specific pathologic processes that can result in morbidity and mortality. Persons with arterial disease commonly have other underlying disease processes, some of which may contribute to the development of disease and increase the morbidity and mortality rates associated with surgery (Box 36-1). The progression of atherosclerosis, which leads to most vascular surgical procedures, is a systemic disease that affects all arterial beds, including those in the extremities, heart, kidneys, and brain. Venous surgical procedures have also increased in number in the past few years as a result of improvements in technology. This chapter is limited to care of the patient undergoing surgery on blood vessels outside of the heart.

### Diagnostic Procedures

Noninvasive diagnostics, such as the ankle-brachial index (ABI), ultrasonography, computed tomographic (CT) scanning, magnetic resonance angiography and imaging, have contributed greatly to the early treatment of vascular disease. These procedures do not usually require sedation. Arteriography continues to be the gold standard for invasive diagnostic testing and usually requires intravenous (IV) sedation. Arteriography may also be done in conjunction with various treatment methods,

---

| Box 36-1 | Underlying Conditions Common in the Patient with Arterial Disease |
|---|---|

Chronic tobacco use
Chronic obstructive pulmonary disease
Multiple arterial bed involvement: coronary, renal, carotid, extremities
Diabetes
Peripheral neuropathy
Hypertension
Obesity
Advancing age

---

including angioplasty, cryoplasty, atherectomy, and stenting.

### Interventional Procedures

Interventional treatments for peripheral vascular disease include PTA, PTA with stent placement, atherectomy, cryoplasty, and fibrinolytic therapy. These endovascular procedures are performed by a variety of specialists including interventional radiologists, vascular surgeons, and cardiologists. These procedures may require only local anesthetic and IV sedation depending on the patient's condition and physician's preferences. They may also be performed alone or in conjunction with other vascular surgical procedures in the operating room and may be done with local plus IV sedation, epidural, spinal, or general anesthesia.

Percutaneous transluminal angioplasty may be performed on carotid, aortic, renal, iliac, femoral, popliteal, and tibial vessel stenosis. Major complications after PTA include bleeding, hematoma, and intimal tears (disruption of the inner lining of the vessel). This procedure may be used alone or in conjunction with stent placement. Stents are used to compress and hold the plaque against the vessel wall and are associated with longer patency rates of the vessel. They may also be used in treatment of an intimal tear in the vessel wall. Stents with drug coating, such as sirolimus and paclitaxel, are being evaluated for their potential to reduce in-stent stenosis as a result of their effects on smooth muscle cell proliferation. The goal is to increase long-term patency rates. Long-term data will help to determine whether these will be an effective tool for PAD.

Atherectomy is a technique designed for removal of plaque from the vessel wall with a special rotating blade and suction apparatus. Angioplasty or stenting may follow atherectomy. Cryoplasty uses a freezing technique with nitrous oxide inside a balloon for the opening of occluded vessels.

After these procedures, patients are monitored for recovery from IV sedation and for bleeding and hematoma formation at the puncture site. Distal pulses are assessed bilaterally to detect any change in blood flow that may be related to formation of an embolism or thrombus for procedures that involve the abdominal vessels or extremities. These pulses should be compared with the baseline pulses documented before the procedure. Intake and output should be monitored closely and adequate hydration maintained after any procedure with IV contrast. IV contrast can be toxic to the renal system, and additional treatments such as additional

IV fluids, N-acetylcysteine, diuretics, sodium bicarbonate, and fenoldopam may be used to provide additional protection against postprocedural nephropathy. Bed rest is maintained for 6 to 8 hours after the procedure with the extremity in a straight position to prevent bleeding at the puncture site. If a closure device is used at the puncture site, the patient may be allowed out of bed sooner. Any patient who undergoes an arteriogram, angioplasty, or stenting that involves the carotid or cranial circulation should undergo frequent neurologic assessment after the procedure. Special protection devices are used during angioplasty and stenting to trap any free-floating particles of plaque or thrombus that may be dislodged during the procedure. These devices serve to minimize postprocedural complications such as stroke.

Fibrinolytic therapy is used when an embolus or thrombus has occluded a vessel. Special catheters are placed in the area of the thrombus, and agents such as urokinase, tissue plasminogen activator (tPa), or tenectaplase (tKa) are used to lyse the clot. This process is done via infusion and may take hours for complete lysis of the thrombus. These patients need close observation throughout the infusion for signs of bleeding, such as hematoma at the puncture site and hematuria. Frequent assessment of the limb is also needed as reperfusion occurs. As the limb reperfuses, pain may actually worsen initially as microemboli break away from the thrombus and move distally to smaller vessels. As the infusion continues, pain improves as these emboli are dissolved. Frequent laboratory work includes serial monitoring of fibrinogen, prothrombin time (PT), partial thromboplastin time (PTT), hemoglobin, and hematocrit. Periodic assessment in radiology is done to follow the progress of the lytic agent. The infusion is discontinued when lysis is complete, fibrinogen levels drop to less than 100, bleeding occurs that necessitates transfusion, or no response to the agent is found.

### Other Medications Used in the Patient for Vascular Surgery

Among the most commonly used medications in the treatment of the patient for vascular surgery are anticoagulants. Unfractionated heparin (UH) may be administered before, during, and after surgery. Its actions occur at multiple points in the coagulation cascade to ultimately inactivate thrombin and prevent conversion of fibrinogen to fibrin. Heparin may be administered intravenously or subcutaneously. It has a short 60-minute to 90-minute half-life. The response to heparin is measured with the activated partial thromboplastin time (aPTT) and is targeted at 1.5 to 2.5 times normal to obtain a therapeutic response and prevent thromboembolism. Complications associated with the use of heparin include increased risk of bleeding and heparin-induced thrombocytopenia (HIT). Platelet counts should be monitored for decrease of 40% to 50% from baseline or any decrease to less than 100,000. If HIT develops, heparin must be discontinued and alternative anticoagulants used. Protamine is the antidote for heparin; its action occurs within 5 minutes of administration. Care must be taken to avoid too rapid administration of protamine. When administration is too rapid, side effects can include hypotension, pulmonary hypertension, shortness of breath and flushing. The usual target dose for reversal is 1 mg of protamine for every 90 units of heparin.

Low–molecular weight heparins (LMWHs), such as enoxaparin, dalteparin, and tinzaparin, may also be used in the care of the patient for vascular surgery. These drugs have a significantly lower molecular weight than does unfractionated heparin, which gives them improved predictability in the dose response and a longer half-life. This advantage greatly reduces the need for laboratory monitoring. The LMWHs are administered subcutaneously and have a significantly lower incidence rate of HIT associated with their use. They are primarily used in the prevention of thromboembolism after surgery but are also approved in the treatment of deep vein thrombosis (DVT) and pulmonary embolism (PE). Complications are similar to those of unfractionated heparin. Patients still need monitoring for HIT, although it occurs much less frequently with the use of LMWH.

Warfarin is an anticoagulant that inhibits vitamin K–dependent coagulation factors and the anticoagulant proteins C and S. It has a half-life of 36 to 42 hours. Monitoring of warfarin is done with the prothrombin time (PT) and the international normalized ratio (INR). The prothrombin time is laboratory dependent, and specific methods vary among institutions. Caregivers should be familiar with institutional methods. Warfarin is used to treat a variety of thromboembolic disorders and is used in promoting long-term patency of infrainguinal bypass grafts. Complications include increased risk of hemorrhage and skin necrosis. Patients on warfarin must be counseled to discontinue the drug several days before any invasive procedure to allow time for the PT levels to decrease to normal. Some patients may need the use of LMWH or UH in the interim between discontinuation of warfarin and surgery to prevent thromboembolic complications.

Direct thrombin inhibitors act at the active site of thrombin. These drugs provide an alternative to heparin in the patient with HIT. Current drugs available in this category are lepirudin, desirudin, bivalirudin, and argatroban.

Factor X inhibitors are the newest category of anticoagulants available. This category currently includes only fondaparinux. It activates antithrombin III, leading to inactivation of factor X. It is administered subcutaneously and requires no laboratory monitoring. Its primary usage is in prevention of DVT and treatment of acute coronary syndromes.

Antiplatelet agents, such as aspirin, clopidogrel, and ticlopidine, may also be used in the patient with vascular disease as a preventative measure for myocardial infarction and stroke and as a treatment for patients after placement of infrainguinal bypass grafts, carotid endarterectomy, or peripheral and carotid stenting. The most commonly used drug is aspirin. These drugs exhibit an irreversible permanent effect on the platelet for its lifespan and produce a qualitative effect on the platelet that is measured with the bleeding time. Platelet counts are not affected by these agents. Patients should be counseled regarding the discontinuation of these drugs 7 to 10 days before invasive procedures to decrease the risk of bleeding.

### Arterial Surgical Procedures: Extremity Vessels and Extraanatomic Procedures

Arterial surgical procedures that involve the extremities include bypass, endarterectomy, embolectomy, and thrombectomy. A bypass is performed to reroute blood flow around an area of stenosis and is named for the vessels it arises from and connects into. Examples of these in the lower extremities are femoral-popliteal, femoral-tibial, and femoral-peroneal. The distal anastomosis for femoral-popliteal bypass procedures may be above the knee or below the knee depending on the location of the stenosis (Fig. 36-1). Bypass procedures may also be performed in the upper extremities but are much less common and may include bypass to circumvent lesions of the axillary artery, such as carotid-axillary bypass. Extraanatomic bypass procedures route blood in a more unusual fashion and may be done based on a patient's condition or inability to tolerate a more major procedure. Examples of these types of bypass include axillofemoral, axillary-axillary, and femoral-femoral (Fig. 36-2). Endarterectomy may be done alone or in conjunction with a bypass and involves removal of plaque from a stenotic vessel. Embolectomy and thrombectomy may also be performed to remove the clot from a vessel.

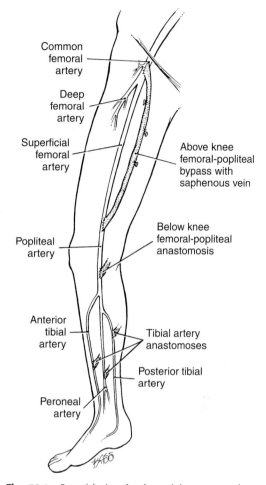

**Fig. 36-1** Potential sites for femoral bypass procedures. *(From McCartny WJ, Williams LR: Femoral artery reconstruction,* Critical Care Quarterly 8:43, 1985. *In Fahey V:* Vascular nursing, *ed 4, Philadelphia, 2004, Saunders.)*

Materials used for bypass procedures may be autogenous (vein) or synthetic (artificial). Use of the greater saphenous vein may be accomplished in a reversed fashion or in situ. In the reverse method, the vein is reversed, and the small end is attached to the proximal artery and the large end to the smaller artery distally. Arm veins may be used but are much less common. Synthetic grafts that may be used include polytetrafluoroethylene (PTFE), which may be with or without supporting rings, and knitted or woven Dacron. PTFE is commonly used in the lower extremities and for other low flow states such as extraanatomic bypass. In some cases, a combination of autogenous and synthetic grafts may be used.

Choice of anesthesia is based on the type of procedure and patient and physician preference. Many procedures that involve smaller incisions or the use of endovascular techniques may be done with local with IV sedation. Epidural and

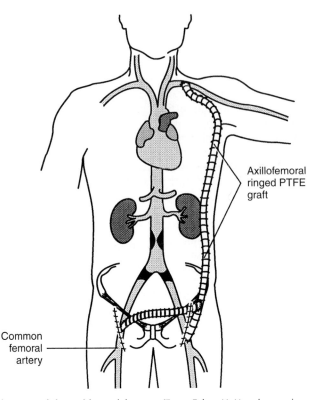

**Fig. 36-2**  Axillofemoral bypass and femoral-femoral bypass. *(From Fahey V: Vascular nursing, ed 4, Philadelphia, 2004, Saunders.)*

spinal anesthesia may be used but in some situations are not the preferred choice because of the effects on the sympathetic nervous system that result in vasodilation of the vasculature in the lower extremities. This vasodilation may lead to hypotension, which places the patient at risk for thrombosis of the graft after surgery.

**Positioning.**  Immediately after surgery, the patient is supine with the head of the bed elevated. Care should be taken to place the limb in a position of comfort. For the patient with lower extremity surgery, care must be taken to prevent compression of the popliteal area. The limb should not be significantly elevated unless edema is present. However, both heels should be protected from pressure and the toes should be protected from heavy bed linens. Bed rest is usually maintained for the first 24 hours after surgery.

**Cardiopulmonary Status.**  Vital signs are monitored at least hourly initially. Because of the atherosclerosis, patients who undergo vascular procedures have much higher mortality rates. Myocardial ischemia is most common in this patient population and occurs more often in the postoperative period than during surgery. Continuous cardiac monitoring and pulse

oximetry are standard monitoring parameters for these patients. Arterial lines and pulmonary artery catheters may be used selectively in this patient population.

**Neurovascular Status.**  The dorsalis pedis pulses and the posterior tibial pulses should be assessed frequently. Recommendations are for every 1 to 2 hours in the first 24 hours after surgery. These results should be compared with baseline pulses documented before surgery. Pulses should be assessed based on a scale of 0 to 3 (Box 36-2). In some cases of distal bypass procedures, the position of the palpable pulse may be in a different location than before surgery. This information should be provided by the physician. A Doppler scan should be available for assessment of pulses because pulses are commonly present but not palpable. Routine

| Box 36-2   Pulse Assessment |
| --- |
| 0: Absent |
| 1: Diminished |
| 2: Normal |
| 3: Bounding |
| D: Doppler |

| Box 36-3 | Obtaining an Ankle Brachial Index (ABI) |
| --- | --- |

1. Obtain the blood pressure in both arms with the patient lying supine.
2. Obtain the blood pressure with a Doppler scan at the dorsalis pedis and posterior tibial pulses on each ankle.
3. Calculate the ABI with the highest ankle pressure divided by the highest arm pressure. (Example: Right blood pressure [BP], 140/80 mm Hg; left BP, 146/88 mm Hg; right DP, 136 mm Hg; right PT, 124 mm Hg; left DP, 128 mm Hg; left PT, 132 mm Hg; right ABI = 136 mm Hg/146 mm Hg [0.93]; left ABI = 132 mm Hg/146 mm Hg [0.90].)

assessment of Doppler scanned pulses also provides a method of early detection of a change in blood flow. Normal blood flow is heard as a triphasic (three whooshing sounds) or biphasic (two whooshing sounds) flow. If assessment indicates a change from a triphasic or biphasic sound to a monophasic sound (one whooshing sound), blood flow may have changed in the extremity and the physician should be notified. Establishment of a baseline includes knowledge of whether the patient had monophasic flow before surgery.

Assessment of ankle-brachial indices (ABI) should be part of the vital sign assessment for the vascular patient. This measurement is an indicator of blood flow to the lower extremities. The steps for assessment of an ABI are listed in Box 36-3.

Assessment is needed for changes in motor and sensory function and the presence of foot drop. These symptoms may be indicative of compartment syndrome. Color and temperature changes should also be assessed. The extremity should be warm and dry and of normal color. Acute ischemia is recognized quickly with assessment for the six P's: pain, paralysis, paresthesia, pulselessness, poikilothermia, and pallor (Box 36-4).

| Box 36-4 | Signs of Acute Ischemia |
| --- | --- |

Pallor
Pain
Pulselessness
Paresthesias
Poikilothermia
Paralysis

***Dressings.*** Dressings should be dry and intact throughout the postanesthesia care unit (PACU) stay. After distal bypass procedures, dressings may extend the full length of the extremity. Frequent observation for bleeding or hematoma at the area of the incisions is critical. Signs of bleeding should be reported to the physician as soon as possible. Bleeding may compromise blood flow through the graft and lead to compartment syndrome.

***Pain Relief.*** Pain and discomfort are common after lower extremity arterial surgery. This pain must, however, be assessed and differentiated from ischemic pain and that of compartment syndrome. Sudden severe pain may be indicative of graft occlusion, especially when located across the foot at the metatarsal heads. Occlusions usually result in pain out of proportion to the usual postoperative pain. Patients may have pain in the thigh and medial aspect of the leg away from the incision that may be characterized as a burning type of pain; this pain is related to neuropathy that may occur as a result of operative injury to the nerve. Most neuropathies resolve after a few months.

***Intake and Output.*** Renal status must be monitored closely after surgery. Intake and output should be monitored every 1 to 2 hours in the first 24 hours. Hydration is important in the patient with vascular disease because of the potential for renal insufficiency; the use of contrast during the procedure increases the risk of postoperative nephropathy. Electrolytes, blood urea nitrogen (BUN), and creatinine values should be monitored closely for changes in hydration status.

### Carotid Vessels

The most common procedure performed on the carotid arteries is endarterectomy. Other procedures performed on the carotid arteries include bypass, angioplasty, and stenting. Endarterectomy is performed for removal of plaque from the carotid artery bifurcation and internal carotid artery. This removal is done to improve cerebral circulation and decrease the risk of embolization to the brain, which may result in a stroke. On completion of the endarterectomy, the carotid artery may be closed in a primary fashion (with suturing of the edges of the artery together) or with a patch graft to leave a larger vessel after surgery.

For lesions located in the common carotid closer to the aortic arch, a bypass to the subclavian artery may be the only means of restoring sufficient blood flow to the brain. A bypass from one carotid to another can also be performed. Angioplasty and stenting are also used

NURSING CARE IN THE PACU

**Table 36-1    Cranial Nerve Assessment**

| Cranial Nerve | Function | Abnormal Response |
|---|---|---|
| Facial (VII) | Facial expression<br>Saliva secretion | Inability to smile symmetrically<br>Contralateral asymmetry indicates possible stroke<br>Nerve injury on ipsilateral side |
| Glossopharygeal (IX) | Swallowing<br>Pharyngeal muscle | Difficulty swallowing with ipsilateral Horner's syndrome (ptosis, exophthalmos, reduced sweating) |
| Vagus (X) | | Minor swallowing problems and fatigued voice |
|   Superior laryngeal branch<br>  Recurrent laryngeal branch | Pharyngeal and laryngeal muscles | Vocal cord paralysis, hoarseness, inadequate gag reflex |
| Spinal accessory (XI) | Shoulder muscles | Ipsilateral weakness in neck and shoulder with shrugging |
| Hypoglossal (XII) | Muscles of tongue | Tongue droops to ipsilateral side, difficulties with speech and chewing, hoarseness, difficulty with high-pitched sounds |

for carotid lesions. Procedure locations and technicians are the same as that for the lower extremities. A major difference in the procedure for carotid angioplasty and stenting is that the procedure uses distal protection devices designed to trap any debris that may be dislodged during the procedure. These devices trap debris in a basket-type apparatus that removes the debris at the conclusion of the procedure as the catheter is withdrawn. This debris, if not trapped, may significantly increase the risk of a stroke.

***Positioning.*** Immediately after the procedure, the patient is positioned supine with the head of the bed elevated. Bed rest is maintained for the initial 24 hours.

***Cardiopulmonary and Circulatory Status.*** Vital signs, including oxygen saturation, and neurologic checks are assessed every hour during the first 24-hour period. Intake and output are initially monitored every 4 hours. Uncontrolled hypertension may threaten the anastomosis, and hypotension may predispose the patient to carotid artery thrombosis. Underlying cardiac disease may also be aggravated by extremes in blood pressure. Vasoactive infusions may be necessary to control blood pressure and maintain the levels at less than 180 mm Hg systolic and 100 mm Hg diastolic after endarterectomy. Patients should also be monitored for respiratory distress and hematoma formation.

***Dressings.*** Immediately after surgery, the incision may be covered with a dressing. Some physicians may use a drain if oozing is seen in the wound bed at the time of surgical closure. Bruising, discoloration, and swelling around the incision are common. However, changes in the patient's respiratory status or increasing hematoma around the incision require immediate attention. Tracheal compression may lead quickly to respiratory compromise. Reoperation may be necessary to locate and correct a suture line bleed and drain the hematoma.

***Pain Relief.*** Most patients need little for pain after endarterectomy. Opioids are avoided as much as possible because of their effects on level of consciousness and interference with accurate assessment of neurologic function. When analgesia is needed, it is usually in the form of acetaminophen or aspirin suppository. Close attention should be paid to symptoms of severe headache because these may indicate hyperperfusion syndrome or cerebral hemorrhage. This complication usually occurs 2 to 3 days after surgery as a result of impaired cerebral autoregulation but may present earlier. Severe cases may need treatment with steroids and vasoconstricting agents for prevention of seizures and stroke.

***Neurologic Function.*** Level of consciousness, movement of extremities, and cranial nerve assessment are included in the assessment of vital signs after endarterectomy. Because of the close proximity of cranial nerves to the operative site, risk of injury during the procedure exists. Cranial nerve assessment is summarized in Table 36-1. Cranial nerve injuries are usually temporary and heal over time as the patient recovers from surgery.

## Large Vessels

Surgical procedures that involve the aorta and iliac vessels may be performed for atherosclerotic disease, aneurysmal disease, dissection, or trauma. Bypass procedures include aorto-iliac and aorto-femoral procedures and those that involve the renal arteries and the mesenteric vessels. Endarterectomy may also be performed on these vessels.

The development of endovascular techniques has led to the use of devices designed to reduce extensive surgical procedures, operative time, blood loss, and anesthesia. Endovascular procedures are now used to repair thoracic and abdominal aortic aneurysms (endografts). Patients must meet certain inclusion criteria to qualify for an endovascular procedure. These devices are made of a nickel-titanium stent with graft material, Dacron or PTFE, attached to the stent. The graft material may be on the outside or the inside of the stent depending on the manufacturer. Some devices are a unibody (one part to the device) design; others are modular in design. Physician preference and individual patient anatomy are used in determination of the best design for each patient. These procedures may be done with local with IV sedation and are performed most often through a cutdown into the femoral arteries in each groin. In some instances, these procedures may be performed percutaneously.

Open abdominal procedures that involve the large vessels usually involve a midline incision. Some procedures may be done from a retroperitoneal approach, and laparoscopic techniques have also been used in procedures that involve the aorta. These procedures usually require general anesthesia. However, supplemental epidural anesthesia may be used to allow a lighter level of general anesthesia.

***Positioning.*** Immediately after the procedure, the patient is positioned supine with the head of the bed elevated. Bed rest is maintained for the initial 24 hours.

***Cardiopulmonary Status.*** Because of the high risk of aortic procedures, cardiopulmonary assessment is of the utmost importance. Many patients receive beta blockers in the perioperative period to decrease left ventricular workload and the risk of myocardial ischemia. Cardiac stress is greatly increased as a result of cross clamping and declamping. Arterial pressure monitoring, electrocardiography, pulse oximetry, arterial blood gas analysis, pulmonary artery pressure, and central venous pressure measurements are all tools that may be used in these patients to monitor during the immediate postoperative period. Normotension reduces the stress on suture lines and decreases the risk of thrombosis in a graft limb. Vasoactive medications may be used to normalize blood pressure. Dysrhythmias may occur as a result of hypoxemia, myocardial ischemia, and electrolyte imbalances.

Some patients may need mechanical ventilation after surgery. Because of underlying pulmonary disease in many vascular patients, pulmonary status must be monitored closely for atelectasis as a result of incisional pain and decreased lung function.

***Circulatory Status.*** The level of cross clamp of the aorta, if necessary during the procedure, influences greatly the potential for complications after surgery. Neurologic checks should be monitored with hourly vital signs for assessment of any signs of paralysis as a result of spinal cord injury related to cross clamp. Lower extremity pulses, color, temperature, and motor and sensory function should be assessed every 4 hours initially. ABIs are the best tool for determination of whether the blood flow to the distal arterial bed of the extremities is adequate after surgery. Ischemia in the lower extremities may occur as a result of embolization, graft occlusion, or hypoperfusion of the extremity.

***Dressings.*** Dry dressings are applied to the abdominal incision for open procedures. For endovascular procedures, dressings may be used on one or both groins at the site of access. Dressings and surgical sites should be assessed for signs of bleeding or hematoma.

***Pain Relief.*** Adequate analgesia is critical to reducing the workload of the heart. Epidural analgesia is commonly used to assist with pain relief.

***Intake and Output.*** Cross clamp above the renal arteries may predispose the renal bed to injury and acute renal failure. Intake and output should be monitored hourly in the first 24 hours after aortic surgery. The patient should be monitored closely for mobilization of fluids in the initial postoperative period. Diuretics may be used to assist in removal of excess fluids and in reduction of the risk of congestive heart failure.

***Temperature.*** Because of the length of open procedures and the exposure of the peritoneal cavity, hypothermia is usually present after surgery. Active rewarming techniques are vital after aortic procedures to return the patient to a normothermic state.

## Sympathectomy

Sympathectomy is performed to interrupt the sympathetic nerve chain and can be performed in the cervical, thoracic, or lumbar region. It may be performed with radiofrequency ablation, electrocautery, chemical injection, or dissection and excision of a segment of the sympathetic chain. Newer techniques used for sympathectomy include the use of laparoscopic and thoracoscopic instruments to allow for minimally invasive surgical options. The procedure is performed to increase blood flow by reducing sympathetic tone in the skin and subcutaneous tissue. Results have been mixed. Some patients obtain benefit; others receive little to no benefit. In arterial occlusive disease, pain relief is one indication for sympathectomy. The procedure may be useful in improving rest pain but does not usually provide sufficient blood flow to heal an ulcer because no increase in muscle circulation exists. The relief of pain is also believed to be accomplished by interruption of the afferent sensory nerve fibers in the sympathetic chain. A dry dressing is placed over the surgical site. Mild analgesics are usually sufficient to manage pain.

***Cervical and Thoracic.*** Sympathectomy in this region may be used to treat upper extremity conditions, such as Raynaud's phenomenon (hyperactive response to cold exposure or emotional stress) and hyperhidrosis (excessive sweating of the hands, axilla, or face). It involves excision of the lower portion of the stellate ganglion and T2 and T3 ganglion. The primary complication is Horner's syndrome, which results in ptosis and miosis with decreased sweat production of the side of the face. Other complications include phrenic nerve damage with paralysis of the hemidiaphragm, pneumothorax, bleeding, and impaired functioning of the hand muscles as a result of injury to the first thoracic nerve.

***Lumbar.*** Lumbar sympathectomy most often involves the ganglion from L2 to L4. L1 may also be involved. Areas of the lower extremity affected include the leg below mid thigh, including the foot (L2, L3) and the buttocks, thigh, and parts of the leg (L1). Complications may include damage to the vena cava or ureter, paralytic ileus, and postsympathectomy neuralgia. Endoscopic procedures may involve injury to the bowel from the trocar, bleeding from injury to blood vessels, or emboli to lower extremities from retraction of the aorta.

## Amputation
The leading causes of amputation are diabetes and peripheral arterial disease. Although amputation is often seen as a failure of medical and surgical management of disease, this procedure is the critical beginning for rehabilitation and is essential to maximizing the status of the patient

| Box 36-5   Types of Amputations |
| --- |
| Toe amputation (ray amputations) |
| Transmetatarsal (incision made across the center of the metatarsal bone) |
| Transtibial (below knee) |
| Transfemoral (above knee) |
| Hip disarticulation |

and enhancing quality of life. Amputations may be done at many levels depending on the patient's level of disease, infectious processes, joint function, and blood supply. Types of amputations are listed in Box 36-5. The more tissue preserved, the higher the functioning of the patient and the lower the morbidity and mortality rate.

***Postoperative Care.*** Immediately after the procedure, the patient is positioned supine with the head of the bed elevated. The limb may be elevated to assist with edema control and pain management. Adequate analgesia is critical. Initial pain is from the surgical incision and postoperative edema. Epidural analgesia may be used to assist with pain relief. Some pain may also be related to phantom limb sensations that may require long-term pain management. Dressings and surgical sites should be assessed for signs of bleeding or hematoma and kept clean and dry. Patients who undergo amputation may also have multiple comorbidities that require close observation of cardiopulmonary and renal status.

## Venous Surgical Procedures
Venous disease is more complex and is not as amenable to surgical treatment as is arterial disease. Venous insufficiency occurs when valves within the veins of the lower extremities become incompetent, leading to an increase in the venous pressure in the lower extremities. This condition may develop as a result of venous obstruction as from DVT, primary valvular incompetence, or failure of the calf muscle pump. Varicose veins often develop as a result of chronic venous insufficiency. Traditional procedures for the treatment of venous disease include high ligation of the greater saphenous vein with stab avulsion, stripping of the vein, and perforator vein ligation. These procedures may be performed alone or in combination with each other. They are typically performed in the operating room. Advances in the treatment of venous disease have added procedures that include liquid and foam sclerotherapy, ambulatory phlebectomy, radiofrequency closure, and

endovascular laser. These procedures are usually performed in an outpatient setting and may be done in the physician's office. Many patients undergo more than one type of procedure because of the complexity of the venous disease.

Ligation of the greater saphenous vein is performed to limit pressure on the distal saphenous vein to decrease the risk of further incompetence and distal varices. Ligation is performed at the level of the saphenofemoral junction; the vein may then be removed through stripping of the vein from the groin to the knee or to the ankle if the distal portion of the vein is involved. Individual varicose veins may be treated with stab avulsion, a technique in which individual varicose veins are removed through tiny incisions at the point of valvular reflux. Complications include wound infection, DVT, nerve injury that results in numbness in the lateral foot, and hematoma formation.

Perforator vein ligation is performed to interrupt incompetent perforator veins and may be performed as an open procedure or with a minimally invasive endoscopic technique. Perforator veins serve to channel blood from the superficial to the deep veins and may become incompetent, leading to reflux of blood into the superficial veins. Interruption of these incompetent perforators decreases the pressure in the superficial system and may be performed in conjunction with other procedures. Many patients with incompetent perforator veins also have ulcers in the lower extremities. This procedure may enhance wound healing as a result of the decreased venous pressure over the gaitor area where most venous ulcers are located.

Sclerotherapy is most commonly used for the treatment of veins less than 4 mm in diameter. A sclerosing agent is injected directly into the vein, which causes the vessel to swell and seal itself. This action prevents blood from reentering the vessel. Foam sclerotherapy has advantages over traditional sclerotherapy in that it has fewer side effects, requires fewer treatments, and usually yields better results. This technique involves the mixing of oxygen into the sclerosant to produce the foam. The foam forces blood from the vein, and as the oxygen bubbles dissolve, the vein deflates. Agents commonly used include hypertonic saline solution, sodium tetradecyl sulfate, and polyiodinated iodine. Associated complications include allergic reaction, intraarterial injection, multiple needle punctures, pigment discoloration, hematoma, and ulceration.

Ambulatory phlebectomy is a technique that is performed with tumescent anesthesia, which is produced by diluting lidocaine. It is performed with a phlebectomy hook, and large varicosities are removed through small incisions that do not require suturing. This procedure is preferred in more tortuous vessels. Complications include excessive hemorrhage, superficial hematoma, blisters, hyperpigmentation, nerve injury, scarring, contact dermatitis, and superficial phlebitis.

Radiofrequency (RF) closure of varicose veins can be performed with local or tumescent anesthesia and involves the use of RF energy through an endovenous electrode that causes controlled heating of the vessel. This action produces collapse of the vessel from heat-induced vasospasm and collagen shrinkage as the electrode is slowly withdrawn from the vessel. This procedure may not be used if thrombus exists in the vein segment to be treated. Complications associated with this procedure include skin burns, phlebitis, vessel perforation, thrombosis, pulmonary embolism, hematoma, infection, and paresthesias.

Endovenous laser therapy uses laser energy with an electrode and is painless and bloodless and shorter in length of procedure than is RF. No scarring and a shorter recovery period are seen with this procedure. The shorter exposure time with the electrode minimizes collateral damage. Rather than shrinking the vessel wall, this procedure leads to thrombotic occlusion from heating of the blood components and thermal damage to the endothelium. Complications with this technique are much lower than with RF. Less postoperative pain and less risk of DVT are seen.

***Postprocedure Care.*** After venous procedures, most patients are placed in a compression dressing with elastic bandage. Standard postanesthesia care for patients who undergo general anesthesia is used. The dressings should be assessed for signs of bleeding. Circulation should be assessed to ensure adequate blood flow and to be certain that the elastic bandages are not wrapped too tightly. Elevation of the extremities may be used to assist in the management of edema. Ambulation is encouraged as soon as possible after surgery.

## Vena Caval Filters

Inferior vena caval (IVC) filters are placed to prevent PE, which is a life-threatening complication of DVT. Indications for IVC filter placement are listed in Box 36-6. This procedure may be performed percutaneously in the operating room or in the radiology suite with fluoroscopy and local anesthesia. Traditionally, these filters were placed permanently. A new generation of devices now allows some devices to be removed

## Box 36-6   Indications for IVC Filter

Anticoagulation therapy is contraindicated
Free-floating DVT/PE occurred during
   anticoagulation therapy
Pulmonary embolectomy has been performed
Major surgery needed after relatively recent DVT
Trauma
Paralysis, prolonged immobilization
History of DVT/PE
Advanced malignant disease

after the high risk period is over, usually 14 to 21 days, although some devices may remain reportedly for up to 3 months. Safe indwelling times are still under evaluation. Placement of an IVC filter does not eliminate the need for concurrent means of prophylaxis for thromboembolic events. Complications of filter placement include perforation of the vena cava with retroperitoneal bleeding, migration of the filter, and improper deployment of the filter. Occlusion of the vena cava as a result of a large embolus is also a possibility.

## SUMMARY

The patient for vascular surgery presents many challenges to the perianesthesia nurse. Most patients have multiple comorbidities that require extensive preparation before surgery and critical thinking to prevent complications after surgery. Improved medications and technology have enabled these patients to survive longer with higher quality of life than ever before. The perianesthesia nurse plays a vital role in the care and survival of these patients.

## BIBLIOGRAPHY

Barrett B, Parfrey P: Preventing nephropathy induced by contrast medium, *N Eng J Med* 354(4):379-386, 2006.

Bozkurt A, Besirli K, Koksal C, et al: Surgical treatment of Buerger's disease, *Vasc* 12(3):192-197, 2004.

Burton K, Lindsay T: Assessment of short-term outcomes for protected carotid angioplasty with stents using recent evidence, *J Vasc Surg* 42(6):1094-1100, 2005.

Bush R, Kougias P, Guerrero M, et al: A comparison of carotid artery stenting with neuroprotection versus carotid endarterectomy under local anesthesia, *Am J Surg* 190:696-700, 2005.

Comerota A: Retrievable IVC filters: a decision matrix for appropriate utilization, *Pers Vasc Surg Endovasc Ther* 18:11-18, 2006.

Coventry B, Walsh J: Cutaneous innervation in man before and after lumbar sympathectomy: evidence for interruption of both sensory and vasomotor nerve fibres, *Anz J Surg* 73:14-18, 2003.

Creager M: *Atlas of vascular disease*, ed 2, Philadelphia, 2003, Current Medicine.

Davies M, Waldman D, Pearson T: Comprehensive endovascular therapy for femoropopliteal arterial atherosclerotic occlusive disease, *J Am Coll Surg* 201(2):275-296, 2005.

Dooner J, Lee S, Griswold W, et al: Laparoscopic aortic reconstruction: early experience, *Am J Surg* 191:691-695, 2006.

Fahey V: *Vascular nursing*, ed 4, Philadelphia, 2004, Saunders.

Fletcher L: Management of patient with intermittent claudication, *Nurs Stand* 20(31):59-65, 2006.

Goldenburg I, Matetzky S: Nephropathy induced by contrast media: pathogenesis, risk factors and preventive strategies, *CMAJ* 172(11):1461-1471, 2005.

Gordon P: Effects of diabetes on the vascular system: current research evidence and best practice recommendations, *J Vasc Nurs* 22(1):2-11, 2004.

Gramse C: Hyperperfusion syndrome after carotid endarterectomy, *J Vasc Nurs* 21(2):72-73, 2003.

Hirsch A, et al: ACC/AHA 2005 practice guidelines for the management of patients with peripheral arterial disease (lower extremity, renal, mesenteric, and abdominal aortic), *J Am Coll Card* 147:1-192, 2006.

Karthikeyan G, Bhargava G: Managing patients undergoing non-cardiac surgery: need to shift emphasis from risk stratification to risk modification, *Heart* 92:17-20, 2006.

Kertai M, Klein J, Bax J, et al: Predicting perioperative cardiac risk, *Prog Cardiovasc Dis* 47(4):240-257, 2005.

MacVittie B: *Vascular surgery*, St Louis, 1998, Mosby.

Mekako A, Bryce H, Heng M, et al: Combined endovenous laser therapy and ambulatory phlebectomy: refinement of a new technique, *Eur J Vasc Endovasc Surg* 32(6):725-729, 2006.

Moore W: *Vascular and endovascular surgery: a comprehensive review*, Philadelphia, 2006, Saunders.

Murphy M, Ghosh J, Khwaja N, et al: Upper dorsal endoscopic thoracic sympathectomy: a comparison of one-and two-port ablation techniques, *Eur J Cardiothor Surg* 30:223-227, 2006.

Niesen W, Rosenkranz M, Eckert B, et al: Hemodynamic changes of the cerebral circulation after stent-protected carotid angioplasty, *Am J Neuroradiol* 25:1162-1167, 2004.

Noble K: Stroke is no joke, *J Perianesth Nurse* 21:1, 2006.

Pearce W, Astleford P: What's new in vascular ultrasound, *Surg Clin North Am* 84:1113-1126, 2004.

Puggioni A, Kalra M, Carmo M, et al: Endovenous laser therapy and radiofrequency ablation of the great saphenous vein: analysis of early efficacy and complications, *J Vasc Surg* 42(3):488-493, 2005.

Rempher K: Cardiovascular sequelae of tobacco smoking, *Crit Care Nurs Clin North Am* 18:3-20, 2006.

Rothrock J: *Alexander's care of the patient in surgery*, ed 13, St Louis, 2007, Elsevier.

Rutherford R: Prophylactic indications for vena cava filters, *Semin Vasc Surg* 18:158-165, 2005.

Sadick N: Advances in the treatment of varicose veins: ambulatory phlebectomy, foam sclerotherapy, endovascular laser, and radiofrequency closure, *Dermatol Clin* 23:443-455, 2005.

Teruya T, Ballard J: New approaches for the treatment of varicose veins, *Surg Clin North Am* 84:1397-1417, 2004.

Treiman G: Subintimal angioplasty for infrainguinal occlusive disease, *Surg Clin North Am* 84:1365-1380, 2004.

Tsetis D, Belli A: Guidelines for stenting in infrainguinal arterial disease, *Cardiovasc Intervent Radiol* 27:198-203, 2004.

Van den berg J: A close look at closure devices, *J Cariovasc Surg* 47:285-295, 2006.

Wiesinger B, Beregi J, Oliva V, et al: PTFE-Covered self-expanding nitinol stents for the treatment of severe iliac and femoral artery stenoses and occlusions: final results from a prospective study, *J Endovasc Ther* 12:240-246, 2005.

NURSING CARE IN THE PACU

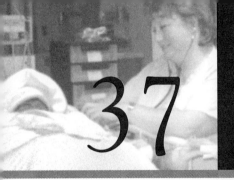

# 37

# CARE OF THE ORTHOPEDIC SURGICAL PATIENT

*Nancy M. Saufl, MS, RN, CPAN, CAPA*

Orthopedics (also spelled orthopaedics) is a specialty of health care that is concerned with the prevention and correction of disorders of the musculoskeletal system of the body. Orthopedic surgery is concerned with the treatment of the musculoskeletal system mainly with manipulative and operative methods. Perianesthesia nursing care of the orthopedic patient can be challenging and rigorous. In this highly technologic age, the care needed by the orthopedic patient requires both vigilant general perianesthesia care and a sound knowledge of orthopedic surgical procedures. Familiarity with orthopedic procedures and the anticipated patient outcomes helps the perianesthesia nurse provide high quality postoperative care. The perianesthesia nurse must possess astute nursing observation and assessment skills to ensure a low incidence rate of morbidity in this patient population. The psychosocial challenges are generally more evident within this group because, more commonly, the goal of the surgery is focused on restoring mobility and relieving pain and disability. The nurse must be sensitive to heightened anxieties and empathetic to individual needs.

## DEFINITIONS

**Anesthesia:** Local or systemic loss of sensation caused by trauma or injury.
**Arthrodesis:** Surgical fixation or fusion of a joint.
**Arthroplasty:** Reconstruction of joints for restoration of motion and stability.
**Arthroscopy:** Surgical examination of the interior of a joint with the insertion of an optic device (arthroscope) capable of providing an external view of an internal joint area.
**Arthrotomy:** Surgical exploration of a joint.
**Articulation:** The connection of bones at the joint.
**Cineplastic (Kineplastic) Amputation:** An amputation that includes a skin flap built into

a muscle; a portion of the prosthetic mechanism is activated by the muscle.
**Disarticulation:** Amputation at a joint.
**Diskectomy (Discectomy):** Removal of herniated or extruded fragments of an intervertebral disk.
**External Fixators:** Equipment used in the management of open fractures with soft-tissue damage (provides stabilization for the fracture while it permits treatment of soft-tissue damage).
**Fasciotomy:** Surgical separation of the fascia (a fibrous membrane that covers, supports, or separates the muscles) for relief of muscle constriction or reduction of fascia contracture.
**Harrington Rods:** Equipment used in spinal fixation for scoliosis and for some spinal fractures.
**Hemiarthroplasty:** Replacement of the femoral head with a prosthesis.
**Internal Fixation:** The stabilization of a reduced fracture with the use of metal screws, plates, nails, and pins.
**Joint Replacement:** The substitution of joint surfaces with metal or plastic materials.
**Laminectomy:** Removal of the lamina for exposure of the neural elements in the spinal canal or relief of constriction.
**Lordosis:** Abnormal anterior convexity of the lower part of the back.
**Luque Rods:** Spinal fixation that applies transverse force in treatment of scoliosis.
**Meniscectomy:** Surgical removal of the damaged knee joint fibrocartilage.
**Open Reduction:** The reduction and alignment of a fracture through surgical dissection and exposure of the fracture.
**Osteoporosis:** Diminished amount of calcium in the bone.
**Osteotomy:** Surgical cutting of the bone.
**Paresthesia:** Numbness and a tingling sensation.
**Scoliosis:** Lateral curvature of the spine.
**Sequestrectomy:** Surgical removal of necrotic bone.
**Spinal Fusion:** A fusion of the cervical, thoracic, or lumbar region of the spine with an

iliac or other bone graft that primarily fuses the laminae and sometimes the joints, most often through the posterior approach.

**Syme's Amputation:** Modified ankle disarticulation (below-the-ankle) amputation of the foot.

**Volkmann's Contracture:** The final state of unrelieved forearm compartment syndrome; contractures of tendons to wrist and hand.

## GENERAL PERIANESTHESIA CARE

Specific nursing care related to the patient for orthopedic surgery that begins in the postanesthesia care unit (PACU) includes positioning, neurovascular assessment, care of immobilization devices, wound care, range-of-motion exercises, and observation for complications.

### Positioning

After the initial assessment of the patient is made, attention is turned to positioning. Proper body alignment is important for all these patients and requires a sound knowledge of operative procedure and body mechanics. Each surgeon generally has specific directives for positioning, but general guidelines apply to all patients. The goal is optimal comfort and safety for the operated limb. The upper extremities should be held close to the body; elevation should be achieved without undue pressure on the elbow or shoulder. The lower extremities are in a neutral position, with support provided for the entire length, and heels are off the bed.

Elevation of operative limbs is usually indicated to increase venous return, reduce swelling, and promote comfort. In elevation of a hand or arm, the hand must be higher than the heart and no pressure should be placed on the elbow. This position can be achieved with the use of a stockinette device for suspension on an intravenous (IV) pole. The stockinette is measured from the elbow to approximately 12 inches beyond the fingertips; a piece is cut double this length. That piece is then folded in half, with the elbow resting in the fold. With safety pins, the sides are closed around the limb to form a tube, while ensuring that the fingers are exposed (for assessment of neurovascular status). With the excess material, a knot is tied and suspended from the IV pole. The elbow should be properly supported. If a pillow is used for elevation, the arm should be allowed slight flexion for maximum comfort and provide additional support for the elbow and shoulder.

Lower extremity elevation is most effective if the toes are above the heart. If the limb is not in an immobilization device, it is kept in a position of extension. This position is achieved by elevating the foot of the bed rather than with the use of pillows. The entire length of the limb should be supported if pillows are used and the heels kept off the bed.

Shoulder immobilization can be accomplished with a sling or shoulder immobilizer. An airplane splint may be applied for rotator cuff repairs. If a sling is used, the patient is instructed to keep the arm close to the chest with the wrist and elbow supported. The shoulder immobilizer requires special care to pad areas where skin contacts skin.

The patient with a hip pinning is positioned with proper body alignment, and the legs are in a proper neutral position. Care is given to avoid stress to the operative area with exaggerated flexion or rotation. A pillow is placed between the knees during turning to prevent adduction and rotation. For the patient with a total hip replacement, proper body alignment is achieved with placement of an abduction pillow between the knees at all times. Most important with these patients is to avoid flexion and adduction of the newly placed joint. If the abduction pillow straps are not in use, support of the lateral aspect of the leg is necessary to avoid external rotation and can be accomplished with the use of rolled towels or sheets.

The perianesthesia nurse should also be familiar with various types of orthopedic equipment that may be used and that can affect positioning. Often, patients with total knee replacement and those with more extensive knee arthrotomy are placed in a continuous passive motion (CPM) machine. The purpose of CPM is to enhance the healing process by providing CPM to the joint, thus increasing circulation and movement. Traction may also be used with various patients to immobilize and align a specific area. The perianesthesia nurse is not usually involved in setting up the traction but should be aware of some basic principles for maintenance: (1) the traction must be continuous; (2) the patient is centered in bed in good alignment to maintain the line of pull in line with the long bone; (3) weights should hang freely and not resting on the floor or bed; and (4) the pulley ropes should be in alignment and free of knots. One type of traction is depicted in Fig. 37-1.

### Neurovascular Assessment

Critical to the care of the patient for orthopedic surgery is assessment of the neurovascular status of the operative limb. Any alteration in blood flow to the extremity or nerve compression requires immediate intervention. Assessment is recommended every 30 minutes because

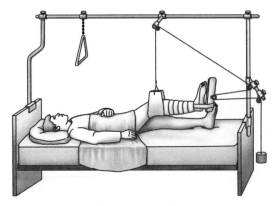

**Fig. 37-1**   Russell skin traction (single) with overhead frame and trapeze.

problems can occur as soon as 2 to 4 hours. Baseline neurovascular indicators should be noted in the admission nursing assessment. These can be used to establish any deleterious effects from the surgery and to avoid the masking of potential complications. Both the affected and unaffected limbs are assessed.

The hallmarks of neurovascular changes from constriction and circulatory embarrassment are pain, discoloration (skin that is pale or bluish), decreased mobility, coldness, diminished or absent pulses, altered capillary refilling, and swelling. Pain is common with patients for orthopedic surgery, and the approach to treatment must be individualized. Pain unrelieved with conventional methods, such as elevation and repositioning and the administration of opioids, must be further assessed. Color indicates circulatory compromise. Cyanosis suggests venous obstruction; pallor suggests arterial obstruction. Mobility is assessed by determining the range of motion of the fingers or toes and strongly indicates neural compromise. Fingers are flexed, extended, spread, and wiggled. Toes should be dorsiflexed, plantarflexed, and wiggled. An inability to move the fingers or toes, pain on extension of the hand or foot, or coldness of the extremity is indicative of ischemia. Sensation is described as normal, hypesthetic (dulled), paresthetic, or anesthetic. Alteration in sensation suggests nerve compression or circulatory compromise. Limb perfusion is further assessed with the presence of peripheral pulses and capillary refilling. Capillary refilling is assessed with compression of the nail bed, which causes blanching; when the compression is released, color briskly returns. Compromise delays the filling time. With the development of pulse oximetry, a more reliable method of perfusion assessment is available. With placement of the oximeter sensor on a finger or toe

of the affected limb, the pulsation is sensed and oxygen saturation displayed. This method is more reflective of perfusion than capillary refilling and is valuable when pulses cannot be assessed because of the presence of a cast or dressing.

### Care of Immobilization Devices (Cast Care)

Immediate assessment of the patient after orthopedic surgery in the PACU should include the type of immobilization device applied. The soft knee immobilizer should be checked for proper placement and closure and the surgical dressing checked for drainage. For care that involves traction, refer to the previous section on positioning in this chapter.

The cast is a rigid immobilization device molded to the contours of the part to which it is applied. The cast has a dual purpose: immobilization in a specific position and provision of uniform pressure on the encased soft tissue. The cast should be inspected for visibility of fingers and toes for neurovascular assessment. If the cast is bivalved, the edges should be inspected for roughness to avoid discomfort and potential skin breakdown. When the patient arrives in the PACU, the cast is probably still wet, and special care must be taken to prevent indentations. A wet cast must be handled carefully with the palms of the hand to avoid pressure from fingertips. The cast should be supported on a pillow, and hard flat surfaces should be avoided. Improper handling and flat surfaces can cause indentations that may lead to the development of pressure sores. More frequently, a fiberglass cast is applied with quicker drying properties, but the same general principles still apply. Any drainage noted on the cast should be circled, and the time should be noted. This documentation can provide a guide for postoperative blood and fluid loss and can alert the nurse if the drainage appears to be excessive. Note that orthopedic wounds tend to ooze and may bleed more than other surgical wounds.

### Wound Care

All surgical dressings should be checked for drainage and closure. Patients with orthopedic surgery are highly susceptible to infection; therefore, strict asepsis in changing dressings or handling drains is required. Drains may be placed in the wound to minimize blood accumulation and the possibility of infection. Care must be taken to attend these drains to maintain suction.

A patient with total joint replacement may commonly have a large amount of blood loss in the immediate postoperative period. This loss can be as great as 250 to 300 mL in the first hour. The retrieval of this blood for reinfusion (autotransfusion), when coupled with preoperative autologous blood donation, has substantially reduced the need for homologous transfusions. Autotransfusion is accomplished with the use of self-contained disposable systems that are designed for easy setup and safe use.

### Range-of-motion Exercises

Range-of-motion exercises can be initiated in the PACU as soon as the patient is alert and cooperative. Flexion, extension, and rotation of joints distal to the operative area assist in stimulating circulation and strengthening muscles. Prevention of venous stasis decreases the incidence rate of thromboembolism, and early movement of joints promotes healing and stabilization.

### Observation for Complications

Postoperative complications for the patient after orthopedic surgery include deep vein thrombosis, pulmonary embolism, fat embolism syndrome, compartment syndrome, shock, and urinary retention.

*Deep Vein Thrombosis.* Thrombosis is the formation of a blood clot associated with three conditions outlined by Virchow in 1846: venous stasis, altered clotting mechanism, and altered vessel wall integrity. Immobilization and the insult of the surgical procedure place the orthopedic patient at high risk. Immobilization impairs the leg muscle action needed to move the blood sufficiently, and the surgical procedure injures vessel walls that activate and alter clotting mechanisms. An inflammation process begins within the vessel wall and leads to deep vein thrombosis. The patient usually has pain and tenderness. Signs include swelling and sometimes localized redness. Palpation of the calf reveals firmness or tension of the muscle. A positive Homans' sign may be seen.

Venous complications can usually be prevented with early initiation of exercise, but if they occur, exercise should cease; anticoagulant therapy is usually initiated. Anticoagulant therapy is routinely begun after surgery on patients at higher risk, such as those with total joint replacements. Antiembolism stockings or pneumatic hose should be used on all patients who will not be ambulatory, who have hip or lower extremity injury, who are elderly, or who have a history of thrombophlebitis. These stockings provide compression that enhances venous flow rates. The pneumatic stockings (alternating–pressure gradient stockings) automatically provide a consistent compression-decompression system. These stockings are growing in popularity and should be considered for patients at higher risk from total hip replacement and spinal surgery.

*Pulmonary Embolism.* The most serious sequela of deep vein thrombosis is pulmonary embolism. If the patient has been inactive and movement has been restricted before surgery, the risk of clot formation is greatly enhanced. Embolization of this clot leads to pulmonary embolism. The severity of symptoms depends on the size and number of clots. Symptoms range from none if the clot is small to a myriad that may include, with increasing severity, anxiety, dyspnea, tachypnea, hemoptysis, substernal pain, stabbing pleuritic pain, tachycardia, cough, signs and symptoms of cerebral ischemia, fever, elevated sedimentation rate, shock, and sudden death. Immediate nursing care involves administration of oxygen and relief of pain. Medications usually include heparin-bolus doses with continuous infusion or other antithrombolytic agents.

*Fat Embolism Syndrome.* Fat embolism syndrome is a condition that leads to respiratory insufficiency and is related to multiple fractures, especially of the long bones. It is caused by fat droplets released into the circulation from the bone marrow and local tissue trauma. Similar to pulmonary embolism, these fat globules migrate to the lungs, where they cause occlusions. The fat globules break down into acids and irritate vascular walls and cause extrusion of fluids into the alveoli. The lung involvement alters ventilation and leads to hypoxemia. Fat embolism syndrome may lead to adult respiratory distress syndrome. The symptoms related to lung involvement include tachypnea, tachycardia, anxiety, chest discomfort, petechiae over the chest, $PO_2$ less than 60 mm Hg, fever, pallor, and confusion. Brain involvement is evidenced by agitation, confusion, delirium, and coma. Immediate nursing care of this sometimes-fatal complication includes administering oxygen, keeping the patient quiet, and preventing motion at the fracture site.

*Compartment Syndrome.* Compartment syndrome is a condition in which increased pressure within a muscle compartment causes circulatory compromise and leads to tissue necrosis and diminished function of the limb. Left undetected, the compression may cause permanent damage to the extremity. The compartment is described as a fascial sheath that encloses bone, muscle, nerves, blood vessels, and soft tissue. The two main causes of increased pressure to this space are: (1) constriction from the outside, such as a cast or bandage that decreases the size of the compartment; or (2) increased pressure within the compartment, such as swelling. The hallmark symptoms of compartment syndrome include intense pain unrelieved with conventional methods, paresthesia, and sharp pain on passive stretching of the middle finger of the affected arm or the large toe of the affected leg. Progressive symptoms include decreased strength, decreased sensation (numbness and tingling), and decreased capillary refilling; peripheral pulses are not generally compromised. Immediate intervention includes elevation of the extremity, application of ice, and release of restrictive dressings. Fasciotomy may be required within 4 to 6 hours of onset of symptoms if conservative measures are unsuccessful.

**Shock.** Because of the highly vascular composition of bone and secondary injury to the soft tissue, hemorrhage is always a potential risk in patients after trauma and orthopedic surgery. Vigilant observation of the operative area and blood pressure and pulse alerts the perianesthesia nurse to any impending danger. Immediate nursing measures include keeping the patient warm and flat in bed, monitoring vital signs, and replacing fluid volume. The surgeon is notified immediately, and more definitive treatment is initiated (see Chapter 54, Care of the Shock Trauma Patient).

**Urinary Retention.** Urinary retention refers to the inability to void despite the urge or desire. This condition may occur in adult patients on whom hip or back surgery has been performed. The retention may be the result of spinal anesthesia or possibly the inability to void in the supine position. These patients should be monitored for bladder distention and pain in the lower abdomen. The surgeon should be notified if distention occurs or if the patient is unable to void within 8 hours after the surgery is completed.

## PERIANESTHESIA CARE AFTER HAND SURGERY

The patient with hand surgery usually is admitted to the PACU with a large bulky dressing in place on the hand and forearm. An elastic bandage for application of pressure may also be in place outside the dressing. The hand should be elevated above the level of the heart at all times for prevention of edema and hemorrhage. The hand may be placed on pillows on the chest of the patient or suspended from the bed frame or IV pole with stockinette. The elbow should be supported with a pillow. Support under the shoulder and wrist aids in decreasing pressure to the elbow. If a drain is present, it should be checked to ensure that it is activated, or it

may be connected to a vacuum blood tube. The drain is placed to minimize the bleeding into the wound and to reduce the possibility of infection. Drains should be checked every 1 or 2 hours to maintain a proper vacuum, and the output should be recorded on the intake and output records. The tips of the fingers should be visible, and the neurovascular status should be assessed every 30 minutes for signs of change. Hand surgery is often done with the use of an axillary block, and sensation and movement may not fully return for several hours after surgery. Baseline neurovascular indicators should be noted in the admission nursing assessment and can be used to establish any deleterious effects from the surgery.

## PERIANESTHESIA CARE AFTER ARM AND FOREARM SURGERY

Postanesthesia care of the patient who is recovering from arm and forearm surgery centers on elevating the extremity, observing for excessive bleeding, and monitoring for neurovascular changes. The radial pulse should be taken every 30 minutes and compared with that of the unaffected limb. If pulses cannot be assessed because of a dressing or cast, the pulse oximeter sensor should be placed on a finger of the affected arm; the pulsation reflects perfusion to the limb. Any decrease in intensity of the pulse or in bilateral strength of the hand, any excessive bleeding, and any changes in neurovascular status should be reported to the surgeon. Symptoms of excessive pain, weakness, or decreased sensation, especially on passive extension of the fingers, usually indicate compartment syndrome, which constitutes an orthopedic emergency. Patients should be encouraged to perform active range-of-motion exercises with the wrists and hands.

## PERIANESTHESIA CARE AFTER SHOULDER SURGERY

Shoulder surgery may include arthroscopy, arthrotomy, or total shoulder joint replacement. The patient is admitted to the PACU with a bulky pressure dressing in place along with a sling-style shoulder immobilizer. The immobilizer should not interfere with chest expansion because this inhibits adequate respiratory exchange. The surgical dressing should be inspected for bleeding because the shoulder is a vascular area in which hemorrhage is difficult to manage.

Inspection should include checking to see whether any skin surface is in contact with another. If this situation occurs, a protective pad should be inserted between the two skin surfaces. The radial pulse should be monitored because flexion of the arm in the immobilizer can reduce blood flow to the hand. The immobilizer should be checked for areas that might be causing pressure to the shoulder and arm. The elbow and wrist should be supported to prevent any undue pressure to the ulnar and radial nerves. Again, neurovascular observations are a critical part of the postanesthesia assessment of these patients. The patient should be encouraged to perform active range-of-motion exercises with that hand.

## PERIANESTHESIA CARE AFTER HIP OR FEMORAL SURGERY

Hip replacement surgery removes the arthritic ball of the upper femur and the damaged cartilage from the hip socket. The ball is replaced with a metal or ceramic ball that is solidly fixed to a stem inserted into the femur. The socket is replaced with a metal cup, which is fixed to the acetabulum, or socket. The implants are designed to create a new smoothly functioning joint that prevents painful bone-on-bone contact. A minimally invasive surgical technique is available for hip replacement. The minimally invasive technique reduces the incision from 6 to 8 inches to 3 to 4 inches and reduces the extent of soft tissue disruption in the hip. The decreased trauma to the muscles, ligaments, and tendons results in less postoperative pain. Other advantages of the minimally invasive hip replacement include shorter hospital stays, earlier mobilization, quicker rehabilitation, less blood loss, and a faster return to productivity and normal activities.

When the patient who has had hip or femoral surgery is admitted to the PACU, nursing assessment should include pulmonary and neurovascular function, body alignment, and the amount and type of bleeding from the surgical incision. Because of long bone trauma and the often advanced age of this group of patients, these patients represent the highest risk group for postoperative orthopedic complications.

Preexisting medical conditions and the effects of anesthetic agents may compromise respiratory function. Coughing and deep breathing, sustained maximal inspirations, and position changes, when possible, are of utmost importance. The incentive spirometer can be used to facilitate good lung expansion. Any change in pulmonary dynamics should be reported to the anesthesia provider.

Because swelling at the operative site can reduce blood flow to the feet, neurologic signs along with pulses of the affected foot should be monitored and compared with those of the unaffected foot. The dorsalis pedis pulse can be palpated on the dorsum of the foot and lateral to the extensor tendon of the great toe. The posterior tibial pulse can be palpated just behind and slightly below the medial malleolus of the ankle. The extremity is elevated where indicated.

The body should be aligned as normally as possible. The legs and feet are maintained in a neutral position, elevated as indicated, and supported to avoid rotations of and pressure on the heels. Traction may be applied and has been discussed previously in this chapter. Any patient with lower limbs wrapped in elastic bandages or strapped as in an abductor pillow should be observed for peroneal nerve compression. Compression may occur where the peroneal nerve crosses the knee at the head of the fibula. Decreased sensation over the dorsum of the foot, tingling, extremity weakness, and an inability to bring the foot up are signs indicative of this injury, which is a common cause of foot drop. The patient should be encouraged to perform active range-of-motion exercises of the ankle to enhance venous return.

The patient with total hip replacement has an abduction pillow placed between the knees at all times. This position must be maintained to avoid adduction and internal rotation of the newly placed joint. The patient should not be allowed to flex the hips at a greater than 30-degree to 40-degree angle or to adduct the leg of the affected side. The muscle groups are weakened, and dislocation of the joint is a potential risk. If turning is necessary, the patient may be turned to the unoperated side no more than 45 degrees, with hip abduction maintained and total leg support provided. The head of the bed may be elevated no more than 45 degrees.

An autotransfusion system or other drain with suction, such as a Hemovac, is usually inserted at the operative site to facilitate the removal of blood; the color and amount should be inspected frequently. Autotransfusion is a technique that salvages red blood cells lost by the patient at the wound site and reinfuses that blood into the same patient. Autotransfusion may be used if the patient is expected to lose enough blood during the perioperative period to require transfusion and can reduce or eliminate the need for allogeneic transfusion. The perianesthesia nurse should know how to operate any device that is used for drainage or autotransfusion and the hospital policies and procedures that apply (Fig. 37-2).

If the color of the drainage is bright red or is more than 300 mL in an 8-hour period, the surgeon should be notified. The patient with total

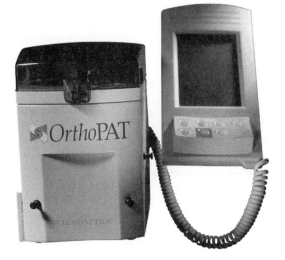

**Fig. 37-2** Photograph of Orthopat orthopedic perioperative autotransfusion system (Haemonetics Corporation). *(Used with permission of Haemonetics Corporation.)*

hip replacement may have a large blood loss, which becomes a problem if the loss is sustained or if it increases.

## PERIANESTHESIA CARE AFTER KNEE SURGERY

Total knee replacement (arthroplasty) is a surgical procedure to replace the worn surfaces of the knee. Knee replacement implants include a metal alloy on the bottom of the femur and polyethylene (plastic) on the top of the tibia and underneath the kneecap. The implant is designed to create a new smoothly functioning joint that prevents painful bone-on-bone contact. Surgeons may elect to replace all or part of the knee, depending on the patient's condition and the extent of the arthritis affecting the knee. In patients with only limited knee arthritis, surgeons may choose to perform a unicompartmental or partial knee replacement. Unlike total knee replacement that involves removal of all the knee joint surfaces, a unicompartmental knee replacement replaces only one side of the knee joint. Usually knee osteoarthritis occurs first in the medial compartment of the knee because this side of the knee bears the most weight. If the knee is otherwise healthy, a unicompartmental approach allows the outer compartment and the ligaments to remain intact, which may help the joint bend better and function more naturally. The partial knee replacement is done through a small incision, with minimal trauma to surrounding tissue. Many patients leave the hospital on the same day of or on the day after the surgery. Patients also have less postoperative pain, earlier

mobilization, and less blood loss, which results in a faster return to productivity.

Postanesthesia care of the patient who has had surgery of the knee involves observation for complications and proper knee positioning. The surgical procedure may involve repair of ligaments and tendons or removal of all or of a portion of the meniscal cartilage. Patients may undergo a total knee replacement when degenerative processes have caused the knee joint to become nonfunctional.

The knee joint is formed by the articulation of rounded condyles of the femur with shallow depressions in the tibia, also called condyles. At the periphery of the articulation between the femoral and tibial condyles are the wedge-shaped meniscal cartilages that function primarily in joint lubrication and in cushioning. Located within the joint capsules, the medial and lateral cruciate ligaments are primarily responsible for lateral stability, and the anterior and posterior cruciate ligaments within the intercondylar notch are primarily responsible for anteroposterior stability. Externally, the joint is strengthened by the tendons of the quadriceps muscle, which is stabilized by the patella.

After knee surgery, the patient arrives in the PACU with a bulky compression dressing in place. Ice over the surgical site may be ordered to provide comfort and minimize swelling. The leg should be elevated and positioned in full extension, which can be facilitated by elevation at the ankle so that maximum extension of the leg can be accomplished. Pressure to the heel needs to be avoided. An effective means of providing compression and cold is the use of the CryoCuff (Fig. 37-3). The CryoCuff is a large vinyl bladder that fits over the knee. The cuff, anchored by Velcro straps to the leg, is then filled with ice water via a portable canister. When filled, safe cooling and compression are provided to the operative area.

Assessments of neurovascular status should be performed every 30 minutes. Any decrease in sensation over the dorsum of the foot should be noted because this can represent compression of the peroneal nerve where it crosses the fibula at the knee. The surgeon should be notified if any neurologic or circulatory change is found because early detection and correction prevent permanent nerve deficit or ischemic muscular injury. If the patient received a spinal anesthetic, the nurse cannot initially assess the patient's motor function.

These patients should be encouraged to flex, extend, and rotate the ankles as soon as possible to improve circulation. Knee-strengthening exercises may also be started in the PACU.

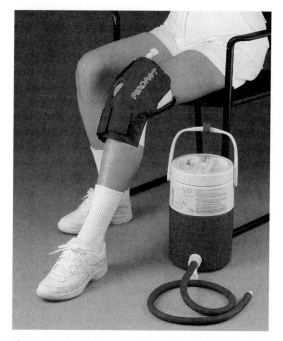

**Fig. 37-3**   CryoCuff system (Aircast, Summit, NJ). (*Courtesy of Aircast, Summit, NJ.*)

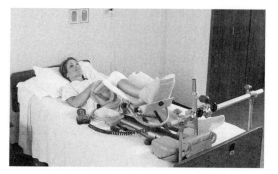

**Fig. 37-4**   OptiFlex Knee CPM with bed mount (Chattanooga Group, Inc, Hixson, TN). (*Courtesy Chattanooga Group, Inc, Hixson, TN.*)

Isometric exercises and quadriceps sets aid in healing the muscle and providing stability to the joint. Isometrics involve a 6-second contraction of the entire leg followed by relaxation. The quadriceps sets require contraction of the quadriceps muscle while pressing the knee to the bed for 5 to 10 seconds and then relaxation.

Arthroscopic examination of the knee is done to facilitate minor repairs and the diagnosis of more extensive damage to the knee; in general, fewer postoperative complications occur because this procedure is less invasive. However, neurovascular assessment remains an important part of the postanesthesia care of these patients.

The patient with total knee replacement and the patient who has undergone extensive arthrotomy knee repair are sometimes placed in a continuous passive motion (CPM) machine (Fig. 37-4). This device provides a safe method of elevation, comfort, and continuous range-of-motion to the operative knee. The CPM promotes healing by increasing circulation and movement of the knee joint. The machine should be inspected to ensure proper positioning of the limb. The flexion and extension settings of the machine should be determined by the physician and are generally 0 to 30 degrees at slow speed initially.

Extensive knee procedures generally have large amounts of drainage. An autotransfusion device or Hemovac drain is present to facilitate removal of drainage from the wound. The Hemovac drain is emptied and reactivated as necessary. Drainage amounts of 250 to 300 mL in 1 to 2 hours are not uncommon. See the section on Hip Replacement Surgery for a discussion of autotransfusion.

## PERIANESTHESIA CARE AFTER FOOT SURGERY

The patient who has had a surgical procedure performed on the foot has either a cast or a bandage over the operative site. The amount and color of bleeding should be noted. Neurovascular signs should be monitored every 30 minutes. The extremity should be elevated above the level of the heart, with pillows supporting the entire length of the leg.

## PERIANESTHESIA CARE AFTER SPINAL SURGERY

Several types of spinal procedures exist. The important features of the postoperative assessment relate mostly to the surgical area of the spine. Patients who have had a cervical procedure should be monitored for neurologic signs of the upper extremities. Symptoms such as weakness and radiating pain should be reported to the surgeon. Patients in halo traction should be monitored for any deficiency in the sixth cranial (abducent) nerve. Any decrease in the lateral movement of the eye is indicative of injury to the abducent nerve.

If the surgical procedure involves C3, C4, or C5, respiratory movements should be monitored because the diaphragm muscle is innervated by the spinal outflow from these vertebrae. The patient with this nerve deficit has a lack of diaphragmatic excursion and shortness of breath and the use of intercostal and accessory muscles in breathing. If these symptoms appear, oxygen should be administered and assistance in ventilation may be necessary.

Patients who have had midthoracic or lower spinal surgery may have an ileus develop. This complication is signaled by abdominal distention, diminished or absent bowel sounds, and tympany on percussion of the abdomen. The usual treatment is to withhold oral food and fluids and to decompress the stomach with a nasogastric tube.

Patients who have had lumbar or sacral spinal surgery should be observed for loss of strength in the lower extremities and bladder distention. Bladder distention may be indicated by diaphoresis, hypertension, tachycardia, tachypnea, and a feeling of distress. If the patient has a catheter in place, it should be irrigated to remove any obstruction. If the patient has no urinary catheter and cannot urinate, the surgeon should be notified.

Patients with progressive curvature of the spine (scoliosis) may undergo a Harrington or Luque rod insertion for correction or stabilization of the spine. The procedure entails a spinal fusion followed by rod placement. The postanesthesia assessment entails those features included in the assessment of the patient after thoracic and lumbosacral spine surgery.

Patients who have surgery on the spine should also be observed for bleeding from the site of the operation. The patient should be turned from side to side to help reduce stasis of fluids in the lungs. The technique for turning the spinal patient is called log rolling. All parts of the patient's body should move in unison. To facilitate this action, a pillow is placed between the patient's knees and the knee opposite the side the patient is turned to should be flexed. Use of a draw sheet can also help to facilitate turning in one smooth motion. Pillows should be placed to support the length of the back and buttocks along with the pillow between the patient's knees. This method of turning the patient puts the least amount of pressure on the spine. With the advent of microdisk surgery, disturbance to the stability of the spine is minimal, and these patients are generally allowed activity as desired and often go home on the first postoperative day.

All spinal patients with restricted movement should have antiembolism or pneumatic stockings on, and ankle pumping and rotation should be encouraged to decrease the stasis of blood in the lower extremities. The patient should be encouraged to use the incentive spirometer every hour to reduce the stasis of fluids in the lungs. Neurovascular evaluation is performed every 30 minutes to assess any improvements or deficiencies. Pain is a relative experience for the patient after spinal surgery. In many instances, the relief from nerve compression pain is so dramatic that the operative site pain is minimized. In other instances, the pain from spinal fusion is often difficult to manage. As discussed previously in this chapter, the pain experience must be individualized and treated appropriately. The perianesthesia nurse's goal is to help the patient perceive the pain as something that can be controlled rather than a fearful unrelenting burden.

## PERIANESTHESIA CARE AFTER LIMB AMPUTATION

Patients who have had an amputation of the leg are admitted to the PACU with a dressing or a cast applied to the extremity. A cast is used to provide uniform pressure to the soft tissue, to control swelling, and to position the limb to avoid contracture. See cast care discussed previously in this chapter in the section on immobilization devices. To prevent hip contracture, elevation of the lower extremity with a soft compression dressing should be achieved by elevating the foot of the bed rather than using a pillow. The patient with an amputation of the arm usually has a bulky compression dressing in place. The dressing should be assessed for drainage. The extremity should be elevated, and ice may be applied to reduce postoperative edema and discomfort.

## POSTOPERATIVE PAIN MANAGEMENT FOR THE PATIENT AFTER ORTHOPEDIC SURGERY

Pain management for the orthopedic patient involves conventional pain protocols and may include the insertion of an epidural catheter or use of a patient-controlled (PCA) pump (see Chapter 31, Pain Management in the PACU). The PCA pump administers a predetermined intravenous dose of the prescribed pain medication. It can be set to allow a continuous infusion of analgesic and bolus administration when the patient finds it necessary. Nonopioid analgesics such as acetaminophen, aspirin, and nonsteroidal antiinflammatory drugs may also be used, with the possibility of gastrointestinal irritation, renal and hepatic toxic effects, and the inhibition of platelet aggregation kept in mind. Opioids such as hydromorphone, morphine, and fentanyl may be administered via intravenous drip, epidurally, or intrathecally to promote analgesia. Increasingly, orthopedic surgeons are using single-use systems that provide continuous

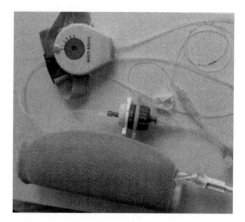

**Fig. 37-5** SmartInfuser Pain Pump.

delivery of local anesthetic through a small catheter inserted directly into the surgical site to decrease postoperative pain (Fig. 37-5). The catheter is secured at the operative site with the dressing and with tape. Often times, the patient is discharged home with this type of pain management. Also of note is the increased use of peripheral nerve blocks for postoperative pain management. These blocks are well tolerated by the patient and greatly increase patient satisfaction.

The perianesthesia nurse must collaborate with the surgeon and the anesthesia provider to determine an individualized plan of care to provide the patient with appropriate and effective pain management. In addition to pain medications, other comfort measures must be used (see the American Society of PeriAnesthesia Nurses [ASPAN] Pain and Comfort Guideline, available at www.aspan.org).

## SUMMARY

Postanesthesia care unit nurses are highly skilled to assess, plan, and care for patients as they recover from surgery and anesthesia. When caring for the patient after orthopedic surgery in the PACU, the patient must be provided with appropriate care related to the surgical treatment received for a specific musculoskeletal disorder. These procedures can vary from outpatient hand and foot surgeries to more major joint and spine surgeries. Regardless of the complexity of the surgery, the patient is susceptible to joint stiffness and skin breakdown from impaired physical mobility, neurovascular compromise from pressure on major blood vessels or nerves caused by compartmental edema or immobilization devices, infection of the surgical site, and general discomfort and pain. The PACU nurse

who has a basic understanding and knowledge of orthopedic procedures and associated nursing care is able to provide the patient with safe and efficient care in the immediate postoperative period.

## BIBLIOGRAPHY

Alspach JG: *Core curriculum for critical care nursing*, ed 6, St Louis, 2006, Saunders.

Altizer L: Compartment syndrome, *Orthopaedic Nurs* 23:391-396, 2004.

Altizer L: Neurovascular assessment, *Orthopaedic Nurs* 21(4):48-50, 2002.

American Society of Perianesthesia Nurses: *ASPAN pain and comfort guideline*, available at http://www.aspan.org/PDFfiles/pain&comfort.pdf, accessed March 2007.

Atlee J: *Complications in anesthesia*, ed 2, Philadelphia, 2007, Saunders.

Barash PG, Cullen BF, Stoelting RK: *Clinical anesthesia*, ed 5, Philadelphia, 2005, Lippincott Williams & Wilkins.

Biomet: *Information for patients and caregivers*, available at www.biomet.com, accessed March 2007.

Brunton L, Lazo J, Parker K: *Goodman and Gilman's the pharmacological basis of therapeutics*, ed 11, New York, 2005, McGraw-Hill Professional.

DeFazio-Quinn D, Schick L: *PeriAnesthesia nursing core curriculum*, St Louis, 2004, Saunders.

Fleisher LA: *Anesthesia and uncommon diseases*, ed 5, Philadelphia, 2006, Saunders.

Ganong W: *Review of medical physiology*, ed 21, New York, 2005, McGraw-Hill Professional.

Guyton AC, Hall JE: *Textbook of medical physiology*, ed 11, Philadelphia, 2006, Saunders.

Harvey CV: Complications, *Orthopaedic Nurs* 25:410-412, 2006.

Hohler SE: Looking into minimally invasive total hip arthroplasty, *OR Nurse* 1(1):32-37, 2007.

Katzung BG, editor: *Basic and clinical pharmacology*, ed 10, Los Altos, Calif, 2006, Lange McGraw Hill.

Lake C, Hines R, Blitt C: *Clinical monitoring: practical applications for anesthesia and critical care*, St Louis, 2001, Mosby.

Longnecker D, Murphy F: *Dripps/Eckenhoff/Vandam introduction to anesthesia*, ed 9, Philadelphia, 1997, Saunders.

McCaffery M, Pasero C: *Pain: clinical manual*, ed 2, St Louis, 1999, Mosby.

Medical Flow Systems: *Innovative infusion technologies for home therapies*, available at http://www.mfs-medical.com/generalpump.asp, 2007. Accessed 03-04-07.

Miller RD, editor: *Anesthesia*, ed 6, New York, 2005, Churchill Livingstone.

*Mosby's medical, nursing & allied health dictionary*, ed 6, St Louis, 2002, Mosby.

Mulroy MF: *Regional anesthesia: an illustrated procedural guide*, ed 3, Philadelphia, 2002, Lippincott, Williams & Wilkins.

Nagelhout J, Zaglaniczny K: *Nurse anesthesia*, ed 2, Philadelphia, 2001, Saunders.

Rothrock J: *Alexander's care of the patient in surgery*, ed 13, St Louis, 2007, Mosby.

Shugars RA, More RC: Arthroscopic hip surgery, *AORN J* 82(6):975-976, 978-984, 986-992, 2005.

Stoelting R, Hillier SC: *Pharmacology and physiology in anesthetic practice*, ed 4, Philadelphia, 2005, Lippincott Williams & Wilkins.

Stoelting RK, Miller RD: *Basics of anesthesia*, ed 5, New York, 2007, Churchill Livingstone.

Swank ML, Lehnert IE: Orthopedic roles in the OR for computer-assisted total knee arthroplasty, *AORN* 82(4):631-640, 2005.

Tetzlaff J: *Clinical orthopedic anesthesia*, Boston, 1995, Butterworth-Heinemann.

Townsend CM, Beauchamp RD, Evers BM, et al: *Sabiston textbook of surgery: the biological basis of modern surgical practice*, ed 17, Philadelphia, 2004, Saunders.

Warner C: The use of the orthopaedic perioperative autotransfusion (OrthoPAT$^{TM}$) system in total joint replacement surgery, *Orthopaedic Nurs* 20(6):29-32, 2001.

# 38

# CARE OF THE NEUROSURGICAL PATIENT

*Cecil B. Drain, PhD, RN, CRNA, FAAN, FASAHP*

As shown in Chapter 10, the physiology of the nervous system is extremely complex. Because of the specific type of care needed in the perioperative period, many neurologic care units have emerged. Also, special education on the physiology, pharmacology, and nursing care is necessary to facilitate appropriate outcomes for the neurosurgical patient. Because the postanesthesia care unit (PACU) is able to render very specialized nursing care to these patients, most facilities require that these patients first recover from anesthesia in the PACU before return to the neurologic care unit or a routine care unit. Neurosurgical patients, or those with underlying neurologic conditions, present a challenge to the perianesthesia nurse. In addition to familiarity with routine perianesthesia care, the nurse must have a basic understanding of the nervous system and pathologic conditions or injuries that may affect this system and must be able to translate this knowledge into the skills necessary to assess, provide care for, and evaluate the neurosurgical patient. This chapter is divided into two sections: cranial surgery and spinal surgery. The division is made solely for this discussion because some aspects of care related to each topic are common to both areas. In addition, disease or injury in any portion of the nervous system may also affect other organs and systems of the body. In caring for the neurosurgical patient, the nurse must consider each structure of the nervous system (see Chapter 10) as it relates to the individual as a whole.

## DEFINITIONS

**Atony:** Decreased or absent muscle tone.

**Babinski's Reflex:** A reflex that is normal in newborns but abnormal in adults; in adults, it indicates a lesion in the pyramidal tract. The reflex is elicited with firm stroking of the lateral aspect of the sole of the foot, which normally elicits dorsiflexion of the big toe with extension and fanning of the other toes.

**Baroreceptor:** A sensory nerve cell aggregate present in the wall of a blood vessel that is stimulated by changes in blood pressure.

**Compliance:** The ability of the brain to yield when a pressure or force is applied.

**Cranial Surgery:** Surgery classified by infratentorial and supratentorial location.

**Craniectomy:** Removal of a portion of the skull without a replacement.

**Cranioplasty:** Repair of the skull with replacement of a part of the cranium with a synthetic material.

**Craniotomy:** A surgical opening of the skull.

**Crepitus:** A crackling sound produced by the rubbing together of fractured bone fragments or by the presence of subcutaneous emphysema.

**Cushing's Reflex:** An elevated systolic blood pressure, bradycardia, and widening pulse pressure.

**Decompensation:** The inability of the heart to maintain adequate circulation because of an impairment in brain integrity.

**Diabetes Insipidus:** A metabolic disorder caused by injury or disease of the posterior lobe of the pituitary gland (the hypophysis).

**Focal Deficit:** Any sign or symptom that indicates a specific or localized area of pathologic alteration.

**Infratentorial:** The area below the tentorium that includes the brain stem, cerebellum, and posterior fossa. This approach is used for lesions in the brain stem and cerebellum region.

**Laminectomy:** Excision of the posterior arch of a vertebra to allow excision of a herniated nucleus pulposus.

**Phrenic Nucleus:** A group of nerve cells located in the spinal cord between the levels of C3 and C5. Damage to this area abolishes or alters the function of the phrenic nerve.

**Pyramidal Signs:** Symptoms of dysfunction of the pyramidal tract, including spastic paralysis, Babinski's reflex, and increased deep tendon reflexes.

**Queckenstedt's Test:** The veins of the neck are compressed on one or both sides. In a healthy person, the cerebrospinal fluid (CSF) pressure rises rapidly and then quickly returns to normal when the pressure is taken off the neck. In a patient with spinal cord obstruction, little or no increase in pressure is found. This test is diagnostically accurate for most cord compressions; however, false-negative results may be obtained if the lesion is located high in the cervical spine area. This test is not performed in patients with known or suspected increased intracranial pressure (ICP).

**Rhizotomy:** Surgical interruption of the roots of the spinal nerves within the spinal canal.

**Spinal Shock:** A state that occurs immediately after complete transection of the spinal cord. It may sometimes occur after only partial transections. All sensory, motor, and autonomic activities are lost below the level of the transection, and reflexes are absent. Paralysis is of a flaccid nature and includes the urinary bladder. Autonomic activity gradually resumes as spinal shock subsides. Once autonomic activity has returned, bladder and bowel training programs may be begun. Flaccid paralysis may develop into varying degrees of spastic paralysis, as evidenced by spasms of flexor or extensor muscle groups. The presence of autonomic activity also allows for episodes of autonomic hyperreflexia.

**Subarachnoid Block:** The injection of a local anesthetic into the subarachnoid space around the spinal cord.

**Subluxation:** Partial or incomplete dislocation.

**Supratentorial:** The area above the tentorium that includes the cerebrum. The supratentorial approach is used for frontal, temporal, parietal, and occipital lobe lesions.

**Tonoclonic Movements:** Tense muscular contractions that alternate rapidly with muscular relaxation.

**Valsalva Maneuver:** Contraction of the thorax in forced expiration against the closed glottis; results in increases in intrathoracic and intraabdominal pressures.

## CRANIAL SURGERY

### Diagnostic Tools

Techniques used to ascertain the presence and extent of cranial injury or disease include invasive and noninvasive techniques. A brief discussion of invasive and noninvasive diagnostic procedures is included to familiarize the PACU nurse with the techniques and special considerations necessary in the care of these patients. Many interventional neuroradiology procedures with general anesthesia are now done; these patients go to the PACU after the procedure is completed. The specific PACU care is

presented; if information on types of sedation (usually dexmedetomidine) for these patients is needed, please see Chapter 21.

***Conventional Radiography.*** Skull films are not ordered as often as computed tomographic (CT) scans and magnetic resonance imaging (MRI) scans. They are most often ordered for diagnosis of the presence of a skull fracture; information about the size, shape, and integrity of the skull and facial bones and any unusual calcification; and presence of air.

***Computed Tomography.*** Computed tomographic scanning creates a cross-sectional picture that separates various densities in the brain by means of an external x-ray beam. A computer-based apparatus allows the assessment of brain-emitted radiation and stores this information in the computer. The computer performs thousands of simultaneous equations on the radiation input and output data stored on its tapes and delivers an accurate detailed picture of the brain and of any abnormalities. The computer images correlate to tissue density. The dense structures, such as bone, appear white in color. Air and CSF appear as black area because they have much less density. The radiologist looks at the structures, changes in density, and any abnormalities in shape, size, or location of structures.

Contrast material may be used to enhance images. An iodinated radiopaque material is injected intravenously. Scans are usually taken before and after the administration of the radiopaque material. CT scanning has the advantages of accuracy and rapidity; both are essential in emergency situations. The entire procedure may last 15 to 20 minutes and may be difficult to use in an agitated, confused, or restless patient.

The CT scan is most helpful in diagnosis of hematomas, subarachnoid hemorrhage, hydrocephalus, cerebral atrophy, and tumors.

Care before the CT scan should include an assessment of the patient's allergies, specifically allergies to shellfish, iodine, or contrast dye. Blood urea nitrogen and creatinine levels should be checked to assess kidney function. Some patients may have a headache, feeling of warmth, salty taste in the mouth, or nausea or vomiting when given contrast dye. After the procedure, the patient must be well hydrated to help excrete the contrast dye.

***Magnetic Resonance Imaging.*** Also known as nuclear magnetic resonance imaging, MRI is a technique for obtaining cross-sectional pictures of the human body without exposure of the patient to ionizing radiation. MRI yields anatomic information that is comparable in many ways with the information supplied by a CT scan but often more accurately discriminates between healthy and diseased tissues. MRI is excellent in detection of soft tissue changes. It can detect necrotic tissue, small malignant tumors, and degenerative diseases.

The patient is placed within a cylindric high-powered magnet. Body tissues are then subjected to a magnetic field, which causes some of the hydrogen ions to align themselves with the field. A burst of low-energy radio waves is then applied to knock atomic protons within the tissues out of alignment. When the radio waves are discontinued, these protons release tiny amounts of energy that are "read" by a computer. Then, the MRI generates an image based on this information, thus yielding a detailed picture of the structural content and contours of the internal organs.

Contraindications for MRI include claustrophobic, agitated, or obese patients and patients with metallic devices or fragments present in the body.

***Positron Emission Tomography.*** Positron emission tomographic (PET) scanning is used most often in major research facilities. The PET scan measures glucose uptake and metabolism, cerebral blood flow patterns, and oxygen uptake to ascertain the functioning of the tissues or organs. The patient is injected with a glucose analogue that is tagged with a radionuclide. As the radionuclide decays in the tissue, the protons emitted are recorded with detectors and a computerized picture is generated. PET scans have been helpful in identification of schizophrenia, Alzheimer's disease, epilepsy, cardiovascular disease, head trauma, and other brain disorders.

***Electroencephalography.*** An electroencephalogram (EEG) is the tracing and recording of the electric activity at the surface of the brain. Aberrations in the rate and amplitude signal the presence of tumors, abscesses, scars, hematomas, or infection and may aid in the localization of such lesions.

***Cerebral Angiography.*** Arteriography, or angiography, is the diagnostic tool for aneurysms, arteriovenous malformations, and other cerebrovascular abnormalities. A cannula is introduced into the femoral or axillary artery and threaded to the level of the common carotid artery. Radiopaque dye is then injected, and radiographs record its path through the cerebral vasculature (Fig. 38-1). During and after arteriography, the patient may have an allergic reaction to the dye that may range from mild urticaria to anaphylaxis. Resuscitative equipment must be immediately available until the danger of allergic reaction has passed.

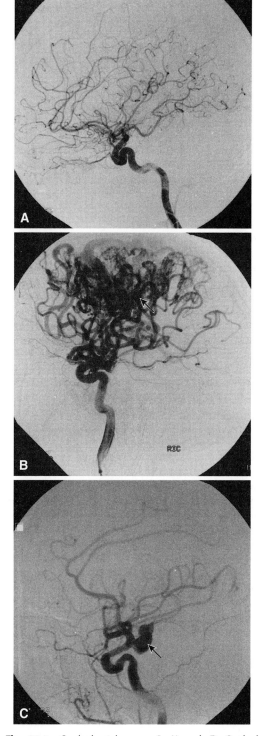

**Fig. 38-1** Cerebral angiograms. **A,** Normal. **B,** Cerebral hemorrhage. **C,** Cerebral aneursym. *(From Bucher L, Melander S: Critical nursing, Philadelphia, 1999, Saunders.)*

Irritation brought on by use of the dye may manifest itself in altered states of consciousness, hemiparesis, or speech difficulties that are usually transient. The site of injection must be examined closely at frequent intervals for the presence of bleeding that may occur beneath the skin and may defy casual detection. The effects of the local anesthetic agent often last for several hours and prevent the patient from detecting and reporting the pain caused by hemorrhage. Routine postprocedure care includes bedrest, observation of the puncture site for signs of bleeding, and monitoring of vital signs and neurologic signs. Intravenous fluids are maintained until the danger of untoward reaction has passed and the patient no longer has the transient nausea that occasionally occurs.

*Brain Scanning.* A radioactive compound is injected intravenously and is taken up by brain tissue. The pattern of this uptake is detected with a scintillation scanner, and a visual record is made. Uptake may be altered at the site of a disorder and may reflect the presence of cerebral neoplasms, hematomas, abscesses, and arteriovenous malformations (AVMs).

### Injuries and Pathologic Conditions of the Brain

*Types of Injuries.* When a head injury occurs, the most crucial concern is the extent of injury to the brain itself. Linear skull fractures in and of themselves are of little significance. The injury becomes more severe when the fracture involves depression of fragments into the brain, penetration of a foreign object, leakage of CSF, expanding hematomas, or signs and symptoms of herniation. The primary goal is to protect the brain and facilitate the patient's return to an optimal level of functioning.

Skull fractures are categorized as linear, depressed, or basilar. They are often described as simple, comminuted, or compound. The linear skull fracture is the most common. Most linear skull fractures are not depressed and do not require treatment. A depressed skull fracture is an inward depression of the skull and is classified as open or compound. Infection is a primary concern, and surgery may be necessary to remove bony fragments, clean the wound, and elevate the depressed bone. Basilar skull fractures occur in the base of the skull and are difficult to diagnose with radiographs. Diagnosis is confirmed with clinical data. Patients often have "raccoon's eyes," periorbital ecchymosis; or Battle's sign, ecchymosis around the mastoid process; or CSF otorrhea.

Concussion is caused by a violent jar or shock to the skull, such as rapid acceleration-deceleration. The patient may be dazed, "see stars," or have a period of impaired consciousness. When consciousness is regained, these patients may have posttraumatic amnesia and remember nothing of the injury itself or the events immediately preceding the injury.

Contusion is a bruising of the brain or hemorrhage on its surface. The extent of severity depends on the site and degree of brain injury. Consciousness may or may not be lost, but coma indicates diffuse injury. Laceration is the tearing of the brain. Laceration and contusions of the brain are usually found in the frontal and parietal lobes.

*Consequences of Injury.* Traumatic head injury can cause hemorrhage beneath a skull fracture or from a shearing of the veins or cortical arteries and results in epidural, subdural, subarachnoid, or intraventricular hemorrhage (Fig. 38-2). The signs and symptoms of brain ischemia and increased ICP vary with the speed at which the functions of vital centers are altered. A small clot that accumulates rapidly may be fatal. On the other hand, the patient may survive a slowly developing much larger hematoma through effective compensatory mechanisms.

An epidural hematoma, or extradural hematoma, accumulates in the epidural space (between the skull and the dura mater) and is arterial. Often the cause is the rupture or laceration of the middle meningeal artery, which runs between the dura and the skull in the temporal region. Epidural hematomas may also be seen in the frontal, occipital, and posterior fossa regions. Epidural hematomas need rapid emergency surgery. The patient usually loses consciousness, after which a lucid period and then rapid deterioration occur. The hemorrhage may be massive, and treatment consists of evacuation of the clot through burr holes made in the skull.

Subdural hematoma may result from trauma and the shearing of the bridging veins. Venous blood usually accumulates beneath the dura and spreads over the surface of the brain. A subdural hematoma may be acute, subacute, or chronic, depending on the size of the vessel involved and the amount of blood present. Patients with acute subdural hematomas have a rapid deterioration in condition and are critically ill.

Subacute subdural hematomas fail to show acute signs and symptoms at onset. Brain swelling is not great, but the hematoma may become large enough to produce symptoms. Progressive hemiparesis, obtundation, and aphasia often appear 4 to 21 days after injury. The degree of ultimate recovery depends

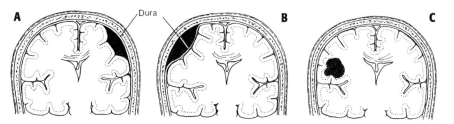

**Fig. 38-2** Types of hematomas. **A,** Subdural hematoma. **B,** Epidural hematoma. **C,** Intracerebral hematoma. *(From Luckman J, Sorensen KC: Medical-surgical nursing: a psychophysiologic approach, ed 3, Philadelphia, 1987, Saunders.)*

on the extent of damage produced at the time of injury.

Chronic subdural hematomas are seen most often in older adults. A history of head injury may be lacking because the causative injury is often minimal and long forgotten or deemed insignificant by the patient. The history is usually one of progressive mental or personality changes with or without focal symptoms as blood slowly accumulates and compresses the brain. The blood itself becomes thicker and darker within 2 to 4 days and within a few weeks resembles motor oil in character and color. Papilledema may be present. Chronic subdural hematomas may mimic any disease that affects the brain or its coverings. Treatment consists of evacuation of the defibrinated blood through multiple burr holes or a craniotomy incision.

Intracerebral hematomas are more commonly found in the elderly, often after a fall, but are also seen as a result of spontaneous rupture of a weakened blood vessel. Hemorrhage may be scattered or isolated. Surgical evacuation of an isolated or well-defined clot may be attempted, but the mortality rate remains high.

Subarachnoid hemorrhage may occur as the result of traumatic brain injury. Bleeding into the subarachnoid space may result in a vasospasm. A vasospasm is the narrowing of the blood vessel lumen and places the patient at risk for a delayed ischemic event. The risk of develoment of vasospasms is greatest 3 to 7 days after the bleed.

Intraventricular hemorrhage is bleeding into the ventricles caused by brain trauma such as penetrating wounds.

Supratentorial herniation is regarded as an emergency more severe than an epidural hematoma. The tentorium is an extension of the dura mater, which forms a transverse partition or shelf that divides the cerebral hemispheres from the cerebellum and brain stem. The superior portion of the brain stem passes upward through an aperture in the tentorium known as the tentorial hiatus. No space-occupying mass or lesion that expands within the cerebral hemispheres can escape upward or outward because of the confinement of the skull. Consequently, expansion within and compression of the hemispheres cause herniation of its contents (usually a portion of the temporal lobe known as the uncus) through the tentorial hiatus.

Uncal herniation is accompanied by compression of the lateral brain stem on the same side, which thus shuts off its blood supply and suppresses certain basic functions. The third cranial nerve (oculomotor) is in close proximity to the herniated uncus, and the pupil on the injured side becomes fixed and dilated. The reticular-activating system located in the brain stem that is responsible for waking and alertness becomes affected, and the patient rapidly becomes less and less responsive. Displacement of the midbrain causes compression of the pyramidal tract and results in contralateral hemiparesis or hemiplegia and plantar extensor responses (Babinski's reflex). The respiratory center in the medulla may be affected, which results in changes in the respiratory pattern or cessation of respiration altogether.

In addition to these changes, the cerebellum itself may be so compressed that the cerebellar tonsil herniates inferiorly through the foramen magnum. This condition usually results in immediate death because the centers vital to life are compressed or sheared. The best treatment for supratentorial herniation is prevention through early detection and treatment of increased ICP and its causes.

If efforts to minimize edema and increased ICP fail, surgical intervention, if possible, is necessary as a life-saving measure.

***Types of Pathologic Conditions.*** Cerebral aneurysms are round dilations of the arterial wall that develop as a result of weakness of the wall from defects in the media layer of the artery. Most cerebral aneurysms occur at bifurcations close to the circle of Willis and usually involve the anterior portion. Common bifurcations include those with the internal carotid, the middle cerebral, and the basilar arteries and in relation to the anterior and posterior communicating arteries. The exact cause or precipitating factor is not well defined but may be related to congenital abnormality, arteriosclerosis, embolus, or trauma. Aneurysms are usually asymptomatic and present no clinical problem to the patient unless rupture occurs, which results in neurologic deficits. Ruptured cerebral aneurysm is the major cause of subarachnoid hemorrhage. Intracerebral hemorrhage may occur alone or with the subarachnoid bleed. Morbidity and mortality rates are high because of rebleeding of the aneurysm and cerebral vasospasm of adjacent arteries. Surgical intervention involves identification and clipping of the aneurysm through a craniotomy.

Arteriovenous malformation is a vascular network that appears as a tangled mass of dilated vessels that create an abnormal communication between the arterial and venous systems. The communication may be singular or multiple and resembles an arteriovenous fistula in that no connecting capillary system between the arteries and the veins exists. AVMs most commonly occur in the supratentorial structures and usually involve the vessels of the middle cerebral arteries. AVMs are usually present at birth as the result of congenital abnormalities but may have a delayed age of onset; symptoms most commonly occur between the ages of 10 and 20 years. These symptoms may include headache, seizures, altered level of consciousness (LOC), and intracranial hemorrhage with resultant increased ICP. The treatment of choice is complete surgical excision via dissection or obliteration with ligation of feeder vessels. Radiation is used to treat AVMs that are not surgically accessible.

Intracranial tumors are space-occupying lesions that destroy brain tissue and nerve structures with invasion, infiltration, and compression and that produce increased ICP.

Intracranial tumors can be primary or metastatic. Primary tumors are classified as primary intracerebral (intraaxial) tumors, which originate from glia cells, or primary extracerebral (extraaxial) tumors, which originate from supporting structures of the nervous system. Metastatic tumors most commonly arise from breast malignant disease in women and lung malignant disease in men. Clinical manifestations can be both localized and generalized in nature. Local pathophysiologic changes, such as focal neurologic deficits, seizures, visual disturbances, cranial nerve dysfunction, and hormonal changes, result from the tumor itself destroying tissue at a particular site in the brain. Generalized pathophysiologic changes result from the effects of increased ICP. The treatment for cerebral tumors is surgical excision or surgical decompression if total excision is not possible. Surgery is often performed before, during, or after radiation treatment and chemotherapy.

Hydrocephalus in and of itself is not a disease entity but rather a clinical syndrome characterized by excess fluid within the cerebral ventricular system, the subarachnoid space, or both. Hydrocephalus occurs because of abnormalities in overproduction, circulation, or reabsorption of CSF. Hydrocephalus can be classified into two categories: noncommunicating (obstructive) or communicating (nonobstructive). Noncommunicating hydrocephalus is the result of an obstruction in the ventricular system or the subarachnoid space that prevents the flow of CSF to the location of the arachnoid villi, where reabsorption occurs. The obstruction may be caused by congenital abnormalities or space-occupying lesions. Communicating hydrocephalus occurs when the flow of CSF is normal but impaired absorption of the fluid at the arachnoid villi is impaired. Common causes of communicating hydrocephalus include inflammation of the meninges, subarachnoid hemorrhage, congenital malformation, and space-occupying lesions.

## Intracranial Pressure Dynamics

Intracranial pressure is pressure that is exerted against the skull by its contents: solid brain matter and intracellular water, CSF, and blood. These contents are essentially noncompressible, and a volume change in any compartment requires a reciprocal change to occur in one or both of the other compartments if the ICP is to remain constant (Monro-Kellie hypothesis). Because of the communications between the intracranial and extracranial compartments, CSF and blood can be translocated extracranially in partial compensation for increased ICP. These compensation capabilities are limited because of the small amount of CSF that the spinal subarachnoid space can hold, and total displacement of cerebral blood results in cerebral ischemia. Normal ICP is 0 to 15 torr. Intracranial hypertension occurs when a sustained increased ICP at the level of the head occurs and exceeds 15 torr.

Volume may be added to any of the cerebral compartments and results in increased ICP when the compensatory capacity is exceeded. Brain volume can be increased by a tumor, a hematoma, or edema. Blood volume can be increased through dilation of the vascular bed. CSF volume can be increased through obstruction in the ventricles, resistance to reabsorption, or, in rare instances, increased production of the CSF. Large brain tumors increase pressure by their mass, by blocking the rate of CSF reabsorption, or both. If the tumor is near the surface of the brain, it can cause inflamed meninges that may exude large quantities of fluid and protein into the CSF, thus increasing ICP. Hemorrhage or infection also causes increases in ICP. Large numbers of cells suddenly appear in the CSF and can almost totally block CSF absorption through the arachnoid villi. Regardless of the mechanism, when the volume added exceeds the volume that can be displaced, intracranial compliance is greatly reduced and ICP begins to increase.

Fig. 38-3 illustrates the relationship between intracranial volume and pressure. Phase I shows the success of compensatory mechanisms in maintenance of a constant ICP despite early increases in volume. In phase II, the limited capability of compensatory mechanisms has been exceeded and ICP begins to rise. In phase III, even a slight increase in volume causes a dramatic rise in ICP and thus results in complete decompensation and death. The shape of the curve may be altered by the rate at which the volume increases. Slowly developing increases in volume broaden the curve, whereas rapid increases narrow it.

Perianesthesia care for the patients with the potential for increased ICP requires an understanding of cerebral blood flow (CBF) and the factors that affect it; these factors become defective during increased ICP and are manipulated to reduce ICP. CBF is directly proportional to cerebral perfusion pressure (CPP) and inversely proportional to cerebrovascular resistance. CPP is the difference between the mean arterial pressure (MAP) and the right atrial pressure. When ICP is greater than right atrial pressure, the CPP is determined with the difference between the MAP and ICP:

$$CPP = MAP - ICP$$

and

$$CBF = (MAP - ICP)\ CVR$$

in which CVR is cerebrovascular resistance.

Consequently, any increase in ICP or reduction in MAP reduces CPP and resultant CBF. Normal CBF is 45 to 60 mL/100g/min. The CBF below which cerebral ischemia occurs has been termed the critical CBF, which is a flow rate of 16 or 17 mL/100g/min. Normal CPP is 80 to 100 torr. CBF begins to fail at a CPP of 30 to

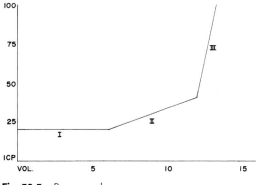

**Fig. 38-3** Pressure-volume curve.

40 torr. Irreversible hypoxia occurs at a CPP less than 30 torr. When ICP equals MAP, CPP equals zero and CBF ceases.

Factors that influence CBF regulation are partial pressure of oxygen in arterial blood ($PaO_2$) and partial pressure of carbon dioxide in arterial blood ($PaCO_2$; metabolic regulation), arterial blood pressure and autoregulation, and venous blood pressure. Metabolic regulation works in two ways. The first is regulation of blood flow based on the tissue needs for metabolic substrates: oxygen and glucose. As the activity of neuronal and glial cells in the brain increases, the demand for oxygen and glucose increases. The increased demand causes vasodilatation of arterioles, which increases CBF. Likewise, if the metabolic demand decreases, vasoconstriction occurs and CBF decreases.

The second, and most significant, way metabolic regulation affects CBF is the presence of metabolic byproducts, specifically carbon dioxide. Carbon dioxide is the most potent vasodilator of cerebral blood vessels. Normal cerebral vessels respond to changes in carbon dioxide by dilating when carbon dioxide increases and constricting when carbon dioxide decreases. The relationship between CBF and carbon dioxide is linear, and changes in CBF are in direct proportion to changes in carbon dioxide. A decrease of 1 mL/100g/min in CBF occurs for every 1 torr decrease in carbon dioxide. In treatment of elevated ICP, carbon dioxide levels of 30 to 35 torr are used to lower CBF.

Autoregulation is the ability of the cerebral vasculature in normal brain tissue to alter its resistance so that CBF remains relatively constant over a wide range of CPP. This mechanism causes vasoconstriction when perfusion pressure increases and vasodilation when perfusion pressure decreases. The limits of autoregulation are at a CPP of approximately 60 torr at the lower end and 160 torr at the upper end. Beyond the limits of autoregulation, CBF becomes passively dependent on CPP. When CPP increases to more than the upper limit of autoregulation, it exceeds the ability of the vasculature to constrict; CBF becomes directly related to and possibly dependent on CPP.

The lower limit of CBF autoregulation is the blood pressure below which vasodilatation becomes inadequate and CBF decreases. When CPP decreases to less than 60 torr because of increases in ICP, autoregulation ceases to be beneficial or effective in regulation of CBF. Defective autoregulation aggravates pressure increases and creates critical or irreversible levels of ICP by increasing the blood volume within the cranium in an effort to maintain CBF. Defective autoregulation generally occurs when ICP exceeds 30 to 35 torr. Eventually, autoregulation ceases altogether, and blood flow fluctuates passively with changes in arterial pressure, regardless of metabolic activity or regulation.

When ICP is increased, CPP and CBF are reduced, which renders the tissues ischemic. Ischemic cerebral tissue releases acid metabolites that cause a relatively fixed reduction in cerebrovascular tone. Autoregulation ceases, and any increase in MAP causes further increase in cerebral blood volume and elicits a further increase in ICP. CPP is reduced and thus causes ischemic areas (such as those that surround an expanding intracranial mass) to enlarge. As can be seen in Fig. 38-4, a pathologic cycle ensues in which ICP and MAP eventually equilibrate, the CPP drops to zero, CBF stops, and death occurs.

***Neurosurgical Procedures.*** With further developments in technology, neurosurgeons have more options in the treatment of patients. Surgical procedures that use instrumentation, lasers, and radiation therapy have increased the surgeon's ability to treat neurologic disorders.

***Stereotaxis.*** Stereotaxis is the precise location of deep brain lesions. A stereotactic frame is applied to the patient's head, and the target tissue is located with the stereotactic frames coordinates and CT scanning. Stereotaxis is also used for destruction of intracranial sensory pathways and is especially useful in the treatment of intractable chronic pain.

***Stereotactic Radiosurgery.*** The most common approaches to stereotactic radiosurgery (SR) are gamma knife and medical linear accelerator units (LINAC). Stereotactic radiosurgery can destroy deep and surgically inaccessible areas. The goal of SR treatment is the delivery of high-dose radiation to a specific target area without delivery of the radiation to surrounding tissue. Regardless of the type of SR, a stereotactic frame is secured to the patient's head for accurate determination of target location. The

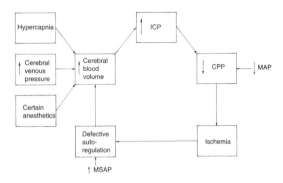

**Fig. 38-4**  Intracranial pressure dynamics with failed compensatory mechanisms.

placement of the stereotactic frame necessitates local anesthesia. Complications after SR may not appear for months to years later. Potential complications include permanent neurologic deficit, rebleeding, and worsening clinical symptoms.

***Laser Surgery.*** The benefit of laser surgery is that it enables the neurosurgeon to access areas that were surgically inaccessible with conventional surgery. With laser surgery, the surgeon can dissect a structure without trauma to the surrounding tissue, shrink tumors, and coagulate blood vessels. See Chapter 47 for a complete discussion on laser surgery.

***Anesthetic Agents and Intracranial Pressure.*** Anesthetic agents alter ICP by increasing or decreasing CBF and cerebral metabolic rate. In addition to the effects on ICP, some of these agents may also reduce systemic blood pressure and cause cerebral ischemia as a result of inadequate CPP.

***Inhalation Anesthetics.*** The inhalation anesthetic agents generally decrease blood pressure and may increase ICP in the patient for cranial surgery. They produce a clinically significant degree of cerebrovascular vasodilation and metabolic depression and can modify autoregulation. In fact, high dosages of volatile anesthetic agents can cause a total loss of autoregulation. The resulting increase in CBF ultimately leads to increased ICP. In patients with decreased intracranial compliance from neurologic disease, anesthetic agents that increase CBF may produce marked changes in ICP.

Isoflurane (Forane) at normocarbia has been shown to increase ICP. The initiation of hyperventilation simultaneously with the introduction of isoflurane prevents the increase in ICP that occurs at normocarbia. Isoflurane does not alter production of CSF and actually decreases resistance to absorption. It does not cause excitation of the central nervous system. Isoflurane produces reductions in cerebral metabolic rate, and autoregulation is not impaired to any degree. The greater decrease in cerebral metabolic rate may explain why CBF increases are minimal at low concentrations.

Desflurane and sevoflurane have essentially the same characteristics as isoflurane. During normocarbia, desflurane and sevoflurane cause cerebral vasodilation with resultant increases in CBF and ICP. The cerebrovascular response to $CO_2$ is maintained; therefore, the increase in CBF can be attenuated with hyperventilation. The cerebral metabolic rate is reduced in a dose-dependent manner similar to that of isoflurane, and no neuronal excitation is seen. Both agents cause cardiovascular depression and can be used with caution for controlled hypotension to reduce CBF. Desflurane, unlike sevoflurane, may result in an increase in MAP and heart rate when used for induction or at initially high concentrations. This effect may be attenuated with the use of narcotics or beta blockers. Both desflurane and sevoflurane have relatively low blood/gas partition coefficients that allow for rapid elimination of the agent, which makes them desirable for use because of the more rapid recovery.

Nitrous oxide has become controversial for use during intracranial surgical procedures. When used alone, nitrous oxide can cause an increase in CBF, ICP, and cerebral metabolic rate at normocarbia. These effects, however, are attenuated with the use of barbiturates, benzodiazepines, narcotics, and hyperventilation. To a small extent, nitrous oxide is a cerebral vasodilator and does not interfere with autoregulation of the CBF. For neurosurgical patients in whom increased ICP is not a problem, nitrous oxide may be an acceptable choice when combined with other agents to benefit from its rapid onset and elimination. However, it should be used cautiously in patients with increased ICP.

***Intravenous Anesthetics.*** Intravenous anesthetic agents (with the exception of ketamine) are usually the anesthetics of choice in cranial surgery.

Barbiturates, such as thiopental (Pentothal), are potent cerebral vasoconstrictors that can reduce CBF with subsequent reduction in elevated ICP. Cerebral vasoconstriction that is produced by barbiturates and the impact on CBF and ICP are dose-related. The reduction in CBF produced by barbiturates is even greater if hypocarbia is also present and is maintained at a constant level. Deep thiopental anesthesia during normocarbia results in about a 50% reduction in both cerebral metabolic rate and CBF.

Benzodiazepines, such as diazepam (Valium) and midazolam (Versed), produce sedation and amnesia by stimulating specific receptors in the brain. The benzodiazepines produce dose-related reductions in cerebral metabolic rate and CBF. When central benzodiazepine receptors are pharmacologically saturated, these drugs may decrease cerebral metabolic rate by as much as 40%.

Narcotics, such as fentanyl, morphine, and meperidine, are typically classified as cerebral vasoconstrictors, with resultant reductions in CBF. This effect is readily abolished by vasodilation that can accompany narcotic-induced ventilatory depression and the resultant increase in $PaCO_2$. With conditions maintained at normocarbia, fentanyl does not alter CBF. During normocarbia, the combination of nitrous oxide and morphine does not significantly alter CBF or autoregulation. Fentanyl causes a reduction in CBF and ICP in patients with normal CSF pathways. Alfentanil and sufentanil may in fact cause an increase in ICP in patients with compromised cerebral compliance.

Etomidate (Amidate) produces a maximal 45% decrease in cerebral metabolic rate and CBF; like the barbiturates, it can produce complete EEG suppression and appears to be comparable with lowering of ICP. Unlike the barbiturates, etomidate has less effect on MAP and offers greater stability in patients with hemodynamic compromise.

Propofol (Diprivan) reduces cerebral metabolic rate, CBF, and ICP and increases cerebrovascular resistance in a dose-dependent manner. The use of propofol in patients with elevated ICP may not be appropriate because of the substantial decrease in MAP and resultant decrease in CPP.

Ketamine (Ketalar, Ketaject) can rapidly increase ICP and often reduce CPP, despite mild increases in blood pressure. Ketamine is generally contraindicated for use in neurosurgical patients unless the fontanelles are open, CSF aspiration is instituted, or ventilatory control is maintained.

The use of controlled ventilation to produce $PaCO_2$ levels in the range of 25 to 30 torr and administration of nitrous oxide and oxygen and possibly low concentrations of isoflurane, together with narcotics and muscle relaxants, is a generally accepted anesthetic technique for the neurosurgical patient.

### Adjunctive Drugs Used to Reduce Intracranial Pressure

**Diuretics.** Mannitol and furosemide (Lasix) are diuretics often used to control increased ICP.

Mannitol, an osmotic diuretic, is the agent of choice for ICP reduction. Mannitol is administered intravenously in doses of 0.25 to 1g/kg in a 15% to 25% solution over 30 to 60 minutes, with maximal effects in 1 or 2 hours. Urine output can reach 1 or 2 L within 1 hour. Appropriate infusion of crystalloid and colloid solutions is often necessary to prevent adverse changes in plasma concentrations of electrolytes and intravascular fluid volume because of the rapidity of diuresis.

Potential complications of the use of mannitol include hyperosmolarity, electrolyte loss, changes in blood viscosity and coagulation, transient intravascular hypervolemia, and rebound or secondary elevation of ICP.

Furosemide is a loop diuretic. Furosemide is administered intravenously at a dose of 1 mg/kg to patients with normal ICP who are undergoing craniotomy and is more effective in reducing ICP than is mannitol. Furosemide is the drug of choice in patients with congestive heart failure.

Furosemide, when combined with mannitol, has been shown to potentiate the ICP-reducing effects of mannitol at the cost of rapid loss of intravascular volume and electrolytes. The ICP effects of these drugs are lost after 1 or 2 hours.

**Corticosteroids.** The drugs most commonly used are dexamethasone and methylprednisolone. Steroids are effective in lowering increased ICP because of localized vasogenic cerebral edema associated with mass-type lesions, such as neoplasm, abscess, and intracerebral hematoma. Usage is controversial with head trauma and cerebral infarctions with edema. The mechanism for the beneficial effect of corticosteroids is not known but may involve stabilization of capillary membranes, reduction in CSF production, blood-brain barrier repair, prevention of lysosomal activity, enhanced cerebral electrolyte transport, improved brain metabolism, and promotion of water and electrolyte excretion.

**Barbiturate Therapy.** Initiation of barbiturate therapy is the last medication adjunct used in treatment of intracranial hypertension. The patient must have an intracranial pressure–monitoring device, usually started when ICP is more than 30 mm Hg for 30 minutes and CPP is less than 70 mm Hg. The most common barbiturate is pentobarbital, which lowers the ICP by inhibiting free radical mediated lipid peroxidation, altering vascular tone, and suppressing metabolism.

**Intracranial Pressure Monitoring.** The most precise indicator of the pressure state within the cranium is the CSF pressure. Monitoring of ICP is the standard of care for patients at risk for intracranial hypertension. Measurement of this pressure may be obtained from the lateral ventricles, subarachnoid space, epidural or subdural spaces, or the intraparenchymal. Values from these areas are meaningful indicators of ICP only if pressure is freely transmitted between these compartments. Because injury and disease of the brain often create obstruction in CSF flow, the most accurate values are those obtained from the ventricle.

Lumbar puncture values reflect only a relative index of the actual ICP. These values depend on the state of the spinal canal and all the factors that affect it. On the other hand, measurement of the ventricular fluid pressure gives a direct and absolute value of the ICP, regardless of the influence or condition of the spinal canal. Lumbar puncture has other limitations. Its use is limited to those patients without suspected intracranial mass or to those whose ICP is not elevated or is elevated only slightly. In patients with these conditions, herniation of the brain tissue with the removal of CSF is a risk. ICP monitoring does not present this risk and can be used in a variety of conditions.

The ICP monitoring devices are categorized into two primary categories. The first category includes devices that use fluid or hydrostatic coupling to transmit to an external transducer. Ventricular catheters, subarachnoid bolts or screws, and subdural catheters fall into this group. The second group uses a transducer to directly monitor ICP. These intracranial devices use fiberoptics to transmit ICP pressures (Fig. 38-5).

The subarachnoid bolt or screw was developed in 1973 and requires only a twist-drill hole in the skull and a nick in the dura for insertion. As the name implies, the sensor lies in the subarachnoid space. The advantages of this type of monitoring device are less risk of infection and use in patients with small ventricles. However, in the presence of moderately severe cerebral edema, a small piece of brain tissue may be driven into and occlude the proximal end of the screw, thus rendering it useless.

The intraventricular catheter (IVC) is introduced into a CSF-containing ventricle via a twist-drill burr hole and is connected to an external transducer that converts the hydrostatic pressure force into a graph and numeric readout. The advantages of the IVC are that it provides a direct ICP reading and is easily kept patent. Another advantage is that CSF can be drained through the catheter for treatment of ICP elevations. In this way, it may serve as a temporary artificial extension of the CSF-shunting compensatory mechanism. Intracranial compliance

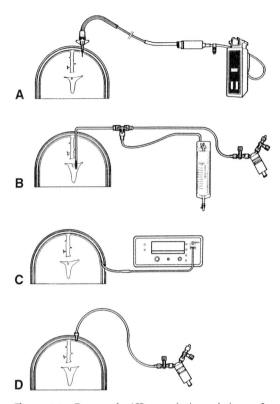

**Fig. 38-5** Types of ICP monitoring devices. **A,** Intraparenchymal monitoring system. **B,** Intraventricular monitoring system. **C,** Epidural monitoring system. **D,** Subdural monitoring system. *(Sole ML, Lamborn ML, Hartshorn JC: Introduction to critical care nursing, ed 3, Philadelphia, 2001, Saunders. Courtesy Integra NeuroSciences, Camino, San Diego, Calif.)*

can also be tested with injecting fluid into the cranium and reading the responding pressure. If an abrupt and steep rise in ICP occurs, one can assume that compliance no longer exists and that the volume-pressure curve is a steep one. When the patient's arterial pressure is monitored simultaneously, exact CPP can be calculated at any time. The ventricular catheter also has the advantage of allowing instillation of contrast media or air for study of the size and patency of the ventricle. The principal disadvantage of the IVC is the risk of infection and hemorrhage.

The fiberoptic catheter uses the fiberoptic transducer-tipped probe and can be placed in the ventricles and in subarachnoid, subdural, and intraparenchymal sites. The advantages are its easy placement and lack of relation to ventricular size. The major disadvantages are its expense, its inability to allow for CSF sampling or drainage, its possible need for probe replacement, and the fragility of the fiberoptic cable, which breaks easily.

Intracranial pressure monitoring is a valuable tool in assessment of the efficacy of nursing interventions that are intended to decrease ICP and is essential in determination of accurate assessments of the pressure state within the cranium and in treatment of elevations in ICP before the patient's condition deteriorates.

***Pressure Waves in Increased Intracranial Pressure.*** Pressures waves are abnormal spontaneous variations in ICP. Three patterns have been identified. The first and most significant type is the A wave, which is more commonly called a plateau wave. These waves are associated with increases in ICP between 50 and 100 torr that last for 5 to 20 minutes. They are seen only in advanced stages of increased ICP (the last phase of the volume-pressure curve) and superimpose themselves when the baseline ICP is elevated and exceeds 20 torr. Early increases in MSAP do not accompany plateau waves, and autoregulation is impaired. Thus, plateau waves signal hypoxia of brain cells and a decrease in CPP. They may cause both transient and irreversible damage to the brain and may be premonitory signs of acute incidents. The cause of plateau waves is not fully understood, but they probably result from a combination of transient blood volume alterations and CSF obstruction. Hypoventilation (with accumulating carbon dioxide and increasing intracranial blood volume) may be the cause, and the high ICP causes ischemia of the respiratory centers and thus results in irregular breathing.

The second type of pressure wave pattern is called the B wave. These waves are sharp rhythmic oscillations with a sawtooth pattern that occurs every 30 seconds to 2 minutes. These waves may indicate increases in ICP as much as 50 torr and are more commonly seen in patients with unstable increases.

The third type of pattern is the C wave. These waves are smaller rhythmic oscillations in ICP that occur every 4 to 8 minutes, and they indicate increases in ICP by as much as 20 torr. They are associated with respiratory influence on the blood pressure, but their significance is questionable.

**Intracranial Pressure Assessment**
With the availability of high-resolution noninvasive imaging techniques such as CT scanning and MRI, these studies themselves may be the chief determining factor in the decision to initiate ICP monitoring. Some of the indications for ICP monitoring are expanding intracranial tumors, hydrocephalus, benign intracranial hypertension, trauma, vascular anomalies, certain cases of metabolic coma with cerebral edema, certain cases of

viral hepatitis or fulminant hepatic encephalopathy, and patients in a controlled barbiturate coma for status epilepticus.

Continuous ICP monitoring is the only accurate method of assessment of ICP at any given time. This method has two advantages: (1) it provides an ongoing record of the ICP; and (2) it provides a means of assessment of intracranial dynamics. The clinical signs of increased ICP are numerous. The early signs are often vague and overlooked, and research has shown the unreliability of these signs in determination or recognition of increased ICP.

Early signs of increased ICP are increasing restlessness, confusion, and severe headache. Nausea, vomiting, paralysis, visual field deficits, conjugate deviation of the eyes, sensory loss, and nuchal rigidity are also early signs. The presence of these signs may or may not confirm a diagnosis of increased ICP.

The late signs of increased ICP are decreasing responsiveness and LOC; pupillary changes; increased systolic blood pressure; bradycardia; widening pulse pressure; alteration in respiratory pattern; decorticate or decerebrate posturing; and absence of or decrease in cough, gag, corneal, and deep tendon reflexes. A positive Babinski's reflex is normal in infants younger than 18 months of age but indicates increased ICP in those older than 18 months.

Most of these signs are manifestations of brain shift, with resultant dysfunction of the reticular-activating system, brain stem, and medulla. Pressure either has to elevate quite rapidly or be sustained at high levels to affect these structures so dramatically. Primary injury to these structures may elicit the same signs without appreciable increases in ICP. In this situation, they may well indicate the level of brain function and the gravity of the situation but not reflect the pressure dynamics that exist at that moment.

Just as these signs may be present without increase in ICP, ICP may be dangerously high with few, if any, signs. Classic brainstem signs (reflecting changes in cardiac, respiratory, or vasomotor function) usually occur late, after the onset of intracranial hypertension, if at all. The most important factor in determination of the degree of secondary brain damage incurred by elevated ICP is the effect of altered CPP on the brain. Clinical research has shown that the level of CPP is the best indicator of outcome from severe head injuries. CPP lower than 40 torr has been associated with poor outcomes. CPP needs to be maintained no lower than 50 to 60 torr to provide a minimally adequate blood supply to the brain.

Most hospitals with the capacity for cranial surgery also have the capacity for continuous ICP monitoring. Recognition of signs and symptoms of intracranial hypertension without the assistance of an ICP monitor is still important. Thus, the traditional signs and symptoms of increased ICP are discussed here, although they are not precise or infallible as indicators of increased ICP. At the least, they indicate that "something is not right" and that constant vigilance and further investigation are necessary. Even the transient appearances of these pressure signs are important. They indicate development of a highly delicate and unstable intracranial situation, a sign that the patient may be having plateau waves.

### Perianesthesia Nursing Management

The following four major areas of assessment are necessary in PACU care of the cranial surgical patient: vital signs, LOC, motor and sensory functioning, and pupillary signs. These areas should be routinely assessed at least every 15 minutes for the first 2 hours after surgery. Then, if results are within normal limits or unchanged since surgery, the areas should be assessed every 30 minutes. If the patient's condition is unstable or deteriorating or if the surgeon specifies, assessments should be made more frequently. If the patient's ICP is monitored, correct calibration of the monitor must be ensured, ICP value recorded, and waveform described. The same approach is used for arterial pressure recording.

Reports should be taken from both the anesthesiologist and the surgeon. Of particular importance are surgical procedure, pathologic findings, bone flap presence, allergies, preexisting medical problems, anesthetics, and any problems that occurred during surgery. Special positioning orders or restrictions, the presence of drains, and known CSF leaks must be noted. The Glasgow Coma Scale (GCS; Table 38-1) is a widely used neurologic assessment tool because of its simplicity, consistency, and reliability between raters who use it. However, the GCS cannot be used to assess subtle changes in the patient's neurologic status. When the GCS is used, the patient's responses are scored on a scale of 3 to 15. A score of 3 indicates coma, and a score of 15 indicates a fully alert oriented person with all neurologic functions intact.

***Vital Signs.*** Assessment of vital signs includes blood pressure, pulse, respirations, and ICP (if monitored). Changes in vital signs may indicate increasing ICP, shock, hemorrhage, electrolyte imbalance, or other disturbances. The perianesthesia nurse should keep in mind that the

**Table 38-1  Glasgow Coma Scale**

| Category | Response | Score |
|---|---|---|
| Eye opening | Spontaneous | 4 |
| | To speech | 3 |
| | To pain | 2 |
| | None | 1 |
| Best verbal response | Oriented to person, place, and time | 5 |
| | Confused | 4 |
| | Inappropriate words | 3 |
| | Incomprehensible sounds | 2 |
| | No response | 1 |
| Best motor response | Obeys commands | 6 |
| | Localizes to pain | 5 |
| | Withdrawal from pain | 4 |
| | Abnormal flexion | 3 |
| | Abnormal extension | 2 |
| | Flaccid | 1 |

injured patient may have other pathophysiologic processes unrelated to the head injury. Temperature is always monitored, and an elevation usually represents an infectious process, most often in the respiratory or urinary tract. Infrequently, elevations are attributable to direct damage to the temperature-regulating center in the hypothalamus. Temperature elevation also increases the metabolic rate of the brain, which may further increase ICP.

Airway patency is ensured, and the rate, depth, and rhythm are noted. If the rhythm is irregular, its pattern should be determined. Changes in the respiratory pattern may indicate injury to the respiratory center of the brain and the severity of the neurologic injury (Table 38-2). If the patient is on a ventilator, the machine should be checked for proper functioning and settings. However, mechanical ventilation may mask changes in the respiratory pattern.

For many years, the nursing literature has documented a relation between changes in blood pressure and pulse and increases in ICP. These changes are often referred to as Cushing's reflex, Cushing's triad, or Cushing's response. Cushing's reflex is described as elevated systolic blood pressure, bradycardia, and widening pulse pressure. Further increases in ICP may lead to Cushing's triad, which is described as bradycardia, hypertension, and bradypnea. Cushing's reflex and triad are late clinical signs of increased ICP and may indicate brain stem

herniation. Patients with head injury often have a higher than normal blood pressure and heart rate that may be the result of pain, hypoxia, and agitation or the release of endogenous catecholamines.

*Level of Consciousness.* The most important indicator of brain function is the LOC, but it is not necessarily indicative of altered ICP. A decreased LOC in the PACU may be caused by the lingering effects of the anesthesia or by neuromuscular-blocking agents sometimes used with patients on positive-pressure ventilation. A change in LOC may also be the result of hypoxia, hypoglycemia, vitamin deficiency, or fluid and electrolyte imbalances. Other underlying pathologic changes may cause alterations in LOC. For assessment of LOC, a description of the patient's response is best instead of vague terms such as stuporous, semiconscious, or unconscious. A standard assessment form such as the GCS (see Table 38-1) should be available for assessment of the LOC. A change in LOC may also be indicative of deterioration or improvement in the patient's condition.

*Motor and Sensory Functioning.* Assessment of motor and sensory function is part of an ongoing neurologic assessment and is performed to note changes from the baseline assessment. It can also provide clues to extending hemorrhage or expanding edema. Focal changes, such as decreased hand strength unilaterally or an inability to move one side of the body, often accompany these events. Sensations may be decreased because of brain involvement, not just spinal cord injury (SCI). Observe whether the patient can move all four extremities. Check both hand grasps simultaneously. Are they weak or strong; equal or unequal? Foot strength can be tested by having the patient push or pull against the nurse's hands. (Be sure the patient uses only the foot and ankle, not the entire leg.) If the patient does not respond to simple commands, test to see whether a painful stimulus such as a pin prick or pinch induces movement. (Test both sides to determine sensory impairment.) If the patient does not respond to pain, test for motor function by raising both arms or both legs and letting them fall together. A paralyzed limb falls to the bed more quickly than an unaffected one. To further check leg motor ability, flex both of the patient's knees with the feet flat on the bed; release them at the same time. The healthy leg maintains its position momentarily and then resumes the original position. The affected limb abducts while falling and maintains knee flexion.

Facial muscle movement should also be tested. If possible, ask patients to wrinkle the

| Table 38-2   **Respiratory Patterns** | | |
|---|---|---|
| Pattern | Description | Location of Injury and Other Causes |
| Cheyne-Stokes respirations | Regular increase in rate and depth of breathing that peaks and is followed by decreasing rate and depth of breathing, which progresses to apnea; cycle then repeats itself | Bilateral dysfunction of cerebral hemispheres Midbrain and upper pons |
| Central neurogenic hyperventilation | Deep, rapid, and regular pattern of breathing | Low midbrain and upper pons Increased ICP with head trauma |
| Apneusis breathing | Pause at full inspiration occurs; may see prolonged inspiratory pause that alternates with prolonged expiratory pause | Mid and low pons Hypoglycemia, anoxia, and meningitis |
| Cluster breathing | Periodic breathing with frequent apneic episodes | Low pons and high medulla |
| Ataxic breathing | Irregular breathing with shallow deep respirations and irregular apneic episodes; usually slow in rate | Medulla |

forehead, shut the eyes tightly, smile, and show the teeth. Any asymmetry should be noted. If the patient is not responsive to verbal commands, noxious stimulation may elicit a grimace or other facial movement. The presence of a Babinski's reflex is pathologic and indicates pyramidal tract dysfunction in any person older than 18 months of age. Starting at the heel and using a moderately sharp object, such as the rounded tip of a bandage scissors or the tip of a retracted pen, stroke the lateral sole and proceed to the ball of the foot. Firm pressure is necessary to elicit an accurate response. The Babinski's reflex is present when the great toe dorsiflexes (bends toward the head) and the remaining toes "fan out." The Babinski's reflex is not present when the stimulus elicits a plantar or downward flexion of the great toe.

Motor response to a painful stimulus may be one of decerebrate or decorticate rigidity, or these postures may exist in the absence of any stimulation. Decerebrate posturing is characterized by rigidity and contraction of all the extensor muscles. The legs are stiffly extended with the feet plantar flexed. The arms are extended and hyperpronated. Decerebrate rigidity is usually the result of upper brain stem damage, which means that the cerebral hemispheres are functionally cut off. Decorticate posturing indicates that function has been cut off at a lower level and that the entire cortex is physiologically cut

off. In this instance, the legs are extended and internally rotated, and the feet are plantar flexed. The arms are flexed at all joints, and the hands are often held beneath the chin.

***Pupillary Activity.*** Pupillary reactions are controlled by the third cranial nerve. In assessment of the pupils, the perianesthesia nurse should examine both simultaneously for shape, size, and equality. Normal pupils are round and, at a midpoint diameter, within the range of 1 to 9 mm. Instead of use of terms like constricted or dilated, measurement of the diameter directly with a pocket millimeter ruler is more precise. Test the direct light reflex of each pupil with a small bright flashlight. Normally, the pupil constricts briskly. If it reacts sluggishly or not at all, the reaction is abnormal. To test the consensual light reflex, hold both eyelids open, shine the light in one eye, and observe the other pupil. The opposite pupil should constrict simultaneously with the lighted one, although perhaps not to the same degree.

Normal pupillary size and reactivity can be altered by some medical situations and by certain drugs. Previous surgery or direct injury to the eye may alter or abolish reactivity. Blindness abolishes reactivity to light because the sensory part of the reflex pathway is absent.

Unusual eye movements should be noted. Normal gaze in a person who is awake and alert is straight ahead, with no involuntary movements. This condition is generally true of unresponsive patients, although the eyes may rove slowly and in random fashion. (In detection of this movement, do not be misled into thinking that the patient is actually following you or your movements.) The eyes should move together in the same direction (conjugate gaze). If the eyes are disconjugate, they move in a jerky oscillatory fashion (nystagmus) or the gaze deviates from the midline. These ocular movements are abnormal and should be detailed in the nursing notes.

### Nursing Care in the Postanesthesia Care Unit

The PACU nurse has three primary responsibilities in the care of the neurosurgical patient: (1) to institute measures of care to sustain optimal physiologic function in the perianesthesia patient; (2) to recognize and prevent conditions that increase ICP beyond normal limits; and (3) to detect and communicate signs and symptoms of the patient's condition to the physician (Box 38-1).

## SPINAL SURGERY

The goal of surgical intervention is minimization of complications related to SCIs, spinal cord tumors, or developmental abnormalities.

Complete or incomplete SCI, bony fragments in the canal, unstable dislocation, and evidence of cord compression are some indications for immediate surgical intervention.

### Diagnostic Tools

Several methods are used in diagnosis of injury or disease involving the spine or spinal canal.

Conventional radiography and fluoroscopy are used to identify fractures and fracture-dislocations. Narrowing of an intervertebral space is sometimes evident as a result of a herniated nucleus pulposus, or "slipped disk." Fluoroscopy is used to show instability of the injured part on manipulation. Splintered or displaced bone fragments and radiopaque foreign bodies (such as bullets or other metal fragments) are also seen on radiographs. Radiographs also show abnormalities such as scoliosis and osteoporotic and arthritic changes. Tumors may be evidenced by erosion, calcium deposits within the mass, increased interpediculate distance, enlargement of an intervertebral foramen, or collapse of a vertebra.

Computed tomographic scanning is used to delineate mass lesions that exist in the same plane as the spine and spinal cord. Large blood clots may also be localized with this method.

Magnentic resonance imaging is being used increasingly for accurate detection and

---

### Box 38-1 Postanesthesia Nursing Management

**Maintain patent airway**
Encourage deep breathing and use of incentive spirometer
Encourage avoidance of coughing to help prevent increased ICP
Administer oxygen
Provide ventilatory assistance if indicated
Monitor pulse oximetry
**Monitor $PO_2$ and $PCO_2$**
Provide oral and nasal airways as indicated
Position to prevent aspiration and obstruction
Suction as necessary
Monitor vital signs
Provide for baseline data
Investigate changes from baseline
Monitor for any signs of restlessness and evaluate for underlying cause
**Maintain proper position of supertentorial craniotomy and head**
Elevate head of bed 30 to 45 degrees to facilitate venous return, promote CSF circulation, and reduce cerebral edema
Maintain neutral head position and avoid neck flexion
Turn side to side; may position supine
Position on nonoperative side as indicated by specific surgical procedure and physician orders to:
**Prevent shifting and displacement of intracranial contents**
Infratentorial craniotomy

NURSING CARE IN THE PACU

*Continued*

---

**Box 38-1   Postanesthesia Nursing Management—cont'd**

Keep flat or slightly elevated
Position body in neutral position
May be turned side to side; do not position on back
Transsphenoidal surgery
Elevate head of bed 30 to 45 degrees
Position body in neutral alignment
**Maintain skin and mucous membrane**
Provide mouth care frequently
Turn every 2 hours and monitor bony prominences
Maintain body alignment with the use of positioning aids
For periorbital edema, use cool compresses to eyes
Instill artificial tears, normal saline solution, or lubricate to prevent corneal damage
Use an eye shield if necessary to prevent corneal abrasions
**Prevent infection**
Observe dressing for signs of CSF drainage
Observe for halo or ring sign (lighter colored rings on dressing or linen with blood in the center)
Check drainage for glucose (mucus does not contain glucose; CSF does)
Use sterile technique when changing dressings
Provide urinary catheter care, if present, with soap and water; prevent undue stress on catheter
**Monitor fluid and electrolyte balances**
Maintain accurate I/O
Monitor serum osmolarity (290 to 320 mOsm/kg)
Maintain urine output greater than 30 mL/h
Monitor urine specific gravity
Monitor skin turgor
Administer antiemetic to prevent vomiting and increased ICP
Maintain normothermia
Hyperthermia
Remove excessive layers of clothing or bed covers
Administer antipyretics
Administer sponge baths with tepid water
Use hypothermia blanket
Prevent shivering (shivering increases ICP); administer chlorpromazine if indicated for shivering
**Provide for pain relief and comfort**
Administer analgesics as ordered (do not mask neurologic signs; usually codeine or acetaminophen)
Do not cluster nursing activities together
Elevate head of bed to help prevent headache
Reduce environmental stimulation by keeping light low; reduce noise
**Prevent thrombophlebitis**
Apply thigh-high elastic stockings and sequential compression boots
Inspect legs daily
**Provide emotional and psychosocial care**
Explain all procedures and offer psychologic support and reassurance
Communicate with family and involve in plan of care
Speak quietly

Adapted from Shpritz DW: The neurosurgical patient. In Litwack K, editor: *Core curriculum for perianesthesia nursing practice,* Philadelphia, 1999, Saunders.

assessment of space-occupying lesions of the spine, such as herniated nucleus pulposus and tumors.

Electromyography is used in evaluation of muscle function as a means of detecting the nature and location of motor unit lesions. Tumors and herniated nucleus pulposus that compress the cord or motor nerve roots affect the function of the muscle groups they innervate.

Myelography is one of the most valuable tools available in diagnosis of compression of the spinal cord caused by tumor, fracture-dislocation, or herniated nucleus pulposus. A lumbar puncture is performed, at which time a Queckenstedt's test may also be done. The myelogram consists of the injection of a radiopaque dye into the CSF canal and the fluoroscopic observation of its flow in the suspected area. Cord compression is evidenced by an interruption in the contour of the spinal cord. Disruption of the contours of the spinal nerve roots may also be found.

### Injuries and Pathologic Conditions of the Spine

*Injuries of the Spine.* The spine protects the spinal cord and the terminal nerve roots. Injuries to the spine and spinal cord occur as a result of flexion, hyperextension, rotation with both flexion and extension, compression, and penetrating wounds (Fig. 38-6). Head injuries often accompany injuries to the spine and vice versa. The cervical spine is extremely mobile and therefore particularly susceptible to injuries that hyperflex or hyperextend the neck. Propulsion may occur anteroposteriorly or laterally. The spinal cord is relatively large in the cervical area and sustains damage fairly easily after injury. This area is unique in that the superior portion of C2 lacks a vertebral body. Instead, the neck has a dens, or projection, called the odontoid. Many injuries to the odontoid

extend into C1, or atlas, which has no vertebral body at all.

The thoracic spine is fixed by the ribs, but the lumbar spine is not; thus, an increased incidence rate is seen of injury to the thoracic, lumbar, or sacral regions of the spine. Motor vehicle accidents are the leading cause of spinal cord injuries.

Consequences of injury to the spine are the result of the mechanical insult or biochemical and hemodynamic changes. Mechanical insult includes the direct injury and changes to the cord structure, motion stress on the cord, and continuous compression to the cord. This physical injury to the cord results in the primary or initial spinal cord dysfunction. Edema of the cord, which causes cellular changes and ischemia, may occur in the hours after the initial injury. This process is called secondary injury and may last up to 5 days.

The primary goal in the early treatment of spinal cord injuries is prevention of further compromise of spinal cord tissue from secondary injury. If the damage to tissue as the result of the direct injury cannot be altered, an attempt is made to protect the remaining tissue by alleviation of compression and movement of the spinal cord. Spinal cord immobilization, surgical intervention to alleviate cord compression, and pharmacologic therapies to reduce edema are used as immediate therapies.

**Complete Spinal Cord Lesion.** The extent of injury to the spinal cord is described as complete or incomplete lesion. In a complete SCI, no motor or sensory function is seen more than three levels below the level of injury. When this type of injury lasts more than 24 hours, no recovery of distal function is indicated. Clinical findings during the acute phase after total cord transection include the following:

1. Immediate loss of all sensory, motor, autonomic, and reflex functions below the level

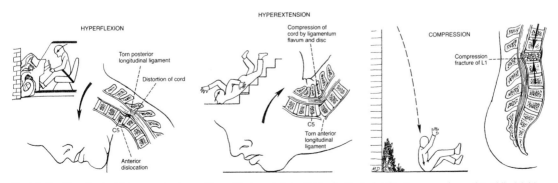

**Fig. 38-6**  Closed spinal injury mechanisms. *(From Clochesy J, Breu C, Cardin S, et al: Critical care nursing, ed 2, Philadelphia, 1996, Saunders. In Luckman J, Sorensen KC: Medical-surgical nursing: a psychophysiologic approach, ed 3, Philadelphia, 1987, Saunders.)*

of the injury from spinal shock. Spinal shock may persist for days or weeks, depending on the injury and the patient's general state of health. It usually lasts 4 to 8 weeks.

2. Urinary retention as a result of bladder sphincter paralysis.
3. Paralytic ileus with progressive abdominal distention.
4. Respiratory insult or cessation. Injury to the lower cervical or upper thoracic spine results in cessation of intercostal function. In this event, respiration is under the sole stimulus of the phrenic nerve, and breathing is diaphragmatic. Injury to the cord at the levels of C3 to C5 affects the phrenic nucleus and thus paralyzes the diaphragm and causes respiratory failure.
5. Loss of sweating below the level of the lesion.
6. Point tenderness over the injured part. Crepitus may or may not be present.

Initial therapeutic efforts are directed at preservation of life. Mechanical stability, protection of nervous tissue, and freedom from pain are long-term therapeutic goals.

**Incomplete Spinal Cord Lesion.** Incomplete spinal cord lesion indicates residual motor or sensory function more than three segments below the level of injury. Indications of incomplete lesion are sensation, sense of position, or voluntary movement of the legs; sensation around the anus; voluntary rectal sphincter contraction; and voluntary toe flexion.

Various syndromes or types of incomplete lesions may result from the injury. Incomplete lesions include central cord syndrome, Brown-Séquard's syndrome, anterior cord syndrome, and posterior cord syndrome.

Central cord syndrome (CCS) is the most common type of incomplete lesion. CCS occurs more commonly in older adults as a result of a hyperextension injury, such as a blow to the face or forehead. CCS from sports injuries is also seen in younger patients.

The center of the cord is contused and may hemorrhage, thus resulting in bilateral upper extremity weakness and a burning sensation. If CCS is caused by a contusion, lower extremity function usually returns first, then bladder function, upper extremities, and lastly, finger movement.

Brown-Séquard's syndrome may occur after injuries that transect the cord, such as knife or gunshot wounds, epidural hematoma, herniated cervical disc, spinal cord tumor, spinal AV malformation, and cervical spondylosis. Clinical signs are ipsilateral loss of motor, touch, pressure, and vibration below the lesion and contralateral loss of pain and temperature below the lesion. This type of lesion has the best functional recovery rate; many patients regain independent ambulation.

Anterior cord syndrome usually occurs as the result of compression of the anterior portion of the cord and loss of blood supply from the anterior spinal artery. Clinical signs are loss of motor function, pain, temperature, and sensation below the level of injury. Touch, position, and vibration sensation are still intact. Anterior cord syndrome is usually caused by flexion injuries in the cervical area.

Posterior cord syndrome is a rare disorder. Clinical signs are pain and paresthesias in the neck, upper arms, and torso. Mild paresis of the upper arms may occur.

### Surgical Intervention for Spinal Cord Injuries

Surgeons differ in opinions about the optimal timing for surgical decompression and fusion. Early surgical intervention is indicated to decompress the spinal canal from bone or disk fragments, provide stabilization, and repair damage caused by penetrating objects.

Patients who need surgery may have exploration, insertion of Harrington rods or stabilization instruments, or decompression laminectomy procedures. Procedures may be performed through an anterior or posterior approach, depending on the cord lesion. Fusion is accomplished with the placement of a bone graft taken from tibial or iliac bone into the involved interspace or of a fixation device. External immobilization is often used after surgery until osseous union is complete.

General contraindications to surgery are the existence of associated life-threatening injuries, depressed respiratory function caused by high cervical injuries, lack of skilled personnel and necessary equipment, and improved neurologic status.

### Perianesthesia Nursing Care for the Patient with Spinal Cord Injury

In the United States alone, more than 10,000 people annually have SCIs. Of these people, 36% sustain injuries to the spinal cords in motor vehicle accidents. Permanent injuries of this nature are devastating to the patient and the patient's family. The nursing responsibilities are great during the acute, rehabilitative, and chronic phases. Patients with SCI may be sent to the PACU in any of these phases, and care requires special consideration and knowledge of SCI pathophysiology.

The initial assessment of the patient with SCI in the PACU needs to focus on airway patency, adequate respiration, and maintenance of systemic and spinal cord perfusion. Vital signs should be assessed every 15 minutes until the condition is stable. Baseline neurologic assessment including motor and sensory evaluation should be completed with the initial and ongoing assessments.

Immobilization is a primary intervention to help prevent the process of secondary injury. The standard of care for immobilization is placement of the neck in a neutral position and in a rigid cervical collar. Stabilization of fractures may be accomplished with several devices that promote alignment.

Current pharmacologic treatments to help reduce spinal cord edema and secondary injury include the administration of methylprednisolone. The current standardized treatment for patients with SCI treated within 8 hours is a bolus and continuous intravenous (IV) infusion. Improvement in motor function has been directly associated with the administration of methylprednisolone.

### Complications Associated with Spinal Cord Injury

**Spinal Shock.** Spinal shock is a form of neurogenic shock characterized by a loss of motor, sensory, autonomic, and reflex activity below the level of the lesion and resulting in flaccid paralysis and paralytic ileus. The classic signs and symptoms of spinal shock include systemic hypotension, bradycardia, and hypothermia. Spinal shock is a condition that occurs immediately after injury and may last hours to months, depending on severity of the injury. Average recovery from spinal shock is 1 to 6 weeks.

**Hypotension.** Hypotension is not uncommon because of vasodilation of the vessels below the level of the injury. The goal of treatment is maintenance of systemic and renal perfusion. Bradycardia may accompany the hypotension. Dopamine is indicated for the treatment of hypotension and bradycardia. Other causes of hypotension, such as a gastrointestinal (GI) hemorrhage, must be considered and ruled out. Hypotension is usually not caused by hemorrhagic shock; therefore, the patient volume status should be monitored closely and not overloaded with intravenous fluids.

**Bradycardia.** Bradycardia is associated with spinal shock and nursing interventions such as manipulation of an endotracheal tube, suctioning, turning, and insertion of a nasogastric tube, which may elicit a vasovagal response that leads to bradycardia. Nursing interventions should closely monitor for and provide prevention from a vasovagal response.

**Thrombosis.** Conditions are optimal for the development of deep vein thrombosis and pulmonary embolus because of venous pooling and loss of movement below the level of injury. Calf measurements, use of antiembolism stockings, compression devices, low-dose heparin, and low–molecular weight heparin are used to prevent these complications.

**Autonomic Dysreflexia.** Autonomic dysreflexia usually occurs after the resolution of spinal shock and the return of reflex activity. It results from reflex stimulation of the sympathetic nerves below the level of injury. Causes of the reflex stimulation include bladder distension, fecal impaction, and noxious stimuli. Symptoms of autonomic dysreflexia are pounding headache, hypertension, profuse sweating and flushed skin above the level of injury, pallor and goose bumps below the level of the injury, anxiety, and visual disturbances. Treatment is aimed at removal of the noxious stimulus and prevention of complications from hypertension.

The PACU nursing care centers around the routine prevention of known precipitants of autonomic dysreflexia. For example, the bladder must not become distended, and skin breakdown must be prevented. If signs and symptoms appear, the stimulus must be sought and removed as rapidly as possible. If the symptoms cannot be alleviated, the nurse should notify the physician, elevate the head of the bed (if not contraindicated), and monitor the blood pressure every 5 minutes. Severe cases can require treatment with spinal anesthesia and the administration of ganglionic-blocking agents. For chronic problems, subarachnoid blocks or rhizotomy may be necessary.

***Pain Management.*** Patients may have pain in areas about the level of injury. The pain may be described as sharp, dull, or burning and often is associated with muscle spasms. Morphine for pain or Valium, Flexeril, or other antispasmodic agents may be ordered. Intramuscular medications should never be administered below the level of the lesion because they only cause local inflammation and tissue breakdown and absorption is negligible.

***Concomitant Head Injury.*** Every patient with acute injury to the spine must be observed for signs and symptoms that indicate head injury. Evaluation of cranial status should be done at the same intervals as the vital sign measurements. An abnormal neurologic "check" should be reported to the physician immediately because it may indicate injury to the brain or increased ICP that results from the upward expansion of cord edema.

*Respiratory Complications.* Respiratory insufficiency or failure is the most serious complication of SCI. Respiratory complications can be independent of the level of injury. C4 and higher injuries require mechanical ventilation because of the direct involvement of the phrenic nerves. Assessment of a patient's ventilation should include the following parameters: status, rate, depth, pattern, and oxygen saturation. Evaluation of pulmonary function should include tidal volume, inspiratory force, and vital capacity. Changes in pulmonary function are early indicators of deterioration in respiratory status and may necessitate ventilator support. Intubation of the patients may depend on the ability to clear secretions and to maintain adequate gas exchange. A program of chest physiotherapy and the use of pressure support ventilation and positive end-expiratory pressure assists with the prevention of atelectasis. Auscultation of lung sounds should also be performed routinely to assess the presence of abnormal lung sounds. Chest radiographic examinations and arterial blood gas determinations should be monitored routinely and ordered immediately if signs of deterioration occur. Potential respiratory complications that result from SCI include pneumonia, aspiration, pulmonary edema, and pulmonary embolism. Rotational beds before surgical stabilization facilitate the mobilization of secretions and help prevent respiratory complications (Fig. 38-7). A team approach by nursing staff, physicians, respiratory therapists, and physical therapists is necessary in treatment of SCI. Because of the rapid onset of pulmonary complications, the PACU nurse must be aggressive in caring for the patient with SCI.

*Skin Breakdown.* As with the patient for cranial surgery, skin care for the patient with SCI is an important aspect of PACU nursing care. Skin breakdown is one of the most obvious, costly, and detrimental complications that a patient with SCI can have. The patient must be turned and repositioned at least every 2 hours to prevent skin breakdown and damage to underlying body tissues. A specialty surface such as an air mattress or alternating pressure mattress may be necessary to prevent skin breakdown.

*Bone Demineralization.* Long-term immobility causes demineralization of bone tissue. Calcium is freed into the circulation and results in osteoporosis, or "silent fractures," and renal calculi.

*Gastrointestinal Complications.* Generalized atony and loss of motility render the stomach and intestine distended and highly susceptible to fecal impactions and obstructions.

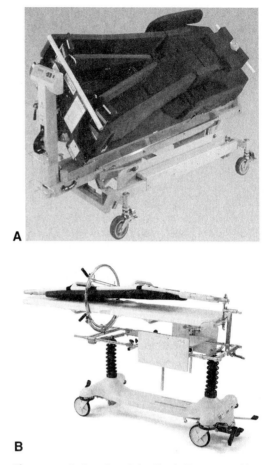

**Fig. 38-7   A,** Roto Rest Delta Kinetic Treatment Table. **B,** Stryker Wedge Turning Frame, Model 965. (**A,** *Courtesy of KCI, San Antonio, Texas.* **B,** *Courtesy of Stryker Corporation, Kalamazoo, Mich. Used with permission of Stryker Corporation.*)

Distention is relieved with intermittent nasogastric suction. Programs of bowel training are initiated within 24 hours of admission.

A high incidence rate of stress ulcers is seen among these patients, especially in those with quadriplegia. Here, parasympathetic vagal action is unopposed because of sympathetic block from the ascending and descending visceral nerve paths, and gastric acid secretion by the parietal cells of the stomach is increased. This stressful situation is further compounded by the administration of corticosteroids used to reduce cord edema that are singularly capable of inducing hyperacidity of gastric juices. Antacids or a histamine$_2$ antagonists, or both, are given prophylactically to prevent stress ulcers. If gastric juices are accessible through a nasogastric tube, gastric pH can be monitored as a guide to treatment. Serial hematocrit determinations establish a baseline and may be the first indication of "silent" gastrointestinal hemorrhage.

**Urologic Complications.** After transection of the spinal cord, the bladder sphincter becomes paralyzed and urinary stasis develops. Indwelling urinary catheterization is necessary to prevent bladder distention during the acute phase.

Long-term catheterization, osteoporosis, decreased muscle tone, fluid and electrolyte abnormalities, alterations in cardiovascular dynamics, anemia, and catabolism contribute to urologic complications. Stasis, calculi and fistula formation, and chronic urinary tract complications that lead to septicemia make urologic complications the leading cause of death in patients with paraplegia and quadriplegia.

**Anesthetic Considerations.** The most influential factors in the anesthetic management of the patient with SCI are the duration of the injury (acute or chronic), fluid and electrolyte status, airway management, and autonomic hyperreflexia.

The use of a depolarizing muscle relaxant (succinylcholine) for intubation purposes in the patient with SCI is conservatively contraindicated because of the release of potassium. The succinylcholine-induced release of potassium is the result of proliferation of cholinergic receptors in muscle tissue below the level of transection. The resultant hyperkalemia, often as high as 14 mEq/L, can lead to ventricular fibrillation and cardiac arrest. The release of potassium caused by succinylcholine administration can be seen as early as 1 day after injury and as long as 9 months later. The degree of muscle involvement, not the dosage of succinylcholine, is the determining factor in the amount of potassium released.

Patients with SCI may have some degree of hypotension because of a relative hypovolemia that results from sympathetic nervous system depression. The degree of the hypotension depends on the level of transection and the duration of the injury with regard to whether the patient still has spinal shock. The patient must be adequately resuscitated with fluids, and measures must be taken to monitor fluid status and ensure adequate organ perfusion.

Airway management is a significant problem in patients with SCI whose injuries involve the cervical spine. Endotracheal intubation must be performed without manipulation of the cervical spine to avoid further irreversible damage. Intubation may be accomplished with awake blind oral or nasal approach, fiberoptics, or retrograde intubation. When the airway obstruction is severe, tracheostomy or cricothyrotomy may be necessary. Patients may arrive in the PACU with the endotracheal tube in place and not undergo extubation until adequate management of the airway and ventilation are ensured.

## Herniated Nucleus Pulposus

Herniated nucleus pulposus (Fig. 38-8) may occur in any of the intervertebral disks but is most commonly found in one of the last two lumbar interspaces. Pain and some degree of compromise in sensory or motor function along the distribution of the involved nerve are common preoperative findings. Before surgical intervention is undertaken, diagnostic confirmation is sought and the suspected herniated nucleus pulposus is differentiated from tumor, subluxation of the facets, or rheumatoid spondylitis.

Surgery consists of partial hemilaminectomy and removal of the diseased disk. If fusion is necessary to prevent recurrence of pain or deformity, a bone graft is removed from the iliac crest or tibia and placed as a bridge over the defective space. Spinal fusion lengthens the operative procedure and requires a second operative wound site. Therefore, a greater potential for postoperative complications exists and the recuperative phase may be lengthened. The threat of shock is also greater because of increased blood loss and pain.

Movement restrictions in the PACU are determined by the surgeon and depend on the extent of the surgery and whether a fusion was done. If a fusion was not done, the patient is often allowed to stand at the bedside and ambulation is allowed as soon as the effects of the anesthetic have subsided. If the spine is fused, mobility restrictions are more severe. Usually, turning is allowed if done in the log-rolling fashion.

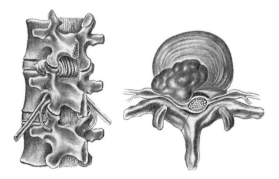

**Fig. 38-8** Herniated nucleus pulposus and laminectomy. *(From Thompson JM, McFarland G, Kirsch J, et al: Mosby's clinical nursing, ed 5, St Louis, 2002, Mosby.)*

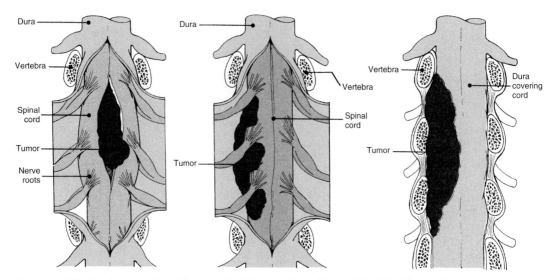

**Fig. 38-9**   Spinal cord tumors. *(From Thompson JM, McFarland G, Kirsch J, et al: Mosby's clinical nursing, ed 5, St Louis, 2002, Mosby.)*

As in all spinal procedures, sensory function and motor strength of the extremities should be assessed along with the vital signs in the PACU. Evidence of CSF leaks must be sought on dressings and bed linens.

### Intraspinal Neoplasms

Intraspinal neoplasms may occur at any level of the cord from the foramen magnum to the sacral canal. Most of the tumors are found in the thoracic region because this is the longest subdivision of the spine. Cord compression and neurologic deficit produce symptoms similar to those produced by displaced fracture of the spine, but they usually develop and progress at a slower pace. Neurologic examination, myelography, and tomography are used to determine the exact location of the lesion.

Intraspinal tumors may arise from the cord or its coverings, from fibrous tissue, or as a result of metastatic disease (Fig. 38-9). For descriptive purposes, they are placed in the following subdivisions:

- Intramedullary tumors: Those that arise solely from the substance of the cord.
- Extradural-extramedullary tumors: Those that arise outside the dura, either in the epidural space, vertebrae, or surrounding tissues.
- Intradural-extramedullary tumors: Those that arise within or under the dura but do not invade the cord.
- Dumbbell tumors: Those that arise within the spinal canal and extend extraspinally along the nerve through the intervertebral foramen.

Early diagnosis and treatment are essential to prevent irreversible damage to the spinal cord. Eighty-five percent of intraspinal neoplasms are benign. The remainder are either primarily malignant or caused by metastasis. The decision to intervene surgically is made after the patient's general condition and life expectancy are considered. Also considered are other metastases and the type and location of the primary tumor.

Treatment consists of laminectomy, surgical exploration, and excision of the mass. Most benign tumors can be excised completely. Prognosis depends on the location of the tumor, the severity and duration of the preoperative neurologic deficit, and whether the tumor is completely removable. Intramedullary tumors are associated with a more guarded prognosis because they can rarely be excised without increasing the neurologic deficit.

### Postoperative Care for Spinal Cord Injury Surgical Interventions

Perianesthesia care of patients for lumbar surgery should include keeping the head of the bed flat and log rolling the patient to help maintain proper body alignment, promote skin integrity, and minimize discomfort. The surgical site should be inspected for drainage and hematoma, and if spinal fusion was performed, the donor site should also be inspected. Assessment of the patient's comfort should be performed frequently because of muscle spasms that are often associated with lumbar surgery. The neurologic examination should include assessment of sensation in the lower extremities and notation of the presence of tingling, numbness, or paralysis. The pedal pulses, color, temperature, and capillary refill of the lower extremities should also be assessed.

## SUMMARY

Perianesthesia care of the neurosurgical patient can be quite complex. However, the introduction of modern drugs and monitors and our improved understanding of patient's physiology should facilitate the removal of many of the challenges in the care of these patients. Consequently, for a neurosurgical procedure or central nervous system trauma that necessitates radiologic studies with anesthesia, the anatomy and physiology (see Chapter 10) and pathophysiology have been described to include the monitoring equipment that can be used, all in an effort to ensure that outcomes are as favorable as possible. Besides the basic principles of PACU nursing management, which include airway management, ventilatory assistance, and hemodynamic support, the neurosurgical case entails unique preparation and management. This chapter has provided an in-depth discussion of the perianesthesia care of the neurosurgical patient in an effort to facilitate favorable outcomes.

## BIBLIOGRAPHY

Aitkenhead A, Smith G, Rowbotham D: *Textbook of anaesthesia*, ed 5, 2007, Churchill Livingstone.

Alspach J: *Core curriculum for critical care nursing*, ed 6, Philadelphia, 2005, Saunders.

Atlee J: *Complications in anesthesia*, ed 2, Philadelphia, 2007, Saunders.

Barash P, Cullen B, Stoelting R: *Clinical anesthesia*, ed 5, Philadelphia, 2005, Lippincott Williams & Wilkins.

Barker E: *Neuroscience nursing*, ed 3, St Louis, 2007, Mosby.

Baumann C: Image guided surgery in the treatment of malignant brain tumors, *J Neurosci Nurs* 30(6):362–363, 1998.

Brunton L, Lazo J, Parker K: *Goodman and Gilman's the pharmacological basis of therapeutics*, ed 11, New York, 2005, McGraw-Hill Professional.

Buckley DA, Guanci MM: Spinal cord trauma, *Nurs Clin North Am* 34(3):661–687, 1999.

Chulay M, Burns S: *AACN essentials of critical care*, St Louis, 2005, AACN.

Cottrell J, Smith D: *Anesthesia and neurosurgery*, ed 4, St Louis, 2001, Mosby.

DeFazio-Quinn D, Schick L: *PeriAnesthesia nursing core curriculum*, Philadelphia, 2004, Saunders.

Dodson B: Pharmacology of anesthetic agents and adjuncts used in neuroanesthesia, *Anesthesia Today* 6(2):15–19, 1995.

Duffy C, Matta B: Sevoflurane and anesthesia for neurosurgery: a review, *J Neurosurg Anesthesiol* 12(2):128–140, 2000.

Evers A, Maze M: *Anesthetic pharmacology: physiologic principles and clinical practice*, Philadelphia, 2004, Churchill Livingstone.

Fisher L: *Benumof's anesthesia and uncommon diseases*, ed 5, Philadelphia, 2007, Saunders.

Fleisher L: *Anesthesia & perioperative complications*, ed 5, St Louis, 2006, Mosby.

Gallager C, Issenberg B: *Simulation in anesthesia*, Philadelphia, 2007, Saunders.

Ganong W: *Review of medical physiology*, ed 22, New York, 2005, McGraw-Hill Medical.

Grande C, editor: Textbook of trauma anesthesia and critical care, St Louis, 1993, Mosby.

Guyton A, Hall J: *Textbook of medical physiology*, ed 11, Philadelphia, 2006, Saunders.

Hickey J: *The clinical practice of neurological and neurosurgical nursing*, ed 4, Philadelphia, 1997, Lippincott-Raven.

Hilton G, Frei J: High-dose methylprednisolone in the treatment of spinal cord injuries, *Heart Lung* 20(6):675–680, 2001.

Juarez VJ, Lyons M: Interrater reliability of the Glasgow coma scale, *J Neurosci Nurs* 27(5):283–286, 1995.

Kajs-Wyllie M: Antihypertensive treatment for the neurological patient: a nursing challenge, *J Neurosci Nurs* 31(3):141–151, 1999.

Kirkness CJ, Mitchell PH, Burr RL: Intracranial pressure waveform analysis: clinical and research implications, *J Neurosci Nurs* 30(5):271–277, 2000.

Lake C, Hines R, Blitt C: *Clinical monitoring: practical applications for anesthesia and critical care*, Philadelphia, 2001, Saunders.

Leith B: Pharmacological management of pain after intracranial surgery, *J Neurosci Nurs* 30(1):220–224, 1998.

Longnecker D, Murphy F: *Dripps, Eckenhoff, Vandam introduction to anesthesia*, ed 9, Philadelphia, 1997, Saunders.

Longnecker D, Tinker J, Morgan G: *Principles and practice of anesthesiology*, ed 2, St Louis, 1998, Mosby.

Luchka S: Working with ICP monitors, *RN* 54(4):34–37, 1991.

Lucke KT: Pulmonary management following SCI, *J Neurosci Nurs* 30(2):91–103, 1998.

McCance K, Huether S: *Pathophysiology: the biologic basis for disease in adults and children*, ed 5, St Louis, 2006, Mosby.

Miller R, editor: *Anesthesia*, ed 6, Philadelphia, 2005, Churchill Livingstone.

Minton MS, Hickey JV: A primer of neuroanatomy and neurophysiology, *Nurs Clin North Am* 34(3):555–572, 1999.

NURSING CARE IN THE PACU

Nagelhout J, Zaglaniczy K: *Nurse anesthesia*, ed 3, St Louis, 2005, Saunders.

Neatherlin JS: Foundation for practice, *Nurs Clin North Am* 34(3):573–592, 1999.

Newfield P, Cottrell J: *Handbook of neuroanesthesia*, Philadelphia, 1999, Lippincott Williams and Wilkins.

Nikas DL: The neurologic system. In Alspach J, editor: *AACN's core curriculam for critical care nursing*, ed 5, Philadelphia, 1998, Saunders.

Pendergast V, Sullivan C: Acute spinal cord injury, *Crit Care Nurs Clin North Am* 12(4):499–508, 2000.

Pope W: External ventriculostomy: a practical application for the acute care nurse, *J Neurosci Nurs* 30(3):185–190, 1998.

Schultz DL: The role of neuroscience nurse in lumbar fusion, *J Neurosci Nurs* 27(2):90–95, 1995.

Shpritz DW: The neurosurgical patient. In Litwack K, editor: *ASPAN: core curriculam for perianesthesia nursing practice*, ed 4, Philadelphia, 1999, Saunders.

Shpritz DW: Neurodiagnostic studies, *Nurs Clin North Am* 34(3):593–606, 1999.

Stoelting R: *Pharmacology and physiology in anesthetic practice*, ed 3, Philadelphia, 1999, Lippincott-Raven.

Stoelting R, Miller R: *Basics of anesthesia*, ed 5, Philadelphia, 2007, Churchill Livingstone.

Sullivan J: Positioning of patients with severe traumatic brain injury: research-based practice, *J Neurosci Nurs* 32(4):204–209, 2000.

Tempelhoff R: The new inhalation anesthetics desflurane and sevoflurane are valuable additions to the practice of neuroanesthesia, *J Neurosurg Anesthesiol* 9(1):69–71, 1997.

Thompson JM, McFarland G, Hirsch J: *Mosby's clinical nursing*, ed 5, Philadelphia, 2002, Mosby.

White CL, Pokrupa RP, Chan MH: An evaluation of the effectiveness of patient-controlled analgesia after spinal surgery, *J Neurosci Nurs* 30(1):225–232, 1998.

White P: *Perioperative drug manual*, ed 2, Philadelphia, 2005, Saunders.

Young W: Effects of desflurane on the central nervous system, *Anesthesia Analgesia* 75:S32–S37, 1992.

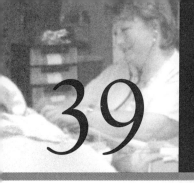

# 39

# CARE OF THE THYROID AND PARATHYROID SURGICAL PATIENT

Matthew D. Byrne, RN, MS, CPAN
Joni M. Brady, RN, MSN, CAPA

Surgery of the thyroid gland was first performed around 500 AD, and the first successful removal of goiter occurred in 1000 AD. By the 1800s, numerous thyroidectomies had been performed; however, nearly half of the patients died after surgery as a result of tetany. This morbidity rate was secondary to the removal of the parathyroid glands, whose function was not well understood at the time. In the early 1900s, a greater understanding of the role of the parathyroid glands promoted the subtotal thyroidectomy procedure, which significantly reduced postoperative complications. In the late 1990s, the endoscopic thyroidectomy and minimally invasive radio-guided parathyroidectomy techniques further reduced perioperative and postoperative complications. These techniques are performed on an outpatient basis for many patients. The type of thyroid surgical procedure chosen depends on the patient's age, tumor cell type and size, presence of encapsulated or extracapsular tumor, and any invasion of adjacent structures (Fig. 39-1).

## DEFINITIONS

**Bilateral Subtotal Thyroidectomy:** Removal of most of the thyroid tissue in both lobes, with a small remnant of thyroid tissue left at the back portion of the thyroid to protect the parathyroid glands and prevent recurrent laryngeal nerve damage, a potential complication associated with total thyroidectomy.

**Endoscopic Thyroidectomy:** Minimally invasive surgical removal of small (< 3 cm) single-nodule thyroid lesions or cysts that show no evidence of malignant disease on biopsy results. Uses three to four small incisions that produce less pain, a faster return to normal activity, less scarring, and a magnification of the surgical site with the use of an endoscope. May be performed on an outpatient basis.

**Minimally Invasive Radio-Guided Parathyroidectomy (MIRP):** Pioneered in 1996; a technique of minimal invasiveness for removal of diseased parathyroid lobe with intraoperative nuclear mapping. Because 90% of patients have only one diseased lobe, this technique allows for preservation of the remaining healthy tissue and minimizes potential postoperative complications. May be performed with local anesthesia on an outpatient basis.

**Near Total Thyroidectomy:** Removal of the thyroid gland with the exception of a very small portion that remains on the opposite side of the thyroid.

**Parathyroidectomy:** Excision of one or more diseased parathyroid glands.

**Thyroidectomy:** Total excision of the thyroid gland, with the parathyroid glands left intact. Total thyroidectomy is normally only performed in patients with medullary malignant disease because total thyroidectomy renders the patient immediately unable to produce any thyroid hormone, thus requiring supplementation with thyroid hormone for the remainder of the patient's life. Those patients who are not candidates for radioablation may also be considered for thyroidectomy.

**Thyroid Lobectomy With Isthmisectomy:** Removal of one lobe of the thyroid and the isthmus that connects the two lobes.

## ANESTHESIA

Surgery on the thyroid and parathyroid glands is commonly performed with general anesthesia. Postoperative care indicated for a patient receiving general anesthesia is instituted in the postanesthesia care unit (PACU). Minimally invasive radio-guided parathyroidectomy is performed with local anesthesia, which minimizes the recovery requirements of these patients.

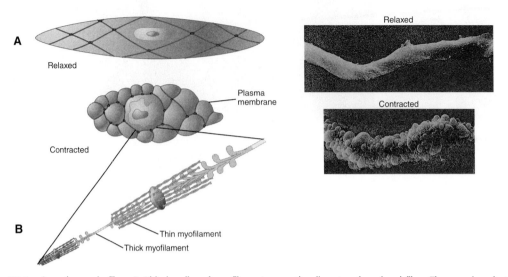

**Fig. 39-1**    Smooth muscle fiber. **A,** Thin bundles of myofilaments span the diameter of a relaxed fiber. The scanning electron micrograph *(right)* shows that the surface of the cell is rather flat when the fiber is relaxed. **B,** During contraction, sliding of the myofilaments causes the fiber to shorten by "balling up." The micrograph shows that the fiber becomes shorter and thicker and exhibits "dimples" where the myofilament bundles are pulling on the plasma membrane.

## PERIANESTHESIA NURSING CARE

### Positioning

If the patient's condition is minimally responsive on arrival to the PACU, the patient should be placed in a side-lying position to protect the airway. Once the patient is responsive, or if the patient is responsive on admission, a semi-Fowler's position of at least 30 degrees elevation is used to promote venous return. The nurse must position the patient with specific attention given to supporting the head and neck to prevent undue tension on the suture line. The patient is instructed to support the head and neck during position changes by placing both hands behind the neck.

### Cardiopulmonary Assessment and Care

Immediate postoperative observations include close attention to respiratory function, which may be compromised by hemorrhage, venous oozing, or laryngeal edema. The nurse should carefully monitor the airway, respiratory rate, breath sounds, and pulse oximetry. Signs and symptoms of impending respiratory obstruction, such as tracheal deviation, stridor, air hunger, or falling oxygen saturations, should be immediately reported to the anesthesia provider and surgeon. In some situations, immediate reintubation or tracheostomy may be necessary, and the associated reintubation or tracheostomy equipment should be readily available.

Humidified oxygen can help to ease a sore throat encountered after endotracheal intubation, airway surgery, and general anesthesia. Hypertension and transient elevations of blood pressure should be avoided to decrease stress on sutures lines and to avoid hematoma and hemorrhage. The prevention and management of heavy coughing, nausea, vomiting, or dry retching are essential.

### Pain Management

Pain may be minimal after thyroidectomy and parathyroidectomy surgeries performed on an outpatient basis. Postoperative analgesia requirements are greater in the open procedure population. Small doses of an opioid such as fentanyl or morphine may be needed in the first 24 hours for patients admitted to a facility. Severe pain is an abnormal finding that may indicate unexpected bleeding or nerve damage and is a risk factor for unwanted hypertension. Severe pain requires an immediate report to the attending surgeon.

### Dressings and Drains

Postoperative dressings are minimal, and drains are generally not required. Some disagreement exists about surgical drains: namely, whether or not they can be useful in both identification and prevention of hematomas.[1,2] Drains are generally indicated only when a large space is left after removal of a tumor or goiter.

Postoperative drainage is minimal and should not visibly soak through the dressing. The perianesthesia nurse should assess the patient for usual symptoms of hemorrhage, watch for swelling of the neck, and assess the back of the neck for drainage. Any excess bleeding requires immediate reporting to the surgeon.

## Intake and Output

As with any surgical patient, monitoring of intake and output is important in the evaluation of cardiovascular stability. Because many thyroid surgeries are performed on an outpatient basis, ensuring that the patient is capable of tolerating oral fluids before discharge is particularly important. Routine phonation and swallowing evaluations serve to rule out laryngeal nerve damage that could precipitate aspiration. Many facilities require the patient to void before discharge or within a specified number of hours after discharge.

## Complications

As knowledge of thyroid and parathyroid function and interventional surgical techniques has improved, postoperative complication rates have decreased and now reportedly occur in less than 1% of patients. Complications are largely attributed to surgeon skill level, type and invasiveness of tumor, anatomic visualization during the procedure, and the patient's preoperative thyroid state.

*Bleeding and Airway/Respiratory Compromise.* As surgical techniques have become more refined and less invasive, the risks of postoperative bleeding have significantly reduced. However, postoperative bleeding may cause tracheal compression and subsequent airway obstruction. Excessive bleeding, as previously discussed, should be reported to the surgeon immediately. Respiratory difficulties that range from dropping oxygen saturations to stridor may result from airway obstruction or compromise from bleeding, vocal cord and laryngeal nerve damage, laryngeal edema, or pneumothorax in cases that involve extensive dissection. Neck swelling; pain, pressure, or fullness in the neck; and dysphonia or hoarse voice can be specific indications of bleeding and the potential for airway/respiratory compromise.

*Recurrent Laryngeal Nerve Injury.* The recurrent laryngeal nerve may be injured from clamping, compression, severing, or stretching during surgery. Symptoms of bilateral recurrent laryngeal nerve injury may indicate life-threatening airway obstruction and may necessitate immediate intervention, including the potential for reintubation and tracheostomy. Unilateral recurrent laryngeal nerve injury may present as voice changes and a weak cough, but in some cases, no outward signs may appear that this damage has actually occurred. Aspiration is a potential risk. Nerve injury is generally transient and may be treated with time or corticosteroids.

*Hypoparathyroidism and Hypocalcemia.* Hypoparathyroidism is a complication that may occur after total thyroidectomy or total parathyroidectomy. The condition may be caused by intentional removal of the parathyroid glands or inadvertent or unavoidable damage during thyroidectomy. This complication manifests as hypocalcemia and is usually transient. Signs and symptoms of hypocalcemia, which are caused by neuromuscular irritability, rarely occur in the immediate postoperative period but may present 24 to 72 hours after surgery. Symptoms include numbness and tingling of the fingers and toes and around the mouth, muscle cramps (tetany), and spasm. If calcium levels are not restored, seizures and laryngeal stridor are imminent.

Assessment of any patient who verbalizes tingling symptoms includes testing for the presence of Chvostek's sign (the development of a lip twitch or facial spasm when the cheek is tapped over the facial nerve) and Trousseau's sign (the development of a carpal spasm when a blood pressure cuff is applied and circulation transiently occluded). Laboratory findings, Chvostek's sign, and an evaluation of carpopedal spasms (clonus in the feet when dorsiflexed) are preferred to assessing for Trousseau's sign, which can sometimes be painful. Definitive treatment involves intravenous administration of calcium. Although both calcium chloride and calcium gluconate may be used, calcium gluconate is preferred for its greater bioavailability and less arrhythmogenic potential. If intravenous calcium is administered, it is given via slow push with continuous electrocardiographic monitoring before, during, and after the infusion.

*Thyroid Storm.* Thyroid storm or thyrotoxic crisis is a rare complication that may occur after surgical manipulation of a hyperactive thyroid. Rapid diagnosis of the cause for an apparent postoperative hypermetabolic state is critical for appropriate treatment of the problem. Malignant hyperthermia (another potential cause for postanesthetic hypermetabolic state) and thyroid storm must be differentiated because these disorders have significantly different treatment algorithms.

With ideal conditions, an overactive thyroid is controlled before surgery with medications and the patient arrives in the preoperative setting in a euthyroid state. Thyroid storm more commonly occurs in a patient with hyperthyroidism and thyrotoxicosis who is seen for an emergent procedure or in circumstances when an inadequate preoperative time period is available to bring down thyroid levels. The patient may have fever and tachycardia develop during surgery. After surgery, additional symptoms in the hypermetabolic state may include agitation, disorientation, hypertension, tachycardia, and heart failure that may proceed to shock. Treatment should focus on bringing down the patient's thyroid levels, maintaining cardiopulmonary integrity, and reducing the other signs and symptoms of hypermetabolism, most notably hyperthermia. Treatment generally includes the administration of beta blockers, iodine, vasopressors, fluid support, oxygen, salicylates, cooling measures, and steroids.

**Infection.** Disagreement exists about the need for routine antibiotics because the incidence of postoperative infection in patients who have undergone thyroid and parathyroid surgery is rare. Any symptoms of postoperative infection should be investigated and treated with appropriate antibiotic therapy and wound care.

# SUMMARY

Increased knowledge of the thyroid and parathyroid functions and improved surgical techniques significantly decreased the length of stay and postoperative complication rates in the thyroid surgical population. Surgery on the thyroid and parathyroid glands is commonly performed with general anesthesia, and postoperative nursing care is focused on the recovery of a patient from general anesthesia. Selected procedures performed with local anesthesia minimize postoperative recovery requirements and length of stay.

Postoperative nursing assessment and treatment focuses on the potential for cardiopulmonary compromise from hemorrhage, venous oozing or laryngeal edema, pain management, proper positioning to minimize suture line stress, and ongoing assessment of the operative dressing and intake and output status. Although rare, possible complications of thyroid surgery include inferior or superior laryngeal nerve damage with possible vocal cord paralysis; laryngeal stridor; airway and respiratory compromise; bleeding that causes cervical or neck hematoma and requires surgical evacuation; hypocalcemia; tetany, seizures, and mental disturbances; thyroid storm; and infection. Recognition of potential complications and implementation of appropriate and rapid treatment interventions are essential for good postoperative outcomes.

# REFERENCES

1. Carty, SE: Prevention and management of complications in parathyroid surgery, *Otol Clin North Am* 37:897-907, 2004.

2. Fewins J, Simpson CB, Miller FR: Complications of thyroid and parathyroid surgery, *Otol Clin North Am* 36:189-206, 2003.

# BIBLIOGRAPHY

AACE/AME Task Force on Thyroid Nodules: American association of clinical endocrinologists and associazione medici endocrinologi medical guidelines for clinical practice for the diagnosis and management of thyroid nodules, *Endocrine Pract* 12:63-102, 2006.

De Manicor NA: Primary hyperparathyroidism: a case study, *J PeriAnesthesia Nurs* 19:334-344, 2004.

Holcomb S: Thyroid diseases: a primer for the critical care nurse, *Dimens Crit Care Nurs* 21:127-133, 2002.

Johnson K: Laparoscopic or open removal of parathyroid? *Intern Med News* 38:28, 2005.

Langley RW, Burch HB: Perioperative management of the thyrotoxic patient, *Endocrinol Metabolism Clin North Am* 32:519-534, 2003.

Mazzaferri EL, Harmer C, Mallick UK, et al: *Practical management of thyroid cancer: a multidisciplinary approach*, New York, 2005, Springer.

McKennis A, Waddington C: *Nursing interventions for potential complications after thyroidectomy*, available at at http://www.sohnnurse.com/thyroidectomy.html; accessed November 14, 2006.

Noble KA: Thyroid storm, *J PeriAnesthesia Nurs* 21:119-125, 2006.

Oertli D, Udelsman R, editors: *Surgery of the thyroid and parathyroid glands*, New York, 2007, Springer.

Patel M, Rohit G, Rice DH: Fibrin glue in thyroid and parathyroid surgery: is under-flap suction still necessary? *Ear, Nose Throat J* 85:530-532, 2006.

Randolph G: *Surgery of the thyroid and parathyroid glands*, Philadelphia, 2003, Saunders.

Sonner JM, Hynson JM, Clark O: Nausea and vomiting following thyroid and parathyroid surgery, *J Clin Anesthesia* 9:398-402, 1997.

Takesuye D, Breathauer S, Thiringer JK, et al: Practice analysis: techniques of head and neck surgeons and general surgeons performing thyroidectomy for cancer, *Qual Manage Health Care* 15:257-262, 2006.

Thyroid Carcinoma Task Force: AACE/AAES medical/surgical guidelines for clinical practice: management of thyroid carcinoma. *Endocrine Pract Official J Am Coll Endocrinol Am Assoc Clin Endocrinologists* 7:202-220, 2001.

Watkinson JC, editor: British Thyroid Association: The British thyroid association guidelines for the management of thyroid cancer in adults, *Nucl Med Commun* 25:897-900, 2004.

Zarnegar R, Brunaud L, Clark OH: Prevention, evaluation, and management of complications following thyroidectomy for thyroid carcinoma, *Endocrinol Metabolism Clin North Am* 32:483-502, 2003.

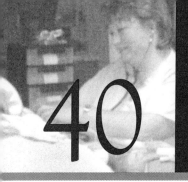

# 40

# CARE OF THE GASTROINTESTINAL, ABDOMINAL, AND ANORECTAL SURGICAL PATIENT

*Denise O'Brien, MSN, APRN,BC, CPAN, CAPA, FAAN*

Care of the patient after abdominal surgery or surgery on the gastrointestinal tract is an extremely broad subject. Surgical intervention within the abdominal cavity is generally directed toward restoration of normal function and therefore involves repair of congenital abnormalities, reconstruction of deformities, removal of obstructions to restore patency of the gastrointestinal tract and the biliary tract, treatment of malignant disease, and maintenance of the integrity of related organs, such as the liver, pancreas, and spleen (Fig. 40-1).

## DEFINITIONS

**Antrectomy:** Removal of the lower part of the stomach.

**Appendectomy:** Removal of the vermiform appendix, performed with an open or laparoscopic technique.

**Cholecystectomy:** Removal of the gallbladder; the procedure may be performed with an open or a laparoscopic approach.

**Cholecystostomy:** Establishment of an opening into the gallbladder to permit drainage of the organ and the removal of stones. This procedure is performed infrequently except to provide relief in a patient with an extremely debilitated and unstable condition. This procedure is usually performed percutaneously in the radiology suite.

**Colostomy:** Opening of the colon onto the abdomen; may be permanent or temporary, single or double lumen. May be performed with either an open procedure or a laparoscopic approach.

**Diverticulum:** A "herniation" of mucosa/submucosa through a weakness in a muscular wall, most commonly in the sigmoid colon, although one may be found anywhere in the gastrointestinal (GI) tract.

**Endoscopic Retrograde Cholangiopancreatography (ERCP):** A side-viewing fiberoptic endoscope is used to cannulate pancreatic and biliary ducts through the ampulla of Vater for cholangiography, pancreatography, stone removal, and invasive manipulation such as sphincterotomy.

**Endoscopy:** Visualization of a body cavity with a lighted tube or scope. Most commonly performed to visualize the inside of the esophagus, stomach, and duodenum or colon.

**Esophagogastroduodenoscopy (EGD):** Passage of a fiberoptic endoscope, usually with topical anesthesia and intravenous sedation, to view the esophagus, stomach, and duodenum. Biopsies or control of bleeding may also be performed with this procedure.

**Esophagoscopy:** Direct visualization of the esophagus and cardia of the stomach by means of a lighted instrument (esophagoscope). Esophagoscopy may be used to obtain a tissue biopsy or secretions for study to aid in diagnosis.

**Gastrectomy:** Removal of the stomach. If a subtotal gastrectomy is done, in which only part of the stomach is removed, the procedure is typically expressed as a percentage (usually 60% to 80%; can be much as 95%), also called gastric resection (Fig. 40-2, A). Total gastrectomies are most commonly performed for cancers in the proximal part of the stomach.

**Gastroplasty:** Procedure to reduce the digestive capacity of the stomach by shortening the small intestine or shrinking the stomach's effective size for weight reduction. The three most common bariatric procedures performed include laparoscopic adjustable gastric banding, vertical banded gastroplasty, and Roux-en-Y gastric bypass. Laparoscopic banding procedure requires no alteration or removal of the stomach; an adjustable band is placed around the proximal stomach to reduce gastric size, creating a small pouch. Vertical banded gastroplasty includes the creation with staples of a small stomach pouch in the proximal stomach and placement of a Marlex (polypropylene mesh) band to restrict the stomach size. Roux-en-Y gastric bypass is a malabsorptive and restrictive procedure in which the stomach is stapled and transected into two compartments; the smaller proximal stomach pouch is anastomosed to the jejunum, bypassing

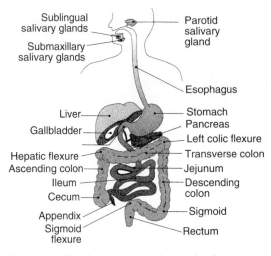

**Fig. 40-1**   Digestive system and its associated structures. *(From Sole ML, Klein D, Moseley M: Introduction to critical care nursing, ed 4, Philadelphia, 2005, Saunders.)*

the distal stomach, duodenum, and proximal jejunum. Vertical banded gastroplasty and Roux-en-Y gastric bypass procedures may be performed either laparoscopically or as open procedures.

**Gastroscopy:** Direct inspection of the stomach with possible removal of a tissue specimen by means of a lighted instrument (gastroscope); bleeding can also be controlled with this procedure.

**Hemorrhoidectomy:** Surgical excision of dilated veins of the rectum.

**Hernia:** The displacement of any viscus (usually bowel) or tissue through a congenital or acquired opening or defect in the wall of its natural cavity, most commonly the muscular wall of the abdomen. Usually, this term is applied to protrusion of abdominal viscera; however, it is actually the defect itself through which abdominal contents have protruded.

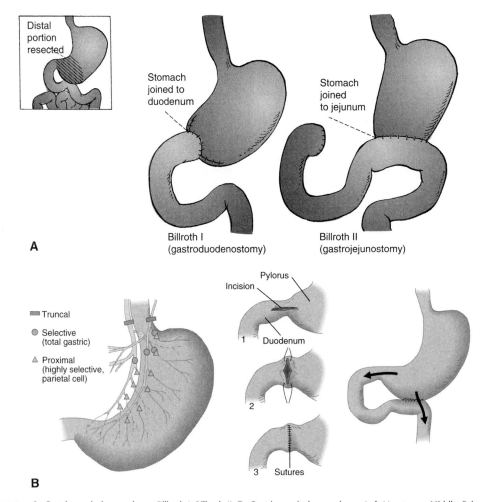

**Fig. 40-2   A,** Gastric surgical procedures: Billroth I, Billroth II. **B,** Gastric surgical procedures. *Left*, Vagotomy. *Middle*, Pyloroplasty. *Right*, Gastroenterostomy. *(From Black JM, Hawks JH: Medical-surgical nursing: clinical management for positive outcomes, ed 7, St Louis, 2005, Saunders.)*

**Herniorrhaphy:** Repair of a hernia. Hernias are classified according to anatomic site and condition of the viscus that has protruded. Reducible hernias are those in which the bowel or contents of the hernia sac can be replaced into the normal cavity. An irreducible, or incarcerated, hernia is one in which the contents cannot be replaced. A strangulated hernia is one in which the blood supply to the protruding segment of bowel is obstructed. When a segment of bowel becomes strangulated, it rapidly becomes necrotic. A strangulated hernia constitutes a surgical emergency. Hernias can be repaired with an open or laparoscopic technique.

**Herniorrhaphy, Diaphragmatic:** Replacement of abdominal contents that have entered the thorax through a defect in the diaphragm and repair of the diaphragmatic defect.

**Herniorrhaphy, Epigastric and Hypogastric:** Repair and closure of the abdominal wall defect.

**Herniorrhaphy, Femoral:** A defect in the region of the femoral ring, which is located just below Poupart's (inguinal) ligament and medial to the femoral vein. Femoral hernias are seldom found in children and occur most often in women.

**Herniorrhaphy, Incisional:** Repair of a defect in the abdominal wall that was a prior site of placement of a surgical incision. These types of repairs commonly involve placement of prosthetic (synthetic) mesh (e.g., Marlex, Gore-Tex, Prolened).

**Herniorrhaphy, Inguinal:** Repair of a defect in the inguinal region; may be direct (through Hesselbach's triangle) or an indirect (through the internal ring) inguinal hernia (Fig. 40-3). These repairs also commonly use some type of prosthetic mesh.

**Herniorrhaphy, Umbilical:** Reconstruction of the abdominal wall beneath the umbilicus (umbilical ring); usually occurs in pediatric patients and is most common in African-American infants. The condition often closes spontaneously in infants before 2 years of age; therefore, these repairs should generally not be performed until after the age of 2 years.

**Ileostomy:** Opening of the ileum to the surface of the abdomen. Most commonly used to treat inflammatory conditions of the bowel, such as ulcerative colitis and regional enteritis, and to provide a permanent or temporary stoma after emergency surgery for obstruction or cancer.

**Intussusception:** Telescoping of the bowel into itself.

**Laparoscopy (Peritoneoscopy):** Direct visualization of the peritoneal cavity by means of a lighted instrument (often connected to a color

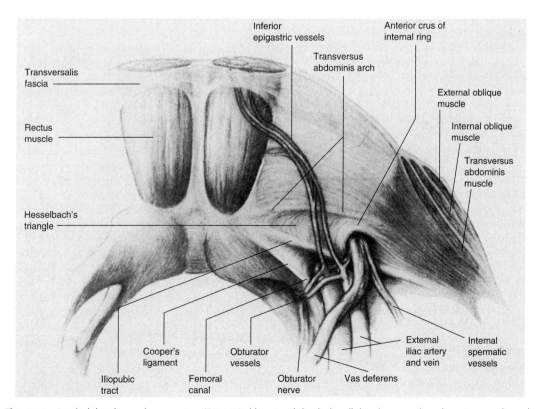

**Fig. 40-3** Inguinal hernia repair: anatomy. *(From Madden JL: Abdominal wall hernias: an atlas of anatomy and repair, Philadelphia, 1989, Saunders.)*

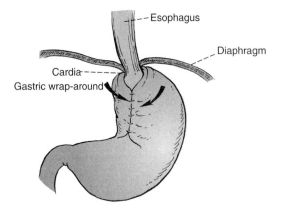

Fig. 40-4    Hiatal hernia repair with gastric wrap (Nissen fundoplication). *(From Black JM, Hawks JH: Medical-surgical nursing: clinical management for positive outcomes, ed 7, St Louis, 2005, Saunders.)*

video monitor) inserted through the abdominal wall via a stab wound. An increasing number of abdominal procedures are performed assisted via laparoscopy (lap-assisted). Gastrointestinal or abdominal procedures currently performed via laparoscopy include cholecystectomy, truncal vagotomy, gastrojejunostomy, splenectomy, Nissen fundoplication (Fig. 40-4), inguinal herniorrhaphy, appendectomy, jejunostomy, colostomy, colectomy, and ileocolectomy.

**Laparotomy (Celiotomy):** An opening made through the abdominal wall into the peritoneal cavity, usually for exploratory purposes. If an abnormality is found, the operation is usually named according to the procedure or procedures carried out.

**Pancreaticoduodenectomy (Whipple Procedure):** Removal of the head of the pancreas, the entire duodenum, the gallbladder, a portion of the jejunum, the distal third of the stomach, and the lower half of the common bile duct, with reestablishment of continuity of the biliary, pancreatic, and gastrointestinal systems. The procedure, which is used primarily for the treatment of malignant disease of the pancreas and duodenum, is associated with a 2% to 5% risk of mortality. Sometimes a pylorus-sparing procedure is performed, which leaves the entire stomach intact.

**Percutaneous Endoscopic Gastrostomy (PEG):** Endoscopic procedure for the insertion of a tube into the stomach, either for the purpose of decompression or feeding, performed with local anesthesia and intravenous sedation.

**Pyloromyotomy (Fredet-Ramstedt Operation):** Enlargement of the lumen of the pylorus with longitudinal splitting of the hypertrophied circular muscle without severing of the mucosa; used as treatment for pyloric stenosis. Pyloric stenosis is most common in firstborn male infants.

**Pyloroplasty:** A longitudinal incision made in the pylorus (full-thickness) and closed transversely to permit the muscle to relax and establish an enlarged outlet. Heineke-Mikulicz is the most common type of procedure (Fig. 40-2, *B*).

**Splenectomy:** Removal of the spleen.

**Transduodenal Sphincterotomy:** Partial division of the sphincter of Oddi and exploration of the common bile duct for treatment of recurrent attacks of acute pancreatitis caused by formation of calculi in the pancreatic duct or blockage of the sphincter of Oddi. May also be used in treatment of biliary stones.

**Vagotomy:** Division (usually with frozen section) of branches of the vagus nerve that innervate the stomach to reduce acid secretion (see Fig. 40-2, *B*). Rarely done any more. Previously used as part of the surgical treatment of peptic ulcer disease. Since the discovery of *Helicobacter pylori*, virtually all peptic ulcer disease is now treated medically. Surgical treatment of peptic ulcer disease is now reserved only for its complications and is rarely necessary.

**Volvulus:** Intestinal obstruction as a result of twisting of the bowel.

## GENERAL CARE AFTER ABDOMINAL SURGERY

Abdominal or gastrointestinal surgery may be performed with local, regional, or general anesthesia. The choice of anesthesia varies with the type of procedure, the patient's cardiac and pulmonary status, and the surgeon's need for muscle relaxation. Usually, only short simple procedures are performed with local or regional (spinal or epidural) anesthesia. Diagnostic procedures such as endoscopy, biopsy, and percutaneous gastrostomy often are performed with local anesthesia with appropriate sedation. Inguinal or femoral herniorrhaphies are often performed with local, spinal or epidural, or general anesthesia. Most other abdominal surgical and laparoscopic procedures are performed with general anesthesia. Virtually all laparoscopic procedures require general anesthesia because of the need for relaxation of the abdominal wall and the need to control the patient's respirations.

A number of abdominopelvic incisions have been developed and are commonly used (Fig. 40-5). An ideal incision ensures ease of entrance, maximal exposure of the operative site, and minimal trauma. It should also provide good primary wound healing with maximal wound strength.

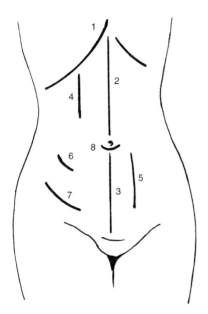

**Fig. 40-5** Commonly used abdominal incisions. *1*, Kocher's incision: *right side*, gallbladder and biliary tract surgery; *left side*, splenectomy. *2*, Upper abdominal midline incision: rapid entry to control bleeding ulcer. *3*, Lower abdominal midline incision: female reproductive system. *4*, Upper paramedian incision: *right side*, biliary tract surgery, cholecystectomy; *left side*, splenectomy, gastrectomy, vagotomy, hiatal hernia repair. *5*, Lower paramedian incision: *right side*, appendectomy, small bowel resection; *left side*, sigmoid colon resection. *6*, McBurney's incision: appendectomy. *7*, Inguinal incision: inguinal herniorrhaphy. *8*, Infraumbilical: umbilical herniorrhaphy.

The reader should review Chapters 26 through 31 for general care after surgery.

## Perianesthesia Care

As with any procedure, the surgeon and anesthesia care provider should give the perianesthesia nurse a full report on the anesthesia used and the procedure performed. With complicated abdominal procedures, especially those that involve extensive resection or rerouting of the gastrointestinal tract, the surgeon may draw a diagram of the procedure performed, along with the incisions and drainage tubes that are present. This action assists those who are caring for the patient in an assessment of the wounds, dressings, and expected drainage. The surgeon can draw this diagram on the nursing care plan, which should be initiated on the patient's admission to the postanesthesia care unit (PACU), so that continuity of information is ensured.

*Positioning.* After abdominal surgery, patients are often positioned on the side until laryngeal reflexes have started to return. They are then placed in a semi-Fowler's position to ease the tension on suture lines and to promote

respiratory effort. After some procedures on the esophagus, however, patients should be kept flat to avoid tension on the suture line. After hemorrhoidectomy, patients may assume any position of comfort, which is most likely on the right or left side.

*Dressings and Drains.* All dressings should be checked. The nurse must know what kind of incision was used and whether any drains are in place. If drains are in place, considerably more drainage can be expected. Drains are discussed in more detail in the specific procedures. Drainage should be assessed for character, volume, and odor. The nurse should determine who can or should remove the dressing if needed. Some surgeons reinforce the abdominal incision and dressing with a binder. They believe that this gives the incision valuable support. Others, however, believe that binders restrict respiratory effort and that this disadvantage outweighs the limited advantage of incisional support.

Because drainage is often copious after gastrointestinal surgery, frequent reinforcement of dressings may be necessary. Ask the surgeon for anticipated or expected amounts of drainage for the patient and procedure. If drainage becomes excessive (more than expected from the particular procedure), the surgeon should be notified and the incision directly inspected.

All tubes should be connected to the appropriate drainage devices, usually straight-gravity or suction drainage, as the surgeon specifies. Maintenance of the patency of these tubes is one of the most important nursing functions after gastrointestinal surgery. Irrigation of nasogastric tubes after esophageal or gastric surgery should be directed by the surgeon's orders.

*Respiratory Function.* The promotion of good respiratory function is a nursing priority for the patient who has had abdominal surgery. Painful abdominal incisions cause the patient to restrict chest expansion voluntarily, which is especially true with high abdominal incisions. The patient must be coached often in sustained maximal inspirations, coughing, and changing position to prevent respiratory complications. Assisting the patient with splinting of the incision and judicious use of pain medications aid in deep breathing and coughing and help prevent the development of atelectasis. Coughing and incentive spirometry in the PACU setting are valuable in promotion of respiratory function.

Frequent assessment of breath sounds during the postoperative period can alert the nurse to impending respiratory problems. An accidental nick into the diaphragm during upper abdominal surgery is possible and can result in respiratory distress. Positive pressure ventilation during anesthesia can also lead to respiratory problems. Breath sounds must be monitored closely to assess for pneumothorax and other respiratory complications.

***Fluid and Electrolyte Balance.*** Fluid and electrolyte shifts or losses can be substantial during gastrointestinal surgery. Losses continue after surgery through gastrointestinal tubes or other drains. For this reason, accurate intake and output records are mandatory. This recording begins with the intake and output report from the anesthesia care provider, which should be the first PACU entry. All drainage from incisions should be included in the assessment of electrolyte balance. Frequent serum electrolyte determinations may be necessary if losses are great. Intravenous fluids are used for replacement for at least the first 24 hours after surgery and at least until the nasogastric tube is removed. See Chapter 14 for a discussion of the specific problems in electrolyte loss from the gastrointestinal tract.

Urinary retention may become a problem after abdominal surgery because of incisional pain, opioid analgesics, anesthetics, and physiologic splinting. Urine output should be checked frequently, and accurate records should be kept. The nurse should also check for bladder distention and document the findings; the patient may not recognize the need to void, particularly after spinal or epidural anesthesia. Ultrasound scan examination of the bladder with a bedside scanner can aid in assessment of bladder status. The patient should void within 6 to 8 hours after surgery. If the patient has not voided by the time of discharge from the PACU, the receiving unit should be notified to check specifically for urinary retention. If permissible, the male patient may benefit by standing to void. If urinary retention causes pain, distends the abdomen, or becomes prolonged, urinary catheterization may become necessary. Patients who have had extensive surgery often return to the PACU with a urinary catheter in place. Accurate output records should be maintained.

## Care of the Patient with Nasogastric or Intestinal Tubes

Anesthesia and manipulation of the viscera during surgery cause gastric and colonic peristalsis to diminish or disappear completely for up to 5 days after surgery. Nasogastrointestinal or nasogastric tubes are commonly used after surgery to prevent the sequelae of this hypomotility. Edema at the operative site also can result in temporary obstruction. Decompression of the stomach, with removal of accumulated fluid and air, not only prevents vomiting and eases tension on the abdominal suture line but also increases the area's vascularity and thus improves its nutrition and reduces the risk of gastric anastomotic leak.

If gastric decompression is needed, short tubes are generally used today; long intestinal tubes are no longer used. Short tubes used include the Levin and the plastic Salem sump, which is a double-lumen nasogastric tube and is the most commonly used tube. The double lumen prevents excessive negative pressure from developing when the tube is connected to suction.

When the patient returns from the operating suite with a nasogastric tube in place, the nurse must ascertain why the tube was placed, where it was placed, and whether it should be connected to suction or to straight-gravity drainage. The physician often orders the tube to be connected to low-pressure intermittent suction (20 to 80 mm Hg). Usually only low-pressure intermittent suction is used because excessive negative pressure in either the stomach or the bowel pulls the mucosa into the lumen of the tube and can cause traumatic ulcers. For double-lumen nasogastric tubes, continuous suction at 40 to 60 mm Hg is usually ordered and is necessary for the tube to function properly. Keeping the open lumen above the midline improves functioning of the double-lumen tube.

***Tube Patency.*** Patency of the tube must be ensured. The nurse should observe for drainage from the tube. All characteristics of the drainage must be noted: consistency, color, odor, quantity, and any deviations from the expected drainage. After gastrointestinal surgery, initial drainage is bright red in small volumes but should become dark after 24 hours. Bloody drainage should not be expected from a nasogastric tube placed only for decompression of the stomach after biliary tract, liver, or splenic surgery. If no drainage is present, if the patient's abdomen becomes distended, or if the patient vomits around the nasogastric tube or has nausea, the tube may be clogged or the suction apparatus may be malfunctioning; check both. For maintenance of the patency of the nasogastric tube, irrigation with 20 to 30 mL of normal saline solution may be done every hour, or more frequently if necessary. Before irrigating the tube, check with the surgeon regarding the permissibility of nasogastric tube irrigation. Plain water in 20-mL amounts may be used to irrigate the tube without creation of electrolyte abnormalities. Larger amounts of plain water should not be used when irrigating for gastric bleeding because of the large volume and the risk of electrolyte alterations. Frequent irrigations increase the loss of electrolytes from the gastrointestinal system. Some surgeons advocate the use of air to irrigate the nasogastric tube to maintain patency.

*Irrigation.* The amount of irrigating solution instilled should be recorded as such, unless its equivalent is aspirated via syringe. All gastrointestinal drainage should be accurately measured and recorded. If irrigations do not increase drainage, the tubing should be checked for clogs by milking it toward the suction container to dislodge any obstruction. The suction apparatus is checked by disconnecting the nasogastric tube at the junction of the nasogastric tube and the drainage tube that leads to the container. With the suction turned on, the end of the drainage tube is placed in a glass of water; if the water is sucked up, the suction device is functioning. If these measures fail, gastric mucosa may be occluding the lumen of the tube or the tube may be kinked. In this instance, the patient or the tube may need to be repositioned. If the patient has had gastric, pancreatic, or esophageal surgery, the tube should not be manipulated; the surgeon should be notified of the malfunctioning tube. In general, unless ordered by the surgeon, checking with the surgeon before manipulating or replacing a nasogastric tube is always prudent.

*Patient Comfort.* The presence of a nasogastric tube is a most uncomfortable experience for the patient. However, appropriate nursing care can relieve sore throat, dry mouth, hoarseness, earache, sore nose, and dry lips. The tube should be taped securely and properly (hypoallergenic tape is best or use of a specially designed tube securement device) in a position to prevent pressure on the naris. The tube may be secured to the upper lip or nose in the position it naturally assumes. The tube should not be taped to the patient's nose and then to the forehead. This causes pressure on the underside of the nostril and can cause tissue necrosis. To lessen the pressure and pull on the patient's nose, the tube can be taped or pinned to the gown.

Petrolatum ointment is applied to the tube where it enters the nose and around the nares. The outside portion of the tube is kept free of mucus or other drainage, which prevents encrustations from forming and reduces irritation of the nostril. Petrolatum ointment, cream, or lip balm is applied to the lips to keep them soft and to prevent cracking. Good frequent mouth care is essential for the comfort of the patient and prevention of parotitis. Moistened swabs, mouthwash, or even a toothbrush may be used to provide mouth care for the patient. The nurse should ensure that the patient understands not to swallow any of the material used. This, of course, is not fatal but could be detrimental to fluid and electrolyte balance.

Gargles with warm tap water or warm saline solution (or with viscous lidocaine or applications of a local anesthetic spray) relieve the patient's sore throat. A physician's order should be provided for these measures. Some surgeons allow patients to suck on isotonic ice chips or hard candy or to chew gum. Anesthetic throat lozenges, if allowed, are comforting to the patient. All patients with a gastrointestinal tube in place are given essentially nothing by mouth until the tube is removed. The only exception may be certain medications, given orally or through the tube, or ice chips, less than 200 mL every 8 hours. Some surgeons believe that allowing patients ice chips increases comfort and also helps to keep the tube patent by having the melted ice chips frequently sucked out of the stomach by the tube.

## DIAGNOSTIC STUDIES

Invasive diagnostic procedures are occasionally done at the patient's bedside on the nursing unit, but they are more commonly done in a special procedures room, often located within the surgical suite. They require local anesthesia and appropriate sedation or sometimes general anesthesia. Patients may be sent to the PACU for a brief observation period. Care after endoscopy includes all the general care afforded a perianesthesia patient. After esophagoscopy and gastroscopy, the nurse should be alert for the return of the gag reflex. When pharyngeal reflexes have returned, the patient may be started on liquids and may progress to a regular diet as tolerated unless contraindicated by diagnosis or in anticipation of further surgery. Rest is the most important treatment for this patient. Bleeding, swelling, or dysfunction of the involved area may occur and are indications of complications from the procedure.

Patients who have had laparoscopy have only small bandages or tape strip closures (Steri-Strips) over the stab wounds used for entry of the scope and its accessories. These bandages should remain clean and dry. The patients are probably apprehensive regarding discovery about conditions during the diagnostic procedure; the surgeon should give accurate information after the procedure. The nurse should be familiar with what the patients have been told regarding findings of the diagnostic laparoscopy so that information can be interpreted or repeated for the patient, if necessary.

## CARE AFTER SURGERY ON THE GASTROINTESTINAL TRACT

### Esophagus

Surgery on the esophagus includes repair of hiatal hernia and various forms of tracheo-esophageal fistulas, excision of esophageal diverticula, treatment of stenosis of the lower end of the esophagus, esophagomyotomy, esophagectomy, antireflux procedures, and cardiomyotomy.

Postoperative care depends on the kind of incision used to expose the operative site: abdominal, thoracic, or laparoscopic. Surgery on the esophagus frequently involves a thoracic incision. Care for the patient after a thoracic incision is discussed in Chapter 34. Procedures on the esophagus are performed with general anesthesia. A tracheostomy often is performed (see Chapter 32 for care of the patient after tracheostomy).

On arrival to the PACU, the patient should be placed in a semi-Fowler's position. This position aids in the drainage of blood from the pleural space and prevents tension from impinging on the suture lines. The incision is generally long (from the tip of the scapula to the seventh or eighth rib area) and painful. Analgesics must be given in adequate doses to promote rest and adequate respiratory effort. An interpleural or epidural catheter often is in place for postoperative analgesia. Patient-controlled analgesia may be used.

A nasogastric tube is in place and should be cared for as previously discussed. The nurse should not manipulate the tube. Chest tubes should be managed as discussed in Chapter 34. A large sterile dressing should be in place and should be checked frequently for drainage and reinforced as necessary. Excessive bloody drainage should be reported to the surgeon.

### Stomach

Surgery on the stomach involves procedures to treat the complications of ulcers (antrectomy and vagotomy, gastric resection, gastrectomy), removal of portions of the stomach for malignant disease, and rerouting of the gastrointestinal system at this point to treat pyloric obstruction. In addition, gastric restrictive procedures for the treatment of clinically severe obesity (bariatric surgery) are also now commonly performed; these procedures can be conducted as both open and laparoscopic procedures. All postoperative care of the patient is generally the same, and anesthesia is general.

The patient after surgery should be placed in a semi-Fowler's position to relieve tension on the suture line and to promote drainage. Once the condition is hemodynamically stable, the patient after bariatric surgery may benefit from positioning in a reverse Trendelenburg's position at 45 degrees to maximize respiratory effort and decrease the impact of the abdominal weight interfering with adequate ventilatory effort. For open procedures, the abdominal incisions are fairly high, long, and painful; particular attention must be paid to pulmonary toilet. This patient must be encouraged more often than any other to expand the lungs and to cough and must generally have assistance to change position. Assistance in splinting the wound with the hands or with a firm pillow is most appreciated by the patient. These procedures generally produce considerable postoperative pain, and analgesics should be used generously but judiciously. Patient-controlled or epidural analgesia may be effective for upper abdominal incisional and visceral pain. Patients after bariatric surgery may have obstructive sleep apnea or obesity hypoventilation syndrome and be extremely sensitive to opioid analgesics. Cautious administration and vigilant monitoring are essential especially in these patients to avoid respiratory depression and complications.

A nasogastric tube is in place and should be cared for as previously discussed. Small volumes of bright bloody drainage from the nasogastric tube can be expected for the first 2 to 3 hours because bleeding at the anastomotic site is not uncommon in these procedures. However, bright bleeding that does not decrease after this period or bleeding that becomes excessive (more than 75 mL/h) should be reported immediately to the surgeon. Observe the nasogastric tube and its drainage closely because blood easily clots and clogs the tube; notify the surgeon immediately if the tube stops draining or appears obstructed with blood. Because blood loss may be highly significant in this patient, cardiovascular status must receive careful scrutiny. Vital signs are checked frequently. If hypotension and tachycardia persist or maintain a downward trend, the surgeon should be notified.

Blood replacement may have to be instituted. Hemoglobin and hematocrit levels should be determined 4 to 6 hours after surgery, and the surgeon should be notified if they are significantly lower than previous determinations. Little or no drainage should be expected from the incision unless drains are in place. If drainage does appear, the dressing should be reinforced and the surgeon notified. The nurse in the PACU should not replace the initial dressing unless so directed by the surgeon. Drains with copious output may need a drainage device applied over them to protect the patient's skin and allow for accurate measurement of drainage.

Urinary retention is commonly a problem; many surgeons prefer to insert an indwelling balloon-tipped catheter while the patient is in the operating room. Accurate measurements of output should be ascertained. If a urinary catheter is not in place, the patient should be checked frequently for bladder distention, which may indicate an overfull bladder and urinary retention. If the patient is unable to void, a catheterization order should be obtained.

***Perforated Ulcer.*** Perforation of an ulcer is usually a surgical emergency, and neither the patient nor the family members are adequately prepared, either physically nor emotionally, for the surgery. This situation concerns the perianesthesia nurse because complications, especially hypovolemia and shock, may more readily occur in this patient.

***Pyloric Stenosis.*** Specific care for infants after surgery for pyloric stenosis is detailed in pediatric texts. However, the perianesthesia nurse should be aware of general care. Position is important. The infant should be kept either on the right side or on the abdomen until the danger of vomiting and aspiration has subsided and then should be placed in an upright position. Careful placement of the diaper is important to avoid contamination of the wound. Application of a pediatric urine collector may also be helpful not only to prevent contamination of the wound with urine but also to determine accurate output. Feedings are usually begun for these infants 4 to 6 hours after surgery, but the surgeon's instructions should be explicitly followed.

After bariatric gastroplasty and gastric bypass procedures, the nurse should also be aware of the risk of leaks that occur with anastomoses. Anastomotic leaks may occur and can be fatal if unrecognized. Symptoms of leaks range from abdominal tenderness, left shoulder pain, tachycardia, decreased urine output, fever, elevated white blood cell counts, oxygen desaturation, or a patient's "sense of impending doom." The surgeon should be notified immediately.

## Small Bowel
Operations on the small bowel include exploratory laparotomy with lysis of adhesions and resection for obstruction or perforation. Care after these procedures is essentially the same as that already mentioned. No excessive drainage from incisions should be noted unless drains have been placed. Fluid and electrolyte balance must be monitored carefully. Remember that the loss of sodium and bicarbonate ions is great, which results in imbalance, and that fluid losses during surgery may be significant, but fluid overload must be avoided.

The patient with an ileostomy enters the PACU with a bag in place over the stoma. Returns may be expected almost at once and should be recorded. Particular attention must be paid to this stoma, the drainage, and the collection device; no leakage onto the skin should be allowed because this causes significant skin damage. Under the collection device, the peristomal skin is protected with a skin barrier that includes pectin-based and karaya-based wafers or paste.

## Large Bowel
Surgery on the large bowel includes appendectomy, colostomy, various types of colonic resection for removal of tumors or correction of other problems, total proctocolectomy with ileostomy or ileoanal anastomosis (Fig. 40-6), and abdominoperineal resection with permanent colostomy (Fig. 40-7). Most of these surgical procedures are performed with general anesthesia. On return to the PACU, patients are kept flat and on one side until the reflexes have returned; they may then assume a position of comfort unless otherwise specified by the surgeon. Postoperative care is essentially the same as for small bowel surgery.

If the patient returns from surgery with a colostomy, some special care is required. The colostomy usually does not start functioning immediately after surgery; however, spillage must be prevented from contaminating the incision or excoriating the skin. A pouch or

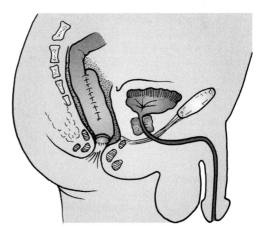

**Fig. 40-6** Ileoanal anastomosis with J-pouch for treatment of ulcerative colitis. *(From Black JM, Hawks JH: Medical-surgical nursing: clinical management for positive outcomes, ed 7, St Louis, 2005, Saunders.)*

**NURSING CARE IN THE PACU**

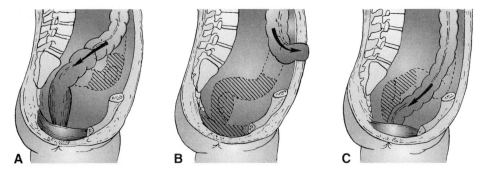

**Fig. 40-7** Large bowel procedures for resection of malignant disease. **A,** Anterior resection with primary anastomosis. **B,** Abdominoperineal (anteroposterior) resection with permanent colostomy. **C,** Proctosigmoidectomy with "pull through." *(From Black JM, Hawks JH: Medical-surgical nursing: clinical management for positive outcomes, ed 7, St Louis, 2005, Saunders.)*

collection device may be in place over the colostomy. The skin around the stoma should be protected with an appropriate skin barrier if drainage is present. The color and appearance of the stoma (it should be bright red and moist) should be assessed and documented in the nursing record.

Fluid and electrolyte balance must be monitored carefully. Some blood-tinged urine may be expected after colectomy because retractors used in surgery may have caused contusions of the bladder; however, gross blood may indicate that the bladder was more severely injured. Dressings should remain dry, unless drains were placed in the wound. If drains were placed, some bloody drainage may be expected and dressings should be reinforced as necessary. Drainage that soaks through the dressings is considered excessive and must be reported to the surgeon.

Incisions may be left open to heal with delayed primary closure or secondary intent. Abdominal wounds for bowel surgery may be contaminated (e.g., traumatic penetrating injuries, colostomies) with an increased risk of infection. For a delay primary closure, the wound is left open, protected with moist gauze, and, when it is clean and red, closed with sutures that were placed during the original surgery and left slack. The cleanliness of the wound and the health of the granulation tissue in the wound generally determine the best time for closure.

### Abdominoperineal Resection.

Abdominoperineal resection for cancer of the rectum is a major procedure that results in permanent colostomy and two separate incisions. Vital signs are monitored carefully, and any adverse trend is reported. Perineal drains are in place and should be noted on the patient's chart and nursing care plan. The perineal dressings often become saturated with bloody drainage and must

be reinforced. If drainage remains bright and obviously new bleeding occurs and if frequent dressing changes are necessary, the surgeon should be notified. If sump catheters are used to drain the perineal wound, they may be attached to a grenade or bulb (Jackson-Pratt) device and an accurate measurement of drainage may be obtained.

The patient who has undergone abdominoperineal surgery has a colostomy. Check the blood supply to the stoma frequently because impaired blood supply is an early and serious complication. Pain may be severe and should be relieved with adequate doses of opioid analgesics or use of an epidural catheter for analgesia to ensure comfort of the patient and promote respiratory sufficiency.

### Appendectomy and Herniorrhaphy.

Patients who have undergone surgery for appendectomy or herniorrhaphy usually return to the PACU almost fully awake and without serious postoperative complications. No nasogastric tube, indwelling urinary catheter, or drain is in place, and recovery is generally uneventful. However, patients who have large ventral hernia repairs with mesh may have nasogastric tubes and drains in place. Patients may assume a position of comfort as soon as pharyngeal reflexes have returned, and they may start on a progressive diet as tolerated unless a nasogastric tube is in place. All the postoperative care outlined in Chapters 26 through 31 is applicable. When the laparoscopic approach is used, general anesthesia usually is given. Patients may have shoulder pain or bloating because of insufflation of air. They may also have sore throat from intubation and the neuromuscular blocking agents. Monitor fluid intake and replace fluid losses appropriately. Dressings should remain dry and intact, and any postoperative incisional bleeding or drainage should be reported to the surgeon.

The most important postoperative complication is bleeding. The nurse should also watch for urinary retention. If the patient has undergone inguinal hernia repair, the nurse should watch for development of scrotal edema or hematoma, which may indicate slow bleeding from the operative site.

### Lower Rectum and Anus

Surgery on the lower rectum and anus includes excision of pilonidal cysts, rectal fissures, fistulas, rectal abscesses, tumors, and hemorrhoids. Perianesthesia nursing care is the same as for any patient who undergoes anesthesia, either local, regional, or general. Dressings should be checked frequently for excessive drainage and bleeding. The incisions may be closed but often are packed to facilitate drainage of infected material and aid in healing. Urinary retention may be a problem because the proximity of the bladder and operative site may make urination difficult. Pain can be severe, but patients are often embarrassed by the location of the operative site and may not ask for analgesia. The nurse should be alert to signs and symptoms of pain and discomfort and administer analgesia as necessary for relief.

## SURGERY ON RELATED ORGANS WITHIN THE ABDOMINAL CAVITY

### Liver

Surgery on the liver includes biopsy, excision of tumors, major resection, repair of traumatic lacerations, and hepatic transplant.

Percutaneous liver biopsy is a common procedure that is usually performed in the endoscopy suite, although the patient may be taken to the operating suite and may return to the PACU for a short period of observation. Postoperative care depends on the type of anesthesia used; anesthesia is usually local but may involve other types if the patient cannot or will not cooperate. The patient should remain positioned on the right side for at least 2 hours after the procedure. Vital signs should be determined frequently: every 10 to 15 minutes for the first hour and every 30 minutes for the second hour. Complications include hemorrhage from penetration of a blood vessel and peritonitis from accidental puncture of the bile duct. If the patient's vital signs begin a downward trend and if the patient reports severe abdominal pain or becomes febrile, the surgeon should be notified immediately.

Open surgery on the liver for the excision of tumors or the repair of lacerations is done with general anesthesia and involves a fairly long upper abdominal vertical or bilateral subcostal oblique (chevron) incision. All care previously discussed for patients after general anesthesia and upper abdominal incisions applies. Respiratory care is of paramount importance. The liver is an extremely vascular and friable organ. It is difficult to suture; gross bleeding is common and often involves large blood losses, especially when surgery is necessitated by traumatic injury or large resection. Large drains of the Penrose or suction (grenade or bulb) type are placed in the region of the laceration or excision of the tumor and are brought through separate sites to the skin surface. For the first 8 hours, expect approximately 100 to 250 mL of sanguineous drainage from the drains.

Coagulation studies must be performed frequently and monitored closely because many patients have coagulation abnormalities develop during and after liver surgery. Specific coagulation factors may be administered, according to the results of the coagulation tests.

Vital signs must be assessed frequently, and any downward trend should be reported to the surgeon at once. Blood replacement or hemostasis may be inadequate. Rapid infusions of fluid replacements may be needed, especially after extensive liver resection or transplant. Occasionally, this patient also has a T-tube in place in the common bile duct (Fig. 40-8). This tube should be attached to straight-gravity

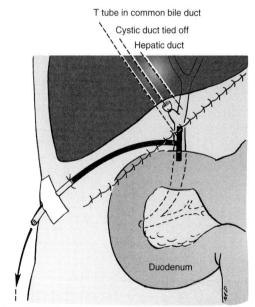

**Fig. 40-8** T-tube placement in common bile duct. *(From Black JM, Hawks JH: Medical-surgical nursing: clinical management for positive outcomes, ed 7, St Louis, 2005, Saunders.)*

drainage, and accurate measurements of the output should be made. A nasogastric tube is in place and should receive care as discussed previously. Pain is usually severe, and opioid analgesics or epidural analgesia are necessary to promote rest and respiratory effort.

## Spleen

Surgery on the spleen involves general anesthesia and removal of the organ, with either an open or laparoscopic technique. The spleen is removed because of rupture from trauma; accidental trauma from associated surgery; diseases that cause damage, such as mononucleosis and malaria; a variety of hematologic malignant diseases; left-sided portal hypertension; and hypersplenism. If the procedure is done with an open technique, a midline or left subcostal incision is used. Postoperative care for the patient after splenectomy is the same as that for the patient after repair of a lacerated liver. Dressings should remain dry and intact. A drain may be placed in the subdiaphragmatic space to prevent the collection of blood under the diaphragm and to detect unrecognized injury to the pancreas that may have occurred.

The perianesthesia nurse should know the circumstances that lead to the patient's splenectomy. If it was necessitated by trauma, the nurse must be particularly alert for signs that indicate development of unrecognized complications from the accident. Vital signs should be determined frequently, and trends watched, especially those that indicate progressive bleeding. Neurologic signs should be checked, and the patient should be assessed carefully for any signs of injury to the extremities. Any dysrhythmia should be reported because this may indicate cardiac injury.

## Pancreas

Surgery on the pancreas is difficult and technically demanding. It involves general anesthesia, and care for these patients is the same as for other postoperative patients. If the operative procedure done is for removal of malignant tumors, a mortality rate of 2% to 7% is not unreasonable because of extensive resection and poor general condition of the patient.

Postoperative care of the patient after a pancreaticoduodenectomy (Whipple or modified Whipple procedure) is a challenge. All postoperative care for the abdominal surgery patient applies. Particular attention must be paid to drains and catheters. Surgeons should augment their reports to the nurse by explaining exactly what procedure was performed, where drains or wound catheters were placed, and how to care

for them. Surgeons should brief the nurse on expected drainage and what should be considered excessive. As with all abdominal surgeries, intravenous lines and intravenous therapy have already been initiated. Because of the generally poor nutritional status of these patients, hyperalimentation may be started almost immediately after surgery.

All respiratory, cardiac, and renal functioning must be monitored carefully, and the surgeon should be notified of any untoward signs. Assisted ventilation may be necessary for at least 24 hours after this procedure (this type of care is discussed in Chapter 28). If frequent arterial blood gas analysis is needed for this patient, an arterial line should be in place for this purpose. Blood gas analysis yields valuable information about the patient's respiratory acid-base status. Urine output should be determined hourly, and at least 0.5 to 1 mL/kg/h should be expected.

Frequent assays of blood glucose levels should be ordered on all patients after pancreatic surgery. Most of these patients need to receive intravenous insulin during the postoperative period. Insulin doses are titrated to maintain the blood glucose levels at less than 110 mg/dL in the critical care setting and at less than 180 mg/dL in the noncritical care setting. The insulin aids in the prevention of hyperglycemia.

Large fluctuations in serum glucose levels or acid-base balance can precipitate electrolyte abnormalities in these patients. Potassium and calcium levels, in particular, should be monitored closely.

## Biliary Tract

Surgery on the biliary tract includes exploration for removal of stones from the gallbladder and the ducts and removal of the gallbladder. It may also include repair of biliary tract injuries and resection for malignant disease or benign strictures. Anesthesia is general, regional, or a combination of both. The procedure is performed with a laparoscope, and the patient has an umbilical incision and three or four abdominal stab wounds for instruments (Fig. 40-9). The open incision is either a right subcostal or a midline incision. On return to the PACU, the patient is placed in a semi-Fowler's position. All tubes must be cared for appropriately. A nasogastric tube is placed during surgery and is often removed when the operative procedure ends. A T-tube is placed in the common bile duct if the common duct was opened during surgery. This tube is usually connected to straight-gravity drainage to a bile bag. Careful attention must be paid to maintaining the patency of this

After laparoscopic cholecystectomy, the patient may have one of the most stable conditions of any seen in the PACU. Any patient with unexplained pain, oliguria, or hypotension should be immediately discussed with the surgeon. Complications of gas embolism, deep vein thrombophlebitis, subcutaneous emphysema, injuries to major vessels and intestine, and bile leakage all have been reported after laparoscopic procedures.

## SUMMARY

This chapter discussed the care involved after surgery on the gastrointestinal tract, including the esophagus and the anus, and the accessory organs: the liver, gallbladder, pancreas, and spleen. Surgery on the female reproductive organs, which are also contained within the abdominal cavity, is reviewed in Chapter 42. The care common to all patients undergoing abdominal surgery was discussed, and only the most important variations related to specific procedures were included.

## BIBLIOGRAPHY

ACE: Position Statement on Inpatient Diabetes and Metabolic Control, *Endocr Prac* 10(1):77-82, 2004.

Black JM, Hawks JH: *Medical-surgical nursing: clinical management for positive outcomes*, ed 7, St Louis, 2005, Saunders.

Etala E: *Atlas of gastrointestinal surgery*, Baltimore, 1997, Williams & Wilkins.

Owens TM: Bariatric surgery risks, benefits, and care of the morbidly obese, *Nurs Clin North Am* 41:249-263, 2006.

O'Brien D: The gastrointestinal surgical patient, *Perianesthesia nursing core curriculum*, St Louis, 2004, Saunders.

O'Brien D, Walter V, Burden N: Special procedures in the ambulatory setting, *Ambulatory surgical nursing*, Philadelphia, 2000, Saunders.

Palmer TJ: Hepatobiliary and gastrointestinal disturbances, *Nurse anesthesia*, ed 2, Philadelphia, 2001, Saunders.

Phippen ML, Wells MP: *Patient care during operative and invasive procedures*, Philadelphia, 2000, Saunders.

Schmieding NJ, Waldman RC: Gastric decompression in adult patients, *Clin Nurs Res* 6(2):142-155, 1997.

Smith CE: Gastrointestinal surgery, *Alexander's care of the patient in surgery*, ed 13, St Louis, 2007, Mosby.

Thompson JM, McFarland GK, Hirsch JE, et al, editors: *Mosby's clinical nursing*, ed 5, St Louis, 2002, Mosby.

Townsend CM, Beauchamp D, Evers BM, et al, editors: *Sabiston textbook of surgery: the biological basis of modern surgical practice*, ed 17, Philadelphia, 2004, Saunders.

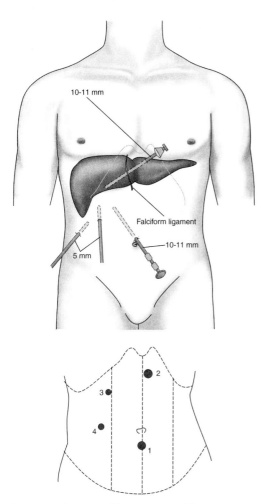

**Fig. 40-9** Placement of laparoscope and instrument ports for laparoscopic cholecystectomy. *(Redrawn from Malt RA: The practice of surgery, Philadelphia, 1993, Saunders.)*

tube and its attachment to the patient; the surgeon needs to be called immediately if the tube is dislodged.

Bile drainage should be carefully measured and accurately reported. Between 200 and 500 mL of bile drainage can be expected within a 24-hour period. Dressings should remain dry and intact and should be reinforced as necessary to keep the surrounding skin dry.

As with all upper abdominal incisions, pain is a challenge, and analgesics (intermittent, continuous, or patient-controlled), epidural analgesia, and relaxation exercises should be used to promote rest and respiratory effort. Any downward trend in vital signs, excessive bleeding from the incision, or bleeding noted in the bile drainage from the T-tube should be reported to the surgeon. Bleeding from the cystic artery is a serious complication and can lead to rapid deterioration in the patient's status.

NURSING CARE IN THE PACU

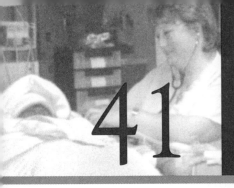

# CARE OF THE GENITOURINARY SURGICAL PATIENT

*Candace Taylor, BSN, RN, CPAN*

Genitourinary surgery involves procedures performed on the kidneys, ureters, bladder, urethra, and male genitalia. The genitourinary system can be the host of multiple problems, either congenital or acquired. In caring for patients undergoing genitourinary surgeries, the perianesthesia nurse should have an understanding of anatomic location and normal function of this system.

Adrenalectomy is included in this chapter for convenience and because of the proximity of the adrenal glands to the kidneys.

## DEFINITIONS

**Adrenalectomy:** Partial or total excision of one or both adrenal glands.

**Bladder Neck Operation (Y-V Plasty):** A plastic repair of the bladder neck for correction of stricture.

**Chordee:** Downward bowing of the penis as a result of congenital malformation or hypospadias with fibrous bands.

**Circumcision:** Excision of the foreskin (prepuce) of the glans penis.

**Cystectomy:** Excision of the bladder and adjacent structures; may be partial (excision of a lesion) or total (excision of a malignant tumor). This operation usually involves the additional procedure of ureterostomy.

**Cystolithotomy:** Opening of the bladder for removal of stones.

**Cystoscopy:** Direct visualization of the urethra, prostatic urethra, and bladder by means of a tubular lighted telescopic lens.

**Cystotomy:** An incision into the bladder.

**Epididymectomy:** Excision of the epididymis from the testis. This procedure is rarely done but may occasionally be indicated for treatment of persistent infection.

**Epispadias:** Urethral meatus situated in an abnormal position on the upper side of the penis. Surgical correction involves plastic repair.

**Extracorporeal Shock Wave Lithotripsy:** Use of shock waves through a liquid medium into the body to disintegrate stones.

**Heminephrectomy:** Partial excision of the kidney.

**Hydrocelectomy:** Excision of the tunica vaginalis of the testis for removal of a hydrocele (a fluid-filled sac).

**Hypospadias:** A deformity of the penis and malformation of the urethral wall in which the urinary meatus is located on the underside of the penis, either short of its normal position at the tip of the glans or on the perineum or scrotum. This condition is often associated with chordee. Surgical correction involves plastic repair; penile straightening and urethral reconstruction (urethroplasty) are usually done in two or more stages.

**Kidney Transplant:** Removal of a donor kidney with nephrectomy and ureterectomy, followed by transplantation of the donor kidney into the recipient's iliac fossa.

**Nephrectomy:** Removal of a kidney; used in treatment of some congenital unilateral abnormalities that cause renal obstruction or hydronephrosis; sometimes necessitated by the presence of tumors or severe injuries.

**Nephrostomy:** An opening into the kidney for temporary or permanent drainage.

**Nephrotomy:** An incision into the kidney.

**Nephroureterectomy:** Removal of a kidney and the entire ureter that drains it.

**Orchiectomy:** Removal of the testis or testes. This procedure renders the patient sterile.

**Orchiopexy:** Suspension of the testis within the scrotum. This procedure is used in treatment of an undescended or cryptorchid testis to bring it into the normal intrascrotal position.

**Penile Implant:** A penile prosthesis implanted for treatment of organic sexual impotence.

**Percutaneous Nephrolithotomy:** Removal or disintegration of renal stones with passage of a nephroscope through a percutaneous nephrostomy tract.

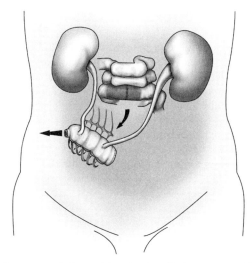

**Fig. 41-1** Ileal conduit, showing ileal segment with anastomosed ureters. *(Redrawn from LeMaitre GD, Finnegan JA: The patient in surgery: a guide for nurses, ed 4, Philadelphia, 1980, Saunders.)*

**Phimosis:** Tightness of the foreskin so that it cannot be drawn back from over the glans; also, the analogous condition in the clitoris.

**Prostatectomy:** Enucleation of prostatic adenomas or hypertrophied masses.

**Pyeloplasty:** Revision or reconstruction of the renal pelvis.

**Pyelostomy:** An incision into the renal pelvis for drainage or for irrigation of the renal pelvis.

**Pyelotomy:** Incision into the renal pelvis.

**Spermatocelectomy:** The removal of a spermatocele, which usually appears as a cystic mass within the scrotum, attached to the upper pole of the epididymis. A spermatocele is usually caused by an obstruction of the tubular system that conveys the sperm.

**Transurethral Surgery:** Piecemeal resection of the prostate gland and of tumors of the bladder and bladder neck and fulguration of bleeding vessels and of tumors with a resectoscope passed into the bladder via the urethra.

**Ureterectomy:** Complete removal of one or both of the ureters.

**Ureterolithotomy:** Incision into the ureter and removal of stones.

**Ureteroneocystostomy (Ureterovesical Anastomosis; Vesicopsoas Hitch Procedure):** Division of the ureter from the urinary bladder and reimplantation of the ureter into the bladder at another site.

**Ureteroplasty:** Reconstruction of the ureter.

**Ureterostomy, Cutaneous (Anastomosis of Transplant; Bricker's Operation; Ureteroileostomy):** Diversion of the urinary stream with anastomosis of the ureters into an isolated loop of ileum that is brought out through the abdominal wall as an ileostomy (Fig. 41-1).

**Urethral Dilatation and Internal Urethrotomy:** Gradual dilation of the urethra and lysis of a urethral stricture.

**Urethral Meatotomy:** Incisional enlargement of the external urethral meatus for relief of stenosis or stricture.

**Urethroplasty:** Reconstructive surgery of the urethra.

**Urethrovesical suspension (Pubovaginal Slings):** Suspension of the urethra with a permanent polypropylene mesh tape for the treatment of stress incontinence.

**Varicocelectomy:** Ligation and partial excision of dilated veins in the scrotum.

**Vasectomy:** Excision of a section of the vas deferens. This procedure is carried out electively for birth control or before prostatectomy to prevent the spread of infection from the urethra to the epididymis.

**Vasoepididymostomy:** Anastomosis of the vas deferens to the epididymis.

**Vasovasostomy:** Anastomosis of two separate segments of the vas deferens for reversal of a vasectomy.

**Vesicourethral suspension (Marshall-Marchetti Operation):** Suspension of the bladder neck to the posterior surface of the pubis in women for treatment of stress incontinence.

## NURSING CARE AFTER DIAGNOSTIC PROCEDURES

Several invasive diagnostic procedures are performed on patients with genitourinary disease. If patients require monitored anesthesia care (MAC), spinal anesthesia, or general anesthesia, they are admitted to the postanesthesia care unit (PACU) for postanesthesia care.

### Renal Angiography

For a renal angiographic examination, a small catheter is threaded through the femoral artery into the aorta or renal artery, radiopaque dye is instilled, and radiographs are made. Local anesthesia is usually all that is needed; however, general anesthesia may be used for children or patients who cannot cooperate during the procedure. When the patient is admitted to the PACU, the groin area is inspected for bleeding. A pressure-type dressing usually is present and may be replaced with a simple bandage after a few hours. Pedal pulses should be checked to ensure that no interruption of blood supply to the extremities has occurred. If possible, the leg should be kept straight. Fluids should be encouraged to facilitate excretion of the dye.

NURSING CARE IN THE PACU

### Renal Biopsy

Renal biopsy is usually performed at the bedside with only local anesthesia, although general anesthesia may be used for children. The patient should maintain bed rest in a flat supine position for as long as 4 hours. A small pillow may be positioned under the head for comfort. Vital signs are monitored, and the site of biopsy is checked for bleeding. Coughing and other activities that increase abdominal venous pressure should be avoided. Fluids should be increased to 3000 mL daily, and the urine should be observed for occult blood.

### Cystoscopy

Diagnostic cystoscopy may be performed in a special-procedures room with only local anesthesia and appropriate sedation. Children and patients who cannot or do not cooperate during the procedure may need general anesthesia. This procedure may also be performed with spinal anesthesia.

On admission to the PACU, the patient is placed in a side-lying position if general anesthesia was used. The patient may have to lie flat on the back if spinal anesthesia was used, with a gradual increase in the head of bed if tolerated and allowed by physician orders. After the effects of anesthesia have been eliminated, the patient may assume a position of comfort. The patient may have back pain, a feeling of bladder fullness, and bladder spasms. These symptoms may become severe enough to necessitate analgesia. Belladonna and opium suppositories or intravenous opioids may be administered to relieve patient discomfort.

Oral fluid administration should be encouraged and started as soon as the effects of anesthesia are gone. Urine output should be monitored carefully. The patient can expect frequency of urination and a burning sensation because of trauma to the mucous membranes from the procedure; this condition may inadvertently cause voluntary retention. The urine may be pink tinged for several voidings, which is to be expected. Bright blood or clots in the urine, however, should be reported to the surgeon. Severe abdominal pain should be reported because it may indicate accidental ureteral or bladder perforation or internal hemorrhage.

The patient should be observed for signs of sepsis because infection may spread throughout the urinary tract or into the blood stream after a cystoscopy. If symptoms of sepsis, such as chills, tachycardia, tachypnea, flushing, and temperature elevation, are noted, the surgeon should be notified.

## GENERAL POSTOPERATIVE CARE

Assessment of the patient after genitourinary surgery involves particular attention to fluid and electrolyte balance. Intake and output records are especially important and must be accurately maintained. Postoperative care is directed primarily at urinary tract function, which is second in importance only to cardiorespiratory function. Maintenance of patency of the urinary tract often depends on the use of catheters, which come in a variety of shapes and sizes (Fig. 41-2).

Urethral catheters are used to drain urine from the bladder for decompression and accurate measurement of urine output. A retention catheter may be used after surgery and left in place until the patient's condition is stable and the surgeon orders its removal. The catheter is attached to a sterile closed gravitational-drainage collection system. The urine collection

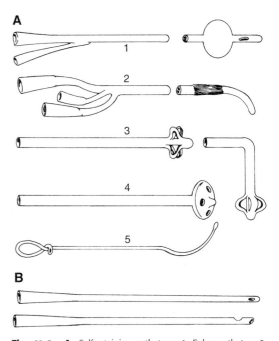

**Fig. 41-2   A,** Self-retaining catheters: *1,* Foley catheter; *2,* three-way Foley catheter; *3,* Malecot catheter; and *4,* Pezzer catheter. Self-retaining protuberance at tip of Malecot and Pezzer catheters must be elongated with a stylet *5,* which is passed through lumen before insertion. After insertion, stylet is removed and protuberance secures catheter in place. **B,** Straight catheters. Straight catheter may have single eye or many eyes; it may have round tip or whistle tip. These catheters are not self retaining and must be secured with adhesive tape when used as indwelling tubes. *(From Whitehead S: Nursing care of the adult urology patient New York, 1970, Appleton-Century-Crofts.)*

reservoir may be a large (usually 2000-mL) container or a small calibrated chamber that can be emptied into a large reservoir after timed urine output volumes have been determined and recorded (Fig. 41-3).

The catheter should be anchored securely to the patient's thigh with tape and the tubing brought over the leg. The catheter should be looped over once before taping to prevent undue tension on the urinary meatus. The connecting tubing should be attached to the bed linens so that no proximal loops of tubing lie below the distal tubing; this is a straight gravity drainage system. The tubing should never be under the patient because compression of the tubing obstructs the flow of urine. The tubing should be checked frequently for kinks. The urine receptacle should always be kept below the bladder level to prevent urine reflux up the tubing. Particular attention must be paid to this principle during the transfer of patients.

For collection of a urine specimen from the closed system, a sterile syringe and needle is used. Some catheters have a small specially constructed port from which to draw specimens. On those catheters that do not have such a port, the distal part of the catheter, close to the drainage tubing, is used. The area is cleansed with alcohol

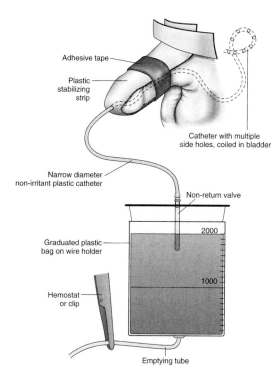

**Fig. 41-3** Closed drainage of bladder. *(Redrawn from Douglas AP, Kerr DS: A short textbook of kidney disease, London, 1968, Pitman Medical.)*

Adhesive tape

Plastic stabilizing strip

Catheter with multiple side holes, coiled in bladder

Narrow diameter non-irritant plastic catheter

Non-return valve

2000

Graduated plastic bag on wire holder

1000

Hemostat or clip

Emptying tube

or povidone-iodine (Betadine), the needle inserted, and a specimen withdrawn.

Mucus or blood, or both, can clog the tubing and prevent urine flow. Irrigations should be administered only according to the surgeon's orders. All irrigations are sterile procedures and can be either continuous or intermittent. For intermittent irrigation, a large sterile Toomey syringe and sterile irrigating solution (usually normal saline solution alone or with a selected antibiotic) are used. Care must be taken to keep all parts of the drainage system sterile. This action may be accomplished with placement of a small sterile plastic cover on the drainage tubing while the irrigation is performed. Irrigations should never be given with pressure. When the bladder is irrigated, no more than 30 mL should be instilled at one time, unless ordered otherwise by the surgeon.

After transurethral resection of the prostate (TURP), continuous irrigation is usually preferred. With continuous irrigation, normal saline solution is typically connected with a three-way urinary catheter. Nursing care should include vigilant monitoring of patients for hyponatremia and the development of TURP syndrome. The report from the perioperative nurse should include the amount of intraoperative irrigation and the duration of the procedure. During the immediate postanesthesia phase, patient confusion should be monitored and differentiated from confusion as a result of amnesiacs, opioids, or hyponatremia (see also the Prostatic Surgery section in this chapter).

If hyponatremia is diagnosed, treatment may include the administration of hypertonic saline solution for a gradual increase in the patient's serum sodium level. Care includes monitoring for signs of intracellular to extracellular fluid shifts. As fluid moves back into the extracellular space, pulmonary edema and heart failure can occur quickly.

## Suprapubic Catheters

Suprapubic catheters are used to drain residual urine from the bladder. A temporary catheter can be placed into the urinary bladder via a stab wound through the lower abdomen and into the anterior bladder wall. The catheter is sutured in place, and a dressing is applied (usually a type of dressing that allows direct observation of the puncture site). The catheter is connected to a straight gravitational drainage system. Care of the suprapubic catheter is similar to that of the Foley catheter. The catheter should be securely taped with a loop made to prevent tension on the bladder wall or the abdomen. The skin around the puncture site should be kept clean and dry. The catheter tubing should be checked periodically for kinks and to ensure that the stopcock valve is open to allow the urine to drain from the bladder.

A suprapubic catheter can also be placed into the urinary bladder via abdominal incision and cystostomy. This procedure is typically done for more permanent or long-term use of the suprapubic catheter. The surgeon may choose this method if conventional methods of treatment for urinary incontinence fail, as with spinal cord injury or neurogenic bladder. The care of the catheter is the same as with the puncture wound, but the nurse should also apply nursing care that relates to the abdominal incision.

### Ureteral Catheters

Ureteral catheters are used to drain urine or splint the ureters while they heal. They may be placed through the urethra or through abdominal or flank incisions. Care of these catheters is essentially the same as that for urethral catheters. Attention to patency must be especially scrupulous because the renal pelvis can hold only 5 mL without overdistension and damage to the kidneys.

Sterile irrigations are undertaken only as ordered by the physician. Only 5 mL of fluid should be used for the irrigation via gravitational flow. Irrigations should never be given with pressure, such as with a syringe and plunger. The nurse must be sure to avoid situations that may cause dislodgement or displacement of these catheters, which could be disastrous to the outcome of the surgery. Special care must be taken during patient transfer to ensure that these catheters stay in place. One person should be assigned this responsibility during the transfer. If the catheters should become dislodged in spite of all the precautions taken, the surgeon must be notified immediately.

### Intake

Optimal fluid intake is exceptionally important for the patient after surgery; increased fluids are the general rule. Fluids should be given orally if the patient can tolerate this preferred route, and intake should be increased to total 3000 mL in a 24-hour period. Parenteral fluid therapy is indicated for a short time until the effects of anesthesia have passed and is continued only if the oral route of intake is inadequate.

### Dressings

Care of dressings varies according to the procedure. Dressings applied after urinary tract surgery often become soaked with blood and urine. They should be reinforced as necessary, and the surrounding skin should be kept clean and dry to prevent unnecessary excoriation and breakdown. (Excessive staining that is unexpected for a particular procedure and indicates a complication is so indicated in the discussion of the specific procedure later in this chapter.) Excessive bleeding and hemorrhage are ever-present dangers of this surgery because the kidneys and prostatic bed are extremely vascular. Vital signs must be monitored closely, and all avenues of output, especially the incisions and drainage tubes, should be evaluated frequently for bleeding.

### Abdominal Distention

All patients should be assessed for abdominal distention after surgery that involves abdominal and flank incisions (see Chapter 40 for care of the patient after an abdominal incision because the same care applies after genitourinary surgery). These patients often arrive with nasogastric tubes, the care for which is discussed in Chapter 40. In addition, the patient should be assessed for distention caused by overfilling of the bladder because of an inability to void or a malfunction of the catheters.

Bladder ultrasound scan is a noninvasive method to assess bladder volume for determination of bladder distention or postvoid residual urine. This portable battery-operated devise can be used at the bedside as a noninvasive replacement to intermittent catheterization. This painless procedure eliminates discomfort, embarrassment, and risks associated with catheterization. Data from the bladder ultrasound scan can be printed off and become part of the patient's chart. Depending on the volume and whether or not the patient is capable of voiding, straight catheterization should be performed to relieve urinary retention; this procedure is typically done with volumes greater that 300 mL. Bladder ultrasound scan can be repeated as necessary and has been shown to decrease the risk of urinary tract infections associated with intermittent catheterization.

### Management of Discomfort and Pain

Discomfort after genitourinary surgery may be relieved with the administration of opioids, including intravenous morphine, belladonna, and opium suppositories. The physiology of the "need to void" should be explained to the patient before surgery. The patient should be instructed not to attempt to void around the catheter because exertion of pressure causes the bladder muscles to contract and results in painful bladder spasms. The avoidance of straining around the catheter and of intake of excessive fluids decreases bladder irritability and spasms. As the nerve endings become fatigued, the frequency and severity of the spasms diminish.

## NURSING CARE AFTER SPECIFIC PROCEDURES

### Renal and Ureteral Surgery

Procedures that involve the kidneys and ureters include excision of tumors and obstructions to urine flow (such as stones), reconstruction of urine outflow tracts, repair of lacerations, correction of deformities, excision of a kidney, and total organ transplant.

General anesthesia is commonly used for surgery on the kidneys and ureters. The kidneys are usually approached posteriorly through an incision that requires resection of the 11th or 12th rib. The surgical approach to the ureters is made through muscle-splitting flank incisions (Fig. 41-4). The perianesthesia course for these patients is usually smooth and involves general care and maintenance of urinary tract function. The patient should be placed in a position that avoids tension on suture lines or as indicated by the surgeon.

All surgical patients are at risk for fluid volume deficit from the intake restrictions before surgery and from the decreased intake after surgery, possibly related to postoperative nausea or vomiting. Maintenance of exceptionally accurate intake and output records is important. Low urine output should be reported to the surgeon.

Dressings should remain dry and intact unless drains are used, in which case dressings should be weighed when they are removed to determine output via this route. With determination of output from the dressings, the dressings should be weighed before application and again at

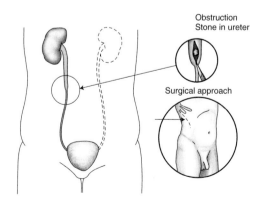

**Fig. 41-4** Right hydroureter from obstructing calculus. Inset shows incision in ureter for removal of stone. *(Redrawn from LeMaitre GD, Finnegan JA: The patient in surgery: a guide for nurses, ed 4, Philadelphia, 1980, Saunders.)*

removal and the difference subtracted (1 g equals 1 mL of output). Patients with drains or stomas may need a small plastic bag over the area for collection of drainage that consists primarily of urine. Drainage bags should be emptied frequently; if the bags are allowed to fill to capacity, the continual flow of urine is interrupted.

Skin care for these patients is important. Urine should not be allowed to remain on the skin. Plain water should be used to cleanse the skin, which should be carefully dried. No powders, lotions, or harsh skin preparations should be applied to the skin. If an ureteroileostomy has been performed, the stoma must be inspected frequently to ensure adequate vascularization. If skin turns a bluish hue, the surgeon should be notified immediately.

A Foley catheter is often in place and receives care as previously discussed. Fluid intake is increased both orally and parenterally to keep blood clots from forming in the ureters or bladder. Intestinal decompression may be necessary and is accomplished via nasogastric tube (see Chapter 40). Decompression is essential when an ileal conduit procedure (ureterostomy) is performed to allow healing of the intestinal anastomosis. Any evidence of abdominal distention should be reported to the surgeon immediately.

***Extracorporeal Shock Wave Lithotripsy.*** After extracorporeal shock wave lithotripsy, the patient may be admitted to the PACU for a brief period of observation. Vital signs should be monitored as with any renal or ureteral surgery. Fluids should be increased, and intake and output monitored carefully. Initially, the color of the urine may be cherry red to pink because of trauma from surgery; this condition may take several hours to clear. Petechiae, redness, and bruising may be seen on the skin at the site of lithotripsy. This petechiae should be documented by the perianesthesia nurse on assessment in the PACU. The patient may have pain from the force of the shock waves. This pain is usually localized to the skin and may be relieved with ice packs. Renal colic pain may also be experienced as the fragments of pulverized stones pass through the lower urinary tract.

***Ureteroscopy.*** Since the 1980s, rigid ureteroscopy has been used for the removal of distal ureteral calculi. Today, flexible and rigid ureteroscopy are used for the diagnosis and treatment of stones, fulguration of epithelial tumors, analysis of gross hematuria, and management of ureteral strictures. Complications are rare but include perforation of the ureter; therefore, close observation of color and amount of urine output should be maintained. All urine should

NURSING CARE IN THE PACU

be strained, and any calculous fragments should be collected for inspection and identification. Ureteral stents are commonly placed during this procedure to facilitate urine flow and prevent obstruction or ureteral colic caused by edema. If the surgeon has elected to externalize the stent suture, patients should be educated on its care.

***Percutaneous Nephrolithotomy.*** Large stones that are not easily removed with ureteroscopy can be removed through a percutaneous tract into the renal collecting system. Local anesthesia or moderate sedation is used to establish the percutaneous nephrostomy tract with the guidance of fluoroscopy or ultrasound scan. A plastic sheath is left in place through which a rigid or flexible nephroscope can pass. Stones smaller than 1 cm can be manually removed with a grasping forceps. General anesthesia is used for the surgical procedure itself. For stones greater than 71 cm, lithotripsy is used according to the surgeon's preferred method and location of the stone.

Postoperative nursing care should include the consideration of surgical complications and all postanesthesia considerations. Blood loss from damage to an intrarenal artery is the most significant complication of percutaneous nephrolithotomy. Extravasation of the irrigation solution used during surgery is another complication. Rare complications include damage to the surrounding organs caused by perforation with the placement of the percutaneous nephrostomy tube. The nephrostomy tube may be left in place for 1 to 5 days. Pain at the nephrostomy site may require management with opioids. As with all genitourinary surgeries, adequate fluid intake is encouraged.

***Kidney Transplantation.*** The kidney is the most commonly transplanted organ and the only one that can be preserved in a viable state for some time (Fig. 41-5). The kidney is relatively easy to remove and implant. Most people have two functioning kidneys and need only one to sustain life; therefore, kidney transplantation is done only for patients who need the organ to replace a diseased or nonfunctioning solitary kidney. Transplantation can be accomplished two, three, or even more times in the same patient, with the use of hemodialysis when a functioning kidney is not in place.

Kidney grafts come from two sources: cadaver donors and living donors. Most living donors are a close blood relative of the recipient. Ideally, an identical twin is the best donor. The closer the recipient and donor in blood line, the better the chances for survival of the kidney graft. Although the living related donor is best,

cadaver donors are the most common source of kidney graft.

General anesthesia is the preferred method of anesthesia for both the donor and the recipient in renal transplantation. After surgery, care of the living donor is essentially the same as that for the patient who has undergone nephrectomy. All care considered previously for the urologic patient applies, as does care for the patient after abdominal incision. If the laparoscopic approach was used (for the living donor), four to five stab wounds are found from the trocars used during surgery. Postoperative priorities include accurate intake and output, fluid volume and electrolyte replacement, adequate pulmonary perfusion, and pain and comfort measures.

Because postoperative care is routine, the donor patient often feels forgotten. Before surgery, the patient was considered heroic and received a generous helping of attention and glory; after surgery, attention is directed primarily to the organ recipient. The donor patient feels this even in the PACU. For this reason, the perianesthesia nurse must be aware of the needs of the postoperative donor and show concern for the patient's physical and psychologic well being. The care of these patients should be assigned to separate teams, if possible. In addition to normal self concern, the donor is concerned about the recipient and should receive factual information.

For the renal transplant patient, the commonly used immunosuppressive agents are nonspecific and suppress the entire immune system. However, immunosuppressive therapy is vital to the treatment for the renal transplant patient to prevent rejection of the donor kidney.

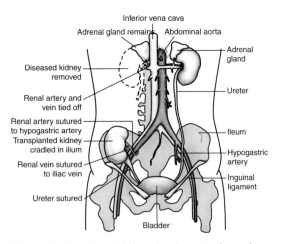

**Fig. 41-5** Transplanted kidney in place. *(Redrawn from Bergersen BS, et al, editors: Patients with kidney transplants, Curr Concepts Clin Nurs 1:1967.)*

Calcineurin inhibitors, which block production of interluekin-2 in the T-cell lymphocyte, purine inhibitors, and steroids are the first-line medications given for immunosuppression. A transplant patient receives one drug from each category. Sometimes, an antibody agent directed against T cells is given (Box 41-1). PACU nurses should know the specific agents and transplant protocols used by their hospitals. Wound infections are among the common causes of death after kidney transplantation. Meticulous aseptic technique is therefore imperative with these patients to prevent the introduction of infection.

On admission to the PACU, the recipient should be kept in a flat position for 12 hours, which allows the kidney to set. The head of the bed may be elevated 30 degrees to provide comfort and respiratory care. After 12 hours, the patient may turn to the side of the transplant. Turning to the opposite side may dislodge the graft. All vital signs are monitored continuously. Many renal transplant patients need antihypertensive medications after surgery. Blood pressures are more easily controlled as the fluid status becomes stable.

A Foley catheter is in place, and all urine should be carefully monitored for volume and specific gravity. During the immediate postoperative period, the renal allograft is extremely sensitive to hypovolemia and even a transient period of poor renal perfusion may result in oliguric renal failure. The kidney from a living

donor may start to function almost immediately after transplantation, and diuresis occurs. The volume of urine output may be great enough to warrant measurement every 15 minutes. The cadaver kidney, on the other hand, reacts more slowly, depending on the cold ischemic time spent during transportation.

Urine samples are generally collected hourly to ascertain electrolyte content, creatinine level, and osmolarity. Once daily, the total 24-hour urine collection (minus the small samples sent hourly) is sent to the laboratory for creatinine clearance test and culture. Urine output less than 1 mL/kg/h should be reported to the surgeon because any decrease in urine output may be a sign of early rejection or complications of the anastomosis site. Likewise, any gross hematuria should be reported immediately. A baseline postoperative weight should be ascertained as soon as feasible.

Other nursing considerations include care of the nasogastric tube that provides intestinal decompression and receives care as previously discussed. A central venous pressure line is present to further assess the patient's cardiovascular status. Monitoring of these systems is imperative to ensure adequate renal perfusion and prevent fluid overload. Skin integrity should be maintained, and the dressing over the incision site should evidence a minimal amount of drainage. The recipient may have a stenting catheter from the renal pelvis out through the urethra along with the Foley catheter for the first 36 to 48 hours to ensure ureteral patency.

Intravenous fluids provide most of the intake for these patients until the nasogastric tube can be removed. Intravenous replacement fluid composition is determined by the serum and urine electrolyte content, the hematocrit, and the clinical course of the patient. Volume is determined from necessary fluid requirements of the patient in normal status plus replacement on a volume-to-volume basis of drainage from the Foley catheter, nasogastric tube, ureterostomy, and cystostomy. For the first 72 hours after operation, the major source of output is from the ureterostomy. Meticulous handling of the closed urinary drainage system is mandatory to prevent the introduction of infection.

Vigorous pulmonary toilet should be instituted immediately to prevent atelectasis. The patient may be turned to the side of the kidney graft and back every 30 minutes to provide for change of position. The painful flank incision can be splinted either with the nurse's hands or with a firm pillow or a rolled blanket to assist the patient with coughing.

---

**Box 41-1  Immunosuppression Medications**

**Induction** (administered in the first week after transplantation)
  Antibody agents
  Steriods
  Purine inhibitors (azathioprine/mycophenolate mofetil)
  Calcineurin inhibitors (cyclosporine/tacrolimus)
**Maintenance** (administered during the first week and maintained throughout viability of transplant)
  Steroids
  Purine inhibitors (azathioprine/mycophenolate mofetil)
  Calcineurin inhibitors (cyclosporine/tacrolimus)
**Rejection** (administered when rejection is identified, often the first 2 to 4 weeks after transplant)
  High-dose steroids
  Antibody agents

From Barone CP, Lightfoot ML, Barone GW: The postanesthesia care of an adult renal transplant recipient, *J Perianesth Nurs* 18:32-41, 2003.

NURSING CARE IN THE PACU

The threat of graft rejection is ever present; therefore, the health care professional must observe closely for signs of rejection. Hyperacute allograft rejection can occur within minutes of the completion of the vascular anastomosis or in the first few postoperative hours. Signs and symptoms of hyperacute rejection are noted in Box 41-2. For prevention of irreversible damage to the kidney, treatment of a threatened rejection immediately is of the utmost importance.

The patient may have a strong fear of rejection while still in the PACU. Many patients view this surgery as the last chance to live a normal life after facing numerous physical, psychologic, and socioeconomic stressors. The perianesthesia nurse may need to reassure the patient often that the kidney is functioning.

After discharge from the PACU, the patient is usually transferred to the surgical intensive care unit for several days after surgery for close observation and intensive care.

### Bladder Surgery

The bladder is a smooth muscle storage tank that holds urine until a reflex, normally with voluntary control, releases the urine to pass through the urethra to be eliminated. Surgical procedures on the bladder include the removal of stones, foreign bodies, and tumors; the repair of strictures at the bladder neck and of injuries, such as lacerations; and the removal of the bladder itself.

Anesthesia for these procedures may be either spinal or general. On admission to the PACU, the patient is placed in a supine position. The head of the bed may be raised 30 degrees as

---

**Box 41-2   Signs and Symptoms of Allograft Rejection**

Irritability
Anxiousness
Restlessness
Lethargy
Swollen tender kidney
Decreased urine output
Fever, may be low-grade
Increased blood pressure
Weight gain
Anorexia
Increased blood urea nitrogen and serum creatinine levels
Decreased creatinine clearance
Increased urine protein and lysozyme activity
Lymphocytes in the urine

---

soon as feasible. The removal of stones or foreign bodies and the resection of selected tumors may be accomplished via cystoscopy, which was discussed previously. After the repair of lacerations or after cystotomy for removal of stones, the patient is admitted to the PACU with a Foley catheter and a urinary diversion, such as a suprapubic cystostomy, usually in place. Urine from these drainage systems is pink tinged but should not become grossly bloody. Dressings should remain dry and intact, fluids should be increased, and oral fluids should be started as soon as the effects of anesthesia have passed.

**Cystectomy.** Lacerations or ruptures of the bladder are often the result of accidental trauma. They require emergency surgery, and the postoperative patient should be assessed carefully for any unrecognized associated injuries. Pain should be minimal for these patients and easily controlled with mild analgesics. The presence of severe pain may represent a complication, such as internal hemorrhage and damage to a ureter, and should be reported to the surgeon.

Cystectomy may be performed as a result of trauma or underlying pathology, such as muscle invasive bladder cancer. Whether the cystectomy is partial or radical (includes hysterectomy and anterior vaginectomy in females and prostatectomy in males), urinary diversion is necessary. Care for an ileal conduit was discussed in the section on ureteral surgery. Other forms of urinary diversion include Koch pouch, cutaneous continent ileocecal reservoir, and ileocolic neobladder and orthotopic bladder substitution. The type of urinary diversion is specific for each patient with consideration to age, height and weight, surgical history, and medical history.

Postanesthesia care includes all the principles of surgical nursing along with special consideration to drains and catheters specific to type of diversion. The PACU nurse should observe the patient for potential complications that include stricture of the anastomosis site, rupture of the reservoir with neobladder or Koch pouch, infection, and any metabolic complications. Irrigation of the urethral catheter with 50 mL of saline solution 0.9% every 6 hours while the suprapubic catheter is freely draining is started immediately after surgery to prevent mucous from clotting the catheter.

Patients may awaken in the PACU with questions regarding the surgeon's ability to remove the cancer in its entirety. Patients should be allowed to discuss fears and feelings. The nurse should pay close attention to patient concerns for changes in body image and fears for loss of intimacy with a partner.

### Bladder Neck Suspensions.
Quality of life challenges are significant in patients with incontinence. Bladder neck suspensions in a variety of techniques are done to correct urinary stress incontinence. Postoperative complications for all techniques include urinary retention, wound infection, urinary tract infection, continued incontinence, retroperitoneal hemorrhage, and organ perforation.

Sling procedures including the Tension-free Vaginal Tape (TVT Sling) are a recent development for the correction of urinary stress incontinence caused by pelvic floor relaxation in women and are considered a first-line surgical intervention. This procedure can be done with local anesthetic and MAC. Potential complications include postoperative voiding difficulties, bowel perforation, and erosion of the tape into the bladder, urethra, or vagina.

Immediate postoperative care includes monitoring of patients depending on the level of sedation after MAC. Pain medication should be administered as ordered. Close monitoring of voiding status ensures that bladder overdistention does not occur. Once the patient is able to void, postvoid residual should be assessed with bladder ultrasound scan. If the patient is unable to void or postvoid residual is greater than 100 mL, an indwelling urinary catheter may be ordered. Nursing care then includes patient teaching on care of the catheter at home and instructions on follow-up with the surgeon for voiding trial.

### Artificial Urinary Sphincter.
Another treatment for urinary incontinence is the placement of an artificial urinary sphincter (AUS). This invasive procedure is a method to restore control over urinary function. AUS is a prosthetic device that consists of three parts: a balloon pressure reservoir, a control pump that is implanted in the scrotum or labia, and a cuff that occludes the urethra. This prosthetic device substitutes for the sphincteric mechanism and prevents the loss of urine. Indications for this procedure include postprostatectomy urinary leakage, congenital disorders of the bladder, and unsuccessful reconstructive surgery of the urethra.

Postanesthesia care includes principles of care for patients receiving general anesthesia. Specific assessment for this procedure includes observation for signs of hematoma along the plane of dissection for the pump in the scrotum or labia. Bladder ultrasound scan can be used to assess for urinary retention that may result from edema around the cuff site.

Along with use of opioid analgesics to control pain, ice packs to the scrotum or labia and perineal areas provide comfort and prevent swelling.

The patients arrive in the PACU with an indwelling catheter, and traction on the urethral catheter should be avoided to avoid increased pressure on the cuff of the sphincter.

## Prostatic Surgery
The prostate gland is a small walnut-sized male reproductive organ. Its sole function is to manufacture a secretion that becomes part of the semen; the prostate gland is a nonessential organ. Surgical procedures performed on the prostate gland include the excision of tumors and the resection or total removal of the gland.

The preferred anesthesia is spinal, although general anesthesia may be used. Several different approaches are common in surgery on the prostate. Most common is the transurethral approach, especially if only minor obstructive lesions or small portions of the gland are to be removed. A resectoscope is introduced through the urethra, and the surgeon excises the tissue with a moveable tungsten wire that operates on high-frequency current controlled with a foot pedal.

When the patient is admitted to the PACU after transurethral resection of the prostate (TURP), a three-way Foley catheter may be in place (see Fig. 41-2, A). One lumen allows filling of the retention balloon, one lumen allows outflow of the urine and irrigation fluid from the bladder, and one lumen is attached to the irrigation fluid system. Irrigation fluid, which is usually normal saline solution at room temperature, is available in 3000-mL plastic bags and may be regulated like intravenous solutions. To avoid creation of a hypothermic state with irrigation of the bladder with this solution, the saline solution should be warmed before administration and the patient's temperature should be monitored. The triple-lumen catheter is advantageous in that blood clots do not regularly form and block the system when the flow is continuous. The irrigation rate should be regulated so that drainage remains a light-pink watermelon color. If drainage becomes bright red, speed up the irrigation; if the returning fluid is clear, slow down the irrigation. Some institutions use a Y-connecting system with one arm of the Y connected to the irrigating fluid and the other to straight-gravitational drainage from the bladder. In either instance, because the prostatic bed is highly vascular, a fair amount of bleeding can be expected after TURP. This bleeding may also increase as the spinal anesthesia wears off and may require frequent irrigation to prevent clogging of the drainage tube. If the catheter becomes clogged, irrigation with a piston syringe and the same normal saline irrigating solution may be necessary. If patency of the catheter cannot be reestablished, the surgeon must be notified.

The patient's vital signs should be monitored closely. Observe for signs and symptoms of post-TURP syndrome (hyponatremia) that may occur from venous absorption of the irrigation fluid through the venous sinuses. Serum sodium and potassium levels should be checked during the postoperative period because changes in fluid balance may affect these electrolytes. Signs and symptoms of hyponatremia are a low serum sodium level, tachypnea, shortness of breath, nausea, vomiting, hypertension, bradycardia, increased pulse pressure, restlessness, apprehension, and mental disorientation. If this syndrome occurs, the perianesthesia nurse should notify the anesthesia provider and surgeon, administer oxygen to the patient, monitor blood loss and electrocardiographic and fluid and electrolyte status, and administer intravenous fluid (hypertonic saline solution 3% or 5% in 100 mL/h increments until the serum sodium level is satisfactory) and diuretics to mobilize the edema.

Oral fluids should be started and increased as tolerated as soon as possible. Diet may be progressed as tolerated in the absence of any postoperative nausea. Intravenous fluid replacement should be maintained until adequate oral fluids are maintained.

Pain should be minimal and easily controlled with mild analgesics. Analgesics or tranquilizers may be administered to control the discomfort of bladder spasms and of the presence of the catheter, which makes the patient feel an urgency to void although the bladder is being emptied. Symptoms of abdominal pain, abdominal rigidity, increase in pulse rate, and other signs of shock should alert the nurse to the possibility that the bladder wall or the capsule of the prostate was accidentally perforated during surgery; these symptoms should be reported to the surgeon immediately.

Other approaches to prostatic surgery include retrograde or suprapubic, perineal, and retropubic incisions. When the suprapubic approach is used, a midline vertical incision is made in the lowest part of the abdomen, the bladder is incised, and the tumors are removed. This procedure is the choice when 60 g or more of tissue is to be removed. The patient is admitted to the PACU with a Foley catheter, which may or may not be attached to an irrigation system. If it is not connected to an irrigation system, the catheter has to be irrigated frequently via syringe to prevent clots from clogging the drainage system. The patient also has a suprapubic catheter that should be connected to straight-gravitational drainage in place; output should be measured carefully (Fig. 41-6). In addition, a small Penrose drain is inserted in the suprapubic space and brought out through a separate stab wound. A dressing of several layers of 4 × 4 sponges should cover the incision and the drain. A moderate amount of serosanguineous drainage can be expected because of the presence of the drain. This dressing should be reinforced as necessary to keep the skin clean and dry. If excessive bright-red bleeding occurs, the surgeon must be notified.

The surgeon may apply traction to the Foley catheter by taping the catheter to the inner thigh. Because the traction puts tension against the vesical outlet and promotes hemostasis, it may produce painful bladder spasms that may be relieved with the use of intravenous opioids such as meperidine or belladonna and opium suppositories. After the traction is removed, a small increase in bleeding may be expected for a short time.

The perineal approach, used for removal of large amounts of tissue, is the approach of choice for prostatic cancer. A V-shaped incision is made above the rectum in this approach. The patient is admitted to the PACU with a Foley catheter and a perineal drain. Because of the perineal drain, a moderate amount of serosanguineous drainage can be expected, and the dressing should be reinforced as necessary. No instrumentation, including thermometers, should be placed in the rectum during the immediate postoperative period.

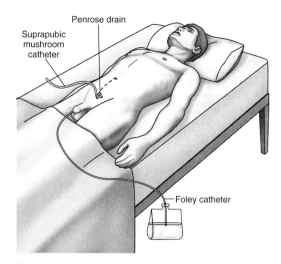

**Fig. 41-6** Postoperative positions of drainage tubes after suprapubic prostatectomy. *(Redrawn from LeMaitre GD, Finnegan JA: The patient in surgery: a guide for nurses, ed 4, Philadelphia, 1980, Saunders.)*

When a retropubic approach is used, a small incision is made above the pubis and a capsular incision is made into the upper surface of the prostate. This approach is used in the nerve-sparing radical prostatectomy for patients whose carcinoma is confined within the prostate. This approach is preferred because of the decreased risk of postoperative complications of long-term incontinence and impotence.

On the patient's arrival to the PACU, a Foley catheter is in place and a small drain may be present that was inserted in the incision or brought out through a stab wound lateral to the incision. As with all urologic patients, accurate intake and output records must be maintained after prostatic surgery. The perianesthesia nurse must be sure to indicate in the output data whether irrigation solution is included. Output should be documented hourly. Color and appearance of urine should be monitored closely and documented.

Most prostatic surgery is performed on adult men older than 50 years of age because prostatic hypertrophy most commonly occurs after 40 years of age. Therefore, assessment of cardiorespiratory status should be performed frequently. Oxygen should be administered and weaned with pulse oximetry. All patients should be placed on a cardiac monitor for assessment of changes. Astute observation of vital signs is imperative to monitor cardiovascular function because postoperative bleeding may impair it. Observe carefully for decreasing blood pressure and increasing pulse rate, which may indicate impending shock.

One of the most common postoperative complications after the nerve-sparing radical prostatectomy is pulmonary embolism. For this reason, the surgeon may order low-dose heparin. Care in the PACU should include deep-breathing exercises and position changes along with passive or active movement of the extremities. Some type of antiembolism stocking should be used.

## Scrotal Surgery

The scrotum is a sac separated into two pouches: externally by the median raphe and internally by the dartos tunic. Each pouch contains a testis, an epididymis, and a spermatic cord. The vas deferens, which is continuous with the epididymis at the lower end of the testis, and the arteries, veins, nerves, and lymphatic vessels that are held together by spermatic fascia form the spermatic cord. Operations on the scrotum include excision of masses and tumors, correction of deformities, and excision of diseased or abnormal structures that interfere with normal function.

Anesthesia for scrotal surgery may be local, general, or spinal. Spinal anesthesia is commonly used for adult patients, whereas general anesthesia is usually preferred for children younger than 12 years of age. Local anesthesia is often used for simple procedures, such as vasectomy and epididymectomy.

The PACU course after surgery on the scrotal structures is usually uneventful. Care is dictated primarily by anesthesia agent and its method of administration. The patient may assume a position of comfort after surgery. Any dressings present should remain dry and intact. Oral food and fluids may be reinstituted as soon as the patient tolerates them. A Bellevue bridge commonly is applied to provide scrotal support and elevation (Fig. 41-7). This device is suspended from thigh to thigh with a tight sling across the expanse on which the scrotum is supported. A T-binder may also be used (Fig. 41-8).

The application of a light crushed-ice bag helps relieve scrotal edema, enhances hemostasis, and promotes comfort. Scrotal enlargement with apparent tension should be reported to the surgeon immediately. Progressive inguinal swelling may denote lymphatic obstruction after a varicocelectomy, and the surgeon must be notified. Pain should be minimal after these procedures and easily controlled with mild analgesics. Severe pain that is not controlled with mild analgesia should be reported to the surgeon.

As with any genital surgery, the patient's body image concerns and questions of fertility in particular may be of paramount importance. These concerns are not usually addressed in the PACU, but the nurse must be sensitive to

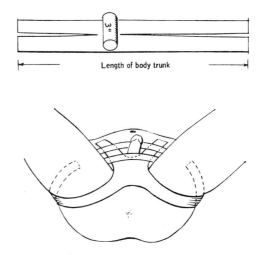

**Fig. 41-7** Bellevue bridge for scrotal support. *(From Sutton AL: Bedside nursing techniques in medicine and surgery, ed 2, Philadelphia, 1969, Saunders.)*

Length of body trunk

NURSING CARE IN THE PACU

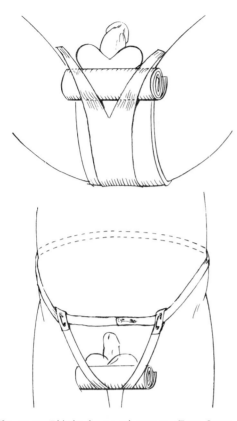

**Fig. 41-8**   T-binder for scrotal support. *(From Sutton AL: Bedside nursing techniques in medicine and surgery, ed 2, Philadelphia, 1969, Saunders.)*

them and prepared to assist the patient with factual information and reassurance. Often, these patients feel an urgency to inspect the operative site and should be assisted, if necessary, to do so.

The patient may be embarrassed by this type of surgery, may be reluctant to ask the nurse for assistance or to report pain, and may hesitate to allow the nurse to inspect the incision area. A matter-of-fact attitude on the part of the nurse and efficient care promote a sense of well being for the patient and may help alleviate these feelings. The nurse should keep in mind that preadolescent and adolescent boys are especially sensitive about the genital area. If at all possible, a male nurse should be assigned to these patients to alleviate anxiety.

### Penile and Urethral Surgery
Surgery on the penis and urethra involves removal of tumors or obstructions to urinary flow, plastic repair of deformities, and circumcision or excision of the foreskin. Partial or total amputation of the penis is rarely necessary but may be performed for malignant disease, which is essentially skin cancer. Laser technique is generally effective for the treatment of

condyloma acuminata and squamous cell carcinoma of the penis.

Anesthesia for these procedures may be local, general, or spinal. The PACU course is usually smooth, and care is determined primarily by the type of anesthesia. Physical care of the patient who has had a plastic repair of hypospadias or epispadias is dictated by the surgeon. Care for the patient after cystoscopy was discussed at the beginning of this chapter; the same care applies for patients who undergo cystoscopy for the resection of tumors.

After circumcision, which may be performed for correction of phimosis or for elective reasons, the nurse should check for bleeding. Usually, only a small band of petrolatum-impregnated gauze is applied as a dressing around the glans and is changed as directed. Bleeding that soaks this dressing is excessive and should be reported.

Patients who have undergone surgery on the penis should avoid erection during the PACU phase and at least a week after surgery. Patients with penile prostheses should be admitted to the PACU with the penis in a flaccid state; the prosthesis should remain deflated. Inflation of the prosthesis should be avoided until after the first postoperative visit to the surgeon.

Pain may be significant but should not be severe. Scrotal and penile support with a Bellevue bridge and the application of a light ice pack provide some relief; however, analgesia with small doses of opioids may be necessary. Food and fluids may be restarted as soon as the patient tolerates them. Urine output should be checked and recorded. Low abdominal distention on palpation may be caused by voluntary retention, which is not uncommon because of fear that micturition creates pain. The patient should be reassured and informed that overdistention of the bladder causes an increase in discomfort and possible complications.

### Adrenalectomy
Adrenalectomy involves the removal of one or both of the adrenal glands, which are situated on top of the kidneys. Adrenalectomy, an extensive and shock-producing procedure, may be performed for several reasons, including metastasized cancer from the reproductive organs, hyperfunction caused by hyperplasia of the organ, and adrenal tumors. The following two adrenal tumors are of major consequence: pheochromocytoma, a usually benign tumor that causes hyperfunction and results in severe symptoms; and neuroblastoma, a malignant tumor that is a leading cause of death in childhood.

General anesthesia is used for adrenalectomy and may include the use of cortisone titrated to maintain catecholamine levels and blood pressure. Cortisone is usually necessary only when bilateral adrenalectomy is performed or when the uninvolved adrenal gland has poor function. The administration of cortisone, which is continued in the PACU, is an extremely important nursing procedure. The anesthesia provider and surgeon should give specific instructions for titration of the solution. Failure to maintain postoperative levels of cortisone leads to hypovolemic and hyponatremic shock. Perianesthesia care of these patients is a nursing challenge; observations must be especially astute.

The surgical approach for adrenalectomy may be lateral, anterior, or posterior. On admission to the PACU, the patient is placed in the sidelying position until reactive from anesthesia, at which time the patient is placed in a semi-Fowler's position. The surgeon may prefer the patient to be positioned on the operative side so that the perinephric space is obliterated to discourage bleeding. Assessment is aimed primarily at the cardiovascular status of the patient because hemorrhage and shock are the two most common and most disastrous complications. Profound shock may develop because of the reduction of circulating catecholamines that is precipitated by removal of the glands and the effects of the drugs used for preoperative control of hypertension. The effects of these drugs usually last for a few hours after surgery. Because most of these drugs produce vasodilation, they are usually a factor in postoperative hypotension. Therefore, a fluid challenge usually is given in an attempt to treat hypotension. If fluid is not successful in increasing the blood pressure, then vasopressor drugs are used. Epinephrine or norepinephrine in an intravenous solution may be titrated to maintain blood pressure, according to the surgeon's instructions.

Shock may also result from hemorrhage because the adrenal glands are extremely vascular. Intravenous fluids, including hypertonic saline solutions, blood, plasma, dextran, and glucose in water, may be used to maintain blood volume and prevent shock. Dressings over the bilateral incisions should remain relatively dry even though drains are placed. If these dressings become soaked, the surgeon should be notified because this represents excessive bleeding. If the patient has abdominal pain, abdominal distention, nausea, or vomiting, development of an abdominal hematoma may be indicated; these signs should be reported to the surgeon.

Other parameters of the patient's status that may give clues to the development of shock should also be assessed. Dehydration (increased urine specific gravity) and restlessness may indicate developing shock. Central venous pressure should be checked. A Foley catheter is in place, and urine output should be monitored hourly. The development of oliguria or output of less than 1 mL/kg/h may indicate shock and subsequent renal shutdown. Serum and urine electrolyte levels, especially sodium, should be determined hourly.

All care outlined for the patient after high abdominal incisions in Chapter 40 is applicable to this patient. Good pulmonary toilet should be instituted immediately in the PACU. A nasogastric tube often is necessary until normal intestinal peristalsis returns. Incisional pain may require the use of opioid analgesics. Because many opioids have a hypotensive effect, they should be titrated judiciously; blood pressure must be monitored continuously for at least 30 minutes after their administration.

The patient often is placed in protective isolation to avoid the introduction of infection. Meticulous sterile technique must be used when changing or reinforcing dressings. Because of extreme lability, which lasts for approximately 48 hours, these patients should be transferred to the surgical intensive care unit for continuous monitoring.

## SUMMARY

This chapter has discussed the perianesthesia care of the patient who undergoes genitourinary surgery. The perianesthesia nurse should have an understanding of anatomic location and normal function of this system and the important postanesthesia nursing concerns for this type of patient. Adrenalectomy was included in this chapter because of the proximity of the adrenal glands to the kidneys.

## BIBLIOGRAPHY

Alspach JG: *Core curriculum for critical care nursing,* ed 6, St Louis, 2006, Saunders.

Atlee J: *Complications in anesthesia,* ed 2, Philadelphia, 2007, Saunders.

Barash PG, Cullen BF, Stoelting RK: *Clinical anesthesia,* ed 5, Philadelphia, 2005, Lippincott Williams & Wilkins.

Barone CP, Lightfoot ML, Barone GW: The postanesthesia care of an adult renal transplant recipient, *J Perianesth Nurs* 18:32-41, 2003.

Bickley LS, Szilagyi PG: *Bates' guide to physical examination and history taking,* ed 9, Philadelphia, 2005, Lippincott Williams & Wilkins.

Brunton L, Lazo J, Parker K: *Goodman and Gilman's the pharmacological basis of therapeutics*, ed 11, New York, 2005, McGraw-Hill Professional.

Cottrell J, Smith D: *Anesthesia and neurosurgery*, ed 4, St Louis, 2001, Mosby.

DeFazio-Quinn D, Schick L: *Perianesthesia nursing core curriculum*, St Louis, 2004, Saunders.

Eaton J: Detection of hyponatremia in the PACU, *J Perianesth Nurs* 18(6):392-397, 2003.

Fleisher LA: *Anesthesia and uncommon diseases*, ed 5, Philadelphia, 2006, Saunders.

Ganong W: *Review of medical physiology*, ed 21, New York, 2005, McGraw-Hill Professional.

Guyton AC, Hall JE: *Textbook of medical physiology*, ed 11, Philadelphia, 2006, Saunders.

Hanson K: Minimally invasive and surgical management of urinary stones, *Urol Nurs* 25:458-464, 2005.

Katzung BG, editor: *Basic and clinical pharmacology*, ed 10, Los Altos, Calif, 2006, Lange McGraw Hill.

Krapp K, Gale T, editors: Bladder ultrasound, Encyclopedia of Nursing & Allied Health, 2002, eNotes.com. 2006. Available at http://health.enot es.com/nursing-encyclopedia/bladder-ultrasound, Accessed July 15, 2007.

Lake C, Hines R, Blitt C: *Clinical monitoring: practical applications for anesthesia and critical care*, St Louis, 2001, Mosby.

Longnecker D, Murphy F: *Dripps/Eckenhoff/Vandam introduction to anesthesia*, ed 9, Philadelphia, 1997, Saunders.

Nagle GM: Genitourinary surgery. In JC Rothrock, editor: *Alexander's care of the patient in surgery*, ed 13, St Louis, 2007, Mosby.

Nagle GM: Renal/genitourinary surgery. In DM Quinn, and L Schick, editors: *Perianesthesia nursing core curriculum, preoperative, phase I and phase II PACU nursing*, St Louis, 2004, Saunders.

Nagelhout J, Zaglaniczny K: *Nurse anesthesia*, ed 2, Philadelphia, 2001, Saunders.

Miller RD, editor: *Anesthesia*, ed 6, New York, 2005, Churchill Livingstone.

Overstreet DL, Sims TW: Care of the patient undergoing radical cystectomy with a robotic approach, *Urol Nurs* 26(2):117-125, 2006.

Perimenis P, Koliopanou E: Postoperative management and rehabilitation of patients receiving an ileal orthotopic bladder substitution, *Urol Nurs* 24(5):383-386, 2004.

Polt CA: Taking the pressure off for women with stress incontinence, *Nursing* 36(2):49-51, 2006.

Quallich SA, Ohl DA: Urinary sphincter, part I: overview, *Urol Nurs* 23(4):259-268, 2003.

Quallich SA, Ohl DA: Artificial urinary sphincter, part II: patient teaching and perioperative care, *Urol Nurs* 23(4):269-273, 2003.

Stoelting R, Hillier SC: *Pharmacology and physiology in anesthetic practice*, ed 4, Philadelphia, 2005, Lippincott Williams & Wilkins.

Stoelting RK, Miller RD: *Basics of anesthesia*, ed 5, New York, 2007, Churchill Livingstone.

Townsend CM, Beauchamp RD, Evers BM, et al: *Sabiston textbook of surgery: the biological basis of modern surgical practice*, ed 17, Philadelphia, 2004, Saunders.

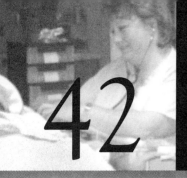

# 42

# CARE OF THE OBSTETRIC AND GYNECOLOGIC SURGICAL PATIENT

*Wendy K. Winer, RN, BSN, CNOR*

Surgery on organs of reproduction usually involves an adult patient. However, the perianesthesia nurse may encounter pediatric or adolescent female patients who undergo gynecologic surgery for repair or correction of congenital or traumatic deformities or incapacitating pelvic pain (from causes such as endometriosis, ovarian cyst, or appendicitis). Surgery on the female genitalia may be conveniently divided into three major categories: (1) obstetric; (2) lower genital and vaginal; and (3) abdominal gynecological surgery. Abdominal surgery is then subdivided into either traditional surgery in the form of a laparotomy or into the category of operative laparoscopy. The area of operative laparoscopy in gynecologic surgery is expanding to such an enormous extent that most benign gynecologic surgery is moving in that direction. If the surgeon and operative team have the proper training, most benign surgeries, except obstetric surgeries, can be done in this way with many benefits for the patient. For this reason, the perianesthesia nurse must be aware of how the care of the patient differs with these procedures.

## DEFINITIONS

### Obstetric Surgery

**Cerclage Procedure:** Procedure for the treatment of incompetent cervix. The McDonald procedure involves the placement of a purse-string suture on the cervix at the level of the internal os; the Shirodkar's procedure involves placement of a fascia lata (from the thigh) or a surgical band at the level of the internal os.

**Cesarean Hysterectomy:** Incision of the abdomen and the uterus, extraction of the infant and the placenta, and performance of a hysterectomy.

**Cesarean Section (C-section):** Delivery of an infant through an incision made in the abdominal and uterine walls.

**C-section, Classic:** A midline incision between the umbilicus and the symphysis pubis and an anterior incision through the uterine wall.

**C-section, Low Segment:** An incision in the lower part of the uterus made after an abdominal incision.

**Ectopic Pregnancy:** Implantation of the fertilized ovum in any site other than the upper half of the uterus (Fig. 42-1).

**Uterine Aspiration (suction curettage):** Dilation of the cervix and vacuum removal of the uterine contents.

### Lower Genital Surgery, Vaginal Surgery, Abdominal Surgery (Laparotomy and Laparoscopy)

**Bartholin's Duct Cyst:** A cyst that results from chronic inflammation of one of the major vestibular glands at the vaginal introitus (Fig. 42-2).

**Bartholinectomy:** Removal of a Bartholin's duct cyst.

**Cervical Conization:** Removal of abnormal cervical tissue via scalpel, electrosurgical current, or laser.

**Colporrhaphy:** Repair of the vaginal wall. May be anterior, as for cystocele repair, or posterior, as for rectocele repair or enterocele repair specifically for vaginal prolapse.

**Culdoscopy:** An operative diagnostic procedure in which an incision is made into the posterior vaginal cul-de-sac, through which a tubular instrument similar to a cystoscope is inserted for the purpose of visualization of the pelvic structures, including the uterus, fallopian tubes, broad ligaments, uterosacral ligaments, rectal wall, sigmoid colon, and sometimes, the small intestine. A newer technique for this procedure is transvaginal hydrolaparoscopy, which uses normal saline solution and a camera attached to a small-diameter rigid endoscope.

**Cystocele:** Prolapse of the bladder into the anterior vaginal wall.

**Dilation of the Cervix and Curettage of the Uterus (D&C):** Introduction of instruments (dilators) through the vagina into the cervical

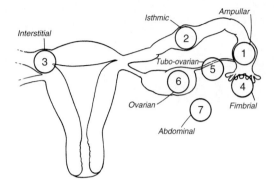

**Fig. 42-1** Ectopic pregnancy. Diagram shows various implantation sites, numbered in order of decreasing frequency of occurrence. *(From Townsend CM: Sabiston textbook of surgery: the biological basis of modern surgical practice, ed 16, Philadelphia, 2001, Saunders.)*

canal and scraping of the uterus with a curette for removal of substances, including blood. This procedure is used for diagnostic purposes and for treatment of conditions such as incomplete abortion, abnormal uterine bleeding, and primary dysmenorrhea.

**Enterocele:** Defect in the continuity of the endopelvic fascia most commonly seen after posthysterectomy when the anterior pubic fascia is not attached to the denoviellers fascia.

**Hysterectomy:** Removal of the uterus; can be vaginal (with or without laparoscopic assistance) or abdominal (via laparotomy).

**Hysteroscopy:** Direct visualization of the canal of the uterine cervix and cavity of the uterus with an endoscope called a hysteroscope.

**Procidentia:** Herniation of the uterus beyond the introitus.

**Prolapse of the Uterus:** Downward displacement of the uterus. Vaginal hysterectomy is often recommended for a prolapsed uterus when childbearing is no longer desired or when marked prolapse is present.

**Rectocele:** Prolapse of the rectum into the posterior vaginal wall.

**Trachelorrhaphy:** Removal of torn surfaces of the anterior and posterior cervical lips and reconstruction of the cervical canal.

**Urethrocele:** Prolapse of the urethra into the anterior vaginal wall.

**Vaginal Plastic Operation (Anterior and Posterior Repair):** Reconstruction of the vaginal walls (colporrhaphy), the pelvic floor, and the muscles and fascia of the rectum, urethra, bladder, and perineum. Used to correct a cystocele or rectocele, restore the bladder to its normal position, and strengthen the vagina and the pelvic floor.

## ABDOMINAL GYNECOLOGIC SURGERY (LAPAROTOMY AND LAPAROSCOPY)

**Abdominal myomectomy:** Removal of leiomyomas; laparoscopy endoscopic visualization of the peritoneal cavity through a small incision in the anterior abdominal wall after the establishment

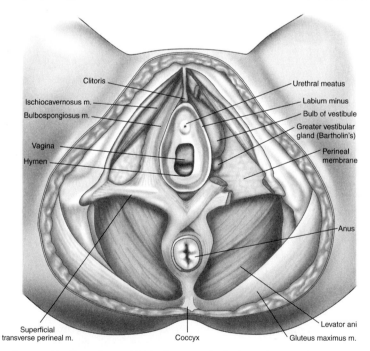

**Fig. 42-2** Female perineum with skin and superficial fascia removed. *(Redrawn from Jacob SW, Francone CA, Lossow WJ: Structure and function in man, ed 5, Philadelphia, 1982, Saunders.)*

of a pneumoperitoneum. A videocamera is attached to the eye piece of the laparoscope so that the surgeon and team can visualize the procedure from a video monitor and have an enhanced magnified view of the pelvis.

**Oophorectomy:** Removal of an ovary.

**Oophorocystectomy:** Removal of a cyst on the ovary.

**Radical Hysterectomy:** Removal of the uterus, the uterosacral and uterovesical ligaments, the upper third of the vagina, and all the peritoneum.

**Salpingectomy:** Excision of the fallopian tube.

**Salpingoophorectomy:** Removal of the fallopian tube and the associated ovary.

**Salpingostomy (Tubal Plasty):** Removal of the obstructed portion of the fallopian tube and opening of the tube to establish patency. Tubal plasty or tubal reanastomosis is used for removal of an obstructed portion of the tube and reconnection of each normal end of the tube after the obstruction has been removed to establish patency. Note: Tubal reanastomosis increases the risk of ectopic pregnancy.

**Total Abdominal Hysterectomy:** Removal of the uterus, including the corpus and the cervix (with or without the adnexa), through an abdominal incision.

**Tubal Ligation:** Interruption of fallopian tube continuity, which results in sterilization. The most common technique is the Pomeroy's procedure, which is done through a laparoscope. A segment of the fallopian tube is ligated and excised. Reversal procedures are now performed with microsurgery.

## OBSTETRIC SURGERY

Obstetric surgery involves procedures on pregnant women to promote full-term pregnancy, to provide an alternative means of delivery when normal vaginal delivery is not feasible for reasons of fetal or maternal well being, and to interrupt pregnancy.

### Care After Specific Procedures

*Cesarean Section.* Cesarean sections are performed on both an emergency and an elective basis. These patients have special physical and psychologic needs. A selection of articles is included in the bibliography at the end of this chapter to assist the reader who provides care for families who experience cesarean birth.

Cesarean sections are indicated for dystocia (usually caused by cephalopelvic disproportion); antepartum bleeding; some toxemic conditions; certain medical complications, especially diabetes mellitus; and previous cesarean section. The low-segment cesarean section is usually the procedure of choice. Anesthesia may be general inhalation, spinal, or local infiltration of the operative field.

Postoperative care after cesarean section includes all care rendered to a patient who undergoes abdominal surgery and postpartum care.

On admission to the postanesthesia care unit (PACU), a report is given by the circulating nurse who transports the patient with the anesthesia provider to the PACU area. The patient's vital signs should be monitored regularly in keeping with the PACU guidelines in the facility. As soon as condition permits, the patient can assume any position of comfort. Oxygen should be delivered and monitored with the use of pulse oximetry.

Parenteral fluids are usually administered during the first 24 hours after surgery, but oral fluids can usually be resumed as soon as bowel sounds are audible and the patient desires. Intravenous fluids often contain oxytocin to increase uterine muscle tone and stop excessive blood flow. Usually 10 to 20 units of oxytocin are added to 1000 mL of Ringer's lactate solution and infused at 125 mL/h. Side effects with oxytocin are not common. Serious side effects include an allergic reaction (shortness of breath; closing of the throat; hives; swelling of the lips, face, or tongue; rash; or fainting), difficulty in urination, chest pain or irregular heart beat, difficulty in breathing, confusion, sudden weight gain or excessive swelling, severe headache, rash, excessive vaginal bleeding, or seizures. Other, less serious, side effects may be more likely to occur and include redness or irritation at the injection site; loss of appetite; and nausea or vomiting. The physician should be notified if any side effects occur. Perianesthesia nurses should be familiar with potential side effects. Intake and output should always be monitored appropriately in the PACU regardless of what medications are given. A progressive diet is advised, pending the return of bowel sounds.

The patient has an abdominal dressing and a perineal pad; both should be inspected for drainage. The abdominal dressing should remain dry and intact. A moderate amount of lochia rubra is normal, but saturation of two or more perineal pads with blood during the first hour is considered excessive. The area underneath the buttocks should be checked for pooling of blood.

The fundus should be checked frequently to ensure that it is firmly contracted. Checking of

NURSING CARE IN THE PACU

the fundus is an uncomfortable procedure for the patient; therefore, careful explanation should be provided before it is performed. The patient should be encouraged to relax the abdominal muscles as much as possible. Slow deep breathing with an open mouth facilitates relaxation of those muscles. If the uterus is firmly contracted, it need not be massaged, and in fact should not be massaged, because massage may cause uterine muscle fatigue and subsequent relaxation and bleeding. If the uterus is soft and "boggy," it should be gently but firmly massaged through the abdominal wall to stimulate contraction. The patient may be instructed to do this herself with supervision, which may allay anxiety and be more comfortable. Oxytocin often is administered intravenously and titrated to maintain the uterus in a state of contraction. If oxytocin is used, the uterus should be checked for firmness but usually does not need frequent massage.

A full bladder is one cause of uterine atony. An indwelling urethral catheter commonly is left in place for the first 12 postoperative hours. A fundus palpated above the umbilicus or to the side of the abdomen (usually the right side) may indicate a nonfunctioning catheter. The catheter should be positioned for gravitational drainage and avoidance of kinks. The urine should be monitored for volume and color.

Many patients have transient trembling or shivering after delivery. Several theories have been proposed with regard to this sense of chilling, although the actual cause remains unknown. This trembling is generally not associated with an elevation of temperature. Warmed blankets or warm-air therapy should be available as a comfort measure.

Many hospitals have separate PACUs for postpartum patients; thus, the special considerations for the cesarean section patient pose no significant problems. The nurse who cares for the cesarean section patient within the general PACU must be judicious and often innovative to meet the needs of not only the mother but also the new family. The mother, the neonate, and the father should be together as soon as possible to allow for the bonding experience. This experience may be accomplished with using a quiet corner of the unit (if such a place exists), drawing curtains around the family, or expediting the discharge process to transfer the patient to the postpartum unit. The mother and father are anxious to review the details of the birth together, and the perianesthesia nurse should be prepared to answer questions. Consistent communication between the surgical nurse and the perianesthesia nursing staff makes answering these questions much easier.

***Ectopic Pregnancy.*** Faulty implantation of the ovum may take place in the fallopian tube (in approximately 98% of all ectopic pregnancies), in the ovary, in any part of the abdominal cavity, or in the uterine cervix. Until recently, the treatment of choice for an ectopic pregnancy in the fallopian tube was laparoscopy (or laparotomy) with removal of the ectopic pregnancy and most often with preservation of the fallopian tube. In cases in which bleeding cannot be controlled or the physician feels the fallopian tube poses too much of a risk for the patient, removal of the fallopian tube at the time of surgery may be necessary. Obviously, the patient must give proper consent before surgery, and all of these possibilities are thoroughly discussed between the surgeon and the patient. More recently, however, patients with the early diagnosis of an unruptured ectopic pregnancy can receive intravenous (IV) methotrexate and not undergo surgery. Regardless of the treatment, these patients must have proper follow-up with their physicians to ensure successful treatment, which involves follow-up quantitative HCG studies and possibly ultrasound scans as well.

If laparoscopy is performed, the ovary preferably is not resected or removed. However, this procedure may be necessary if the ovary is involved with the ectopic pregnancy. If implantation occurs in the cervix, a hysterectomy is usually indicated to control hemorrhage. If abdominal implantation has occurred, the fetus is removed and the placenta often is left within the cavity to be reabsorbed.

Laparoscopy (or laparotomy) is performed with general anesthesia. The perianesthesia nurse should be especially observant for signs of intraabdominal hemorrhage and shock because these are not uncommon complications of ectopic pregnancy, especially one that has ruptured before surgery. All patients with ectopic pregnancy should have complete typing and cross-matching for whole blood, which should be kept available in the laboratory for 24 hours. Women who are Rh-negative should receive RhoGam to prevent sensitization.

***Cerclage Procedures.*** The McDonald or Shirodkar's procedure is used in treatment of an incompetent cervix and is fairly successful in maintenance of pregnancy. The suture is usually placed between the 14th and 18th week of gestation. These procedures may be accomplished with general, spinal, or regional anesthesia.

On admission to the PACU, hospital guidelines are followed regarding patient admission to the PACU and care of the patient (see Chapters 27 and 28).Oxygen should be administered and weaned with pulse oximetry. Food and fluids may be resumed as soon as the patient is conscious and the laryngeal reflexes have returned. A perineal pad should be kept in place. Only a minimal amount of bloody spotting is normal. Pain should be minimal and easily controlled with a simple analgesic such as acetaminophen. Any gross vaginal bleeding or abdominal cramping should be reported to the surgeon because this procedure may induce labor and expulsion of the uterine contents. The surgeon may order an external fetal monitor to assess the presence of uterine contractions and fetal heart tones. If labor begins, the suture must be removed immediately.

**Uterine Aspiration.** Uterine aspiration is used in termination of early pregnancy (i.e., first trimester) or in treatment of incomplete spontaneous abortion. It is a type of dilation of the cervix and curettage of the uterus (D&C). A general anesthetic may be used, but the trend has been toward the use of paracervical block and sedation only. Nursing care in the PACU is essentially the same as after D&C by conventional means. The woman who is Rh-negative should receive Rho-Gam to prevent sensitization. Complications from this procedure include incomplete evacuation and hemorrhage, which may be treated with oxytocin. Uterine perforation may occur and must be treated surgically.

## GYNECOLOGIC SURGERY

Certain problems are inherent in gynecologic disease processes and the surgical procedures that deal with them. Because of prolonged or heavy menstrual periods, the patient is often more chronically anemic than even the peripheral blood indices indicate. Moreover, large amounts of blood may have accumulated within the pelvic organs at the time of the operation and may not be reflected in the external blood loss. Although the procedures are elective, many gynecologic operations are associated with significant blood loss, depending on the approach taken. One of the potential benefits of a well-trained laparoscopic team is a decrease in intraoperative complications and blood loss and a significant reduction in postoperative morbidity. For example, in the case of a hysterectomy or large fibroids, the uterine vessels are large vascular pedicles that need to be carefully and thoroughly controlled to ensure hemostasis during surgery. For this reason, regardless of the approach (laparoscopic, vaginal, or laparotomy), these vessels must be identified and coagulated or ligated effectively. In addition, because of the proximity of the female organs to the urinary tract, great care must be taken during surgery to identify the ureters and bladder and provide proper follow-up during the observation period after surgery to ensure the integrity of this system. Therefore, in addition to overall assessment and general care of these patients, the perianesthesia nurse should direct specific attention toward the patient's cardiovascular status, renal function, and fluid balance.

### Laparoscopy

Operative laparoscopy commonly is performed as outpatient surgery for treatment of benign gynecologic problems and may involve advanced operative laparoscopic procedures for more significant problems that involve the pelvic organs. A small incision (approximately 1 cm) is made at the subumbilical site for insertion of the primary trocar (typically 10 to 12 mm in diameter), which houses the laparoscope with attached video camera for visualization of the procedure (Fig. 42-3). After pneumoperitoneum is established, the surgeon can visualize the organs within the peritoneum. The video camera enables the surgeon, first assistant, scrub

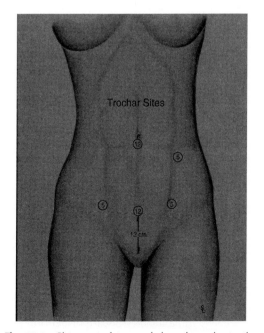

**Fig. 42-3** Placement of trocars during advanced operative laparoscopy. Trocar in upper left quadrant is optional and only recommended in cases in which primary trocar is not sufficient because of severe adhesions. Laparoscope needs to be placed off to one side or the other for taking down adhesions.

NURSING CARE IN THE PACU

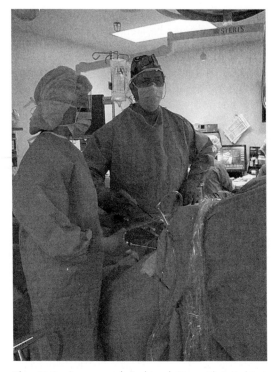

**Fig. 42-4** Surgeon and Registered Nurse First Assistant (RNFA) and the rest of the team are able to benefit from improved resolution attainable with high-definition cameras and monitors. *(Photo courtesy of Wendy Winer.)*

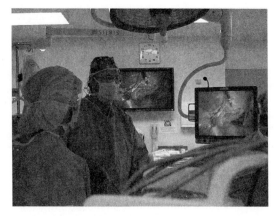

**Fig. 42-5** High-definition cameras and monitors used for laparoscopic surgery at Northside Hospital in Atlanta. (Photo courtesy of Wendy Winer.)

technician, and entire team to view the procedure on the video monitor. (Fig 42-4). The video camera provides excellent resolution and visualization of the pelvis.

Advances in digital technology with high-definition (HD) cameras and monitors provide better resolution than ever before (Fig. 42-5). The surgeon is able to operate from HD monitors with instruments that are typically 5 mm in diameter (sometimes the instruments are as small as 3 mm in diameter or as large as 12 mm in diameter, depending on the procedure). In addition, an angled laparoscope may be used for improved visualization in the case of a large uterus. The surgeon can thoroughly examine the ovaries, fallopian tubes, and uterus after placement of a second and third incision suprapubically in the right and left lower quadrant of the abdomen for additional instrumentation. Generally, a fourth incision along the midsuprapubic area is used as well. During operative laparoscopy, the surgeon may differentially diagnose pelvic inflammatory disease or perform relatively simple procedures, such as aspiration of an ovarian cyst, lysis of adhesions, tissue biopsy, and tubal ligation. In addition, more advanced laparoscopic procedures may be done, including extensive lysis of adhesions, excision of severe

endometriosis, myomectomy, hysterectomy, salpingectomy, salpingoooophorectomy, removal of an ovarian remnant, ureterolysis, burch or colposuspension procedures, repair of pelvic floor relaxation (including sacral culpopexy with nonabsorbable mesh or paravaginal repairs), appendectomy; fimbriolysis, and tubal reanastomosis (see Fig. 42-6). Various types of laparoscopic hysterectomy include laparoscopic supracervical hysterectomy (LSH), in which the cervix is preserved; laparoscopic-assisted vaginal hysterectomy (LAVH); and total laparoscopic hysterectomy (TLH).

Closure of the skin wound involves only a few sutures to close the fascia at the subumbilical site and possibly sutures at the ancillary sites, depending on size (incisional sites that house instrumentation 5 mm in diameter or less often may not need to be sutured and may only be closed with SteriStrips to approximate the edges of the skin incision). Typically, any incisions larger than 5 to 7 mm need to have the fascia closed to prevent the development of a postoperative hernia. SteriStrips are used over all incision sites after a liquid adhesive is applied. Dressings include an eye pad at the subumbilical site with clear adhesive type bandages over the other sites to allow the patients to shower. Some serous type drainage from these incision sites occurs and may last for a couple of days. If any heavy bright red bleeding occurs from any of these sites, the physician should be notified immediately. Initial pain in the PACU area should be minimal to moderate and is generally successfully controlled with antiinflammatory agents or mild opioids. Severe pain may indicate a more severe condition, and the surgeon should be notified immediately. A firm abdomen could indicate abdominal bleeding

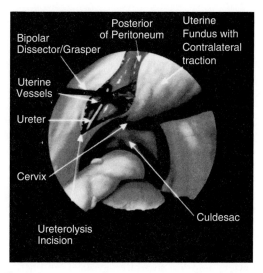

**Fig. 42-6** Laparoscopic anatomy as seen through laparoscope. Figure shows bipolar instrument used for uterine occlusion. *(Courtesy Center for Women's Care and Reproductive Surgery, Atlanta.)*

that is not normal; severe pain, nausea, or vomiting could indicate a bowel perforation. If any of these conditions occur, the surgeon should be notified immediately. Postoperative care instructions, including an explanation of the possibility of referred chest or shoulder pain, should be discussed with the patient and a significant other. Instructions should always be written as well and given to the patient for review after discharge.

A follow-up phone call to the patient within 24 to 48 hours is recommended. Special care for the patient who undergoes outpatient surgery is outlined in Chapter 46.

## Lower Genital and Vaginal Surgery
The conditions that require this type of surgery occur most often in parous and older women. They are caused most commonly by exaggeration of the normal relaxation of the pelvic ligaments and support that occurs during childbirth and after menopause. A number of specific procedures, named after their developers, may be encountered and include the following:

- Baldy-Webster procedure: Shortening of the round ligaments and changing of the direction of their pull by attaching them to the back of the uterus.
- Fothergill-Hunter procedure: Complete repair of the vaginal wall, from above downward toward the vulva, to correct faulty supportive structures of the pelvic floor.
- Gilliam's procedure: Shortening of the round ligaments by attaching them to the abdominal wall.

- Le Fort's operation (colpocleisis): Closure of the vagina with approximation of the anterior and posterior vaginal walls with or without attendant vaginal hysterectomy.
- Radical vulvectomy: Abdominal and perineal dissection of the superficial and deep inguinal nodes and portions of the saphenous veins, reconstruction of the vaginal walls and pelvic floor, and closure of the abdominal wounds.
- Vulvectomy: Removal of the labia majora, labia minora, and possibly the clitoris and perianal area, with a Z-plasty closure. Used in treatment of leukoplakia vulva, carcinoma in situ of the vulva, and Paget's disease of the vulva.

Other vaginal surgical procedures include fistula repairs, correction of urinary stress incontinence (various sling procedures with nonabsorbable transobturator tape), and vaginal reconstruction to repair congenital or acquired defects developed during childbirth. Many of the pelvic floor repair procedures can be done laparoscopically if the surgeon is comfortable with laparoscopic suturing and is a well-trained laparoscopist. The pelvic floor procedures are done with nonabsorbable sutures and mesh for optimal long-term results. The role of the operative team in these procedures cannot be overemphasized in enabling the surgeon to focus on the surgery at hand. The entire team can play an integral part in large part thanks to the video cameras and monitors now used during laparoscopic surgery

## General Perianesthesia Care
Anesthesia for lower genital and vaginal surgery may be local, general, or regional, depending on the amount of pelvic relaxation necessary to perform the procedures. Routine guidelines are followed when the patient is admitted to the PACU. Once alert, the patient may assume a position of comfort and be encouraged to move about frequently as part of antiembolism care. After a general assessment of the patient's condition, all dressings should be checked carefully. Vaginal packing may be in place with some vaginal procedures, or a perineal pad only may be used vaginally in the case of laparoscopy. Intake and output is monitored as per routine. Saturation of the vaginal packing may be expected after any vaginal surgery; however, saturation of the perineal pad when vaginal packing is in place should be considered excessive bleeding and should be reported. Vaginal and groin wounds often have drains, and care must be exercised to avoid dislodgement. If drains are in place, a moderate amount of drainage may be expected.

Food and fluids may be safely resumed after the minor procedures, such as D&C and bartholinectomy, once the pharyngeal reflexes have returned. After more extensive procedures, the patient is usually not given anything by mouth until peristalsis is reestablished; intake is supplied with intravenous fluids. Urine output should be monitored carefully for amount and for the presence of blood. Oftentimes, patients have a urinary catheter in place until they are ambulatory, and securing the catheter is important so no tugging or pulling may cause irritation after its removal.

Pain must be carefully evaluated and may be alleviated with appropriate analgesics. Abdominal cramping is common after gynecologic surgery. For these patients, relaxation exercises are often helpful if they have been learned before surgery. Warm blankets over the abdomen may also aid in relaxation. Because the patient is often drowsy from the anesthesia, coaching is needed, especially during the first hour. If cramping is not relieved with relaxation exercises, analgesics, or other comfort measures, the surgeon should be notified because this may indicate a perforated uterus or more severe problem. After removal of tumors or cysts from the vaginal area, ice may be applied to reduce edema and provide comfort.

## ABDOMINAL GYNECOLOGIC SURGERY

Abdominal gynecologic surgery may be performed alone or in conjunction with vaginal surgery.

### General Postoperative Care

Postoperative care after abdominal gynecologic surgery involves all the care and considerations rendered to the patient who undergoes any type of abdominal surgery. Anesthesia is most often general.

Overall assessment of the patient, with special emphasis on the cardiovascular status, should be undertaken as soon as the patient is admitted to the PACU.

The most common and dangerous complications of any obstetric or gynecologic surgery are excessive hemorrhage and shock; therefore, the perianesthesia nurse should direct assessment to a complete evaluation of the patient's circulatory status at frequent intervals. All dressings should be checked for drainage. Pain should be evaluated, and appropriate comfort measures and analgesics should be administered.

After total abdominal hysterectomy or major abdominal procedures, the patient is usually not given anything orally until peristalsis has

returned and nausea has subsided. Intake is supplied with intravenous fluids. Occasionally, the patient is admitted to the PACU with a nasogastric tube for prevention of abdominal distention. If abdominal distention develops, nasogastric and rectal tubes may be used to relieve it.

A Foley catheter is often in place, and its patency must be ensured. The perianesthesia nurse should accurately document the amount of urinary output and the presence of blood. A possible complication of hysterectomy is accidental perforation or ligation of a ureter. Inadvertent injury to the bladder wall or the bowel may also occur.

For prevention of vascular disorders, especially in the lower extremities, the patient's position should be changed frequently. A high Fowler's position should be avoided, and active and passive range-of-motion exercises of the lower extremities should be instituted in the PACU as soon as possible.

If a hysterectomy is done laparoscopically and the uterus is removed vaginally (i.e., LAVH), whether the vaginal cuff is repaired vaginally or laparoscopically, vaginal packing typically is not used. In addition, patients encounter some vaginal bleeding after LAVH and also after most laparoscopies because a uterine manipulator is used during the procedure. Patients who have undergone a hysteroscopy likely have postoperative vaginal bleeding as well. However, in all of these cases, the bleeding should not be heavier than that from a menstrual period; if heavier bleeding occurs, the surgeon should be notified immediately. After surgery, patients should be instructed to refrain from sexual intercourse and from vaginal insertion of foreign objects, including tampons; these instructions may vary among physicians. On discharge, patients should be provided with written home instructions that outline specific guidelines to follow. These guidelines should include a telephone number for the patient to be able to contact the surgeon or the physician on call 24 hours a day. Many of the patients who undergo laparoscopic procedures are discharged within 24 hours after surgery; therefore, they must know who to call. Patients may have vaginal discharge in some form for several weeks after these procedures. After laparoscopic surgery, the surgeon typically has the patient return for a postoperative checkup 2 weeks after surgery.

After laparoscopic surgery, patients should begin to feel significantly better within 48 to 72 hours. If they still have a great deal of discomfort or if they begin to feel better and then start to feel much worse a couple of days later, the surgeon should be notified immediately.

This condition could indicate a postoperative complication that could involve an injury to the bowel, bladder, or ureter. A bowel injury often does not present itself until the patient has gone home. The injury could be serious, and the physician must identify and recognize it as soon as possible. All of these criteria should be outlined in the written home instructions. Many facilities that discharge patients within 24 hours after surgery follow up by calling patients within 24 to 48 hours to see how they are doing. As much as anything, this call is a courtesy call; if a problem is found, the patient is generally encouraged to contact the physician.

## SUMMARY

This chapter discussed gynecologic surgery for repair or correction of congenital or traumatic deformities or incapacitating pelvic pain. The chapter discussed female surgery of three major categories: obstetric; lower genital and vaginal; and abdominal gynecologic surgery. Abdominal surgery can be traditional surgery in the form of a laparotomy or in the category of operative laparoscopy. This chapter also discussed the area of operative laparoscopy in gynecologic surgery because it is expanding to such an enormous extent that most benign gynecologic surgery is moving in that direction. The perianesthesia nurse can combine knowledge about the procedures with knowledge of postanesthesia care of the patient undergoing gynecologic surgery to provide the best care for the patient.

## BIBLIOGRAPHY

Adolph A, Lyons TL, Winer W: Laparoscopic supracervical hysterectomy for the large uterus, *J Am Assoc Gynecol Laparosc* 11(2):170-174, 2004.

Donnelly AJ, Baughman VL, Gonzales GP, et al: *Anesthesiology and critical care drug handbook*, ed 7, Lenexa, Kan, 2007, American College of Clinical Pharmacology.

Lyons TL, Adolph A, Winer W: Ovarian remnant with bilateral duplicate ureters, *J Am Assoc Gynecol Laparosc* 10(3):407-408, 2003.

Lyons TL, Lee T, Winer WK: Laparoscopic removal of a bladder leiomyoma, *J Am Assoc Gynecol Laparosc* 5(4):423-426, 1998.

Lyons TL, Winer WK: An innovative bipolar instrument for laparoscopic use, *J Soc Laparoendosc Surg* 9(1):39-41, 2005.

Lyons TL, Winer WK: Laparoscopic treatment of urinary stress incontinence. In Tulandi T: *Atlas of laparoscopic and hysteroscopic techniques for gynecologists*, ed 2, Philadelphia, 2000, Saunders.

Lyons, TL, Winer, W, Stepanian, AA: Laparoscopic hysterectomy. In *UpToDate*, Rose, BD (editor), UpToDate, Waltham, MA 2005.

Lyons TL, Winer W, Woo A: Appendectomy in patients undergoing laparoscopic surgery for pelvic pain. *J Am Assoc Gynecol Laparosc* 8(4):542-544, 2001.

McEwen DR: Gynecologic and obstetric surgery, *Alexander's care of the patient in surgery*, ed 13, St Louis, 2007, Mosby.

Monahan FD, Sands JK, Neighbors M, et al: *Phipps' medical-surgical nursing*, ed 8, St Louis, 2007, Elsevier.

O'Brien D: Gynecologic and reproductive surgery, *Perianesthesia nursing core curriculum*, St Louis, 2004, Saunders.

Winer WK: Core curriculum for the RN first assistant, section VIII: gynecology and obstetrics, *AORN* 197-212, 2005.

Winer WK: Laparoscopic procedures: innovations and complications, *Today Surg Nurse* 21(1):15-19, 1999.

Winer WK, Seifert PC, editors: *Advances in minimally invasive gynecology, perioperative nursing clinics*, vol 2, no. 4, Philadelphia, 2006, Saunders.

NURSING CARE IN THE PACU

# 43

# CARE OF THE BREAST SURGICAL PATIENT

*Nancy M. Saufl, MS, RN, CPAN, CAPA*

Breast cancer is a malignant tumor that has developed from cells of the breast. The disease occurs mostly in women. Although breast cancer in men is rare, it does occur. With the newer forms of treatment of cancer of the breast, including improved forms of diagnosis, surgical procedures on the breast have increased. However, with earlier breast cancer diagnosis and with the advent of enhanced radiation and chemotherapy protocols, surgical procedures performed on the breast may not be as extensive as in years past. All women are at risk for breast cancer. The two most significant risk factors are female gender and older age. The risks increase with age, and early detection is the best defense. Breast surgery is most commonly performed on women; however, procedures are occasionally performed on men and children. In addition, nondisease breast procedures may be performed for cosmetic purposes. Breast cancer is the most common cancer among women, other than skin cancer. It is the second leading cause of death for women after lung cancer. Chances of women having breast cancer are one in eight. Chances of dying from breast cancer are about one in 33. Breast cancer is also the most common cause of cancer in African-American women and the second leading cause of death in African-American women, exceeded only by lung cancer. Approximately one in 100 men is expected to develop breast cancer in a lifetime. As the patient's advocate, the perianesthesia nurse must be supportive, caring, and reassuring to the patient having breast surgery. Positive support is the start of the patient's rehabilitation process.

## DEFINITIONS

**Adenocarcinoma:** A general type of cancer that starts in glandular tissues anywhere in the body. Nearly all breast cancers start in glandular tissue of the breast and therefore are adenocarcinomas. The two main types of breast adenocarcinomas are ductal carcinomas and lobular carcinomas.

Benign breast lesions are the most commonly excised lesions (fibrocystic changes and fibroadenomas).

**Augmentation Mammoplasty:** Surgery to enlarge or augment the size of the female breast with a breast implant; the most popular cosmetic procedure.

**Breast Biopsy:** Excision of breast tissue. The specimen is sent to the pathology laboratory for frozen section. Also, a needle localization can be performed when a suspected lesion is identified with mammogram results. The procedure involves placement of a thin needle or guide into the breast with mammographic visualization. The lesion is then excised and taken to the pathology laboratory for a frozen section for determination of diagnosis.

**Breast Reconstruction (Mammoplasty):** The breast is reconstructed after mastectomy.

**Ductal Carcinoma In Situ (DCIS):** Ductal carcinoma in situ (also known as intraductal carcinoma) is the most common type of noninvasive breast cancer. Cancer cells are inside the ducts but have not spread through the walls of the ducts into the fatty tissue of the breast. Nearly all women diagnosed at this early stage of breast cancer can be cured. The best way to find DCIS is with a mammogram. With more women getting mammograms each year, diagnosis of DCIS is becoming more common. DCIS is sometimes subclassified based on its grade and type to help predict the risk of return of cancer after treatment and to help select the most appropriate treatment. Grade refers to how aggressive cancer cells appear with a microscope. Several types of DCIS exist, but the most important distinction among them is whether tumor cell necrosis (areas of dead or degenerating cancer cells) is present. The term comedocarcinoma is often used to describe a type of DCIS with necrosis.

**Infiltrating (or Invasive) Ductal Carcinoma (IDC):** With a start in a milk passage, or duct, of the breast, this cancer has broken through the wall of the duct and invaded the fatty tissue of the breast. At this point, it has the potential to metastasize, or spread, to other parts of the body through the lymphatic system and bloodstream. Infiltrating ductal carcinoma accounts for about 80% of invasive breast cancers.

**Infiltrating (or Invasive) Lobular Carcinoma (ILC):** ILC starts in the milk-producing glands. Similar to IDC, this cancer has the potential to spread (metastasize) elsewhere in the body. About 10% to 15% of invasive breast cancers are invasive lobular carcinomas. ILC may be more difficult to detect with mammogram than IDC.

**Inflammatory Breast Cancer:** This rare type of invasive breast cancer accounts for about 1% of all breast cancers. In inflammatory breast cancer, the skin of the breast looks red and feels warm, as if it were infected and inflamed. The skin has a thick pitted appearance that doctors often describe as resembling an orange peel. Sometimes the skin develops ridges and small bumps that look like hives. Doctors now know that these changes are not caused by inflammation or infection, but the name given long ago to this type of cancer still persists. Cancer cells that block lymph vessels or channels in the skin over the breast cause these symptoms.

**In Situ:** This term is used for an early stage of cancer in which it is confined to the immediate area at which it began. Specifically in breast cancer, in situ means that the cancer remains confined to ducts (ductal carcinoma in situ) or lobules (lobular carcinoma in situ). It has not invaded surrounding fatty tissues in the breast nor spread to other organs in the body.

**Lobular Carcinoma In Situ (LCIS):** Although not a true cancer, LCIS (also called lobular neoplasia) is sometimes classified as a type of non-invasive breast cancer. It begins in the milk-producing glands but does not penetrate through the wall of the lobules. Most breast cancer specialists think that LCIS itself does not become an invasive cancer but that women with this condition have a higher risk of developing an invasive breast cancer in the same or the opposite breast. For this reason, women with LCIS should have physical examinations two or three times a year and an annual mammogram.

**Lumpectomy:** Only the tumor and surrounding tissue of a "breast lump" are excised. The rest of the breast remains intact. The procedure includes dissection of the axillary lymph nodes. The lump is generally smaller than 4 cm in diameter.

**Mastopexy (Breast Lift):** Reshaping (uplifting) the sagging breasts with surgical tightening of the skin (Figs. 43-1 and 43-2).

**Medullary Carcinoma:** This special type of infiltrating breast cancer has a relatively

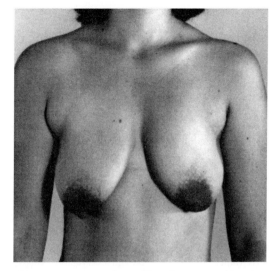

**Fig. 43-1** Mastopexy (breast lift). Before surgery, this patient had sagging (ptosis) of the breasts.

well-defined distinct boundary between tumor tissue and normal tissue. It also has some other special features, including the large size of the cancer cells and the presence of immune system cells at the edges of the tumor. Medullary carcinoma accounts for about 5% of breast cancers. The outlook, or prognosis, for this kind of breast cancer is better than for other types of invasive breast cancer.

**Modified Radical Mastectomy:** Removal of the entire breast and axillary lymph nodes; the pectoralis major muscle is left intact. In some instances, the pectoralis minor muscle is excised.

**Mucinous Carcinoma:** This rare type of invasive breast cancer is formed by mucus-producing

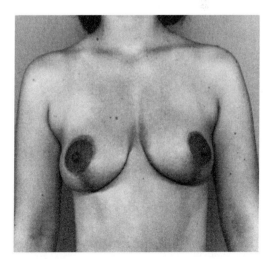

**Fig. 43-2** Mastopexy, showing same patient in Fig. 43-1 several weeks after surgery. Scars are beginning to fade.

cancer cells. The prognosis for mucinous carcinoma is better than for the more common types of invasive breast cancer. Colloid carcinoma is another name for this type of breast cancer.

**Paget's Disease of the Nipple:** This type of breast cancer starts in the breast ducts and spreads to the skin of the nipple and then to the areola, the dark circle around the nipple. It is a rare type of breast cancer and occurs in only 1% of all cases. The skin of the nipple and areola often appears crusted, scaly, and red with areas of bleeding or oozing. Women may notice burning or itching. Paget's disease may be associated with in situ carcinoma or with infiltrating breast carcinoma. If no lump can be felt in the breast tissue and the biopsy shows DCIS but no invasive cancer, the prognosis is excellent.

**Phyllodes Tumor:** This rare type of breast tumor forms from the stroma (connective tissue) of the breast, in contrast to carcinomas, which develop in the ducts or lobules. Phyllodes (also spelled hylloides) tumors are usually benign but rarely malignant (with the potential to metastasize). Benign phyllodes tumors are successfully treated with removal of the mass and a narrow margin of normal breast tissue. A malignant phyllodes tumor is treated with removal along with a wider margin of normal tissue or with mastectomy. These cancers do not respond to hormonal therapy and are not so likely to respond to chemotherapy or radiation therapy. In the past, both benign and malignant phyllodes tumors were called cystosarcoma phyllodes.

**Radical Mastectomy:** Removal of the entire breast, skin, nipple, areolar complex, and pectoralis major and minor muscles with axillary node dissection (Figs. 43-3 and 43-4).

**Tubular Carcinoma:** Tubular carcinomas are a special type of infiltrating breast carcinoma and account for about 2% of all breast cancers. They have a better prognosis than usual infiltrating ductal or lobular carcinomas.

## PERIANESTHESIA CARE AFTER SPECIFIC PROCEDURES

### Breast Biopsy

Breast cancer is often first suspected when a lump is felt or an abnormal area is found on mammogram results. Lumps in the breast often are discovered during monthly self examination or with routine mammograms, breast ultrasound scans, or magnetic resonance imaging. A biopsy is done when the results of these other tests suggest breast cancer. The biopsy is the only way to know for sure. The lumps or masses are aspirated or excised and sent for definitive diagnoses.

In approximately half of all female patients who undergo a biopsy, the diagnosis is fibrocystic disease. Fibrocystic disease describes a variety of benign and localized tumors or swelling within the breast tissues. Other nonfibrocystic conditions also may cause breast lumps. Inflammatory conditions, such as breast abscesses, fat necrosis, and lipomas of the skin (e.g., sebaceous cysts), may cause breast lumps.

A breast biopsy can be a one-step (biopsy and mastectomy, if needed) or two-step procedure. Two-step procedures are now the most common practice. The two-step procedure allows the patient to be educated about the choices and given the opportunity to make an informed decision regarding the type of surgery to be performed in the event of a positive biopsy finding. The short delay between the biopsy and further treatment has not been shown to affect survival rates. If, however, more extensive surgery is planned in the event of a positive biopsy result, the patient must have given preoperative informed consent for the definitive surgical procedure.

The patient is usually admitted as a same-day surgery patient. The patient may undergo needle biopsy, incisional biopsy, or excisional biopsy. A needle biopsy includes the introduction of a disposable cutting type needle through the mass to entrap a core of tissue. The needle is withdrawn, and the specimen is sent to the pathology laboratory. In an incisional biopsy, a portion of the mass is surgically excised along a curved incision line. An excisional biopsy may be needed to remove the entire mass and some of the adjacent tissue around it for examination. Because of the patient's natural apprehension, the patient may receive intravenous moderate (conscious) sedation along with local anesthesia. Monitored anesthesia care may also be indicated.

If the patient meets phase I discharge criteria while still in the operating suite, the patient may bypass the phase I postanesthesia care unit (PACU). Otherwise, the patient is usually awake on arrival in the PACU but drowsy because of the sedation. Routine admission procedures are accomplished. The head of the bed may be elevated 45 degrees.

The dressing is usually a 4 × 4 sponge held in place with the patient's bra. It should be inspected for excessive drainage, which occurs only rarely. The patient can resume fluid and food intake as soon as the cough and gag reflexes have fully returned and nausea has subsided. Pain should be minimal, if any, and easily controlled with minor analgesics.

If midazolam has been administered, the patient may repeatedly ask the same questions.

SURGICAL MANAGEMENT OF BREAST CANCER

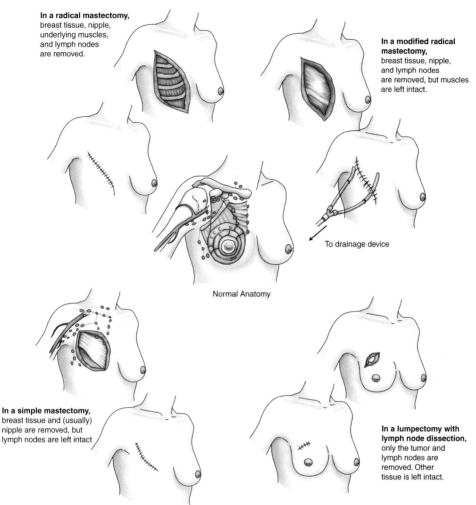

**In a radical mastectomy,** breast tissue, nipple, underlying muscles, and lymph nodes are removed.

**In a modified radical mastectomy,** breast tissue, nipple, and lymph nodes are removed, but muscles are left intact.

To drainage device

Normal Anatomy

**In a simple mastectomy,** breast tissue and (usually) nipple are removed, but lymph nodes are left intact

**In a lumpectomy with lymph node dissection,** only the tumor and lymph nodes are removed. Other tissue is left intact.

**Fig. 43-3**   Surgical choices for treatment of breast cancer. *(Redrawn from Ignatavicius DD, Workman ML:* Medical-surgical nursing: critical thinking for collaborative care, *ed 4, Philadelphia, 2002, Saunders.)*

The perianesthesia nurse must patiently repeat the answers and also ensure that the person who accompanies the patient at discharge understands the home care instructions.

### Surgical Choices for the Treatment of Cancer

Most women need some type of surgery to treat the breast tumor and remove as much of the cancer as possible. Advances in early diagnosis and modifications in surgical techniques have increased the number of surgical choices in the treatment of breast cancer (see Fig. 43-3). Surgical treatment may range from breast-conserving techniques (lumpectomy) to modified radical mastectomy that involves the breast and the axillary nodes.

***Lumpectomy.*** Lumpectomy, also called breast-conserving therapy, is the surgical treatment of choice when the breast tumor is well defined and less than 5 cm in diameter. In landmark clinical trials reported in 1988, the National Surgical Adjuvant Breast Cancer Project reported that lumpectomy followed by radiation therapy produced 8-year disease-free survival rates equal to those of modified radical mastectomy.

Lumpectomy is usually performed with general anesthesia. Only the breast tumor and a margin of surrounding normal tissue are removed. Surgery may also be done to determine whether the cancer has spread to the lymph nodes. A sentinel lymph node biopsy may be done to look at the lymph nodes without having to remove them first. A radioactive dye is injected near the tumor and is carried by the lymph system to the first (sentinel) node to receive lymph from the tumor. This lymph

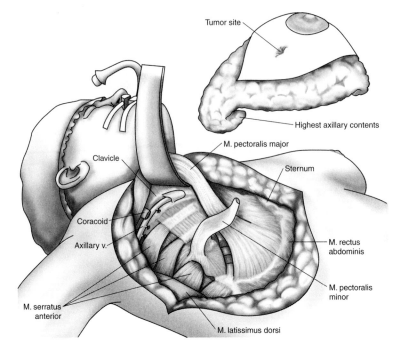

**Fig. 43-4**   Mastectomy.

node is most likely to contain cancer cells if the cancer has spread. Once this node is found, it is removed and examined. If it is free of cancer, further surgery may not be needed. An axillary node dissection may also be performed to see whether breast cancer has spread to the lymph nodes under the arm. It is done through a separate incision and involves a sample of 10 to 15 lymph nodes lateral and inferior to the pectoralis minor muscles for pathology. This procedure helps the patient and provider to choose adjuvant postoperative therapy and helps guide treatment options. A possible side effect from the removal of the lymph nodes is lymphedema or swelling of the arm (seen in 1 to 3 of 10 women).

When the patient is admitted to the PACU, all the initial assessment measures should be accomplished. The blood pressure cuff should be placed on the arm opposite the operative side. The arm on the operative side should be elevated on a pillow because the removal of lymph nodes increases the risk of lymphedema. The operative-side arm should be assessed frequently for circulatory adequacy with monitoring of color, temperature, capillary refill, and the presence and strength of the radial pulse. Venipunctures and injections should not be performed on the operative-side arm.

Dressings should be small, and bleeding or drainage should be minimal. A Hemovac or Jackson-Pratt closed-drainage system may be connected to drains placed at the incision site.

Nursing personnel should be aware that although this procedure allows the patient to keep the breast, it does not eliminate fear of the cancer diagnosis or concerns about whether the procedure was successful; thus, the nurse must provide factual reassurance.

### *Mastectomy*
**Partial (Segmental) Mastectomy.** The partial mastectomy involves the removal of more of the breast tissue than in the lumpectomy and is usually followed by radiation therapy.

**Simple Mastectomy.** The simple mastectomy is the removal of the entire breast but not the lymph nodes under the arm. Both breasts may be removed if the patient is at an increased risk for breast cancer. Most patients go home the next day.

**Modified Radical Mastectomy.** The modified radical mastectomy is the most commonly performed surgery for elimination of breast cancer. The entire breast and axillary nodes are removed. This procedure differs from the Halsted's radical mastectomy in that the pectoralis major muscle is left intact.

**Radical Mastectomy.** The radical mastectomy is rarely performed in the United States because the modified radical mastectomy has been found to be just as effective for the patient and less disfiguring, with fewer side effects.

The radical mastectomy involves the extensive removal of the entire breast, lymph nodes, and chest wall muscles under the breast. Refined techniques for diagnosis and surgery, radiation therapy, and chemotherapy have made it unnecessary in most instances. Radical mastectomy may be performed in women (primarily elderly women) who do not desire adjuvant therapy (radiation or chemotherapy).

Nursing care after either modified radical or radical mastectomy is essentially the same, except that, of course, the radical mastectomy involves more gross excision of tissue and demands more detailed observation of viability of remaining tissue.

Mastectomy is performed with general anesthesia. The patient is admitted to the PACU with the head of the bed elevated 30 to 45 degrees. All admission assessments should be made, oxygen administered per protocol, and respiratory sufficiency determined with pulse oximetry and observation.

Dressings are usually bulky and should be checked frequently for excessive serosanguineous drainage and for constriction. The most important postoperative complication is hematoma below the skin flaps. Attention to the drains and the maintenance of free drainage within the vacuum system prevent this occurrence. Drains are usually placed under the skin flaps to remove excess blood and serum that ordinarily collect under the wound site, thus causing edema, infection, and sloughing of the skin graft. The drains may be connected to Hemovac or Jackson-Pratt devices or some other closed suction device. Generally, additional vacuum is needed the first 8 postoperative hours, and the Hemovac is connected to vacuum pressure of 20 to 30 mm Hg. These drains should be monitored for excessive bleeding, which must be reported to the surgeon. Dressings are necessarily snug but should not impair respiration or circulation to the upper extremity. The arm on the operative side should be supported and elevated on a pillow; it must be checked frequently for cyanosis or pallor, and the pulse must be palpated for intensity. If signs of respiratory distress or impaired circulation arise, the surgeon should be notified to rearrange the dressing. Unless an emergency arises, the perianesthesia nurse should not attempt to loosen the dressing because skin grafts may inadvertently be disrupted.

When a radical mastectomy is performed, extensive excision and skin grafting are usually required (see Chapter 44). Donor sites (usually the thigh) should be checked for drainage and treated according to hospital policy.

The patient should be advised to avoid excessive motion in the immediate postoperative period and should not strain the pectoral girdle by levering on the bed with the arms to change position. These patients usually need intravenous fluid augmentation for the first 24 postoperative hours. Oral feeding is allowed after cough and gag reflexes have returned and if nausea is not present. Small sips of fluids may be offered and taken as desired, and diet resumed as tolerated. Postoperative pain can be moderate to severe and can usually be controlled with opioids such as meperidine and morphine. With the increased preoperative use of paravertebral nerve blocks for breast surgery patients, pain management has been greatly enhanced, resulting in less need for opioids and improved patient satisfaction. Hypothermia may be a problem because of prolonged exposure in the operating room, and rewarming should be accomplished with additional warmed blankets or a forced warm air device. Postoperative instructions for patients who have axillary node dissections should include hand and arm care instructions. Consistent education and support are necessary. Emotional support may be sought through support groups such as the "Reach to Recovery" program (American Cancer Society: on the web, www.cancer.org/; or phone 800-ACS-2345).

***Breast Reconstruction.*** The loss of a breast from cancer can be devastating to women and the changes in body image may be difficult to manage. One of the advances made in breast surgery during recent years is the availability of effective means of reconstructing the breast after removal for cancer. Breast reconstruction may be accomplished in conjunction with mastectomy or at a later time, depending on each patient's individual decision and preference and the need for chemotherapy or radiation.

Breast reconstruction may be performed in a variety of methods in which the surgeon, in collaboration with a plastic surgeon, tailors the operation to the patient's individual irregularity.

Breast reconstruction may be performed with three different techniques: available tissue with an implant, the use of tissue expanders, and the use of flaps. Use of the available tissue is the simplest procedure, but often times sufficient tissue is not left after mastectomy. If enough tissue is available, an appropriately sized implant is placed under the remaining skin flap or muscle. The other breast may have its size adjusted with either a reduction mammoplasty or a mastopexy to achieve symmetry if necessary and the patient desires to do so.

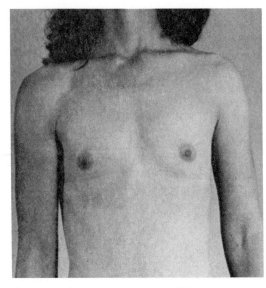

**Fig. 43-5**   Appearance of patient before breast augmentation.

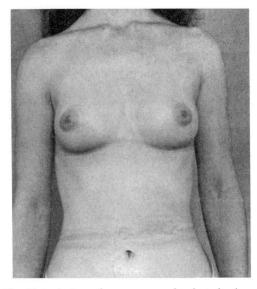

**Fig. 43-6**   Postoperative appearance of patient after breast augmentation with silicone bag prostheses.

Mastectomy can leave a shortage of enough skin tissue to create a breast mound. For these patients, a breast reconstruction technique with available tissue and implants is used to stretch the normal tissue to create extra tissue. A pocket is made under the remaining tissues into which a soft silicone bag is made to simulate the natural contour (Figs. 43-5 and 43-6). The pocket can be made at the time of surgery or before the surgery with an inflatable tissue expander. The expander method requires the administration of several injections of gradually increasing volumes of saline solution over a period of weeks. When the desired amount of stretch has been reached, the temporary tissue expander is removed and replaced with a permanent breast implant.

Myocutaneous flap reconstruction (Figs. 43-7 and 43-8) involves moving nearby muscle and skin into the area of the mastectomy to replace the significant tissue deficiency after mastectomy. Commonly used muscle and skin flaps include the latissimus dorsi and rectus abdominis muscles with attached skin. Nipple-areola reconstruction may be accomplished with small portions of the labia and grafting to the selected location.

Postoperative care is generally the same as for the patient who undergoes other types of breast surgery, with attention to graft and flap donor sites (see Chapter 44).

These operations have provided a measure of comfort to patients whose body image has been significantly disrupted by mastectomy. Patients report return of a sense of femininity and confidence. Many women do not choose to undergo additional surgery after mastectomy, but knowledge that the operation is available is reassuring.

***Mastopexy (Breast Lift).*** Breast ptosis (sagging) is defined by the position of the nipple areolar complex related to the inframammary crease. The reshaping process differs from reduction mammoplasty in the amount of tissue removed. Generally less than 300 g of tissue removed is considered a mastopexy procedure.

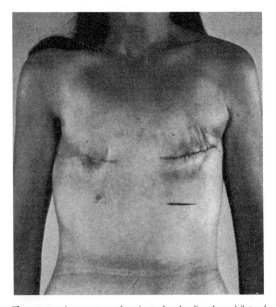

**Fig. 43-7**   Appearance of patient after healing from bilateral mastectomies for cancer.

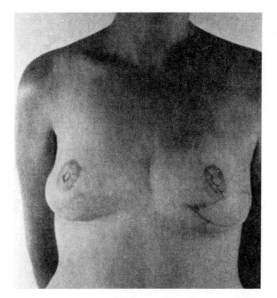

**Fig. 43-8** Appearance of same patient in Fig. 43-7 after muscle-skin flap (latissimus) and nipple reconstructions. Patient has gained considerable weight, and later she delivered a healthy baby. She is free of disease 6 years after the mastectomy.

Mastopexy is commonly performed as a same-day procedure, and postoperative care after mastopexy is generally not demanding. General anesthesia is most commonly used, and only minor adjustments in breast tissue are made.

The patient is positioned on the back after surgery and may assume a semi-Fowler's to high-Fowler's position for comfort as soon as she awakens. The motion of the arms is restricted to below shoulder level.

Postoperative dressings are minimal, and drains are rarely necessary because the entire procedure, with the exception of nipple release, is at the level of the dermis. Drainage should be minimal, and if frank bleeding occurs, the surgeon should be notified. Pain is usually not a problem, and discomfort can be controlled with mild analgesics. Food and fluids may be resumed as tolerated after nausea has disappeared.

***Augmentation Mammoplasty.*** Breast augmentation is done for hypomastia, to correct breast asymmetry, to recreate the breast after mastectomy, or for the patient's desired enhancement of breast size. Incisions may be inframammary, axillary, or semicircular around the lower half of the areolar outline. The inframammary approach is the simplest, but the axillary incision provides the least visible scar after surgery. Breast implants can be placed beneath the mammary tissue or under the muscle layer of the chest. Many surgeons believe that positioning the implants beneath the muscle provides the

patient with the most natural appearance. Breast augmentation can also be accomplished endoscopically with transluminal breast augmentation (TUBA) in which a small incision is made inside the navel. These patients have self-adhesive wound strips over the umbilical incision and are fitted with an elastic bandage.

Breast augmentation patients usually receive general anesthesia, but local anesthesia with sedation is a viable consideration. The patients may have compression dressings in place on admission to the PACU, but some physicians have a brassiere placed on the patient immediately after surgery. The patients usually go home the same day and see the physician in the office the following day to change the dressing. Incisional drains are rarely used with breast augmentation. Patients may need aggressive pain management in the initial phase I PACU, but generally can be comfortable with the use of oral analgesics. Patients should be encouraged to gently move the arms to prevent stiffness and discomfort.

***Reduction Mammoplasty.*** Reduction mammoplasty is the surgical method to correct gigantomastia or macromastia in which patients have back pain, breast pain, postural changes, or shoulder strap discomfort from the weight of the breasts. These women may also have an inability to participate in physical activities such as jogging, aerobics, and horseback riding. Breast reduction is performed with general anesthesia. Breast tissue and skin are excised; the nipple areolar complex is elevated superiorly on the new breast mound. Reduction mammoplasty is a lengthy procedure in which significant fluid and blood loss is anticipated. Because of the prolonged anesthesia and surgery time, some providers use a team approach to reduce the surgical time. Some patients donate autologous blood before this surgery, but all patients should be typed and screened before surgery. Often times, however, intravenous crystalloids are all that is necessary for fluid replacement.

A new method in reduction mammoplasty is the laser deepithelialization technique. When the carbon dioxide laser is used to remove the epidermis from the inferior pedicle, reduction mammoplasty can be performed with little blood loss. The inferior pedicle technique is a commonly used approach to reduction mammoplasty. When the inferior pedicle technique is used, the laser simplifies skin removal. The laser is preferred for pedicle deepithelialization in all patients, especially patients who have large ptotic breasts, because rigid stabilization is not necessary.

NURSING CARE IN THE PACU

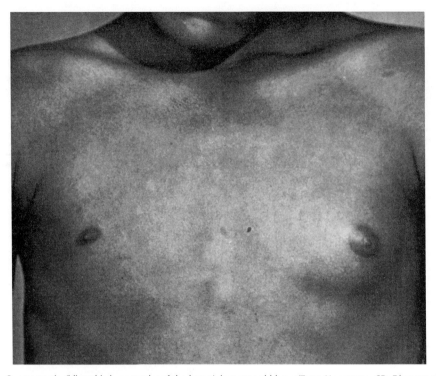

**Fig. 43-9**    Gynecomastia (idiopathic hypertrophy of the breast) in 8-year-old boy. *(From Haagensen CD: Diseases of the breast, ed 3, Philadelphia, 1986, Saunders.)*

On admission to the PACU, the patient is positioned on the back; as soon as the condition warrants, the patient is placed in a low-Fowler's position. Dressings may be of any variety, but most often wide strips of Elastoplast, which readily conform to the patient's new skin contours, are used. A Velpeau bandage should be in place to restrain the patient from raising the arms, and the patient should be advised of this. Drains are rarely necessary, and drainage should be minimal. If drains are present, they should be connected to a vacuum source, such as the Hemovac. Because of the length of the surgery and the fluid volume loss, special attention should be paid to urine output, pulse rate, and blood pressure. Rewarming may be necessary to prevent or reduce hypothermia. Initially, parenteral opioids may be needed after surgery, followed by oral analgesics. Light ice packs may be used to relieve discomfort and minimize tissue swelling. Most patients spend one night in the hospital after surgery. As after mastectomy, the patient should be advised to not do anything that puts strain on the pectoral girdle.

### Surgery in Gynecomastia

Gynecomastia, or benign hypertrophy of one or both breasts in boys and men, is relatively common (Fig. 43-9). The condition may be bilateral or unilateral. The causes may be hormonal, systemic disease-oriented, drug-related, or idiopathic.

In extreme instances or in cases in which gynecomastia causes problems in psychologic adjustment, this excess tissue can be excised or removed with suction lipectomy. Suction lipectomy is useful when the gynecomastia is caused primarily by fat. Optimal cosmetic results can be obtained. The surgical procedure is similar to that of breast reduction in women. A periareolar incision is made, and tissue is removed. Suction drainage of the incision site is usually necessary and may be conveniently accomplished with a Hemovac.

Postoperative care is essentially the same as that for women who undergo breast surgery. If no drains are necessary, the patient can be discharged the day of surgery once reflexes have returned, nausea has subsided, and food and fluids can be taken.

## SUMMARY

Breast cancer is most commonly diagnosed in women, and the risk of development of breast cancer increases with age. All women are at risk for breast cancer, and one in eight women is predicted in the United States to have breast cancer develop at some point in life. Early detection with self examination or mammography is key and may be the reason for the slowly declining increase in breast cancer mortality rates. Surgical procedures on the breast are performed to establish a definitive diagnosis when cancer is a possibility or to treat a breast cancer. These surgeries range from biopsy to mastectomy. In addition, a sentinel node biopsy may be performed to help establish a diagnosis. Axillary node dissection may be necessary. Other breast surgeries include mastopexy, augmentation mammoplasty, and reduction mammoplasty.

After breast surgery, patients need emotional support and encouragement to express concerns and fears. Patients should be provided with accurate and complete information in a hopeful and positive manner, yet they should not be given unfounded or unreasonable hopes and promises. The web site for the American Cancer Society (www.cancer.org) can provide the patient with an abundance of information regarding breast cancer after care and support groups.

# BIBLIOGRAPHY

Alspach JG: *Core curriculum for critical care nursing*, ed 6, St Louis, 2006, Saunders.

American Cancer Society: *Cancer facts and figures: cancer reference information*, Atlanta, 2007, American Cancer Society.

Atlee J: *Complications in anesthesia*, ed 2, Philadelphia, 2007, Saunders.

Barash PG, Cullen BF, Stoelting RK: *Clinical anesthesia*, ed 5, Philadelphia, 2005, Lippincott Williams & Wilkins.

Bickley LS, Szilagyi PG: *Bates' guide to physical examination and history taking*, ed 9, Philadelphia, 2005, Lippincott Williams & Wilkins.

Burden N, DeFazio-Quinn D, O'Brien D, et al: *Ambulatory surgical nursing*, ed 2, Philadelphia, 2000, Saunders.

DeFazio-Quinn D, Schick L: *Perianesthesia nursing core curriculum*, St Louis, 2004, Saunders.

Fisher B, Redmond C, Poisson R, et al: Eight-year results of a randomized clinical trial comparing mastectomy and lumpectomy with or without radiation in the treatment of breast cancer, *N Engl J Med* 320:822-828, 1989.

Fleisher LA: *Anesthesia and uncommon diseases*, ed 5, Philadelphia, 2006, Saunders.

Ganong W: *Review of medical physiology*, ed 21, New York, 2005, McGraw-Hill Professional.

Gutowski KA: Aesthetic and functional breast surgery, *Clin Obstet Gynecol* 49:337-345, 2006.

Guyton AC, Hall JE: *Textbook of medical physiology*, ed 11, Philadelphia, 2006, Saunders.

Katzung BG editor: *Basic and clinical pharmacology*, ed 10, Los Altos, Calif, 2006, Lange McGraw Hill.

Lake C, Hines R, Blitt C: *Clinical monitoring: practical applications for anesthesia and critical care*, St Louis, 2001, Mosby.

Longnecker D, Murphy F: *Dripps/Eckenhoff/Vandam introduction to anesthesia*, ed 9, Philadelphia, 1997, Saunders.

Miller RD editor: *Anesthesia*, ed 6, New York, 2005, Churchill Livingstone.

Nagelhout J, Zaglaniczny K: *Nurse anesthesia*, ed 2, Philadelphia, 2001, Saunders.

Rothrock J: *Alexander's care of the patient in surgery*, ed 13, St Louis, 2007, Mosby.

Stoelting R, Hillier SC: *Pharmacology and physiology in anesthetic practice*, ed 4, Philadelphia, 2005, Lippincott Williams & Wilkins.

Stoelting RK, Miller RD: *Basics of anesthesia*, ed 5, New York, 2007, Churchill Livingstone.

Susan B. Komen Breast Cancer Foundation: available at www.komen.org, 2007. Accessed July 15, 2007.

Townsend CM, Beauchamp RD, Evers BM, et al: *Sabiston textbook of surgery: the biological basis of modern surgical practice*, ed 17, Philadelphia, 2004, Saunders.

# 44

## CARE OF THE PLASTIC SURGICAL PATIENT

*Joni M. Brady, RN, MSN, CAPA*
*Matthew D. Byrne, RN, MS, CPAN*

The field of plastic surgery encompasses cosmetic and reconstructive surgery. The procedures and techniques have continuously evolved over the past decade. This discipline is growing exponentially as consumer demand for cosmetic surgical procedures increases and the ability to achieve aesthetic reconstructive surgical outcomes improves.

Plastic surgery derives its name from the Greek word *plastikos*, which means to mold or give shape. The first successful tissue transfers are said to have originated in India more than 2500 years ago. Modern grafting techniques were explored in 19th century Germany. Reconstructive procedures involve much more than the correction of acquired and congenital deformities. They are also performed to correct defects related to tumors, trauma, infection, or disease. Ideally, these procedures represent interconnected therapy that strives to restore normal function and appearance with maintenance or improvement in psychologic comfort.

Few absolutes exist in plastic surgical techniques or in the associated preoperative or postoperative care. Perianesthesia nurses may encounter a variety of plastic surgical techniques, from simple to complex, depending on the type of facility in which the procedures are performed. Only the basic aspects of postoperative plastic surgery patient care are presented in this discussion. Elements of nursing care related to the specific treatment of an affected area during plastic surgery procedures are discussed in allied chapters. The reader is advised to refer to the appropriate related chapter for more details.

## DEFINITIONS

**Abdominoplasty:** Surgical removal of abdominal fat and skin.

**Allograft (Homograft):** Grafting between two nongenetically linked individuals.

**Augmentation Mammoplasty:** Surgical procedure performed to enhance the size and shape of a breast.

**Autograft:** Tissue transplantation from one site to another on the same person.

**Blepharoplasty:** Procedure to correct deformities of the upper or lower eyelid with excision of redundant skin or protruding fat.

**Composite Graft:** Tissue grafting that involves multiple germ layers; may include skin, subcutaneous tissue, cartilage, or mucosa.

**Dermabrasion:** Surgical planing of the skin with removal of the epidermis and portions of the superficial dermis for removal of high spots or other irregularities in an uneven skin surface.

**Free Cartilage Graft:** Transplantation of cartilage for restoration or maintenance of anatomic function or likeness.

**Full-thickness Skin Graft:** Use of all underlying dermis and epidermis and a small amount of subcutaneous tissue.

**Inosculation:** Vessel invasion from either host to graft, or graft to host, that allows for revascularization.

**Isograft:** Graft donation between individuals that are genetically similar.

**Lipectomy:** Surgical removal of fatty tissue.

**Otoplasty:** Surgical procedure done to reduce prominence of the ears.

**Pedicle Flap:** A preferred flap for wound tissue that is somewhat avascular, such as cartilage, bone, and tendon, or in the presence of avascular scar tissue and radiation-affected tissue. This type of flap is used to provide soft tissue closure while allowing blood vessels to remain intact.

**Reduction Mammoplasty:** Surgical removal of glandular tissue, fat, and skin from the breasts to achieve lighter, smaller, and firmer breast proportions.

**Rhinoplasty:** Reshaping or reconstruction of the nose when its shape has been altered as a result of trauma or when the patient is unhappy with its form.

**Rhytidectomy:** Surgical tightening of facial and neck muscles with removal of excess skin; commonly called a face lift procedure.

**Split-thickness Skin Graft:** Tissue grafting that is classified as thin, medium, or thick based on tissue thickness.

**Tissue Expansion:** Insertion and positioning of a temporary inflatable balloon or implant device under the skin, which is periodically increased in size through instillation of normal saline solution, to promote expansion of the skin for reconstructive purposes.

**Transverse Rectus Abdominis Musculocutaneous (TRAM) flap:** This procedure is performed after a mastectomy and involves the reconstruction of a breast with autografting of lower abdominal skin and adipose tissue.

**Tumescent Liposuction:** A dilute solution of lidocaine, used in combination with epinephrine, is injected into the adipose tissue layer to facilitate the vacuum removal of fat cells via a small cannula.

**Xenograft:** Grafting from a nonhuman species.

## PERIANESTHESIA NURSING CARE

Preanesthetic concerns for the patient undergoing skin grafting, flap repair, or any type of tissue grafting should include evaluation of smoking status and smoking cessation education; assessment for vascular concerns that may threaten the healing process, such as diabetes; identification of peripheral vascular disease or hypertension; nutritional assessment of the patient; and patient education regarding the postoperative need for wound site immobilization, effective pain management, intensive care monitoring if necessary, and avoidance of straining or strenuous activities that may cause shearing of new grafts or increase the risk for hematoma development.

Basic plastic surgery techniques include excision of skin lesions, closure of skin wounds, and placement of skin grafts and skin flaps. Many minor plastic surgical procedures are performed with local anesthesia and require minimal postoperative nursing care, primarily involving close observation of the surgical site. When the patient receives general anesthesia, postoperative nursing care includes all of the considerations discussed for general care of the postoperative patient in addition to careful surgical site observation. Postoperative vital signs provide an important baseline for assessment for possible complications related to an untoward immunologic reaction.

## SKIN GRAFTS

Skin grafting is the most common method for covering open areas that result from incomplete wound healing, trauma, burns, or large surgical incisions. Grafting involves the removal of a skin layer of varying thickness that is then transplanted to a host site. Transplanted skin layers may originate from the individual, be synthetic in origin, or be an artificially enlarged portion of the host's own skin.

Revascularization generally takes 3 to 5 days and requires growth of vessels from the host or the recipient tissue via a process called inosculation. For cosmetically pleasing results, the color, texture, thickness, and hair-bearing nature of the skin used for grafting should be chosen to match the recipient site. As a rule, the closer the donor skin is located to the recipient area, the better the match. The major types of grafts are outlined in Box 44-1.

Factors that influence graft survival include adherence to the recipient tissue; adequate vascularity signs, which include color and capillary refill of site; close monitoring of graft tissue for early identification of complications; and strict management of vital signs, thermoregulation, pain control, and positioning.

Monitoring and assessment for serum or blood in the graft site is important during the first 24 postoperative hours. Excess fluid may cause the graft to lift from its bed and must be removed. The donor site should be kept clean and heals with a new layer of skin. Many variations exist in wound dressings used, required positioning of the patient, use of ice or antibiotic ointments, use of pressure dressings, and handling of donor sites.

Every effort should be made to keep the patient calm and still and to prevent touching, removal, or shifting of dressings. Some dressings, such as the bolster dressing shown in Fig. 44-1, may actually be sutured in place. Generally, the grafted area should be elevated and protected from both pressure and motion. The patient should be positioned to prevent any pressure on, or other trauma to, the graft or the donor site. The surgeon may order cold packs to reduce metabolic requirements of the graft and enhance its chances of survival. Dressings over grafts should be observed closely for drainage. Any excess drainage should be reported to the physician.

Full-thickness donor sites may be sutured closed and treated as a surgical wound if the donor site is small. If a large area is used for full-thickness grafting, grafting the donor site with split-thickness grafts may be necessary (Fig. 44-2).

## Box 44-1   Major Types of Skin Grafts

1. A *full-thickness graft* includes all underlying dermis and epidermis and a small amount of subcutaneous tissue. These grafts, used to cover areas such as the nasal tip, dorsum, ala, and sidewall of the lower eyelid and ear, are more prone to necrosis.
2. A *split-thickness graft* includes a portion of the underlying dermis and the entire epidermis. This graft is the least durable. It may be thin, medium, or thick, depending on the amount of dermis included.
3. A *composite graft* comprises two or more tissue components and often includes skin and subcutaneous tissue, cartilage, or mucosa that may be used to reconstruct a patient's ear, nose, or eyelid.
4. A *free cartilage graft* involves a portion of cartilage that is harvested and reimplanted to provide structure and support to the site. One example is the use of rib cartilage to create an ear structure in a patient with microtia.
5. *Autograft* indicates that the donor and the recipient are the same person.
6. *Isograft* signifies that the donor and the recipient are genetically identical.
7. *Allograft* or *homograft* means that the donor and the recipient are of the same species; this procedure may entail the use of cadaver tissue.
8. *Xenograft* indicates that the donor and the recipient are of different species (e.g., porcine or bovine sources).
9. *Bioengineered skin and skin substitutes* may be animal, human, or host hybrids. Apligraf (Organogenesis; Novartis) is derived from bovine collagen and tissue-cultured infant foreskin. Dermagraft (Smith & Nephew, Inc.) is derived from human dermal cells that are implanted onto an absorbable matrix. Both substances have been proven not to invoke an immune response because of their processing, and each represents a growing number of bioengineered hybrid skin substitutes.

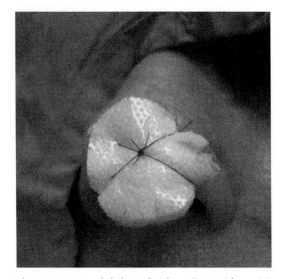

**Fig. 44-1**  Sutured bolster dressing. *(From Adams DC, Ramsey ML: Grafts in dermatologic surgery: review and update on full- and split-thickness skin grafts, free cartilage grafts, and composite grafts, Dermatol Surg 31:1055-1067, 2005.)*

vascularity from the original location of harvest, unlike transplantation, which implies complete separation from original vascular site.

### Local Flaps

Flaps (Fig. 44-3) are the preferred surgical treatment method for covering of wounds with inadequate vascularity to support a skin graft; reconstruction of full-thickness defects of specialized body parts such as ears, eyelids, nose and lips; and concealment of gliding tendons. Reconstructions that require tissue bulk, such as decubitus ulcer closure, are also done with flaps.

### Microvascular Tissue Transfer and Free Flaps

Microvascular tissue transfer is one of the most important advances in the field of reconstructive surgery. It requires the use of a high magnification operative microscope for reestablishment of vasculature. Regardless of the type of flap used, the newly positioned tissue is kept under constant observation by perianesthesia nursing personnel. Postanesthesia nursing management of the patient who has undergone microsurgery is consistent with established care requirements for the principal procedure, with emphasis on notation of color changes in the skin at the operative site.

The most serious complication in a microvascular tissue transfer procedure is tissue necrosis. Tissue death occurs when the artery or the vein that supplies the flap develops a thrombus.

## FLAPS

The term "flap" commonly refers to a skin flap. However, because of recent advances in reconstructive surgery, flaps are not limited to skin tissue. Flaps are classified by anatomic composition: skin with muscle fascia or bone, or both; skin alone; omentum; or a composite of these tissues. The term flap implies maintenance of

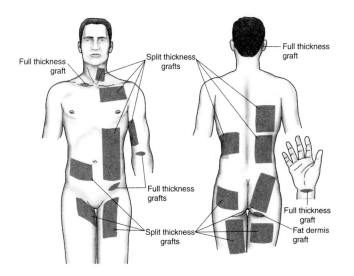

**Fig. 44-2** Available donor sites of skin grafts. *(Redrawn from Converse JM: Reconstructive plastic surgery, vol 1, ed 2, Philadelphia, 1977, Saunders.)*

Arterial thrombosis can result in complete flap failure within 4 hours of onset. Arterial occlusion is characterized by a pale cool flap that does not bleed when stuck with a needle.

Venous thrombosis is more commonly encountered, but it is not an immediate threat. Thrombosis is characterized by a congested warm mottled flap that continuously oozes dark blood. Objective assessment of the flap is possible with fluorometry, transcutaneous oxygen tension, thermometry, laser Doppler scan, temperature monitoring, buried Doppler probe, or photoplethysmograph disk for monitoring of blood flow. Any change in skin color from the normal baseline or monitoring findings that indicates imminent occlusion should be reported to the surgeon immediately. Pain at the skin graft or flap site is usually minimal. The donor sites typically generate more painful stimuli. Pain management should be individualized and based on the patient's self-reported pain levels. Nursing care should include administration of analgesics and attention to comfort measures as needed.

### Transverse Rectus Abdominis Musculocutaneous Flap

Breast reconstruction has become a routine part of breast cancer treatment. The TRAM flap procedure, which can be performed after mastectomy, involves the reconstruction of a breast with autografting of lower abdominal skin and adipose tissue. Breast reconstruction accomplished with autologous grafting does not adversely affect cancer survival rates and can serve to enhance the patient's psychologic

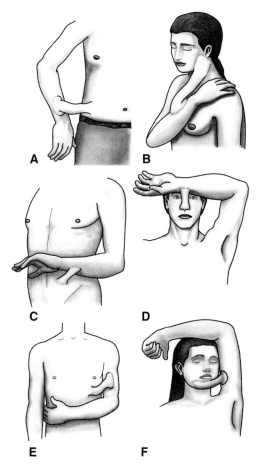

**Fig. 44-3** Various methods of transfer of tubed pedicle flaps. **A** and **B,** Transfer via wrist. **C** and **D,** "Salute" position of Kilner. **E** and **F,** Transfer via arm (Schuchardt). *(Redrawn from Converse JM: Reconstructive plastic surgery, vol 1, ed 2, Philadelphia, 1977, Saunders.)*

state. As with all postoperative flap procedures, nursing care centers on observation of the graft site in addition to general perianesthetic breast surgery patient care (see Chapter 43).

## BONE GRAFTS

After bone grafting has been performed, the graft site must be immobilized and excessive movement of the patient avoided. The donor site is generally the greater source of postoperative discomfort over the graft site. Pain should be anticipated and aggressively managed with opioid analgesics. If split-rib grafts are used, the patient should be placed in a low-Fowler's position. Respiratory status should be frequently assessed, and any signs of possible pneumothorax, such as tachycardia and tachypnea, should be immediately reported to the surgeon. Ice often is applied for reduction of swelling and pain management, and the graft site may necessitate elevation.

## SURGICAL REPAIR OF FACIAL BONE INJURIES

The facial bones often are fractured during motor vehicle accidents, falls, fights, and sporting events because of their protrusion and prominence. Fractures differ in location and complexity, and repair may vary from closed reduction to internal fixation with plates and screws, interosseous wiring, and bone grafting. Repair of facial bones often requires general anesthesia. If the damage is extensive and airway obstruction or concomitant cranial or intrathoracic injury is present, a tracheostomy must be performed. All patients who have facial, jaw, or neck surgery need the placement of a tracheostomy tray at the postanesthesia care unit (PACU) bedside in the event an airway emergency should occur.

On admission to the PACU, the patient who has undergone repair of the facial bones is placed in a low-Fowler's position as soon as the condition warrants. This position helps to minimize the development of head and neck edema. The nurse must maintain close airway monitoring with careful performance of oral and endotracheal tube suctioning if needed. Frequent suctioning of secretions may be necessary in the early postoperative period. In the case of a patient with a wired jaw, treatment with antiemetics is essential for the prevention of vomiting and aspiration.

When interdental wire fixation is performed, opening of the jaws may become necessary if an airway emergency develops (see Chapter 32 for care of the patient with interdental fixation). A pair of wire clippers should be clearly visible and affixed to the head of the bed to facilitate rapid opening of the jaws if needed. Good oral hygiene is a priority for these patients, and petrolatum ointment should be applied to the lips to prevent drying and cracking.

## SURGICAL REPAIR OF CLEFT LIP AND PALATE

Cleft lips and palates are common congenital defects that occur in as many as 1 in 800 births in the United States. Children born with these defects may have many associated problems, including facial growth abnormalities, dental irregularities, speech difficulties, ear diseases, psychologic disorders, and cosmetic challenges. The infant with a cleft palate has difficulty nursing and swallowing.

Repair of the cleft lip (Figs. 44-4 and 44-5) is usually accomplished when the "rule of 10" is met: 10 weeks of age, a body weight of at least 10 lbs, and a hemoglobin level of at least 10 g/dL. Repair is accomplished with general anesthesia. The infant is placed in a semiprone position on admission to the PACU, and the arms should be restrained to avoid disruption of the newly repaired lip. Measures should be taken to minimize crying because it puts excessive tension on the newly repaired lip. When possible, the parents should be allowed in the PACU to facilitate soothing the child. Postoperative pain medication or sedation may be needed to comfort the infant.

In addition to prevention of trauma to the lip, the most important nursing activity is airway management. Humidified mist should be used at least 12 hours after surgery to promote general respiratory well being and aid in clearing of secretions. In some cases, a nasal trumpet is used to maximize oxygenation and may be

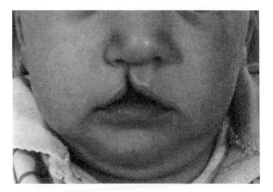

**Fig. 44-4**   Preoperative appearance of unilateral cleft lip.

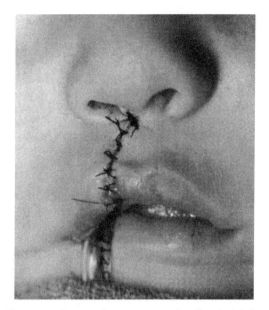

**Fig. 44-5** Postoperative appearance of unilateral cleft lip. Incision is covered with antibiotic ointment to prevent crusting.

sutured to the nare to prevent dislodgement. Hemorrhage, although rare, is a possible complication. Because loss of even a few milliliters of blood in an infant can be significant, any bleeding requires definitive control. Once the child is fully awake from the anesthesia, small sips of clear fluids may be given. Pain is difficult to assess in an infant. Iced normal saline solution–soaked gauze may be applied to the suture areas to reduce swelling and promote comfort. Analgesia should be provided when indicated, and oral analgesics such as acetaminophen can be used.

### Cleft Palate
Depending on the extent of the palate defect and accompanying lip defect, if present, repair may be completed when the child is 6 to 18 months of age. Optimization of speech and feeding is often a priority. The repair can be phased, requiring multiple procedures that include palatoplasty with bone grafts and orthodontic inserts. Certain procedures, such as nasoseptal reconstructions, may be delayed until the child becomes a teenager. On admission to the PACU, the child is placed in the semiprone or "tonsil" position with careful attention given to airway maintenance. As in cleft lip repair, the child's arms should be restrained and crying avoided. The head should not be flexed because this position tends to occlude the airway.

Suctioning of secretions may be necessary but must be performed gently and only if the nurse's view is unobstructed. The catheter, plastic dental suction tip, or Yankauer suction tip should be passed over the dorsum of the tongue, and only minimal vacuum pressure should be used. A mist tent or cold-mist humidifier should be used after surgery for at least 12 hours to aid in the elimination of tenacious secretions. Hemorrhage is a possible complication. Any active bleeding requiring control should be recorded and reported to the surgeon. Pain should be assessed and managed with appropriate analgesics.

## COSMETIC SURGERY

Men and women seek cosmetic surgery to enhance their physical appearance and emotional well being. Millions of cosmetic surgical procedures are performed each year in the United States. Most of these cosmetic procedures are performed on an outpatient basis. The anesthetic course depends on the selected procedure and the individual patient and can involve local, local with sedation, or general anesthesia. Nursing assessments and nursing care should be adjusted to the type of anesthesia administered and then individualized for each patient's needs.

### Blepharoplasty
Blepharoplasty is a procedure to correct deformities of the upper or lower eyelid with excision of redundant skin or protruding fat. The procedure is usually performed with local anesthesia with supplemental intravenous sedation. Iced compresses minimize swelling and bleeding. The patient may resume a regular diet after surgery; however, hot liquids are contraindicated for 24 hours to prevent vasodilation and bleeding. Activities such as bending and heavy lifting should be avoided. Pain should be assessed and managed with appropriate analgesics. Drugs that increase bleeding time should be avoided. Antibiotic ointment may be used for lubrication (see Chapter 33).

### Dermabrasion
Dermabrasion is the surgical planing of the skin, with removal of the epidermis and portions of the superficial dermis, for removal of high spots or other irregularities in an uneven skin surface. Enough of the dermal and epidermal elements are preserved to allow reepithelialization, and the result is smooth healing and blending of the scarred areas with the surrounding skin surface.

Usually the dermabraded areas are treated with the open method, and postanesthesia care includes protection of those areas from abrasion caused by rubbing on pillows or bed clothing. Facial edema, especially of the eyelids, may be expected, and the patient must be reassured that this subsides rapidly. The dermabraded area should be observed closely for the development of moisture. If moisture develops, it should be dried with a heat lamp or a warm hair dryer. This procedure may produce an uncomfortable burning sensation for the patient and may be minimized by holding the lamp or dryer a considerable distance from the area to be dried. Appropriate analgesics should be administered to manage burning-type pain sensations.

### Liposuction

Suction lipectomy (liposuction) removes subcutaneous fat to improve facial or body contours. It may be used in conjunction with other techniques. Anesthesia may be local or general. Liposuction is commonly performed on a same-day surgical basis. However, if more than 2500 mL of fat is removed, an overnight stay and fluid replacement may be required.

In the tumescent liposuction approach, pain should be minimized because of local lidocaine infiltration. However, if large areas are treated, an opioid analgesic could be required and intravenous fluid replacement is needed. Drugs that increase bleeding time should be avoided. The patient can usually start oral fluids and a progressive diet as soon as pharyngeal reflexes have returned. Postoperative bleeding and infection are possible complications.

### Otoplasty

Otoplasty is performed to reduce prominence of the ears. The patient has a head dressing for support. Generally, patients have mild postoperative discomfort that lasts approximately 12 hours. Pain of a longer duration suggests a possible hematoma or other complication and should be reported to the surgeon.

### Rhinoplasty

Rhinoplasty is performed to reshape or reconstruct the nose when its shape has been altered as a result of trauma or when the patient is unhappy with its form. Rhinoplasty may be performed with local anesthesia with supplemental opioids and intravenous sedation or general anesthesia. On admission to the PACU, the patient's head is elevated 30 to 45 degrees. Humidified oxygen is administered. In addition to routine assessment, the nasal area is assessed for swelling and bleeding. Nasal drip pads may be lightly taped under the nostrils.

### Rhytidectomy

The face lift operation is usually done with local anesthesia with supplementary sedation. Although some "lift" is accomplished around the cheek areas, the most important and long-lasting change is in the loose skin of the neck. The facial-neck skin is freed from the underlying tissues and pulled upward and backward toward the postauricular scalp. Excess skin is trimmed off, and meticulous suturing is performed. The procedure takes from 2 to 5 hours, and the patient arrives in the PACU with a large bandage over the neck and cheeks. Sedation, a quiet atmosphere, and continued elevation of the head of the bed are important measures in the prevention of complications. Pain should be assessed and appropriately treated. Pain located only on one side is unusual and may indicate a potentially serious bleeding complication, which is more commonly found in patients with hypertension. The surgeon should be notified immediately if bleeding occurs.

## SUMMARY

As the plastic surgery discipline and related plastic surgical techniques continue to grow and evolve, the critical thinking, astute judgment, keen assessments, and targeted interventions of the perianesthesia nurse are paramount to quality patient outcomes. The perianesthesia nurse may encounter a variety of plastic surgical techniques, which can require simple local anesthetic outpatient education and treatment to technologically advanced surgical intensive care. Perianesthesia nurses should become knowledgeable about the type and scope of plastic surgery care performed in the facility where care is delivered.

Primary postoperative concerns for this patient population include viability of flaps or transplanted tissue, minimization of and assessment for postoperative bleeding, conservative management of surgical sites and dressings, and aggressive pain control to facilitate healing and the patient recovery process. Psychosocial concerns and cosmetic outcomes are often a unique priority in this patient population. This personalized focus may significantly impact the course of care, the perianesthetic treatment and education performed, and the psychosocial integrity of the postoperative patient. Positive procedural outcomes, regardless of the surgical site, technique, or technology, require preparation, vigilance, and prompt intervention on the part of the perianesthesia nurse.

## BIBLIOGRAPHY

Adams DC, Ramsey ML: Grafts in dermatologic surgery: review and update on full- and split-thickness skin grafts, free cartilage grafts, and composite grafts, *Dermatol Surg* 31:1055-1067, 2005.

American Society of Plastic Surgeons: *Reconstructive procedures*, available at http://www.plasticsurgery.org/patients_consumers/procedures/, accessed March 2, 2007.

Boyce ST, et al: Cultured skin substitutes reduce requirements for harvesting of skin autograft for closure of excised, full-thickness burns, *J Trauma* 60:821-829, 2006.

Boynton JF, Cohen BE, Barrera A: Rhytidectomy and parotidectomy combined in the same patient, *Aesthetic Plast Surg* 30:125-131, 2006.

Chiu TW: *Key topics in plastic and reconstructive surgery*, London, 2005, Taylor & Francis.

Choi CM, Bennett RG: Laser dopplers to determine cutaneous blood flow, *Dermatol Surg* 29:272-280, 2003.

Connor NP, et al: Augmented blood removal after medicinal leech feeding in congested tissue flaps, *J Rehabil Res Develop* 39:505, 2002.

Dolan R, editor: *Facial, plastic, reconstructive, and trauma surgery*, London, 2003, Informa Healthcare.

Francis A: Nursing management of skin graft sites, *Nurs Stand* 12:41-44, 1998.

Fujiwara M, Nakmura Y, Sano A, et al: Delayed rectus abdominis myocutaneous flap for anterior chest wall reconstruction, *Aesthetic Plast Surg* 30:120-124, 2006.

Haskins N: Intensive nursing care of patients with a microvascular free flap after maxillofacial surgery, *Intens Crit Care Nurs* 14:225-230, 1998.

Khan MN, Davies CG: Advances in the management of leg ulcers-the potential role of growth factors, *Int Wound J* 3:113-120, 2006.

LoGiudice J, Gosian AK: Clinical overview pediatric tissue expansion: indications and complications, *Plast Surg Nurs* 24:20-27, 2004.

Maillard GF, Garey L: Plastic surgery after ablative cancer surgery, *Aesthetic Plast Surg* 30:47-52, 2006.

Marston WA, Hanft J, Norwood P, et al: The efficacy and safety of Dermagraft in improving the healing of chronic diabetic foot ulcers, *Diabetes Care* 26:1701-1705, 2003.

Mulliken JB, Wu JK, Padwa BL: Repair of bilateral cleft lip: review, revisions, and reflections, *J Craniofacial Surg* 14:609, 2003.

Nordstrom H, Stange K: Plasma lidocaine levels and risks after liposuction with tumescent anesthesia, *Acta Anaesthesiol Scand* 49:1487-1489, 2005.

O'Brien M, Moiemen N: Use of tissue expanders in trauma, *Trauma* 7:69-75, 2005.

Papel ID, editor: *Facial plastic and reconstructive surgery*, ed 2, New York, 2002, Thieme Medical Publishers.

Phillips JC: Understanding hyperbaric oxygen therapy and its use in the treatment of compromised skin grafts and flaps, *Plast Surg Nurs* 25:72-82, 2005.

Sandberg DJ, Magee WP, Denk MJ: Neonatal cleft lip and cleft palate repair, *AORN J* 75:488-508, 2002.

Sarwer DB, Pruzinsky T, Cash TF, et al: *Psychological aspects of reconstructive and cosmetic plastic surgery: clinical, empirical and ethical perspectives*, Philadelphia, 2005, Lippincott Williams & Wilkins.

Snyder RJ, Doyle H, Delbridge T: Applying split-thickness skin grafts: a step-by-step clinical guide and nursing implications, *Ostomy Wound Manage* 47:20-26, 2001.

Thomas PC: Multidisciplinary care of the child born with cleft lip and palate, *J Soc Otorhinolaryngol Head-Neck Nurses* 18:6-16, 2000.

Wang HJ, et al: The application of new biosynthetic artificial skin for long-term temporary wound coverage, *Burns* 31:991-997, 2005.

Yoho RA, Romaine JJ, O'Niel D: Review of the liposuction, abdominoplasty, and face-lift mortality and morbidity risk literature, *Dermatol Surg* 31:733-743, 2005.

Yuen JC: Techniques of external monitoring of buried free flaps, *Ann Plast Surg* 55:460-465, 2005.

Yüksel F, Silit E, Bahattin C: Reliance on double pedicle TRAM flap technique in breast reconstruction based on mammographic evidence, *Indian J Plast Surg* 37:44-50, 2004.

NURSING CARE IN THE PACU

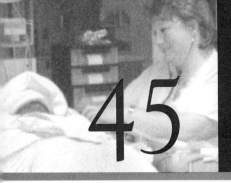

# 45

## CARE OF THE THERMALLY INJURED PATIENT

*Mary Bryant Ford, MSNA, CRNA*

A serious burn is one of the most devastating injuries that a human can sustain. It affects the skin and every organ system of the body, with the magnitude of the effect proportionate to the extent of the burn. As the fifth most common cause of unintentional-injury death in the United States, thermal injury is a major health problem in that an estimated 1 million people seek medical attention annually for thermal injuries. This number represents a significant decline from estimates reported in the last decade. Approximately 45,000 are hospitalized, and an estimated 4500 die of the direct effects or complications associated with these injuries.[1] Nursing care for the thermally injured patient requires collaboration between members of a multidisciplinary health care team. Knowledge of the local and systemic manifestations of thermal injury is necessary to ensure a thorough assessment of the patient's condition and an evaluation of the patient's response.[1]

## DEFINITIONS

**Deep-Dermal Partial-Thickness Burn Injury:** Burn injury in which the entire epidermis and most of the dermis is destroyed, with only the epithelial lining of the hair follicles and sweat glands left intact; dark red or waxy white in appearance with wet serous exudates.

**Dermatome:** Device used in removal of a portion of the patient's epidermis with a partial layer of dermis from a region of unburned tissue that serves as a skin graft.

**Full-Thickness Burn Injury:** Burn that involves the destruction of both layers of the skin to the level of hypodermis or subcutaneous tissue and may involve fat, fascia, muscle, and bone; dry, charred, or pearly white in appearance with a leathery texture.

**Rule of Nines:** Guideline used for quick estimate of the percentage of body surface area involved in a burn injury based on the concept that various body regions represent multiples of 9% of the total body surface area.

**Superficial Burn Injury:** Painful burn that involves the outermost layer of the epidermis; commonly caused by prolonged sun exposure; the skin appears dry and erythematous, usually without blisters, and has a rapid capillary refill.

**Superficial Partial-Thickness Burn Injury:** Painful burn that involves the epidermis with sparing of most dermal appendages: pink or mottled red in appearance with possible blister formation or wet serous exudate.

**Vacuum-Assist Closure Devices:** Device used for healing wounds covered with split-thickness skin grafts with use of a sponge and occlusive dressing to create continuous negative pressure in the sealed wound bed.

## INTEGUMENTARY SYSTEM

A review of the anatomy of the skin (Chapter 17) is important in understanding the physiologic reactions to a thermal injury. The skin is more than a simple covering for the body. It is a combination of tissues that form the largest organ of the body and provides a buffer between the internal and external environments. Skin is the body's first line of defense for protection against infection, prevention of loss of fluids, regulation of temperature, and provision of sensory input through the sense of touch.

The anatomic layers of the skin are the epidermis and the dermis. The epidermis is the outermost layer and is composed of stratified squamous epithelial tissue that varies in depth from 0.07 to 0.12 mm, with the deepest areas on the palms of the hands and the soles of the feet.[2] Histologically, the epidermis can be subdivided into five layers, the most important of which are the stratum corneum and the stratum germinativum. The stratum corneum, which is constantly shed, is composed of densely packed dead cells, keratin, and surface lipids. The major function of this layer is to provide a barrier to prevent the loss of body fluids or the invasion of microbes or noxious agents from the environment. The stratum germinativum constantly undergoes subdivision to form new cells that replace those shed from surface layers. Only in the germinativum layer do cells undergo mitosis and generate new epithelium.

The dermis ranges in thickness from 1 to 2 mm and lies below the epidermis. This layer is composed of collagen, connective tissues, smooth muscle, blood vessels, nerves, lymphatics, and glandular structures. Within the dermal layer, the sweat glands and hair follicles are lined with epithelial cells that generate epithelium to assist in the closure of partial-thickness wounds. The dermis provides nutrients and structure for the epidermis. Under the dermis lies the hypodermis, which contains fat, smooth muscle, and areolar tissue. This layer acts as a heat insulator and shock absorber.

## THERMAL INJURY CLASSIFICATION

The classification of thermal injuries is based on the depth of the injury, which is directly related to the temperature and duration of exposure to the thermal energy.[3] The longer the tissue is in contact with a high temperature or heat source, the deeper the tissue destruction. Formerly, the depth of injury was identified as first, second, or third degree. The preferred nomenclature for reporting depth of injury is superficial, partial-thickness, and full-thickness injury. Superficial injury involves the outermost layer of the epidermis and is usually caused by prolonged exposure to the sun. Superficial burns are painful; the skin appears dry and erythematous, and usually without blisters; and has a rapid capillary refill. Systemic involvement is limited, with complete healing in 5 to 7 days. The magnitude of the physiologic response ranges from a minor alteration of the evaporative barrier to edema formation. The major debilitating symptom is pain. Patients with superficial injury usually do not need hospitalization.

Partial-thickness injury can be subdivided into superficial partial-thickness and deep-dermal partial-thickness injuries. These injuries are characterized by damage that involves the epidermis and varying depths of the dermis. The superficial partial-thickness injury involves the epidermis with sparing of most dermal appendages. On presentation, the skin is pink or mottled red, has formed blisters, or is wet with serous exudate. A decreased rate of capillary refill is seen, and the wound is extremely painful. The margin of the wound is raised relative to adjacent uninjured tissue because of the edema within the wound. This level of

partial-thickness injury usually heals without skin grafting. Deep-dermal partial-thickness injury destroys the entire epidermis and most of the dermis, with only the epithelial lining of the hair follicles and sweat glands left intact. On examination, the skin appears wet with serous exudate, is dark red or waxy white in color, and has a decreased sensitivity to touch. Because of the structures involved and the compromised perfusion that occurs in deep-dermal injury, mechanical trauma or infection may convert this injury to a full-thickness level.

Full-thickness injury involves the destruction of both layers of the skin to the level of hypodermis or subcutaneous tissue and may involve fat, fascia, muscle, and bone. All epithelial elements are destroyed. These wounds present as dry, charred, or pearly white and have a leathery texture. The wound is depressed relative to uninjured tissue or adjacent partial-thickness injury because of the lack of circulation, loss of elasticity, and coagulation necrosis. With the destruction of the dermal elements, these wounds lack sensation and require autografting wound closure.

## EXTENT OF INJURY

Two methods are used to estimate the body surface area (extent) of thermal injury. The most commonly used method for rapid estimation for an adult victim is the Rule of Nines. This guideline reflects the fact that various body regions represent 9% or multiples of 9% of the total body surface area. The head and neck area represents 9%; the anterior and posterior trunk each represent 18%; each upper extremity represents 9%; each lower extremity represents 18%; and the perineum and genitalia represent 1% (Fig. 45-1). With determination of the portion of each region involved, one can quickly estimate the percentage of body surface area injured. Because the percentage of the various regions differs with age, an age-adjusted tool is needed for infants and children. A more precise prediction can be accomplished with the Lund and Browder chart, which is an age-adjusted surface area chart (Fig. 45-2).

## TYPES OF THERMAL INJURY

Thermal injury may result from contact with heat, cold, chemicals, or electricity. Most thermal injuries are caused by flames, hot liquids, heated metals, or steam. Cold injuries may occur with immobility of body parts, even at temperatures above freezing when the humidity is high. Frostbite is characterized by the

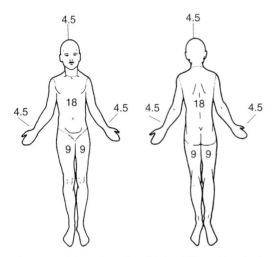

**Fig. 45-1** Schematic outline of Rule of Nines. Use of rule provides rapid method for determination of percentage of body surface burned but is of limited accuracy. *(From Sabiston DC Jr: Davis-Christopher Textbook of surgery: the biological basis of modern surgical practice, ed 11, Philadelphia, 1977, Saunders.)*

formation of intracellular fluid crystals. In patients with severe frostbite, regional ischemia is seen with necrosis of the epidermis, the dermis, or the underlying structures. Because the nursing management and wound care for frostbite are similar to the treatment for heat-related injuries, these patients may be treated in burn centers.

Chemical injury is caused by exposure to acids, alkali, or organic compounds. Acids and alkali are frequently used in industry for cleansing, curing, extracting, and preserving purposes. In the home, chemicals are commonly found in drain cleaners and cleaning solvents that, when used, may cause tissue damage. Most exposures to organic compounds are associated with use of fertilizers, pesticides, or petroleum products. The depth of chemical injury is the result of the concentration of the chemical and the duration of exposure. The proper use of protective clothing decreases the risk of dangerous exposure. After a chemical exposure, initial intervention should include removal of all dry chemical and then immediate irrigation with copious amounts of water to dilute and remove the agent. The chemical neutralization of acids or alkali compounds is contraindicated because of the delay in treatment and risk of an exothermic reaction when acids and bases are combined.[4] Patients exposed to chemical agents should be monitored for systemic toxicity, such as pulmonary insufficiency and hepatic or renal failure.[5]

Electric injuries are subdivided into low-voltage (less than 1000 V) and high-voltage

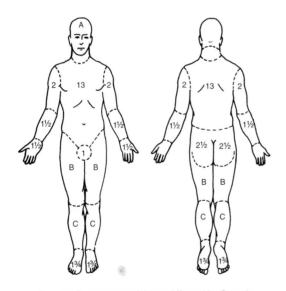

**Fig. 45-2** Classic Lund and Browder chart. Best method for determination of percentage of body surface burn is marking areas of injury on chart and then computing total percentage according to patient's age. Every emergency department should have such a chart for plotting of burned area soon after patient is admitted. *(From Sabiston DC Jr: Davis-Christopher Textbook of surgery: the biological basis of modern surgical practice, ed 11, Philadelphia, 1977, Saunders.)*

### Relative Percentages of Areas Affected by Growth
(AGE IN YEARS)

|  | 0 | 1 | 5 | 10 | 15 | ADULT |
|---|---|---|---|---|---|---|
| A : ½ of head | 9½ | 8½ | 6½ | 5½ | 4½ | 3½ |
| B : ½ of thigh | 2¾ | 3¼ | 4 | 4¼ | 4½ | 4¾ |
| C : ½ of leg | 2½ | 3½ | 2¾ | 3 | 3¼ | 3½ |

Total Per Cent Burned _____ 2° + _____ 3° = _____

(more than 1000 V) types. Electric injury is caused by the passage of electric current through the body, with the conversion of electric current to heat.[6] Electric current follows the path of least resistance, with the extent of injury related to the intensity of the current and the duration of contact time. Specific tissue resistance is irrelevant with high-voltage electric injury; the body acts as a volume conductor.[6] The contact points may be the only visible wounds, yet deep tissue damage is often sustained. The extent of injury is often difficult to assess immediately after injury and necessitates sequential assessment for appreciation of the amount of tissue involved. Surgical exploration may be needed if any indication of deep tissue damage exists as assessed with palpation of the muscle compartments. Associated injuries such as fractures; cardiac dysrhythmias; soft tissue, vascular, and head injuries; cataracts; and neuropathies may occur from electric current passage or associated falls.[7]

## PATHOPHYSIOLOGY OF THERMAL INJURY

During the first 48 hours after thermal injury, systemic consequences are associated with a hypodynamic stage followed by a hyperdynamic stage.[6,7] Organ system involvement, magnitude, and duration are proportional to the extent of the burn and reach a plateau when the injury is approximately 50% to 60% of the total body surface area.[6,7] The hypodynamic stage is characterized by an acute decrease in metabolic rate and a decrease in cardiac output of roughly 50%.[8] Individuals with an injury that involves more than 25% of total body surface area have immense fluid shifts from the intravascular space into the surrounding tissue because of changes in capillary permeability.[9] The initial changes in capillary integrity permit even large protein molecules to pass freely into the interstitium. For this reason, colloid-containing fluids are usually withheld until capillary integrity is restored around 24 hours after injury. Tissue edema occurs in both injured and uninjured tissue because of the changes in capillary permeability and hypoproteinemia and the volume and pressure effects of fluid resuscitation. Redistribution of body water, electrolytes, and protein associated with the increased capillary permeability creates a decrease in the circulating blood volume. This intravascular depletion is accompanied by a sudden abrupt decrease in cardiac output that does not correlate with the gradual reduction in blood volume. Peripheral vascular resistance increases as a result of the neurohormonal stress response after injury. This increase in afterload contributes to the decreased cardiac output and reduces perfusion to major organ systems.

Cardiac output and organ perfusion improve with adequate fluid resuscitation. Within 36 hours after injury, cardiac function becomes supranormal. This hyperdynamic phase lasts until the burn wound is closed.[9] In a setting of adequate fluid resuscitation, the hyperdynamic stage correlates with an increase in metabolic rate that peaks between 7 and 12 days after injury and lasts until the burn wound is closed.[2,9]

Fluid management of the patient with thermal injury requires attention to detail to prevent the potential morbidity associated with either underresuscitation or overresuscitation. Failure to deliver enough fluid may result in inadequate organ perfusion. Overresuscitation may lead to pulmonary or wound edema. Wound edema in a circumferentially injured extremity may decrease perfusion of uninjured tissue in the distal portion of that extremity.

During the early postinjury period, the individual may have symptoms of modest pulmonary hypertension. Even an individual without inhalation injury may have decreased lung compliance, impaired gas exchange, and increased pulmonary vascular resistance.[8,10] The mechanisms of these associated lung injuries are not completely understood but are thought to be the result of direct damage from complex inflammatory processes.[8] In addition, burn patients have pneumonia develop approximately 50% of the time and as a result commonly need mechanical ventilation.[8] Barotrauma and other pulmonary morbidity may be the direct result of mechanical ventilation in this patient population.[8] In the early stages of resuscitation, the minute ventilation may be decreased in a patient with hypovolemia but commonly increases in proportion to the extent of burn as the resuscitative phase progresses.[7] These changes in minute ventilation parallel alterations in metabolic rate associated with the injury.

The kidneys have a similar hypodynamic-hyperdynamic pattern. The consequences of diminished intravascular volume, plasma flow, and glomerular filtration rate result in decreased urine output. Acute renal failure, although rare, may result if fluid resuscitation is delayed. Approximately 24 hours after injury, vascular integrity is restored and fluid requirements decrease. This period is followed by the shift of interstitial fluid to the intravascular compartment, with an ensuing diuresis that occurs 48 to 72 hours after injury.[2]

The gastrointestinal tract shows decreased activity in patients with injuries that involve more than 25% of total body surface area.[11]

A nasogastric tube should be inserted to decrease the risk of gastric dilation, emesis, and aspiration. After adequate fluid resuscitation, normal functioning of the gastrointestinal system returns. Endoscopic studies have shown that gastrointestinal ulcerations occur in 80% of critically ill patients with thermal injury if some form of prophylactic therapy is not used. Because of the potential risk of acute stress ulcers, preventive modalities are used for all thermally injured patients with total body surface area involvement of 35% or more.[9] Gastric pH levels are maintained between 3.5 and 4.5 with antacid or histamine blocker therapy.

Several hematologic changes follow a thermal injury. Although the number of red blood cells decreases after injury, the hematocrit level is usually elevated because of hemoconcentration from the fluid shifts that occur immediately after the injury. Some red blood cells are lysed because of direct thermal injury; however, continued hemolysis may last for several days. Blood loss related to wound débridement, phlebotomy, or alterations in the coagulation system, such as thrombocytopenia, thrombocytosis, and disseminated intravascular coagulation, should be monitored closely.

The thermally injured patient is highly susceptible to infection because of alterations in host-defense mechanisms. The primary and secondary lines of defense against infection are limited with the loss of integument. A depressed responsiveness of lymphocytes is seen in thermally injured patients, and immunosuppressive substances can be isolated in the sera.[3] These changes occur immediately after injury and continue until the wound is closed. The immune response at the cellular level is unclear, and whether changes are caused by the introduction of organisms or a deficiency in components can only be hypothesized. What have been described are alterations in T-cell function, the humoral B-cell system, and nonspecific host defenses.[10] The immunologic responses result from complex interactions of multiple factors, including the thermal injury, nutritional deficits, stress, microbial products, and treatment.

Extensive thermal injury results in catabolism characterized by a significant elevation of the metabolic rate and loss of lean body mass.[11-13] Thermally injured patients manifest a negative nitrogen balance in response to the injury. The rate of catabolism may be further increased with infection. Aggressive nutritional support is needed to meet energy requirements, replace the protein losses, and promote wound healing.[11] Blood glucose levels increase in response to a stressful critical injury or illness. Wilmore[14] reported that increased gluconeogenesis accounts for this hyperglycemia. The gastrointestinal tract is the preferred route for feeding the thermally injured patient once return of gastrointestinal function has been established. Maintenance of a functional gastrointestinal tract helps maintain the intestinal barrier to prevent translocation of intestinal bacteria throughout the body.[8] In this manner, enteral feeding promotes nutrition and reduces concomitant infection.[8] With facial injury, altered levels of consciousness, or gastric ileus, oral intake should be limited; initiation of tube feedings should be considered.[7] Total parenteral nutrition should be considered when enteral feeding is contraindicated.

## WOUND MANAGEMENT

Twenty-five years ago, patients with extensive thermal injuries had a limited chance of survival. Those who survived the resuscitative phase often died of overwhelming infection. Although wound treatment modalities are initiated at the time of admission, they become the focus of care during the acute phase. The goals of wound management are the prevention of infection, the preservation of tissue, timely wound closure, and the maintenance and restoration of function. Nursing care rendered in the postanesthesia care unit (PACU) is important in the attainment of these goals.

All the energies invested in the care of the thermally injured patient are directed at a single outcome: the transformation of a contaminated open wound to a clean closed wound. The open wound is associated with the hypermetabolic and physiologic stress responses that do not become corrected until the wound is closed.[6] Current wound management after resuscitation involves excision of the necrotic tissue and coverage of the wound.[3] Advantages of early excision include early mobilization, reduction of pain, early wound closure, reduced risk of infection, and reduced length of hospital stay. Disadvantages include exposure to surgical stress in the early postresuscitation period and the risk of excision of viable tissue that might heal.[6]

The necrotic tissue, foreign material, and cellular debris are mechanically removed from the burn wound with either tangential or full-thickness excision. Tangential excision is the sequential removal of thin layers of necrotic tissue until viable tissue with an adequate blood supply is reached. This débridement technique may be used for both superficial and deep-dermal partial-thickness injury.[6]

Full-thickness excision involves the removal of nonviable tissue to the level of viable tissue, usually down to subcutaneous fat or fascia, with scalpel or electrocautery techniques. Excision of an area of thermal injury that exceeds 20% of the total body surface at one time is not recommended because of surgical stress and the magnitude of blood loss. Each operative procedure is limited to 20% of the total body surface area or 2 hours of operative time. Time between procedures allows for recovery and reepithelialization of donor sites.[15]

After the excision is complete, hemostasis must be achieved. Topical thrombin may be sprayed onto the excised bed, followed by the placement of warm moist laparotomy pads. An alternative method is the application of gauze sponges soaked in 1:10,000 epinephrine solution to the wound bed.[3] Pressure is then applied with application of a circumferential gauze dressing. After approximately 10 minutes, the pressure dressing is gently removed. Specific sites of bleeding are identified and cauterized or ligated.

Many skin grafting techniques are available to the surgeon who manages the care of the thermally injured patient. For the purposes of this chapter, only the definitive closure of the wound is addressed. Once the necrotic tissue is removed, the exposed underlying tissues must be covered to provide protection and prevent infection. The definitive covering is autograft skin. A portion of the patient's epidermis with a partial layer of dermis is removed from a region of unburned tissue with a dermatome. This tissue is referred to as a split-thickness skin graft and can be applied as an intact sheet or an expanded meshed sheet to the wound bed. A full-thickness skin graft is one in which a segment of full dermis and epidermis is transplanted to a recipient site.[3,12,13] The skin graft is secured in place with fibrin glue, staples, sutures, an immobilizing dressing and splints, or a combination of these methods.

Split-thickness grafts typically vary in thickness from 0.01 to 0.035 inches. Sheet grafts are preferred when the wound location has cosmetic or functional importance, such as the face, neck, hands, and feet. In the postanesthesia period, nurses must assess the healing grafts for the presence of hematoma or seromas, which may prevent graft adherence.

Meshed autograft skin is indicated for patients with extensive thermal injury because meshing allows for maximum coverage of wounds from limited donor sites. The mesh graft's interstices allow the escape of blood and plasma, thus decreasing the risk of interference with graft vascularization. The meshed autografts are usually expanded one and a half to four times the normal size. A layer of fine-mesh and course-mesh gauze soaked in an antimicrobial or saline solution is applied directly over the grafts and is secured with roller gauze. This dressing prevents the desiccation of the exposed wound bed until the interstices are closed with epithelial migration.

Vacuum-assist closure devices have been used to facilitate healing of wounds covered with split-thickness skin grafts.[16] These devices, commonly referred to as wound vacs, consist of a sponge over the wound, covered with an occlusive dressing that is open to suction to create continuous negative pressure in the sealed wound bed.[16] Application of such devices has been shown to decrease the incidence rate of graft failure and thus decrease the requirement for repeat grafting.[16] This type of negative pressure dressing promotes the formation of granulation tissue and accelerates wound reepithelialization to enhance wound healing.[16] In addtion, creation of a negative pressure environment around the wound removes fluid and prevents the development of hematomas and seromas. Vacuum-assisted closure devices also help stabilize the graft and decrease shear stress on the wound.[16]

The donor site selection may be limited because of the extent of the injury, but cosmetic or functional outcomes should be considered, if possible. After the harvesting of the skin grafts, the newly created partial-thickness wound at the donor site must be protected against maceration and infection. Management of these wounds includes the application of various types of dressings or temporary coverings.[12,13] Fine-mesh gauze is often applied directly over the donor site. Blood is evacuated from beneath the gauze with a straight edge such as scissors or scalpel handle, and the dressing is allowed to dry. Donor site care in the PACU includes the application of radiant heat to begin drying this dressing. Any insult, such as mechanical trauma, heat or cold injury, and infection, may convert this surgically created partial-thickness wound to a full-thickness injury.

Most operative procedures on thermally injured patients are performed with general anesthesia. Ketamine may be administered to the thermally injured patient for anesthesia or analgesia. The advantages of ketamine induction include the production of intense analgesia and maintenance of normal pharyngeal and laryngeal reflexes.

Regional anesthesia may be used for local débridement. If grafting is to be completed after the excision, regional anesthesia may not be adequate to allow harvest of donor sites from areas remote from the excision. For additional information on anesthetics, see Section III.

## POSTANESTHESIA NURSING CARE

In health care facilities that have a specialty care unit for the treatment of thermally injured patients, postanesthesia care is typically provided in that unit. If a thermally injured patient must be cared for in a PACU, selected factors in addition to standard postanesthesia care must be considered. Ambient room temperature should be maintained at 85°F for prevention of hypothermia. Infection control policies, including isolation procedures, handwashing techniques, and a strict dress code, should be developed for the PACU for this unique patient population.

Postanesthesia nursing care for thermally injured patients includes recovery from anesthesia, proper positioning, immobilization to prevent autograft disruption, use of restraints as appropriate, prevention of hypothermia, inspection of dressings for signs of hemorrhage, and adequate pain management. Assessment and documentation are critical components of nursing management during the postanesthesia period. Assessment must be directed primarily toward the maintenance of a patent airway and adequate respiration and circulation. Standard procedures for the management of patients recovering from anesthesia should be used. The secondary assessment focuses on the donor and graft sites. Documentation should include a review of systems plus the location of graft and donor sites, the appearance of the dressings, patient position, and all medications administered.

Specific wound care depends on the type of operative procedure and the location of the operative site. The most frequent cause of graft loss is mechanical shear from movement of the grafted body part. Immobilization of the joint above and below the grafted region is necessary. Most split-thickness mesh grafts are dressed with a nonadherent material, covered with course-mesh gauze, and secured with roller gauze. Immobilization is accomplished with the application of splints over the dressings. Although hemostasis is achieved during surgery, postoperative increases in blood pressure and movement may cause bleeding at the operative sites. If bleeding occurs, the surgeon should be notified.

Sheet skin grafts are generally not dressed to allow direct visualization. Sheet grafts must be assessed for the accumulation of blood or serum under the graft. Formation of hematomas or serous blebs between a graft and the wound bed requires evacuation to prevent graft loss. Fluid accumulations beneath the graft may be aspirated with a small syringe and needle. The surgeon may make a small incision near a bleb to allow the fluid to be expelled or use a cotton-tipped applicator to "roll" the fluid to the edges of the graft.[7]

In the immediate postanesthesia period, the donor sites should receive heat and aeration to promote drying. The nurse must ensure that donor sites remain clean, dry, and free from pressure. With proper care, multiple skin grafts can be harvested from the same location.

Thermal injuries are one of the most painful forms of trauma that one can have, and pain management provides a major challenge for the PACU nurse.[17] Astute nursing assessment and evaluation are needed to differentiate restlessness as a result of pain from other causes such as hypoxia and bladder or gastric distention. Pain can be reduced with frequent intravenous administration of small doses of morphine sulfate (3 to 5 mg in adults).[2] Intramuscular injections should be avoided during the postoperative period because the normal fluid shifts may impair soft-tissue circulation, rendering analgesia ineffective. As circulatory integrity is restored, opioids previously deposited in the muscles and subcutaneous tissue may be mobilized and possibly lead to an overdosage. Continuous infusion of intravenous opioids may be an effective technique to produce a constant level of analgesia but requires careful monitoring for undesirable physiologic effects, including respiratory depression.[11]

## SUMMARY

The nursing care of the thermally injured patient provides an exciting challenge for the PACU nurse. With the advent of successful resuscitation formulas, new surgical techniques, improved nutritional delivery systems, and innovative wound management interventions, the survival rate of patients with major thermal injury has greatly improved. However, the nurse must continue to understand the rationale for intervention to provide optimal monitoring and evaluation of these patients in the postanesthesia period. Outcomes are enhanced when all members of the health care team provide collaborative care for the severely injured patient.

## REFERENCES

1. Burn Foundation: *Burn incidence and treatment in the US: 2000 fact sheet*, available at www. ameriburn. org/pub/factsheet.htm. Accessed December 5, 2006.

2. Sheridan RL: Evaluating and managing burn wounds, *Dermatol Nurs* 12:17-31, 2000.

3. Funke DJ: Thermal injury and anesthesia. In Nagelhout JJ, Zaglaniczny KL, editors: *Nurse anesthesia*, ed 2, Philadelphia, 2001, Saunders.

4. Bates N: Acid and alkali injury, *Emerg Nurs* 7:21-26, 1999.

5. Chandler SK: Plastic and reconstructive surgery. In Rothrock JC, editor: *Alexander's care of the patient in surgery*, ed 13, St Louis, 2007, Mosby.

6. Pruitt BA Jr, Goodwin CW Jr: Thermal injuries. In Davis JH, Drucker WR, Foster RS, editors: *Clinical surgery*, St Louis, 1987, Mosby.

7. Pruitt BA Jr, Treat RG: The burn patient. In Dudrick SJ, Bave AE, Eiseman B, et al, editors: *Manual of preoperative and postoperative care*, Philadelphia, 1983, Saunders.

8. Marko P, Layon AJ, Caruso L, et al: Burn injuries, *Curr Opin Anaesthesiol* 16:183-191, 2003.

9. Cummings J, Purdue GF, Hunt JL: Objective estimates of the incidence and consequences of multiple organ dysfunction and sepsis after burn trauma, *J Trauma* 50:510-515, 2001.

10. Arturson MG: The pathophysiology of severe thermal injury, *J Burn Care Rehabil* 6:129-146, 1985.

11. Romito RA: Early administration of enteral nutrients in critically ill patients, *AACN Clin Issues* 6:242-256, 1995.

12. Gueugniaud PY, Carson H, Bertin-Mayht M, et al: Current advances in the initial management of major thermal burns, *Intens Care Med* 26:848-856, 2000.

13. Kao CC, Garner WL: Acute burns, *Plast Reconstruct Surg* 10:2482-2493, 2000.

14. Wilmore DW: Metabolic changes after thermal injury. In Boswick JA, editor: *The art and science of burn care*, Rockville, MD, 1987, Aspen.

15. Kravitz M: Thermal injuries. In Cardona VD, Hurn PD, Bastnagel Mason PJ, et al, editors: *Trauma nursing: from resuscitation through rehabilitation*, Philadelphia, 1994, Saunders.

16. Scherer LA, Shiver S, Chang M, et al: The vacuum assisted closure device: a method of securing skin grafts and improving graft survival, *Arch Surg* 137:930-934, 2002.

17. Weinberg K, Birdsell C, Vail D, et al: Pain and anxiety with burn dressing changes: patient self report, *J Burn Rehabil* 21:155-161, 2000.

## BIBLIOGRAPHY

Bishop JF: Burn wound assessment and surgical management, *Crit Care Clin North Am* 16(1):145-177, 2004.

Harrison M: Discussion on wound care in the 21st century, *Br J Nurs* 15(19):S12-16, 2006.

How S, Chan HH, Ying SY, et al: Skin care in burn patients: a team approach, *Burns* 27:489-491, 2001.

Hunt JP, Calvert CT, Peck MD, et al: Occupational-related burn injuries, *J Burn Care Rehabil* 21:327-332, 2000.

Linneman PK, Terry BE, Burd RS: The efficacy and safety of fentanyl for the management of severe procedural pain in patients with burn injury, *J Burn Care Rehabil* 6:519-522, 2000.

Rose DD, Jordan EB: Perioperative management of burn patients, *AORN J* 69:1211-1226, 1999.

Still JM Jr, Law EJ: Primary excision of burn wounds, *Clin Plast Surg* 27:23-47, 2000.

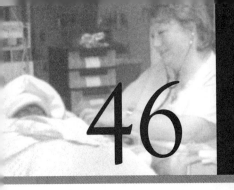

# 46

## CARE OF THE AMBULATORY SURGICAL PATIENT

*Nancy Burden, RN, MS, CPAN, CAPA*

Ambulatory surgery continues as an area of growth, both in number of patients and in advancement of knowledge and technology. A significant number of procedures continues to migrate to the outpatient setting each year, with inpatient numbers decreasing slightly. Baby boomers are now hitting their 60s, and we are seeing the beginning effects of their needs on health care. Not only will this huge generation place demands on health care providers simply because of their numbers; the baby boomers also bring demands for the best and fastest care, as typical of their generation. The great mobility of the population in the United States brings another challenge as families are scattered and the stronger family support systems of years past are reduced.

A variety of factors drives the move toward outpatient surgery. Foremost, experience over the past 30-plus years has shown the process to be successful and safe. Overall clinical outcomes have not suffered from shortened postoperative hospitalization in appropriate cases. In fact, avoidance of a hospital stay can reduce the opportunity for health care–associated infection and medical errors.

## DEFINITIONS

**Ambulatory Surgery Center (ASC):** A facility that is separate from a hospital and may be on the same campus as or separate from other medical facilities.
**Freestanding Ambulatory Surgery Center (FASC):** Term used interchangeably with ASC.
**Hospital Outpatient Department (HOPD):** An area within a hospital that provides perioperative care for surgery patients who are discharged on the same day. These departments often function as a same-day admitting area for other surgical patients.
**Joint Venture Surgery Center:** An ambulatory surgery center that has more than one ownership entity, such as a corporation and physicians, a hospital and physicians, or a combination of all three.

**Third-Party Payers:** Payers that include insurance companies, health maintenance organizations, and the federal government; generally mandate that surgical procedures be performed in the appropriate lowest cost setting for payment eligibility. Thus, the trend has been to push procedures from hospitals to outpatient settings to physician offices. Ambulatory surgery and hospital industry organizations continually work with federal agencies to lobby for appropriate placement of procedures. Federal payment decisions often result in managed care companies following suit; so this is an important focus for administrators in all levels of health care settings.

## AMBULATORY SURGERY ISSUES

A discrepancy still exists in government reimbursement for the same procedures done in a hospital outpatient department (HOPD) versus a freestanding ambulatory surgery center (FASC), with the hospital department financially favored. Although most procedures are reimbursed by the Centers for Medicaid and Medicare Services (CMS) at a higher rate in the hospital setting, in 2007, the 275 codes that had been paid higher in the freestanding setting were now capped at the hospital rate as part of the federal Deficit Reduction Act. CMS has plans to further significantly change the ASC reimbursement system in 2008. Financial pressures on physicians are also driving the trend toward physician-owned or joint-ventured surgery centers and specialty hospitals as a way of securing a portion of the technical (facility) fee to supplement diminishing professional fees.

In addition to the financial pressures of identification and use of the most cost-effective site for surgical procedures, other factors have contributed to the trend of same-day admission and early postoperative discharge. Technologic advances in instrumentation and equipment allow more complex procedures to be done with less invasiveness and physical trauma. Examples include lithotripsy and laparoscopic, endoscopic, and arthroscopic approaches in a multitude of surgical specialties from sinus surgery to orthopedics, urology, gynecology, and more.

Innovative procedures have come on the market but remain self-pay procedures because Medicare does not approve payment. They are performed in the HOPD, FASC, or physician offices. Examples include orthotripsy, similar in concept to lithotripsy but for treatment of heel spurs, and cosmetic procedures such as new approaches to eliminate unsightly veins. The merits of some of these procedures remain controversial in medical circles.

The pharmacologic industry has developed shorter-acting anesthetic agents and adjunctive drugs that allow quicker return to alertness and self care with fewer unpleasant side effects. Also, consumers are more educated and sophisticated than in past generations, and current fast-paced lifestyles lend themselves to "in and out" care.

In response to the special needs of patients who require nursing care in a much shortened time span, ambulatory perianesthesia nurses place emphasis on rapid yet comprehensive patient assessment along with complete understandable patient and family education. Ambulatory surgical nurses encourage the patient's self care and self responsibility for pre-admission and postdischarge compliance with the planned medical and nursing care and then must assess the patient's ability, desire, and intentions to comply. In addition, these nurses emphasize the patient's early ambulation and return to normal life activities, patient teaching, and family involvement in the patient's care.

Recognizing and addressing the social, emotional, and educational needs of patients as well as the physical needs is important. Many people ask all the questions they have, but in some cases, unspoken questions linger for patients and their families. These questions may relate to the final outcome of the procedure and concerns about health and well being, financial burdens, doubts about the availability and quality of postoperative support at home, vulnerability, and whether full preoperative life activities can resume and how quickly. Nurses should provide open doors for these types of questions and discussions.

Home support is essential because the patient returns home so quickly after surgery. Involvement of the family or another responsible adult is integral to the overall plan of care. Postoperative complications such as nausea and vomiting might be considered minor or merely unpleasant for hospitalized patients who have nursing support. For ambulatory surgical patients, however, these problems become serious deterrents to discharge and can lead to a costly prolonged hospital stay, unplanned hospitalization, or unpleasant home recuperation.

The ambulatory surgery nurse's assessment of the patient's medical, surgical, and social needs may lead to a referral to a home health provider for general medical care, infusion therapy, pain management, physical therapy, or equipment-related needs. If needs are known before the day of the procedure, this referral can be in place, with equipment and supplies delivered to the patient's home to ensure its availability as soon as the patient arrives there.

The basic tenet of nursing care in this setting is the promotion of wellness and self care to the degree possible. Patients should be continually encouraged to think positively and to provide self care as is appropriate and possible. Orem's[1] general theory of nursing, the Self-Care Deficit Nursing Theory, can be used to describe nursing planning and intervention appropriate to the ambulatory surgical patient. The nurse calculates the patient's self-care demand and shares with the patient what must be done to regain or promote health in relation to postoperative recovery. Nursing actions revolve around teaching the patient and family, gaining acceptance of the prescribed actions, and then assessing the degree to which the nurse feels the patient can and will comply.

The concept of a self-fulfilling prophecy is a tool often used by managers to motivate a team. Nurses can use the concept to help patients expect success and comfort. This concept can be summarized with four key points:

- We form certain expectations of people or events.
- We communicate those expectations with various cues.
- People tend to respond to these cues by adjusting their behavior to match them.
- The result is that the original expectation becomes true.[2]

Thus, according to the principles of a self-fulfilling prophecy, an outcome is more likely to happen just because the patient expects it. The outcome is "preprogrammed" by the patient's outlook; thus the nurse's programming of wellness and uneventful recovery can be an important tool to shape the mindsets of the patient and caregiver in a positive direction.

Whether the patient has surgery in a hospital setting, a freestanding ASC, or a physician's office, the basic nursing needs remain the same. That care combines both critical assessment and monitoring during periods of high dependence, such as immediately after general anesthesia or sedation, with periods when the patient is encouraged and taught how to assume responsibility for self care. This care often is provided through a two-phase recovery process: the initial post-anesthesia care unit (PACU) and a less care-intensive second-phase unit from which the patient is eventually discharged.

The ambulatory surgical patient population has changed during the past 30-plus years. More complex procedures are performed on sicker and older patients. Services such as 23-hour admission units, recovery care centers, and surgical specialty hospitals have provided a safety net of lengthier postoperative nursing care after more complex procedures, such as percutaneous spinal procedures, laparoscopically assisted vaginal hysterectomy, laparoscopic bariatric procedures, and open shoulder procedures. Some physicians discharge patients a few hours after these advanced procedures. Early discharge after more complex procedures becomes more common as we gain more history of patient outcomes, the frequency and extent of complications, and the level of patient acceptance based on experience and research.

Without several shifts of nurses to prepare and educate patients and families before ambulatory surgery or to tend to the patient's postoperative needs, ambulatory surgical nurses must possess certain characteristics. Foremost, clinical assessment skills must be accurate and rapid. Nurses must be self motivated and able to communicate both in professional terms with peers and physicians and in lay terms with patients. Documentation skills and the forms used in the facility should allow for precise documentation of findings in minimal time. Probably most important from the patient's viewpoint, the nurse working in ambulatory surgery should present a positive calm demeanor and show genuine concern for and interest in patients and their families.

## ASSESSMENT AND PREPARATION OF THE PATIENT

Careful preoperative selection and preparation of patients for outpatient surgery help to reduce the risks of perioperative complications. Nonetheless, many patients may be less than physically, emotionally, or socially ideal candidates, yet they return home soon after surgery or other procedures because of insurance requirements. In addition to systemic illnesses that limit their ability to care for themselves and possibly increase the risk of perioperative complications, many people have limited social or family support. Nurses are especially challenged to prepare these more complex patients for an early transition to home.

The ultimate goals of complication-free recovery and early discharge are supported by what occurs before surgery. Proper patient selection, preparation, and education all contribute significantly to eventual patient outcome. Nursing preparation must be comprehensive. Physical assessment, history taking, and evaluation of the patient's social, emotional, and cognitive status are all essential to that care. The challenge for the ambulatory surgical nurse, however, is completing all those evaluations in a condensed time frame.

Nursing care also must reach beyond the facility into the patient's home setting. This care includes preoperative education that helps encourage preparation of a safe home setting for postoperative recuperation. Although nurses cannot be responsible for the actions of patients outside the facility, nurses do provide education, coaching, and suggestions for the patient's preoperative and postoperative care at home. The need to gain the patient's confidence and cooperation and to ensure the involvement of a responsible adult cannot be overstated.

Before the day of surgery, an on-site preadmission assessment is ideal for the nurse to establish a rapport with the patient, secure the patient's history, complete a physical assessment, help reduce patient anxiety, provide comprehensive preoperative instructions, identify potential risk factors, and take steps to reduce those risk factors on or before the day of surgery. However, a telephone contact before the day of the patient's procedure is much more common today. The industry has come to this more streamlined approach for a number of reasons, including the busy lifestyles of the patient population, the economic restrictions of health care providers, the trend toward little or no diagnostic testing, and our current comfort with a telephone process borne out by history. Although a physical assessment or facility tour cannot occur via telephone, all other components of the preadmission care can be provided.

Patients at high risk can be identified and may be asked to come to the facility for physical examination and anesthesia consultation. Early identification of significant risk factors allows time to correct any deficiencies or, if necessary, to reschedule the surgery to avoid day-of-surgery cancellations or unexpected postoperative complications and overnight admissions that are more costly to the institution, upsetting to the patient and physician, and generally time consuming. A report by the American College of Cardiology and American Heart Association has identified major, intermediate, and minor clinical predictors of increased perioperative risk.

- Unstable coronary syndromes, such as acute or recent myocardial infarction (MI) or unstable angina, decompensated congestive heart failure, and severe dysrhythmias or valvular disease, are major predictors of perioperative risk.

- Intermediate risk factors include mild angina, prior MI determined with history or Q waves, compensated or prior heart failure, diabetes mellitus, and renal insufficiency.
- Minor risks include advanced age, abnormal electrocardiogram (ECG) results, dysrhythmias, low functional capacity, history of stroke, and uncontrolled hypertension.[3]

These factors should be considered before any surgery but especially before elective surgery that could wait until a more stable status can be attained.

Specific instructions necessary before the day of the procedure include arrangements for transportation and adult support, the projected length of stay, and, in general, expectations on the day of surgery. The patient also should be instructed in the proper clothing to wear for ease of dressing after surgery, preparation of the home environment, physical restrictions after surgery, and any equipment or supplies to purchase or secure before arrival for surgery.

With the emphasis on safety in the perioperative period, involvement of the patient as fully as possible in safety practices is prudent. Information such as that in Boxes 46-1 and 46-2 is one way to raise the patient's understanding and consciously set expectations that the patient and family will be part of the overall safety plan.

The Internet has become a common source of information. Nurses should be prepared to evaluate the value and accuracy of such information and advise the patient toward appropriate sites. An example of a valuable site for those who are considering surgery is the Agency for Healthcare Research and Quality at www.ahrq.gov. See Box 46-3 for content information. Other valuable Internet sites for patient information include the following:

- American Society of Anesthesiologists (www.asahq.org)
- American College of Surgeons (www.facs.org)
- Society for Ambulatory Anesthesia (www.sambahq.org)
- Institute for Healthcare Improvement (www.ihi.org)
- The Joint Commission (www.jointcommission.org)
- Society of Gastroenterology Nurses and Associates (www.sgna.org)
- American Association of Nurse Anesthetists (www.aana.com)
- Association of PeriOperative Registered Nurses (www.aorn.org)
- American Society of PeriAnesthesia Nurses (ASPAN; www.aspan.org).

The ASPAN site provides patient information on the following:
1. Preanesthetic interview and testing
2. Expectations for the day of surgery
3. Preoperative holding area
4. Expectations for the operating room
5. Expectations for the postanesthesia care unit

---

**Box 46-1  10 Tips to Keep You Safe in the Outpatient Setting**

1. Be sure that everyone who cares for you knows who you are by asking you to say your name or birth date and by checking your name band.
2. If you have any questions or concerns, ask a team member. Ask a family member or friend to speak for you if you are not able to do so.
3. If you feel you are not steady on your feet, please ask us to help you. We do not want you to fall.
4. When you are asked about the medicines you take, please tell us about every medicine. Be sure to include creams, vitamins, herbs, diet supplements, and all prescription and over-the-counter medicines, including street drugs.
5. Tell us about all of your allergies. Include allergies to medicines, tape, latex, shellfish, and anything else you may have reacted to in the past.
6. If you have a new prescription given to you while you are here, be sure you know what it is for, how to take it, and any possible side effects.
7. If you have any questions about a test or procedure, please ask your nurse, doctor, or any health care team member.
8. Ask team members who have direct contact with you if they have washed their hands. It is the best way to prevent the spread of germs, and our team members will be glad you asked.
9. Be sure you know and understand how to take care of yourself when you go home.
10. If you notice any other safety concerns, please tell a team member so that we can work to make our outpatient center a safer place for all.

---

### Box 46-2   Having an Outpatient Procedure?

Here are 10 things you can do to help prevent an infection.

**BEFORE YOUR PROCEDURE**
1. Shower or bathe with an antibacterial soap before your procedure.
2. Do not shave the skin near your incision area before surgery to prevent cuts in the skin that could harbor bacteria.
3. Do not apply creams or lotions near the incision area on the day of your procedure.

**BEFORE AND AFTER YOUR PROCEDURE**
4. Take care of yourself to enhance healing with adequate rest, plenty of fluids, and good nutrition: a diet high in protein and vitamin C, if not contraindicated by your health.
5. Avoid close contact with anyone who has an obvious infection, cold, or the flu.

**AFTER YOUR PROCEDURE**
6. Feel free to ask health care workers if they have washed their hands before caring for you. Do not be embarrassed to ask, we want to keep you safe.
7. Keep any dressing, bandage, or cast clean and dry. If it gets wet and you have been instructed not to remove or change it, tell your physician immediately.
8. If antibiotics are prescribed, take all of the pills and take according to directions.
9. Wash your hands before touching your bandage or caring for catheters and drains.
10. Do not put anything on your incision area that is not prescribed.

---

### Box 46-3   Quick Tips: When Planning for Surgery

The single most important way you can stay healthy is to be an active member of your own health care team. One way to get high-quality health care is to find and use information and take an active role in all of the decisions made about your care. This information helps you when planning for surgery.

No surgery is risk-free. Learning about the possible benefits and risks involved in the surgical procedure you are about to have is important. Research has shown that patients who are informed about their procedures can better work with their doctors to make the right decisions.

A second opinion is important. Your doctor, surgeon, health plan, or local medical society can help you find someone who can give you a second opinion. Before you seek a second opinion, be sure your health plan covers this expense.

Before you have surgery, ask your physician these questions:
- What operation are you recommending?
- Why do I need the operation?
- Are there alternatives to surgery?
- What are the benefits of having the operation?
- What are the risks of having the operation?
- What will happen if I do not have this operation?
- Where can I get a second opinion?
- What has been your experience in doing the operation? How many have you performed?
- Where will the operation be done?
- What kind of anesthesia will I need?
- How long will it take me to recover?
- How much will the operation cost?

Remember, quality matters, especially when it comes to your health.

Taken from AHRQ: *Quick tips—when planning for surgery,* AHRQ Publication No. 01-0040d, May 2002, Rockville, Md, 2002, Agency for Healthcare Research and Quality. Also available at http://www.ahrq.gov/consumer/quicktips/tipsurgery.htm, accessed December 12, 2006.

| Box 46-4    Medications Generally Continued until the Time of Surgery |
| --- |
| Antihypertensives<br>Cardiac antiarrhythmics<br>Coronary artery dilators<br>Bronchodilators<br>Respiratory inhalants (should be brought on the day of surgery) |

6. Admission to a facility
7. Outpatient surgery
8. Expectations for going home on the day of surgery
9. Pain management

Patients who take routine medications need instructions by the attending physician or anesthesiologist about which medications should be taken on the morning of surgery, usually with a small sip of water. Medications most often continued until the time of surgery are listed in Box 46-4. Precise instructions regarding insulin and diet on the day of surgery for patients with diabetes can help avoid wide swings in glucose levels. Although medication instructions are the responsibility of the physician, they are often confirmed, reinforced, and clarified by nursing personnel.

Patients should be encouraged to fill prescriptions for postoperative medications before the day of surgery even if they believe they may not actually need analgesic medication after surgery. If patients have not yet received any prescriptions, they should know to bring money or insurance cards to obtain medications if it is likely that prescriptions will be given on the day of surgery.

Parents of small children are asked to have two adults accompany the child, one to drive and the other to attend to the child in transit to home. In some institutions, supporting adults are instructed that they must remain at the facility throughout the patient's stay. In others, only parents of minors or special needs adults are required to remain on site. Patients and families should be told about such expectations ahead of time.

## Admission of the Patient

The preparation of patients immediately before surgery is essentially the same as for all surgical patients. Physical assessment includes at least vital signs, breath sounds, peripheral pulses as indicated, baseline oxygen saturation levels, skin condition at the site of surgery or regional anesthetic injection, and other appropriate assessments. Essential safety practices include a valid, correct, and signed consent; verification of the fasting period; home support and driver; and

careful preoperative identification of the patient with two consistent identifiers, neither of which should be the patient's bed or room location. Meticulous operative site identification begins with the scheduling of the patient, but during the time of admission, the site, side and procedure must be confirmed with the patient and any discrepancies immediately investigated and clarified.

Current pressure from government, industry, consumer, and other groups to reduce medical errors and improve overall patient safety is shown by a Sentinel Event Alert regarding wrong site surgery published in December 2001 by The Joint Commission. In the database of 150 reported cases of wrong site/person/procedure surgery collected from August 1998 through December 2001, the commission noted that 58% of errors had occurred in HOPDs and FASCs. Seventy-six percent involved surgery on the wrong body part or site; 13% involved surgery on the wrong patient; and 11% involved the wrong surgical procedure. Of the 126 cases, 41% relate to orthopedic or podiatric surgery.[4] Later clarification assigned a small percentage of those errors to FASC locations.

## Fasting Before Surgery

Fasting requirements as defined per facility by the department of anesthesia are decidedly more lenient that in the past. Traditional guidelines for "nothing after midnight" have been challenged and are now rarely used. Studies have found that prolonged fasting can result in thirst, headache, irritability, hunger, and nonadherence and fails to reduce gastric volume and acidity as was formerly thought.[5] Brady, Kinn, and Stuart[6] analyzed the literature for the results of 22 trials of generally healthy adults and concluded that "there was no evidence to suggest a shortened fluid fast results in an increased risk of aspiration, regurgitation or related morbidity compared with the standard 'nil by mouth from midnight' fasting policy. Permitting patients to drink water preoperatively resulted in significantly lower gastric volumes."[6]

The American Society of Anesthesiologists advocates the following fasting guidelines for elective procedures that involve anesthesia and sedation.[7]

| Ingested Material | Minimum Fasting Hours |
|---|---|
| Clear liquids | 2 |
| Breast milk | 4 |
| Infant formula | 6 |
| Light meal (e.g., toast and clear liquid) | 6 |
| Nonhuman milk | 6 |
| Meal with fried or fatty foods or meat | 8 |

In the ambulatory surgical population, ensuring the required fasting period can be more challenging because the nurse has decidedly less opportunity to teach and less ability to control the patient who is not admitted to a hospital bed overnight. Adult patients and parents of pediatric patients must be thoroughly educated about the specifics of the fasting period. They should know that in addition to food and beverages, they should avoid water, gum, candy, coffee, and cough drops immediately before surgery. An explanation in lay terms may be helpful that although gum and hard candy are not swallowed, they stimulate the stomach to produce acids that may be harmful if aspirated. Although scare tactics are not appropriate, all patients must understand the seriousness of breaking the fasting period and of accurate reporting of non-adherence.

Parents should carefully monitor children at home and in the automobile so that the child does not eat or drink without the parent's knowledge. Adolescents also may be at particular risk because of their tendency to resist authority and their misguided sense of immortality. On the day of surgery, the nurse must strive to elicit truthful and accurate verification of the patient's actual adherence.

### Diagnostic Testing

Required preoperative diagnostic tests vary widely from one institution to another and are a matter both of clinical judgment by individual physicians and the policies set by the medical board that administers the ambulatory surgical program. Current trends are toward performing no or only essential diagnostic tests that are aimed at providing the basic information necessary for safe anesthesia and surgical interventions. The American Society of Anesthesiologists supports the concept that no routine or screening testing is necessary. Routine refers to tests performed without regard to clinical indications for an individual patient. Screen refers to efforts to detect disease in asymptomatic patients in unselected populations.[8] The use of generic screenings without clinical evidence of patient appropriateness has a significant financial impact on health care. Institutional policies prevail; however, patients should be informed before any diagnostics of any expectation that their insurance will not cover specific testing (e.g., an Advanced Beneficiary Notice for Medicare recipients).

Continued controversy exists regarding routine preoperative pregnancy testing in women of childbearing age. Not only does a difference of opinion exist on whether testing is necessary for all patients, significant practice differences also exist regarding the need for the patient's consent to have this test performed.[9]

Nurses responsible for preparing patients for surgery should carry out the policies of the facility for all diagnostic testing and ensure that results of any tests are included in the medical record. Abnormal results should be provided to the physician before the patient is medicated or transferred to surgery. Test results should be secured and the physician notified of abnormal values before the day of surgery whenever possible.

### Preoperative Medications

Some providers prefer to avoid all premedications in the ambulatory surgical patient and may even encourage patients to walk to surgery to promote a sense of normalcy and self control. Others believe that certain goals can be met pharmacologically to smooth the anesthetic course.

Preoperative medications may be given to decrease salivation; reduce anxiety; promote calmness before induction of general anesthesia; and, for children, reduce the fear and stress of separation from parents. Antiemetic and gastrokinetic medications may be used to reduce the risk of vomiting and subsequent aspiration. Occasionally, opioids may be added to the regimen before painful procedures, although their penchant to promote nausea and vomiting often precludes their preoperative use.

When premedications are given, intravenous (IV) administration is certainly the trend. This route spares the patient from the pain of intramuscular injections and helps avoid prolonged sedative effects that can delay eventual postoperative discharge. Children particularly dread and fear shots and for many years may recall an injection more negatively than the surgical procedure itself. Also, many patients do not arrive at the surgical facility long enough before surgery to be given intramuscular medications and obtain the most effective results.

After the administration of any preoperative medications, patients should be monitored for allergic, atypical, or untoward drug reactions, such as respiratory or cardiac depression. Appropriate interventions to correct such situations should be initiated immediately with concurrent notification of the physician.

## EMOTIONAL SUPPORT

Emotional support also helps reduce patient anxiety and potentially associated complications, such as hypertension, tachycardia, vomiting, aspiration, and increased postoperative pain related to fear. The emotional component of nursing care while the patient is prepared for surgery cannot be overstressed. All words spoken to the patient should be positive. Questions or statements should imply the positive aspects of recovery, particularly the ability to go to a familiar and comfortable home soon after the surgery. The nurse also teaches the family directly and by example to speak in similar positive terms to encourage the patient's confident attitude. This approach supports a climate of wellness and positive outcome.

### Preoperative Goals

The primary goals of patient preparation for ambulatory surgery are focused on identifying and reducing the potential risks related to surgery and anesthesia and promoting each patient's quick return to self care. This preparation includes a significant shift of responsibility to the patient and family by educating them and then encouraging and evaluating their actions. Although patient preparations may not necessarily be identical for inpatients and outpatients, they should meet the same quality standards of care. Nurses who admit and prepare patients for surgery must be thorough in their assessments; instructions must be prepared personally and with adequate equipment to intercede effectively in emergencies.

## INTRAOPERATIVE PERIOD

Intraoperative care of the ambulatory surgical patient basically parallels that of all surgical patients. Specific nursing responsibilities include maintaining asepsis; properly preparing the operative site; providing for patient safety in identification, transfer, and positioning; assisting the anesthesia team; maintaining confidentiality; protecting the patient's dignity; maintaining a safe environment; handling specimens; and documenting and reporting the intraoperative care and events. A time out period should be enforced in which every participant in the operating room stops what they are doing and focuses on the identification of the correct operative site, side, procedure, patient, and implants.

Because of the trend to reduce or eliminate preoperative sedative medications and because a significant number of ambulatory surgical patients are given regional or local anesthesia, the perioperative nurse may care for more patients who are awake and aware of their surroundings than for those with general anesthesia. This trend increases the importance of monitoring and controlling the appropriateness of any discussions that occur near the patient.

Also, the increased use of registered nurse (RN)–administered sedation/analgesia demands competency of the perioperative nurse in monitoring, dysrhythmia detection, medication effects and side effects, and effective reversal agents. The nurse's knowledge base should also include related cardiac and respiratory anatomy and physiology, airway management, and resuscitative techniques. The availability of emergency supplies and support personnel must be ensured before the procedure begins. In particular, flumazenil and naloxone, specific reversal agents for benzodiazepines and opioids, respectively, should be immediately available for treatment of serious respiratory or cardiac depression related to the sedative drugs. The procedural physician responsible for patient care during nurse-monitored sedation and analgesia should show competency in the appropriate physiologic and pharmacologic concerns, including rescue methods and drugs and the preprocedural assessment and documentation of the airway.

### Anesthesia Considerations

Anesthesia for the ambulatory surgical patient incorporates the traditional goals of adequate analgesia, muscle relaxation, amnesia, and, in the event of general anesthesia, loss of consciousness to accomplish the intended procedure. Because the ambulatory surgical patient is discharged soon after the procedure, the anesthesia plan should promote reduced postoperative hangover and complications. Both general and regional anesthesia approaches are used and sometimes combined. Regional and local techniques are favored by many clinicians because the patient does not lose consciousness, can usually be discharged sooner after the procedure, and often has prolonged pain relief at the operative site or extremity.

The ongoing development of new and shorter-acting general anesthetic agents has significantly reduced complications such as

NURSING CARE IN THE PACU

postoperative nausea and vomiting and has encouraged rapid return to alertness, thus making general anesthesia as likely to be used as other techniques.

## POSTANESTHESIA PERIOD

Recovery of ambulatory surgical patients often occurs in several stages. After general or major regional anesthesia or after intraoperative complications in any patient, a two-phase recovery is typical. Phase I begins when the patient arrives in a fully equipped and staffed PACU. Once the patient regains consciousness, lucidity, and physiologic stability and meets PACU discharge criteria, transfer to a less-intensive care unit is appropriate. Phase II of recovery is usually completed in a department equipped with lounge chairs and more homelike surroundings where families reunite and where the patient's self care is encouraged. After local or regional anesthesia, which has a limited effect on physiologic stability, the patient is often transferred from the operating room (OR) directly to the phase II level of care as long as they meet predetermined criteria for care in that setting.

### Postanesthesia Care Unit

After a report from the OR and anesthesia personnel, the nurse applies all the usual parameters of PACU care to the ambulatory surgical patient. Airway and respiratory management are paramount. The patient is closely observed for untoward cardiac, respiratory, or other effects from anesthetic agents. The operative site and any related areas are monitored for bleeding, and any existing parenteral fluids are maintained. Further nursing duties include oxygen delivery, monitoring of vital signs and oxygen saturation, and periodic stir-up of the patient to move and deep breathe. Observation for any complications of surgery or anesthesia is coupled with rapid and appropriate nursing interventions if problems are identified.

These parameters are essential to the care of all patients in the PACU, but certain specific needs of ambulatory surgical patients must be met as well. Nursing care should be planned in a manner that not only identifies, reports, and treats complications in the early stages but that also reduces the risk of unpleasant complications that delay the patient's discharge to home. For instance, the speed of progressive head elevation should be paced to the individual patient's responses. Faintness, lightheadedness, hypotension, pallor, nausea, or vomiting implies the need to lower the patient's head and begin the process again. Adequate parenteral hydration

before the patient sits upright may reduce the patient's risk of development of gastrointestinal symptoms related to hypovolemia or hypotension. Oral fluids are given slowly, with adequate time between drinks, to assess the patient's tolerance.

Pain should be managed aggressively and immediately, not only because it is humane and kind to do so but also because prevention of pain is easier than control of pain when it has become severe. Again, intramuscular injections may be unpleasant and, for some patients, can interfere with the goal of imminent discharge. Patients who have more complex procedures may benefit from the long action of an intramuscular injection, but for most patients, the IV or oral route is the first choice because of its immediate effects and the shortened observation time for related complications such as respiratory depression. Provision of adequate analgesia with oral medications and general comfort measures is usually attained before the patient is transferred to the phase II recovery area.

The goal of adequate patient comfort is supported when the patient knows, before surgery, that the nurse is concerned about and eager to provide adequate pain relief. Patients should be encouraged to discuss their usual tolerance for pain and should not be judged in that regard based on the attitudes and prior experiences of the staff. The use of an objective pain scale helps in determination of the patient's need for intervention, and patients should be educated on that scale before procedures. They should also know that although total absence of postoperative discomfort may not be a realistic goal, acute pain should be reported and treated. Patient comfort, supported by positive thinking, general comfort measures, and oral analgesics, is one of the criteria with which eventual discharge readiness is measured, and this goal must be addressed even in the early stages of recovery.

In pediatric patients, some potential postoperative problems include bleeding, croup, nausea and vomiting, and fever of unknown origin, any of which can result in unplanned hospitalization. Children need gentle care and strong emotional support. The presence of one or both parents in the PACU can be quite reassuring to both the child and the parents. On the other hand, emotional parents can precipitate anxiety and distress in the child, so support and guidance of the parents becomes an adjunctive nursing responsibility.

Emergence delirium is more common in children than in adults. The child who is agitated and thrashing should be gently restrained to prevent self injury. Parents who observe this behavior need explanation and support. In both children and adults, accurate differentiation is essential of the restlessness associated with emergence delirium from other physiologic complications, such as hypoxia, bladder distention, and pain, that must be treated appropriately.

## Progressive or Phase II Care

Patients who do not require the intensity of PACU care are transferred to the phase II unit of the ambulatory surgical facility. This area is generally furnished with lounge chairs, and the decor is more homelike than in the PACU to encourage a sense of wellness and normalcy. The phase II area includes a nourishment center, patient bathrooms and changing areas, and ready access to an outside door for patient discharge. As in all acute health care settings, emergency equipment and support personnel must be readily available.

The goals of nursing care in this setting address the patient's physical, emotional, social, educational, and spiritual needs. These needs are summarized in Box 46-5. The comprehensive goals also include meeting the needs of the family or other responsible adult. Close nursing observation for potential complications is ongoing during the patient's stay. Expediting a safe discharge and complication-free recuperation is the ultimate objective of all nursing and medical interventions.

Specific areas of concern in the phase II unit include observation of cardiorespiratory status and other vital signs to ensure stability in relation to the patient's preoperative normal levels. Other goals are to ensure adequate nutrition and fluid status, provide effective pain management, avoid

unpleasant gastrointestinal symptoms, observe the operative site and associated symptoms, and encourage ambulation. Observation of the patient sitting up and then walking without orthostatic hypotension, faintness, or dizziness provides some element of confidence that the patient will be able to maneuver in a similar manner at home. Patients should be able to show proper use and care of ambulatory aids such as walkers, crutches, and casts. Existing parenteral fluids or IV access ports should be maintained until the patient is able to ambulate without faintness and discharge readiness is attained.

The tradition of a certain level of oral intake before discharge has come under scrutiny. Certainly the patient's level of hydration must be considered, but forced oral intake on someone who has no desire or interest can be self defeating and result in poor tolerance. The patient's appetite and desire to eat or drink are often considered the best indicators of readiness. In the decision of whether to delay discharge until the patient can tolerate oral fluids, the physician considers the patient's overall condition. This decision includes gastrointestinal status, the amount of IV fluid replacement given, the level of home support, and the patient's likeliness to report and to handle any inability to tolerate food or fluids at home. Extensive nausea or vomiting should be effectively treated before the patient is discharged.

Most often, the phase II unit is where patients reunite with family members or the responsible adults who will accompany and care for them at home. Early reunion should be encouraged, and nurses in this setting must purposefully involve such support people. The responsible adult may

---

### Box 46-5 Goals of Nursing Care in Phase II Recovery Unit

1. To provide close assessment of and attention to the patient's physical, emotional, and educational needs in the postoperative period.
2. To provide an environment and personnel who are prepared for emergency interventions at all times.
3. To provide family-oriented care that stresses the concept of wellness and acknowledges the integral relationship of the patient and family or other supporting adult.
4. To encourage the patient toward as much self sufficiency as possible, given the type of surgery and anesthesia performed.
5. To respect the patient's right to confidentiality, privacy, and respectful compassionate nursing care.
6. To maintain accurate records of patient-related care and environmental preparedness.
7. To interact with physicians and other health care providers in a professional manner that results in high-quality patient care.
8. To provide patients and families with a resource for questions, comments, and nursing information during their stay and in the immediate period after discharge.
9. To offer an environment that encourages the professional growth of nursing personnel.

Adapted from Smith S: Progressive postanesthesia care: phase II recovery. In Burden N, DeFazio D, O'Brien D, et al, editors: *Ambulatory surgical nursing*, ed 2, Philadelphia, 2000, Saunders.

need to learn how to care for the patient's physical needs, such as changing a dressing, observing extremity circulation, or emptying drains. Encouraging a return demonstration of manual skills or having the caretaker repeat information is a good way to reinforce learning and to evaluate the person's ability to provide support. Concerns about violation of the patient's privacy with a companion or family member should not be a deterrent to the discussion of care needs. The nurse should focus on the information specifically needed to provide care and not divulge extraneous health information.

The nurse also helps the responsible adult understand that the patient should perform self care to the extent of the patient's ability and that encouraging such behavior is in the best interest of the patient for both a speedy recuperation and a positive mental outlook.

Discharge of patients to home after anesthesia and invasive procedures is a serious responsibility. Planning for that discharge should begin well before the actual time of discharge, hopefully at the time the patient is scheduled for surgery. Still, the discharging nurse is the one who ensures that all those plans come together. Ensuring patient safety at home and in transit may require the nurse to discuss problems with the physician and enlist the assistance of home health agencies or transportation sources. Whatever is necessary, the nurse is ethically obliged to intervene for the patient's safety before discharge.

The physician is ultimately responsible for the decision to discharge a patient; however, the nurse's application of written discharge criteria that have been previously approved by the physician staff must meet the standards of The Joint Commission.

Specific written criteria that patients must attain before discharge are included in the policies of the institution. In most facilities, application of the discharge criteria that have been ratified by the medical oversight board now is within the scope of the nurse's job description. Any special concern about the patient's actual condition or ability to safely recuperate at home should prompt the nurse to solicit direct physician involvement in the discharge process. Various areas of concern typically included in discharge criteria include vital signs; level of consciousness; comfort (pain, nausea, use of oral analgesics); activity level; surgical site; instructions; the support of a responsible adult and driver; and to a lesser degree, nourishment, hydration and ability to urinate.

Any patient who does not meet the facility's predetermined discharge criteria requires a specific physician's order for discharge. The nurse's notes should reflect why or how the patient did not meet existing criteria and what was done about it. For example, the criteria may require that all patients void before discharge, but a patient is eager to leave, cannot void after several hours of recovery, and has been discharged by the physician without meeting the criterion. The nurse should document the involvement of the physician, notification of the responsible adult about the problem area, an assessment of the patient's abdomen, the specific guidelines and instructions given to the patient about what symptoms might indicate a full bladder, the importance of avoiding overdistention of the bladder, how long to wait at home without voiding before seeking care, telephone numbers given to the patient for obtaining medical assistance, and any other specific instructions given.

The eventual closure of documentation also should include a nursing notation regarding the patient's status related to unmet discharge criteria on the following day or later that day as ascertained via telephone contact. This last portion of comprehensive care and documentation is possible only if the person who makes the postdischarge telephone call is aware of such an issue. Therefore, a mechanism must be in place for communication of information from one nurse to the next or discharging nurses must be personally responsible for the eventual postdischarge follow-up of patients in their care.

Before discharge, written and verbal instructions for home care should be provided. Anxiety, discomfort, and the amnesic effects of many medications given to patients can result in poor or absent recall of information from the day of surgery; therefore, whenever possible, instructions should be given both to the patient and to the adult responsible for the patient after discharge.

Most facilities have developed preprinted discharge instruction sheets with carbonless copies that remain on the chart after being signed by the patient, the accompanying adult, or both, as proof that the instructions were given. In addition to the usual instructions about eating, hygiene, wound care, ambulation, return physician visit, and telephone numbers for assistance, the patient should receive a description of what symptoms may be usual and what should be reported to the physician. For instance, knowledge that a slight sore throat or generalized sore muscles may follow general anesthesia helps the patient avoid worry. When those same discharge instructions have been followed by suggestions for alleviating possible minor symptoms, the patient has an even greater chance of recuperating comfortably. The patient's list of usual medications should be reconciled with any medications given in the center that have a prolonged effect into the home recuperative period and with medication prescriptions given. This reconciliation is simply a review of the medications to identify contraindications, misunderstandings, and potential for duplication of medication. For instance, consider the patient who routinely takes the brand name drug Lasix at home who is given a prescription for furosemide. Without the physician or nurse reviewing the lists with the patient, a duplication could occur with serious ramifications.

The individual patient's specific needs must be addressed as well. The nurse should ensure that the physician's discharge instructions have included areas such as the following:

When should the diabetic patient resume taking insulin, and how much?

When should oral medications be resumed?

When can the patient drive, watch television, have a glass of wine?

Although the patient or partner may not verbalize this question, many patients also want to know whether sexual intercourse should be avoided and for how long and why. Inclusion of this information in the general instructions as appropriate to the patient and procedure avoids the need for the patient to ask. Comprehensive discharge instructions mean individualization of information for each patient.

## POSTDISCHARGE FOLLOW-UP

Mechanisms should exist for assessing and documenting patient outcomes and patient and family satisfaction with the care provided by the ambulatory surgical unit. Telephone calls and written surveys that can be returned by mail are two means of providing that follow-up. Written surveys most often address satisfaction issues, but evaluation of the patient's recuperation from anesthesia and surgery requires a more aggressive and timely approach.

In many communities, the standard of care is that patients are telephoned on the day after surgery to ascertain their clinical condition, safety, and comfort level. Such a contact can serve as a valuable resource for patients who may have symptoms that should be evaluated by their physicians or questions about which they are embarrassed or reluctant to telephone and ask their physicians. Not only is the patient's safety and medical condition supported, but the nursing staff also can identify the

effectiveness of current modes of care. Other reasons for a postdischarge call include promotion of the facility's caring attitude, identification and reduction of medicolegal issues, marketing, the meeting of accrediting and regulatory standards, and closure and a sense of job satisfaction for the nurse.

In some instances, a second call may be made at a date several weeks after the patient's discharge for the goal of assessing a particular concern related to a quality improvement or risk management study, for instance a study on postoperative infection. Documentation of patient contacts via telephone should become a permanent part of the medical record. This level of follow-up after the patient's discharge closes the loop of the evaluation phase of the nursing process in the ambulatory surgery setting.

## SUMMARY

The number of patients who have surgery in the outpatient setting has continued to increase. Sicker patients and more complex procedures are performed in these settings. The ambulatory surgery nurse must be cognizant of special requirements for preparation and discharge of the ambulatory surgery patient and must also be prepared for any complications that can occur in the PACU setting. This chapter provided an overview of care of the ambulatory surgery patient. Details of the care of patients who are in the PACU, those requiring care for complications or those undergoing specific procedures may be found in the appropriate chapters in the book.

## REFERENCES

1. Orem D: *Nursing: concepts of practice*, ed 6, St Louis, 2001, Mosby.
2. ACCEL Team: *Better management by perception*, available at http://www.accel-team.com/pygmalion/prophecy_01.html, accessed December 12, 2006.
3. Eagle KA, Berger PB, Calkins H, et al: ACC/AHA guideline update for perioperative cardiovascular evaluation for noncardiac surgery: Executive summary: a report of the American College of Cardiology/American Heart Association Task Force on Practice Guidelines, *Circulation* 105:1257-1267, 2002.
4. Joint Commission on Accreditation of Healthcare Facilities: *Sentinel event alert*, issue 24, Chicago, 2001, JCAHO. Also available at www.jcaho.org, accessed December 12, 2006.
5. Green CR, Pandit SK, Schorck MA: Preoperative fasting time: are the traditional guidelines changing? *Anesth Analg* 83:123-128, 1996.

6.  Brady M, Kinn S, Stuart P: Preoperative fasting for adults to prevent perioperative complications, *Cochrane Database System Rev* 4:CD004423, DOI:10.1002/14651858.CD004423, 2003.

7.  American Society of Anesthesiologists, Inc: Practice guidelines for preoperative fasting and the use of pharmacologic agents to reduce the risk of pulmonary aspiration: application to healthy patients undergoing elective procedures, Park Ridge, Ill, American Society of Anesthesiologists, *Anesthesiology* 90:896-905, 1999.

8.  American Society of Anesthesiologists: *Statement on routine preoperative laboratory and diagnostic screening: approved by House of Delegates October 14, 1987: last amended October 15, 2003*, Park Ridge, Ill, 2003, ASA.

9.  Bierstein K: Preoperative pregnancy testing: mandatory or elective? *Am Soc Anesthesiologists Newslett* 70(7):37, 2006.

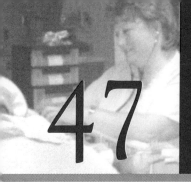

# 47 CARE OF THE LASER/LAPAROSCOPIC SURGICAL PATIENT

*Vallire D. Hooper, MSN, RN, CPAN, FAAN*

The evolution of laser and laparoscopic procedures over the last decade or so has greatly changed the face and pace of perianesthesia nursing care. More and more procedures are conducted on an outpatient basis. Patients who undergo procedures that 15 years ago required lengthy hospitalizations are now discharged within 24 to 48 hours. Much of this increase in ambulatory surgery and rapid hospital discharge has been driven by reimbursement and insurance issues. Anesthetic innovations such as bispectral index (BIS) monitoring, improved inhalational agents and muscle relaxants, advances in pain management, and regional anesthetic and analgesic techniques have also had a positive impact. Technologic advances in surgical techniques, however, have had the greatest impact because these advances allow more complex procedures with less trauma to the patient. Laser and laparoscopic techniques form the foundation for many of these surgeries.

This chapter provides an overview of laser and laparoscopic technologies and how use of this technology affects perianesthesia patient care. Details of the care of patients who undergo specific procedures may be found in the appropriate systems chapters throughout the book.

## DEFINITIONS

**Absorption:** The action of the tissue taking up the laser energy, which causes a reaction within the tissue.

**Coherence:** A state in which all of the waves travel in the same phase and direction and all of the peaks and troughs of the waves are synchronized.

**Collimation:** A state in which light waves travel parallel to each other and do not diverge or spread, which reduces the loss of power and allows for better focus and precision.

**Laparoscopic Surgery:** A form of endoscopic surgery with a fiberoptic laparoscope inserted into the peritoneum for surgical assessment or treatment of a wide and continually expanding range of conditions.

**Laser:** An acronym for light amplification by stimulated emission of radiation. A process by which energy is converted into a light form or light energy.

**Monochromatic:** Light composed of one color or wavelength.

**Pneumoperitoneum:** Created when gas is insufflated into the abdominal cavity with puncture of the abdominal wall with a Veress needle and then use of a mechanical insufflator with a pressure-limiting function for inflation of the peritoneum. Allows the surgical team to visualize the abdomen and perform the indicated procedure.

**Reflection:** Occurs when the direction of the laser beam is changed after it comes in contact with an area.

**Scattering:** Process in which the light beam is distributed in many different paths after striking a surface.

**Transmission:** Occurs when the laser beam passes or is transmitted through a medium such as fluids or tissue with little or no thermal effect.

## LASER SURGERY

The term *laser* is actually an acronym for *l*ight *a*mplification by *s*timulated *e*mission of *r*adiation. It describes a process by which energy is converted into a light form or light energy. The theory on which laser technology is based was developed by Albert Einstein in 1917. Schawlow and Townes further explored this theory and developed the LASER principle in 1958; the first true laser device was built by Dr. Theodore H. Maiman in 1960. Laser devices, although initially controversial, revolutionized surgical procedures; technology and use continue to expand.[1,2] The benefits of laser-assisted surgery are many (Box 47-1).[2-4]

### Laser Light

Ordinary light travels in waves that have four distinct properties: wavelength, amplitude, velocity, and frequency. Laser light differs from

**Box 47-1    The Benefits of Laser Surgery[2-4]**

- Seals small blood vessels, possibly reducing intraoperative and postoperative blood loss
- Often decreases postoperative edema and the chance of the spread of malignant cells with sealing of lymphatics
- Sometimes seals nerve endings, thus reducing postoperative pain in certain procedures
- Sterilizes tissue as a result of the heat generated by the laser
- Decreases scarring through the possible reduction of postoperative stenosis
- Laser beam precision usually minimizes tissue damage
- Usually decreases operative and anesthesia time
- Increased use of local anesthetic techniques as opposed to general anesthesia
- More procedures can be done on an ambulatory basis
- Often quickens recovery and return to activities of daily living

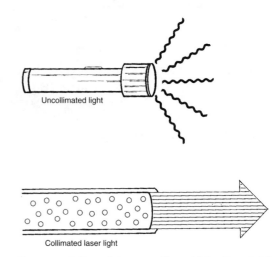

**Fig. 47-1**   Collimated versus uncollimated light. *(From Ball K: Lasers: the perioperative challenge, ed 2, St Louis, 1995, Mosby.)*

**Fig. 47-2**   Coherent versus incoherent light. *(From Ball K: Lasers: the perioperative challenge, ed 2, St Louis, 1995, Mosby.)*

ordinary light in three ways that make it both unique and effective in the surgical setting.[1,4-6]

1. Ordinary light is polychromatic, which means that it comprises a multiple array of colors or wavelengths. Laser light, on the other hand, is monochromatic and thus is all one color or wavelength. This pure color of the laser beam can determine how it reacts with certain tissues.
2. Laser light is also collimated. The light waves travel parallel to each other and do not diverge or spread. Ordinary light spreads out in space as it travels (Fig. 47-1). Collimation reduces the loss of power and allows for better focus and precision.
3. Laser light is coherent. All of the waves travel in the same phase and direction, and all of the peaks and troughs of the waves are synchronized. Ordinary light, on the other hand, is incoherent as its waves travel out in random directions (Fig. 47-2). This coherence gives the laser beam its power.

### Tissue Interaction

Four different interactions can occur when laser energy comes into contact with human tissue (Fig. 47-3). These interactions include reflection, scattering, transmission, and absorption. The extent of this interaction is dependent on the wavelength of the laser, power settings, spot size, contact time of the laser beam with the tissue, and the characteristics of the tissue.

These interactions can have both positive and negative effects.[1,2,4-6]

1. *Reflection.* Reflection occurs when the direction of the laser beam is changed after it comes in contact with an area. This direction change can be intentional or accidental and thus can have both positive and negative effects. Mirrors can be used to intentionally reflect the laser beam to direct the beam to a

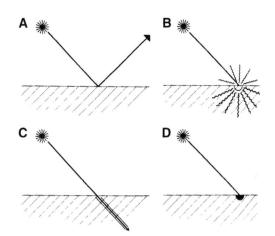

**Fig. 47-3** Laser tissue interaction. **A,** Reflection. **B,** Scattering. **C,** Transmission. **D,** Absorption. *(From Ball KA: Surgical modalities. In Meeker MH, Rothrock JC, editors: Alexander's care of the surgical patient, St Louis, 1999, Mosby.)*

| Table 47-1 | Tissue Changes With Temperature Increases[1,2,4-6] | |
|---|---|---|
| Temperature | Visual Change | Biologic Change |
| 37°C-60°C | No visual change | Warming, welding |
| 60°C-65°C | Blanching | Coagulation |
| 65°C-90°C | White/gray | Protein denaturization |
| 90°C-100°C | Puckering | Drying |
| 100°C | Smoke plume | Vaporization, carbonization |

hard-to-reach area. This action must be done carefully, however, to prevent an inadvertent strike and possible damage to a nontargeted area. Reflection can also occur if the laser beam hits an obstacle (such as a surgical instrument) and then is inadvertently reflected to another area, thus causing a tissue burn.

2. *Scattering.* The laser beam can also scatter as it comes into contact with certain tissues. This scattering causes the beam to disperse over a large area and weakens its strength. Backscattering can also occur as the beam scatters backward up the endoscope, thus causing damage to the operator's eye or the optics or distal end of the scope.

3. *Transmission.* Transmission occurs when the laser beam passes or is transmitted through fluids or tissue with little or no thermal effect. Transmission depends on the active medium of the laser and the tissue with which it comes in contact. For example, an argon laser beam can be transmitted through the clear structures and solutions of the eye to coagulate a bleeding vessel on the retina. This action occurs because the argon energy is not absorbed by clear structures and solutions; therefore, no thermal effect is noted on these tissues.

4. *Absorption.* Thermal effects and tissue response occur only when tissue absorbs the energy of the laser that contacts it. The amount of absorption and penetration depends on the beam's wavelength and power, the characteristics of the contact tissue (color, consistency, and water content),

the duration of the beam exposure, and the beam spot size. As the tissue absorbs the laser energy, a thermal response occurs and the target cells are heated. The degree of tissue change or thermal damage depends on the temperature to which the cells are heated. This temperature change is purposely regulated to effect the desired tissue response (Table 47-1).

## Types of Lasers

Lasers are classified by the four active mediums (gas, solid, liquid, and semiconductor crystals) used to generate the laser energy. In a gas medium, electric energy is pumped through a gas (such as argon) to produce the laser energy. A solid medium uses a special rod doped with an element that is activated with exposure to flash lamps to create the laser energy. Liquid mediums are organic dyes that produce a wide range of wavelengths when activated with another laser beam. Semiconductor crystals are used in the medical field and in consumer products and fiberoptic communication systems. Experimental mediums that are currently being explored include metal vapor and free electrons. The actual laser name is usually derived from the medium substance that is used to generate the laser energy.[1,2,4-6] A summary of the various lasers currently in use can be found in Table 47-2.

## Preoperative Care

Preoperative care, as with any procedure, focuses on adequate preoperative assessment and preparation of the patient. Although procedure-specific issues are addressed in other chapters, certain issues unique to laser surgery must be addressed in this discussion. One of those issues is appropriate patient selection. Procedure-specific requirements and contraindications must be evaluated.

**Table 47-2 Summary of Laser Types and Uses[1,2,4-6,8,14]**

| Name | Wavelength (nm) | Active Medium | Special Characteristics | Uses |
|---|---|---|---|---|
| Ruby laser | 694 | Solid | First successful medical laser<br>Has been replaced by newer technology | Tattoo and hair removal |
| Nd: YAG | 1064-1318 | Solid | Transmitted through clear fluids and structures and more highly absorbed by darker tissue<br>Can be focused to precise diameter for precise procedures in tight areas such as middle ear<br>Provides good penetration depth, although energy is not highly focused and laser light tends to scatter, thus causing thermal damage to approximately 5 mm<br>Can be delivered in contact and noncontact mode | Primary function is coagulation<br>Special pulsed mode also used in ophthalmology<br>Used for skin rejuvenation and removal of pigmented lesions and tattoos in dermatology<br>Interstitial laser prostatectomy<br>Various applications also used in gastroenterology, pulmonary, oral surgery, and gynecology |
| Erbium: YAG | 2900 | Solid | Highly absorbed by water<br>Shallow depth of penetration | Used for oral surgery, ophthalmic surgery, dermatology<br>Used with endoscopes |
| Holium: YAG | 2100 | Solid | Produces vapor bubble to transmit beam to tissue in fluid environments<br>Shallow depth of penetration<br>Ablates tissue precisely<br>Can be conducted through flexible fiber | Transmyocardial revascularization<br>Oral surgery<br>Fragmentation of stones<br>Many other applications in surgical arena |
| Frequency- doubled (KTP) YAG | 532 | Solid | Depth of penetration dependent on wavelength | Used with flexible or rigid endoscopes<br>Used for general surgery, urology, gastroenterology, neurosurgery, otorhinolaryngology, dermatology, and cosmetic surgery |
| $CO_2$ | 10600 | Gas | Most versatile laser<br>Can be operated in continuous or pulsed modes<br>Different tissue and thermal effects can be created by varying length and frequency of each pulse<br>Highly absorbed by water<br>Requires articulating arm system for delivery | Performs coagulation, cutting, and vaporization functions<br>Transmyocardial revascularization<br>Popular for use in cutaneous laser resurfacing<br>Also used in following surgical specialties: general, gynecology, ENT, neurosurgery, plastic surgery, dermatology, and oral surgery |

| Type | Wavelength (nm) | Medium | Characteristics | Uses |
| --- | --- | --- | --- | --- |
| Argon | 488-514 | Gas | Transmitted through clear structures and solutions; Moderate depth of penetration; Highly selective to pigmented tissue such as hemoglobin, melanin, and other similar tissues; Because of high selectivity of beam to pigmented tissues, adjacent tissue injury is significantly reduced | Used with rigid endoscopes; Well suited for ophthalmic surgery; Used in dermatology for ablation of vascular and pigmented lesions; Also used in gastroenterology, gynecology, and otology |
| Krypton | 531-647 | Gas | Used in ophthalmology as alternative to argon laser | Effective for selective photocoagulation procedures; Used primarily in ophthalmology; Also used for removal of pigmented lesions |
| Dye | 400-1000 | Liquid | Can emit different wavelengths (400-1000 nm) depending on dye used; Can be used in continuous or pulsed modes | Used primarily in ophthalmology and dermatology; Fragmentation of stones; Limited applications such as photodynamic therapy and for vascular lesions; Used with flexible or rigid endoscopes |
| Excimer | 193-351 | Excited dimmer | Complex delivery system; Gases are extremely toxic and require appropriate laser housings and exhausts; Larger units need more floor space | Excellent cutting capabilities with no significant damage to adjacent tissue; Has been used successfully to sculpt corneas for refractive purposes and to ablate plaque in arteries; Also used for phototherapeutic keratectomy procedures; Other uses in orthopedics and dermatology also being explored |
| Diode | 193-351 | Semiconductor crystals | Extremely compact efficient crystals | Often used in consumer products such as video disc players and computers; Now being used for surgical lasers primarily in ophthalmic and urologic applications such as interstitial laser prostatectomy; Other applications, including pain management, oral surgery, and treatment of leg vein telangiectasia, are being explored |
| Free electron | — | Relativistic electron beam | Large experimental laser consisting of magnetic field; Great versatility in emitting variety of wavelengths with high precision capability | Currently under investigation |

*ENT*, Ear, nose, and throat; *YAG*, yttrium-aluminium-garnet; *ND*, neodymium; *KTP*, potassium titanyl phosphate.

For example, transmyocardial laser revascularization (TMLR) is generally limited to patients with advanced cardiovascular disease who have hemodynamically stable conditions and are not candidates for traditional bypass surgery. Several thallium-201 scans must be conducted before surgery to differentiate healthy and ischemic tissues and determine the number of channels needed.[1,7] Dermatologic procedures may require extensive skin preparation at home, preoperative administration of prophylactic antibiotics or antivirals, multiple treatments, and extensive postoperative skin care regimens that may last up to a month or more.[1,2,8-10] Preoperative care must include education concerning these issues and must be used to determine whether the patient will be able to comply with the treatment regimen.

The patient must also be prepared for expectations both during and after surgery. Many of these procedures are conducted without any anesthesia or with moderate sedation. The patient must be prepared for the sights, smells, and other sensations that will be experienced. Eye protection must be provided. Odors may include the smell of flesh burning or vaporizing. The patient may also have burning or stinging types of painful sensations with certain procedures.[1,2,11-13]

### Intraoperative Issues

Intraoperative issues with laser procedures primarily concern safety. Lasers are considered a class III medical device and, as such, are subject to US Food and Drug Administration (FDA) jurisdiction. Many other regulatory, industry, and professional bodies also address the safe use of lasers. Regulations addressed include the registration of laser devices, training requirements, laser safety officer responsibilities, and safety rules.[1,11,14]

Lasers must be classified by the manufacturer according to their potential to cause biologic harm and their inherent level of hazard. The classification system is based on the laser output power, wavelength, exposure duration, and emergent beam exposure. The classification system ranges from I to IV, and the higher the class, the greater the potential hazard. Most lasers used in surgery are classified as a class IV and can damage eyes and skin and present a fire hazard.[1,11,12] Because of the many provider and patient risks associated with laser use, a laser safety program should be in place in any facility in which laser procedures are conducted. This includes freestanding ambulatory facilities and physician's offices. A laser safety committee complete with a laser safety officer should be established and responsible for guiding and overseeing all laser use in the facility. Issues that should be addressed include staff education, physician credentialing, and the monitoring of quality and safety issues. All staff involved in laser use must receive appropriate education before using or being involved in laser procedures. Topics included in these special training classes include laser biophysics, laser equipment, laser-tissue interaction, safety procedures, and clinical applications. Knowledge and skills should be verified through a competency-based credentialing program, and the skills should be reassessed and updated on a regular basis.[1,2,11,12] The three most important areas of safe laser use include eye protection, smoke evacuation, and fire safety.

The eyes are susceptible to damage from laser radiation. The damage may occur acutely or may go unnoticed and develop gradually over time. The type of damage also varies with the type of laser. Anyone who enters an operating room in which a laser is in use (including the patient) is at risk for eye damage and therefore should wear protective eyewear specific to the laser in use. Filtering devices should also be placed on operative microscopes and endoscopes. The patient's eyes should be protected with either the appropriate eyewear or moist gauze pads.[1,2,11,12,14]

Another major safety concern with the use of laser technology is the control of the smoke that the laser produces. This smoke is called the laser or surgical plume and can contain particles of vaporized tissues, toxins, and steam that are extremely small and capable of coating the alveoli over time, thus leading to respiratory conditions and complications. Even short exposure may be related to headaches, nausea, myalgia, rhinitis, and conjunctivitis. Patients may also have these symptoms. As such, a smoke evacuation system with high-efficiency particulate air filters should be used whenever a smoke plume is generated. This system should be maintained as close to the laser-tissue impact site as possible. All persons in the room should also wear high-filtration masks to protect against any residual plume in the air because routine surgical masks do not provide adequate filtration.[1,2,11,12,14]

Whenever a laser is in use, risk of fire is also increased. A fire can be triggered anytime a reflected laser beam or a direct beam comes in contact with a dry combustible item. The oxygen, anesthetic gases, and vapors from alcohol-based preparation solutions also contribute to the possible danger. All members of the laser team must be trained in fire safety and be able to respond quickly should a fire occur. All combustibles near the laser tissue impact site should be kept wet to prevent ignition. Use of flammable draping materials and skin preparation solutions should be avoided. Sterile water or saline solution should be immediately available to douse any small fires that may occur. Airway fires are of particular concern because polyvinyl chloride (PVC) endotracheal tubes (ETT) are highly flammable, particularly when combined with the high oxygen flows that run through them during anesthesia. Specific laser-retardant ETT or special ETT protective wraps should be used during oral, tracheal, or esophageal laser procedures that require general anesthesia, and the cuffs should be inflated with sterile saline solution to provide a heat sink and retard a fire.[1,2,11,12,14]

### Postoperative Care

A laser procedure does not in and of itself require any technique-specific postoperative care. Patient management should include routine postanesthesia care unit (PACU) and phase II care that is geared to the type of anesthesia administered and the given procedure. Specific surgical procedure issues are addressed in the systems-appropriate chapters throughout this book.

## LAPAROSCOPIC SURGERY

Laparoscopic surgery is a form of endoscopic surgery with a fiberoptic laparoscope inserted into the peritoneum for surgical assessment or treatment of a wide and continually expanding range of conditions.[15] This surgical approach affords many benefits to the patient and surgeon, including smaller incisions, decreased hospital stays and recovery time, and better visualization and magnification of surgical anatomy and pathology.[16] To understand the history of laparoscopy, one must first examine the origins of endoscopy, which began in ancient times and were driven by the innate human curiosity to peer inside body cavities. Speculums were first developed and used to examine various areas of the body such as the rectum and vagina as early as 400 BC. An Arabian physician first used a mirror to reflect light and examine the cervix in 1012 AD. The first crude endoscope was developed in 1585 and used the sun as a light source for examination of the nasal cavity.[4,14,17,18]

The 1800s saw the addition of more reliable, but crude, light sources to these endoscopic examinations. An Italian physician, Phillip Bozinni, developed a device that used a candle for illumination to examine the urethra of a living patient. Later devices used alcohol lamps and a wick. Edison's development of the incandescent light bulb in 1880, however, truly spurred the evolution of modern endoscopy and laparoscopy as we know it today.[4,14,18]

True laparoscopy was first accomplished by George Kelling in 1901, when he viewed the abdominal viscera of a living dog with a cystoscope. Kelling is also credited with performing the first pneumoperitoneum with this procedure. Equipment and techniques continued to evolve, and the first laparoscopic tubal ligation was performed in 1941. By 1973, more than 500,000 gynecologic laparoscopic procedures had been performed. Laparoscopic cholecystectomy procedures all but replaced open procedures within 3 years of its introduction in 1987. The technology continues to expand today into multiple therapeutic and diagnostic procedures across most surgical specialties.[4,14,18]

### Preoperative Issues

Preoperative care should be focused on the adequate assessment and preparation of the patient. Routine diagnostics and assessments that are conducted for all general anesthesia or surgical patients should be completed. Special attention should be paid to establishing the appropriateness of a laparoscopic procedure for this patient because laparoscopy, and the creation of a pneumoperitoneum, brings its own inherent risks and problems. A recommended preoperative checklist should include the following[18]:

- History and physical examination
- Evaluation of medical problems
- Thorough evaluation of the cardiac and respiratory systems
- Normalization of fluids and electrolytes
- Antibiotics
- Deep vein thrombosis prophylaxis
- Genitourinary system evaluation
- Appropriate laboratory and radiologic studies
- Informed consent

Numerous relative and absolute contraindications to laparoscopic procedures (Table 47-3) are well established, and the patient should be closely evaluated with regards to these issues. Previous abdominal surgery should be thoroughly evaluated because possible scarring or adhesions may impact the performance of the laparoscope or limit the surgeon's view of the surgical field. A comprehensive evaluation of the cardiovascular and pulmonary systems is mandated before any laparoscopic procedure because a pneumoperitoneum may greatly stress these systems; patients with significant pulmonary disease are at particular risk for development of respiratory acidosis from the build up

| Table 47-3 Contraindications to Laparoscopic Surgery[16,19-22] | |
|---|---|
| Relative | Absolute |
| Prior abdominal or pelvic surgery | Hypovolemic shock |
| Previous peritonitis or pelvic fibrosis | Large pelvic or abdominal mass |
| Obesity | Severe cardiac decompensation |
| Diaphragmatic hernia | Hemodynamic instability |
| Umbilical abnormality | Massive bleeding |
| Abdominal/iliac aneurysm | Inability to tolerate laparotomy |
| Severe pulmonary disease | Inexperienced surgeon |
| Bowel obstruction | Condition unfit for general anesthesia |
| Intolerance to positioning | |
| Abdominal wall hernia | |
| Uncorrected coagulopathies | |
| Portal hypertension | |
| Late pregnancy | |
| Severe acute cholecystis | |
| Ductal calculi | |
| Sepsis | |
| Thickened gallbladder, > 4 mm | |
| Jaundice | |
| Acute pancreatitis | |

of insufflation carbon dioxide in the system. Large abdominal wall hernias, diaphragmatic defects, and previous scars may affect trocar placement. Pregnancy was once considered an absolute contraindication to laparoscopic surgery; however, these procedures have now been shown to be safe and effective well into the second trimester. Obese patients should also be closely evaluated with specific attention to cardiac and pulmonary status.[16,19-22]

### Intraoperative Issues

The primary difference between laparoscopic surgeries and their open counterparts are patient positioning and the creation of a pneumoperitoneum, both of which can create patient management challenges during the operative and recovery phases.

*Pneumoperitoneum.* The creation of a pneumoperitoneum involves the insufflation of the abdomen with a gas. The most commonly used gas for insufflation is $CO_2$ because of its relatively low risk of venous gas embolism and noncombustibilty. Other gases that have been evaluated in clinical and experimental settings include nitrous oxide, helium, and argon as described in Table 47-4.[16,23,24]

A pneumoperitoneum is used during laparoscopic surgery to allow the surgical team to visualize the abdomen and perform the indicated procedure. Unfortunately, however, the creation and maintenance of this pneumoperitoneum can

have varying effects on the patient and is associated with many of the complications generally associated with laparoscopic surgery. The patient's position during surgery can exacerbate these adverse affects.[16,19,24]

The pneumoperitoneum is created when gas is insufflated into the abdominal cavity with puncture of the abdominal wall with a Veress needle and then use of a mechanical insufflator with a pressure-limiting function for inflation of the peritoneum. Normal insufflation pressures are 15 to 18 cm $H_2O$. Insufficient pressure produces an inadequate pneumoperitoneum and impairs surgical visualization. Excessive pressure creates even greater cardiovascular and respiratory compromise than that commonly associated with the procedure.[14]

*Cardiovascular Changes.* A wide variety of hemodynamic effects have been reported with the insufflation of a $CO_2$ pneumoperitoneum. The increased abdominal pressure compresses veins within the abdominal cavity and results in an initial increase in preload; however, true preload is ultimately decreased because of impaired venous return. Afterload is also increased as a result of the increased abdominal pressure and the resultant neurohumoral reflexes. The most common net effects from these changes include increases in heart rate, systemic vascular resistance (SVR), and central venous pressure (CVP). Cardiac output (CO) drops, and mean arterial pressure (MAP) may

**Table 47-4   Advantages and Disadvantages of Insufflation Gases[23]**

| Gas | Advantages | Disadvantages |
|---|---|---|
| Carbon dioxide | Low risk of gas embolism<br>Noncombustible | Hypercarbia<br>Acidosis<br>Pain |
| Nitrous oxide | Low risk of gas embolism<br>Decreased pain | Supports combustion |
| Helium | Stable acid-base status<br>Does not support combustion | Subcutaneous emphysema<br>Unknown risk of venous gas embolism |
| Argon | Stable acid-base status<br>Does not support combustion | Possible cardiac depression |

From Corwin CL: *Pneumoperitoneum, Society of American Gastrointestinal Endoscopic Surgeons, Primary Care Physician's Resource Center*, available at www.sages.org/primarycare/chapter5.html, accessed online January 23, 2007.

increase, decrease, or remain unchanged, depending on the relative changes in CO and SVR. Hemodynamic monitoring may be used to monitor for pressure changes and myocardial compromise in patients at extremely high risk. Pneumoperitoneum can cause dysrhythmias to include sinus tachycardia, bigeminy, and premature ventricular contractions. Once pneumoperitoneum has been established, a resultant increase in the abdominal pressure causes vagal stimulation that can lead to severe bradycardia and possible asystole.[16,18,19,24]

**Respiratory Changes.** The creation of a $CO_2$ pneumoperitoneum also has several adverse effects on the respiratory system. Oxygenation may be impaired because of reductions in lung volume and the associated atelectasis that results from an elevated diaphragm. Ventilation may also be impaired and result in $CO_2$ retention and hypercarbia. Other untoward effects include reduced pulmonary compliance, increased airway resistance, and reduced vital capacity. All of these effects are exacerbated by the commonly used Trendelenburg's position. These respiratory changes are also further exacerbated by the following conditions: surgery that lasts more than 4 hours, a history of chronic obstructive pulmonary disease (COPD), age, obesity, and an American Society of Anesthesiologists (ASA) physical status of III or greater.[16,18,19,24] A summary of these effects can be found in Table 47-5.

**Other System Effects.** In addition to the extensive cardiopulmonary changes affected by the creation of a pneumoperitoneum, various other body systems may be impacted as well. The patient should be closely monitored for the development of hypothermia, and preventative measures should be taken to prevent this

complication.[25] Hypercarbia may lead to increased cerebral blood flow with a net result of increased intracranial blood pressure, possible cerebral edema, and potential brain stem herniation. Renal failure may result from the impaired renal blood flow caused by the increased abdominal pressure (IAP) or hypercarbia. IAP also compromises venous return and puts the patient at risk for development of deep vein thrombosis (DVT). Stress hormones are also elevated because of peritoneal distention, increased anesthetic time, pain, decreased venous return, and acidosis. The release of epinephrine, norepinephrine, and plasma cortisol may all contribute to numerous adverse effects.[18,26] Concerns about the effect of a pneumoperitoneum on the implantation and spread of tumor cells also arise. The role of laparoscopic surgery for the treatment of cancer remains controversial; however, animal studies have shown no increase in the spread of tumor cells as a result of the laparoscopic versus open surgical approach.[27,28]

**Gasless Laparoscopy.** Several systems are currently being evaluated for use in gasless laparoscopy. These systems work with various slings and retractors to lift the abdominal wall away from the intraabdominal contents and create a surgical space in which the procedure can be performed. The primary advantage of this technique, of course, is the elimination of the need for a pneumoperitoneum. Disadvantages center around the inability to establish adequate surgical field exposure. Patient indications for gasless laparoscopy essentially parallel those for similar open and pneumoperitoneum cases. The gasless approach is better suited to lower abdominal cases, however, because greater abdominal distension can be accomplished in this area, particularly with women.[18]

NURSING CARE IN THE PACU

## Table 47-5  Cardiopulmonary Effects of a Pneumoperitoneum[16,18,19,24]

| | Elevated | Reduced |
|---|---|---|
| Respiratory | Respiratory rate | pH |
| | $PaCO_2$, mixed venous $CO_2$ tension, alveolar volume | Forced expiratory |
| | | Forced vital capacity |
| | $CO_2$ tension | Functional residual capacity |
| | Arterial-venous $CO_2$ difference | Total lung capacity |
| | Peak airway pressure | Compliance |
| | Plateau airway pressure | |
| | Intrathoracic pressure | |
| | Airway resistance | |
| | Atelectasis | |
| Cardiovascular | Heart rate with initial insufflation | Stroke volume |
| | Systemic blood pressure | CO |
| | MAP | Venous return unchanged or reduced |
| | CVP | Bradycardia with maintenance of pneumoperitoneum |
| | Pulmonary artery pressure | |
| | SVR | |
| | Myocardial oxygen demand | |

***Patient Positioning.*** Exaggerated surgical positions are often necessary with laparoscopic surgery to affect adequate organ exposure. The two most commonly used positions are the Trendelenburg's, or head-down, position for bowel surgery and the reverse Trendelenburg's, or head-up tilt, position for upper abdominal procedures. Both positions result in changes in cardiac filling pressures and lung volumes that affect ventilation, oxygenation, and lower extremity venous stasis. These changes are exacerbated with the addition of a pneumoperitoneum (Table 47-6).[18]

### Postoperative Issues

Care of the patient immediately after any laparoscopic procedure should include basic PACU care and monitoring specific to the procedure and type of anesthesia administered. Postoperative pain management is typically easier after laparoscopic procedures than after open procedures and can often be accomplished with a small amount of opioids in combination with nonsteroidals and local anesthetics. Visceral discomfort is often more difficult to treat and more unpredictable. This pain is triggered by the retained gas in the peritoneal cavity and the resulting irritation of peritoneal surfaces. It commonly presents as shoulder pain and may persist for several days after surgery. The patient should be prepared for this discomfort as a part of the preoperative education. The pain can generally be managed with oral analgesics.[18,19]

Postoperative nausea and vomiting can pose a significant problem with any intraabdominal surgery. Routine drainage of the stomach at the end of the case before removal of the nasogastric (NG) tube helps to reduce the incidence but does not completely eliminate it. Prophylactic treatment with an antiemetic is not indicated for all laparoscopic cases, although it may be appropriate when multiple risk factors for postoperative nausea and vomiting are present.[19,29]

In addition to basic PACU care, careful attention should be paid to monitoring the patient for any complications associated with laparoscopic intervention. Laparoscopic procedures are remarkably safe when correctly performed; their major complication rate is less than 1%, and the overall mortality rate is 4 to 8 deaths per 1000 procedures.[18] Complications can occur, however, and are divided into two categories: those associated with the procedure and those associated with the pneumoperitoneum.

***Pneumoperitoneum Complications.*** The complications associated with the creation of the surgical pneumoperitoneum are directly related to the physiologic changes associated with this procedure. Most complications occur during the initiation and maintenance of the pneumoperitoneum; however, the perianesthesia nurse may be the one who picks up on the complication or is responsible for the continued care and management of the patient. Table 47-7 provides a summary of pneumoperitoneum complications

**Table 47-6    Physiologic Effects of Patient Position during Laparoscopic Surgery[16,18,19,22,24,33]**

| System | Trendelenburg's | Reverse Trendelenburg's |
|---|---|---|
| Cardiovascular | Increased central filling pressures | Decreased central filling pressures |
|  | Increased MAP | Decreased MAP |
|  | No change in CO | Decreased CO |
| Pulmonary | No change in oxygenation | No change in oxygenation |
|  | No change in ventilation | No change in ventilation |
| Venous stasis | No change in lower extremity venous blood flow | No change in lower extremity venous blood flow |

and their causes. Care should be based on the complication presented.

***Laparoscopy Complications.*** Complications associated with laparoscopic technique are usually trocar-related injuries and involve the bowel, vasculature, or bladder.[16,18,19,24] Early recognition and treatment in the operating room, of course, results in the best outcome; however, up to two thirds of injuries may go unrecognized at the time of surgery[30]; thus, vigilant PACU assessment and care and thorough discharge teaching are essential to positive patient outcome.

**Bowel Injuries.** Bowel injuries are most troubling because they tend to go unrecognized at the time of surgery. The most common bowel injury involves perforation of the small intestine. Injury to the colon, duodenum, and stomach also occur. Nearly 50% of these injuries go unrecognized for at least 24 hours.[16] Perforations that go unrecognized in the operating room may be seen as peritonitis sometime

after discharge. Delayed onset of sepsis is also quite common with these injuries. The mortality rate associated with unrecognized bowel injuries can be as high as 5%.[16,18] These injuries may go unrecognized in the PACU because the patient may be asymptomatic at the time. Discharge teaching that emphasizes reporting of unrelieved pain, nausea and vomiting, and unresolved fever is particularly important in the recognition and resolution of this complication.

**Vascular Injuries.** Although rare (0.02% to 0.03%), vascular injuries carry a significant mortality rate of 15%.[16] Vascular injuries are most commonly associated with pelvic procedures and tend to occur in the vicinity of the distal aorta and its branches, the inferior vena cava, or iliac veins. Abdominal wall hemorrhage may also occur from inadvertent trocar insertion. Major vascular injury during laparoscopic procedures is rare. Most injuries are generally rapidly recognized and repaired in the operating room with direct suture ligation, although a patch or

**Table 47-7    Pneumoperitoneum Complications[16,18,19]**

| System | Complication | Possible Mechanism |
|---|---|---|
| Cardiovascular | Tension pneumothorax | Diaphragm injury |
|  |  | Dissection near esophageal hiatus |
|  |  | Barotrauma |
|  | Myocardial infarction | Inadequate perfusion to meet increased demand |
|  | Metabolic acidosis | Inadequate tissue perfusion from reduced CO |
|  | Visceral organ ischemia | Hypercarbia |
|  | Venous stasis/thromboembolism | Impaired visceral blood flow |
|  |  | Impaired lower extremity venous return |
|  |  | Endothelial damage from increased IAP |
| Pulmonary | Hypoxia | Atelectasis and reduced lung volume |
|  | Hypercarbia | $CO_2$ retention |
|  | Respiratory acidosis | Hypercarbia |
|  | Aspiration | Increased risk of regurgitation of gastric contents from increased IAP |
| Other | $CO_2$ gas embolus | Entry of $CO_2$ bubbles through injured blood vessels |

NURSING CARE IN THE PACU

synthetic graft may be necessary for more extensive damage.[16,18,24] Injuries that go unrecognized in the operating room again pose the greatest challenge to the perianesthesia nurse. Unresolved tachycardia and hypotension must be closely evaluated as possible signs and symptoms of hemorrhage. Unresolved or extremely severe postoperative pain and abdominal distension are also possible signs and symptoms. Recognition of surgical hemorrhage and immediate surgical evaluation are critical to a positive patient outcome.

**Bladder Injuries.** The risk of bladder injury can be decreased with the routine insertion of a Foley catheter and decompression of the bladder with all laparoscopic procedures. Even with the routine insertion of a catheter, however, occasional bladder perforation occurs. The risk of perforation is greatest in those patients with previous abdominal or bladder surgery; risks are also elevated in patients with congenital anomalies. The most common signs and symptoms are the appearance of air in the Foley bag or unexplained urinary tract bleeding during the procedure. Diagnosis can be confirmed with a retrograde cystogram, and surgical repair can be pursued.[16,18]

**Other Complications.** Other complications of interest include postoperative infection and laparoscopic electrosurgery complications. Antibiotic prophylaxis is a well-established standard for all laparoscopic procedure and all types of surgical procedures.[31] Studies show that wound infection rates range from 0.1% for diagnostic laparoscopy to as high as 1% for laparoscopic cholecystectomies.[16] Electrosurgery has replaced laser energy as the preferred power supply during laparoscopic surgery because it is less expensive and provides for better tissue coagulation. This technique, however, has been associated with secondary thermal injuries that may go unrecognized because they occur outside of the surgeon's view through the laparoscope. As with bowel perforations, these injuries often are seen days to weeks after surgery as peritonitis or sepsis, which again highlights the importance of thorough discharge instructions regarding the signs, symptoms, and management of postoperative infections.[1,32]

## SUMMARY

Technologic advances in surgical techniques have had a significant impact on surgical procedures and perianesthesia care as more complex procedures can be conducted with less trauma to the patient. Laser and laparoscopic techniques form the foundation for many of these surgeries. Laser devices, which convert energy into a light form or light energy, have revolutionized surgical procedures as technology and use continue to expand. Laparoscopic surgery, a form of endoscopic surgery with a fiberoptic laparoscope inserted into the peritoneum for surgical assessment or treatment of a wide range of conditions, also continues to expand into multiple therapeutic and diagnostic procedures across most surgical specialties. This chapter provided an overview of laser and laparoscopic technologies and how use of this technology affects perianesthesia patient care. Details of the care of patients who undergo specific procedures may be found in the appropriate systems chapters throughout the book.

## REFERENCES

1. Ball KA: *Lasers: the perioperative challenge*, ed 3, Denver, 2004, AORN.
2. Houck PM: Comparison of operating room lasers: uses, hazards, guidelines, *Nurs Clin North Am* 41(2):193-218, 2006.
3. Redmond MC: General surgery. In Quinn DMD LS, editor: *PeriAnesthesia nursing core curriculum: preoperative, phase I, and phase II PACU nursing*, St Louis, 2004, Saunders.
4. Ball KA: Surgical modalities. In Rothrock JC, editor: *Alexander's care of the patient in surgery*, ed 12, St Louis, 2003, Mosby.
5. Coluzzi DJ: Fundamentals of dental lasers: science and instruments, *Dental Clin North Am* 48(4):751-770, 2004.
6. Stratigos AJ, Dover JS: Overview of lasers and their properties, *Dermatol Ther* 13(1):2-16, 2000.
7. Lindsay MR: Transmyocardial laser revascularization revisited, *Crit Care Nurs Q* 26(1):69-75, 2003.
8. Liew SH: Laser hair removal: guidelines for management, *Am J Clin Dermatol* 3(2):107-115, 2002.
9. McBurney EI: Side effects and complications of laser therapy, *Dermatol Clin* 20(1):165-176, 2002.
10. Romero P, Alster TS: Skin rejuvenation with cool touch 1320 nm Nd:YAG laser: the nurse's role, *Dermatol Nurs* 13:122-127, 2001.
11. Andersen K: Safe use of lasers in the operating room—what perioperative nurses should know, *AORN J* 79(1):171-188, 2004.
12. Piccione PJ: Dental laser safety, *Dent Clin North Am* 48(4):795-807, 2004.

13.  Bing J, McAuliffe MS, Lupton JR: Regional anesthesia with monitored anesthesia care for dermatologic laser surgery, *Dermatol Clin* 20(1):123-134, 2002.

14.  Miller G: Minimally invasive surgery, laser, and other technologies. In Burden N, editor: *Ambulatory surgical nursing*, ed 2, Philadelphia, 2000, Saunders.

15.  Venes D, editor: *Taber's cyclopedic medical dictionary*, ed 20, Philadelphia, 2005, F.A. Davis.

16.  Wadlund DL: Laparoscopy: risks, benefits and complications, *Nurs Clin North Am* 41(2):219-229, 2006.

17.  Ball KA: *Endoscopic surgery*, St Louis, 1997, Mosby.

18.  Soper NJ, Swanstrom LL, Eubanks WS editors: *Mastery of endoscopic and laparoscopic surgery*, ed 2, Philadelphia, 2004, Lippincott Williams & Wilkins.

19.  Gerges FJ, Kanazi GE, Jabbour-khoury SI: Anesthesia for laparoscopy: a review, *J Clin Anesthesia* 18(1):67-78, 2006.

20.  Hooper VD: *Laparoscopic hernia repair*, Carrolton, Tex, 2000, Health & Science Television Network.

21.  Jobe BA, Hunter JG: Minimally invasive surgery. In Brunicardi FC, Andersen DK, Billiar TR, et al editors: *Schwartz's principles of surgery*, ed 8, New York, 2005, McGraw Hill.

22.  Lamvu G, Zolnoun D, Boggess J, et al: Obesity: physiologic changes and challenges during laparoscopy, *Am J Obstet Gynecol* 191(2):669-674, 2004.

23.  Corwin C: *Pneumoperitoneum*, available at www.sages.org/primarycare/chapter5.html, accessed January 23, 2007.

24.  Steuer K.: Pneumoperitoneum: physiology and nursing interventions, *AORN J* 68:410-436, 1998.

25.  ASPAN: Clinical guideline for the prevention of unplanned perioperative hypothermia, *JOPAN* 16:305–314, 2001.

26.  Targarone EM, Balague C, Knook M: Laparoscopic surgery and surgical infection, *Br J Surg* 87:536-544, 2000.

27.  Gutt C, Riemer V, Kim Z: Impact of laparoscopic colonic resection on tumour growth and spread in an experimental model, *Br J Surg* 86:1180-1184, 1999.

28.  Tsivian A, Shtabsky A, Issakov J: The effect of pneumoperitoneum on dissemination and scar implantation of intra-abdominal tumor cells, *J Urol* 164:2096-2098, 2000.

29.  ASPAN: ASPAN's evidence-based clinical practice guideline for the prevention and/or management of PONV/PDNV, *JOPAN* 21:230-250, 2006.

30.  Ferriman A: Laparoscopic surgery: two thirds of injuries initially missed, *BMJ* 321:784, 2000.

31.  MedQIC: *Infections CMS measures: SCIP INF 1*, available at http://www.medqic.org/dcs/Content Server?cid = 1107196776637&pagename = Medqic%2FMeasure%2FMeasureTemplate&c= Measure, accessed January 23, 2007.

32.  Wu MP, Ou CS, Chen SL, et al: Complications and recommended practices for electrosurgery in laparoscopy, *Am J Surg* 179(1):67-73, 2000.

33.  Henny CP, Hofland J, Henny CP, et al: Laparoscopic surgery: pitfalls due to anesthesia, positioning, and pneumoperitoneum, *Surg Endosc* 19(9):1163-1171, 2005.

NURSING CARE IN THE PACU

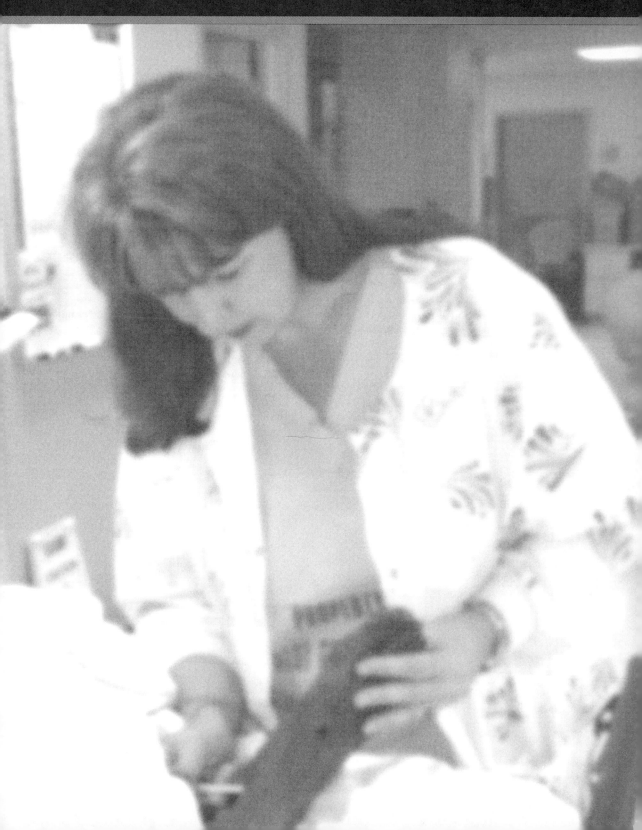

# 48

## CARE OF THE PATIENT WITH CHRONIC DISORDERS

Cecil B. Drain, PhD, RN, CRNA, FAAN, FASAHP

Patients in the perioperative phase of hospitalization need extensive nursing care, before, during, and after surgery. A well known fact is that if the patient's overall health can be enhanced before surgery, the chance of a positive outcome after the surgical experience is much better.

Patients with chronic obstructive pulmonary disease (COPD) can have significant preoperative respiratory dysfunction, of which some improvement can be accomplished with intense and knowledgeable nursing care. COPD is a serious condition that starts to develop up to 30 years before significant symptoms; it affects more than 25 million Americans and is responsible for about 80,000 deaths per year. These patient's have significant risks for anesthesia and surgery. Appropriate preanesthesia nursing interventions, such as establishment of better pulmonary function, optimal blood volume, and appropriate pharmacologic therapy, ensure that the patient has the best chance for a positive surgical outcome.

## DEFINITIONS

**Acetylcholine (ACh) Receptors:** Cholinergic neurotransmitter receptors.

**Anticholinesterases:** Drugs that act to block the cholinesterase enzyme.

**Asthma:** A lung disease characterized by constriction and spasms of the muscles of the small airways. A component of COPD.

**Atelectasis:** Collapse of a lung or portion of the lung.

**Bronchospasm:** Muscle spasm in the bronchi that causes constriction and a reduction in airflow. A component of COPD.

**Cardiomegaly:** Enlargement of the heart.

**Chronic Bronchitis:** Lung disease usually caused by chronic infections in the lungs characterized by increased pulmonary secretions.

**Cor Pulmonale:** Right heart failure as a result of primary lung disease.

**Diplopia:** Double vision.

**Dynamic Compliance:** Elasticity of the lungs over the tidal volume range.

**Dyspnea:** Patient's perception of difficulty in breathing.

**Emphysema:** A disease of the lungs characterized by a physical breakdown of the pulmonary tissue and a disease component of COPD.

**$FEV_1$:** Forced expiratory volume in the first second.

**Glycosuria:** Glucose in the urine.

**Hemolyze:** Breakdown of red blood cells that causes a release of hemoglobin.

**Hypercarbia:** Abnormally high levels of carbon dioxide in the blood.

**Hypervolemia:** An increase in the volume of circulating blood.

**Hypoglycemic Agent:** A synthetic drug that lowers the blood glucose level for treatment of type 2 diabetes.

**Hypovolemia:** A decrease in the volume of circulating blood.

**Immunosuppressants:** Agents that significantly interfere with the ability of the immune system to respond to antigenic stimulation with inhibiting cellular and humoral immunity.

**Microangiopathy:** A disease of the small blood vessels.

**Miosis:** Contraction of the sphincter muscle of the iris that causes the pupil to become smaller.

**Myasthenic Syndrome:** Called the Eaton-Lambert syndrome; chronic fatigability and muscle weakness, especially in the face and throat.

**Plasmapheresis:** Removal of plasma from previously withdrawn blood via centrifugation, reconstitution of the cellular elements in an isotonic solution, and reinfusion of this solution into the donor or another person who needs red blood cells rather than whole blood.

**Polycythemia:** Increased number of red blood cells.

**Ptosis:** Abnormal condition in which the upper eyelids droop because of muscle weakness.

**Rales:** Crackling sound made inside the lungs during auscultation.

**Rhabdomyolysis:** A disease of the skeletal muscle characterized by the presence of myoglobin in the urine.

**Rhonchi:** Sound made inside the lungs during auscultation.

**Sustained Maximal Inspirations (SMI) Maneuver:** Part of the modified stir-up regime that consists of a breathing maneuver in which the patient is encouraged to take a deep breath and hold it for 3 seconds.

**Thalassemia:** Microcytic, hypochromic, and short-lived red blood cells caused by deficient synthesis of hemoglobin.

**Thymectomy:** Surgical removal of the thymus gland.

**Tracheostomy:** An opening through the neck into the trachea through which an indwelling tube may be inserted to facilitate the movement of air in and out of the lungs.

# CHRONIC OBSTRUCTIVE PULMONARY DISEASE

Chronic obstructive pulmonary disease (COPD) describes bronchial obstructive respiratory diseases. It is characterized by dyspnea with or without cough and sputum. The two major clinical manifestations of COPD are airway obstruction and airway destruction. The magnitude of the various disease entities that the term COPD includes is great; therefore, individual elaboration on the diseases is difficult because each deserves separate attention. Rather, this chapter briefly describes the overall characteristics of COPD and general care required in the postanesthesia care unit (PACU). Variations between patients with COPD exist. The perianesthesia nurse must consult with the physician about the specific nursing care to be administered to the patient with COPD. For discussion of specific COPD diseases, see the bibliography at the end of the chapter.

## Description of COPD
The hallmark of COPD is the evidence of a productive cough and a progressive decrease in the patient's exercise tolerance. Three major diseases are part of COPD: asthma, emphysema, and chronic bronchitis. All are characterized by airway obstruction. These diseases may have medically reversible components, such as bronchospasm, or they may have irreversible components, such as alveolar septal destruction. Some of the reversible components of asthma, such as retained secretions, bronchospasms, and infections, can be corrected with the interaction of the physician, nurse, physical therapist, and respiratory therapist. The treatment of asthma may include oxygen therapy, bronchodilators, chest physiotherapy, and proper hydration.

Chronic bronchitis is associated with chronic cigarette smoking. The nurse can contribute greatly to the patient's future health with strong influences to refrain from smoking. Other therapy for the reversible components may include the use of bronchodilators, chest physiotherapy, and oxygen.

The patient with emphysema usually has airway destruction that is irreversible. As the alveolar septa are destroyed, insufficient alveolar ventilation ensues and eventually leads to hypercarbia. As the disease progresses, carbon dioxide cannot be expelled from the lungs and is retained there. The patient usually increases minute ventilation to try to compensate for the hypercarbia. Respiratory acidosis develops slowly as the various acid-base buffer systems try to neutralize the accumulated acid. In this compensated state, the patient usually has a near-normal pH, high plasma bicarbonate, low chloride concentration, and high total carbon dioxide levels. The $PaCO_2$ usually is low because some inspired oxygen is unable to cross into the blood from the lungs because of the decreased respiratory diffusion membrane surface area in the lungs. Pulmonary hypertension usually appears as the disease progresses. Cor pulmonale may develop, and because of the pulmonary venous engorgement, the right heart may begin to fail. The patient with emphysema who has irreversible destruction may be treated with chest physiotherapy, bronchodilators, and steroids.

## Cigarette Smoking as a Precursor to the Development of COPD
Cigarette smoking has been well established as one of the major precursors to chronic bronchitis and emphysema, two of the three disease components of COPD. Cigarette smoking affects the manner in which a patient recovers from an anesthetic. The perianesthesia nurse should be aware of the diverse reactions that smoking can have on the patient who is emerging from an inhalation anesthetic. Studies on the relationship between smoking and its effects on anesthesia indicate an increase in the risk factor in the patient who smokes. Although the incidence rate of smoking is decreasing slowly, it continues to be on the rise in the teenage population.

## Respiratory Effects of Smoking
A growing body of convincing scientific literature suggests that almost all pulmonary disease

is related in some way to the inhalation of infectious or irritant particulate material. Cigarette smoke in its gaseous phase contains nitrogen, oxygen, carbon dioxide, carbon monoxide, hydrogen, argon, methane, hydrogen cyanide, ammonia, nitrogen dioxide, and acetone. In the particulate phase, cigarette smoke contains nicotine, tar, acids, alcohol, phenols, and hydrocarbons. The bottom line is that cigarette smoke contains oxidants and the oxidants can damage cells and the extracellular matrix components of the lung, all leading to significant damage to the tissue in the lungs. Smokers who inhale nicotine from a cigarette into the lungs actually receive 25% to 30% of the nicotine contained in the cigarette. Thirty percent is destroyed with combustion, and 40% is lost in the side stream. Therefore, if a person inhales the smoke from a cigarette that contains 2.5 mg of nicotine, 1 mg of nicotine is actually absorbed by the lungs. Also, filters are known to make little difference in this absorption. Contrary to some opinions, the smoking of cigars and pipes also presents a risk for pulmonary disease. Carbon monoxide combines with the hemoglobin molecule at the same point as oxygen does. It has an affinity for this receptor point that is 210 times greater than that of oxygen. Therefore, the oxygen-carrying capacity of hemoglobin is reduced, and the end result is that less oxygen is given up to the tissues by the hemoglobin. When carbon monoxide combines with hemoglobin, a compound called carboxyhemoglobin is formed. The amount of carboxyhemoglobin in the blood is especially important in the patient who has a diseased myocardium because myocardial oxygenation is limited by the flow of the blood through the coronary arteries. During stress, such as in surgery and anesthesia, the amount of carboxyhemoglobin saturation could lead to severe myocardial hypoxia in patients who smoke heavily and have coronary artery disease because the diseased coronary arteries cannot increase the flow significantly. The only means of prevention of hypoxia is an increase in the extraction of oxygen from the hemoglobin. Small amounts of carboxyhemoglobin may hinder the uncoupling of the oxygen and thus result in yet more oxygen retention at any given tension. This effect clearly is greater when the oxygen tension is further reduced by local ischemia and any additional vasoconstriction associated with smoking.

Smoking is an important causative factor in chronic pulmonary disease, especially the obstructive type. The pulmonary function alterations characteristic of smokers usually include a reduction in vital capacity, an increase in residual volume to total lung capacity, an uneven distribution of inspired gas, a decrease in dynamic compliance, and an increase in nonelastic resistance. Most critically, chronic cigarette smoking ultimately causes the $FEV_1$ to be less that 80% of normal, a critical sign of COPD.

Chronic bronchitis is the disease most often associated with smoking and is seen often by the perianesthesia nurse. Hypertrophy of bronchial mucous glands with production of excessive mucus is the hallmark of this disease. A vicious cycle develops as this failure to remove the mucus leads to retention of pathogenic organisms and irritants. The resulting distorted alveolar septa and the increased pressure on the alveoli from chronic bronchitis can lead to emphysema.

Cigarette smoke can cause a progression from hyperplasia to metaplasia to neoplasia in the lungs. Sometimes associated with bronchial carcinoma is the Eaton-Lambert syndrome, often called the myasthenic syndrome because its symptoms resemble those of myasthenia gravis (MG). This syndrome in some way affects neuromuscular transmission, and patients have the classic symptoms of muscle weakness. These patients are especially sensitive to the skeletal neuromuscular blocking agents used in clinical anesthesia. If the anesthetist is unaware of this syndrome and administers the normal dosage of skeletal muscle relaxants, the patient will probably be unable to ventilate spontaneously on emergence from anesthesia even when pharmacologic reversal of the muscle relaxant is attempted. In this situation, postoperative mechanical ventilation is necessary.

### Cardiovascular Effects of Smoking

The correlation between vascular disease and smoking is strong. Smoking may influence thrombosis, and because thrombi and platelets contribute to the development of arteriosclerosis, smoking can contribute to arteriosclerosis and its complications.

Inhalation of nicotine produces a release of catecholamines, activates the carotid and aortic chemoreceptor bodies, and directly stimulates the muscles of the vessel walls. As a result, the immediate effects of smoking even a small number of cigarettes can be fairly marked, with production of increases in heart rate, peripheral resistance, cardiac workload, and blood pressure. Each of these actions causes a greater myocardial oxygen demand. Furthermore, because the smoker's hemoglobin can provide less oxygen to the myocardium, that smoking can cause cardiac arrhythmias, either through myocardial anoxia or epinephrine release, is unsurprising.

## Surgical Considerations

The incidence rate of pulmonary complications in patients who have undergone abdominal or thoracic surgery is high. Changes occur in the pulmonary status of the patient who undergoes anesthesia and surgery. In the postoperative phase, these changes are characterized by gradual or abrupt alveolar collapse. The patient with COPD, when subjected to surgery, then represents an even higher risk for postoperative complications. These patients must be given meticulous preoperative care so that they are in the best possible health when they enter surgery. This preoperative medical treatment usually includes hydration, nutrition, chest physiotherapy, bronchodilators, and prophylactic antibiotics if an infection is present. Serial pulmonary function tests and arterial blood gas determinations are used to monitor the progression of the preoperative treatment.

When the patient's pulmonary function reaches a peak before surgery (i.e., when the pulmonary function test and arterial blood gas test results no longer show continued improvement), surgery is considered because the patient has reached optimal pulmonary status.

## Care of the COPD Patient

Perianesthesia care centers on prevention of complications. The modified stir-up regimen should include frequent cascade coughing, sustained maximal inspirations (SMIs), and repositioning of the patient (see Chapters 12 and 28). An appropriately implemented modified stir-up regimen is of great importance, especially in patients who are recovering from upper abdominal or thoracic operations. Surgery at these sites can cause decreased ventilatory effort and a complete absence of sighs by the patient. Given that the patient already has compromised respiratory function, the possibility of retained secretions and atelectasis is magnified. Hence, these patients represent a significant challenge to the perianesthesia nurse.

When the patient is completely reactive from anesthesia, the use of the incentive spirometer may be helpful in reducing the incidence of atelectasis. Consequently, the perianesthesia nurse who is responsible for supportive measures should assist and encourage the patient in using the SMI with or without the incentive spirometer. On the basis of subjective research findings, if the perianesthesia nurse explains the rationale of the SMI

maneuver and properly instructs the patient in the use of the technique before surgery, the patient is more likely to correctly use the SMI maneuver after surgery with or without coaching. The performance of the SMI maneuver, with or without mechanical devices, should be monitored by the nurse to ensure proper production of a sustained inspiration with a 3-second inspiratory hold. The perianesthesia nurse should also encourage and monitor the patient's performance of the cascade cough to facilitate early secretion clearance.

Patients with COPD have some component of reactive airways disease. Consequently, the airway becomes compliant and can become compressed during a forced expiratory maneuver. This dynamic compression of the airways is a function of the equal pressure point theory, as discussed in Chapter 12. To reduce the amount of dynamic compression of the airway during exhalation, the patient should be encouraged to use pursed-lip breathing. Breathing through pursed lips during exhalation can be the same as adding 5 to 10 cm $H_2O$ of positive end-expiratory pressure. Increasing the pressure inside the airway during exhalation reduces the amount of dynamic compression of the airways and decreases the amount of air trapping that commonly occurs in patients with COPD.

The cardiac status should be monitored meticulously because of the frequent involvement of the heart in the pathologic disorders of these patients. Kidney function should also be monitored because it may be altered, especially in patients with fluid retention and edema of the extremities.

The patient with severe COPD who has marked hypercarbia can present difficulties in the PACU. Patients who have severe emphysema usually fit into this category. Their ventilatory effort is stimulated by the hypoxic drive, in which lack of oxygen stimulates ventilation. Hypoxia indirectly stimulates the respiratory center by means of chemoreceptors in the carotid bodies located at the bifurcation of the carotid artery. When the patient receives 100% oxygen to breathe in the PACU, oxygen tensions rise in the inspired gas; the carotid and aortic chemoreceptors cease to function; and the patient quickly becomes apneic. The patient's respiratory status should be assessed carefully and the physician consulted before 100% oxygen is administered. Mist therapy after surgery aids in liquefying the secretions and helps in the all-important maintenance of a patent tracheobronchial tree. If excessive bronchial drainage is not removed, it provides a convenient avenue for bacteria and might also obstruct the airways, thus leading to insufficient alveolar ventilation and hypoxia.

The patient with COPD should be under constant surveillance for signs of cardiopulmonary decompensation, including shallow rapid gasping respirations, severe dyspnea, substernal retraction, and disorientation. Blood pressure may be elevated or low, but the patient usually has tachycardia, fever, and muscle rigidity. Cyanosis may or may not be present.

Patients who are cigarette smokers have significant postanesthesia risks. Cigarette smokers who have smoked for a long period of time and have a $FEV_1$ less that 80% usually have an increased risk of pulmonary complications in comparison with nonsmokers. Patients who smoke more than two packs of cigarettes a day are especially prone to perianesthetic complications. Also, patients who have had a long history of smoking (> 20 pack years) and are presently in a nonsmoking situation still can have pulmonary complications. Many of these complications develop when cigarette smokers have a preexisting chronic respiratory disease, usually bronchitis. The major postoperative complications associated with smoking are infection, atelectasis, pleural effusion, pulmonary infarction, and bronchitis.

Complications associated with chronic cigarette smoking revolve around the inability of the patient to clear secretions. The goal of nursing care in the PACU centers on clearing the tracheobronchial tree, which necessitates frequent suctioning, cascade coughing, and the SMI maneuver. If rales and rhonchi are heard on auscultation, percussion and postural drainage should be initiated.

Because cardiovascular disease is associated with a long history of cigarette smoking, the patient should have continuous electrocardiographic monitoring. Arrhythmias, such as premature ventricular contractions, should be sought because they may be the first signs of decreased myocardial oxygenation in the cigarette smoker.

Respiratory depressant drugs, such as narcotics, should be given in low dosages, or if the COPD is severe, they should be avoided completely. Repositioning of the patient and splinting of the incision site, in addition to reducing the anxiety usually seen in these patients, reduces the need for narcotic drugs. Some form of regional analgesia may be beneficial for these patients.

## MYASTHENIA GRAVIS

The patient with myasthenia gravis (MG) deserves special consideration in the PACU because of the respiratory dysfunction and possible pharmacologic ramifications of the disease. MG is a chronic disease characterized by progressive muscle weakness and easy fatigability. MG is the prototype autoimmune disease because its pathophysiology involves the postsynaptic ACh receptors at the myoneural junction. The causative factor is an immune-mediated destruction or blockage that leads to an inactivation of the postsynaptic ACh receptors. Interestingly enough, the presynaptic ACh receptors in the myasthenic continue to be normal. More specifically, patients with MG have developed antibodies to muscle acetylcholine receptors. The antibody does not bind exactly on the site that binds the ACh, but it does bind close to it. The acetylcholine receptors are steadily destroyed, with a resulting reduction in the binding of acetylcholine at the postsynaptic myoneural junction. The patient with myasthenia sometimes has a lesion in the myocardium that is a spotty focal necrosis accompanied by an inflammatory reaction. An alteration in the S-T segment and T wave is sometimes seen in these patients.

The incidence rate of MG has been estimated to be between 1 in 7500 and 1 in 10,000. MG occurs twice as often in females than in males and at earlier ages. The main symptoms are weakness in one or more of the muscle groups, fatigability on effort, and at least some partial restoration of muscle function after rest.

Ptosis of the eyelid is the most common sign of the disease. Ptosis is usually accompanied by diplopia, blurred vision, or nystagmus. Ocular signs and symptoms often are worsened by bright light. The patient may also have myasthenic facies, which is caused by weakness of the facial muscles and can progress to dysphagia and difficulties in speech.

Respiration is often affected in the patient with myasthenia. Dyspnea can be either inspiratory, if the diaphragm is involved, or expiratory, if the intercostal and abdominal muscles are affected. The patient may also have emotional disturbances caused by anxiety and depression.

Diagnosis of MG is made on the clinical symptoms and the characteristic electromyographic results. The clinical symptoms can be assessed with the neostigmine test or the edrophonium test, both of which involve anticholinesterases that increase the strength of the myasthenic muscle. Should these tests show that MG may be present, serum levels of anti-AChR antibodies can be drawn. These antibodies are usually present in 85% to 90% of patients with myasthenia.

Treatment for this disease consists of various pharmacologic interventions designed to enhance neuromuscular transmission and slow the progression of the disease. Therefore, the treatment may include cholinesterase inhibitors, corticosteroids, specific immunosuppressants, plasmapheresis, intravenous immunoglobulin, and thymectomy.

Anticholinesterase drugs, which slow down the enzymatic destruction of acetylcholine at the neuromuscular junction, are commonly used. Oral pyridostigmine is the anticholinesterase of choice. Patients with myasthenia seem to favor pyridostigmine over other anticholinesterases because its length of action is 3 to 4 hours when administered orally. Steroids and other immunosuppressive agents may be used in some patients to reduce antibody production responsible for the disease. Plasmapheresis, a plasma exchange, arrests severe refractive MG by reducing the concentration of circulating antibodies. Like the use of intravenous immunoglobulin, plasmapheresis is a short-term treatment.

Thymectomy seems to be an appropriate therapeutic mode because the thymus gland appears to be intimately involved in the disease process. About 75% of the patients with myasthenia who do not have thymoma have improvement after thymectomy. On the other hand, about 20% of the patients with myasthenia with thymoma show improvement in the disease process after thymectomy.

Because thymectomy has been used as a therapeutic intervention in the treatment of MG, the perianesthesia nurse will probably render nursing care to many patients with MG. Because of the location of the incision, the myasthenic patient does not usually receive any intraoperative skeletal muscle relaxants. Patients with myasthenia can have an exacerbation of symptoms in the PACU. Hence, critical monitoring of the patient's ventilatory status should be the primary focus of the perianesthesia nursing care. Patients with myasthenia who are recovering from any type of surgical procedure and who have been administered any form of anesthesia (general, inhalation, or regional) can have exacerbated symptoms and myasthenic crisis develop in the PACU. Consequently, respiratory support should always be available for these patients.

### Care of the Patient with Myasthenia

During surgery, the patient has the neuromuscular blockade reversed, if a muscle relaxant is given. After reversal in the operating room, the patient must have a complete sustained return of skeletal muscle strength before extubation. If the patient does not meet the criteria for extubation, the endotracheal tube remains in place and the patient is taken to the PACU for ventilatory support. Also, *in MG patients, the skeletal muscle strength may appear to be appropriate immediately after surgery but may deteriorate a few hours thereafter.*

The patient with MG can have various difficulties because of an impaired respiratory system, possible poor nutrition, susceptability to infection, altered psychiatric status, and possible altered response to drugs used during anesthesia. The patient should be placed in a quiet area, where no direct light shines in the eyes. The patient's respiratory effort and exchange should be monitored continuously. Oxygen should be administered with humidification, and secretions should be removed with frequent suctioning and postural drainage. Oxygen saturation levels for these patients should be maintained at more than 96%. Any change in respiratory status should be reported to the physician immediately.

Because cardiac mechanisms may be responsible for some sudden deaths in this patient population, cardiac monitoring should be instituted for every patient with myasthenia in the PACU. Monitoring of the fluids administered to patients with myasthenia is also important. Hypovolemia and hypervolemia must be avoided because of their deleterious effects on the already compromised heart and lungs.

The patient should be kept as pain free as possible to facilitate good respiratory exchange. Morphine and other narcotics are often potentiated by anticholinesterases. Therefore, the initial narcotic dose should be reduced to half the normal dose and then increased if necessary. If the patient is receiving continuous mechanical ventilation, the normal amount of medication can be given without compromising the patient's respiratory status.

The PACU nurse should monitor for a myasthenic crisis, which is a severe exacerbation of the symptoms associated with MG. It can occur when an anticholinesterase is underdosed and does not reduce the amount of muscle weakness sufficiently. On the other hand, a cholinergic crisis can occur when too much anticholinesterase is administered, resulting in a surplus of acetylcholine at the myoneural junction and causing a depolarizing type block that leads to skeletal muscle weakness, which could be severe. Hence, for all the previous reasons, during PACU care of the patient with MG in the immediate postoperative phase, *airway equipment must be kept at the patient's bedside.* Along with the skeletal muscle weakness, muscarinic side effects occur, such as abdominal cramping, miosis, bradycardia, salivation, and diarrhea.

Please see Chapters 10, 11, 23 on muscle relaxants, which provide the reader an in-depth discussion of the myoneural junction and nicotinic and muscarinic effects.

The emotional status of the patient with myasthenia is of considerable importance. As few clinicians as possible should be responsible for this patient throughout the emergent phase because the patient is likely to be distrustful of anyone he or she does not know. Communication is important, and the patient should be informed about any nursing procedure to be performed. If the patient with myasthenia has a tracheostomy, paper and pencil should be used to facilitate communication between nurse and patient.

## DIABETES MELLITUS

Diabetes mellitus is a chronic metabolic disease associated with insulin deficiency or insensitivity, hyperglycemia, and glycosuria. It occurs in about 6% of the general population or about 18 million people. Diagnosis of diabetes mellitus is made when the fasting plasma glucose (FPG) level is 126 mg/dL or more. One important aspect of this disease is an associated degeneration of the small blood vessels (microangiopathy) that is most marked in the retina, kidneys, and nervous system.

The focus of the physiologic activity of insulin is to "open the door" of the cell to let glucose enter. In the diabetic state, the patient has an elevated blood glucose level because of a defect in the cellular response to insulin and the "door" remains closed. Sources of the excess glucose are dietary carbohydrate, liver glycogen, and glucose formed by the fatty acids metabolized to acetone, or beta-hydroxybutyric acid. These three products are known as ketone bodies. The patient's degree of insulin deficiency is reflected by hyperglycemia, glycosuria, and ketoacidosis.

The two forms of diabetes mellitus are insulin-dependent and non–insulin-dependent diabetes mellitus. Insulin-dependent diabetes mellitus (IDDM) is also called type I diabetes and was formerly called juvenile-onset diabetes. It may be genetic in predisposition and is characterized by the patient's entire dependence on exogenous insulin therapy. The actual cause of IDDM is a vigorous autoimmune destruction of the β-cells of the islets of Langerhans in the pancreas. The onset of IDDM is usually before the age of 40 years; however, IDDM can develop at any age. When the symptoms become evident in the patient with IDDM, about 90% of the β-cells have been destroyed, with the remaining 10% destroyed over the next 2 to 3 years.

About 10% of the patients with diabetes mellitus have this form.

The other form of diabetes mellitus is called non–insulin-dependent diabetes mellitus (NIDDM). Formally called type II or maturity-onset diabetes, it effects about 90% of the diabetic population. This type of diabetes is characterized by impaired insulin secretion or peripheral insulin resistance and therefore has some degree of endogenous insulin production but not at a level sufficient to produce normal carbohydrate homeostasis. Most of the patients with NIDDM are more than 40 years and have a family history of the disease, and 80% are obese. This type of diabetes has an insidious onset, and more than half of the population with NIDDM is estimated to not even be aware of it. Treatment for this type of diabetes consists primarily of oral hypoglycemic agents, injectable hypoglycemics, and diet therapy.

### Anesthesia and Diabetes

Of all the endocrine diseases, diabetes mellitus is the most common seen in surgical patients. The most common types of surgery include cataract removal, kidney transplants, vascular repair, amputation of extremity, and ulcer debridement. The goal of perianesthetic management of the patient with diabetes is maintenance of the serum glucose level at less than 200 mg/dL and prevention of hypoglycemia and severe fluid loss. Clinician stances regarding specific methods to accomplish these goals differ. One method is to withhold the usual dose of long-acting or intermediate-acting insulin. Two liters of 5% dextrose, with 10 to 15 units of crystalline regular insulin added to each liter, are given to the patient during surgery. In another method, the patient is administered 5% dextrose in Ringer's lactate at 125 mL/h. Regular insulin, in 5-unit increments, is administered as needed to keep the patient's blood glucose level at or above 200 mg/dL. A more widely used method consists of giving half the daily dose of insulin on the morning of surgery or one third of the daily dose if the surgery is scheduled later in the day. The patient is given 500 to 1000 mL of 5% dextrose and water before surgery and at least 1000 mL of 5% dextrose and water during surgery. This method avoids hypoglycemia during surgery but increases the need for careful nursing attention in the PACU.

These methods are used in the patient who is undergoing elective surgery. Emergency surgery for the patient with uncontrolled diabetes is an entirely different situation. Before the patient undergoes anesthesia and surgery, treatment of the diabetes should be instituted, if possible.

Blood glucose and blood urea nitrogen levels often are determined to indicate the proper amount of regular insulin to be administered during surgery on a sliding scale. Intravenous solutions are given to treat dehydration.

## Care of the Patient with Diabetes

The patient should be monitored for fluid and electrolyte balance and degree of glycosuria. Most authors agree that mild glycosuria is more desirable than glucose-free urine. Hypoglycemia should be avoided. Patients who have had a stressful problem relieved (e.g, the removal of an intraabdominal abscess) may have reduced postoperative insulin requirements. This reduction may be as much as 50% in the first 24 hours. However, because of the stress of surgery, postoperative insulin requirements are usually increased. A balancing act exists in regard to insulin administration in the PACU. Certainly the medical emergency to avoid is diabetic ketoacidosis (DKA), in which the patient is hyperglycemic. DKA occurs mostly in insulin-dependent diabetes. Stress, such as the stress of surgery, stimulates the release of hyperglycemic counterregulatory hormones such as glucagon, growth hormone, epinephrine, and cortisol. In insulin-dependent diabetes, the inability exists to secrete insulin to counterbalance the excess glucose, free fatty acids, and ketone bodies that are produced by these hyperglycemic hormones. If no exogenous insulin is administered, the patient may have severe ketoacidosis, dehydration, and acute metabolic decompensation. If the patient has a blood glucose level above 250 mg/dL, electrolyte depletion, hypovolemia, ketonemia, nausea, vomiting, abdominal pain, and extreme lethargy are all indicators of DKA. Because the patient has acidosis, the breath has a fruity odor from the acetone; the respiratory center is stimulated by the low pH, and the resulting rapid deep breathing that occurs is called Kussmaul's respiration. If these signs and symptoms appear, the attending physician should be notified. The management of a patient with DKA usually involves restoring intravascular volume, correcting electrolyte imbalance, improving acid-base balance, and reducing blood glucose levels.

A glucose meter and other accurate and rapid methods of monitoring blood glucose levels should be available in the PACU. The use of the Clinitest method does not monitor the blood glucose level directly but provides a rough indicator of insulin requirements. Consequently, because the urinary glucose concentration is considered a late indicator of blood glucose levels, it should not be used in patients

with significant insulin-dependent diabetes. Blood glucose levels can be monitored closely in the PACU by obtaining a plasma glucose measurement and are probably the most accurate methods to determine plasma glucose levels. Blood glucose laboratory determinations should be done at least twice daily for 2 to 3 postoperative days. A sliding scale can be used to determine the amount of insulin to be administered, and the Dextrostix method can be used, as can the Clinitest; however, the plasma glucose level is the most accurate monitor of the glucose level. A sample sliding scare for urine glucose is shown in Table 48-1. The objective during the PACU period is to prevent hypoglycemia and to accept mild hyperglycemia, with the aim of maintaining the blood glucose concentration between 100 and 180 mg/dL, especially for type I diabetes. Because of the stress of surgery, the plasma glucose determinations are preferred over Clinitest and Dextrostix. Many patients with type I and II diabetes are handled with various techniques that basically require plasma glucose measurements throughout the PACU experience and treatment of hyperglycemia with insulin on a sliding scale; or if the patient has severe type I diabetes, frequent blood glucose determinations are made and the patient may have an infusion pump to administer insulin.

Respiratory acidosis should be prevented by aiding the patient to cough and breathe deeply to promote adequate pulmonary ventilation and carbon dioxide elimination. Metabolic acidosis must be prevented with the administration of fluid and electrolytes; therefore, strict monitoring of intake and output measurements should be instituted on every patient with diabetes admitted to the PACU.

The patient with diabetes is likely to receive an insulin preparation in the PACU. The types of insulin and their times of onset, peak effects, duration of action, and route of administration are summarized in Table 48-2.

Observation of the patient with diabetes for possible diabetic coma (as a result of

| Table 48-1 | Sliding Scale for Insulin Determinations | |
| --- | --- |
| Urine Glucose (Trace %) | Regular Insulin Dose (Units) |
| 0.25 | 5 |
| 0.50 | 8 |
| 1 | 10 |
| 2 | 15 |

| Table 48-2 | Types of Insulin and Times of Onset, Peak Effects, Duration of Action, and Route of Administration | | | | |
|---|---|---|---|---|
| Insulin Type | Onset of Action | Peak Activity | Duration | Route |
| **SHORT-ACTING** | | | | |
| Regular | 30-60 min | 1-2 h | 5-12 h | IV, SC, IM |
| **RAPID-ACTING** | | | | |
| Aspart (Novolog) | 10-30 min | 30-60 min | 3-5 h | SC |
| Lispro (Humalog) | 10-30 min | 30-60 min | 3-5 h | SC |
| **INTERMEDIATE-ACTING** | | | | |
| NPH/Lente | 1-2 h | 4-8 h | 10-20 h | SC |
| **LONG-ACTING** | | | | |
| Ultralente | 2-4 h | 8-20 h | 16-24 h | SC |
| Glargine | 1-2 h | No peak | 24 h | SC |

*IV*, Intravenous; *SC*, subcutaneous; *IM*, intramuscular; *NPH*, neutral protamine Hagedorn. Time course is based on subcutaneous administration. From Nagelhout J, Zaglaniczny K: *Nurse anesthesia*, ed 3, St Louis, 2005, Saunders.

hyperglycemia) or insulin reaction ensures proper emergence from anesthesia. The symptoms of each complication are summarized in Table 48-3. It cannot be said enough that detection of hyperglycemia or hypoglycemia with symptoms is sometimes difficult when a patient is recovering from an anesthetic. Therefore, frequent tests of blood and urine glucose are most helpful in determining the patient's state.

Also, any patient who arrives in the PACU, especially in the older age groups, may have undiagnosed diabetes. Consequently, in the diabetic and older patients, the PACU nurse should ensure that careful positioning and padding is provided because these patients probably have a decreased tissue perfusion and peripheral sympathetic neuropathy, all of which can contribute to the development of tissue breakdown and ulceration.

## RHEUMATOID ARTHRITIS

Rheumatoid arthritis is a relatively common disease that affects the connective tissue of the body. The clinical course varies, but it tends to be progressive and lead to characteristic deformities. Many patients become incapacitated over time. The disease affects more women than men, and its incidence rate in temperate climates is about 3%. The cause is not completely understood, but the disease is thought to be an autoimmune phenomenon. The outstanding clinical feature of this disease is proliferative inflammation. The patient often appears chronically ill, undernourished, and anemic.

These patients often undergo surgery to correct restrictive deformities caused by the disease process (Table 48-4). On arrival in the PACU, they require comprehensive nursing management. Some of the hazards to be aware of in patients with rheumatoid arthritis are listed in Table 48-5.

### Care of the Patient with Rheumatoid Arthritis
*Airway.* Extubation is often deferred in these patients until they are unquestionably able to maintain their own airways. This deference is

| Table 48-3 | Characteristics of Diabetic Complications | |
|---|---|---|
| Category | Diabetic Coma | Insulin Reaction |
| Onset | Slow | Sudden |
| Skin | Flushed, dry, hot | Pale, moist |
| Behavior | Drowsy | Excited |
| Breath | Acetone (sweet) | Normal |
| Respirations | Kussmaul's (air hunger) | Normal-rapid, shallow |
| Pulse | Rapid, weak | Normal-slow, full bounding |
| Blood pressure | Low | Normal |
| Vomiting | Present | Absent |
| Hunger | Absent | Present |
| Thirst | Present | Absent |
| Urine glucose level | Large amount | Absent |

| Table 48-4 | Corrective Surgery for Rheumatoid Arthritis |
|---|---|
| **Operative Site** | **Common Operative Procedure** |
| Neck | Atlantoaxial arthrodesis |
| Shoulder | Synovectomy and partial excision of acromion |
| Elbow | Synovectomy and radial head excision; resection arthroplasty |
| Wrist | Synovectomy and excision of distal ulna |
| Hand | Metacarpal phalangeal arthroplasty and flexor and extensor tenosynovectomy |
| Hip | Cup or total replacement, arthroplasty |
| Knee | Synovectomy (often bilateral), arthroplasty |
| Foot | Resection arthroplasty (often bilateral) |

From Jenkins LC, McGraw RW: Anaesthetic management of the patient with rheumatoid arthritis, *Can Anaesth Soc J* 16:408, 1969.

of prime importance because these patients are often extremely difficult to intubate and are prone to airway obstruction.

**Lungs.** The patient with rheumatoid arthritis usually has pulmonary dysfunction, such as diffuse interstitial fibrosis, granulomatous lesions, or large silicotic nodules. These pulmonary dysfunctions lead to stiff lungs, and these patients are prone to atelectasis, hypoxemia, and hypercarbia in the PACU (see Chapter 12). Postoperative blood gas analysis and good pulmonary support are therefore important. Respiratory depressant narcotics should be given with caution, if at all. Deaths in patients with rheumatoid arthritis have resulted from drug-induced respiratory failure during this period.

**Heart.** Disease of the pericardium, myocardium, endocardium, and coronary vessels is usually associated with rheumatoid arthritis. Therefore, cardiovascular status should be monitored continuously in the PACU. Hypotension should be avoided because it may lead to left ventricular decompensation and acute heart failure.

**Blood.** The patient with arthritis usually has anemia, most commonly of the hypochromic microcytic variety. In most instances, this type of anemia can be treated with blood transfusion. Postoperative hematocrit and hemoglobin levels should be determined when the patient arrives in the PACU. Blood loss should be extensively monitored, including observation of the stools for blood. The contents recovered from the nasogastric tube (if present) should be checked for blood because these patients may have a bleeding peptic ulcer from long-term aspirin and steroid therapy.

**Fluid Balance.** Renal function is usually impaired in the patient with chronic rheumatoid arthritis; therefore, drugs that are primarily

| Table 48-5 | Perianesthesia Hazards in Patients with Rheumatoid Arthritis |
|---|---|
| **Area of Concern** | **Complication** |
| **RESPIRATORY SYSTEM** | |
| Airway | Hypoplastic mandible restriction, cervical spine motion, atlantoaxial subluxation, laryngeal tissue damage |
| Ventilation | Rheumatoid nodules in lung, chronic diffuse interstitial fibrosis, costovertebral joint disorder that inhibits ventilation, thoracic vertebrae flexion deformity that inhibits ventilation, tuberculous lung |
| **CARDIOVASCULAR SYSTEM** | Pericardial, myocardial, coronary artery disorders, aortic valve regurgitation, arrhythmias |
| **HEMOPOIETIC, HEPATIC, AND RENAL SYSTEMS** | Anemia, leukopenia, bleeding tendency (decreased platelets), renal amyloidosis |
| **MISCELLANEOUS** | Skin fragility; postoperative chest complications, such as atelectasis, hypercarbia, and hypoxia; multiple joint disease |

Modified from Jenkins LC, McGraw RW: Anaesthetic management of the patient with rheumatoid arthritis, *Can Anaesth Soc J* 16:408, 1969.

excreted by the kidneys should be avoided, and urinary output should be monitored at regular, perhaps hourly, intervals.

## OBESITY

Obesity, the most common nutritional disorder in the world today, in fact is a disease that affects more than a third of the adult population in the United States. It presents many difficulties to the perianesthesia nurse. Many definitions of obesity can be found in the literature. The American Life Insurance Company states that a person is obese if he or she exceeds the expected or ideal weight, corrected by age and gender, by more than 10%. Morbid obesity is a term that denotes a weight twice as much as that predicted for age, gender, body build, and height. Patients with morbid obesity can be divided into two groups. Obesity with normal levels of arterial carbon dioxide tension is called simple obesity and includes 90% to 95% of morbidly obese patients. The other group, which represents 5% to 10% of obese patients, has the obesity-hypoventilation (pickwickian) syndrome. This syndrome is characterized by extreme obesity, episodic somnolence, and hypoventilation (increased $PaCO_2$ level) with twitching, plethora, edema, periodic respiration, secondary polycythemia, right ventricular hypertrophy, and right ventricular failure.

The most useful anthropometric index for determination of obesity is the body mass index (BMI). This measurement uses the person's weight (in kilograms) divided by height squared (in meters):

$$BMI = weight\,(kg)/height\,(m)^2$$
$$Or$$
$$BMI = (body\ weight\,[pounds]/height\,[inches])$$
$$\times\ 703$$

The patient with a BMI of 27 (25% to 30% overweight) usually presents minimal risks in the perioperative period. A BMI higher than 30 is associated with an increased perioperative mortality rate and is considered obesity. Certainly, patients in the obese and morbidly obese categories come to the PACU for surgery on a number of conditions. Now, with the advent of the resectional gastric bypass (RGB) and gastric banding surgical procedures, these patients are seen in the PACU with increased frequency.

### Physiologic Considerations in Obesity

***Respiratory System.*** Preoperative evaluation of obese patients reveals that 85% have exertional dyspnea and some degree of orthopnea. Periodic breathing, especially when sleeping, may also be present.

Obese patients tend to develop some degree of thoracic kyphosis and lumbar lordosis because of a protuberant abdomen. In addition, the layers of fat on the chest and abdomen reduce the bellows action of the thoracic cage. The overall lung-thorax compliance is reduced and thus leads to increased elastic resistance of the system. Usually the diaphragm is elevated, and the total work of breathing is increased as a result of the deposition of abdominal fat. Because of these factors, the oxygen cost of breathing is three or more times that of normal, even at rest.

The primary respiratory defect of obese patients is a marked reduction in the expiratory reserve volume. The reason for the decrease in expiratory reserve volume and other lung volumes is that the obese patient is unable to expand the chest in a normal fashion. Therefore, diaphragmatic movement must account for the changes in lung volume to a much greater extent than thoracic expansion does. As previously discussed, the diaphragmatic movement is moderately limited by the anatomic changes of obesity, which account for the decreased lung volumes.

In the obese patient, the functional residual capacity may be below the closing capacity in the sitting and supine positions; therefore, the dependent lung zones may be effectively closed throughout the respiratory cycle (see Chapter 12). Consequently, inspired gas is distributed mainly to the upper or nondependent lung zones. The resulting mismatch of ventilation to perfusion produces systemic arterial hypoxemia (Fig. 48-1).

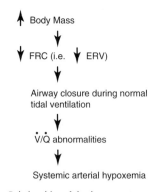

**Fig. 48-1**  Relationship of body mass to systemic arterial hypoxemia. *FRC,* Functional residual capacity; *ERV,* expiratory reserve volume; *V/Q,* ventilation/perfusion. *(From Drain C, Vaughan R: Anesthetic considerations of morbid obesity, AANA J 47:556–565, 1979.)*

The hypoventilation and ventilation-perfusion abnormalities that contribute to systemic arterial hypoxemia also contribute to retained carbon dioxide and thus lead to hypercarbia, which can be observed in the pickwickian syndrome.

In about 5% of the morbidly obese population, obstructive sleep apnea (OSA) occurs. OSA can occur in patients with redundant pharyngeal tissue. Obstructive sleep apnea is characterized by excessive episodes of apnea (about 10 seconds) and a 50% reduction in airflow or a reduction sufficient to lead to a 4% decrease in oxygen saturation during sleep as a result of a partial or complete upper airway obstruction. Clinically significant apnea episodes of more than five episodes in one hour or 30 per night will result in hypoxia, hypercapnia, systemic and pulmonary hypertension, and cardiac arrhythmias. Adult patients with severe OSA may need a tracheostomy with local anesthesia before a general anesthetic is administered. Should a patient with OSA arrive in the PACU and become obtunded, an emergency tracheostomy may be performed.

**Cardiovascular System.** Thirty pounds of fat are estimated to contain 25 miles of blood vessels, and the increased body mass in obesity leads to increased oxygen consumption and carbon dioxide production. That the cardiac output and the total blood volume are increased in the obese state is not surprising. This increase in cardiac output is a result of an increase in stroke volume rather than an increase in heart rate; the latter usually remains normal.

The transverse cardiac diameter has been shown to be greater than normal in approximately two thirds of obese patients. A linear relationship seems to exist between cardiac diameter and body weight.

Obesity has been suggested to predispose to electrocardiographic changes. The Q-T interval is often prolonged, and the QRS voltage is reduced (because of the increased distance between the heart and the electrodes). Finally, likelihood of ventricular arrhythmias is increased in the obese patient.

A positive correlation exists between an increase in body weight and increased arterial pressure. A weight gain of 28 lbs can increase the systolic and diastolic blood pressure by 10 and 7 torr, respectively. The increase in blood pressure is probably caused by the increased cardiac output.

Chronic heart failure, although uncommon, can occur in persons with long-standing morbid obesity with or without hypertension.

It is usually characterized by high output and biventricular dysfunction, with the left ventricle predominating. Clinically, heart failure may be difficult to diagnose because pedal edema may be chronically present.

Cerebral blood flow in obese persons does not differ significantly from that in persons of normal weight. Oxygen uptake of the brain remains normal in the obese person. However, the fraction of the total body oxygen represented in the cerebral metabolism is less than normal because the total body oxygen requirement is increased. Although the kidneys of obese subjects weigh more than those of nonobese counterparts, renal blood flow is the same as or slightly lower than that of patients of normal weight.

**Pregnancy.** Problems associated with obesity in pregnancy occur relatively commonly. Studies indicate that patients who weigh at least 250 lbs have a 35% chance of operative obstetrics. In fact, some form of obstetric complication may be observed in 63% of obese patients. Seven times more toxemia, five times more pyelonephritis, and 10 times more diabetes mellitus occur in obese patients than in similar groups of nonobese pregnant patients.

**Other Disorders.** Diabetes mellitus has been associated with obesity. It is the third most prevalent preoperative pathologic condition found in obese patients. Adult patients with diabetes are often obese, and an improved glucose tolerance test follows weight reduction. Other associated problems that may be clinically present include abnormal liver function tests, fatty infiltration of the liver, gallstones, hiatal hernia, and varicose veins.

### Care of the Obese Patient

Because these patients can be quite large, two PACU beds may be needed for the morbidly obese patient. Also, padding should be used to avoid pressure injuries that result in neurologic injury or rhabdomyolysis. Because of problems associated with central lines in these patients, checking with the anesthesia care team to see what monitoring equipment is being used is important so that it can be continued in the postanesthesia phase.

**Respiratory.** Significant problems arise in the PACU phase of the perioperative care of the obese patient. In fact, the problems associated with obesity are becoming more apparent to all perianesthesia nurses since the advent of the jejunoileal bypass and gastric stapling procedures for the treatment of morbid obesity. A direct correlation exists between the incidence rate of postoperative pulmonary complications and the

SPECIAL CONSIDERATIONS

degree of obesity. The mortality rate after upper abdominal operations in obese patients is 2.5 times that of the nonobese counterparts.

The functional residual capacity (FRC) decreases with increasing BMI, the expiratory reserve volume (ERV) decreases, and the residual volume (RV) stays the same. Thus, the FRC is reduced (ERV + RV = FRC) and the result is that the closing volume (CV) is increased, which leads to an increase in the alveolar-arterial oxygen (a-A $PO_2$) difference, resulting in hypoxemia. Therefore, the a-A $PO_2$ increases as the BMI increases (please see Chapter 12).

Positioning can be a valuable therapeutic tool for improvement of arterial oxygenation. Position has been shown to significantly affect $PaO_2$ levels for 48 hours after surgery. The obese patient should be cared for in a semi-Fowler's position unless cardiovascular instability exists. *Routine use of the supine position should be avoided because the functional residual capacity can decrease below the closing capacity and thus reduce the number of ventilated alveoli, which ultimately leads to hypoxemia.* Another position that aids in relief of pressure on the diaphragm is the head-elevated laryngoscopy position (HELP), which is a modified semi-Fowler's position with elevation of the head and upper body with pillows to create a horizontal line between the sternum and ear that also improves the view for reintubation (if needed). Moreover, early ambulation in the PACU is of great value in enhancement of lung volumes of the obese patient.

In the postanesthesia period, the position of the operative incision is a factor because obese patients with a vertical incision have been shown to have a more marked postoperative hypoxemia than obese patients who receive a transverse incision. Therefore, supplemental inspired oxygen may be necessary after surgery for 3 to 4 days in patients with a vertical incision. Serial arterial blood gas determinations can serve as a guide to supplemental oxygen administration. Moreover, after the patient's arterial line is in place, arterial blood gas determinations should be done to provide a baseline guide for proper ventilation. If the patient arrives in the PACU with the endotracheal tube in place, the patient should be started on a ventilator. The nurse should then auscultate for bilateral breath sounds to ensure proper placement of the endotracheal tube. Because of the many technical difficulties associated with tracheal intubation of the obese patient, the perianesthesia nurse should constantly monitor the patient for proper placement of the tube. If the tube becomes displaced, the patient should be ventilated with a bag-valve-mask system, and the

anesthesia personnel should be summoned immediately.

Adult patients with severe OSA may need a tracheostomy with local anesthesia before a general anesthetic is administered. If a patient with OSA arrives in the PACU and becomes obtunded, an emergency tracheostomy may be performed.

Cardiovascular pathophysiology may reduce cardiac reserve, especially in the older obese patient. A reduction in arterial oxygen tension caused by incision site or postoperative position causes an increase in cardiac output to facilitate tissue oxygen delivery, which could lead to cardiac decompensation in an already compromised cardiovascular system. Arterial hypoxemia should be avoided because many obese patients cannot compensate for the increased cardiac output demand and the concomitant pulmonary vasoconstriction caused by the reduced arterial oxygen tension.

Early postoperative ambulation is important not only in enhancing lung volumes but also in helping reduce the incidence of venous thrombosis. Indeed, relatively immobile obese persons are particularly susceptible to the development of pulmonary emboli.

**Cardiovascular.** The obese patient has a higher incidence rate of hypertension, coronary artery disease, myocardial infarction, and cardiomegaly. Therefore, careful electrocardiographic monitoring should be used. If an arterial line was not used during surgery, a blood pressure cuff that covers one third to half the length of the upper arm should be used. A baseline blood pressure measurement when the patient arrives in the PACU proves valuable in comparison with the intraoperative measurements for assessment of the accuracy of the blood pressure reading. The PACU nurse may need a forearm blood pressure cuff, especially if used before and during surgery, and those readings provide a baseline blood pressure measurement.

**Fluid Dynamics.** Because fatty tissue is 6% to 10% water (in comparison with lean tissue, which comprises 70% to 80%), alteration in fluid requirements is likely to occur in the obese patient. In the healthy person, body water is 65%; in the obese person, the body water is about 40% of total weight. Calculations of fluid requirements must be adjusted to compensate for this reduction in total body water.

**Psychologic Aspects.** Psychologic support of the obese patient should not be overlooked when perianesthesia care is administered. Many of these patients have become obese because of repeated episodes of emotional stress. Body image, along with the ability to interact with others, may be a problem for obese patients; they may appear to be demanding and aloof from others. The perianesthesia personnel must establish a positive rapport with the obese patient before surgery. Also, the perianesthesia staff must not express any negative feelings about the patient or about morbid obesity in general. The added psychologic support serves to minimize fear and anxiety and ultimately improve the outcome of the obese patient.

## SICKLE CELL DISEASE

Sickle cell disease is an inherited type of hemolytic anemia. It is a chronic disease marked by exacerbations. The clinical manifestations are based entirely on sickling of the red blood cells and its consequences.

More than 100 abnormal hemoglobins have been described in humans. When these hemoglobins are exposed to low oxygen tensions, this particular form of hemoglobin causes the red blood cell to distort its shape (sickle) and cause infarction and other complications. Normal hemoglobin is labeled hemoglobin A, whereas this sickling hemoglobin is labeled hemoglobin S.

Hemoglobin S is thought to have arisen in Arabia in Neolithic times and from there to have spread eastward and westward; it is found today in parts of India, east and west Africa, and the West Indies and among African Americans.

The common sickle cell disorders are sickle cell trait (SA), homozygous sickle cell disease (SS), sickle cell-hemoglobin C disease, and sickle cell-thalassemia. A combination of thalassemia and sickle cell anemia occurs in sickle cell-beta thalassemia.

Sickle cell trait is found in about 8% to 12% of the African-American population, which is heterozygous for sickling, and represents a combination of sickle hemoglobin (SA) and normal hemoglobin (AA). The red blood cells of such persons contain from 20% to 40% hemoglobin S but are not misshapen in normal living conditions. The person may have sickling with exposure to any conditions that cause hypoxia, such as depressed respiratory function from anesthetics in the PACU.

The most common form of sickle cell disease is the homozygous sickle cell disease. It occurs in about 1 in 400 to 500 African Americans. These persons have inherited sickling genes from both parents, and they usually have 80% to 100% hemoglobin S. Sickling is present all the time, and minor reductions in oxygen tension can

cause a sickle cell crisis. The onset of symptoms occurs around the age of 2 years; rarely do these persons live past the age of 40 years.

Sickle cell-hemoglobin C disease is caused by the presence of the gene for sickle hemoglobin and the gene for hemoglobin C. The course of the disease is usually milder than that of the homozygous sickle cell disease, although the person has discomfort and occasional sickle cell crises.

Sickle cell-thalassemia, which occurs in persons who have traits for sickle cell-thalassemia and beta-thalassemia, has a less severe course and symptoms in comparison with the other forms of these diseases. The sickle cell crises are not seen as commonly in this disease.

### Pathogenesis of Sickle Cell Disease
To understand the pathogenesis of this disease, knowledge of what happens to the red blood cell when sickling occurs is helpful. If oxygen tension is lowered, long crystals called tactoids are formed within the red blood cells because of rearrangement of the amino acid chains or polymers. The cell membrane becomes distorted by the twisting of the polymers. The result is the sickle cell shape for which the disease is named. The process can be reversed if the oxygen tension is increased.

The actual pathologic action of sickling occurs in the microcirculation. Because of increased viscosity and the distortion of the red blood cells with the formation of tactoids, which prevents the cells from molding to the size and structure of the capillaries, the sickled cells are wedged in the capillary bed and thus occlude normal flow. As the cells aggregate, a thrombus is formed. Symptoms depend on whether the thrombus becomes an embolus and, if so, on where it becomes lodged; infarctive episodes are caused in that tissue. Areas of infarctive crisis are the spleen, myocardium, kidney, liver, mesentery, bone marrow, and brain.

Oxygen tension causes sickling, but several other precipitating factors are also involved, such as acidosis, hypotension, regional vasodilation, dehydration, hemoconcentration, stasis of blood, hypothermia, sepsis, decreased cardiac output, and respiratory impairment.

### Sickle Cell Anemia and Anesthesia
Anesthesia is not generally believed to be hazardous to patients with sickle cell trait. Nevertheless, keep in mind that sufficiently adverse hypoxic conditions can precipitate a sickling crisis. Definite hazards arise with anesthesia in patients with sickle cell and sickle cell–hemoglobin C disease. Because of its ability

to cause the intravascular sickling syndrome, general anesthesia has been the subject of much research. The most important factor in this syndrome is hypoxemia, which generally occurs during the emergent period rather than during surgery. Local anesthesia or nerve block is the technique of choice. Epidural and spinal techniques should be avoided because of the possibility of hypotension with these two methods.

### Care of the Patient with Sickle Cell Disease

Prevention of sickle cell crisis is the main objective in the PACU phase. A general guideline for preoperative preparation is a hemoglobin A level of at least 50% and a hematocrit value of 35%. A recent study indicated that a conservative transfusion regimen is effective as an aggressive regimen in prevention of postoperative complications. If diagnostic procedures are not available or if emergency surgery prevents testing for the sickling trait, all African-American patients should be treated as possible carriers of the trait because the incidence rate of this disease is relatively high among African Americans.

In the patient with sickle cell disease, the postoperative period is critically important because incisional pain, analgesics, pulmonary infections, and low arterial oxygen partial pressures all are predisposing factors to the formation of sickle cells. Hence, in the PACU, supplemental humidified oxygen, along with appropriate monitoring of intravascular volume and core temperature, is of utmost importance for ensuring positive outcomes.

Temperature regulation is important for the patient with sickle cell disease. Although cold reduces tactoid formation, it also reduces body metabolism, which may lead to crisis. Hyperthermia causes excess sweating, however, and may lead to dehydration, which can also cause sickling. Temperature monitoring and the use of hypothermia and hyperthermia blankets can allow maintenance of body temperature in the optimal range of 36° C to 37° C.

Cardiac monitoring is important because the occurrence of arrhythmias, such as extrasystole and prolonged P-R interval, in patients with sickling is high. Vasodilators or vasoconstrictors should be avoided, if possible, because the dilators may cause hypotension and the vasoconstrictors may cause circulatory stasis.

Respiratory rate and volume should be monitored closely so that hypoxia can be avoided. Oxygen saturation or arterial blood gas monitoring can aid in assessment of respiratory status, and postoperative pain should be managed with drugs that do not depress respiratory function.

Kidney function should be monitored because the renal tubules become blocked by the hemolyzed red blood cells if crisis occurs and infarcts may occur in some areas of the kidney. Insertion of a urinary catheter to monitor urinary output at regular intervals has proven useful.

## SICKLE CELL CRISIS

The types of crisis seen in sickle cell anemia are vasoocclusive, aplastic, sequestration, and hemolytic. The vasoocclusive crisis is the most common type and is characterized by tissue ischemia, infarction, and necrosis. The bones, tendons, synovia, spleen, liver, and intestine are common sites of occlusion. Infections, dehydration, high altitudes, extreme physical exertion, and emotional upsets can trigger this type of crisis.

The aplastic crisis is most grave and constitutes a medical emergency. It is characterized by a sudden drastic decrease in red blood cell production. The patient initially appears weak and has signs of cardiac decompensation.

The spleen is involved in sequestration crisis. A large amount of blood becomes trapped in the spleen and thus causes hypovolemia and shock, which constitutes a medical emergency. Clinically, the patient's blood pressure decreases and the pulse rate increases. Palpation and percussion reveal an enlarged mass in the right upper quadrant of the abdomen.

Bacterial infections, poisons, and medications, such as phenothiazines and sulfonamides, aspirin in large quantities, and quinine, can produce hemolysis of the red blood cell. The patient also has an enzyme deficiency (glucose-6-phosphodehydrogenase) in this type of sickle cell anemia.

If crisis occurs, the following modes of treatment are recommended: keep the patient warm; treat infections; and maintain oxygenation, hydration, and alkalinization. Heparin may be administered to reduce the risks of embolus formation, and magnesium sulfate may also be indicated for its vasodilator and anticoagulant properties.

## SUMMARY

Patient's with various chronic disorders present the perianesthesia nurse with significant pathophysical challenges throughout the perianesthesia phase of hospitalization. The number of patients with COPD is increasing exponentially. These patients have altered lung mechanics; with the appropriate knowledge base for reversal of the altered lung mechanics, these patients have an excellent outcome during recovery from anesthesia. Also, patients who have a history of cigarette smoking present significant challenges to the perianesthesia nurse. These patients often have COPD and usually need special care in the PACU because of chronic bronchitis. Perianesthesia nursing care was presented with a focus on the maintenance of a patent airway and enhanced use of the modified stir-up regime.

Another chronic disease that is becoming a national health issue is diabetes. As described in this chapter, these patients usually need enhanced care in regard to fluid and electrolytes and insulin management. Another chronic disease that is receiving a significant amount of media attention is obesity. The number of patients who are considered obese is rising and is predicted to become a national epidemic. Chronic obesity was discussed at length in this chapter, and the various pathophysiologic concerns and methods of nursing care in the PACU for these patients were presented. Another chronic disease, sickle cell disease, was presented with a focus on identification of possible clinical problems and appropriate nursing interventions during the perianesthesia phase.

# BIBLIOGRAPHY

Aitkenhead A, Smith G. Rowbotham D: *Textbook of anaesthesia*, ed 5, Philadelphia, 2007, Churchill Livingstone.

Alspach J: *Core curriculum for critical care nursing*, ed 6, Philadelphia, 2005, Saunders.

*American Obesity Association Fact Sheet*, available at http://www.obesity.org/subs/fastfacts/obesity_US.html, accessed March 10, 2007.

Aronson R, Weiss S, Ben R, et al: Association between cigarette smoking and acute respiratory tract infections in young adults, *JAMA* 248:181-183, 1982.

Atlee J: *Complications in anesthesia*, ed 2, Philadelphia, 2007, Saunders.

Austin R: Cigarette smoking and chronic bronchitis, *Br Med J* 2(6046):1261, 1976.

Barash P, Cullen B, Stoelting R: *Clinical anesthesia*, ed 5, Philadelphia, 2005, Lippincott Williams & Wilkins.

Bayes J: Asymptomatic smokers: ASA I or II? *Anesthesiology* 56:76, 1982.

Benumof J.: Obstructive sleep apnea in the adult obese patient: implications for airway management, *J Clin Anesth* 13:144-156, 2001.

Benumof J, Saidman L: *Anesthesia & perioperative complications*, ed 2, St Louis, 1999, Mosby.

Berman L: Cigarettes, coronary occlusions, and myocardial infarctions, *JAMA* 246:871-872, 1981.

Biddle C, Biddle W: A survey of perianesthetic complications in the asymptomatic smoker, *AANA J* 51(5):481-484, 1983.

Biddle C, Hernandez S: Perioperative control of diabetes mellitus-revised, *AANA J* 51(2):138-141, 1983.

Biring M, Lewis M, Liu J, et al: Pulmonary physiologic changes of morbid obesity, *Am J Med Sci* 318:293-297, 1999.

Brodsky J, et al: Morbid obesity and tracheal intubation, *Anesth Analg* 94:732, 2002.

Brodsky J, et al: Is the super-obese patient different? *Obes Surg* 14:1428, 2004.

Brodsky J, et al: Nitrous oxide and laparoscopic bariatric surgery, *Obes Surg* 15:494, 2005.

Brodsky J, et al: Obesity, surgery, and inhalation anesthetics: is there a "drug of choice"? *Obes Surg* 16:734, 2006.

Brunton L, Lazo J, Parker K: *Goodman and Gilman's the pharmacological basis of therapeutics*, ed 11, New York, 2005, McGraw-Hill Professional.

Burrows B, Knudson R, Quan S, et al: *Respiratory disorders: a pathophysiologic approach*, ed 2, Chicago, 1983, Year Book Medical Publishers.

Cameron L, Kirsch J: Myasthenia gravis pharmacologic management, *Crit Care Rep* 1:157-163, 1989.

Chand B, et al: Perioperative management of the bariatric surgery patient: focus on cardiac and anesthesia considerations, *Clev Clin J Med* 73:S51, 2006.

Cote' C, Todres I, Goudsouzian N, et al: *A practice of anesthesia for infants and children*, ed 3, Philadelphia, 2001, Saunders.

DeFazio-Quinn D, Schick L: *PeriAnesthesia nursing core curriculum*, Philadelphia, 2004, Saunders.

DeFronzo R: Pharmacologic therapy for type 2 diabetes mellitus, *Ann Intern Med* 131:281, 1999.

Drake R, Vogl W, Mitchell A: *Gray's anatomy for students*, Philadelphia, 2005, Churchill Livingstone.

Drain C: Anesthesia care of the patient with reactive airways disease, *CRNA: Clin Forum Nurse Anesthetists* 7(4):207-212, 1996.

Drain C: Physiology of the respiratory system related to anesthesia, *CRNA: Clin Forum Nurse Anesthetists* 7(4):163-180, 1996.

Drain C: Pathophysiology of the respiratory system related to anesthesia, *CRNA: Clin Forum Nurse Anesthetists* 7(4):181-192, 1996.

Drain C, Robinson S: The pharmacology of respiratory disorders related to anesthesia, *CRNA: Clin Forum Nurse Anesthetists* 7(4):193-199, 1996.

Erikssen J, Hellen A, Stormorken H: Chronic effect of smoking on platelet count and platelet adhesiveness in presumably healthy middle-aged men, *Thromb Haemost* 38(3):606-611, 1977.

Estafanous F, Barash P, Reves J, editors: *Cardiac anesthesia: principles and clinical practice*, ed 2, Philadelphia, 2001, Lippincott Williams & Wilkins.

Evers A, Maze M: *Anesthetic pharmacology: physiologic principles and clinical practice*, Philadelphia, 2004, Churchill Livingstone.

Fink D, Raymon R: Rheumatoid arthritis of the cricoarytenoid joints: an airway hazard, *Anesth Analg* 54(6):742, 1975.

Fisher L: *Benumof's anesthesia and uncommon diseases*, ed 5, Philadelphia, 2007, Saunders.

Friedman F: Mortality in cigarette smokers and quitters: effects of baseline differences, *N Engl J Med* 30:1407-1410, 1981.

Frost E: Preanesthetic assessment of the patient with respiratory disease, *Anesthesiol Clin North Am* 8:657-676, 1990.

Gallager C, Issenberg B: *Simulation in anesthesia*, Philadelphia, 2007, Saunders.

Ganong W: *Review of medical physiology*, ed 22, New York, 2005, McGraw-Hill Medical.

Gibson J: Anesthesia for the sickle cell diseases and other hemoglobinopathies, *Semin Anesth* 6(1):27-35, 1987.

Guyton A, Hall J: *Textbook of medical physiology*, ed 11, Philadelphia, 2006, Saunders.

Hemmerling T, Schmid M, Schmidt J, et al: Comparison of a continuous glucose-insulin-potassium infusion versus intermittent bolus application of insulin on perioperative glucose control and hormone status in insulin-treated type 2 diabetics, *J Clin Anesth* 13:293-300, 2001.

Hirsch I, McGill J, Cryer P, et al: Perioperative management of surgical patients with diabetes mellitus, *Anesthesiology* 74:346-359, 1991.

Kaplan J, Slinger P: *Thoracic anesthesia*, ed 3, New York, 2003, Churchill Livingstone.

Kier L, Dowd C: *The chemistry of drugs for nurse anesthetists*, Chicago, 2004, AANA Publishing, Inc.

Lake C, Hines R, Blitt C: *Clinical monitoring: practical applications for anesthesia and critical care*, Philadelphia, 2001, Saunders.

Lemmens H, et al: Anesthetic drugs and bariatric surgery, *Expert Rev Neurother* 6:1107, 2006.

Longnecker D, Murphy F: *Dripps, Eckenhoff, Vandam introduction to anesthesia*, ed 9, Philadelphia, 1997, Saunders.

Longnecker D, Tinker J, Morgan G: *Principles and practice of anesthesiology*, ed 2, St Louis, 1998, Mosby.

Lynch J: Preoperative and intraoperative insulin needs in diabetic patients, *AANA J* 52(3):275-279, 1984.

Maduska A: Sickling dynamics of red blood cells and other physiologic studies during anesthesia, *Anesth Analg* 54(3):361-364, 1975.

Miller R editor: *Anesthesia*, ed 6, Philadelphia, 2005, Churchill Livingstone.

Murray J, Nadel J: *Textbook of respiratory medicine*, ed 4, Philadelphia, 2005, Saunders.

Nagelhout J, Zaglaniczy K: *Nurse anesthesia*, ed 3, St Louis, 2005, Saunders.

National Institute of Diabetes and Digestive and Kidney Diseases of the National Institute of Health: available at http://niddk.nih.gov, accessed March 10, 2007.

Ogden S: *Calculation of drug dosages*, ed 7, St Louis, 2005, Mosby.

Passannante A, et al: Anesthetic management of patients with obesity and sleep apnea, *Anesthesiol Clin North Am* 32:479, 2005.

Schenker M, Samet J, Spiezer E: Effect of cigarette tar content and smoking habits on respiratory symptoms in women, *Am Rev Respir Dis* 125:684-690, 1982.

Shorten G, Browne J, Carr D, et al: *Postoperative pain management: an evidence-based guide to practice*, Philadelphia, 2006, Saunders.

Stoelting R: *Pharmacology and physiology in anesthetic practice*, ed 3, Philadelphia, 1999, Lippincott–Raven.

Stoelting R, Miller R: *Basics of anesthesia*, ed 5, Philadelphia, 2007, Churchill Livingstone.

Thompson J, McFarland G, Kirsch J, et al: *Mosby's clinical nursing*, ed 5, St Louis, 2002, Mosby.

Townsend C, Beauchamp R, Evers B, et al: *Sabiston textbook of surgery: the biological basis of modern surgical practice*, ed 17, Philadelphia, 2004, Saunders.

Traver G, Tremper Mitchell J, Glodquist-Priestley G: *Respiratory care: a clinical approach*, Gaithersburg, Md, 1991, Aspen Publishers.

Vaughan R, Engelhardt RC, Wise L: Postoperative hypoxemia in obese patients, *Ann Surg* 180(6):877, 1974.

Voelker M: Assessing quality of life in gastric bypass clients, *J PeriAnesthesia Nurs* 19(2):89-104, 2004.

Waxman SJ, Waxman SG: *Correlative neuroanatomy*, ed 24, Norwalk, Conn, 1999, Lange Medical Publishers.

White P: *Perioperative drug manual*, ed 2, Philadelphia, 2005, Saunders.

Wightman J: A prospective survey of the incidence of postoperative pulmonary complications, *Br J Surg* 55:81-91, 1968.

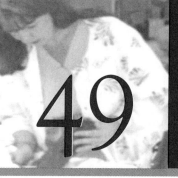

# 49

# CARE OF THE PEDIATRIC PATIENT

*Donna Landriscina, RN, MSNA, CRNA*

Pediatric anesthesia is a subspecialty in the practice of anesthesiology. Pediatric patients are not merely miniature adults. Consideration and application of age-appropriate care is important throughout the perioperative period. Because their immaturity presents various definite physiologic differences, infants and children cannot be regarded as simply small adults. Some of the main differences lie in the respiratory and cardiovascular systems and in the regulation of body temperature.

Anesthetic management of the pediatric patient has been revised in several areas as advancement in knowledge of physiology and pathophysiology are applied to patient care. Along with this increased depth of knowledge, pediatric anesthesiology and perianesthesia care are increasingly more challenging and rewarding. Many nurses may occasionally care for a pediatric patient and therefore may find issues related to perioperative management to be particularly more stressful and challenging. The content within this chapter provides an overview with key take-home points regarding perianesthesia care for children of all ages. The ultimate goal of this chapter is to simplify approaches to managing and caring for our pediatric population in a safe environment and to promote a rewarding and enjoyable experience for both the nurse and patient.

## DEFINITIONS

**Analgesia:** Absence of pain.
**Analgesic:** A drug used to relieve pain.
**Anesthetic:** An agent used to produce anesthesia.
**Anesthesia:** Partial or complete loss of sensation, with or without loss of consciousness; referred to in this chapter as the administration of an anesthetic agent via injection or inhalation.
**Antagonist:** To counteract the action of something else, such as a drug that binds to a receptor site and prevents receptor stimulation.

**Anticholinergic:** A parasympatholytic; blocks the parasympathetic nerve fibers and parasympathetic nerve impulse conduction.
**Antiemetic:** Used to relieve or prevent nausea and vomiting (prevent emesis).
**Anxiolytic:** Used to reduce, relieve, or counteract anxiety.
**Aspiration:** The general use of this term is to draw in or out via suction, however, specifically referred to in this chapter are situations in which an individual is at risk for entry of gastric secretions, oropharyngeal secretions, or exogenous food or fluids into tracheobronchial passages, because of loss of the normal protective mechanisms as occurs with induction of general anesthesia.
**Atelectasis:** A collapse, lack of expansion, or airless condition of the lungs.
**Barotrauma:** An injury caused by a change in atmospheric pressure relative to a potentially closed space within a surrounding area.
**Child:** Younger than 13 years of age; before puberty.
**Conception:** Onset of pregnancy with implantation of a fertilized ovum in the uterine wall; fertilization.
**Delirium:** An acute and reversible condition characterized by agitation, confusion, disorientation, hallucinations or delusions, difficulty focusing attention, and inability to rest.
**Emergence Delirium:** Occurs during initial cessation from general anesthesia to an awake state and initial transfer into the postanesthesia care unit.
**Desaturation:** When oxygen is dissociated from hemoglobin.
**Dissociative:** A type of anesthesia with marked catalepsy, amnesia, and analgesia.
**Dysphoria:** A mood disorder of restlessness without apparent cause, anxiety, dissatisfaction, and discomfort.
**Emergence:** To evolve or rise out of anesthesia to a level of consciousness and status of protective reflexes, motor activity, and orientation.
**Erythropoiesis:** Forming red blood cells.
**Extubation, Extubate:** The act of removal of an endotracheal tube.

**General Anesthesia:** Affecting the entire body with loss of consciousness.

**Gestation:** Period of intrauterine fetal development from conception to birth.

**Hemostasis:** To stop bleeding; stasis refers to standing still.

**Hypercarbia, Hypercapnia:** Elevated above normal levels of carbon dioxide in the blood (> 45 mm Hg).

**Hyperflexion:** Increased flexion of a joint; in this text, refers to the neck.

**Hyperoxia:** Increased levels of oxygen in the blood.

**Hyperthermia, Hyperpyrexia:** An elevated body temperature above the normal range.

**Hypervolemia:** An abnormal increase in circulating blood volume.

**Hypothermia:** A lower body temperature below normal range.

**Hypovolemia:** An abnormal decrease in circulating blood volume.

**Hypoxemia:** Decreased levels of oxygen in the blood.

**Induction:** Anesthetization, onset of general anesthesia.

**Infant:** Includes the neonatal period and extends through 12 months of age.

**Inhalation:** To draw a breathe, vapor, or gas into the lungs.

**Inspiratory Pressure:** An active positive pressure ventilatory maneuver in which a delivered volume of gas is given to a set peak level of pressure before passive expiration.

**Intubation, Intubate:** The act of placement of an endotracheal tube.

**Isotonic:** In this chapter, pertains to an intravenous (IV) solution with the same osmotic pressure as normal body fluid.

**Laryngospasm:** A spasm of the laryngeal muscles.

**Larynx:** The musculocartilaginous organ at the upper end of the trachea, below the root of the tongue, and part of the airway and vocal apparatus.

**Macroglossia:** An abnormally small tongue.

**Maintenance:** Stage of anesthesia in which relaxation of muscles and loss of sensation and consciousness are adequate for the performance of surgery.

**Micrognathia:** Refers to the jaw; abnormal smallness, particularly of the lower jaw.

**Neonatal Period:** The first 28 days of life.

**Newborn or "Newly Born":** Younger than 72 hours old.

**Occiput:** The back part of the skull.

**Opioid:** A synthetic narcotic.

**Parenteral:** Any route of administration for a medication other than alimentary; such as IV, subcutaneous, intramuscular, or mucosal.

**Pediatrics:** The medical science specific to the care of children and treatment of diseases that occur in childhood.

**Pharynx:** Refers to the passageway from the nasal and oral cavity to the larynx and esophagus.

**Postconceptual Age:** Postgestational age (number of weeks since birth) plus conceptual age (number of weeks at delivery).

**Premature Newborn:** Birth before 37 weeks of gestation.

**Rebreathing:** Inhalation of a gas or gases previously exhaled.

**Retrognathia:** When the mandible lies behind the frontal plane of the maxilla.

**Thermogenesis:** Heat production; nonshivering thermogenesis is a physiologic response of the newborn infant during periods of hypothermia with stimulation of the sympathetic catabolism of brown fat with release of energy in the form of heat. Brown fat is primarily located in the neck and chest of the infant.

**Trachea:** A cartilaginous tube from the larynx to the bronchi; windpipe.

**Ventilation:** The movement of air into and out of the lungs.

## ANATOMIC AND PHYSIOLOGIC CONSIDERATIONS

### Respiratory System

Newborns are usually obligate nose breathers and are prone to airway obstruction because the newborn has small nares, a large tongue, a small mandible, a short neck, and a large amount of upper airway lymphoid tissue.[1-3] Consequently, with ventilation of a newborn via a face mask, the nurse should be careful not to apply too much pressure over the soft tissue of the neck because pressure of this kind can easily obstruct the airway. Also, the epiglottis is at the level of the first cervical vertebra (C1) in the neonatal period.[3] By 6 months of age, the epiglottis usually has moved down to the level of C3, which makes oral breathing more feasible.[3]

The vocal cords of the newborn are situated at approximately the level of C4, as opposed to the location at C6 in the adult.[3] The shape of a child's larynx is that of an inverted cone, whereas in the adult it is more cylindric.[3] The opening of the vocal cords in the adult normally is the narrowest portion of the trachea, but in the newborn, the narrowest portion of the trachea is the cricoid cartilage.[3] The clinical implications of this anatomic feature are that if edema around the cricoid cartilage occurs, because of infection or mechanical irritation from an endotracheal tube (ETT), significant narrowing of the airway may occur. Also, because the cricoid ring is the narrowest part of the larynx, the size of the ETT to be used is limited. Until the mid 1990s, an uncuffed ETT was recommended in children younger than 8 to 10 years of age.[3] An uncuffed endotracheal tube should allow a slight leakage (20 to 25 cm of water pressure) around itself when positive pressure is applied with an anesthesia bag. With technologic advancement in cuffed ETTs, inhalational agents available to the anesthetist, and decreased use of prolonged postoperative positive-pressure ventilation, the current trend is toward more routine use of a cuffed ETT in small children.[3]

The epiglottis of the newborn is U-shaped, hard, short, and narrow; it is flatter in the adult. Generally, a straight laryngoscope blade is used for intubation in the postanesthesia care unit (PACU). Finally, the tracheal length is relatively short, particularly in the infant less than 6 months of age, which makes proper placement and taping critical to avoid bronchial intubation or accidental extubation. Once the endotracheal tube position is secured, the nurse should reconfirm the presence of bilateral breath sounds.

Newborns are diaphragmatic breathers because the ribs are situated horizontally in a cylindric thorax, which limits thorax expansion. Consequently, ventilatory efforts are the result almost entirely of the movement of the diaphragm. Because newborns are diaphragmatic breathers, they are susceptible to ventilatory problems, such as hypoventilation when excursion of the diaphragm is impeded. Hence, gastric distention caused by faulty bag and mask ventilation, improper positioning, or bowel obstruction can produce inadequate ventilation. In addition, the sternum and anterior rib cage are compliant, and the intercostal and accessory muscles of respiration are poorly developed. In the premature infant, the sternum may be retracted deeply with each inspiration, which may lead to impaired ventilation. The respiratory rate of infants and young children is faster for multiple reasons. The perianesthesia care provider should be knowledgeable of the normal values of respiratory rate for infants and children (Table 49-1).

As in the adult, the newborn's primary drive to ventilation is carbon dioxide. However, the secondary drive in the newborn is different from that of the adult. The newborn younger than 1 week of age responds to a reduction in the partial pressure of oxygen by transient hyperventilation followed by hypoventilation.[3,4] Therefore, hypoxia does not stimulate but rather depresses ventilation in the newborn.[3] This secondary drive response is aggravated by hypothermia, a condition that can occur in the PACU. The respiratory rate is higher and the tidal volume lower in infants and children. When ventilation equipment, such as a mask, is used, dead space is increased.

The respiratory control center in both full-term and premature infants may easily fatigue; therefore, ventilatory reaction to high carbon dioxide tensions or to low percentage of oxygen is not as rapid in the newborn.[3,4] As a result, the newborn may not be able to compensate for rapid changes in arterial blood gas levels. By 3 weeks of age, hypoxemia induces sustained hyperventilation, as in older children and adults.[3,4] Also, newborns and infants may breathe irregularly because of the lack of a mature respiratory center; periodic breathing is often seen in this age group.[3]

Endotracheal intubation is more widely used in pediatric anesthesia today (Table 49-2). The advantages of endotracheal intubation include decreased dead space, avoidance of laryngospasm and gastric distention, and prevention of aspiration. However, the incidence rate of postintubation edema from trauma and infection may be increased.

| Table 49-1 **Cardiovascular Age-Related Changes in Children** | | | | | | |
|---|---|---|---|---|---|---|
| Age | Respiratory Rate (per min) | Heart Rate Awake (bpm) | Heart Rate Asleep (bpm) | Heart Rate Exercise/Fever (bpm) | Systolic Blood Pressure (bpm) | Diastolic Blood Pressure (bpm) |
| Newborn | 45-60 | 100-180 (140) | 80-160 | <220 | 65 | 40 |
| 12 mo | 40 | 80-160 (120) | 70-120 | <200 | 95 | 65 |
| 3 y | 30 | 80-120 (100) | 60-90 | <200 | 100 | 70 |
| 6 y | 25 | 70-115 (100) | 60-90 | <200 | 90 | 60 |
| 12 y | 20 | 65-90 (80) | 50-90 | <200 | 110 | 60 |

Adapted from Motoyama E, Davis P: *Smith's anesthesia for infants and children*, ed 7, St Louis, 2006, Mosby.

## Table 49-2 Pediatric Airway Equipment

| Age | Weight (kg) | Internal Diameter (mm) | Length Oral (cm) | Length Nasal (cm) | Suction Catheter | LMA Size (#) | LMA Cuff Volume (ML) | Oral Airway Size* |
|---|---|---|---|---|---|---|---|---|
| Premature | 0.7-1.0 | 2.5 uncuffed | 7-8 | 9 | 5F | — | — | 000-00 |
| Premature | 1.0-2.5 | 3.0 uncuffed | 8-9 | 9-10 | 5F | — | — | 000 (30 mm) |
| Newborn | 2.5-3.0 | 3.5 uncuffed | 9-10 | 11-12 | 6F | 1 | 2-5 | 00 (40 mm) |
| 3 mo | 3.5-5.0 | 3.5 uncuffed | 10-11 | 12 | 6F | 1 | 2-5 | 0 (50 mm) |
| 3-9 mo | 5.0-8.0 | 3.5-4.0 uncuffed | 11-12 | 13-14 | 6F | 1.5 | 7 | 0 (50 mm) |
| 9-18 mo | 8.0-11.0 | 4.0-4.5 cuffed | 12-13 | 14-15 | 8F | 1.5 | 7 | 1 (60 mm) |
| 1.5-3 y | 11.0-15.0 | 4.5-5.0 uncuffed | 12-14 | 16-17 | 8F | 2 | 10 | 1 (60 mm) |
| 4-5 y | 15.0-18.0 | 5.0-5.5 uncuffed | 14-16 | 18-19 | 10F | 2 | 10 | 2 (70 mm) |
| 6-7 y | 19.0-23.0 | 5.5-6.0 uncuffed | 16-18 | 19-20 | 10F | 2.5 | 14 | 2 (70 mm) |
| 8-10 y | 24.0-30.0 | 6.0-6.5 cuffed | 17-19 | 24-25 | 10F | 2.5 | 14 | 3 (80 mm) |
| 10-11 y | 30.0-35.0 | 6.0-6.5 cuffed | 18-20 | 22-24 | 12F | 3.0 | 15-20 | 3 (80 mm) |
| 12-13 y | 35.0-40.0 | 6.5-7.0 cuffed | 19-21 | 23-25 | 12F | 3.0 | 15-20 | 3 (80 mm) |
| 14-16 | 45.0-55.0 | 7.0-7.5 uncuffed | 20-22 | 24-25 | 12F | 3.0 | 15-20 | 3 (80 mm) |

LMA, Laryngeal mask airway; ML, milliliters of air for inflation of cuff.

*Oral airway size as a guide. A quick method of determining oral airway size is by placing the airway along the side of the face. The oral airway length should extend from the lips to the angle of the mandible.

Adapted from Motoyama E, Davis P: *Smith's anesthesia for infants and children*, ed 7, St Louis, 2007, Mosby.

## Cardiovascular System

A multitude of factors influence changes in myocardial function in association with age. Normally, the respiratory rate and heart rate decreases with increasing age. Systolic and diastolic blood pressure increase with age and body size. The cardiovascular age-related changes for newborns, infants, and children is summarized in Table 49-1. The newborn heart function is at near peak ventricular function and therefore has little cardiac reserve. Heart rate plays a major role in determination of cardiac function.[3] The newborn is relatively unable to compensate for suboptimal conditions such as hypoxemia, acidosis, or myocardial depression.[3] With the advent of more sophisticated blood pressure monitoring devices, measurements in infants can be taken with greater accuracy. The pediatric patient ordinarily has the usual signs of impending shock or airway obstruction, yet if the problem is not rectified quickly, physiologic status deteriorates rapidly. Hence, the perianesthesia nurse should closely observe children for subtle changes in status; if abnormalities arise, prompt intervention is essential.

Fetal hemoglobin levels are high in the newborn. The hemoglobin level and number of blood cells are high at birth. However, remember that fetal hemoglobin in the newborn has a high oxygen affinity but a low ability to unload oxygen to the tissues. Values then decrease progressively until age 3 months. A physiologic anemia occurs at approximately 3 months of age from reduction in the fetal hemoglobin present at birth and primarily from a decrease in erythropoiesis production.[1,3] Also, increases in plasma volume have a dilutional effect on the hemoglobin level.[2] The rates then rise slowly to normal adult hemoglobin values. During this time, oxygen delivery to the tissues may not necessarily be compromised because the oxyhemoglobin dissociation curve shifts to the right and because concentrations of 2,3-diphosphoglycerate increase.[1,3] These changes help to ensure oxygen delivery to the tissues.

## Composition and Regulation of Body Fluids

The kidney of the newborn matures rapidly. In the neonate, renal function is characterized with obligate salt loss, slow clearance of fluid overload, and an inability to conserve fluid.[5] Consequently, newborns are intolerant of both dehydration and fluid overload. The newborn can conserve sodium to some degree despite a low glomerular filtration rate and limited tubular function[6]; however, premature infants are prone to hyponatremia and water overloading. Dehydration in the neonate of any gestational age has harmful effects on renal function.[3,6] Moreover, decreased renal function can delay the excretion of drugs primarily eliminated with renal clearance. At 20 weeks after birth,

| Table 49-3 | Formula for Hourly Maintenance Fluid Requirements in Infants and Children |
|---|---|
| Body Weight (kg) | Hourly Fluid Requirement |
| 0-10 kg | 4 mL/kg/h for each kg body weight |
| 10-20 kg | 40 mL + 2 mL/kg/h for each kg >10 kg |
| >20 kg | 60 mL + 1 mL/kg/h for each kg >20 kg |

Based on 1 mL of fluid per 1 kcal of caloric expenditure. Adapted from Motoyama E, Davis P: *Smith's anesthesia for infants and children,* ed 7, St Louis, 2006, Mosby.

maturation of glomerular filtration and tubular function is nearly complete.[4]

The blood volume of the newborn younger than 1 month of age is approximately 80 to 90 mL/kg. However, the blood volume of the premature newborn is as high as 100 mL/kg.[1] The estimated blood volume of an infant from 3 months until 3 years of age is 75 to 80 mL/kg. In children older than 6 years of age, the estimated blood volume approximates that of an adult (65 mL/kg in the adult female; 70 mL/kg in the adult male).

Water distribution in the various body compartments is markedly different among the premature newborn, the full-term newborn, the child, and the adult. Water distribution is significant because body water composition impacts the volume of drug distribution. Premature infants have the highest percentage of fluid in the extracellular fluid compartment. A progressive decrease in total body water and distribution to the extracellular fluid compartment is seen during the first year of life. Complete maturation of renal function occurs when the child reaches 2 to 3 years of age (Table 49-3).[4]

***Thermal Regulation.*** Newborns and infants are sensitive to heat loss because they have a relatively large body surface area, a relatively small amount of subcutaneous fat, poor vasomotor control, and a decreased ability to produce heat.[5] The primary mechanism of heat production in a neonate is nonshivering thermogenesis mediated by brown fat.[5] Shivering is of little significance to thermal regulation. When ambient temperature falls ($< 33°$ C), epinephrine is released by the sympathetic nervous system to activate thermogenesis. The preterm newborn needs a higher ambient temperature ($35°$ C) to minimize oxygen consumption.[7] Ordinarily, to

maintain a body temperature within normal limits, they metabolize brown fat, cry, and move about vigorously. Thus, newborns and infants respond to a cold environment by increasing their metabolism, which ultimately leads to an increase in oxygen consumption and the production of organic acids.

## PREMATURITY

A premature newborn is defined as birth before 37 weeks of gestation. The often labile condition of a premature neonate demands meticulous and vigilant perianesthesia care. Careful attention must be given to airway maintenance, medication dosage, fluid management, and temperature regulation. Premature infants and infants younger than 6 months of age are prone to airway obstruction and apneic episodes. Most infants in whom postanesthesia apnea develops are less than 46 weeks of postconceptual age. However, apnea has been reported in infants up to 60 weeks of postconceptual age.[4] In addition to apneic spells, pulmonary complications include hyaline membrane disease and bronchopulmonary dysplasia. Also, the premature neonate is immunocompromised and at greater risk for postoperative infection. In the sick premature neonate, the likelihood of blood transfusions, artificial ventilation, and the need for parenteral nutrition is greater.[4] The risk of apnea in the PACU may be decreased with intravenous administration of caffeine (10 mg/kg).[2] In neonates, the half-life of caffeine is between 37 to 231 hours.[2] By 4 months of age, the half-life of caffeine drops dramatically to approximately 6 hours and is similar to that of an adult. Also, several authors cite the initial discovery of xanthine derivatives, such as theophylline or aminophylline, as a respiratory stimulant that may be used to decrease the frequency of apneic episodes in the newborn.[2,8]

### Retinopathy of Prematurity

Retrolental fibroplasia is a fibrovascularization and scarring of the retina. Although this disease is associated with hyperoxia, a multitude of other risk factors may be involved, and the role of oxygen therapy is controversial.[2,3] The risk of this retinal disorder is to newborns, especially premature infants who are born before 36 weeks of gestation and weigh less than 1000 to 1500 g.[2] Vascularization of the retina is complete at approximately 44 weeks of gestation.[3] The extreme prematurity may be the single most important factor in the development of retinopathy of prematurity (ROP). The normal $PaO_2$ in neonates is between 60 and 80 mm Hg.

Oxygenation is recommended to be continuously monitored with pulse oximetry, and hyperoxia should be avoided. Thus, a saturation of 90% to 95% results in a $PaO_2$ in the range of 60 to 80 mm Hg.[9] In addition, the pulse oximeter probe must be placed on the right upper extremity or ear lobe, in case of a patent ductus arteriosus. Placement of two pulse oximeter probes on the premature infant may be helpful.[9] Moreover, when an arterial catheter is indicated, it also should be placed in the right upper extremity.

In susceptible patients who are exposed to a hyperoxic environment, blood gas tension should be measured and an oxygen analyzer used to confirm the oxygen concentration. What level of oxygenation, or what exact length of exposure time, may lead to the development of ROP is not known.[2] One must consider that attempts to prevent arterial hyperoxia and visual impairment must be tempered with the realization that unrecognized arterial hypoxemia can result in irreversible brain damage.

### Infant Respiratory Distress Syndrome

Infant respiratory distress syndrome (IRDS), once called hyaline membrane disease, is a severe disorder of the lungs of the newborn. The incidence rate of IRDS increases in premature infants. The basis of the pathogenesis of IRDS is insufficient surfactant levels.[10] Surfactant is beneficial for the following two functions: (1) reduction of surface tension so that less pressure is required to hold the alveoli open; and (2) maintenance of alveolar stability with adjustment of surface tension to changes in alveolar size. Insufficient surfactant levels increase surface tension at the alveolar air-liquid interface, resulting in alveolar collapse, an inordinate increase in the work of breathing, and impaired gas exchange. This impaired gas exchange results in hypoxemia and hypercarbia. Also, the pulmonary vascular resistance is increased and leads to hypoperfusion of pulmonary and systemic circulation. This hypoperfusion, along with hypoxemia, causes tissue hypoxia and metabolic acidosis. An increase in survival with a decrease in serious complications is associated with administration of surfactant into the lungs at birth.[2] As lung compliance improves, a progressive decrease in tidal volume and positive inspiratory pressure helps to prevent further lung injury.

Treatment for neonates with severe IRDS includes oxygen therapy, maintenance of intravenous fluids and nutritional support, temperature regulation, arterial blood gas monitoring, and laboratory sampling.[10] Extremely preterm infants and those with severe disease often need intubation during delivery room resuscitation or shortly after birth.[10] Also, intermittent positive-pressure mechanical ventilation with positive end-expiratory pressure may be necessary to ventilate the exceptionally stiff lungs of these neonates. Chronic air trapping in preterm infants can occur, and excessive inflation pressures must be avoided.[3]

## PEDIATRIC PERIOPERATIVE ANESTHESIA CONSIDERATIONS AND TECHNIQUES

Administration of anesthetic inhalational agents to the pediatric patient has progressed from the technique of open-drop ether, to the nonrebreathing technique, and finally to the pediatric circle system. The Bain system is the coaxial modification of the Mapleson D breathing circuit and was primarily used for the neonate and infant until the development of the pediatric circle system. The Bain system does not have valves and therefore offers the advantages of being light in weight with decreased resistance to breathing. Also, spontaneous ventilation is more easily permitted. A high fresh gas flow rate, two to three times the child's minute ventilation, is required with the Bain system, which is not as economic, particularly for older children. In the PACU, one might expect the pediatric patient's body temperature to be slightly lower in part because of the use of high fresh gas flow rates that lead to a decreased ability to conserve heat loss. Advantages of the pediatric circle system include conservation of potent inhalational agents and body heat, ability to retain humidity, and easy collection and scavenging of waste gases. The pediatric circle system has a smaller diameter than the adult tubing and has a low compression volume[1] that allows for accurate delivery of desired tidal volume. The pediatric circle system can safely be used for the neonate or infant who weighs less than 10 kg if ventilation is controlled.[8]

The laryngeal mask airway (LMA) is widely used for anesthesia in infants and children. The LMA is not a substitute for the endotracheal tube because of its inability to adequately seal off the trachea and therefore is not indicated for use in children at risk for pulmonary aspiration of gastric contents. However, it can maintain upper airway patency, especially in spontaneously breathing patients. The LMA can serve as an emergency airway when the patient cannot be adequately ventilated with a bag and mask system or when intubation is unsuccessful. Successful endotracheal intubation can occur with a Fasttrack LMA, which is designed to facilitate intubation in children with difficult airways, or through a standard

LMA with a fiberoptic bronchoscope. The appropriate LMA size, based on the patient's weight in kilograms, and guidelines for cuff volume inflation are included in Table 49-2.

Children 1 year of age and older benefit from anxiolytic premedication to decrease preoperative anxiety and modify behavioral changes after discharge.[11] Many anesthesia practitioners use oral midazolam premedication in pediatric patients 1 year of age and older, in whom a greater likelihood of uncontrollable separation anxiety exists. Also, midazolam can be given intramuscularly, intravenously, rectally, or intranasally as an alternative route of administration for pediatric premedicant.[12] However, the oral route is generally preferred unless preoperative intravenous access is available. Flumazenil is a competitive antagonist at the benzodiazepine receptor and is used as a reversal agent for midazolam.[9,13] Flumazenil may be administered intravenously at a dose of 10 µg/kg over 15 seconds. If necessary, the dose of flumazenil can be repeated up to four times, at 1-minute to 3-minute intervals. However, the total dose should not exceed 50 µg/kg.[9]

An anticholinergic drug, such as glycopyrrolate or atropine, may be given to protect against bradycardia, which can occur after succinylcholine administration or in association with induction of anesthesia. The most popular inhalation anesthetic agents used for pediatric anesthesia are halothane, sevoflurane, isoflurane, and desflurane. Halothane and sevoflurane are the most common induction inhalation agents. Once the child reaches the maintenance phase of general anesthesia, the anesthetist may switch to either isoflurane or desflurane. All inhalation anesthetic agents offer a relatively rapid emergence. Halothane was the most popular pediatric inhalation agent because of its relative freedom from airway irritation and smooth emergence. Sevoflurane offers a similar smooth induction with a rapid emergence with minimal potential risk and has somewhat replaced halothane in certain circumstances. Although sevoflurane and desflurane offer the advantage of rapid emergence, both may be associated with an increased incidence rate of agitation or delirium on emergence and into the PACU, especially in young children. To prevent emergence delirium, an analgesic base must be in place before this rapid emergence and transfer to the PACU.

Ketamine, a dissociative anesthetic, is sometimes used in pediatrics as an induction agent or for short procedures such as painful dressing changes that do not require muscle relaxation. Emergence time depends on route of administration and whether the drug was repeated during the operation. The most serious disadvantage to ketamine is a high incidence rate of emergence delirium, hallucinations, and possible psychosis. Also, nystagmus may occur. After the use of ketamine, the postanesthesia recovery area should be quiet and conducive to a slow peaceful emergence and recovery.[14] A premedicant with a tranquilizing drug, such as midazolam, can significantly reduce these side effects.[14] Ketamine has the advantage of providing analgesia as well, and caution should be used when additional narcotics are given in the PACU. For uncooperative children or patients with Down syndrome or mental retardation, an intramuscular injection of midazolam combined with ketamine may be helpful.[8]

The narcotic fentanyl can be given as a premedicant in the form of a lollipop called an Oralet (5 to 15 µg/kg).[8] Once the child becomes sedate, the Oralet naturally falls away from the child's mouth. The fentanyl Oralet had fallen out of favor because of the potential for children to associate it with candy. Fentanyl levels continue to rise during surgery and contribute to postoperative analgesia.

The introduction of the intravenous agent propofol has dramatically assisted the anesthesia provider with anesthesia with minimal recovery time. Propofol can be used in remote anesthetizing locations and provides deep sedation for painful or frightening procedures.[9,14] This drug has advanced anesthesia care for children in remote locations such as magnetic resonance imaging or during procedures or therapy for hematology and oncology.[15] Propofol provides rapid onset of action and quick emergence from anesthesia with minimal residual effects.[16] Earlier discharge and decreased recovery time are particularly notable when propofol is the only anesthetic agent used.[17] Maintenance of anesthesia can be accomplished through repeated dosing or continuous infusion.[15] Also, propofol has an antiemetic effect, and postoperative nausea is rare.

## POSTOPERATIVE CARE OF THE PEDIATRIC PATIENT

When children require hospitalization and surgery, an associated potential for organ system dysfunction of respiratory, circulatory, or neurologic function may be present.[4] The greatest vital organ dysfunction predominantly involves the respiratory system. The greatest focus of postoperative care initially should be directed towards respiratory function with the administration of supplemental oxygen delivery and maintenance of a patent airway.

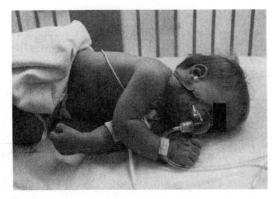

**Fig. 49-1**   An infant is transported to PACU in lateral position. *(From Motoyama E, Davis P: Smith's anesthesia for infants and children, ed 7, St Louis, 2006, Mosby.)*

Ultimately, nutritional support is the primary focus to meet the metabolic needs of the pediatric patient to promote healing and recovery from the stress of surgery and anesthesia. When the pediatric patient arrives in the PACU, the initial assessment should include identification of a patent airway; vital signs, including temperature, should be obtained and recorded. A humidified air-oxygen mixture (high-flow) should be administered and a safe environment secured before report from the anesthetist is given. In a restless child or in one with a history of seizure disorder, side rail pads may be used. The patient is placed in the lateral position in the operating room before transfer to PACU (Fig. 49-1). However, after an intraoral surgical procedure, the patient may be placed in the three-fourths prone position, more commonly known as the tonsillar position, to facilitate adequate drainage of secretions and blood.

During the report, dressings should be checked for drainage and the intravenous infusion line should be checked for patency and for assurance that the line is adequately secured. Also, children's teeth should be checked routinely on admission to the PACU, especially if loose teeth are present, and again before discharge. In the event of tooth loss, all teeth should be saved and given to the parents, if possible.

Over the years, anesthesia techniques have improved; with combined rapid-acting anesthetic agents, the pediatric patient usually arrives in the PACU awake and responsive, with good abdominal muscle tone. These patients are usually quickly responsive to verbal and tactile stimulation. However, about 10% to 15% of pediatric patients who are recovering from general anesthesia have hyperactive behavior. They need constant nursing care to prevent

injury to themselves because they are extremely restless and quite vocal. This agitation or excitement may be related to hypoxemia, the pharmacologic side effects of certain drugs, pain, or awakening in strange surroundings. Therefore, if a pediatric patient has hyperactive behavior, the perianesthesia nurse should assess the patient in the aforementioned areas before providing interventions.

### Psychosocial Considerations

The nurse must address issues of parental and child anxiety, which helps to lessen the stress on the child.[18] The parents should be allowed to be with the child as soon as is practical and preferably before the child awakens.[18] Remember that all surgical procedures and hospitalizations are extremely stressful for a family. When the pediatric patient emerges from anesthesia, the perianesthesia nurse should meet certain emotional needs of all children to facilitate positive outcomes of the perioperative experience. Explanations must be provided to the child in terms that can be understood. Also, the nurse should always be completely honest with the child. The developmental age of the child determines which areas are of greatest concern (Table 49-4). For example, infants can become distressed when physical needs are not met. With the type of surgery and the degree of emergence from anesthesia taken into consideration, the primary care giver should hold or rock the patient, if it is age-appropriate, or do both. This action usually relaxes the patient, and infants especially enjoy being swaddled in a warm blanket, cuddling, rocking, having the head or back rubbed, and hearing the voice of the nurse. In the infant younger than 6 months of age, the nurse is "mom."[3] Because the infant mimics facial expressions, the nurse should smile and use facial expressions of happiness when caring for all children. Another consideration is that the PACU is a strange environment for the child. Often, dolls, teddy bears, and other familiar objects from home are taken to surgery and arrive with the patient in the PACU. These special toys should remain with the child, especially during emergence, to help the child cope with the environmental change.

In the older infant and preschool child, stranger anxiety remains the greatest fear. This stage is a particularly vulnerable one in childhood development. Children at ages 2 to 3 years are at the stage of autonomy versus self doubt. They may exhibit independence that alternates with sudden dependence and the need for periodic cuddling and reassurance. Their greatest fears include separation from

| Table 49-4 | Classic Stages of Development Theories for Children | | |
|---|---|---|---|
| Theory Based on Age | Freud Psychosexual | Erikson Psychosocial | Piaget Cognitive |
| Infancy (0-1 y) | Oral | Basic trust | Sensorimotor (stages 1-5) |
| Toddlerhood (2-3 y) | Anal | Autonomy versus shame and doubt | Sensorimotor (stages V, VI) |
| Preschool (3-6 y) | Oedipal | Initiative versus guilt | Preoperational |
| School age (6-12 y) | Latency | Industry versus inferiority | Concrete operations |
| Adolescence (12-20 y) | Adolescence | Identity versus identity diffusion | Formal operations |

Adapted from Behrman R, Kliegman R, Jenson H: *Nelson's textbook of pediatrics*, ed 16, Philadelphia, 2000, Saunders.

parents, pain, physical harm, strange environments, and the unknown.[3] Often the only mechanism of self expression is crying. Negativism may be the child's means of demonstrating control; thus, "no" may actually mean "yes." Children of this age are prone to temper tantrums, ritualistic behavior, and breathholding spells. The perianesthesia nurse should be sure to differentiate apnea from breathholding spells when assessing the respiratory status of the patient. Three-year-old children are certainly special children, lovable but stormy. They are too young to use their own reason and become impatient at times. Therefore, the perianesthesia nurse must avoid criticism and provide acceptable behavior alternatives to the patient.

Between the ages of 3 and 6 years, the child begins to become independent. However, in the PACU, dependency can occur because of pain, course of disease, or immobilization. Guilt can occur when the child desires to remain dependent.[4] Consequently, the perianesthesia nurse should provide as much opportunity for independence as possible. The nurse can foster independence by allowing the child to select alternatives in care.

The ages of 6 to 12 years coincide with school entrance. These children are striving for approval when tasks are completed and usually do not tolerate failure because it promotes their sense of inferiority and inadequacy. The hospital environment is new to them, and the child may be unprepared to handle the situation and thus have difficulty with impulse control. Because children lose control when they are immobilized or ill, the nurse should allow as much individualization and self care as possible. The nurse should also encourage self expression and compliment the child on accomplishments during recovery from anesthesia. Also, remember that a child of this age has a vivid imagination and could easily distort reality.[4]

The adolescent years of ages 12 to 20 are a transitory time characterized by vacillations between dependence and independence, idealism and realism, confidence and uncertainty. The adolescent may experience anxiety over issues related to privacy, loss of control, autonomy, and competence. Privacy is of utmost importance to these patients; therefore, the adolescent's body should be covered as much as possible to prevent exposure and resulting embarrassment.

Remember that the individual perioperative experience of each child greatly impacts the success of future medical encounters. Addressing the developmental needs of the child and support of parental involvement can go a long way to meet the needs of the child and lead to a positive experience for the whole family. A preoperative program for elective surgical procedures that includes a tour of the postanesthesia care unit can help to reduce preoperative anxiety and minimize postoperative negative behaviors.

## Monitoring

Initially, monitoring in the PACU includes respiratory rate, blood pressure, pulse oximetry, electrocardiogram (ECG), fluid balance, and temperature control.[9] When the vital signs are obtained, the PACU values should be first compared with the preoperative and intraoperative recordings of vital signs. After the initial blood pressure is ascertained, particularly for outpatients, pulse oximetry monitoring may be all that is needed. The pulse oximeter is superior to clinical judgment in providing the earliest warning of a desaturation event.[19] The frequency in measurement of other physiologic parameters depends on the status of the patient and the surgical procedure.[2]

The rate and depth of ventilation should be monitored in the PACU. Respiratory depression occurs with greater frequency if muscle relaxants are used during general anesthesia. Because of the rapid ventilatory changes that can occur in the PACU, an oxygen saturation monitor should be used on all pediatric patients. A variable rate of fraction of inspired oxygen content delivery with supplemental oxygen can occur and is the result of delivery technique and patient depth of ventilation.

The most likely causes of respiratory failure in children with surgical disease include extrathoracic airway swelling and injury, thoracic dystrophy consistent with congenital disease or intraabdominal swelling, respiratory control abnormality such as occurs with congenital anomalies or drug induced, and loss of functional residual capacity that results in atelectasis.[4] The most common etiology involves the extrathoracic airway with swelling of the pharynx, larynx, or trachea. Infants and small children usually have a low incidence rate of postoperative atelectasis because crying from pain or awakening in an unfamiliar environment stimulates ventilation. Older children tend to remain in one position and not move about. They must be encouraged to cough and to perform the sustained maximal inspiration (SMI) maneuver to prevent atelectasis. If the pediatric patient is unable to perform the SMI maneuver, deep breathing should be encouraged.[14]

A change in heart rate of the pediatric patient is one of the first clues of impending physiologic dysfunction. The PACU provider should initially consider hypoxia as the most likely cause of bradycardia. In the PACU, the heart rate of infants and children is influenced by physical activity, fluid volume replacement, and the administration of atropine, glycopyrrolate, and anesthetic agents. Glycopyrrolate (Robinul), an anticholinergic atropine-like drug, may elevate the heart rate mildly, and not to the same degree as atropine. Also, crying, struggling, or pain can increase the heart rate.

In the event of respiratory dysfunction, the designated PACU attending anesthesia provider should be immediately notified. An ongoing airway assessment should be performed, and emergency airway management may be necessary. An oral airway must be of proper size and correct placement to relieve airway obstruction (Fig. 49-2). In addition, correct positioning of the patient assists the anesthesia provider to ventilate and intubate if necessary. However, correct positioning varies depending on the age of the child. For instance, children 6 years of age and older benefit from a folded towel or small pillow placed under the occiput in combination with extension of the head (Fig. 49-3).

This position has often been referred to as the "sniffing" position. In infants and younger children, in most instances, the size of the head is large relative to the trunk and hyperflexion of the neck occurs with lying flat on a bed. Further elevation of the occiput with a folded towel most likely hinders airway management. Mild flexion of the neck, with slight extension of the head, may be accomplished with placement of a shoulder roll. Optimal positioning of the head and neck should assist in maintenance of a patent airway and help to ensure successful bag-mask ventilation when indicated. Excessive elevation of the occiput or exaggerated extension of the head and neck should be avoided.

Reversal agents such as flumazenil (0.1 mg/kg, IV) and naloxone (1 to 10 µg/kg, titrated IV) should be readily available in the event of hypoventilation unresponsive to stimulation and to improve or reverse respiratory depression.[2,8] In addition, the anesthesia care team providers should be notified to offer additional assistance and follow-up care. Pressure cycled ventilators are used in the neonatal intensive care unit to prevent barotrauma.[1] With a pressure cycled ventilator, the risk of pressure trauma to the lungs is reduced by allowing the peak airway pressure to be varied to support optimum ventilation. However, a peak airway pressure alarm and limit must be maintained to decrease the risk of trauma to the lungs. Therefore, in the event of necessary postoperative mechanical ventilation of an infant, the settings is most likely be an intermittent mandatory ventilation rate of 20 to 40 bpm, with a peak positive inspiratory airway pressure set at approximately 20 to 24 cm $H_2O$.[1]

A patent IV line should be maintained in the postoperative care unit. In ambulatory surgery with short-stay recovery rooms, additional IV fluids may not be necessary if the intraoperative total fluid volume is sufficient to cover the initial postoperative recovery. However, in most instances, a patent IV line should be maintained throughout recovery. In the event of postoperative vomiting, additional fluids may be necessary. Initially, the care provider should administer an isotonic maintenance hourly fluid rate based on the kilogram weight of the patient. If the pediatric patient is moderately to severely ill, monitors for central venous pressure, ECG status, urine output, specific gravity, and an arterial line may be used.

The most likely indications for a central venous catheter include the need to monitor central venous pressure, cardiac surgery, inotropic drug administration, neurosurgery (with the potential risk of air embolism), major orthopedic

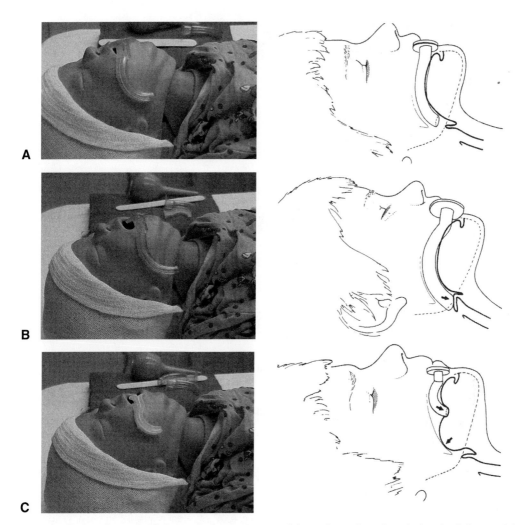

**Fig. 49-2** Identification of correct oral airway selection. **A,** Correct oral airway size can be estimated when tip of airway ends just cephalad to angle of mandible. **B,** If oral airway is too large, tip of oral airway may obstruct glottic opening by pushing down on epiglottis. **C,** If oral airway is too small, tip of airway may lead to obstruction by pushing down on base of tongue. *(Courtesy Department of Nurse Anesthesia, Virginia Commonwealth University. Also adapted from Cote' CJ, Ryan JF, Todres ID, et al: A practice of anesthesia for infants and children, Philadelphia, 2001, Saunders.)*

procedures (such as spinal fusion), and abdominal surgical procedures when massive fluid shifting or blood loss is expected.[9] The central venous pressure line may be inserted via the internal jugular, external jugular, subclavian, femoral, basilic, or axillary veins.[9] This line provides for information on blood volume and serves as an avenue for fluid replacement. Remember, all rapid infusions of blood products or fluids should be warmed before administration. A fluid or blood warming device should have a visible thermometer and an audible warning that indicates excessive heating greater than 42° C.[1] The arterial line, which is inserted through the umbilical (neonate) or radial artery, can measure blood pressure and heart rate and provide for instantaneous blood gas or laboratory sampling. The ECG results

provide information on cardiac rate and rhythm. In the event of circulatory abnormalities, blood pressure and pulse should be ascertained and recorded frequently. Any deviation in the cardiac or pulmonary physiologic parameters should be reported immediately to the attending physician.

Newborns and infants expend a great amount of energy maintaining alveolar ventilation, cardiac output, muscular activity, and an appropriate temperature. Because of these high-energy metabolic processes, glycogen and fat stores may be mobilized and depleted rapidly.[3,4] Consequently, cold, stress, pain, and increased muscle activity compound the need for adequate caloric intake in the PACU. In high-risk situations, plasma glucose concentrations should

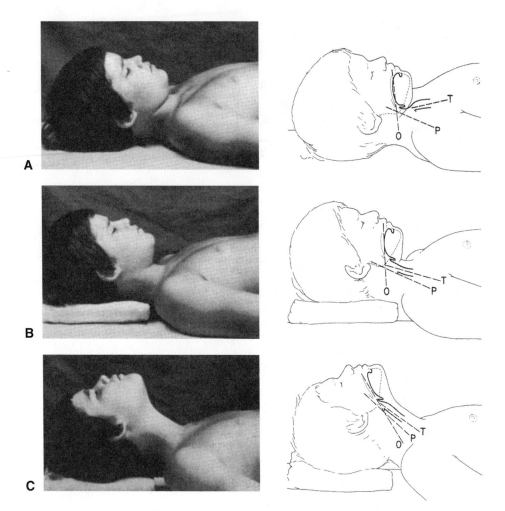

**Fig. 49-3**    Correct positioning for ventilation and tracheal intubation. **A,** When patient is lying flat on bed or stretcher, oral *(O)*, pharyngeal *(P)*, and tracheal *(T)* axes pass through three divergent planes. **B,** When folded sheet or towel is placed under occiput of head, pharyngeal *(P)* and tracheal axes align. **C,** With added extension of atlantooccipital joint, all three planes align to correct positioning for ventilation and tracheal intubation. *(Courtesy Department of Nurse Anesthesia, Virginia Commonwealth University. Also adapted from Cote' CJ, Ryan JF, Todres ID, et al: A practice of anesthesia for infants and children, Philadelphia, 2001, Saunders.)*

be monitored.[13] Also, the patient's clinical condition dictates the final fluid and electrolyte requirements incurred as a result of trauma or complications from surgery. A glucose-containing infusion can be used for postoperative maintenance fluid replacement for children in high-risk circumstances.[4,6,13] However, rapid infusion of glucose-containing solutions should be avoided.[13] During the administration of fluids, the perianesthesia nurse should ensure that the indwelling catheter is patent and not infiltrated and should use a constant infusion pump to facilitate the proper administration of the correct volume and rate of fluids. To prevent inadvertent overhydration, not more than one third of the day's maintenance intravenous fluid volume should be measured into the intravenous bag at any time.

Important considerations for fluid management of the pediatric patient include monitoring for hypervolemia or hypovolemia. Proper administration of fluids must be ensured. When attending to issues related to hydration, additional areas of assessment and monitoring can be helpful and include the following: (1) urine output, specific gravity, and osmolality; (2) temperature; (3) ECG status, pulse, and blood pressure; (4) hydration of the mucosa; (5) assessment of the fontanelle, in the newborn, for bulging or depression; and (6) blood loss. An accurate assessment of blood loss must be made during and after surgery because a small miscalculation of a few milliliters can have a serious impact on the total blood volume of an infant.

Permissible blood loss should be defined individually for each patient and is based on the patient's current medical condition, surgical procedure, and cardiovascular and respiratory function.[1] In healthy children with normal cardiovascular function, a lower hematocrit should be tolerated by increasing cardiac output when ventilation is not compromised. A higher inspired oxygen concentration should be provided. In the neonate or child with significant cardiac or pulmonary disease, initiation of blood loss replacement occurs earlier because of the patient's inability to compensate and because of a greater association with increased morbidity. Initially, ongoing blood loss is replaced with isotonic crystalloid at a ratio of 1:3; for every 1 mL of blood lost, 3 mL of isotonic fluid, such as lactated Ringer's solution, is given. When losses are high, the usual blood replacement is such that for each 1 mL lost, 1 mL of packed red blood cells is administered (1:1) to the patient. Alternatively, if a colloid solution is used, it is replaced at the same ratio (1:1) as that for blood products, 1 mL of 5% albumin per 1 mL of blood lost, until the patient's hematocrit level reaches a predetermined critical level that requires packed red blood cells.[3,4,9]

Dressings should be watched for excessive bleeding. Such bleeding should be reported at once to the attending physician because infants and small children have a narrower time span in which to compensate for loss. The leading cause of circulatory abnormalities in the postoperative pediatric patient is hemorrhage. The second most common cause of circulatory abnormality is plasma redistribution. Rarely is the cause cardiogenic in nature. Urine output and specific gravity may yield additional information on kidney function and volume expansion.

### Thermal Regulation in the Postanesthesia Care Unit

Hypothermia can delay emergence from anesthesia and prolong the stay in the postoperative care unit (see Chapter 53). Hypothermia can have a detrimental affect on termination of neuromuscular blockade, metabolic balance, coagulation, and ventilatory control.[13] If an infant or small child arrives in the PACU with inadvertent hypothermia, the nurse should assess the patient for: (1) vital signs (core temperature, pulse, and respiratory rate); (2) pulse oximetry waveform and saturation; and (3) the degree of emergence from anesthesia. If the patient has a delayed emergence from anesthesia, the nurse should protect the patient from aspiration of

gastric contents and from hypoventilation with positioning (see Fig. 49-1) and stimulation. Dysrhythmias and cardiovascular depression are associated with profound hypothermia. Also, hypothermia may lead to a detrimental effect on coagulation, ventilatory control, and metabolism.[13] A child with profound hypothermia should remain intubated and sedate. Continuous ECG monitoring is necessary until the core temperature reaches at least 35° C.[1] Finally, to avoid excess oxygen demand and acidosis associated with hypothermia, newborns and infants should be maintained in a neutral thermal environment in the PACU with the use of incubators, warm blankets, infrared heating lamps, warm-air heating blankets, or elevated room temperature when possible. Care should be taken to minimize environmental exposure during physical assessment, and the head should remain covered.

A word of warning is needed here. If a water mattress is used to rewarm the patient, the temperature setting should be no higher than 37° C and a layer of sheets between the mattress and the skin should aid as a barrier to prevent burns. Also, when a warm-air heating device is used, following the manufacturer's guidelines for proper use is imperative. Only the manufacturer's recommended blanket should be attached to the warm-air tube. Never place the warm-air heating tube between two blankets or directly blowing onto the infant or child because these actions have resulted in burns. Also, overly vigorous warming can cause a burn injury in infants.[2] Whichever rewarming method is used, the temperature of the device should be monitored frequently to prevent overwarming or injury. Records should be kept of core body temperature (rectal, esophageal, or tympanic), room temperature, and device temperature.

### Postoperative Pain Management and Regional Anesthesia

The primary goals of recovery from anesthesia include the ability of the child to maintain the airway and a return to baseline mental status. If the perioperative plan includes hospital admission, more flexibility is afforded in pharmacologic intervention when access to medical personnel is available. Issues related to intravenous hydration and pain management are critical when discharge is planned from the PACU.

The issues related to pain management for children have received increased attention in recent years.[20] Choices for pain management include parenteral narcotics, regional anesthesia, and even patient-controlled analgesia (PCA), depending on the age and maturity of the child. Alternative medications such as non-steroidal antiinflammatory drugs (NSAIDs), and oral or rectal acetaminophen in combination with parenteral narcotics may be helpful for control of pain in the postoperative period as well. In fact, ketorolac in combination with morphine PCA in children has been shown to provide superior analgesia.[21] The overall opioid dose and incidence rate of opioid side effects decreased when combined with NSAIDs.[21] Ketorolac is the only NSAID approved by the US Food and Drug Administration for parenteral use (0.5 mg/kg, IV/intramuscular [IM], every 6 hours [q 6 h]).[9,21] The recommended dosing of ibuprofen is 8 to 10 mg/kg, orally, every 6 hours. Acetaminophen is a nonopioid analgesic and antipyretic that can be given via the oral (10 to 15 mg/kg q 6 h) or rectal (20 mg/kg q 4 h) route.[2]

Opioids are administered for moderate to severe pain. Routes of administration for opioids include oral, rectal, oral transmucosal (under the tongue), intramuscular, intravenous, transdermal, epidural, subarachnoid, and subcutaneous.[13] The most common postoperative parenteral narcotics used in the pediatric population include meperidine (0.5 to 1 mg/kg, IV/IM, q 2 to 3 h) and morphine (0.05 to 0.1 mg/kg, IV/IM, q 2 to 4 h).[9] However, meperidine use is limited because its metabolite normeperidine can cause dysphoria, agitation, and seizures.[13] Meperidine in low doses can be used for the treatment of rigors and shivering in the PACU. As mentioned previously, ketamine has analgesic properties; therefore, preoperative or intraoperative use of ketamine lowers postoperative opioid requirements. Also, extreme caution should be noted with use of the more potent opioids fentanyl or sufentanil in the PACU for fear of severe respiratory depression. Fentanyl and its analogs can produce chest wall rigidity when administered as a bolus, which makes mask ventilation extremely difficult.

Patient-controlled analgesia has been successfully used for children as young as 6 years of age but requires the understanding and cooperation of the patient.[2,8,9,22] The inherent safety of PCA is based on the idea that a child who becomes too sleepy is not able to push the button. Family members and nurses must not push the button for the child. Usually, the PCA has a loading dose that is administered with the medical staff in attendance. By pushing a button, the child is able to deliver a precise opioid dose preprogrammed into the infusion pump. A minimum interval between dosing (a lock-out mechanism) and a maximum dose delivered over a set period of time are also preprogrammed to prevent

overdose. A basal metabolic rate may be preprogrammed into the infusion pump to prevent severe breakthrough pain. In some cases, a basal infusion rate is not suggested for fear of additive sedation and for prevention of respiratory depression. The overall total drug consumption with PCA use is less.[9,22,23] The potential complications associated with PCA include overdose from incorrect programming of parameters and, rarely, mechanical malfunction of the device.[8] The perianesthesia care provider should assess the child for side effects associated with opioids (nausea, vomiting, itching, and ileus). An order should be written to discontinue all previous pain medications. In addition, all pain medication orders should be written by the Anesthesia Pain Service.[9] Children should be instructed on the use of a pain score method, such as the Visual Analogue Scale, and a record for assessment of pain should be included on the vital sign sheet (Table 49-5). Pediatric PCA with morphine has been shown to provide better analgesia with lower pain scores in comparison with meperidine.[24] Morphine most likely is the opioid of choice for postoperative PCA use in children.[24] All nurses should be trained in PCA use.[9]

Regional anesthesia in children can dramatically improve pain management and lower general anesthesia requirements. The most common regional blocks in children include a penile block for circumcision, ilioinguinal block for hernia repair, spinal anesthesia (most often in the neonate who is very ill), and caudal epidural. Caudal block has been used for a variety of surgical procedures, including circumcision, inguinal herniorrhaphy, hypospadias repair, clubfoot repair, anal surgery, and other procedures below the umbilicus and of the lower extremities.[8] A caudal catheter can be threaded to the thoracic epidural space and can provide a thoracic level block for pain relief in small children (particularly useful for control of pain after open heart surgery).

## SELECTED POSTOPERATIVE CONCERNS IN PEDIATRICS

The most common reasons for postdischarge readmission to the hospital are protracted vomiting and surgery-related complications. Recovery room nursing care of children must include constant assessment of airway patency, ventilation, and circulatory stability.[13] In addition, common postoperative concerns in children include the potential for a postanesthetic excitement phase commonly referred to as emergence delirium, and pain management.[13] Because the pediatric patient does not have the physiologic reserves

**Table 49-5** Age-Specific Pain Measurement Tools for Children

| Name | Features | Age Range | Advantages | Limitations |
|---|---|---|---|---|
| Visual Analog Scale (VAS) | Horizontal 10-cm ruler; subject marks between "no pain" and "worst pain imaginable" | ≥ 8 y | Good psychometric properties; gold standard | Cannot be used in younger children or those with cognitive limitations |
| Faces scales (e.g., Wong, Baker, Oucher, Bieri, McGrath) | Subjects compare pain with line drawings of faces or photos of children | ≥ 4 y | Useful for younger ages than VAS | Choice of anchors affects responses (neutral versus smiling) |
| Color analog scales | Horizontal or vertical ruler, on which increasing intensity of red signifies more pain | ≥ 4 y | Useful for younger ages; converges to VAS at older ages | Cannot be used in toddlers or those with cognitive limitations |
| Behavioral or combined behavioral-physiologic scales (e.g., CHEOPS, OPS, FACS, NIPS) | Scoring of observed behaviors (e.g., facial expression, limb movement) and heart rate and blood pressure | Some work for any age; other tests are age-specific | Can be used even for infants and nonverbal children | Overrates fear in toddlers and preschool children; underrates persistent pain Some inconvenient measures that require videotaping and complex processing |
| Autonomic measures (e.g., heart rate, blood pressure, heart rate spectral analyses) | Scores changes in heart rate, blood pressure, or measures of heart rate variability (e.g., vagal tone) | All ages | All ages; useful for patients with mechanical ventilation | Nonspecific; changes can occur unrelated to pain |
| Hormonal-metabolic measures | Plasma or salivary sampling of hormones (e.g., cortisol, epinephrine) | All ages | Can be used at all ages | Nonspecific; changes can occur unrelated to pain Inconvenient; cannot provide real-time information |

Adapted from Behrman R, Kliegman R, Jenson H: *Nelson's textbook of pediatrics*, ed 16, Philadelphia, 2000, Saunders.

of the adult patient, when complications occur, serious untoward sequelae take place. Hence, the perianesthesia nurse must monitor for and react to any complication in a timely fashion.

## Laryngospasm

The larynx is the musculocartilaginous organ located at the upper end of the trachea and part of the airway and vocal apparatus. Laryngospasm is caused by sensory stimulation of the superior laryngeal nerve.[8] A forceful involuntary spasm of the laryngeal musculature occurs. In the PACU, laryngospasm can occur as the child awakens and is usually caused by blood or pharyngeal secretions draining toward the vocal cords.[25] For this reason, children are placed in the three-fourths prone position to promote drainage of oral secretions away from the vocal cords. Posterior oral pharyngeal suctioning can cause additional trauma and should be avoided after the child has been extubated.

Initial treatment of laryngospasm includes positive-pressure ventilation with an Ambu bag and mask (Fig. 49-4). The two-person bag-mask ventilation technique may provide superior ventilation in the event of significant airway obstruction or poor lung compliance. Intravenous lidocaine (1 to 1.5 mg/kg) also can be helpful.[8] If hypoxia develops and the laryngospasm is not relieved from positive-pressure ventilation via mask, then succinylcholine (0.25 to 1 mg/kg) should be given to allow control of ventilation with paralysis of the laryngeal muscles. Succinylcholine is a rapid-acting and ultrashort-duration depolarizing muscle relaxant and is useful in situations that necessitate rapid endotracheal intubation and securing of the airway. A word of caution is needed here because succinylcholine use is associated with many profound side effects such as cardiovascular complications, severe hyperkalemia, increased intraocular pressure, increased intracranial pressure, prolonged apnea, and injured muscle membranes with associated hyperkalemia and can be a trigger for myotonia, masseter spasm, and malignant hyperthermia. The U.S. Food And Drug Administration issued a "box" warning against the elective use of succinylcholine. Because of the combination of a box warning and an increased availability of alternative agents, succinylcholine use is limited to a clear indication such as emergency airway situations.

A perianesthesia care provider should have airway equipment and drugs readily available to facilitate reintubation if necessary. When laryngospasm develops, large intrathoracic pressures are generated. A negative-pressure pulmonary edema can result even in healthy children, and close attention should be given to further respiratory compromise after the laryngospasm has

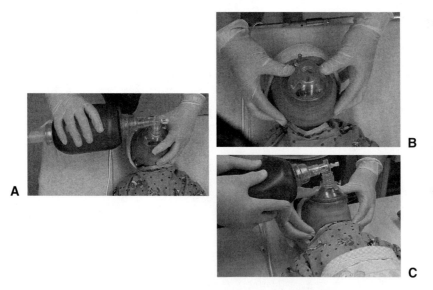

**Fig. 49-4    A,** One-person bag-mask ventilation. **B,** Two-handed technique for mask ventilation may be useful to improve mask fit and therefore ventilation when one-person bag-mask ventilation is difficult or inadequate. Modified jaw-thrust/chin-lift maneuver is shown. Tips of index and ring fingers are applied to ascending ramus of mandible behind pinnae of ear. Thumbs apply downward pressure to facemask to ensure tight seal. Mouth should open, which helps to maintain airway patency. Soft structures of airway should be avoided. **C,** One person uses both hands to open airway and maintain tight mask-to-face seal while assistant compresses ventilation bag. *(Courtesy Department of Nurse Anesthesia, Virginia Commonwealth University.)*

resolved.[8,26] Positive pressure ventilation is used to treat pulmonary edema after a laryngospasm.

## Airway Obstruction

In the PACU, every pediatric patient, particularly children who have been intubated during anesthesia, should be monitored for signs of airway obstruction. Postintubation croup is caused by glottic or tracheal edema. When laryngeal swelling occurs, the diameter of the airway of the infant or small child can become significantly reduced; in fact, 1 mm of edema in the infant's trachea at the cricoid level decreases the diameter of the airway by 75%. The symptoms of laryngeal obstruction, in order of appearance, are croupy cough, hoarseness, inspiratory stridor, and aphonia. These symptoms are accompanied by increasing restlessness, tachypnea, use of accessory muscles of respiration, retraction of the suprasternal notch and intercostal spaces, and drawing in of the upper abdomen.[2] If these symptoms appear, the perianesthesia nurse should act immediately to relieve the obstruction, administer supplemental oxygen, and send someone to notify the PACU anesthesia provider. The progression of these symptoms can be rapid.

Treatment of postintubation croup involves use of a high-humidity atmosphere that is oxygen-enriched. Nebulized racemic epinephrine (0.5 mL of a 2.25% solution in 2.5 mL of normal saline solution) has been useful in the treatment of postintubation croup. Also, corticosteroids such as dexamethasone (Decadron, 0.2 mg/kg, IV) have been useful to decrease the laryngeal inflammation associated with other causes of croup.[7] However, corticosteroid use for postintubation croup remains controversial.[8] If laryngeal edema is allowed to progress, the patient may need reintubation, although this occurs rarely.

## Nausea and Vomiting

Nausea and vomiting (see Chapter 29) is a leading cause of delayed discharge from the PACU. Children who are undergoing tonsillectomy, strabismus, or orchiopexy surgery are at greater risk.[27] The incidence rate of postoperative nausea and vomiting (PONV) varies; anything that can be done to minimize PONV wins the approval of the patient, the parents, and the staff. Early or forced administration of liquids before the child is ready may cause vomiting. If a greater likelihood of postoperative nausea or vomiting exists, administration of prophylactic antiemetics is best whenever possible.[14] In most cases, vomiting can successfully be treated with the use of phenothiazines (rectal promethazine, 0.5 mg/kg), metoclopramide (0.15 mg/kg, IV), or the newer serotonin-3 antagonist ondansetron (0.05 to 0.15 mg/kg, IV; maximum dose, 4 mg). Phenothiazines and metoclopramide can cause dystonic reactions that may be treated with diphenhydramine (0.5 to 1 mg/kg, IV).[13] Ondansetron (Zofran) is safe to use without significant side effects, is approved for use in patients 1 month of age and older, and has been shown to be the most effective drug once PONV is present.[14] In the absence of an IV, ondansetron can be given under the tongue for quick absorption without the need for swallowing.[2] Ondansetron may be less likely given as a preemptive antiemetic because of its higher cost. Propofol used alone for sedation has antiemetic properties, and when it is combined with other drugs for maintaining anesthesia, it may decrease PONV.[27]

## Malignant Hyperthermia

Although a detailed discussion on malignant hyperthermia (MH) is presented in an alternate chapter of this text, a brief description of the condition is given here. The incidence rate of MH is approximately 1:3000 to 1:15,000 in children, in comparison with 1:40,000 to 1:100,000 in adults.[2,3,9,28] Halogenated inhalation anesthetic agents, such as halothane, and the depolarizing muscle relaxant succinylcholine trigger this genetically determined condition. The pathophysiology of the condition centers on the enhanced release and diminished reuptake of calcium in the skeletal muscle, which cause sustained skeletal muscle contraction and ultimately, profound hyperthermia. The muscle cells convert to anaerobic metabolism, and lactic acidosis ensues. Ultimately, muscle cell breakdown occurs. The drug dantrolene sodium effectively treats MH with inhibition of further release of calcium in the skeletal muscle. In most instances, MH occurs in the operating room; however, a patient may first be seen with the disorder in the PACU, or the patient with successfully treated MH may have an exacerbation of MH symptoms later in the recovery process.

The earliest clinical feature of MH is a rising end-tidal carbon dioxide level ($ETCO_2$); however, this feature is not readily apparent in the PACU unless the patient is intubated and an $ETCO_2$ level is being monitored. Therefore, in most cases of MH in the PACU, the first clinical sign is tachycardia with or without other dysrhythmias; tachypnea and a profound increase in tidal volume are then observed in the patient with spontaneous breathing. Generalized muscle rigidity may or may not occur. Hyperthermia is often a late sign. Additional signs include arrhythmias, hypertension, sweating, and mottled skin. Diagnosis of MH in the PACU may be difficult because this syndrome has a variable presentation. For example, fever is often an inconsistent and late sign.

Blood chemistry studies reveal an elevated potassium level and an initially elevated calcium level before it falls. Arterial blood gas levels show a severe fall in bicarbonate and pH and an elevated $PaCO_2$. The $PaO_2$ may be normal, depending on the use of controlled ventilation and the fraction of inspired oxygen content ($FiO_2$). Serum myoglobin, creatine kinase, lactic dehydrogenase, and aldolase levels usually rise.

To facilitate a reversal of this condition, the perianesthesia nurse must understand the pathophysiology of MH and should know exactly where the MH emergency cart is located. If a patient appears to be have developing MH, the nurse should send for help immediately. The nurse should start to assist ventilation of the patient with high-flow 100% oxygen and check to be sure the intravenous line is patent. Once the appropriate personnel arrive, more than one person should mix the dantrolene sodium (20 mg/60 mL of sterile water). A note of warning is needed to ensure that the sterile water does not contain preservatives and that much sterile water will be used. The usual starting dose of dantrolene sodium is 2.5 mg/kg, IV. This dose can be repeated up to 10 mg/kg over 45 minutes or until the patient's condition stabilizes and temperature is reduced.

Once the protocol is initiated, the need for endotracheal intubation and active cooling with frequent temperature monitoring begins. Recognition and treatment of arrhythmias along with correction of the associated acidosis and electrolyte imbalance (hyperkalemia) should be anticipated. Most likely an arterial line, nasogastric tube, and three-way Foley catheter is placed. The most successful outcome occurs when the syndrome is identified and treated early.[8,28] The child is transferred to a pediatric intensive care unit usually for at least 24 hours for close monitoring and continued therapy.

## SPECIAL CONSIDERATIONS

### Otolaryngologic Surgery

The most common surgical procedures performed in pediatrics involve the ear, nose, and throat (ENT). The leading cause of obstructive sleep apnea (OSA) and hypoventilation in children is adenotonsillar hypertrophy.[13] Other anatomic factors that lead to OSA include micrognathia, retrognathia, or macroglossia. Also, morbid obesity in children or a congenitally small airway narrows the nasopharynx. Chronic OSA can disrupt sleep and breathing patterns and lead to impaired daytime

performance and more serious complications such as polycythemia, growth failure, heart failure, pulmonary hypertension, and arrhythmias.[13]

Pediatric patients who have tonsillectomies and other operations on the pharynx, larynx, and esophagus need intensive PACU care because the airway can become obstructed after surgery as a result of surgical manipulation and bleeding. When the patient is admitted to the PACU, the laryngeal and pharyngeal reflexes should be present. The patient should be placed in the tonsillar position, three fourths prone, with the arm and leg flexed and the head turned to the side. This position improves drainage of secretions and blood from the mouth and is helpful in prevention of possible aspiration or laryngospasm. The patient should be kept in this position until the gag reflex has returned completely.

Nausea with vomiting can lead to bleeding and airway compromise in the recovery room. During report, the nurse should note whether a perioperative antiemetic was given. The combination of propofol and ondansetron effectively reduces the incidence of vomiting in children after tonsillectomy. Before emergence and extubation in the operating room, common practice is for the surgeon to suction gastric content and the oral pharynx and to assess for hemostasis. After the child has been extubated, avoidance of deep oral pharyngeal suctioning is best to prevent trauma and bleeding.

### Trauma Victim

Special consideration should be considered with airway management for the child with head or cervical spine injury. When assisted airway support is needed to relieve airway obstruction in the PACU, the jaw-thrust maneuver is indicated to open the airway (see Figs. 49-3 to 49-5).[2,29] An anesthesia provider should be notified at once to offer assistance and airway management. If a second care provider is available, assistance should be placed with emphasis on immobilization of the cervical spine with maintenance of a neutral alignment. The head tilt-chin lift is contraindicated in the presence of cervical spine injury.[29] Once the airway is controlled, a semirigid cervical collar, spine board, linen rolls, and tape can be used to immobilize the child. To support oxygenation and ventilation, intubation may be indicated. Inline traction and spine immobilization are necessary during mask ventilation, laryngoscopy, intubation, and transport.

## DISCHARGE FROM THE PACU

With the advancement in pharmacologic drugs and inhalational agents for general anesthesia,

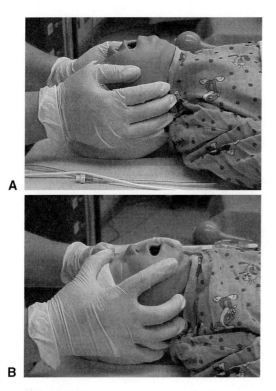

**A**

**B**

**Fig. 49-5   A,** Jaw thrust maneuver. One must elevate the jaw by placing the tips of the index and ring fingers along the ramus of the mandible (on the bony prominences), while avoiding the soft structures overlying the larynx and glottic opening, which potentially can lead to airway obstruction. **B,** Spine immobilization with airway opening in infant with potential head and neck trauma. Combined jaw thrust and spinal stabilization maneuver. *(Courtesy Department of Nurse Anesthesia, Virginia Commonwealth University.)*

rapid recovery with decreased side effects has led to earlier discharge from the PACU for children. Certain criteria must be met for safe transition from the PACU to a short-stay recovery unit or hospital ward; however, the goals of recovery vary depending on the discharge location planned for the patient.[9] In evaluation of a child for possible discharge from the PACU, the perianesthesia nurse should observe for each of the following: (1) an alert and easily arousable child; (2) protective airway reflexes; (3) strong muscle strength; (4) oxygen saturation maintained above 95% on room air or at the baseline preoperative level; (5) normothermia; (6) pain under control; (7) absence of vomiting; (8) no sign of active bleeding; and (9), stable vital signs. Children continue to recover in an ambulatory or short-stay recovery unit after outpatient procedures.

Steward developed a simplified scale to determine when pediatric patients can be discharged from the PACU (Table 49-6).[2,30] This scale scores airway, consciousness, and movement,

**Table 49-6   Steward's Postanesthesia Recovery Score**

| Criterion | Score |
|---|---|
| **CONSCIOUSNESS** | |
| Awake | 2 |
| Responding to stimuli | 1 |
| Not responding | 0 |
| **AIRWAY** | |
| Coughing on command or crying | 2 |
| Maintenance of good airway | 1 |
| Airway requires maintenance | 0 |
| **MOVEMENT** | |
| Limbs move purposefully | 2 |
| Nonpurposeful movements | 1 |
| Not moving | 0 |

From Steward D: A simplified scoring system for the postoperative recovery room, *Can Anaesth Soc J* 22(1):111-113, 1975.

from 0 to 2. The maximal number of points is 6. Discharge depends on the overall functional status of the child. However, after procedures involving the airway, such as tonsillectomies, the child may stay in the hospital for a longer period of time, such as the 23-hour admission for observation.

Factors that delay postoperative recovery in children include residual anesthetic or neuromuscular blockade, hypothermia, hypoxemia, acid-base imbalance, hypocarbia, hypercarbia, hypovolemia, and elevated intracranial pressure.[2] Forcing fluids by mouth to facilitate discharge is never advisable, and indeed, one should wait until the child vocalizes a desire to decrease the likelihood of vomiting. Also, a delay of discharge until the child has voided is not necessary. The anesthesia provider should be notified to assess the child; write the discharge notes, including any findings or recommendations for postoperative care; and sign for discharge from the PACU. The parents or guardian must be instructed concerning discharge care. A phone number should be included with written information on what to do in case of an emergency for further clarification of postdischarge questions or concerns.

## SUMMARY

Skilled nursing care is vital to a smooth perioperative transition of the pediatric patient. In the PACU, the nurse must be able to provide an intensive care unit level of care to the point of assisting in a full resuscitation. In addition, the nurse must be skilled in airway assessment and the provision of basic airway support and management, in the use of oral and nasal airways, bag-to-mask ventilation, and assistance with intubation and extubation as needed. Skilled nursing care includes dealing with emergence delirium, assessing and treating pain, assisting with basic and advanced life support measures, and probably most importantly, being comfortable in providing an age-appropriate level of comfort and reassurance to a frightened child.

## REFERENCES

1. Aker J: Pediatric anesthesia. In Nagelhout J, Zaglaniczny K editors: *Nurse anesthesia*, ed 3, St. Louis, 2005, Saunders.

2. Gregory G: *Pediatric anesthesia*, ed 4, New York, 2002, Churchill Livingstone.

3. Motoyama E, Davis P: *Smith's anesthesia for infants and children*, ed 7, St Louis, 2006, Mosby.

4. Miller R: *Anesthesia*, ed 6, New York, 2005, Churchill Livingstone.

5. Stoelting R, Dierdorf S: *Anesthesia and coexisting disease*, ed 4, New York, 2003, Churchill Livingstone.

6. Ellis D: Regulation of fluids and electrolytes in infants and children. In Motoyama EK, Davis PJ editors: *Smith's anesthesia for infants and children*, ed 7, St Louis, 2006, Mosby.

7. Longnecker D, Murphy F: *Dripps/Eckenhoff/Vandam introduction to anesthesia*, ed 9, Philadelphia, 1997, Saunders.

8. Morgan G, Mikhail M, Murray M: *Clinical anesthesiology*, ed 4, New York, 2006, Lange Medical Books.

9. Badgwell JM: *Clinical pediatric anesthesia*, Philadelphia, 1997, Lippincott-Raven Publishers.

10. Berman S: *Pediatric decision making*, ed 4, St Louis, 2003, Mosby.

11. Eckhenhoff J: Relationship of anesthesia to postoperative personality changes in children, *Am J Dis Childhood* 86:587-591, 1953.

12. Walbergh E: Plasma concentrations of midazolam in children following intranasal administration, *Anesthesiology* 74(2):233-236, 1991.

13. Behrman R, Kliegman R, Jenson H: *Nelson's textbook of pediatrics*, ed 16, Philadelphia, 2000, Saunders.

14. Steward D: *Manual of pediatric anesthesia*, ed 5, New York, 2001, Churchill Livingstone.

15. Martin L, Pasternak L, Pudimat M: Total intravenous anesthesia with propofol in pediatric patients outside the operating room, *Anesth Analg* 74:609-612, 1992.

16. Westrin P: The induction dose of propofol in infants 1-6 months and children 10-16 years of age, *Anesthesiology* 74(3):455-459, 1991.

17. Hannallah R: Propofol: effective dose and induction characteristics in unpremedicated children, *Anesthesiology* 74(2):217-219, 1991.

18. Bevin J, Johnston C, Tousignant G: Preoperative parental anxiety predicts behavioral and emotional responses to induction of anaesthesia in children, *Can J Anaesth* 37:177-182, 1990.

19. Cote C: A single-blind study of combined pulse oximetry and capnography in children, *Anesthesiology* 74(6):980-988, 1991.

20. Mubroy J: Safety and efficacy of alfentanil and halothane in paediatric surgical patients, *Can J Anaesth* 38(4):445-449, 1991.

21. Sutters K, Shaw B, Gerardi J: Comparison of morphine patient-controlled analgesia with and without ketorolac for postoperative analgesia in pediatric orthopedic surgery, *Am J Orthop* 28(6):351-358, 1999.

22. Vesely C: Pediatric-patient-controlled analgesia: enhancing the self-care construct, *Pediatr Nurs Rev* 21(2):124-128, 1995.

23. Gillespie J, Morton N: Patient controlled analgesia for children: a review, *Paediatr Anaesth* 2:51-59, 1992.

24. Vetter T: Pediatric patient-controlled analgesia with morphine versus meperidine, *J Pain Symptom Manage* 7(4):204-208, 1992.

25. Roy W, Lerman J: Laryngospasm in paediatric anaesthesia, *Can J Anaesth* 35:93-98, 1988.

26. Lee K, Downes J: Pulmonary edema secondary to laryngospasm in children, *Anesthesiology* 59:347-349, 1983.

27. Barash P, Cullen B, Stoelting R: *Handbook of clinical anesthesia*, ed 5, Philadelphia, 2005, Lippincott.

28. Hopkins P: Malignant hyperthermia: advances in clinical management and diagnosis, *Br J Anaesth* 85:118, 2000.

29. American Heart Association: *Pediatric advanced life support, circulation*, parts 11-14, 2005; 112:IV-156-200, 2005, available at http://www.circulationaha.org. Accessed February 7, 2007.

30. Steward D: A simplified scoring system for the post-operative recovery room, *Can Anaesth Soc J* 22:111-113, 1975.

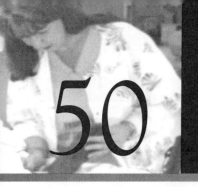

# 50

# CARE OF THE GERIATRIC PATIENT

*Kimberly F. Taylor, PhD*
*E. Ayn Welleford, PhD*

Although chronologic age is an inadequate marker of aging, other markers at present are much too unwieldy and difficult to assess. Many different chronologic markers are used in governmental and programmatic determinations (i.e., age 40 years for age discrimination determination, 50 years for AARP membership, and 65 plus years for Social Security). Therefore, no one definition of old-age, elderly, or geriatric is accepted. Because no biomarkers exist per se, a chronologic definition of when old age begins is difficult because individuals age at different rates than is reflected by chronologic age. Some individuals who are more prudent in lifestyle choices may have little physiologic decline or age-related comorbidities; whereas others may have multiple comorbidities, perhaps at an even earlier age. The growing complexity and diversity of the aging population mandates a holistic interdisciplinary approach to care to move beyond a simplistic chronologic marker toward a more accurate functional assessment. Irrespective of physiologic status, however, individuals aged 65 years or older are generally considered elders.

This geriatric population constitutes 34 million people, which is approximately 13% of the population; projections suggest that by 2030, 69 million individuals will be over the age of 65 years, comprising 19% of the population.[1] This number represents about 25% of surgical patients,[2] which presents a challenge to the perianesthesia nurse because 80% of patients older than 65 years of age have at least one or more chronic diseases when they are seen for anesthesia and surgery.[3]

Care of the geriatric patient is particularly important in the postanesthesia care unit (PACU) because of the normal physiologic changes that occur with aging that may be compounded by multiple comorbid conditions. These conditions include congestive heart failure, insufficient oxygenation of the blood, improper elimination of carbon dioxide, fluid and electrolyte imbalance, diabetes and the associated complications, drug toxicity, nerve palsies, and psychologic changes. Successful anesthesia care of the geriatric patient is highly dependent on the knowledge of the normal physiologic alterations associated with normal aging and the effects of anesthesia on the aged patient. Therefore, the focus of this chapter is primarily on the morphologic changes associated with aging and their translation to functional status, especially of the cardiovascular system.

## PHYSIOLOGIC AGE-RELATED CHANGES

### Cardiovascular System

Some obvious clinical pathologies impact perianethesia decision making and postanesthesia outcomes. Of all of the body systems, the cardiovascular system exerts the most influence on anesthesia and general health outcomes.[4] Annually, more than 1 million surgeries are complicated by adverse cardiac outcomes, such as postsurgical myocardial infarction or death from cardiac disease.[4] This risk can be reduced with a thorough preoperative interview/assessment that examines functional capacity and existing comorbidities and the current treatment regime.[4]

***Cardiovascular Risk Assessment.*** Preoperative risk assessment is an important component in minimization of perioperative morbidity and mortality. This assessment is best achieved through the work of an interdisciplinary team that consists of the patient, the primary care physician, the surgeon, and the anesthesia professional. In addition, geriatric training and expertise is essential to the quality care of geriatric patients. This assessment relies on the evaluation of the interaction of clinical markers, functional capacity, type of surgical procedure, and age. Once risks are identified, measures should be used to minimize the risks before surgery and to improve immediate periprocedural outcomes and long-term clinical outcomes.

## Box 50-1   Clinical Predictors of Perioperative Cardiovascular Risk

| | |
|---|---|
| Major | Unstable coronary syndromes, decompensated CHF, significant arrhythmias, severe valvular disease |
| Intermediate | Mild angina pectoris, myocardial infarction (> 30 d old), compensated or previous CHF, diabetes mellitus |
| Minor | Advanced age, abnormal ECG results, rhythm other than sinus, low functional capacity, history of stroke, uncontrolled systemic hypertension |

CHF, Congestive heart failure; ECG, electrocardiogram.

**Clinical Markers.**  Some markers act as clinical predictors of perioperative cardiovascular risk. These markers can be categorized by the perioperative risk associated with them (Box 50-1) as major, intermediate, and minor perioperative risk.[5]

**Functional Capacity.**  Exercise tolerance in daily life, which can range from habitual physical activity to participation in regular exercise to improve fitness, is the best indicator of the quality of biologic age. It is one of the most important predictors of perioperative outcomes in geriatric patients.[5,6] Poor exercise tolerance reflects low functional capacity and greater severity of disease. Functional status is usually reflected in metabolic equivalent (MET) levels. One MET corresponds to a resting oxygen consumption of 3.5 mL/kg/min. MET scores are multiples of resting metabolism, which are used as a point of reference to describe the oxygen demands of any activity.[7] Box 50-2 provides examples of MET ratings of activities. Functional status can be ascertained during the preoperative screening. Questions concerning daily activities, such as house cleaning, vacuuming, walking, and stair climbing, and any participation in regular exercise should provide adequate information for a subjective assessment of the patient's functional status.[8] Objective assessment can be made via exercise testing. Patients who are unable to regularly meet a 4 MET demand have an increased perioperative cardiac risk.[9]

**Surgery-specific Risk.**  The type of surgery coupled with the degree of hemodynamic stress incurred during the surgery are the major determining factors of perioperative risk.[5,6] Emergency surgeries are particularly high risk, especially in the geriatric patient. Other high-risk surgeries include vascular, cardiac, abdominal, and thoracic surgeries.[10] Box 50-3 categorizes surgery-specific risk according to the incidence rate of cardiac death and nonfatal myocardial infarction for noncardiac surgical procedures.

**Age as a Risk Factor.**  Because no distinct biological or clinical markers indicate when old age has been reached or when a patient is elderly, clarification of age as a risk factor for increased perioperative cardiovascular risk it is difficult. However, with increasing age is an increase in the number of comorbid conditions. Specifically, a geriatric patient is more likely to have more than two comorbid conditions. The Guidelines for Perioperative Cardiovascular Evaluation for Noncardiac Surgery of the American College of Cardiology and the American Heart Association[10] are unclear as to the significance of age as an independent risk factor. However, these same guidelines list emergency surgery in the elderly as high risk and also state that advanced age is a "special risk."

## Box 50-2   Estimated Energy Requirements for Various Activities

| | |
|---|---|
| 1 MET | Can you take care of yourself? |
| | Eat, dress, or use the toilet? |
| | Walk around the house? |
| | Walk a block or two on level ground (2-3 mph)? |
| 4 METs | Perform light housework, such as dusting or dishes? |
| | Climb a flight of stairs or walk up a hill? |
| | Walk on level ground at 4 mph? |
| | Do heavy housework such as scrubbing floors and lifting or moving furniture? |
| | Engage in recreational activities such as bowling, golf, or dancing? |
| >10 METs | Participate in strenuous sports like swimming, singles tennis, basketball, or skiing? |

Adapted from the Duke Activity Status Index[8] and AHA Exercise Standards.[9]

| Box 50-3 | Cardiac Risk* Stratification for Noncardiac Surgical Procedures |
|---|---|

*High (reported risk, ≥ 5%)*
  Emergency major operations
  Aortic, major, and peripheral vascular surgery
  Extensive surgical procedures with large volume shifts or blood loss
*Intermediate (reported risk, ≥ 1% and < 5%)*
  Intraperitoneal and intrathoracic surgery
  Carotid endarterectomy
  Head and neck surgery
  Orthopedic surgery
  Prostate surgery
*Low (reported risk, < 1%)*
  Endoscopic procedures
  Superficial biopsy
  Cataract surgery
  Breast surgery

*Combined incidence rate of cardiac death and nonfatal myocardial infarction. Adapted from Eagle KA, et al.[10]

**Table 50-1**   Changes in Cardiovascular Physiology in Healthy Individuals Between Ages 20 and 80 Years*

| | |
|---|---|
| LV end-diastolic volume | ↑20% males; ↔ females |
| LV end-systolic volume | ↑20% males; ↔ females |
| Ejection fraction | ↔ |
| Stroke volume | ↑20% males; ↔ females |
| Heart rate | ↓10% |
| Cardiac output | ↔males; ↓ 15% females |
| Stroke work | ↑15% |
| Early diastolic filling rate | ↓50% |
| Systolic arterial pressure | ↑15% |
| Systemic vascular resistance | ↔males; ↓ 45% females |

*Adapted from Eagle KA, et al.[10]
LV, Left ventricular; ↔, no change; ↑, increase; ↓, decrease.

With that in mind, age should certainly be considered as a significant factor in evaluation of a patient and assessment of risk before surgery.

### Age-related Cardiovascular Changes

**Heart.** In the heart are many cellular and biochemical changes[11-13] associated with aging. These changes include altered growth-controlling factors, impaired excitation-contraction coupling, impaired calcium homeostasis, increased myocyte apoptosis, and an increase in atrial natriuretic peptide secretion.

As a result of these age-related biochemical and molecular changes, a number of morphologic changes manifest as changes in cardiac function (Table 50-1). Cardiac aging results in a number of functional impairments that include decreased mechanical and contractile efficiency, prolongation of the contraction phase, stiffening of myocardial cells, stiffening of valves and mural connective tissue, decreased number of myocytes, increased myocyte size, increased rate of myocyte apoptosis, and a blunted β-adrenoceptor-mediated ionotropic response.[14-16]

**Vasculature.** Vascular morphology and function are also impacted by aging. Morphologic changes of the arteries include dilation of the large arteries accompanied by thickening of the arterial walls and changes in wall matrix. An increase in elastolytic and collagenic activity and an increase in smooth muscle tone are seen.[12,17-19] As a result of these changes, a decrease is seen in vasodilation through multiple mechanisms, including flow-dependent, endothelial-dependent, atrial natriuretic

peptide–mediated, and β-adrenoreceptor–mediated vasodilation. An accompanying decrease in the production and the effectiveness of nitric oxide is found and results in increased vascular stiffness and decreased vasoreactivity with aging.[12,17,18] Endothelial-dependent vasodilation is altered because of an age-associated increase in plasma concentration of endothelin and an increased vasoconstrictor effect of endothelin-1.[20]

### Cardiac Adaptations to Age-related Changes.
Increased vascular stiffness leads to elevated systolic arterial pressure and pulse wave velocity, early reflected pulse pressure waves, and late peak systolic pressure, which trigger a series of cardiac adjustments (Fig. 50-1). A resultant augmenting of aortic impedance and cardiac mechanical load is seen. These changes can be expected to inhibit cardiac performance and should be considered part of the intrinsic changes associated with aging.[12,17]

Clinically elevated left ventricular afterload causes an increase in myocyte size and thickening of the left ventricular wall.[18] When combined with augmentation of aortic impedance, it prolongs myocardial contraction. This adaptive measure preserves cardiac function by lengthening the amount of time available for the heart to eject blood into stiffened vasculature. The resultant prolonged myocardial contraction delays ventricular relaxation time, which manifests as a decrease in early ventricular filling.[19,21-24]

Between the ages of 20 and 80 years, the rate of early diastolic filling decreases by 50%.[13]

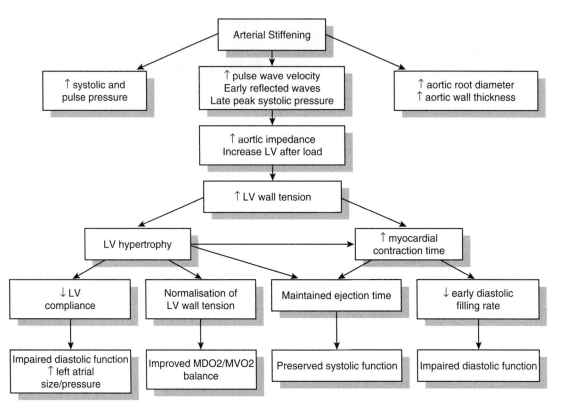

**Fig. 50-1**   Cardiac response to increased flow demand in young and elderly. Young meet increased flow demand primarily with β-adrenoceptor–mediated augmentation of heart rate and contractility, thus preserving preload reserve via Frank-Starling mechanism. In contrast, elderly use primarily preload reserve to augment cardiac performance, thereby losing additional cardiovascular reserve and becoming susceptible to cardiac insufficiency. *V*, End-diastolic volume; *LV*, left ventricular; Δ, change. *(Adapted from Priebe HJ: The aged cardiovascular risk patient,* Br J Anesth *85:763-778, 2000.)*

This decrease may be the result of a prolonged isovolumetric relaxation time between aortic valve closure and mitral valve opening. With aging, alterations in calcium release from the myoplasm to the sarcoplasmic reticulum may contribute to the changes in early diastolic filling.[12,24]

For maintenance of stroke volume, end diastolic filling is increased.[12] The effectiveness of this strategy is dependent on the atrial contribution to end diastolic filling; therefore, left atrial size increase.[21] Enlargement of the atria raises the likelihood of atrial fibrillation in the elderly, thus underscoring the importance of stable hemodynamics to ensure normal sinus rhythm.

Stiffness of the vasculature, atria, or ventricles contributes to increasing risk for the geriatric patient. Vascular stiffness has been shown to contribute to orthostatic hypotension and exaggerated pressure changes in response to sodium intake or diuretics.[25] Atrial and ventricular stiffening may enhance the adverse effects of diastolic autonomic and baroreflex dysfunction on cardiovascular compensatory mechanisms.

Gender differences are found in certain age-related changes in cardiac function.[12] Men seem to have different compensatory mechanisms than women. To maintain stroke volume in the presence of the age-associated decrease in heart rate, men have an increase in left ventricle end-systolic volume and left ventricle end-diastolic volume. This mechanism preserves cardiac output in aging men, whereas a 15% decrease is seen in cardiac output in women. Table 50-2 summarizes cardiac changes that occur with age.[26]

**Age-related Changes of the Cardiovascular Response to Increased Oxygen Demand.**   First, many factors may impose stress or increased oxygen demand on the geriatric patient. One should consider the nature of the stimulus, posture, gender, and cardiovascular health and fitness of the patient, irrespective of age.

In healthy sedentary individuals, maximal oxygen capacity decreases about 10% per decade after the age of 20 years.[13] This decline is influenced by many factors, such as the decrease in maximal heart rate, a blunted heart rate (HR) and ejection fraction response, and peripheral

**Table 50-2   Changes in Cardiovascular Response to Exercise with Comparison of 20 and 80 years***

|  | Peak Response at Age 20 y | Change in Peak Response between 20 and 80 y |
|---|---|---|
| LV end-diastolic volume | ↔,↓ | ↑30% males; ↔ females |
| LV end-systolic volume | ↓ | ↓100% |
| Ejection fraction | ↑ | ↓15% |
| Stroke volume | ↑ | ↔ |
| Heart rate | ↑ | ↓25% |
| Cardiac output | ↑ | ↓25% |
| Stroke work | ↑ | ↑15% males; ↔ females |
| SVR | ↓ | ↑30% |
| Oxygen consumption | ↑ | ↑50% |
| Plasma catecholamines | ↑ | ↑ |
| Myocardial contractility | ↑ | ↓60% |
| β-Adrenergic stimulation | Fully functional | ↓ |

*Adapted from Eagle et al.[10]
LV, Left ventricular; SVR, systemic vascular resistance; ↔, no change; ↑, increase; ↓, decrease.

limitations, such as redistribution of blood flow and oxygen extraction via the muscle.[13,24] The age-associated decline in maximal heart rate and left ventricular contractility during exercise is likely to reflect a diminished β-adrenergic modulation of contractility, chronotrophy, and vasomotor tone.[27,28]

The most clinically relevant age-related changes in cardiovascular function are increased myocardial stiffness and all of the subsequent compensatory actions and blunted β-adrenergic responses. During increased oxygen demand, the most relevant changes in the geriatric patient are autonomic reflex dysfunction and β-adrenoreceptor responsiveness. See Table 50-2 for cardiovascular age-related changes to upright peak exercise. Fig. 50-2 compares myocardial response with increased demand.

### Respiratory System
The structural and age-related changes that occur in the respiratory system are clinically influential to the perioperative care of the geriatric patient. Structurally, an increase in chest wall rigidity increases the work of breathing. By the time an individual is 70 years of age, about a 20% decrease in respiratory muscle strength and endurance and a 15% decrease in alveolar surface area are seen. Older patients have an attenuated response to hypoxemia and hypercapnia. Changes in lung volume include an annual 20 to 40 mL/y decrease in vital capacity, a 30% increase in residual volume by the age of 70 years, increased closing volume, and a 0.05% annual decrease in gas exchange.[29]

These changes in the geriatric patient may hinder the ability of the patient to meet additional postoperative workloads, thus increasing the risk for acute respiratory failure. The geriatric patient is more likely to have apnea develop in response to opioids and benzodiazepines. The blunted response to hypoxia and lower baseline arterial oxygen tension increases the risk of postoperative hypoxemia, which may contribute to myocardial ischemia and infarction.[26]

### Renal System
The kidneys play a crucial role in fluid and electrolyte balance. Age-related changes in renal-function may elevate cardiovascular risk in geriatric patients and make them more prone to hypervolemia and hypovolemia, hypertension or hypotension, and heart failure. By age 70 years, glomerular filtration rate decreases at least 30% and as much as 50%; cortical nephrons are decreased; decreases are seen in renal blood flow, ability to concentrate urine, ability to conserve sodium, and tubular secretion; thirst perception is lowered; and a 10% to 15% reduction in total body water is seen.[30]

The altered thirst, rennin response, and ability to concentrate urine are likely to facilitate sodium and volume depletion, which may disrupt the Starling mechanism and challenge the geriatric patients' ability to maintain cardiac output and arterial pressure during periods of increased demand. Therefore, attention to fluid and electrolyte balance is of the utmost importance in the anesthesia care of the geriatric patient.

### Hepatic
By the time an individual is 80 years old, an approximate 40% reduction in hepatic mass

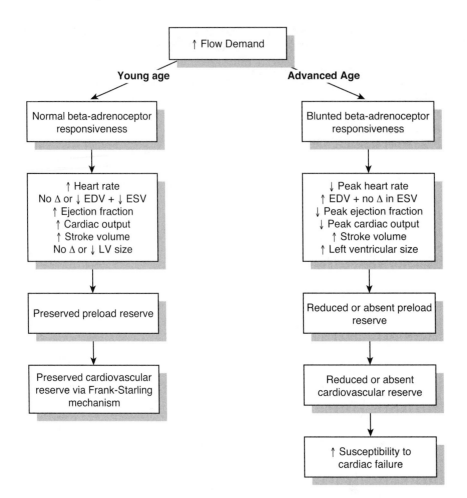

**Fig. 50-2**  Cardiac adjustments to arterial stiffening during aging. *LV*, Left ventricular. *(Adapted from Priebe HJ: The aged cardiovascular risk patient*, Br J Anesth *85:763-778, 2000.)*

and a 40% decrease in hepatic and splanchnic blood flow are seen. With advancing age is also a decrease in the activity of hepatic cholinesterase and microsomal demethylation pathway.[31,32] These changes lead to an impaired ability to meet the increased demands of metabolism, biotransformation, and protein synthesis after surgery. Drugs that rely on hepatic metabolism have a prolonged impact in the elderly. For prevention of hepatic injury from medication, hypoxia, or transfusion, careful attention to appropriate drug dosage and adequate oxygenation should be made.

### Thermoregulation

Age is considered a predisposing factor for perioperative hypothermia,[33-36] which may impose increased demands on the cardiovascular system. Specifically, perioperative hypothermia exerts a number of adverse effects, including prolonged drug action,[37] negative postoperative oxygen balance,[38] immune dysfunction,[39] and subsequent increased incidence of wound infection.[40] Cardiac changes include a leftward shift of the hemoglobin-oxygen saturation curve, increased vascular resistance, cardiac arrhythmias, and up to a four-fold increase in cardiac output and oxygen consumption associated with rewarming and shivering.[41] Special care to maintain normothermia can minimize the risk of postoperative ischemia and angina in geriatric patients.

### Cognitive Impairment

Dementia is a disorder of the brain that seriously affects a person's ability to carry out daily activities, specifically self care. The most common form of dementia among older adults is Alzheimer's disease (AD), which accounts for 60% to 70% of all dementia. Vascular dementia (VAD) is the second most common form of dementia and combined with AD constitutes 90% of all forms of dementia.[42,43]

Initial involvement is in parts of the brain that control thought, memory, and language. Although the exact cause of AD is unknown, autopsies reveal three different types of lesions on patients' brains: senile plaques, neurofibrillary tangles, and vascular lesions. Senile plaques and vascular lesions contain high levels of beta-amyloid protein.

Alzheimer's disease is not a normal part of aging; however, longitudinal studies have identified risk factors for neurodegenerative changes and dementia that are primarily cardiovascular in nature.[44,45] These risk factors may accelerate the onset of dementia, and multiple risk factors may increase stroke and cognitive impairment.[46] Clinically relevant cognitive deficits occur in elderly patients with type 2 diabetes. Several large epidemiologic surveys have reported an increase of incidence rate of AD in patients with type 2 diabetes.[47,48] Moreover, type 2 diabetes occurs in the context of a cluster of metabolic and vascular risk factors that are associated with atherosclerotic cardiovascular disease, ischemic stroke, cognitive decline, and dementia.[42,49,50]

Alzheimer's disease has recently been referred to as type III diabetes.[50] The same risk factors for many other chronic diseases apply to the risk for AD: smoking, impaired fasting glucose, insulin resistance, diabetes, hypertension, elevated lipids, lack of physical activity, high fat, and refined sugar diet and obesity. The important consideration from an anesthesia perspective is that the presence of dementia also indicates that the patient has increased metabolic risk and comorbidities that need to be addressed during preanesthesia and perianesthesia phases.

Normal aging in itself is not necessarily a high-risk proposition; however, when compounded with comorbidities, the amount of risk is dramatically increased. As a general guideline, a 1% annual decline in physiologic function occurs after the age of 30 years[26]; this rate of functional decline is influenced by individual variability, genetics, lifestyle, environment, and comorbid conditions. In assessment of the geriatric patient, not only is consideration of the age-related decline in function important, but so is the decrease in the ability of the organ systems to respond to external demands. The lack of functional reserve, especially in the cardiovascular system, influences preanesthesia and perianesthesia outcomes in the geriatric patient.

## Pharmacology and the Geriatric Patient
Community-dwelling elderly take an average of 2.7 to 4.2 prescription and nonprescription

medications.[51] Geriatric patients at discharge from the hospital take the greatest number of medications.[51] Medication-related problems have many forms often as a result of polypharmacy: overuse of medications, inappropriate prescribing, adverse events, and drug interactions. Hanlon[51] found that 55% of outpatients were taking drugs with no indication, 33% were taking ineffective drugs, and 17% were taking drugs with therapeutic duplications.[52,53] Almost one quarter of community-dwelling elders use medications that should be avoided. Long-acting benzodiazepines, dipyridamole, propoxyphene, and amitriptyline were the most frequently inappropriately prescribed medications.[53] Thirty percent of hospital admissions are linked to medication-related problems; furthermore, medication-related problems are the fifth leading cause of death in the United States.[54] The Beers criteria were created to measure inappropriate prescribing and drugs to be avoided and highlight common drug interactions.[55] These criteria are updated regularly and should be a companion when working with the geriatric patient. Table 50-3 illustrates some possible adverse effects or drug interactions that may take place in the geriatric patient during the perioperative period.

The pharmacokinetic response in the geriatric patient is governed by the drug distribution, hepatic metabolism, and renal excretion, all of which are altered in an unpredictable manner with aging.[56] Pharmacokinetics refers to the concentration of the drug at the site of action. Drug distribution is altered by the age-related decrease in total body water and lean mass, increase in total body fat, decrease in serum albumin, decrease in cardiac output, reduction in blood volume, and increase in $\alpha_1$-acid glycoprotein.[56] Injection of medication into a contracted blood volume produces a higher plasma concentration of drug. High protein–bound drugs may have an exaggerated clinical effect (e.g., lidocaine, propranolol, thiopental, etomidate, profol, alfentanil) because of a higher level of (free) unbound drug. Decreased distribution of water-soluble drugs may cause an adverse reaction because of the initial high plasma concentrations. Conversely, increased distribution of fat-soluble drugs may prolong the action of that medication (e.g., diazepam, midazolam).[56]

Changes in hepatic and renal function influence drug metabolism and excretion. A decrease is seen in hepatic mass, hepatic blood flow, microsomal demethylation pathway, and presystematic metabolism of drugs with a high rate of hepatic clearance, which results in a greater bioavailability of drugs with high hepatic clearance, where the rate limiting step is

| **Table 50-3** | **Adverse Effects or Drug Interactions Associated with the Geriatric Patient** |
|---|---|
| **Drug** | **Adverse Effect or Drug Interaction** |
| Antibiotics | Prolongation of muscle relaxants |
| Antidysrhythmics | Prolongation of muscle relaxants |
| Benzodiazepines | |
|   Diazepam | Decreased metabolism |
|   Chlordiazepoxide | Increased CNS effects |
|   Flurazepam | Prolonged drowsiness |
| Digoxin | Decreased renal excretion with increased CNS disorientation, anorexia, nausea, and cardiotoxicity; blood levels two to three times higher in elderly with any given dose |
| Diuretics | Hypokalemia |
| | Hypovolemia |
| Halothane | Decreased anesthetic requirement |
| Lithium | Clearance decreased by 65% and effective dose by 30% in comparison with patients at age 25 y |
| | Increased side effects of tremor, diarrhea, and edema |
| Meperidine | Markedly elevated plasma levels and decreased red blood cell and plasma binding of drug |
| | Increased incidence rate of nausea, respiratory distress, and hypotension |
| Methyldopa | Enhanced hypotensive effects |
| Pancuronium | Decreased clearance from plasma |
| Propranolol | Plasma level approximately three to four times higher in elderly because of decreased metabolism |
| | Bradycardia, congestive heart failure, bronchospasm, mental confusion, and attenuation of autonomic nervous system activity |
| Tricyclic antidepressants | Increased anticholinergic effects: confusion, agitation, and disorientation |
| | Cardiac conduction disturbances |
| | Increased anesthetic requirements |
| Warfarin | Enhanced sensitivity |

Adapted from Krechel S, editor: *Anesthesia and the geriatric patient*, New York, 1984, Grune & Stratton. And Miller R, editor: *Anesthesia*, ed 5, New York, 2000, Churchill Livingstone.
CNS, Central nervous system.

hepatic flow (e.g., antiarrhythmias, tricyclic antidepressants, most major tranquilizers, lipid soluble β-adrenoreceptor blockers).[56] Renal changes such as reduced renal blood, reduced glomerular filtration rate, reduced tubular secretion flow, and decreased ability to concentrate urine contribute to reduced clearance and volume depletion.[18]

Pharmacodynamics is the ability of the drug to react with a specific receptor and to translate that effect on the receptor into a physiologic response. This reaction may render elders more sensitive to a given concentration of most drugs. However, the opposite is true in regards to β-adrenoreceptor antagonist and agonist and to digoxin. A higher incidence rate of hyperkalemia, renal failure, and death from gastrointestinal bleeding is associated with the use of nonsteroidal antiinflammatories.[18,56]

In assessment of the geriatric patient, one must consider changes in cardiovascular, renal, hepatic, and respiratory function; the compensatory mechanisms; and coexisting comorbid conditions. As a result of marked heterogeneity of drug response in the geriatric patient, no strict age rules can be applied across the entire geriatric population.[26]

## PSYCHOLOGIC AGE-RELATED CHANGES

In addition to the physiologic heterogeneity among an elder population, older adults are also markedly heterogeneous psychologically. Although cohort effects (e.g., being raised during the Great Depression) result in some similarities in terms of preferences from living within one historic time period, many years of lived experience lead to enormous interindividual diversity in capabilities and temperament. Therefore, although guidelines are helpful, person-centered care necessitates taking the time to know the patient to provide the highest quality care.

Psychologic aspects play a significant role in care for our elders. For simplicity, these can be categorized into sense of self, cognition, and mood.

### Sense of Self

At all times, as with all patients, elders' sense of self should be honored and respected. We show respect through our communication, with use of inclusionary and person-first language. Elders' diverse and extensive lived experiences frequently impact health beliefs, which results in a wide variety of understanding, preferences, and knowledge regarding care provision and medical practice. As with all patients, assurance of understanding is essential to quality patient care and is at the foundation of person-centered care. Contrary to the popularly held belief, elders are among the most compliant in regards to care planning. Most frequently, seemingly poor compliance is the result of external barriers (e.g., income restrictions) and lack of understanding from poor communication.

***Sensory Changes.*** Although sensory changes are significantly impacted by lifestyle, by midlife most individuals experience presbyopia (age-associated vision change) and presbycusis (age-associated hearing change). Being mindful of sensory changes improves the care for patients.

Communication with a person with age-associated hearing loss can be improved with:

- Assuming the person understands everything you are saying. Include the patient in the conversation (unless they tell you otherwise).
- Identifying yourself.
- Addressing the person by last name unless asked to do otherwise. Avoid pet names like "honey" and "sweetie" until you have developed a rapport.
- Always approaching the elder from the front. Face the patient when you speak. This action not only enhances the patient's ability to hear you, it also shows interest and respect.
- Using good eye contact. Use a positive friendly facial expression. Elders are much better at interpreting social cues and pick up on negative messages much easier than younger people.
- Using expanded speech and speaking in a lower pitch, rather than raising the voice. This action is helpful because presbycusis is marked by loss of high pitches and raising your voice also raises your pitch. Also, a lower pitch is more calming.
- Using proper enunciation. Loss of "S" and "F" sounds is most frequent.
- Encouraging the patient to wear a hearing aid, if the patient uses one.
- Being certain that the environment is "elder friendly" or a low-distraction/low-noise environment. Presbycusis specifically affects a person's ability to filter out ambient sound.
- Using written instructions if hearing loss is significant.

Communication with a person with age-associated vision loss can be improved with:

- Identifying yourself when you approach and avoiding startling the patient.
- Telling the person your intentions before you begin.
- Using large-print (sans serif high-contrast is best) or recorded material when available.
- Encouraging the patient to wear glasses and keep them clean, if the elder uses glasses.
- Being certain that elders have sufficient time to adjust to light changes and that stairs and walkways are clutter free and clearly marked. Presbyopia specifically affects the ability to adjust between light and dark surroundings and depth perception.

Respectful inclusionary language is foundational to providing quality person-centered care and assisting patients to maintain a sense of self. Frequently, ageist stereotypes lead to inaccurate assumptions regarding compliance and performance. Poor cognitive performance once thought to be the result of age-related cognitive decline is now understood to be the result of extraneous variables such as sensory changes, fatigability, low education levels, hypermotivation, and polypharmacy.

### Cognition

Most older adults perform well cognitively in day-to-day lives throughout late life. However, although cognitive changes do not significantly impact day-to-day functioning, elders in a vulnerable state (e.g., hospitalization, illness, or injury) may show poor concentration, confusion, and disorganized thought patterns. Long-term memory is not altered as a part of normal aging, but attentional abilities and working memory are often affected as part of normal aging by age 80 years.

Compared with younger cohorts, elders do not encode new information as deeply, causing greater difficulty with new information retrieval. This difference is the result of many factors: anatomic changes in the brain, poor sensory encoding, cohort differences in use of memory

SPECIAL CONSIDERATIONS

strategies, and difficulty filtering out irrelevant environmental stimuli and noise. Recent research indicates that elders trained in memory strategies can improve performance on cognitive tasks. Again, although these changes do not typically affect day-to-day functioning, they may impact understanding and compliance to the care plan. Therefore, avoidance of inaccurate assumptions from ageist attitudes and careful communication are essential to quality care.

### Temperament

Temperament and personality are relatively stable across the adult lifespan, barring catastrophic events. Generally speaking, people become more like themselves as they get older (i.e, happy people become happier and grumpy people grumpier). Illness and injury represent significant losses in people's lives and may jeopardize one's sense of identity, sense of self, and temperament. Although losses occur throughout the lifespan, elders may experience the impact of multiple losses that result in compounded grieving (i.e, catastrophic event) that may affect mood or may result in depressive symptomatology.

As health professionals, we see people not at their best but at their most vulnerable. Negative temperament and depressive symptomatology are best interpreted not as the person's normal way of being but as reactive and situationally part of the illness or injury. Just as elders have greater difficulty returning to homeostasis in a physiologic sense, so too do they need greater time in adjusting psychologically to stressful events as a result of greater allostatic load.

## SUMMARY

Perianesthesia nursing care of geriatric patients requires a thorough risk assessment of all body systems and disease states and the psychologic outlook of the patient. When caring for these patients, keep in mind that age is just a chronologic marker of years lived and not of the physiologic, psychologic, or functional status of the geriatric patient.

## REFERENCES

1. US Census Bureau of Census: *Current population survey*, Washington, DC, 2003, U.S. Government Printing Office.
2. Shipton EA: The perioperative care of the geriatric patient, *S African Med J* 63:855-860, 1983.
3. Centers for Disease Control: *Trends in health and aging, Aging and chronic disease statistics branch*, Hyattsville, Md, available at http://www.cdc.gov/index.htm, last updated December 11, 2006.
4. Maddox TM: Preoperative cardiac evaluation for noncardiac surgery, *Mt Sinai J Med* 72(3):185-192, 2005.
5. Eagle KA, Berger PB, Calkins H, et al: ACC/AHA guideline update for perioperative cardiovascular evaluation for non-cardiac surgery: executive summary: a report of the American College of Cardiology/American Heart Association Task Force on Practice Guidelines (Committee to update the 1996 Guidelines on Perioperative Cardiovascular Evaluation for Noncardiac Surgery), *Circulation* 94:1052-1064, 2002.
6. Fleisher LA: Preoperative cardiac evaluation, *Anesthesiol Clin North Am* 22:59-75, 2004.
7. McArdle WD, Katch FI, Katch VI: *Exercise physiology: energy, nutrition and human performance*, ed 3, Philadelphia, 1991, Lea & Febiger.
8. Hlatky MA, Boineau RE, Higginbotham MB, et al: A brief self-administered questionnaire to determine functional capacity, *Am J Cardiol* 64:651-654, 1989.
9. Fletcher GF, Balady G, Froelicher VF, et al: Exercise standards: a statement for healthcare professionals from the American Heart Association, *Circulation*, 104:1694-1740, 2001.
10. Eagle KA: Perioperative cardiac assessment for noncardiac surgery: eight steps to the best possible outcome, *Circulation* 107:2771-2774, 2003.
11. Folkow B, Svanborg A: Physiology of cardiovascular aging, *Physiol Rev* 73:725-764, 1993.
12. Lakatta EG: Cardiovascular aging research: the next horizons, *J Am Geriatic Soc* 47:613-667, 1999.
13. Lakatta EG: Changes in cardiovascular function with aging, *Eur Heart J* II(suppl C):22-29, 1990.
14. Lakatta EG: Cardiovascular mechanisms in advanced age, *Physiol Rev* 73:413-467, 1993.
15. Olivetti G, Melissari M., Capasso JM, et al: Cardiomyopathy of the aging human heart: myocyte loss and reactive cellular hypertrophy, *Circ Res* 68:1560-1568, 1991.
16. Yang B, Larson DF, Watson R: Age-related left ventricular function in the mouse:analysis based on in vivo pressure-volume relationships, *Am J Physiol* 46:HI906-HI913, 1999.
17. Lakatta EG: Aging effects on the vasculature in health:risk factors for cardiovascular disease, *Am J Geriatr Cardiol* 3:11-17, 1994.
18. Lakatta EG, Gerstenblith G, Weisfeldt ML: The aging heart: structure, function and disease, *Heart disease: a textbook of cardiovascular medicine*, ed 5, Philadelphia, 1997, Saunders.

19. Wei JY: Age and the cardiovascular system, *N Engl J Med* 327:1735-1739, 1992.

20. Goodwin AT, Amrani M, Marchbank AJ, et al: Coronary vasoconstriction to endothelin-1 increases with age before and after ischemia and reperfusion, *Cardiovasc Res* 41:554-562, 1999.

21. Klein AL, Leung DY, Murray RD, et al: Effects of age and physiologic variables on right ventricular filling dynamics in normal subjects, *Am J Cardiol* 84:440-448, 1999.

22. Gardin JM, Arnold AM, Bild ED, et al: Left ventricular diastolic filling in the elderly: the cardiovascular health study, *Am J Cardiol* Vol 345–351, 1998.

23. Palka P, Lange A, Nihoyannoupoulos P: The effect of long-term training on age-related left ventricular changes by Doppler myocardial velocity gradient, *Am J Cardiol* 84:1061-1067, 1999.

24. Schulman SP, Lakatta EG, Fleg IL, et al: Age-related decline in left ventricular filling at rest and exercise, *Am J Physiol* 263:H1932-H1938, 1992.

25. Weinbergere MH, Fineberg NS: Sodium and volume sensitivity of blood pressure: age and pressure changes over time, *Hypertension* 18:67-71, 1991.

26. Priebe HJ: The aged cardiovascular risk patient, *Br J Anesth* 85:763-778, 2000.

27. Fleg JL, O'Connor FC, Gerstenblith G, et al: Impact of age on the cardiovascular response to dynamic upright exercise in healthy men and women, *J Appl Physiol* 78:890-900, 1995.

28. Fleg JL, Schulman S, O'Connor F, et al: Effects of acute β-adrenergic receptor blockade on age-associated changes in cardiovascular performance during dynamic exercise, *Circulation* 90:2333-2341, 1994.

29. Carpo RO, Campbell EJ: Aging of the respiratory system. In Fishman AP, editor: *Pulmonary diseases and disorders*, New York, 1998, McGraw-Hill.

30. Shannon RP, Minaker KL, Rowe JW: The influence of age on water balance in man, *Semin Nephrol* 4:346-352, 1984.

31. Shannon RP, Wei JY, Rosa RM, et al: The effect of age and sodium depletion on cardiovascular response to orthostasis, *Hypertension* 8:438-443, 1986.

32. Kampnann JP, Sinding J, Moller-Jorgensen I: Effect of age on liver function, *Geriatrics* 30:91-95, 1975.

33. Woodhouse KW, Mutch E, Williams FM, et al: The effect of age on pathways of drug metabolism in human liver, *Age Ageing* 13:328-334, 1984.

34. Freidl LP, Kronmal RA, Newman AB, et al: Risk factors for 5-year mortality in older adults: the cardiovascular health study, *JAMA* 279:585-592, 1998.

35. Kurz A, Plattner O, Sessler DI, et al: The threshold for thermoregulatory vasoconstriction during nitrous oxide/isoflurane anesthesia is lower in the elderly than in young patients, *Anesthesiology* 79:465-469, 1993.

36. Vaughan MS, Vaughan RW, Cork RC: Postoperative hypothermia in adults: relationship with age anesthesia, and shivering to rewarming, *Anesth Anal* 60:746-751, 1981.

37. Heier T, Caldwell JE, Sessler DI, et al: Mild intraoperative hypothermia increases duration of action and spontaneous recovery of verconium blockade during nitrous oxide-isoflurane anesthesia in humans, *Anesthesiology* 74:815-819, 1991.

38. Carli R, Emery PW, Freemantle CAJ: Effect of preoperative normothermia on post operative protein metabolism in elderly patients undergoing hip arthroplasty, *Br J Anesth* 63:276-282, 1989.

39. Valeri RC, Cassidy G, Khuri S, et al: Hypothermia-induced reversible platelet dysfunction, *Ann Surg* 205:175-181, 1987.

40. Kurz A, Sessler DI, Lenhardt R: The study of wound infection and temperature group: perioperative normothermia to reduce the incidence of surgical wound infection and shorten hospitalization, *N Engl J Med* 334:1029-1035, 1996.

41. Frank SM, Beattie C, Christopherson R, et al: The perioperative ischemia randomized anesthesia trial study group: unintentional hypothermia is associated with post operative myocardial ischemia, *Anesthesiology* 78:468-476, 1993.

42. Kalmijn S, Foley D, White L, et al: Metabolic cardiovascular syndrome and risk of dementia in Japanese-American elderly men: the Honolulu-Asia Study, *Arterioscler Thromb Vasc Biol* 20:2255-2260, 2000.

43. Hebert LE, Scherr PA, Bienias JL, et al: Alzheimer disease in the U.S. population: prevalence estimates using the 2000 census, *Arch Neurol* 60(8):1119-1122, 2003.

44. Katzman R, Aronson M, Fuld P, et al: Development of dementing illnesses in an 80-year-old volunteer cohort, *Ann Neurol* 25:317-324, 1989.

45. Akiyama H, Meyer JS, Mortel KF, et al: Normal human aging: factors contributing to cerebral atrophy, *J Neurol Sci* 152:39-49, 1997.

46. Hofman A, Ott A, Breteler MMB, et al: Atherosclerosis, apolipoprotein E, and the prevalence of dementia and Alzheimer's disease in the Rotterdam Study, *Lancet* 349:151-154, 1997.

47. Stewart R, Liolitsa D: Type 2 diabetes mellitus, cognitive impairment and dementia, *Diabetic Med* 16:93-112, 1997.

48. Ott A, Stolk RP, van Harskamp F, et al: Diabetes mellitus and the risk of dementia: the Rotterdam Study, *Neurology* 53:1937-1942, 1999.

49. Peila R, Rodriguez BL, Launer LJ: Type 2 diabetes, APOE gene, and the risk for dementia and related pathologies: the Honolulu-Asia Aging Study (apolipoprotein E), *Diabetes* 51:1256-1262, 2000.

50. Arvanitakis Z, Wilson RS, Bienias JL, et al: Diabetes mellitus and risk of Alzheimer's disease and decline in cognitive function, *Arch Neurol* 61:661-666, 2004.

51. Hanlon JT, Schmader KE, Ruby CM, et al: Suboptimal prescribing in older inpatients and older outpatients, *JAGS* 4:200-209, 2001.

52. Fick DM, Cooper JW, Wade WE, et al: Updating the Beers criteria for potentially inappropriate medications in older adults: results of a U.S. consensus panel of experts, *Arch Intern Med* 163:2716-2724, 2003.

53. Aparasu RR, Mort JR: Inappropriate prescribing for the elderly: Beers criteria-based review, *Ann Pharomacother* 34:338-346, 2000.

54. Simon SR, Gurwitz JH: Drug therapy in the elderly: improving quality and access, *Clinical Pharmacol Ther* 73:387-393, 2003.

55. Beers MH: Explicit criteria for determining potentially inappropriate medication use by the elderly. An update, *Arch Intern Med* 157:1531-1536, 1997.

56. Montamat SC, Cusack BJ, Vestal RE: Management of drug therapy in the elderly, *N Engl J Med* 304:405-412, 1989.

## SUPPLEMENTAL READINGS

Asher M: Surgical considerations in the elderly, *J PeriAnesthesia Nurs* 19(6):406-414, 2004.

Burden N: Discharge planning for the elderly ambulatory surgical patient, *J PeriAnesthesia Nurs* 19(6):401-405, 2004.

Kuchta A, Golembiewski J: Medication use in the elderly patient: focus on the perioperative/perianesthesia setting, *J PeriAnesthesia Nurs* 19(6):415-427, 2004.

Monarch S, Wren K: Geriatric anesthesia implications, *J PeriAnesthesia Nurs* 19(6):379-384, 2004.

Paynter D, Mamaril M: Perianesthesia challenges in geriatric pain management, *J PeriAnesthesia Nurs* 19(6):385-391, 2004.

Saufl N: Preparing the older adult for surgery and anesthesia, *J PeriAnesthesia Nurs* 19(6):372-378, 2004.

Stevenson J: When the trauma patient is elderly, *J PeriAnesthesia Nurs* 19(6):392-400, 2004.

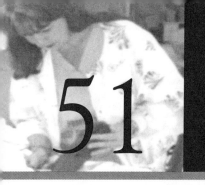

# 51

# CARE OF THE PREGNANT PATIENT

*Joseph F. Burkard, DNSc, CRNA*

The incidence rate of surgery performed on pregnant women for reasons unrelated to the pregnancy itself has been reported to be as high as 50,000 to 75,000 cases per year, with a frequency range from 0.75% to 2%. The most common conditions that require surgical intervention are acute appendicitis, ovarian cysts, and breast tumors, with laparoscopy the most common first-trimester procedure. However, more complicated procedures have been reported and include craniotomy, open-heart surgery, and aneurysm repair that have been performed successfully in pregnant patients.

In care of the pregnant patient after surgery, one must remember that two patients require nursing care and assessment: the mother and the fetus. Perianesthesia nursing care should be directed toward emotional support for the mother and avoidance of uterine stimulation that could produce preterm labor. Also of prime importance are prevention of respiratory depression in the mother and maintenance of normal uterine placental blood flow to ensure adequate fetal supply of oxygen and nutrients.

## DEFINITIONS

**Aortocaval Compression or Scott's Syndrome:** Obstruction of the inferior vena cava and the pelvic veins by the enlarging uterus.

**Aspiration Pneumonitis:** An inflammatory condition of the lungs and bronchi caused by material in the stomach regurgitated into the pharynx and inhaled through the epiglottis into the lungs and bronchi.

**Cesarean Section:** A surgical procedure in which the abdomen and pregnant uterus are incised and the baby is delivered transabdominally.

**Cricoid Pressure (Sellick Maneuver):** Used in rapid sequence intubation of the trachea in which the cricoid cartilage is pushed against the body of the sixth cervical vertebra in a effort to compress the esophagus to prevent passive regurgitation.

**Defasciculation:** Administration of a nondepolarizing muscle relaxant 1 to 3 minutes before the administration of succinylcholine to prevent the muscle twitches that usually occur after the administration of a depolarizing muscle relaxant with the intended outcome of reducing the amount of gastric pressure created by the muscle twitches or fasciculations.

**Esophagitis:** The inflammation of the mucosal lining of the esophagus.

**Gastric Motility:** The spontaneous peristaltic movements of the stomach that move the stomach contents through the pyloric sphincter into the duodenum.

**Gastroesophageal Reflux:** Often referred to as heartburn; a result of a backflow of stomach contents as a result of an incompetent lower esophageal sphincter muscle.

**Hypovolemia:** A reduction from normal in blood volume.

**Laryngoscopy:** With the use of a laryngoscope, the direct observation of the larynx.

**Physiologic Anemia of Pregnancy:** A normal reduction in hemoglobin in the blood as a result of the normal physiologic process of pregnancy.

**Plasma Cholinesterase:** An enzyme in the plasma that is responsible for the metabolic breakdown of acetylcholine to choline and acetate.

**Pruritus:** The symptom of itching of the skin.

**Retained Placenta:** After the birth of the infant, the placenta is usually delivered within 30 minutes; if it is expelled after 30 minutes, it is considered to be a retained placenta.

**Semi-Fowler's Position:** Placement of a patient in an reclined position, with approximately 30 degrees elevation of the head of the bed.

**Sepsis:** Infection or contamination.

**Thromboembolism:** A situation in which a blood vessel becomes obstructed by a clot or thrombus that had been carried by the bloodstream from its site of formation.

## PHYSIOLOGIC CHANGES OF PREGNANCY

Almost every system in the body is affected in some way during pregnancy, either from hormonal changes or from the increasing size of the uterus. The changes that affect perianesthesia nursing care are outlined in Box 51-1 and discussed in the following sections.

### Cardiovascular Changes

*Hemodynamic Alterations.* The cardiovascular system undergoes significant change as pregnancy advances. Cardiac output and heart rate increase progressively during pregnancy until, at 30 to 34 weeks gestation, the cardiac output is 30% to 50% higher than normal and the heart rate is about 15% above the nonpregnant normal level, with electrocardiographic changes and heart sounds possibly developing (Box 51-2). The systolic blood pressure is minimally affected by pregnancy, with a maximum decline of approximately 8% during early to mid gestation and a return to the pregnant level at term. Diastolic blood pressure falls to a greater degree than does systolic pressure, with early to mid gestational decreases of approximately 20%. It also returns to prepregnant level at term.

Perhaps the most significant effect on the cardiovascular system for the nurse to consider in routine postanesthesia management is obstruction of the inferior vena cava and the pelvic veins by the enlarging uterus (Figs. 51-1 and 51-2). This condition, known as aortocaval compression or Scott's syndrome, can develop by the second trimester and cause supine hypotension. Avoidance of the supine position becomes mandatory after surgery because it can significantly aggravate the obstruction. Treatment includes the administration of additional intravenous crystalloid, the placement of the mother in the side-lying position, and the administration of supplemental oxygen (Fig. 51-3).

Collateral circulation for venous return develops through the intervertebral venous plexus and the azygos vein. This condition reduces the volume of the epidural and subarachnoid spaces. Therefore, the amount of drug during regional anesthesia should be decreased. With this in mind, the perianesthesia nurse should assess the patient on admission for a high block and monitor dermatome levels frequently thereafter (see Chapter 25).

In the nonpregnant patient, the sympathetic nervous system plays a role in promoting venous return to the heart from the lower extremities. This sympathetic stimulation of vasomotor tone is enhanced during pregnancy in an effort to counteract the negative effects of uterine

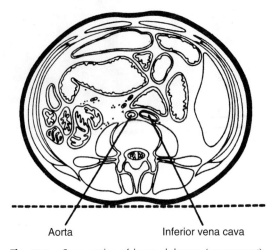

**Fig. 51-1**　Cross section of lower abdomen (nonpregnant). *(From Ostheimer SW: Regional anesthesia techniques in obstetrics, New York, 1980, Breon Laboratories.)*

compression of the vena cava. Clinically, this protective mechanism is abolished with spinal or epidural anesthesia because it acts as a pharmacologic sympathectomy. Without an appropriate preload of fluids (500 to 1000 mL intravenous lactated Ringer's solution), the pregnant patient may have a 30% to 50% decrease in blood pressure during the anesthesia. Therefore, the pregnant patient must receive an appropriate preload of fluids before epidural or spinal anesthesia. Hemodynamic stability can be secured with the infusion of 15 mL/kg of colloid solution or 30 mL/kg of crystalloid solution. If the patient is to receive an inhalation anesthetic agent such as isoflurane or sevoflurane, similar fluid preloading is given because the inhalation anesthetic agents produce peripheral vasodilation.

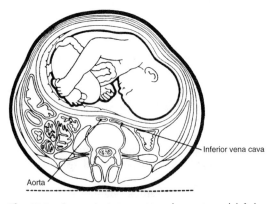

**Fig. 51-2**　Pregnant uterus compressing aorta and inferior vena cava (aortocaval compression). Patient is in supine position. *(From Ostheimer SW: Regional anesthesia techniques in obstetrics, New York, 1980, Breon Laboratories.)*

## Box 51-1  Physiologic Changes in Pregnancy

### CARDIOVASCULAR SYSTEM
- Flow and pressure changes
  - Cardiac output increases from 20% at the end of the first trimester to 40% at term
  - Heart rate at more than 15% of nonpregnant level
  - Stroke volume increases
  - Ejection fraction increases
  - Pulmonary capillary wedge pressure has no significant change
  - Central venous pressure has no significant change
  - Systolic blood pressure decreases to about 10 mm Hg below nonpregnant level at term
  - Diastolic blood pressure decreases by 15 to 20 mm Hg in early gestation through 30 weeks and then returns to pregestation levels at term
- Blood volume and constituents
  - Total blood volume increases to about 45% above nonpregnant levels
  - Total plasma volume increases to about 55% above nonpregnant levels
  - Red blood cell mass increases to about 30% above nonpregnant levels
  - Hematocrit levels decrease to about 36 mg/dL during gestation
  - Hemoglobin levels decrease to about 11.6 g/dL
  - Plasma cholinesterase levels decrease as much as 80% of nonpregnant levels
- Coagulation
  - Prothrombin time and partial thromboplastin time decreases 20%; platelet count decreases 15%; bleeding time decreases 10%

### RESPIRATORY SYSTEM
- Anatomic changes
  - Capillary engorgement of the nasal and oropharyngeal mucosa and larynx
  - Increased circumference of the thoracic cage
  - Elevated diaphragm
- Respiratory system flow, volume, and ventilation changes
  - No change in $FEV_1$
  - No change in flow-volume loop
  - Total pulmonary resistance decreases
  - Tidal volume increases from 20% to 45% above nonpregnant levels
  - Functional residual capacity decreases by 20% to 60% below nonpregnant level
  - Alveolar ventilation increases by 30% to 45% above nonpregnant level
  - Minute ventilation increases by 45% above nonpregnant level
- Changes in blood gases
  - $PaCO_2$ decreases to about 30 mm Hg
  - $PaO_2$ increases to about 103 to 105 mm Hg
  - Arterial pH from 10 week's gestation until delivery is about 7.44
- Metabolic rate and acid-base status
  - Metabolic rate is depressed during first 12 to 16 weeks
  - Metabolic rate is 15% above nonpregnant level at term
  - Oxygen consumption is 35% above nonpregnant level at term
  - Oxygen consumption is 40% above nonpregnant level during first stage of labor
  - Oxygen consumption is 75% above nonpregnant level during second stage of labor
  - Respiratory alkalosis with some metabolic compensation is present

### GASTROINTESTINAL SYSTEM
  - Gastric emptying delays after 34 week's gestation
  - Gastric volume increases
  - Gastric pH decreases
  - Pyrosis (heartburn) is present in about 50% of pregnant women
- Intragastric pressure increases
- Hepatic blood flow and function not altered

*Continued*

SPECIAL CONSIDERATIONS

## Box 51-1    Physiologic Changes in Pregnancy—cont'd

**RENAL SYSTEM**
- Glomerular filtration rate increases
- Urine output increases

$FEV_1$, Forced expiratory volume in 1 second, $PaCO_2$, Partial pressure of carbon dioxide in arterial blood, $PaO_2$, Partial pressure of oxygen in arterial blood.

This increased fluid requirement has significant implications for the perianesthesia care of the pregnant patient. Consequently, the patient's cardiac and hydration status must be monitored closely throughout the emergence phase of regional anesthesia (see Chapter 25).

***Hematologic Alterations.*** Blood volume along with the number of platelets, fibrinogen levels, and the level of activity of several clotting factors (VII, VIII, IX, X, and XII) increases by 15% during the first trimester, rises rapidly during the second trimester to 50% above the pregnant levels, and changes little during the remainder of the pregnancy. However, a smaller rise in the number of circulating red blood cells occurs. This difference results in lower hematocrit and hemoglobin levels (see Box 51-1), although red blood cell mass actually increases. This condition is known as physiologic anemia of pregnancy.

The plasma concentration of the enzyme cholinesterase is decreased during pregnancy, and because plasma cholinesterase is involved in the mechanisms of clotting, the perianesthesia nurse should monitor the pregnant patient for thromboembolism. Plasma cholinesterase is also involved in the destruction of the depolarizing muscle relaxant succinylcholine. The recovery time from succinylcholine is unaltered and in fact may even be somewhat faster in pregnant women, which is explained by the fact that the volume distribution of succinylcholine increases during pregnancy because of an elevation in the plasma volume. In the immediate postpartum period, the plasma cholinesterase concentration and the plasma volume distribution are further reduced.

### Respiratory Changes

***Upper Airway Anatomy.*** During pregnancy, capillary engorgement of the upper respiratory tract includes the nasal and oropharyngeal mucosa and larynx, and pregnant women may have nasal stuffiness. Also, nose breathing is difficult, and nosebleeds can occur. This capillary engorgement of the respiratory mucosa during pregnancy predisposes the upper airways to trauma, bleeding, and obstruction. Gentle laryngoscopy and the use of small endotracheal tubes (6 mm to 6.5 mm) should be used during general anesthesia.

***Lung Mechanics and Ventilation.*** The diaphragm elevates, and the rib cage flares; therefore, at term, 85% of respiratory effort is intercostal and 15% diaphragmatic (normally, approximately 70% is intercostal, and 30% is diaphragmatic). Because of the mechanical changes in the lungs and chest

## Box 51-2    Possible Alterations in Cardiovascular Parameters

- Heart sounds are louder with the development of a split $S_2$
- Short systolic murmur
- More forceful apical impulse
- Inverted T waves in leads III, $V_1$, and $V_2$
- Left axis deviation in months 2 to 6
- Flattened T waves
- Depressed ST segments
- If findings develop during pregnancy, they usually disappear after delivery

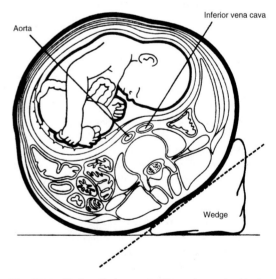

**Fig. 51-3** Uterine displacement with wedge under hip to relieve aortocaval compression. *(From Ostheimer SW: Regional anesthesia techniques in obstetrics, New York, 1980, Breon Laboratories.)*

wall, the lung volumes and capacities do change during pregnancy. Overall, the inspiratory lung volumes and capacities moderately increase, and the expiratory lung volumes and capacities decrease. The inspiratory reserve volume and the inspiratory capacity increase by 5% to 15%. The functional residual capacity (FRC) decreases by approximately 20% to 60%. Also, the residual volume and expiratory reserve volume, which make up the FRC, are decreased. The combination of decreased FRC and increased oxygen consumption promotes rapid oxygen desaturation during periods of apnea.

The tidal volume also increases about 20% to 45%, and the respiratory rate does not change, which leads to a 30% to 45% increase in the alveolar ventilation and the minute ventilation. Therefore, during pregnancy, the arterial oxygen level ranges from 95 to 105 mm Hg and the arterial carbon dioxide level is approximately 30 mm Hg, with an arterial pH of 7.44. Consequently, the pregnant patient has some respiratory alkalosis for which the renal excretion of bicarbonate compensates. Hence, the normal bicarbonate level during pregnancy is about 19 mEq/L, and the base excess is reduced by 2 mEq/L.

In regard to flow rate changes, the forced expiratory volume in 1 second and the flow-volume loop remain unchanged. Also, the closing capacity (see Chapter 12) does not change during gestation. Consequently, the conductance and resistance of the small and large airways do not change during pregnancy.

### Gastrointestinal Changes

*Motility and Secretions.* Gastric emptying slows during pregnancy because the stomach is displaced as the uterus enlarges, which leads to gastroesophageal reflux and esophagitis during pregnancy. All parturients have a gastric pH less than 2.5, and more than 60% have gastric volumes greater than 25 mL. The gastric volume also increases during hours 1 to 8 in the postpartum period. Therefore, the perianesthesia nurse must be cognizant of the potential for vomiting and aspiration, particularly in patients who have had general anesthesia. Muscle relaxants may have been used and may result in the patient's normal protective mechanisms being obtunded. Once again, the side-lying position becomes of significant importance.

*Hepatic System.* Liver function test results are abnormal, but no evidence suggests alteration in liver function. Hepatic blood flow remains constant. Therefore, those anesthetic agents that are metabolized in the liver should have the same duration of effect.

### Renal Changes

Early in pregnancy, the kidneys receive an increased blood flow because of renal vasodilation, so glomerular filtration and urine formation rates increase. This increase is necessary to handle the increased amount of waste products produced. Monitoring of output should reflect this expected increase in volume. Intervention may be necessary for hypovolemia even though the urine output is within ranges acceptable in a nonpregnant patient.

## INTRAOPERATIVE ANESTHESIA CARE OF THE OBSTETRIC PATIENT

Because the effects of anesthesia have such a profound effect on the emergence of the pregnant patient, a complete review of the techniques and procedures of general and regional anesthesia is presented.

### Positioning

Because the supine position causes a reduction in uterine blood flow in the pregnant patient, the semi-Fowler's position is used when possible. For prevention of aortocaval compression, the patient is placed in the lateral decubitus position, and the right hip is elevated with a pillow or the uterus is displaced to the left with devices on the operating table.

### Gastrointestinal Considerations

The pregnant patient has a reduced gastric emptying time and a reduced gastric pH. However, research has shown that gastric volume and acidity in the pregnant patient do not differ significantly from those in the nonpregnant patient. However, many anesthesia clinicians believe strongly that the pregnant patient, especially the patient with pyrosis (heartburn), is at risk of development of aspiration pneumonitis. Consequently, preoperative pharmacologic interventions are usually taken. Drugs that may be administered include a nonparticulate antacid such as 30 mL of 0.3 mmol/L sodium citrate (Bicitra) to increase the gastric pH; cimetidine (Tagamet) or 50 mg ranitidine (Zantac) or granisetron (Kytril), which are histamine-2 receptor blockers that reduce gastric acid secretion; and 10 mg metoclopramide (Reglan), which speeds up gastric emptying time and elevates lower esophageal tone.

### General Anesthesia

*Induction.* Because of the strong full-stomach considerations, the pregnant patient is intubated with a rapid-sequence endotracheal intubation technique (see Chapter 30) that includes intravenous (IV) propofol, etomidate, or ketamine followed by succinylcholine. A defasciculation dose of a nondepolarizing muscle relaxant may be given before the administration of the succinylcholine to avoid the increase in intragastric pressure. Some clinicians do not administer a defasciculating dose of a nondepolarizing muscle relaxant because most pregnant patients do not have fasciculation after succinylcholine. Cricoid pressure (Sellick maneuver) is applied with an assistant's thumb and index fingers exerting downward pressure on the cricoid cartilage to displace the cartilaginous cricothyroid ring posteriorly and thus compress the underlying esophagus against the cervical vertebrae.

The endotracheal tube should be a small tube, usually 7 mm in diameter or smaller, because of increased mucosal engorgement in the nasal and oropharyngeal areas. Also, nasotracheal intubation is not used because of the high risk of tissue trauma.

*Maintenance.* Nitrous oxide in 50% concentration with oxygen is usually administered. Inhalation agents such as sevoflurane, isoflurane, and desflurane can be used. Analgesic concentrations of 0.5 minimum alveolar concentration (see Chapter 20) or less to avoid significant uterine relaxation can be used safely for these inhalation drugs. However, these inhalation agents, particularly sevoflurane, may be used in high concentrations for a short period to produce uterine relaxation for intrauterine manipulation of the fetus or removal of a retained placenta. The clinical implication in the postanesthesia care unit (PACU) for the patient who received a high concentration of an inhalation agent, even for a short period (< 2 minutes) is monitoring for postpartum hemorrhage and maternal hypotension. Also, the uterine response to oxytocic drugs is reduced when high concentrations of these inhalation agents are used.

In regard to skeletal muscle relaxation, succinylcholine infusion or short-acting nondepolarizing muscle relaxants such as rocuronium and vecuronium can be used safely because they lack autonomic side effects and have a low degree of placental transfer. In the immediate postpartum period, the neuromuscular-blocking effects of vecuronium are prolonged.

*Emergence.* At the end of the surgical procedure, the residual effects of the nondepolarizing muscle relaxants are reversed and the inhalation anesthetic agents are discontinued. When the patient is awake, responsive, and able to ventilate without assistance, she is extubated.

### Regional Anesthesia

Regional anesthesia, primarily spinal and epidural, is used extensively for anesthesia in the pregnant patient because it produces analgesia without causing neonatal depression. This technique also reduces the risk of maternal hypoventilation and the need for narcotics and sedatives. Regional anesthesia does not require airway management, preserves airway reflexes, and allows the mother to remain awake during birth. It is contraindicated in patients with severe coagulation problems, severe hypovolemia, sepsis, and infection at the needle insertion site; in situations in which immediate delivery is crucial, such as in fetal distress; and when the patient refuses the procedure.

The level of sensory blockade for either spinal or epidural anesthesia for cesarean section is from T4 to S4. The commonly used local anesthetic drugs for spinal anesthesia are lidocaine and bupivacaine (see Chapter 24). For epidural anesthesia, the commonly used local anesthetic agents are 2-chloroprocaine (Nesacaine), lidocaine with epinephrine, bupivacaine, and ropivacaine, which may be preferable because of possibly less motor blockade and reduced potential for cardiotoxicity.

In comparison with the spinal approach, the epidural approach is the preferred technique because drugs can be administered throughout the surgical procedure via a continuous epidural catheter. The anesthesia clinician then has the ability to control the onset, distribution, and duration of anesthesia. Also, the incidence rate of postdural puncture is much lower in comparison with the spinal technique.

## PERIANESTHESIA CARE OF THE MOTHER AND THE FETUS

Studies have not shown one anesthetic technique to be better than another in the gravid patient. As with nonpregnant patients, the choice of technique is determined by the following:

1. Surgery to be performed
2. American Society of Anesthesiologists' classification of the patient
3. Anesthetist preference
4. Patient preference
5. Underlying disease entities

The care of the pregnant patient after surgery should be the same as for any patient who undergoes that procedure or for one who recovers from that particular anesthetic. However, additions to the routine nursing care must be instituted for all pregnant patients.

### Positioning

To alleviate compression of the vena cava, the uterus should be displaced to the left, either by

**Table 51-1 Fetal Heart Rates**

| Description | Rate (bpm) |
| --- | --- |
| Normal fetal heart rate | 120-160 |
| Moderate tachycardia | 160-180 |
| Marked tachycardia | >180 |
| Moderate bradycardia | 100-120 |
| Marked bradycardia | <100 |

positioning the patient on her left side or by tilting the pelvis with a folded sheet or bath towel under the woman's right iliac crest. Slight elevation of the legs and the use of thigh-high elastic stockings should be standard.

### Psychologic and Emotional Support

The mother's concern for her unborn child is paramount. Constant reassurance is mandatory. If possible, allow the mother to listen to the fetal heartbeat frequently during the recovery phase. Explain all procedures and why they are being done before they are carried out. If the PACU allows visitors, involvement of the father should also be considered.

### Fetal Monitoring

The fetal heart rate must be monitored every 15 minutes if the fetus has reached viability (Table 51-1). If available, an indirect fetal monitoring system should be used for constant assessment of fetal stability (Fig. 51-4).

The second type of monitoring required is close observation of the patient for signs of premature labor. These signs include spontaneous rupture of membranes, increased fetal heart rate, presenting of vaginal mucus plug, uterine palpitations, uterine contractions, and restlessness of the mother.

Initially, the patient may not feel the contractions or be aware of membrane rupture; therefore, palpation of the abdomen and assessment of vaginal discharge must be performed by the nurse. If premature labor begins, transfer of the patient to the labor and delivery area as soon as possible is recommended. A drug may be necessary to stop labor. These drugs should be administered by personnel familiar with proper protocols for administration and side effects.

### Pain Management

***The Patient After Cesarean Section.*** The patient after cesarean section presents unique challenges in regard to pain management. More specifically, more women desire to care for their newborns within the first 24 hours.

Heavy sedation with opioids and IV or epidural catheters inhibits the mother's ability to care for the infant. Also, the infant can be affected through the transfer of the drug in breast milk.

Patient-controlled analgesia (PCA) is becoming quite popular in pain management of the patient after cesarean section (see Chapters 22, 27, and 31). PCA interrupts the pain cycle, gives the patient a feeling of control, hastens the time to ambulation, and reduces the length of stay in the hospital. Morphine is the preferred drug to be administered via PCA. The usual dose is 1 to 1.5 mg, with a lockout of 10 minutes and an hourly limit of 10 to 12 mg.

Epidural administration of opioids is another option that can be used for the control of pain in the PACU. Morphine is the preferred drug because of its demonstrated safety and prolonged duration of action after a single dose of 5 mg. The primary side effects of epidural morphine are pruritus and nausea. Some clinicians have advocated use of the narcotic antagonist naloxone (5 to 10 mcg/kg/h) to treat these side effects. However, problems arise with some reversal of the analgesia. Most clinicians treat the nausea with 2 to 4 mg of odansetron (Zofran) IV and the pruritus with 12.5 mg of IV diphenhydramine (Benadryl).

Fentanyl is an alternative to morphine for epidural analgesia. The difficulty with fentanyl is that its duration of action is less than 5 hours and that it must be administered via continuous infusion or intermittent boluses. The epidural fentanyl technique provides excellent analgesia; however, most women desire to be ambulatory as soon as possible and do not like to be encumbered with the catheter, tape, and pump.

When administered epidurally with opioids, 2-chloroprocaine inhibits the analgesic effects of the opioids. This inhibitory action of 2-chloroprocaine is probably caused by the ethylenediaminetetraacetic acid (EDTA) that is used in the solution of the drug. EDTA is an antioxidant that has analgesic antagonism properties because it is a strong chelator of calcium. Therefore, clinically epidural opioids should be avoided for at least 6 to 8 hours after 2-chloroprocaine has been administered.

A variety of receptor-specific drugs to include opioids, alpha$_2$-adrenergic agonists, and local anesthetics are being evaluated for use via the intraspinal approach. With the refining of the spinal technique to include the use of small needles, this technique is gaining in popularity for post–cesarean section pain relief. Morphine, 0.3 mg administered intrathecally, has a longer duration of action than 4 mg of morphine administered via the epidural route. Some anesthesia clinicians are now adding morphine to

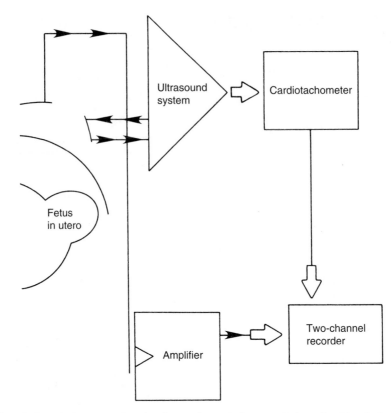

**Fig. 51-4**  Indirect fetal monitoring system. Doppler ultrasound scan device transmits beam for determination of fetal heart rate. When beam strikes moving object within fetus, such as mitral valve leaflet, frequency of transmitted beam is shifted up or down, depending on which way leaflet is moving. This valve movement is counted and displayed as heart rate on recorder.

bupivacaine during surgery, with the outcome of excellent analgesia that lasts well into the post-anesthesia period.

Along with the various opioid analgesics, the patient after cesarean section should be administered supplemental oxygen during anesthesia and for the first 2 hours after surgery, not only to enhance pulmonary function but also to potentially help in the prevention of postoperative nausea and vomiting (PONV). More research is needed to evaluate the effectiveness during the immediate postanesthesia period.

***The Pregnant Patient.*** Because of the growth in consumer awareness, the administration of medication during pregnancy has become a controversial issue that must be addressed on an individual basis. For pain management in the PACU, when the pregnant patient is in a hyper-suggestive state, distraction techniques such as guided imagery and breathing exercises have had favorable results in place of drugs.

If a mild analgesic is needed, the drug of choice is acetaminophen (Tylenol); for moderate pain management, propoxyphene (Darvon) is recommended. Both drugs have been evaluated through prospective studies and have been shown to pose minimal risks to the fetus if used appropriately for short-term pain management. Narcotic analgesia may be warranted for severe pain but must be used judiciously, with the respiratory depressive effects kept in mind.

Ketorolac (Toradol), a prostaglandin synthetase inhibitor, is becoming quite popular in postoperative pain therapy. However, nonsteroidal antiinflammatory agents, such as ketorolac, are not recommended in the parturient because they suppress uterine contractions and promote closure of the fetal ductus arteriosus.

The gravid patient in the PACU is a rare occurrence that requires the nurse to have a great deal of knowledge and the ability to provide continual support during this stressful situation. The nurse must be able to provide a quiet calm reassuring atmosphere for the patient. The objective of the care delivered is an optimal environment for both the mother and the fetus.

## SUMMARY

The perianesthesia nursing care of the obstetric patient who is undergoing a nonobstetric surgical procedure is both challenging and rewarding.

Statistics indicate that about one in 500 pregnancies are complicated by nonobstetric surgical conditions. The intent of this chapter is to provide information on the pregnant patient and fetus undergoing nonobstetric surgery. The physiologic changes, types of surgery, and perianesthesia nursing care were highlighted and should provide the perianesthesia nurse with valuable knowledge to facilitate the appropriate outcomes for the mother and fetus.

## BIBLIOGRAPHY

Abboud T: Nonobstetric surgery during pregnancy, *Semin Anesth* 11(1):51-54, 1992.

Alspach J: *Core curriculum for critical care nursing*, ed 6, Philadelphia, 2005, Saunders.

Atlee J: *Complications in anesthesia*, Philadelphia, 2006, Saunders.

Barash P, Cullen B, Stoelting R: *Clinical anesthesia*, ed 5, Philadelphia, 2006, Lippincott Williams & Wilkins.

Benumof J, Saidman L: *Anesthesia & perioperative complications*, ed 2, St Louis, 1999, Mosby.

Bickley L, Hoekelman R: *Bates' guide to physical examination and history taking*, ed 9, Philadelphia, 2005, Lippincott Williams & Wilkins.

Bowdle T, Horita A, Kharasch E: *The pharmacologic basis of anesthesiology*, New York, 1994, Churchill Livingstone.

Chestnut D: *Obstetrical anesthesia: principles and practice*, ed 3, Philadelphia, 2004, Mosby.

Chichester M: When your patient is from the obstetric department: postpartum hemorrhage and massive transfusion, *J PeriAnesthesia Nurs* 20(3):167-176.

Conklin K: Maternal physiological adaptations during gestation, labor, and the puerperium, *Semin Anesth* 10(4):221-234, 1991.

Coté C, Todres I, Goudsouzian N, et al: *A practice of anesthesia for infants and children*, ed 3, Philadelphia, 2001, Saunders.

Curran C: Perianesthesia care following obstetric emergencies at risk for multisystem organ dysfunction, *J PeriAnesthesia Nurs* 20(3):185-199, 2005.

DeFazio-Quinn D: *Ambulatory surgical nursing core curriculum*, Philadelphia, 1999, Saunders.

Eisenach J: Pain management in the parturient: theoretical and practical aspects, *Semin Anesth* 11(1):55-65, 1992.

Estafanous F, Barash P, Reves J: *Cardiac anesthesia*, ed 2, Philadelphia, 2001, Lippincott Williams & Wilkins.

Fleisher L: *Anesthesia and uncommon diseases*, ed 5, Philadelphia, 2005, Saunders.

Ganong W: *Review of medical physiology*, ed 22, New York, 2005, McGraw-Hill.

Gbods A, Soleimani M, Narimani M: Effect of postoperative supplemental oxygen on nausea and vomiting after cesarean birth, *J PeriAnesthesia Nurs* 20(3):200-205, 2005.

Guyton A, Hall J: *Textbook of medical physiology*, ed 11, Philadelphia, 2005, Saunders.

Hardman J, Limbird L: *Goodman and Gilman's the pharmacological basis of therapeutics*, ed 11, New York, 2005, McGraw-Hill.

Johnson M, Ostheimer G: Airway management in obstetric patients, *Semin Anesth* 11(1):1-12, 1992.

Katzung B, editor: *Basic and clinical pharmacology*, ed 9, Los Altos, Calif, 2003, Appleton & Lange.

Kelly M: Maternal position and blood pressure during pregnancy and delivery, *Am J Nurs* 82:809-812, 1982.

Lake C, Hines R, Blitt C: *Clinical monitoring: practical applications for anesthesia and critical care*, St Louis, 2001, Mosby.

Longnecker D, Murphy F: *Dripps/Eckenhoff/Vandam introduction to anesthesia*, ed 9, Philadelphia, 1997, Saunders.

Longnecker D, Tinker J, Morgan G: *Principles and practice of anesthesiology*, ed 2, St Louis, 1998, Mosby.

Martin J: *Positioning in anesthesia and surgery*, ed 3, St Louis, 1997, Mosby.

Miller R, editor: *Anesthesia*, ed 6, New York, 2004, Churchill Livingstone.

Moran D, Dewan D: Anesthesia for cesarean delivery, *Semin Anesth* 10(4):286-294, 1991.

Morgan E, Mikhail M, Murray M: *Clinical anesthesiology*, ed 4, New York, 2006, McGraw-Hill.

Motoyama E: *Smith's anesthesia for infants and children*, ed 7, St Louis, 2005, Mosby.

Nagelhout J, Zaglaniczny K: *Nurse anesthesia*, ed 3, Philadelphia, 2004, Saunders.

Norris M, editor: *Obstetric anesthesia*, ed 2, Philadelphia, 1999, Lippincott.

Shaver S, Shaver D: Preoperative assessment of the obstetric patient undergoing abdominal surgery, *J PeriAnesthesia Nurs* 20:160-166, 2005.

Shnider S, Levinson G: *Anesthesia for obstetrics*, ed 4, Baltimore, 2002, Williams & Wilkins.

Stoelting R: *Pharmacology and physiology in anesthetic practice*, ed 4, Philadelphia, 2005, Lippincott-Raven.

Stoelting R, Miller R: *Basics of anesthesia*, ed 5, New York, 2006, Churchill Livingstone.

Stone D: *Perioperative care: anesthesia, medicine, and surgery*, St Louis, 1998, Mosby.

Torgersen K: Communication to facilitate care of the obstetric surgical patient in a postanesthesia care setting, *J PeriAnesthesia Nurs* 20(3):177-183, 2005.

Traver G, Tremper Mitchell J, et al: *Respiratory care: a clinical approach*, Gaithersburg, Md, 1991, Aspen Publishers Inc.

Ziadlourad F, Conklin K: Anesthesia for obstetric emergencies, *Semin Anesth* 8(3):222-231, 1989.

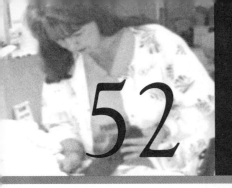

# 52

# CARE OF THE SUBSTANCE USING PATIENT

Cecil B. Drain, PhD, RN, CRNA, FAAN, FASAHP

The great increase in the number of persons who use narcotics, amphetamines, cocaine, hallucinogens, barbiturates, and date rape drugs has created new problems in perianesthesia nursing care.

Drug dependence is the nonmedical use of a drug and consists of the self administration of any drug in a manner that deviates from the approved medical or social practices within a given culture. Physical dependence is an altered physiologic state caused by repeated administration of a drug that necessitates the continued administration of the drug to prevent the appearance of withdrawal or abstinence syndromes characteristic for that drug. Psychologic dependence is habituation-compulsive drug use. In this type of dependence, a drug is used to alter mood and feeling; eventually, dependent people come to believe that the effects of the drug are necessary to maintain an optimal state of well being. Another term that should be defined in discussions of substance dependence is tolerance. Drug tolerance is a state in which, after repeated administration of a drug, a given dose produces a decreased effect or, on the other hand, in which increasingly larger doses are needed to obtain the same effect as that of the original dose.

The pharmacologic agents that are most commonly seen in dependence can be grouped as follows: (1) opioid analgesics; (2) general central nervous system (CNS) depressants, such as alcohol and barbiturates; (3) CNS sympathomimetics, such as amphetamines and cocaine; (4) cannabinoids, such as marijuana; and (5) psychedelics, of which lysergic acid diethylamide (LSD) and phencyclidine are the prototypic drugs (Table 52-1), inhalants, club drugs, and date-rape drugs.

## DEFINITIONS

**Alcoholic:** A person who is excessively dependent on alcohol and who has a noticeable degree of mental, physical, psychologic, or pathologic disorders.

**Alcoholic Cirrhosis (Laennë's Cirrhosis):** A fibrotic form of cirrhosis precipitated by alcohol abuse.

**Anterograde Amnesia:** The inability to form new memories or recall events that occur after the onset of the amnesia.

**Delirium Tremens:** An acute and sometimes fatal psychotic reaction caused by cessation of excessive intake of alcoholic beverages over a long period of time.

**Endocarditis:** Inflammation of the endocardium and heart valves.

**Hallucinations:** A sensory perception that does not result from an external stimulus and that occurs in the waking state.

**Malignant Hyperthermia:** A rare genetic hypermetabolic condition characterized by severe hyperthermia and rigidity of the skeletal muscles.

**Plasma Cholinesterase:** An enzyme in the blood plasma that acts as a catalyst in the hydrolysis of acetylcholine to choline and acetate.

**Potentiated:** A synergistic action in which the effect of two drugs given simultaneously is greater than the sum of the effects of each drug given separately.

**Sensorium:** The part of the consciousness that includes the special sensory perceptive powers and their central correlation and integration in the brain. A clear sensorium conveys the presence of a reasonably accurate memory together with spacial orientation.

**Substance Abuse:** The overuse of stimulant, depressant, or other chemicals or drugs that is detrimental to the patient's physical or mental health.

**Substance Dependence:** The total psychophysical state of one addicted to drugs or alcohol who must receive an increasing amount of the substance to prevent the onset of withdrawal symptoms.

**Substance Use:** A maladaptive pattern of the use of a drug, chemical, or biologic entity that is capable of being abused because of its physiologic or psychologic effects.

**Tremulousness:** Involuntary muscle contraction.

**Table 52-1  Categories of Substance Dependence: Effects and Signs of Dependence and Withdrawal**

| Category | Possible Effects | Signs of Dependence | Signs of Withdrawal |
|---|---|---|---|
| **OPIOID ANALGESICS** | | | |
| Opium<br>Morphine<br>Codeine<br>Heroin<br>Meperidine (Demerol)<br>Sublimaze (Fentanyl)<br>Methadone (Dolophine) | Euphoria, "rush" with IV injection, feeling of detachment, drowsiness, miosis, nausea, respiratory depression<br>Tolerance and physical and psychologic dependence | Injection scars or needle marks, usually on inner surfaces of arms<br>Thrombophlebitis at injection sites, cellulitis<br>Pinpoint pupils<br>Uncoordinated movements<br>Confusion, disorientation<br>Heavy smoking | Watery eyes, runny nose, scratching, yawning, anorexia, irritability, tremors, panic, chills and sweating, muscle pains and cramps, nausea, vomiting, diarrhea |
| **GENERAL CNS DEPRESSANTS** | | | |
| Alcohol | Loss of inhibitions<br>Impaired judgment<br>Carefree mood<br>Impaired motor coordination, concentration, memory<br>Ataxia, incoherence<br>Stupor, coma<br>Tolerance and physical dependence | Reported intake:<br>Heavy drinker*<br>Alcohol-addicted†<br>GI disturbances<br>Malnutrition<br>Heavy smoking<br>Trauma<br>Psychologic problems<br>Social maladjustment | *8 h after abstinence:*<br>Tremors, GI disturbances, anxiety, jittery feeling, and headache<br>*24-72 h or longer of withdrawal:*<br>Increased tremors, hyperactivity, irritability, nervousness, insomnia, delusions, hallucinations, seizures, delirium tremens (DTs), high fever, profuse sweating, tachycardia, hyperventilation, nausea and vomiting |
| **Barbiturates**<br>Amytal<br>Butisol<br>Nembutal<br>Seconal<br>Tunal<br>Phenobarbital | Euphoria, reduced anxiety, dry intoxication (drunken behavior without odor of alcohol)<br>Tolerance and physical and psychologic dependence | Drowsiness, lack of interest, fatigue, irritability<br>Changes in personality and behavior<br>Possession of pills of varying colors and shapes | Range from anxiety, weakness, confusion, anorexia, and mild tremors to delirium, disorientation, hallucinations, and convulsions |

*Continued*

**Table 52-1  Categories of Substance Dependence: Effects and Signs of Dependence and Withdrawal—cont'd**

| Category | Possible Effects | Signs of Dependence | Signs of Withdrawal |
|---|---|---|---|
| **Benzodiazepines**<br>Valium<br>Librium<br>Serax<br>Ativan<br>Versed | Same as barbiturates | Same as barbiturates | Same as barbiturates |
| **CNS SYMPATHOMIMETICS** | | | |
| Amphetamines | Increased alertness, euphoria, anorexia, insomnia, elevated blood pressure, tachycardia, anxiety<br>Tolerance, psychologic dependence | Possession of pills of varying color<br>Injection scars, needle marks<br>Compulsion to talk, extreme activity, chain smoking<br>Frequent nose rubbing or scratching, licking of dry lips, bad breath<br>Changed eating and sleeping habits<br>Projected sense of prowess or capability<br>Possible aggressive or antisocial behavior | "Crashing" (response produced when stimulant effect ends); hunger, extreme lethargy, profound depression, and sleep disturbance |
| Cocaine | Same as amphetamines<br>Possible tolerance, no physical dependence, high psychologic dependence | Same as amphetamines<br>Inflamed nasal mucosa | Same as amphetamines<br>"Crashing" may be profound |

**CANNABINOIDS**

**Marijuana (hashish)**

| Effects | Physical evidence | Abstinence symptoms |
|---|---|---|
| Sense of relaxation and well being | Possession of off-white or brown cigarette papers and coarse brownish-green tobacco | *Reported abstinence symptoms:* Hyperexcitability, insomnia, decreased appetite |
| Distorted orientation to time and space | Conjunctival congestion, dilated pupils | |
| Altered sensory perception | Wearing of dark glasses because of light sensitivity | |
| Occasional excitement and spontaneous (often uncontrolled) laughter | | |
| Increased appetite | | |
| Tolerance and psychologic dependence, degree of physical dependence unknown | | |

**PSYCHEDELICS**

**Lysergic acid diethylamide (LSD)**

**Phencyclidine (PCP)**

| Effects | Physical evidence | Abstinence symptoms |
|---|---|---|
| Illusions | Possession of perforated small squares of blotter paper with colored designs, ampules of clear liquid, or capsules of white or colored powder, or tablets | None reported |
| Distorted perceptions of time, distance, body image, mood, affect | Unusual body odor | |
| Depersonalization and ego dissociation | Marked mood changes | |
| Psychotic behavior | Dreamlike or trancelike state | |
| Tolerance, degree of psychologic dependence unknown | | |

*Heavy drinker: A person who consumes five or more drinks on some occasions and at least 45 drinks a month.

†Alcohol-addicted: A person who consumes approximately 20 drinks of beer, wine, or liquor a day and has developed physiologic tolerance.

From Knor E: Substance dependent. In *Decision making in obstetrical nursing,* Toronto, 1987, BC Decker.

IV, Intravenous; GI, gastrointestinal.

SPECIAL CONSIDERATIONS

## OPIOID ANALGESICS

Opioid analgesics (narcotics) cause strong psychologic dependence. Physical dependence is manifested by the withdrawal syndrome of autonomic storm and CNS irritability. Also, a strong tolerance for these drugs and a cross tolerance with other drugs of the same classification of opioid analgesics develop. Studies indicate that in people who are chronically addicted to opioid analgesics such as morphine, the minimum alveolar concentration of inhalation anesthetics (see Chapter 20) is increased, which indicates that a cross tolerance with general inhalation anesthetics may exist.

Heroin, an opioid analgesic that is derived from morphine, is degraded in the body to morphine about 30 minutes after injection. The most common problem associated with the use of heroin and other opioid analgesics is pulmonary edema; other dysfunctions include superficial bacterial infections, adrenal insufficiency, bacterial endocarditis, liver disease, urinary abnormalities (proteinuria and glycosuria), and false-positive serology. In addition, about 30% of the persons dependent on opiates have positive results on the Venereal Disease Research Laboratory test for syphilis, but only about 25% of these results are true positive when checked with the *Treponema* immobilization test.

Perianesthesia nursing care of a patient who is dependent on an opiate, such as heroin dependency, centers around monitoring the patient for complications. Probably foremost is monitoring for the withdrawal (abstinence) syndrome. The abstinence syndrome after dependence on an opiate occurs in two phases. The acute phase occurs during the first few days. The protracted phase, which is not readily treatable, can persist for as long as 2 to 6 months. The acute opiate abstinence phase is not dangerous to life because it usually is not associated with convulsions and delirium. Instead, the symptoms are anxiety, nervousness, jittery behavior, anorexia, rhinorrhea, hypotension, muscle twitching, insomnia, sweating, pupillary dilation, gooseflesh, and nausea and vomiting. Symptoms during the protracted phase include those of the acute phase, along with convulsions and delirium. Treatment for the acute opiate abstinence phase is accomplished with any narcotic analgesic; reports indicate that clonidine has proved to be most effective in attenuating the symptoms. New research indicates that dexmedetomidine may also be effective in attenuating the symptoms. Treatment for the protracted phase centers around protection of the patient and abatement of the symptoms shown by the patient. If a patient is suspected of dependence on an opiate, narcotic antagonists such as naloxone (Narcan) should not be administered because the withdrawal syndrome can be precipitated. No attempt should be made at withdrawal of the patient who is actively dependent on an opiate during the postanesthesia care unit (PACU) period. Liberal use of morphine or methadone in the PACU appears to be satisfactory. Patients who are formerly dependent on opioids should not receive narcotics; analgesics such as pentazocine (Talwin) and butorphanol (Stadol) should be used in their place.

## GENERAL CENTRAL NERVOUS SYSTEM DEPRESSANTS

The patient dependent on a barbiturate may present only as nervous and anxious before surgery. However, the patient should be monitored after surgery for anxiety, tremors, and hallucinations. These symptoms usually develop on the second or third postoperative day and can be treated with a barbiturate until acute illness has passed. These patients also appear to have an increased tolerance to anesthesia and therefore have an increased chance of anesthetic toxicity.

The dependency rate of persons on benzodiazepine compounds has increased significantly during the last decade. The benzodiazepine drug is usually taken in combination with marijuana or alcohol to obtain a high. Chronic intoxication has been reported with the use of these compounds. The benzodiazepine that produces the most dependency is diazepam (Valium); however, midazolam (Versed) will soon rank at the same level as diazepam. These drugs are becoming popular because of their rapid onset of action coupled with their pleasure-giving effects. The pharmacologic effects of the benzodiazepines are similar to those of the barbiturates. This classification of drugs is somewhat addictive and includes withdrawal syndromes.

For treatment of mild to moderate overdosages of benzodiazepines, the drug physostigmine in an adult dosage of 1 to 2 mg given intravenously can be used. A new antagonist with a longer action and fewer side effects has been introduced into clinical practice. This drug, flumazenil (Romazicon), is a true benzodiazepine receptor antagonist. The usual adult dosage is 0.1 to 0.2 mg given intravenously. As with naloxone for patient dependence on a narcotic, flumazenil must be used with caution with patients who are benzodiazepine dependent. More specifically, reversal of benzodiazepine dependence is associated with precipitating the withdrawal syndrome, including seizures.

Alcoholism has long been widespread, yet it is difficult to define. An alcoholic, for purposes of this discussion, is a person who is excessively dependent on alcohol and who has developed a noticeable degree of mental, physical, psychologic, or pathologic disorders. Alcohol was the first anesthetic; it can produce anesthesia, respiratory depression, and hypotension.

Alcohol affects many of the body's major systems. Cirrhosis of the liver is well known to be quite common in the later stages of alcoholism. This knowledge is of importance to the perianesthesia nurse because the liver detoxifies many drugs administered during the perioperative period (see Chapter 16). Hepatic cirrhosis may produce significant alterations in pulmonary and cardiovascular functions. Hyperventilation and arterial oxygen desaturation are common findings caused by an increase in shunting of blood away from areas in the lung where diffusion of oxygen takes place. Concomitant with this is an increase in blood volume that may lead to cardiac hypertrophy and eventually to congestive heart failure. Fluid balance is affected by the presence of alcohol because alcohol exhibits antidiuretic effects by inhibiting the release of antidiuretic hormone. Alcoholic cirrhosis (Laennëc's cirrhosis) is also associated with portal vein hypertension, renal failure, hypoglycemia, duodenal ulcer, esophageal varices, and hepatic encephalopathy.

The alcoholic, in comparison with the nonalcoholic, usually requires a larger amount of sodium thiopental for induction and a higher concentration of anesthetic agents during surgery. Prediction of the time or the character of emergence from anesthesia is difficult in the alcoholic patient. This patient may be anxious and may have a stormy emergence and postoperative phase.

During the PACU phase, the alcoholic patient should be monitored for withdrawal symptoms. The minor alcohol withdrawal syndrome is characterized by symptoms such as tremulousness, insomnia, and irritability. Because of autonomic nervous system imbalance, signs such as tachycardia, hypertension, and cardiac dysrhythmias are often observed. The minor alcohol withdrawal syndrome can occur within 6 to 8 hours after abstinence by the alcoholic patient. The signs and symptoms of this syndrome usually disappear within 48 hours without treatment.

In about 5% of the alcoholic population, the severe alcohol withdrawal syndrome, or delirium tremens, occurs with abrupt cessation of alcohol ingestion. The mortality rate from this syndrome is about 15%; it is considered a medical emergency. The time of onset of delirium tremens is about 48 to 72 hours after the abrupt discontinuation of alcohol ingestion.

The patient is difficult to manage if withdrawal symptoms are allowed to develop. The severe withdrawal syndrome should be suspected if symptoms, such as restlessness, disorientation, tremulousness, and hallucinations, occur. In addition, because of activation of the sympathetic nervous system, symptoms such as diaphoresis, hyperpyrexia, tachycardia, and hypertension are seen. When any of these symptoms are observed, hypoxia should first be ruled out because the symptoms of withdrawal can be confused with those of hypoxia. The treatment used to control the withdrawal symptoms is sedation with diazepam, along with intravenous fluids and electrolytes, vitamin replacement (i.e., thiamine), and glucose. If deemed necessary by the attending physician, propranolol may be given to suppress the clinical manifestations of the increased sympathetic nervous system activity. Also, if cardiac dysrhythmias occur, lidocaine may be administered intravenously.

## CENTRAL NERVOUS SYSTEM SYMPATHOMIMETICS

Cocaine has a two-pronged effect, vasoconstriction and mood alteration, because it inhibits the reuptake of catecholamines. The mood-altering effect is similar to the psychologic effect produced by amphetamines. Cocaine is steadily becoming one of the most popular drugs among persons dependent on a substance. Patients who are known to be dependent on cocaine should be closely monitored in the PACU for hypertension and cardiac arrhythmias. Also, these patients are quite prone to nosebleeds, so care should be taken in administration of nursing care near or directly to the nose and nasal cavity.

Central nervous system stimulants, which include amphetamines, are becoming extremely popular with the teenage population; they tend to have the pharmacologic effect of long-acting vasopressors. The patient has dilated pupils, tachycardia, palpitations, cardiac arrhythmias, and changes in temperature regulation and appears to be extremely anxious. If the stimulant is wearing off, the patient is lethargic and depressed. Continuous electrocardiographic monitoring for cardiac arrhythmias is necessary and is coupled with frequent blood pressure and pulse measurements. The mental sensorium should also be monitored throughout the patient's stay in the PACU.

## CANNABINOIDS

The hemp plants, of which cannabis is the generic name, contain about 30 active substances that are called cannabinoids. Of these, tetrahydrocannabinol (THC) is the most active. Marijuana is the generic term applied to the hemp plants. The marijuana cigarette contains rolled-up or crushed dried leaves from the hemp plant. Each marijuana cigarette contains about 0.005 g of THC. The cannabinoids are three times more potent when inhaled than when ingested orally. Psychologic changes occur minutes after inhalation of marijuana, and the effects peak in an hour, for as long as 3 hours.

The peripheral effects of THC on the autonomic nervous system include vagal blockade and beta-adrenergic stimulation. Hence, the person dependent on marijuana has tachycardia, peripheral vascular dilation, bronchodilation, conjunctival congestion, and a dry mouth. The actual effects of THC on the CNS are not known.

Because of the rapid effects of the drug, along with the short duration of action and the absence of physiologic dysfunction or changes, patients dependent on marijuana do not seem to present any added problems in the PACU. However, because of the chronic irritation produced by the inhalation of smoke from the marijuana cigarette, chronic dependence should be monitored for chronic bronchitis.

## PSYCHEDELICS

Phencyclidine is the hallucinogen most commonly used today. This drug is a popular veterinary anesthetic agent (Sernylan) and is related pharmacologically to the drug ketamine. It can be ingested, taken parenterally, or inhaled. The sensory effects have a rapid onset and last approximately 1 to 2 hours, and the CNS effects can last for 1 or more days. The CNS activation usually produces sympathetic nervous system activation.

The perianesthesia nurse is unlikely to have much contact with a patient under the influence of this drug. However, if a patient who is dependent on this drug should require perianesthesia care, the nurse must monitor this patient for sympathetic activation; symptoms such as dilated pupils, increased pulse, and elevated blood pressure should be reported immediately to the attending physician.

Lysergic acid diethylamide is a hallucinogen that reached its peak of use in the late 1960s and remained popular through in the 1990s. This drug is ingested orally, and its major effects occur in a dose-related manner. Moderate dosage of the drug causes euphoria, marked sensory distortion (including heightened awareness of sensory stimuli), and occasional visual hallucinations. Large doses of LSD usually lead to frightening hallucinations and a distorted body image, commonly known as a "bad trip." This drug also produces some hypertension, dilated pupils, and increased temperature, by virtue of its stimulation of the central hypothalamic area of the brain. The onset of the psychologic effects of LSD is after about 40 minutes, and the duration is about 2 hours. Some of the milder effects of LSD have been reported to last as long as 8 hours after ingestion.

The primary focus of perianesthesia nursing care for the patient who is in the hallucinogenic state is to prevent self injury and sedation. The "bad trip" effects can be managed with a phenothiazine or benzodiazepine such as diazepam. Other considerations in regard to the patient who has ingested LSD are that the analgesic effects of narcotics are potentiated by LSD and that the plasma cholinesterases are somewhat inhibited by LSD. Hence, narcotic dosage may need to be reduced in these patients, and if succinylcholine is to be administered to the patient, the possibility of prolonged apnea exists (see Chapter 23).

## INHALANTS

Inhalants can make a person extremely dependent and consist of breathable chemical vapors that produce mind-altering effects. Persons who use inhalants can have significant dependence; they are likely to be teenage people because the drugs are easily accessible and inexpensive. Inhalants are classified into three categories: solvents, gases, or nitrates.

The solvents consist of paint thinners or solvents, electronic contact cleaners, and felt-tip marker fluid. The gases consist of such household products and commercial products as butane lighters and propane tanks, whipping cream aerosols, spray paints, hair or deodorant sprays, and fabric protector sprays. Gases used for anesthetic medical purposes, such as isoflurane, sevoflurane, desflurane, and nitrous oxide (see Chapter 20), are now being used and can cause dependency. The nitrates, such as cyclohexyl nitrite and butyl nitrite, which are available to the public, and amyl nitrite, which is only available by prescription, are now being used as substances that can produce dependency.

The inhalants that cause dependency produce effects that are similar to the inhalational anesthetics as described in Chapter 20. Basically, these inhalants cause an intoxicating effect when they are inhaled through the nose or mouth into the lungs. When inhaled in high concentrations, these inhalants can induce heart failure and even death. Some of the irreversible effects of these inhalants can include hearing loss, peripheral neuropathies or limb spasms, central nervous system damage, and bone marrow damage. Some of the serious yet potentially reversible effects include hemoglobin oxygen depletion and liver or kidney damage.

The implications in the perianesthesia care of a patient who is using inhalants can be great. Given the fact that these substances can cause reversible and irreversible effects, each patient should be evaluated individually for use of these drugs. Health care professionals who care for these patients should remember that these inhalants are mainly used by children, with the highest usage between the 6th and 12th grades, and that usage continues to be a significant problem among youth. For perianesthesia nursing, the deliberate misuse of these volatile substances poses a significant risk or considerable morbidity and mortality in the adolescent population in the PACU. All these inhalants basically cause severe dysfunction to the liver and cause it to be unable to detoxify most all drugs used in anesthesia. Consequently, even small doses of opioid or nonopioid drugs have a prolonged length of action. Should the perianesthesia nurse suspect that a patient is dependent on inhalants, the anesthesia care provider must be advised because an entirely new regime of pain relief care has to be developed. Certainly, the lowest dose of any opioid or nonopioid should be considered, and the perianesthesia nurse should monitor for signs of cardiovascular and respiratory depression.

## CLUB DRUGS

Club drugs are most popular in the teenage and young adult population who are part of the nightclub, bar, rave, or trance scenes. Raves and trance parties are usually nightlong events that include adolescents who may not use the specific drugs; however, those who do are attracted to the use of these rather low-cost agents that appear to produce increased stamina and intoxicating highs. Research now shows that these drugs can change critical parts of the brain. Also, because of the different effects on the E-C coupling mechanisms of muscles as opposed to skeletal muscle relaxants (see Chapter 23), these agents are not implicated in malignant hyperthermia (see Chapter 53).

MDMA (Ecstasy) is a psychoactive drug that has both stimulant (amphetamine-like) and hallucinogenic (LSD-like) properties. This drug has many street names such as "Ecstasy," "Adam," "XTC," "hug," "beans," and "love drug." MDMA has many routes of administration, including oral, rectal, intravenous, or inhalation.

The problems associated with MDMA are similar to those found with the use of amphetamines and cocaine, which were discussed previously. The psychologic difficulties may include such phenomena as confusion, depression, sleep problems, severe anxiety, and paranoia. The physical difficulties include such things as muscle tension, involuntary teeth clenching, nausea, blurred vision, faintness, and chills or sweating. Physiologic concerns are that this category of drugs can cause hypertension and tachycardia, and long-term use may result in damage to the brain in the parts that focus on thought, memory, and pleasure.

Research on the impact of MDMA on the patient recovering from anesthesia continues to be desperately needed. The reader is encouraged to review the effects of cocaine because the pharmacologic actions are so similar and consequently the impact of the MDMA category of drugs on emergence from anesthesia could be quite significant, resembling the emergence of the patient with cocaine dependence.

## DATE-RAPE DRUGS

Gamma hydroxybutyrate (GHB) is a euphoric, sedative, and anabolic. It is a widely used drug that was obtained over-the-counter in health food stores until 1992. It has street names of "liquid Ecstasy," "soap," "easy lay," and "Georgia home boy." Coma and seizures can occur after the use of GHB. Combined with alcohol, GHB can cause nausea and dyspnea. GHB has been associated with poisonings, overdoses, date rapes, and deaths. This drug has a short duration of action and is not easily detectable on routine hospital toxicology screening tests. Research needs to be conducted on this drug to determine its long-term effects, and actual dependency has not been established.

Flunitrazepam (Rohypnol) is a benzodiazepine that when mixed with alcohol incapacitates victims and prevents them from resisting sexual assault. This drug, like midazolam, produces anterograde amnesia. This drug is not approved for use in the United States and its importation is illegal. The street names for this drug include "rophies," "roofies," "roach," and "rope," and its illegal use continues to be a problem in the border states, particularly Texas and Arizona.

Ketamine is an intravenous anesthetic drug (see Chapter 21) that is used illegally in the club and rave scenes and has been used as a date rape drug. It can be injected or snorted and is known on the street as "Special K" or "vitamin K." This drug produces a dreamlike state and hallucinations. In high street doses, ketamine causes delirium, amnesia, impaired motor function, high blood pressure, depression, and apnea. The veterinary form of this drug appears to create the most dependency; its frequency of use is steadily increasing.

## SUMMARY

Substance dependence in the United States is increasing at an alarming rate. All ages and people from all walks of life are affected by this problem. Also, this chapter provides evidence that a person can become dependent on a variety of formulations. Even more serious is the number of practitioners on the anesthesia care team who are becoming dependent on drugs that may be readily available

We as health care practitioners must recognize the severity of the addiction trends among our own subsets of professions. We must learn to recognize, report, and prevent this continued escalation of drug dependence. The key feature is that we all must agree that early intervention may save the lives of our colleagues and fellow practitioners.

The intent of this chapter was to provide the reader with an overview of the many drugs and substances that can be used by a person to become dependent. Not all the drugs and substances were identified or discussed because this area is ever changing. The key point presented was the overview of how the perianesthesia practitioner should modify the PACU nursing care with regard to patients who are dependent on a drug or substance category presented. Armed with this knowledge, the outcomes of the perianesthesia patient are enhanced.

## BIBLIOGRAPHY

Aitkenhead A, Smith G, Rowbotham D: *Textbook of anaesthesia*, ed 5, Philadelphia, 2007, Churchill Livingstone.

Alspach J: *Core curriculum for critical care nursing*, ed 6, Philadelphia, 2005, Saunders.

Atlee J: *Complications in anesthesia*, ed 2, Philadelphia, 2007, Saunders.

Barash P, Cullen B, Stoelting R: *Clinical anesthesia*, ed 5, Philadelphia, 2005, Lippincott Williams & Wilkins.

Benumof J, Saidman L: *Anesthesia & perioperative complications*, ed 2, St Louis, 1999, Mosby.

Brouette T, Anton R: Clinical review of inhalants, *Am J Addict* 10(1):79-94, 2001.

Brunton L, Lazo J, Parker K: *Goodman and Gilman's the pharmacological basis of therapeutics*, ed 11, New York, 2005, McGraw-Hill.

Cote' C, Todres I, Goudsouzian N, et al: *A practice of anesthesia for infants and children*, ed 3, Philadelphia, 2001, Saunders.

DeFazio-Quinn D, Schick L: *PeriAnesthesia nursing core curriculum*, Philadelphia, 2004, Saunders.

Drake R, Vogl W, Mitchell A: *Gray's anatomy for students*, Philadelphia, 2005, Churchill Livingstone.

Estafanous F, Barash P, Reves J, editors: *Cardiac anesthesia: principles and clinical practice*, ed 2, Philadelphia, 2001, Lippincott Williams & Wilkins.

Evers A, Maze M: *Anesthetic pharmacology: physiologic principles and clinical practice*, Philadelphia, 2004, Churchill Livingstone.

Fisher L: *Benumof's anesthesia and uncommon diseases*, ed 5, Philadelphia, 2007, Saunders.

Frost E, Seidel M: Preanesthetic assessment of the drug dependent patient, *Anesthesiol Clin North Am* 8(4):829-842, 1990.

Gallager C, Issenberg B: *Simulation in anesthesia*, Philadelphia, 2007, Saunders.

Ganong W: *Review of medical physiology*, ed 22, New York, 2005, McGraw-Hill.

Guyton A, Hall J: *Textbook of medical physiology*, ed 11, Philadelphia, 2006, Saunders.

Huckabee M: Perioperative care of the active substance dependent, *J Post Anesth Nurs* 3(4):254-259, 1988.

Kaplan J, Slinger P: *Thoracic anesthesia*, ed 3, New York, 2003, Churchill Livingstone.

Kier L, Dowd C: *The chemistry of drugs for nurse anesthetists*, Chicago, 2004, AANA Publishing, Inc.

Knor E: *Substance dependent, Decision making in obstetrical nursing*, Toronto, 1987, B.C. Decker.

Kurtzman T, Otsuka K: Inhalant dependent by adolescents, *J Adolesc Health* 28(3):170-180, 2001.

Lake C, Hines R, Blitt C: *Clinical monitoring: practical applications for anesthesia and critical care*, Philadelphia, 2001, Saunders.

Longnecker D, Murphy F: *Dripps, Eckenhoff, Vandam introduction to anesthesia*, ed 9, Philadelphia, 1997, Saunders.

Longnecker D, Tinker J, Morgan G: *Principles and practice of anesthesiology*, ed 2, St Louis, 1998, Mosby.

Luck S, Hedrick J: The alarming trend of substance abuse in anesthesia providers, *J PeriAnesthesia Nurs* 19(5):308-311, 2004.

Miller R, editors: *Anesthesia*, ed 6, Philadelphia, 2005, Churchill Livingstone.

Morgan M: Ecstasy (MDMA): a review of its possible persistent psychologic effects, *Psychopharmacology (Berl)* 152(3):230-248, 2000.

Murray J, Nadel J: *Textbook of respiratory medicine*, ed 4, Philadelphia, 2005, Saunders.

Nagelhout J, Zaglaniczy K: *Nurse anesthesia*, ed 3, St Louis, 2005, Saunders.

Ogden S: *Calculation of drug dosages*, ed 7, St Louis, 2005, Mosby.

Pharm J, Puzantian T: Ecstasy: dangers and controversies, *Pharmacotherapy* 21(12):1561-1565, 2001.

Rogers E: Postanesthesia care of the cocaine dependent, *J Post Anesth Nurs* 6(2):102-107, 1991.

Shorten G, Browne J, Carr D, et al: *Postoperative pain management: an evidence-based guide to practice*, Philadelphia, 2006, Saunders.

Stoelting R: *Pharmacology and physiology in anesthetic practice*, ed 3, Philadelphia, 1999, Lippincott-Raven.

Stoelting R, Miller R: *Basics of anesthesia*, ed 5, Philadelphia, 2007, Churchill Livingstone.

Teter C, Guthrie S: A comprehensive review of MDMA and GHB: two common club drugs, *Pharmacotherapy* 21(12):1486-1513, 2001.

Thompson J, McFarland G, Kirsch J, et al: *Mosby's clinical nursing*, ed 5, St Louis, 2002, Mosby.

Townsend C, Beauchamp R, Evers B, et al: *Sabiston textbook of surgery: the biological basis of modern surgical practice*, ed 17, Philadelphia, 2004, Saunders.

Weiss S: Anesthesia for the alcoholic and addict, *AANA J* 47(3):309-312, 1979.

White P: *Perioperative drug manual*, ed 2, Philadelphia, 2005, Saunders.

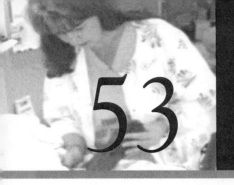

# 53

# CARE OF THE PATIENT WITH THERMAL IMBALANCE

*Vallire D. Hooper, MSN, RN, CPAN, FAAN*

Patients admitted to the postanesthesia care unit (PACU) usually have some form of thermal imbalance. Thermal cimbalance is defined as body core temperature that is outside the normothermic rage of 36° C to 38° C.[1,2] This chapter reviews the physiology of thermoregulation, the concepts of perioperative thermoregulation and hypothermia, malignant hyperthermia (MH), and the impact of these issues on the care of the patient in the PACU.

## DEFINITIONS

**Active Warming Measures:** Forced air convective warming.
**Core Thermal Compartment:** Consists of the organs of the trunk and head, which comprise 50% to 60% of the body mass. Tissues are well perfused and maintain a relatively uniform temperature.
**Malignant Hyperthermia:** A hereditary abnormality of muscle metabolism caused by certain triggering agents and resulting in a life-threatening pharmacogenetic disorder.
**Normothermia:** A core temperature range of 36° C to 38° C.
**Passive Insulation:** Warmed cotton blankets, reflective blankets, circulating water mattress, socks, head covering, and limited skin exposure.
**Perioperative Hypothermia:** A core body temperature lower than 36° C.
**Peripheral Thermal Compartment:** Consists of the arms and legs. Temperature is nonhomogenous and varies over time.
**Preventative Warming:** Initiation of passive insulation or active warming measures to maintain normothermia.
**Thermal Comfort:** A patient's subjective description of temperature comfort level.

## OVERVIEW OF THERMOREGULATION

The body maintains its temperature between the narrow range of 36° C and 38° C.[1-4] Although the peripheral thermal compartment (consisting of the arms and legs) temperatures may vary with environmental and thermoregulatory responses, temperature in the core body compartment is controlled within a 0.2° C range by a balance of heat production and heat loss typically regulated by thermoregulatory mechanisms in the central nervous system (CNS). These mechanisms receive input from various thermoreceptors located in the skin, nose, oral cavity, thoracic viscera, and spinal cord. These thermoreceptors send sensory information in hierarchical order: spinal cord, reticular formation, and primary control in the preoptic hypothalamic region of the brain.[2,3]

The central temperature controls maintain body temperature with two primary responses: physiologic and behavioral. The physiologic thermoregulatory response consists of sweating, shivering, and alterations in the peripheral vasomotor tone. These responses fine-control the regulatory process of body temperature; consequently, heat loss is reduced with vasoconstriction and increased with vasodilation and sweating. They also work by reducing heat production, lowering the metabolic rate, and increasing muscle tone and shivering to enhance heat production. The behavioral thermoregulation is run by subjective feelings of discomfort or comfort. For example, in a hot environment, a person seeks air conditioning; in a cold environment, the person seeks heat. The response mechanism is stronger but does not exhibit fine control as in the physiologic thermoregulatory response system.[2,3]

Body heat is produced by metabolism and has a circadian cycle, with the core temperature lower in the morning than in the afternoon.[5] Body heat is removed with four methods of heat transfer: radiation, conduction, convection, and evaporation, or all of which play a significant role in the development of perioperative hypothermia (Fig. 53-1).

### Radiation
Radiation involves the loss of energy, in this case, heat, through the radiant electromagnetic waves

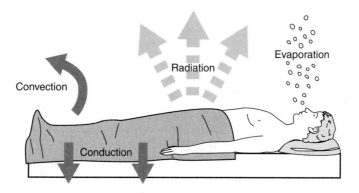

**Fig. 53-1** Mechanisms of heat loss. *(From Sessler DI: Perioperative heat balance,* Anesthesiology *92:583, 2000. In Quinn DMF, Schick L, editors:* Perianesthesia nursing core curriculum, *St Louis, 2004, Saunders.)*

in the infrared spectrum. It involves no direct contact between the objects involved but simply occurs as heat radiates from a warmer object to a cooler one. Radiation heat loss accounts for 40% to 60% of all heat loss and occurs in the operating room (OR) as the uncovered skin of the surgical patient radiates energy away from the patient, resulting in a drop in body temperature. Neonates and the elderly are particularly prone to heat loss via this mechanism.[2,3,6]

### Conduction
Conduction involves the transfer of heat energy through direct contact between objects. Conduction loss accounts for as much as 10% of heat loss in the OR and may occur via several mechanisms, including patient contact with a cold OR table, skin preparation solutions, intravenous (IV) fluids, irrigants, and cold sheets and drapes.[2,3,6]

### Convection
Convection involves the loss of body heat via transfer to the surrounding cooler air and occurs with a temperature gradient between the body and surrounding air. It accounts for 25% to 50% of heat loss in the operating room. This transfer may occur in two ways. Passive movement occurs as a loss of body heat from basic skin exposure as warm air rises. Active movement, which can be facilitated by the laminar flow systems in an OR, occurs as a loss of body heat from a fan or wind blowing across the body surface.[2,3,6]

### Evaporation
Evaporation results in a loss of body heat from the transfer of heat that occurs when a liquid is changed into a gas. Evaporation accounts for up to 25% of heat loss in the OR and can occur via perspiration, evaporation, and exposed viscera during surgery or trauma.[2,3,6]

## TEMPERATURE MEASUREMENT

Patients have rapid core temperature changes during the perioperative period. During such periods of rapid temperature fluctuation, a core temperature measurement provides the most accurate indication of body temperature. Temperature measurement during this period must be accurate and consistent and provide a true reflection of the core temperature measurement. The relationship between temperatures measured at various body sites during this period, however, may differ significantly from a true core reading. Consideration of the best method for obtaining a temperature must also take into account accessibility of the measurement site, patient comfort and safety, and the practitioner's ability to consistently use the device correctly.[1,2,7,8]

The most accurate core temperature measurement is obtained via use of a pulmonary artery (PA) catheter because the artery bathes the catheter with blood from the core compartment and its surroundings. Temperature readings at the site can be impacted by the rapid infusion of large amounts of warmed or cold IV fluids, by respiratory cycles, and by lower limb pneumatic compression devices. Readings from the distal esophagus and nasopharynx provide accurate alternatives to the PA catheter and are commonly used during surgery; however, like the PA catheter, these methods are invasive in nature and are not appropriate outside of the operative setting once the patient has been extubated.[2,7]

Tympanic thermometry (Fig. 53-2) is the preferred instrument for noninvasive core temperature measurement in the perianesthesia setting[9] and is purported to provide a true measurement of core temperature because the tympanic membrane receives blood from the internal carotid artery, which also supplies blood to the

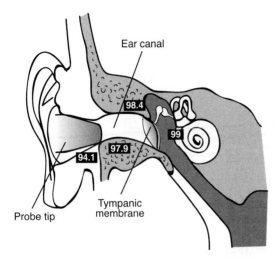

**Fig. 53-2** Tympanic temperature monitoring. *(From Nicoll LH: Heat in motion: evaluating and managing temperature, Nursing 32:S12, 2002. In Quinn DMF, Schick L, editors: Perianesthesia nursing core curriculum, St Louis, 2004, Saunders.)*

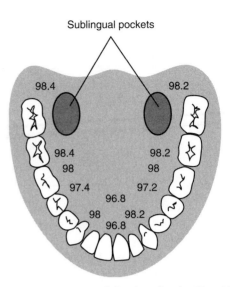

**Fig. 53-3**    Temperature variations in oral cavity. *(From Nicoll LH: Heat in motion: evaluating and managing temperature, Nursing 32:s12, 2002. In Quinn DMF, Schick L, editors: Perianesthesia nursing core curriculum, St Louis, 2004, Saunders.)*

thermoregulatory center of the hypothalamus. Accuracy of tympanic readings, however, can be adversely impacted by common sources of instrument error, including poor operator technique, patient anatomy (site), and the calibration, accuracy, and inherent instrument error of the thermometer used.[2,7,8] The accuracy of tympanic thermometry is further negated by a 2006 integrative review[7] that provided a comprehensive and critical review of the research comparing tympanic, temporal artery, and oral temperature readings with invasive core temperature measurements. This study concluded that the evidence supporting the use and accuracy of tympanic thermometry was of poor quality, outdated, and insufficient.

Temporal artery thermometry, a noninvasive radiation thermometer with use of a scanner probe to scan the forehead and capture the infrared heat from the arterial blood supply and lock in the highest temperature sensed, is also purported to provide a core temperature measurement. Temporal artery thermometry has been found to favorably compare with tympanic and rectal measurements in children but has been shown to be less reliable in adult populations.[7,10-15] Integrative review regarding the accuracy of temporal artery readings as compared with invasive core measurements concluded that an essential lack of evidence exists to support the accuracy of the instrument for core temperature measurement in adults.[7]

Oral temperature measurement with electronic digital thermometers is a popular method of temperature measurement that is easily accessible and less prone to operator error and quickly reflects changes in core body temperature. Oral temperature readings, however, have fallen out of favor in perianesthesia and critical care settings because of concerns with the influence of oxygen therapy, warmed and cooled inspired gases, and respiratory rates.[7,8,16] Oral temperature readings vary based on placement in the oral cavity (Fig. 53-3).[16] Integrative review, however, has confirmed that oral measurement taken in the right or left posterior sublingual (buccal) pocket provides an accurate reflection of core temperature, even in the presence of oxygen therapy, warmed and cooled inspired gases, and varied respiratory rates.[7]

## PERIOPERATIVE HYPOTHERMIA

Perioperative hypothermia is defined as a core body temperature lower than 36° C.[1] As many as 70% of surgical patients have hypothermia in the course of the surgical experience.[6] Risk factors for perioperative hypothermia include[1,2,17,18]:

- Extremes of ages
- Female gender
- Decreased ambient room temperature
- Length and type of surgical procedure
- Cachexia
- Preexisting conditions such as peripheral vascular disease, endocrine disease, pregnancy, burns, and open wounds

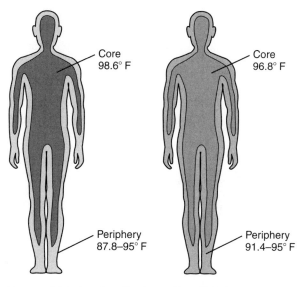

**Fig. 53-4** Core-to-peripheral redistribution after administration of anesthesia. *(From Sessler DI: Perioperative heat balance, Anesthesiology 92:583, 2000. In Quinn DMF, Schick L, editors: Perianesthesia nursing core curriculum, St Louis, 2004, Saunders.)*

- Significant fluid shifts
- Use of cold irrigants
- Use of general or regional anesthesia

Adverse effects associated with perioperative hypothermia include:[1,2,4,17-20]

- Patient discomfort
- Increased adrenergic stimulation
- Untoward cardiac events
- Coagulopathy
- Altered drug metabolism
- Impaired wound healing
- Surgical site infection
- Increased hospital costs

The typical temperature drop associated with perioperative hypothermia is between 1° C and 3° C and depends on the type and dose of anesthesia, amount of surgical exposure, and ambient room temperature. This temperature drop occurs from a loss of normal physiologic thermoregulatory mechanisms that are impaired by anesthetic drugs. As a result, the patient becomes poikilothermic and, without intervention, takes on the cooler temperature of the operative environment.[3,4]

Intraoperative temperature loss typically occurs in a characteristic pattern as a result of core-to-peripheral redistribution (Fig. 53-4). Redistribution occurs as a result of a reduction in the vasoconstriction threshold from the inhibitory impact of general anesthesia, resulting in a drop in core temperature, and peripheral vasodilation triggered by both general and regional anesthesia, which causes an increase in the blood flow to the skin and a resulting

loss in core body heat. An initial heat loss of 1° C to 1.5° C occurs during the first hour of surgery, followed by a slower more linear drop over the next 2 to 3 hours. Core temperature loss generally does not stabilize until 2 to 4 hours into the surgical procedure (Fig. 53-5). Postoperative return to normothermia occurs once the brain anesthetic concentration decreases enough to allow a normal thermoregulatory response. This response may take as long as 2 to 5 hours to kick in and may be inhibited by residual anesthetics and postoperative opioids.[2-4]

Every patient should be assessed for hypothermia on arrival in the PACU, and postoperative care should be provided as per the multidisciplinary American Society of PeriAnesthesia Nurses' (ASPAN) Clinical Guideline for the Prevention of Perioperative Hypothermia[1] (Fig. 53-6). In the case of normothermia, preventative warming measures and passive insulation should be instituted. The ambient room temperature should be increased, and the patient's thermal comfort level should be assessed at least every 30 minutes. In addition to constant observation for the signs and symptoms of hypothermia, the patient's temperature should be reassessed when the thermal comfort level decreases, with any emerging signs or symptoms of hypothermia, and on discharge from the PACU. In addition to the previous measures, active warming should be initiated for any patient with hypothermia who is admitted. In addition, IV fluids should be warmed; all gases

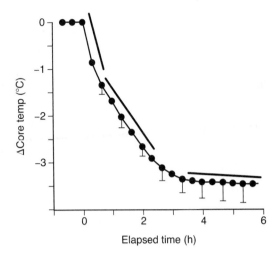

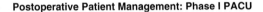

**Fig. 53-5**  Perioperative heat loss over time. *(From Sessler DI: Perioperative heat balance,* Anesthesiology *92:583, 2000. In Quinn DMF, Schick L, editors:* Perianesthesia nursing core curriculum, *St Louis, 2004, Saunders.)*

(oxygen) humidified and warmed; and temperature monitored at least every 30 minutes until normothermia is achieved. The expected outcomes for all patients in phase I PACU include a return to normothermia (minimum discharge temperature of 36.0° C), resolution of the signs and symptoms of hypothermia, and patient verbalization of an acceptable level of warmth. Preventative warming measures and continued assessment for hypothermia should continue at whatever location to which the patient is discharged.[1]

## MALIGNANT HYPERTHERMIA

In the past, reports in the medical literature discussed young healthy persons who, after exercise in hot weather, developed "heat stroke" that was followed by death. Clinical reports of this syndrome continued to appear, especially of patients in the operating room in whom an accelerated

**Postoperative Patient Management: Phase I PACU**

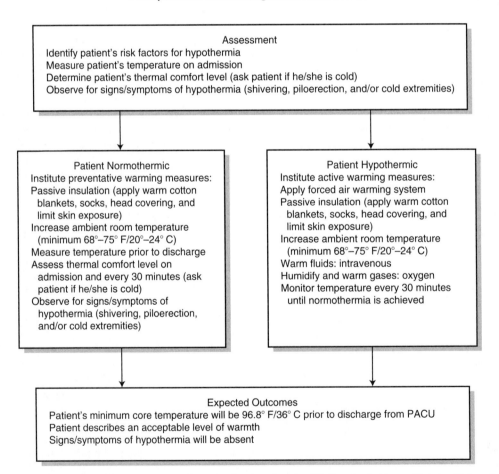

**Fig. 53-6**  Postoperative patient management. *(From the American Society of PeriAnesthesia Nurses:* Clinical guidelines for the prevention of unplanned perioperative hypothermia: ASPAN, 2002 Standards of perianesthesia nursing practice, *Cherry Hill, NJ, 2002, American Society of PeriAnesthesia Nurses.)*

temperature developed during induction of anesthesia. By the 1950s, more information had become available. Because of research, the morbidity and mortality rates from this syndrome have now been reduced. Its cause is a genetically determined condition called malignant hyperthermia (MH). MH is precipitated by certain general inhalation anesthetics, depolarizing skeletal muscle relaxants, and stress.[2,21,22] The incidence rate of MH ranges from 1 in 14,000 to 15,000 in children and 1 in 50,000 in adults.[2,21,23] The onset of MH usually occurs during induction of anesthesia. Once the acute episode is treated in the operating room, the patient may be admitted to the PACU. Reports of MH recurring in the PACU have been made. Because successful management of MH depends on early assessment and prompt intervention, the perianesthesia nurse must be knowledgeable in the pathophysiology and treatment of this syndrome.

## Identification of Patients with Malignant Hyperthermia Susceptibility

*Genetics.* Humans probably inherit susceptibility to MH with more than one gene or more than one group of possible mutational forms of a gene. The pattern of inheritance may range from recessive to dominant, with graded variations in between. The ease of initiation of an episode of MH seems to depend on the degree of genetic susceptibility and on environmental factors, which explains why some patients who are known to be susceptible show no signs of MH when exposed to confirmed MH-triggering agents. A patient with MH susceptibility (MHS) could be given an anesthetic in the presence of trigger agents, and this patient might not experience an acute MH reaction during surgery but could have MH develop in the PACU instead.[21,23]

*Evaluation of Susceptibility.* Before anesthesia is administered, identification of patients who may be susceptible to MH is of major therapeutic importance. On history and physical examination, patients with MHS usually show some subclinical muscle weakness or abnormality, such as deficient fine motor control. Many patients with MHS have muscle cramps that occur spontaneously, during an infectious illness or during or after exercise. When these cramps are present, they may be so severe that they are almost incapacitating. The patient may also describe heat prostration during physical exertion that is associated with environmental heat stress. In addition, a positive patient history or a positive genealogy may go back two generations (i.e., the patient or immediate relatives may show

MH symptoms during an anesthetic experience). Physical examination of the person with MHS may reveal myopathies such as wasting of the distal ends of the vastus muscles and hypertrophy of the proximal femoral muscles of the thigh. Other myopathies that are associated with MH susceptibility are cryptorchidism, pectus carinatum, kyphosis, lordosis, ptosis, and hypoplastic mandible. Electromyographic changes are seen in fewer than half of patients with MHS. Electrocardiographic results of patients with MHS may reveal ventricular or atrial hypertrophy (or both), bundle branch block, myocardial ischemia, and ventricular dysrhythmias. Measurements of blood creatine phosphokinase (CPK) are usually about 70% reliable in estimating susceptibility to MH. The most definitive test for detection of MH susceptibility is the biopsy of skeletal muscle. Samples are obtained from the quadriceps muscle and are subjected to isometric contracture testing. The skeletal muscle of the patient with MHS has an increased isometric tension when exposed to caffeine or halothane.[2,21,23]

A new molecular genetic screening test has recently been developed that detects anywhere from 30% to 50% of those patients at risk for development of MH. A genetic test and DNA analysis is performed with a simply obtained blood sample. Although this method does not detect all people susceptible to development of MH and thus cannot be used to replace the more definitive muscle biopsy testing, the procedure is less costly, does not require the patient to travel to one of the few muscle biopsy testing centers, and shows great promise for future development.[21-24]

Patients at high risk for development of an acute MH crisis have been classified as follows: (1) patients who have an MH-positive muscle biopsy or who have survived an acute MH crisis; (2) patients who have a first-degree relative known to have MHS or to have had a positive muscle biopsy; (3) patients whose family members have a clinically demonstrated muscle abnormality; and (4) patients who are members of a family whose plasma CPK measurements have been found to be elevated in one or more samples (taken on at least three occasions).

## Normal Skeletal Muscle Physiology

Although a complete discussion of skeletal muscle contraction can be found in Chapter 23, a brief synopsis is presented here. The events that lead to the contraction of a skeletal muscle begin with an electric impulse that is transmitted down the axon to the motor nerve terminal, where vesicles that contain acetylcholine are located. On stimulation, the contents of

SPECIAL CONSIDERATIONS

## Box 53-1   Signs and Symptoms of Malignant Hyperthermia

The most consistent indicator of potential MH in the OR is an unanticipated increase (e.g., doubling or tripling) of end-tidal $CO_2$ when minute ventilation is kept constant.

Unexpected tachycardia, tachypnea, and jaw muscle rigidity (masseter spasm) are often common signs of MH that follow the significant $CO_2$ increase.

Respiratory and metabolic acidosis usually indicate fulminant MH. However, metabolic acidosis is not always present before severe temperature increase.

A specific sign of the MH syndrome is body rigidity (i.e., limbs, abdomen and chest).

Temperature elevation is often a late sign of MH. Temperature change during MH is best detected with core temperature measurement (tympanic, nasopharyngeal or oropharyngeal, esophageal, rectal, or pulmonary artery). Forehead skin temperature is less acceptable; it is slower in reflecting changes in core temperature and could be influenced by peripheral vasoconstriction.

Malignant hyperthermia may occur at any time during anesthesia or on emergence from anesthesia, including in the immediate postoperative period.

the vesicles are released. This quantum of acetylcholine crosses the myoneural junction and interacts with its receptor on the postsynaptic membrane. This receptor activation causes a transient increase in the permeability for sodium and potassium ions, which ultimately creates an electric action potential (nerve impulse) that is propagated along the muscle membrane. This action potential electrically excites the sarcolemma and releases into the myoplasm calcium ions that are stored in the sarcoplasmic reticulum. These calcium ions then attach to troponin C, an inhibitory muscle protein that, when stimulated by the calcium, permits the actin and myosin protein filaments to interact and cause muscle contraction. The calcium ions in the myoplasm are then taken up via a reuptake mechanism into the sarcoplasmic reticulum. The process by which the electrically excited sarcolemma is coupled to the calcium released from the sarcoplasmic reticulum is known as excitation-contraction (E-C) coupling.[21]

### Pathophysiology of Malignant Hyperthermia

When a susceptible patient is exposed to a trigger agent, such as halothane, that causes MH to occur, the clinical features are produced by an excess of calcium ions in the myoplasm. Although the exact pathophysiology of MH is not known, in MH the reuptake of calcium from the myoplasm by the sarcoplasmic reticulum appears to be decreased; that the E-C coupling mechanism is defective has also been suggested. With an elevated calcium ion concentration in the myoplasm, the skeletal muscle contraction is intense and prolonged, finally leading to a hypermetabolic state of acid and heat production. More specifically, heat is produced by the accelerated and

continued synthesis and use of adenosine triphosphate (ATP) during glycolysis. The metabolic byproduct of glycolysis, lactic acid, is transported to the liver, where part of it is oxidized to provide the ATP necessary to help make glucose. This glucose, along with glycogen, is released from the liver and transported back to the metabolically active muscle, where the entire cycle repeats. This revolving process liberates much heat and produces a significant amount of metabolic acid. Respiratory and metabolic acidosis develop because of this hypermetabolic state, and symptoms such as tachycardia, tachypnea, ventricular dysrhythmias, and unstable blood pressure appear. Because of intense vasoconstriction, the skin is mottled and cyanotic (Box 53-1). Elevated body temperature can actually be a late sign of MH; for this reason, the nurse should not prolong the assessment of the patient on the assumption that the patient's temperature must be significantly elevated before intervention is attempted. Once the patient's temperature begins to rise, it may increase at a rate of $0.5°$ C every 15 minutes and may approach levels as high as $46°$ C.[2,21,23]

Muscle rigidity occurs in about 75% of the patients with MH, especially after the administration of succinylcholine. In fact, the spasm of the masseter muscles after the injection of succinylcholine may be so severe that the nurse cannot open the patient's mouth to insert an airway. The onset of skeletal muscle rigidity after the administration of succinylcholine could be a sign of the impending development of MH.[2,21-23]

***Triggering of Malignant Hyperthermia.*** Various environmental stimuli and pharmacologic agents can stimulate an acute episode of MH (Box 53-2). The symptoms of heat exertion and heat stroke are similar to MH. However,

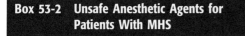

## Box 53-2 Unsafe Anesthetic Agents for Patients With MHS

**INHALED GENERAL ANESTHETICS**

- Chloroform (trichloromethane, methyltrichloride)
- Desflurane
- Enflurane
- Halothane
- Isoflurane
- Methoxyflurane
- Sevoflurane
- Trichloroethylene
- Xenon (rarely used)

**DEPOLARIZING MUSCLE RELAXANTS THAT TRIGGER MH**

- Succinylcholine (suxamthonium)

most patients with heat-related illness are not MH susceptible. In a few cases, MH susceptibility has been diagnosed with muscle biopsy in patients who had heat stroke (nonfatal), and some experts believe that heat stroke may occur more often in individuals with MH susceptibility. This area is an area of intense interest and investigation.

The anesthetic agents that trigger MH seem to affect the sarcoplasmic reticulum or the E-C coupling mechanism, or both. Because of their wide use, halothane and succinylcholine are the most common trigger agents, although all inhalation agents are triggering agents. In patients with MHS or in patients who have had an episode of acute MH in the operating room, all possible trigger agents should be stringently avoided.

***Dantrolene Sodium (Dantrium).*** Dantrolene, the primary pharmacologic agent used in the treatment of MH, is a muscle relaxant that is chemically and pharmacologically unrelated to other muscle relaxants. It is the only known pharmacologic agent that is effective in the treatment of MH. The site of action of this drug is distal to the end plate within the muscle fiber. The main pharmacologic action of dantrolene reduces the release of calcium by the sarcoplasmic reticulum without affecting reuptake. Consequently, the concentration of calcium in the myoplasm is reduced, thus inhibiting the E-C coupling mechanism and causing muscle contraction to cease. When administered orally, dantrolene has a half-life of 8 hours; with intravenous administration, the half-life is 5 hours. When it is used in the treatment of

acute MH, the intravenous dosage is 1 to 2 mg/kg, which can be repeated every 5 to 10 minutes, with a maximal dose of 10 mg/kg. If the acute episode of MH occurs in the operating room and the patient is treated successfully, dantrolene therapy is continued into the recovery (PACU) period to prevent recurrence of MH. After the acute period in the PACU has passed, the patient is given oral dantrolene in four divided doses. Because dantrolene is poorly soluble, it is supplied in vials in the form of a lyophilized powder. To reconstitute a vial of lyophilized powder, 60 mL of sterile water for injection is added to the vial and is shaken until the solution is clear; many compatibility problems arise when dantrolene is mixed with solutions other than sterile water for injection. Also, the sterile water for injection, used to reconstitute the dantrolene, should not contain any bacteriostatic agents because it is not unusual to use more than 2000 mL of diluent during the treatment of acute MH in an adult who weighs 70 kg.[2,21-23]

### Perioperative Management of the Patient with Malignant Hyperthermia Susceptibility

Before surgery, the patient with MHS may be given oral dantrolene in four divided doses of 4 to 7 mg/kg daily for 1 to 3 days before the administration of the anesthetic. The patient is usually well premedicated; however, anticholinergics, such as atropine, should be avoided because they interfere with the normal heat loss mechanisms and, in the case of atropine, can cause tachycardia that may cause confusion in the diagnosis of acute MH. Also, phenothiazines should be avoided in the perioperative period because they may cause a release of calcium from the sarcoplasmic reticulum. Intraoperative anesthesia requires the use of agents that do not trigger an episode of MH (Box 53-3). Although regional anesthesia avoids the use of the general inhalation anesthetic agents and skeletal muscle relaxants, elevated temperatures in patients with MHS have been reported with its use.

Intraoperative monitoring of the patient with MHS includes the electrocardiographic, temperature, arterial blood gas (including acid-base), and precordial stethoscope determinations. These monitoring parameters should be continued into the PACU period (Box 53-4). Because some patients with MHS have had MH triggered in the postoperative period, the patients should be followed for a minimum of 24 hours after surgery and should not be subjected to anxiety or stress. These patients should be reassured that physicians and nurses

## Box 53-3 Drugs that are Considered Safe to Administer to a Patient with MHS

| Barbiturates/Intravenous Anesthetics | Opioids | Anxiety-Relieving Medications |
|---|---|---|
| Diazepam | Alfentanil (Alfenta) | Ativan (Lorazepam) |
| Etomidate (Amidate) | Anileridine | Centrax |
| Hexobarbital | Codeine (Methyl Morphine) | Dalmane (Flurazepam) |
| Ketamine (Ketalar) | Diamorphine | Halcion (Triazolam) |
| Methohexital (Brevital) | Fentanyl (Sublimaze) | Klonopin |
| Midazolam | Hydromorphone (Dilaudid) | Librax |
| Narcobarbital | Meperidine (Demerol) | Librium (Chlordiazepoxide) |
| Propofol (Diprivan) | Methadone | Versed (Midazolam) |
| Thiopental (Pentothal) | Morphine | Paxipam (Halazepam) |
| | Naloxone | Restoril (Temazepam) |
| | Oxycodone | Serax (Oxazepam) |
| | Phenoperidine | Tranxene (Clorazepate) |
| | Remifentanil | Valium (Diazepam) |
| | Sufentanil (Sufenta) | |
| **Inhaled Nonvolatile General Anesthetic** | **Safe Muscle Relaxants** | **Local Anesthetics** |
| Nitrous oxide | Arduan (Pipecuronium) | Amethocaine |
| | Curare (active ingredient is Tubocurarine) | Articaine |
| | | Bupivicaine |
| | Gallamine | Dibucaine |
| | Metocurine | Etidocaine |
| | Mivacron (Mivacurium) | Eucaine |
| | Neuromax (Doxacurium) | Lidocaine (Xylocaine) |
| | Nimbex (Cisatracurium) | Levobupivacaine |
| | Norcuron (Vecuronium) | Mepivicaine (Carbocaine) |
| | Pavulon (Pancuronium) | Procaine (Novocain) |
| | Tracrium (Atracurium) | Prilocaine (Citanest) |
| | Zemuron (Rocuronium) | Ropivacaine |
| | | Stovaine |

## Box 53-4 Suggested Components of Monitoring of Patient with Acute Malignant Hyperthermia

Continuous ECG (consider 12-lead ECG and EEG after acute phase)
Core temperature
Urine output
Arterial pressure line
Pulse and blood pressure
Central venous pressure*
Pulmonary artery catheters*

*Should be considered; however, do not delay treatment if insertion of these monitors is physically or technically difficult.
ECG, Electrocardiogram; EEG, electroencephalogram.

have reliable instruments to monitor for MH and that prompt and effective treatment will be provided if it develops.[9,21,23]

### Treatment of Acute Malignant Hyperthermia in the Postanesthesia Care Unit

The cornerstone of the successful treatment of MH is early detection (see Box 53-1). Box 53-5 lists the suggested equipment and drugs that should be kept in the PACU to be used in the treatment of acute MH. Chapter 1 also provides information on equipment and drugs that should be available for the treatment of acute MH. If the assessment indicates that the patient has developing acute MH, the following steps should be taken:[9,21,23]

1. Discontinue the use of any trigger agent (see Box 53-3) and send for help.
2. Rapidly ventilate the patient with large tidal volumes with a bag-valve-mask system and

## Box 53-5 Suggested Equipment and Drugs to be Used in Treatment of Acute Malignant Hyperthermia

### EQUIPMENT NEEDED

Intravenous lines with assorted cannula gauges
Central venous pressure sets (2)
Transducer kits for arterial and central venous cannulation
Esophageal or other core temperature probes
Pulmonary artery catheter
Laboratory test tubes for blood chemistry analysis
Syringes (60 mL × 5) to dilute dantrolene
Crystalloid solution (10 1000-mL bottles), labeled *for hyperthermia only* and stored in PACU refrigerator
Bucket of cracked ice, labeled *for hyperthermia only* and stored in freezer of PACU refrigerator
Cooling blanket
Nasogastric tubes
Urine meter (1)
Irrigation tray with piston syringe
Fan
Large clear plastic bags for ice

### DRUGS NEEDED

Sodium bicarbonate (8.4%): 50 mL × 5
Furosemide: 40 mg/amp × 4 ampules
Calcium chloride (10%): 10 mL vial × 2
Glucose (2 bottles of 50% strength)
Iced intravenous saline solution (10 1000-mL bottles in refrigerator)
Lidocaine for injection: 100 mg/5 mL or 100 mg/10 mL in preloaded syringes (3)
Amiodarone is also acceptable (ACLS protocol for treatment of cardiac dysrhythmias)
Regular insulin (1 ampule of 100 units; refrigerated)
Dantrolene (Dantrium) intravenous: 36 vials of lyophilized powder with at least 2200 mL of sterile water for injection, USP (without a bacteriostatic agent), to reconstitute dantrolene

Note: All the equipment and drugs listed in the box should be stored in a box or cart in the PACU. The box or cart should be labeled "hyperthermia."

oxygen (total oxygen flow should exceed 15 L/min). Oral endotracheal intubation should be performed if the patient's airway is compromised.

3. Insert arterial and central venous lines and send venous and arterial blood samples to the laboratory for immediate results on electrolyte and arterial blood gas analysis. Also obtain CK, myoglobin, SMA-19, PT/PTT, fibrinogen, fibrin split products, CBC, and platelets.

4. Start reconstituting the dantrolene as soon as possible.

5. Administer the intravenous dantrolene-1 to 2 mg/kg over 1 to 2 minutes, up to 10 mg/kg or until the patient's temperature starts to decrease.

6. Cool the patient. Cover all exposed surfaces with towels soaked in water. Cover the wet towels with ice. Use cooling blankets and fans if possible. Use cold gastric lavage and hydrate with iced intravenous fluids. To avoid hypothermia, discontinue all the cooling interventions when body temperature decreases to 38° C.

7. Administer sodium bicarbonate intravenously at a dosage of 1 to 2 mEq/kg. When results of the arterial blood gas analysis are available, correct the base deficit with sodium bicarbonate according to the following formula:

$$\text{Base deficit} = 0.3 \times \text{weight}\,(\text{kg}) \times \text{base excess}\,(\text{mEq/L})$$

If the $PaCO_2$ is elevated, increase the tidal ventilation of the patient. Do not administer sodium bicarbonate to correct respiratory acidosis because the $PaCO_2$ only increases, which may lead to ventricular fibrillation.

8. Constantly monitor the patient's core temperature, blood pressure, pulse, cardiac rhythm, and pupil size and reactivity and watch for cyanosis (see Box 53-4).

9. The hyperkalemia can be treated with intravenous insulin and glucose (0.25 to 0.5 U/kg of insulin to 0.25 to 0.5 g/kg of glucose) or calcium.

10. If possible, catheterize the bladder and monitor urinary output and appearance. To secure a high urinary output, furosemide (1 mg/kg) or mannitol (1 g/kg) may be given.

11. Avoid calcium channel blockers. Dysrhythmias usually subside with resolution of the hypermetabolic phase of MH. They can be treated with amiodarone, lidocaine, procainamide, adenosine, or other drugs according to the ACLS protocol.

12. Hypotension can be treated with the infusion of cold crystalloid solution.

13. Continue to send arterial and venous blood samples to the laboratory for prompt determination of arterial blood gases and electrolytes.

14. Look for such hopeful prognostic signs as lessening coma, hyperactive tendon reflexes, and stabilization of the temperature. Once

the temperature returns to normal, continue
constant observation of the patient.

### Complications After Acute Malignant Hyperthermia

Renal failure can occur because of myoglobinuria or hypotension. Consumption coagulopathies, such as disseminated intravascular
coagulation, have been reported along with
acute heart failure and pulmonary edema.
Because the brain is the organ most sensitive
to hyperthermia (permanent brain damage at
$\geq 41^\circ$ C), brain deterioration can occur in
patients who are not promptly diagnosed and
treated for MH.[2]

## SUMMARY

Thermal imbalance issues encompass one of the
most common, and one of the rarest, complications experienced by the patient in the PACU.
Perioperative hypothermia, a commonly occurring yet easily preventable complication, can
precipitate many adverse patient events, resulting in increases in both morbidity and mortality.
Malignant hyperthermia, although rare, requires
rapid diagnosis and treatment to avoid certain
death. This chapter has provided an overview
of the physiology of thermoregulation, the
basic concepts of perioperative thermoregulation
and hypothermia, malignant hyperthermia, and
the impact of these issues on the care of the
patient in the PACU. Astute assessment, appropriate prophylaxis, and aggressive patient management by the PACU nurse are critical to
assuring safe quality patient outcomes in the
patient with thermal alterations.

## REFERENCES

1. ASPAN: *Clinical guideline for the prevention of unplanned perioperative hypothermia*, available at http://www.aspan.org/PDFfiles/HYPO THERMIA_GUIDELINE10-02.pdf, accessed March 5, 2007.
2. Hooper VD: Thermoregulation. In Quinn DMF, and Schick L, editors: *PeriAnesthesia nursing core curriculum*, St Louis, 2004, Saunders.
3. Sessler DI: Perioperative heat balance, *Anesthesiology* 92:578-596, 2000.
4. Sessler DI, Akca O: Nonpharmacological pre-vention of surgical wound infections, *Healthcare Epidemiol* 35:1397-1404, 2002.
5. Holtzclaw BJ: Circadian rhythmicity and homeostatic stability in thermoregulation, *Biol Res Nurs* 2:221-235, 2001.
6. Welch TC: AANA journal course, *AANA J* 70(3):227, 2002.
7. Hooper VD, Andrews JO: Accuracy of nonin-vasive core temperature measurement in acutely ill adults: the state of the science, *Biol Res Nurs* 8(1):24-34, 2006.
8. Moran DS, Mendal L: Core temperature mea-surement: methods and current insights, *Sports Med* 32(14):879-885, 2002.
9. Hooper VD: *Perioperative thermoregulation: a survey of clinical practices*, Presented at: ASPAN Consensus Conference on Perioperative Thermoregulation, Bethesda, Md, 1998.
10. Dybwik K, Nielsen EW: [Infrared temporal thermometry], *Tidsskrift for Den Norske Laegeforening* 123(21):3025-3026, 2003.
11. Greenes DS, Fleisher GR: Accuracy of a non-invasive temporal artery thermometer for use in infants, *Arch Pediatr Adolesc Med* 155(3):376-381, 2001.
12. Ostrowsky B, Ober J, Wenzel R, et al: The case of the cold thermometers, *Am J Infect Control* 31(1):57-59, 2003.
13. Roy S, Powell K, Gerson LW: Temporal artery temperature measurements in healthy infants, children, and adolescents, *Clin Pediatr* 42(5):433-437, 2003.
14. Rupp ME, Heermann J, Uphoff ME: Need for a reliable system to measure body temperature, *Am J Infect Control* 32(3):184, 2004.
15. Suleman MI, Doufas AG, Akca O, et al: Insufficiency in a new temporal-artery ther-mometer for adult and pediatric patients, *Anesth Analg* 95(1):67-71, 2002.
16. Nicoll LH: Heat in motion: evaluating and managing temperature, *Nursing* 32(5):s1-s12, 2002.
17. Good KK, Verble JA, Secrest J, et al: Postoperative hypothermia: the chilling consequences, *AORN J* 83(5):1055-1070, 2006.
18. Wagner DV: Unplanned perioperative hypo-thermia, *AORN J* 83(2):470, 2006.
19. Mahoney C, Odom J: Maintaining intraopera-tive normothermia: a meta-analysis of outcomes with costs, *AANA J* 67:155-164, 1999.
20. Sessler DI: Complications and treatment of mild hypothermia, *Anesthesiology* 95:531-543, 2001.
21. Hommertzheim R, Steinke EE: Malignant hyperthermia: the perioperative nurse's role [erratum appears in *AORN J* 83(3):601, 2006], *AORN J* 83(1):151-156, 2006.
22. Rosenburg H: *Malignant hyperthermia syndrome:* 2006, available at http://www.mhaus.org/

NonFB/Slideshow_eng/SlideShow_ENG_files/
frame.htm, accessed March 15, 2007.

23. Naecsu A: Malignant hyperthermia, *Nurs Stand* 20(28):51-57, 2006.

24. Girard T, Treves S, Voronkov E, et al: Molecular genetic testing for malignant hyperthermia, *Anesthesiology* 100(5):1076-1080, 2004.

## BIBLIOGRAPHY

*Malignant Hyperthermia Association of the United States (MHAUS)*, available at www.mhaus.org, accessed March 3, 2007.

*North America MH Registry of MHAUS*, available at www.mhreg.org, accessed March 3, 2007.

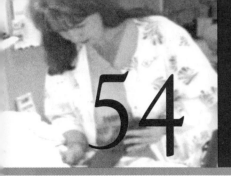

# 54

# CARE OF THE SHOCK TRAUMA PATIENT

*Myrna Eileen Mamaril, MS, RN, CPAN, CAPA*

Swiftly and without warning, traumatic injuries span all ages, cultures, and races and continue to reach epidemic proportions. The postanesthesia nurse's focus includes a primary and secondary assessment for systematic prioritization of nursing interventions and outcomes of care. The mechanism of injury is vital to understanding the pathogenesis of injury and anticipated complications, including shock during the recovery of anesthesia and surgery. Use of trauma scoring systems informs the nurse of the critical nature of the trauma injury. The emphasis of the trauma patient's postanesthesia care is on ensuring vital life functions, promoting safety, and supporting the psychosocial and spiritual needs. Preparedness for emergence delirium from posttraumatic stress disorder (PTSD) assists the nurse in understanding and effectively managing the emergence from anesthesia. Finally, the use of evidence-based practice brings the best available evidence to the practice arena and advances trauma care.

The history of advancements in shock trauma care is directly linked to wars and the military's battlefield medicine. Trauma care always advances in war.[1] During the Vietnam War, the discovery was made of intravascular fluid shifts to the interstitial space related to severe hemorrhagic shock. Consequently, the treatment of shock is now focused on rapid transport and resuscitation within the "Golden Hour."[2] Advances in vascular surgery have led to better patient outcomes. Today, the battlefields in Iraq and Afghanistan have continued to advance shock trauma nursing care and enhance trauma patient outcomes.

## EPIDEMIOLOGY OF TRAUMA

Patients with trauma injuries may enter through the health care setting as an outpatient in a surgery center with minor surgery or may be life-flighted via helicopter transport to a shock trauma center for life-saving surgical care. In the United States, trauma injuries continue to be the fourth leading cause of death, affecting the lives of more than 70 million people each year and resulting in more than 157,000 deaths, more than 430 deaths per day.[3] Furthermore, trauma accounts for more deaths in the United States during the first four decades of life than any other disease and is the fourth leading cause of death in the United States. Surprisingly, fatality rates for older adults are now higher than rates for younger adults.[3] Mortality from trauma is the tip of the iceberg; many patients survive trauma, need surgical intervention, and require lengthy rehabilitation.

Although 50% of all deaths attributed to trauma occur within minutes to hours after the injury, 30% of cases die within 2 days from neurologic injury; the remaining 20% of deaths occur as a result of complications.[3] Overwhelming infection and sepsis result from these traumatic injuries, and trauma patients are at risk for multiple complications, including but not limited to respiratory, circulatory, neurologic, and renal failure. Numerous pathologic conditions and inflammatory derangements may contribute to this high incidence rate of late mortality from sepsis. Trauma patients who need surgery and anesthesia have greater vulnerability to life-threatening conditions and mandate vigilant astute postanesthesia nursing care.

## DEFINITIONS

**Compartment Syndrome:** A pathologic condition caused by the progressive development of arterial compression and consequent reduction of blood supply.

**Injury:** A state in which a patient experiences a change in physiologic or psychologic systems.

**Mechanism of Injury:** The circumstance in which an injury occurs, such as causation from sudden deceleration, wounding with a projectile, or crushing with a heavy object.

**Microvascular:** Pertaining to the portion of the circulatory system that is composed of the capillary network.

**Motor Vehicle Crash:** Many times referred to as MVC; a person becomes injured in a single or multiple vehicle accident.

**Primary Assessment:** The first in order of importance in the evaluation or appraisal of a disease or condition.

**Resuscitation:** Use of emergency measures in an effort to sustain life.

**Secondary Assessment:** Evaluation of a disease or condition with previously compiled data.

**Shock:** An abnormal condition of inadequate blood flow to the body's tissues, with life-threatening cellular dysfunction.

**Shock Trauma:** A sudden disturbance that causes a wound or injury and results in acute circulatory failure.

**Systemic Inflammatory Response Syndrome (SIRS):** Inflammatory disturbance that affects multiple organ systems of the body.

**Trauma:** Tissue injury, such as a wound, burn, or fracture, or psychologic injury in which personality damage can be traced to an unpleasant experience.

## PREHOSPITAL PHASE

During the past 30 years, the ultimate goal of emergency medical services has been to improve the field stabilization, resuscitation, and subsequent transportation of the multitrauma patient to the appropriate-level trauma center.[4] The concept of the "Golden Hour," which was introduced by R. Adams Cowley, MD, former military surgeon, emphasizes the importance of the time in which resuscitation of severely injured patients must begin for survival.[4] It is the window of opportunity in which to institute life and limb measures and can be as varying as minutes for some patients to hours for others.[4] During the prehospital phase, vital information regarding the trauma patient's condition at the scene and mechanism of injury reveals important clues in the clinical finding of how the patient presents in the resuscitation area or later in the postanesthesia care unit (PACU). For example, if the patient had a prolonged extrication period at the scene, the airway may have been compromised; the patient may have had active or uncontrolled bleeding or have been exposed to environmental elements, thus decreasing core temperature.

Other conditions at the scene that may influence the trauma patient's outcome include such considerations as: (1) whether restraint devices were used; (2) whether airbags were deployed during impact; (3) whether the passenger was ejected from the car; (4) what position the patient was found in; (5) whether the car rolled over;

(6) whether the windshield was broken; (7) the speed at which the vehicle was traveling; (8) where the impact was on the car; (9) whether the patient sustained an impaled object; (10) whether the patient wore a motorcycle helmet; (11) whether other fatalities occurred at the scene; and (12) what, if anything, bystanders did to assist the victim. All these observations by the first providers help piece each part of the trauma puzzle together to ensure a comprehensive approach to the management of the trauma patient.

## Mechanism of Injury

Mechanism of injury (MOI) simply refers to the manner in which the trauma patient was injured. For accurate assessment of the trauma patient in the PACU, the nurse needs a basic understanding of the different types of MOI. MOI are related to the categories of the injuring force and the subsequent tissue response. A thorough understanding of these aspects of injury helps in determination of the extent and nature of the potential injuries. Damage occurs when the force deforms tissues beyond failure limits.[5] Injuries result from different kinds of energy (kinetic forces, such as motor vehicle crashes, falls, or bullets) or acute exposure (thermal, chemical, electric, radiation, or high-yield explosives) to the tissues and underlying structures. Some of the major factors that influence the severity of the injury are: the velocity of the objects and the force in terms of physical motion to moving or stationary bodies. The force is the mass of an object times the acceleration. Numerous studies conclude that the mechanism of injury helps identify common injury combinations, predict eventual outcomes, and explain the type of injury sustained.[3] Although a certain pattern of injury may be predictable for specific injuries, trauma patients may sustain other injuries. A thorough assessment for identification of all actual and potential injuries is needed.[6]

Various forms of traumatic injuries are blunt (high-velocity); penetrating, such as those that cut or pierce; falls from great heights; firearms; and chemical, electric, radiant, and thermal burns. Motor vehicle crashes create impressive forces that can fracture extremities, crush organs, and lead to massive blood loss and soft-tissue damage. At the time of a crash, three impacts occur: (1) vehicle to object; (2) body to vehicle; and (3) organs within body (Fig. 54-1). Forces are depicted in relation to acceleration, deceleration, shearing, and compression.[7] Acceleration-deceleration injuries occur when the head is thrown rapidly forward

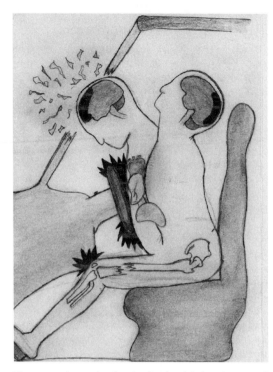

**Fig. 54-1** In acceleration-deceleration injuries, tissues and bones may be injured. Drawing depicts possible coup-contrecoup brain injury, fractured ribs, cardiac and pulmonary contusions, and fractured pelvic and long bones. *(Illustrated by Carolyn A. Dietrich, BSN, RN.)*

or backward, resulting in sudden alterations. The semisolid brain tissue moves slower than the solid skull to collide with the skull, causing injury. The injury where the brain makes contact is called a coup. The brain injury may also occur as the brain tissue is thrown in the opposite direction, causing damage in the contralateral skull surface, which is know as contrecoup injury (see Fig. 54-1). Ever-changing MOI also generate the need for new nursing educational programs and competencies for postanesthesia nurses to stay up to date and advance practice.

**Blunt Trauma.** Blunt trauma is one of the major types of trauma injuries that is best described as a wounding force that does not communicate to the outside of the body. Blunt forces produce crushing, shearing, or tearing of the tissues, both internally and externally.[7] High-velocity motor vehicle crashes and falls from great heights cause blunt-trauma injuries that are associated with direct impact, deceleration, continuous pressure, and shearing and rotary forces.[7] These blunt-trauma injuries are usually more serious and life threatening than other types of trauma because the extent of the injuries is less obvious and diagnosis is more difficult. Because blunt injuries can leave little outward

evidence of the extent of internal damage, the nurse must be extremely vigilant and astute in making observations and ongoing assessments.

When the body decelerates, the organs continue to move forward at the original speed. As the body's organs move in the forward direction, they are torn from their attachments by rotary and shearing forces.[6,7] Furthermore, blunt forces disrupt blood vessels and nerves. This mechanism of injury to the microcirculation causes widespread epithelial and endothelial damage and thus stimulates cells to release their constituents and further activates the complement, the arachidonic acid, and the coagulation cascades that activated the systemic inflammatory response syndrome (SIRS). This unique inflammatory response is covered later in this chapter. Finally, blunt trauma may mask more serious complications related to the pathophysiology of the injury.

**Penetrating Trauma.** Penetrating trauma refers to an injury produced by a foreign object, such as stab wounds and firearms. The severity of the injury produced by a foreign body is related to the underlying structures that are damaged. The mechanism of injury causes the penetration and crushing of underlying tissues and the depth and the diameter of the wound that results from penetrating trauma. Tissue damage inflicted by bullets depends on the bullet's size, velocity, range, mass, and trajectory. Knives often cause stab wounds, but other impaling objects can cause damage. Tissue injury depends on length of the object, the force applied, and the angle of entry. These penetrating wounds cause disruption of tissues and cellular function and thus result in the introduction of debris and foreign bodies into the wound.[8,9] Impaled objects are left in place until definitive surgical extraction is available because of the tamponade effect of vascular injuries. Finally, the insult to the body may occur as local ischemia or may extend to a fulminate hemorrhage from these penetrating injuries.

## Contusion of Tissues

When blunt trauma is significant enough to produce capillary injury and destruction, contusion of tissues occurs. Consequently, the extravasation of blood causes discoloration, pain, and swelling.[7] If a large vessel ruptures, a hematoma may produce a distinct palpable lesion. With a massive contusion or hematoma, an increase in myofascial pressures often results in sequelae known as compartment syndrome.[6] A compartment is a section of muscle enclosed in a confined supportive membrane called fascia; compartment syndrome is a condition in which

| Table 54-1 | AIS Score | | |
|---|---|---|---|
| Region | Injury Description | AIS | Square Top Three |
| Head and neck | Cerebral contusion | 3 | 9 |
| Face | No injury | 0 | |
| Chest | Flail chest | 4 | 16 |
| Abdomen | Minor contusion of liver | 2 | 25 |
| | Complex rupture of spleen | 5 | |
| Extremity | Fractured femur | 3 | |
| External | No injury | 0 | |
| | Injury severity score: | | 50 |

increased pressure inside an osteofascial compartment impedes circulation and impairs capillary blood flow and cellular ischemia, resulting in an alteration in neurovascular function. This syndrome occurs more frequently in the lower leg or forearm but can occur in any fascial compartment. Damaged vessels in the ischemic muscle dilate in response to histamine and other vasoactive chemical substances, such as the arachidonic cascade and oxygen free radicals. This dilation, with resultant leakage of fluid from capillary membrane permeability, results in increased edema and tissue pressure.[8,9] The increased edema and pressure compress capillaries distal to the injury, impeding microvascular perfusion These pathologic changes cause a repetitive cycle within the confined tissues, which increases swelling and leads to increased compartment pressures. Fascial compartment syndrome can be measured if indicated. Normal pressure is more than 10, but a reading of more than 35 suggests possible anoxia.[10] A fasciotomy may be indicated to prevent muscle or neurovascular damage.

## SCORING SYSTEMS

Numerous scoring mechanisms have been designed to assist in measurement of the severity of injuries that try and forecast morbidities, mortalities, and the likelihood of functional outcomes. Many level one trauma center PACUs that are considered critical care PACUs have nurses who use scoring systems. Some of the most notable scoring systems are: the Abbreviated Injury Scale (AIS), which uses 1 as minor injury to 6 as fatal injury (Table 54-1); the Injury Severity Score (ISS), which predicts mortality and outcomes; the Trauma Score (TS); the Revised Trauma Score (RTS); the Glasgow Coma Scale (GCS) Score, which measures best eye opening, best verbal, best motor; and the Trauma and Injury

Severity Score (TRISS), which also is a predictor of mortality and outcomes (correlating TS to ISS). Each scoring system is unique and measures the physiologic status of the patient. Some scoring systems work better for penetrating versus blunt trauma.[11-13] The PACU nurse may record the injury scoring measurement as an initial baseline severity indices. One must remember, however, that accuracy can be limited despite the score.

## STABILIZATION PHASE

The initial assessment, resuscitation, and stabilization processes that are initiated in the emergency department and trauma center (Fig. 54-2) extend into the operating room (OR), the PACU (Fig. 54-3), and the critical care unit. Temperature of the trauma rooms may be increased to prevent hypothermia during resuscitation. Because the most common cause of shock (Table 54-2) in the trauma patient is hypovolemia from acute blood loss, the ultimate goal in fluid resuscitation is prompt restoration

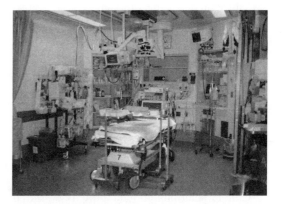

**Fig. 54-2** Trauma resuscitation unit in admitting area at R. Adams Cowley Shock Trauma Center at Maryland Institute of Emergency Medical Services Systems, Baltimore.

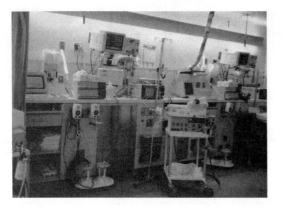

**Fig. 54-3** Patient unit in postanesthesia care unit at Maryland Institute of Emergency Medical Services Systems, Baltimore.

of circulatory blood volume through replacement of fluids so that tissue perfusion and delivery of oxygen and nutrients to the tissues are maintained.[10,14,15] Rapid identification and ensuing correct aggressive treatment are vital for the trauma patient's survival.[15-17] Although hypovolemia is the most common form of shock in the trauma patient, cardiogenic shock, obstructive shock (tension pneumothorax, cardiac tamponade), and distributive shock (neurogenic shock, burn shock, anaphylactic shock, and septic shock) may occur. Rapid-volume infusors deliver warmed intravenous fluids at a rate of 950 mL/min with large-bore intravenous catheters.[10] Many trauma centers initially infuse 2 to 3 L of lactated Ringer's or normal saline solutions and then consider blood products. The fluids should be warmed to prevent hypothermia. Crystalloids, colloids, or blood products may be used for effective reversal of hypovolemia.

Crystalloids are electrolyte solutions that diffuse through the capillary endothelium and can be distributed evenly throughout the extracellular compartment. Examples of crystalloid solutions are lactated Ringer's injection, Plasma-Lyte, and normal saline solution. Although controversy exists between crystalloid versus colloid fluid resuscitation in multiple trauma, the American College of Surgeons' Committee on Trauma recommends that isotonic crystalloid solutions of lactated Ringer's or normal saline solution be used for that purpose. Furthermore, crystalloids are much cheaper than colloids. Administration of crystalloids should be three to four times the blood loss.[15,16]

Colloid solutions contain protein or starch molecules or aggregates of molecules that remain uniformly distributed in fluid and fail to form a true solution.[13-16] When colloid solutions are administered, the molecules remain in the intravascular space, thereby increasing the osmotic pressure gradient within the vascular compartment. Volume for volume, the half-life of colloids is much longer than that of crystalloids. Colloid solutions commonly used are plasma protein fraction, dextran, normal human serum albumin, and hetastarch.

New studies of several human trials have used hypertonic solutions to resuscitate patients in shock. According to Shackford and colleagues,[18] hypertonic saline solution (3% sodium chloride) may be used in resuscitation of the child with a severe head injury because it maintains blood pressure and cerebral oxygen delivery, decreases overall fluid requirements, and results in improved overall survival rates.[16] In addition, patients with low GCS scores from head injuries have improved survival rates in the hospital (Table 54-3).[16]

Although crystalloid and colloid solutions serve as primary resuscitation fluids for volume depletion, blood transfusions are necessary to restore the capacity of the blood to carry adequate amounts of oxygen. Furthermore, blood component therapy is considered after the trauma patient's response to the initial resuscitative fluids has been evaluated.[14] In an emergency, universal donor blood (type O negative for women in childbearing years) packed red blood cells can be administered for patients with exsanguinating hemorrhage. Untyped O negative whole blood can also be given to patients with an exsanguinating hemorrhage. Other blood products, such as platelets and fresh frozen plasma, may need to be given to the trauma patient because of a consumption coagulopathy. Most notable are the leukemic trauma patients with low platelet counts. With fluid resuscitation of these patients with immunosuppression, colloids are contraindicated because of the antiplatelet activity that exacerbates hemorrhaging. Type-specific blood often times is available within 10 minutes and is preferred over universal donor blood. Fully crossmatched blood is preferred in situations that can warrant awaiting type and cross match, which often takes up to 1 hour.[14,15] Finally, the therapeutic goal of all blood component therapy is to restore the circulating blood volume and to give back other needed blood with red blood cells and clotting factors to correct coagulation deficiencies.[14]

In summary, fluid resuscitation of the trauma patient may be administered early and rapidly to ensure that adequate circulating volume and vital oxygen and nutrients are delivered to the tissues. Delay of resuscitation of patients in

| Table 54-2 | Types of Shock | | | |
|---|---|---|---|---|
| **Types** | **Definition** | **Causes** | **Signs** | **Treatment** |
| Hypovolemic | Decrease in intravascular volume | Internal or external hemorrhage, third spacing of fluids, plasma volume loss | Increased HR<br>Decreased BP<br>Decreased CVP<br>Decreased PCWP<br>Increased respirations<br>Visible signs of bleeding or fluid loss<br>Pallor<br>Diaphoresis<br>Anxiety<br>Decreased urine output | Fluids or blood administration |
| Cardiogenic | Circulatory failure from impairment of contractility | Blunt chest trauma<br>Cardiac contusion<br>Injury to heart muscle<br>Myocardial infarction | Decreased BP<br>Cardiac ischemia<br>Anxiety<br>Confusion<br>Tachypnea<br>Decreased pulse pressure<br>Cool and clammy skin<br>Elevated CVP<br>Elevated PCWP | Support cardiac rhythm<br>Increase cardiac output<br>Inotropics<br>Vasoactive drugs<br>Decrease afterload |
| Distributive | *Neurogenic:*<br>Vasodilation from decreased neurogenic tone to vessels<br>*Anaphylactic:*<br>Histamine release into bloodstream after allergic reaction, increased capillary permeability and vasodilation<br>*Septic:*<br>Massive infection resulting in vasodilation and inadequate tissue perfusion | Bacteria<br>Allergens<br>Spinal cord injury<br>Spinal anesthesia | Warm skin<br>Flushed color<br>Increased HR<br>Decreased HR (if neurologic in origin)<br>Increased temperature<br>Decreased BP<br>Increased cardiac output<br>Laryngeal edema with bronchospasm (anaphylaxis) | Treat cause<br>Fluids<br>Antibiotics<br>Vasopressors<br>Steroids<br>Epinephrine<br>Antihistamines |
| Obstructive | Decreased cardiac output from compression to aorta or great vessels that prevents atria from filling and decrease in stroke volume | Cardiac tamponade<br>Tension pneumothorax | Decreased BP<br>Increased HR<br>JVD<br>Tracheal shift<br>Muffled heart sounds<br>Diminished or absent lung sounds<br>Tachypnea | Treat cause<br>Needle decompression and chest tube<br>Pericardial centesis and surgical intervention |

*HR*, Heart rate; *BP*, blood pressure; *CVP*, central venous pressure; *PCWP*, pulmonary capillary edge pressure; *JVD*, jugular venous distension.

| Table 54-3 | Glasgow Coma Scale | | |
|---|---|---|---|
| Eyes | Open | Spontaneous | 4 |
| | | To verbal commands | 3 |
| | | To pain | 2 |
| | | No response | 1 |
| Best motor response | To verbal command | Obeys | 6 |
| | To painful stimulus | Localizes pain | 5 |
| | | Flexion: withdrawal | 4 |
| | | Flexion: abnormal (decorticate rigidity) | 3 |
| | | Extension: (decerebrate rigidity) | 2 |
| | | No response | 1 |
| Best verbal | – | Oriented and converses | 5 |
| | | Disoriented and converses | 4 |
| | | Inappropriate words | 3 |
| | | Incomprehensible sounds | 2 |
| | | No response | 1 |
| Total score | – | | 3-15 |

From Teasdale G, Jennett B: Assessment of coma and impaired consciousness: a practical scale, *Lancet* 2:81, 1974.

patients who are hemorrhagic until the start of surgery has recently been advocated. New studies recognize the "permissive hypotension" that is a protective mechanism of myocardial suppressive factors that conserve homeostasis of fluid shifts. The intent of this protective response is to prevent further hemorrhaging or bleeding out of the red blood cells and clotting factors. By sustaining the hypotension, the blood pressure supports basic perfusion until the patient is in the OR and surgically resuscitated.[15] Early fluid administration has been criticized because it delays transport of the patient. Restoration of blood volume before homeostasis is achieved may have adverse complications of exacerbation of blood loss from increase in blood pressure.[10]

### Diagnostic Studies and Protocols

Diagnostic tests and laboratory studies play a vital role in establishing the patient's baseline and current status. The results of these tests predicate the treatment protocols that are initiated.

Comprehensive diagnostic studies are required to establish an accurate diagnosis and to plan effective treatment of the patient with multiple injuries. The initial routine studies may be arterial blood gas determinations, urinalysis (myoglobinuria), complete blood count, electrolyte levels, lactate, prothrombin and partial thromboplastin times, and type and cross match. Other diagnostic studies that may be ordered for suspected injuries include but are not limited to lateral cervical spine, upright anteroposterior chest, and anteroposterior

pelvic radiographs; computed tomographic (CT) scan; 12-lead electrocardiogram; ultrasound scan; and toxicology laboratory studies. Diagnostic peritoneal lavage is done only on the severely injured patient with hypotension, especially if the abdominal examination is suggestive of injury or is unreliable. Seven pregnancy tests should be performed on all women of childbearing age but should not delay treatment of life-threatening injuries.

### Collaborative Approach

Collaborative practice is essential in the care of the trauma patient. During the initial prehospital phase, vital communication with the trauma team is initiated at the trauma center. Subsequently, when the patient is first admitted to the PACU, a comprehensive approach to patient care is initiated. Together, the postanesthesia nurse, anesthesiologist, respiratory therapist, surgeon, and radiology technician create a collaborative environment so that care becomes focused and directed. This collaborative practice continues through the intraoperative and postanesthesia periods.

The anesthesia provider or OR nurse communicates a comprehensive systems report to the perianesthesia nurse and verbally reviews any definitive findings of the CT scan, including whether generalized edema or lesion is found. Vital nursing information is communicated to the appropriate OR and postanesthesia nurses caring for the trauma patient. The anesthesiologist and trauma surgeon should communicate the significant findings during the intraoperative period that may be problematic during the recovery phase, what the PACU nurse should look for and report promptly to these physicians, and what the PACU nurse should do to prevent harm during the postanesthesia phase of care.[19]

## POSTANESTHESIA PHASE I

Even before the shock trauma patient is admitted to the PACU, the recovery room nurse begins preparing for the PACU admission. When the OR nurse calls the PACU to notify the admitting nurse that the trauma surgeon is beginning to close the patient's surgical site, important prehospital and intraoperative information is communicated. The transfer of care or hands-off communication from the OR nurse to PACU nurse consists of a detailed yet succinct report of all pertinent findings, such as surgical operation, type of anesthesia including opioids, vital signs, oxygen saturation, ventilation settings, hemodynamic monitoring, drains, vasoactive drugs, intravenous (IV) sites with type of solutions, and other pertinent findings so that the PACU nurse can begin to prepare the patient unit.

## PRIMARY ASSESSMENT

The nursing assessment of the shock trauma patient in the PACU begins with evaluation of the ABCDs (airway, breathing, circulation, and disability). Foremost in this vital primary survey is the patency of the airway. This assessment may begin with proper positioning of the patient's head, with cervical spine protection always maintained if injury is suspected. Cervical collars should not be removed unless specifically directed by the trauma or neurosurgeon after confirmation of the absence of spinal cord injury. Also, the patient may need to have the airway cleared with suctioning and removal of secretions or blood. In addition, airway adjuncts, such as oropharyngeal and nasopharyngeal airways, may be needed. If the patient is intubated via endotracheal tube or nasotracheal tube, ventilatory support should be provided with the proper settings to achieve optimal oxygenation and ventilation.

Next, the postanesthesia nurse evaluates the patient's work of breathing. With recalling the mechanism of injury, such as blunt or penetrating trauma to the chest, the nurse should be highly suspicious of pulmonary contusions, fractured ribs, or shearing forces. The nurse assesses spontaneous respirations, respiratory excursion, chest wall integrity, symmetry, depth, respiratory rate, use of accessory muscles, and the work

of breathing. With palpation, the nurse should evaluate for the presence of subcutaneous emphysema, hyperresonance or dullness over the lung fields, and tracheal deviation. With auscultation, the nurse assesses the lungs for bilateral breath sounds and evaluates for adventitious breath sounds. In addition, pulse oximetry and end-tidal $CO_2$ monitoring augment the complete respiratory assessment of the trauma patient.

After thorough evaluation of the airway and breathing, the nurse begins the circulatory assessment. With the use of palpation, the nurse evaluates the circulation, checking the quality, location, and rate of the pulses and comparing the right with the left and the upper extremities with the lower. If the nurse can palpate a radial pulse, the arterial pressure is at least 80 mm Hg. If no radial pulse is palpable, the nurse then palpates the femoral pulse (a situation that indicates a pressure of 70 mm Hg). If only a carotid pulse is palpable, the arterial pressure is approximately 60 mm Hg. The patient's blood pressure and pulse (rate and rhythm) should be monitored via the cardiac monitor. Any changes in the patient's appearance should be investigated and prompt the nurse to reassess. Pulseless electric activity (PEA) may show as electric impulses on the cardiac monitor without the presence of a palpable pulse. PEA may be seen in the trauma patient related to pneumothorax, cardiac tamponade, hypovolemia, or hypothermia, to name a few causes.

Simultaneously, during the palpation of pulses, the nurse assesses the patient's skin temperature, color, and capillary refill. Capillary refill is a good indicator of tissue perfusion, especially in children. Another aspect of circulatory assessment is observation of the patient for any significant or uncontrollable bleeding from the operative site. The nurse should inspect the peripheral, central, and arterial lines to ensure the patency of the lines and healthy intravenous sites. Each line should be identified and labeled with the date and time to distinguish the type of parenteral fluid and medication administration in use.

The final component of the primary survey is the disability or neurologic examination. The patient's mental status should be assessed with the AVPU scale or the GCS. The AVPU is described as follows: A for awake and responding to nurse's questions; V for verbal response to nurse's questions, P for responding to pain; and U for unresponsive.[7-10] The GCS is used in many PACUs for evaluation of neurologic status and prediction of outcomes of severe trauma (see Table 54-3). This neurologic scoring system allows for constant evaluation from field to emergency room to PACU. One must remember that anesthesia blunts the neurologic response; therefore, the response is not as useful in the immediate postanesthesia period. Next, bilateral pupil response is evaluated for equality, roundness, and reactivity: brisk, slow, sluggish, or no response to light and accommodation. Before the primary assessment is complete, the PACU nurse quickly reassesses the ABCDs for stability and then is ready to receive a report from the anesthesiologist.

## ANESTHESIA REPORT

The anesthesiologist's report provides valuable information concerning the trauma patient's presenting status to the perianesthesia nurse. This report includes significant facts that pertain to the mechanism of injury, prehospital phase, admitting and stabilization period, operative report, intubation, anesthetic agents, estimated blood loss, fluid resuscitation, cardiopulmonary status, and treatment abnormalities.

In review of the anesthesia report, the nurse should note any difficulty in intubation of the patient. The nurse should be suspicious if the secretions are pink-tinged or bloody, which may indicate an infectious process, pulmonary edema, trauma, or uncontrolled hemorrhage.

A detailed operative report reveals the surgical insult to the patient. It also presents a comprehensive review of all anesthetic agents that reflects a rapid sequence of induction, balanced analgesia, and heavy use of narcotics, including the time these agents were given and the amount and type of muscle relaxants and reversal agents used.

The anesthesia report should reveal any untoward events that occurred during surgery, such as hypothermic or hypotensive events and significant dysrhythmias, including ischemic changes.

Another important aspect of the anesthesia report is estimated blood loss and fluid replacement, which are carefully monitored through the hemodynamic status of the trauma patient. With the use of arterial lines and pulmonary artery catheters, the anesthesiologist can closely monitor the patient's hemodynamic status. In severe chest injuries, Thora-Drain or other chest drainage units and auto transfusions or Cell Saver blood recovery systems may be used to conserve the vital life-sustaining resource blood. Because the goal of treatment is to keep the patient in a hyperdynamic state, the intraoperative trending should reveal that the patient is volume supported because the body responds hypermetabolically to trauma and achieving that

state ensures the delivery of oxygen and other nutrients to essential tissues in the body. End-organ perfusion is monitored and measured with the urinary output and hemodynamic monitoring. Foley catheters are essential in management of fluids in the trauma patient and assessment of kidney function. Hemodynamic monitoring not only reflects the body's hydration status but also reveals the work of the heart.

## SECONDARY ASSESSMENT

After the anesthesia report is received, a brief initial primary survey is completed and the postanesthesia nurse begins the secondary comprehensive survey with a high degree of suspicion concerning the trauma patient's mechanism of injury for specific perianesthesia problems. The initial surgery often is directed at repair of the major life-threatening injuries, such as a ruptured aorta. Consequently, additional injuries may manifest themselves during this later time in the PACU, after swelling or bruising is allowed to develop. During the comprehensive secondary survey, head-to-toe assessment is performed as the trauma patient is emerging from anesthesia. The perianesthesia nurse may discover other injuries, such as pulmonary, cardiac, or renal contusions and compartment syndrome of different extremities.

The head-to-toe assessment begins with a neurologic assessment, including the patient's level of consciousness; the appropriateness of verbal response; pupillary reactivity, size, and shape; equality of pupillary response to light and accommodation; movement; sensation; and pain response in the extremities. Each aspect is carefully evaluated and documented. Next, the head and face are inspected for abrasions, lacerations, puncture wounds, ecchymosis, and edema. These structures are palpated for subcutaneous emphysema or tenderness. The eyes are assessed for gross vision with asking the patient to identify the number of fingers the nurse is holding up. Furthermore, the eyes are evaluated for ecchymosis, "raccoon's eyes," and possible conjunctival hemorrhage. Extraocular movements are also evaluated with asking the patient to follow the nurse's finger in six directions. The nurse determines whether the patient is wearing contacts. The presence of maxillofacial injuries can be of great concern because of the potential to compromise the patient's airway.

The ears are inspected for Battle's sign (ecchymosis behind the ears). The nose is examined for drainage of blood or clear fluid. Clear fluid draining from the nose or ears should be checked for the presence of cerebrospinal fluid

(CSF). A draining nose or ears should never be packed. If CSF is suspected or Battle's sign is seen, a nasogastric tube should never be inserted through the patient's nose. An oral gastric tube is the placement of choice. Finally, the nurse should immediately report a positive CSF finding to the trauma surgeons.

The neck should be evaluated for edema, ecchymosis, tracheal deviation, pulsating or distended neck veins, and subcutaneous emphysema. As the perianesthesia nurse continues the assessment of the chest, the anterior and the lateral thorax and axilla are inspected for lacerations, abrasions, contusions, puncture wounds, ecchymosis, and edema. The nurse carefully palpates the chest for tenderness and subcutaneous emphysema. The chest wall is observed for symmetry, depth, and equality of expansion and excursion. If the trauma patient has a flail chest from the injury sustained, astute monitoring for effective oxygenation and ventilation should be observed. Again, breathing is observed for rate, degree of effort, use of accessory muscles, or paradoxic chest wall movements. Breath and heart sounds are auscultated, with notation of adventitious lung sounds (such as wheezing, rales, and friction rubs) or murmurs, bruits, and muffled heart sounds. The perianesthesia nurse carefully notes facial expressions or body reactions that may suggest possible cardiac contusions or rib fractures. The operative site and all dressings and drains should be assessed and described. Furthermore, all drains should be labeled, drainage of fluid measured, and color and consistency described. Precise documentation of all fluid output is essential for accurate fluid replacement.

The next areas to be inspected are the abdomen, pelvis, and genitalia. Again, all abrasions, contusions, edema, and ecchymosis are noted. The abdomen is auscultated for bowel sounds before palpation for tenderness and rigidity. The nasogastric tube, jejunostomy, or tube drainage is examined for color, consistency, and amount of fluid. In suspected internal abdominal or retroperitoneal hemorrhage, abdominal compartment measurements should be assessed. Some common etiologies of abdominal compartment syndrome (ACS) are pelvic fractures, hemorrhagic pancreatits, ruptured abdominal aortic aneurysm, blunt and penetrating abdominal trauma, bowel edema from injury, septic shock, and perihepatic or retroperitoneal packing for diffuse nonsurgical bleeding. If intraabdominal hypertension (IAH) or ACS is suspected or considered, the standard of care is measurement of bladder pressures.[20,21] A catheter or similar device is connected to a pressure transducer that is connected to the Foley. The Foley is clamped near the connection, 50 mL of saline solution is instilled to the bladder, the transducer is leveled at the symphysis pubis, and the pressure is measured at end expiration. If the pressure is elevated, a decompression laparotomy should be performed to release the pressure that develops from bowel edema (Table 54-4).[20,21] The abdomen is then left open and covered with a sterile wound vac until the swelling has resolved and the abdomen can be closed.

The pelvis is palpated for stability and tenderness, especially over the crests and the pubis. Priapism, which is persistent abnormal erection, may be noted.[10] In addition, preexisting genital herpes may also be present. The urinary catheter is inspected for color and amount of drainage. Urinary output should be at least 0.5 to 1.0 mL/kg/h in adults and 1 to 2 mL/kg/h in children.[8] Hematuria may indicate kidney or bladder trauma. Furthermore, urinary output must be vigilantly monitored to ensure a minimum of 30 mL/h in adults so that the patient does not develop acute renal failure from rhabdomyolysis, which can occur after traumatic injuries. The vagina and rectum are checked carefully for neurologic function and bloody drainage.

All extremities are examined for circulatory, sensory, and motor functions with range of motion. Because the trauma patient is rushed

| Table 54-4 | **Abdominal Compartment Measurements** | | |
|---|---|---|---|
| Grade | mm Hg | cm H$_2$O | Correlations |
| I | 7-11 | 10-15 | Significant alterations in physiology are evident, but decompression is rarely needed |
| II | 11-18 | 15-25 | Need for treatment is based on patient's clinical condition |
| III | 18-26 | 25-35 | Signs and symptoms of ACS may develop insidiously, but patients usually need decompensation |
| IV | > 26 | > 35 | S/S are overt; patient needs decompression |

*S/S,* Signs and symptoms.

SPECIAL CONSIDERATIONS

to the OR to correct life-threatening injuries, minor soft-tissue injuries often may be missed. Later, however, in the PACU, these soft-tissue and musculoskeletal injuries may develop into compartment syndrome. Again, each extremity must be thoroughly examined for abrasions, contusions, puncture wounds, ecchymosis, and edema. If neurovascular compromise is found, an arteriogram or venogram may be performed as a conclusive diagnostic study.

The patient is then log-rolled onto the side, with maintenance of cervical spine integrity, for assessment of the back, flanks, and buttocks for abrasions, contusions, and tenderness. Rectal tone is noted if spinal cord injury is suspected. Posterior chest assessment is completed as a last step in the head-to-toe assessment. Finally, a detailed succinct description of the primary and secondary assessment is documented.

Preoperative medications given in the emergency department are noted. Included in medications before arrival in the OR may be tetanus prophylaxis, depending on the condition of the wound, and the patient's vaccination history.

### Pain

Assessment and management of pain are important parts of the scope of care provided to the trauma patient in the PACU. The trauma patient may have severe musculoskeletal injuries or even ruptured organs that cause severe pain. Pain may include more than the surgical site. Identification of alcohol or narcotic withdrawal requires a specialized management approach and may be difficult to assess in the patient with multiple traumas during the postanesthesia period. Substance abuse pain assessment scales, such as the CINA (Clinical Institute Narcotic Assessment Scale) and CIWA (Clinical Institute Withdrawal Assessment Scale), are more appropriate to use. The perianesthesia nurse needs to recognize that because pain is subjective, verbal, nonverbal, and hemodynamic, changes that indicate the patient may be exhibiting signs of pain should be noted. Pain can manifest itself with increased heart rate, increased blood pressure, pallor, tachypnea, guarding or splinting, and nausea and vomiting. Pain scales should be used to augment the nursing assessment of pain.

Optimal management of acute pain may use the following techniques: (1) patient-controlled analgesia with intravenous or epidural infusions; (2) intravenous intermittent doses for pain or sedation; and (3) major plexus blocks. Guidance for medications should be based on choosing drugs that minimize cardiovascular depression and intracranial hypertension. A higher incidence rate of substance abuse, both alcohol and recreational or addictive mind-altering drugs, in the trauma patient population may require higher doses of narcotics or analgesics.[22,23] Other complementary techniques, such as music therapy and guided imagery, may be initiated and used as adjuncts when the trauma patient returns for subsequent surgical procedures or wound débridement. Finally, continual pain assessment is vital to the patient's optimal care.

### Nausea

Nausea can be of concern for the trauma patient. Seldom do trauma patients have nothing by mouth (NPO) before the traumatic event; therefore, patients enter anesthesia with a potentially full stomach. Vomiting can lead to aspiration and a host of issues. Extubation of trauma patients should be delayed until the gag reflex returns to avoid aspiration. Many times, nasogastric tubes are present, but if the patient has consumed food before the event, particles may be too large to be evacuated. Nausea needs to be treated after surgery and is seen with a higher incidence rate in the traumatized patient.

### Psychologic Assessment

Often, the psychologic and emotional condition of the trauma patient is not considered a priority because the initial events are life threatening. However, when the patient regains consciousness in the PACU, this aspect of the patient's care may prove to be the most challenging.

### Posttraumatic Stress Disorder

Trauma patients may emerge from anesthesia in a confused or combative state because of pain, disorientation, or posttraumatic stress disorder (PTSD). Emergence delirium or emergence excitement is a recognized complication of patients recovering from anesthesia. Trauma patients are at increased risk for emergence delirium because of PTSD that occurs after the experience or witnessing of life-threatening events, for example military combat, terrorists incidents, natural disaster, or sexual assault.[24] The PACU nurse should be prepared to critically assess the patient on emergence from anesthesia for restlessness, agitation, thousand mile stare, or sudden outbursts when the patient experiences flashbacks from the traumatic event. The nurse must provide a calm, soft, but directive communication, always remembering to orient the recovering patient from anesthesia. Family or friends may be appropriate visitors in PACU phase I to help orient the patient to an unfamiliar hospital environment. In severe cases of

PTSD, the PACU nurse should consider collaborating with an anesthesia consult to resedate the emerging patient. As the patient emerges from anesthesia, the perianesthesia nurse orients the patient to place and time. Because the patient may not even remember or recall the event that caused the accident, the nurse orients the patient to the hospital. Fear of death, mutilation, or change in body image may increase the patient's anxiety. The trauma patient may regain consciousness only to find that the extremities are immobilized or even amputated. Because a high incidence rate of injuries is related to alcohol or substance abuse, the patient may have no memory of events before, during, or after the injury. The patient may have alterations in visual and auditory functions. If the patient was alert at the scene and remembers that loved ones were severely injured or killed, the patient may become upset or hysterical, often reliving the tragic event. Consequently, the patient not only experiences loss of body integrity and control but also the loss of loved ones.

The perianesthesia nurse needs to be supportive but also focused on maintaining the patient's integrity and coping skills. The nurse needs to speak to the patient calmly, slowly, and clearly, with simple language that is easily understood. Often the same information has to be repeated as the patient emerges from anesthesia. The clinician should be honest with the patient. Psychologic aspects of trauma care include the following three concepts, according to the Emergency Nurses Association: (1) need for information; (2) need for compassionate care; and (3) need for hope.[7]

## INFECTION CONTROL

Because trauma patients represent the unknown population, infectious or communicable diseases, such as HIV, hepatitis, venereal diseases, or viruses such as chickenpox, may be transmitted by these patients. The PACU nurse needs to continue to practice vigilant universal precautions (see Chapter 5) to decrease the risk of exposure to pathogens. Gloves, protective eyewear, masks, impervious gowns, and frequent hand washing are important in reducing the risk of exposure to blood and body fluids. The nurse should follow hazardous materials protocols if patients are exposed to unknown substances or if a terrorist threat is suspected.

Infection is the predominant complication that delays recovery and threatens the life of the trauma patient. Wound infections are related to disruption of the skin that compromises the integrity of the skin and consequently results in an infection. At highest risk are massive open soft-tissue injuries, such as traumatic amputations, high-energy fractures, burns, and degloving and avulsion injuries. During surgery, the surgeon classifies the wound contamination, which is determined according to the degree of expected bacterial contamination relative to the surgical procedure.[25] The PACU nurse must be diligent in the timing and documentation of postoperative antibiotics. In addition, the type of antibiotic and the time the antibiotic was given should be communicated in the hands-off transfer of care.

### Nursing Diagnosis

Nursing diagnoses are identified, such as ineffective airway clearance, ineffective gas exchange, alteration in cardiac output, alteration in tissue perfusion, high risk for fluid volume deficit, high risk for hypothermia, high risk for injury, altered comfort, altered thought processes, communication, high risk for anxiety, ineffective coping, disturbance in self-concept, and posttraumatic stress disorder. After nursing diagnoses are formulated, a plan of care is developed and implemented, and patient outcomes are evaluated.

The focus of the nursing care of the trauma patient is on vigilant continuous reassessment. Consequently, treatment priorities are established on the basis of presenting signs and symptoms and of abnormal laboratory values and diagnostic studies. The perianesthesia nurse must be cognizant of the complex pathophysiologic responses to the traumatic injury and should always anticipate that the trauma patient might exhibit subtle or overt signs of shock. Furthermore, if shock progresses, the perianesthesia nurse should be aware of other complications, such as systemic inflammatory response syndrome, which causes a myriad of cascading pathophysiologic etiologies: adult respiratory distress syndrome, clotting derangements (coagulopathies), acute renal failure, and ultimately multisystem organ failure. Nursing care of the trauma patient provides a special challenge because of the unique physiologic responses.

## SHOCK AS A COMPLICATION IN THE PATIENT WITH MULTIPLE TRAUMAS

The most common complication associated with traumatic injuries is shock. Although different types of shock exist, all types exhibit a profound problem with inadequate delivery or utilization of oxygen and nutrients to the cells. Consequently, this anaerobic state results in inadequate tissue perfusion.[26] A measure of the body's overall metabolism is expressed as oxygen consumption ($VO_2$) and oxygen delivery to the cells ($DaO_2$).[26] When $VO_2$ is inadequate, cellular hypoxia evolves. The magnitude of oxygen debt correlates with the lactic acid levels; indeed, this measure quantifies the severity and prognosis in different shock states.[26] Consequently, this complex syndrome of disequilibrium between oxygen supply and demand causes a functional impairment (oxygen debt) in cells, tissues, organs, and eventually, body systems.[26] Vital tissues such as the brain, heart, and lungs require large amounts of oxygen to support their specialized functions. However, other important tissues like the liver, kidney, and gut need essential amounts of oxygen to support their specialized functions. Furthermore, these functions can be maintained only with energy derived from aerobic metabolism, and they cease when oxygen is in short supply.

Unfortunately, ischemia rapidly initiates a complex series of events that affect every organelle and subcellular system in the body. As cells become anoxic, adenosine triphosphate stores are depleted and virtually all energy-dependent functions cease. Protein synthesis is depleted. Changes in ion transport and glycolysis result in the loss of intracellular potassium and the production of lactic acid, which may result in lethal complications for the ischemic heart. Finally, irreversible anoxic cellular injury kills vital tissues.

Clinical manifestations of shock include signs and symptoms of decreased end-organ perfusion: cool, clammy skin; cyanosis; restlessness; altered level of consciousness; altered skin temperature; tachycardia; dysrhythmias; tachypnea; pulmonary edema; decreased urinary output; increased platelet, leukocyte, and erythrocyte counts; sludging of blood; and metabolic acidosis.[26]

### Types of Shock

Many definitions of shock exist; however, in 1870, Dr Samuel Gross defined shock as the "rude unhinging of the machinery of life."[16] The four major types of shock are the following: (1) hypovolemic; (2) cardiogenic; (3) obstructive, and (4) distributed (see Table 54-4). The first and most common type of shock, hypovolemic, results from an acute hemorrhagic loss in circulating blood volume that decreases vascular filling pressure.[26,27] The second type of shock is cardiogenic, which results from an inadequate contractility of the cardiac muscle. It is rare in the trauma patient but may be caused by blunt cardiac injury or myocardial infarction (MI). Distributive shock includes neurogenic, anaphylactic, and septic types. The most common among trauma patients is neurogenic shock

from spinal cord injuries. The third type of shock is obstructive. Obstruction or compression of great vessels or the heart itself is the cause. Both tension pneumothorax and cardiac tamponade can cause obstructive shock.[9] The fourth type of shock is distributive, which causes an abnormality in the vascular system and activation of the systemic inflammatory response syndrome (SIRS) and produces a maldistribution of blood volume.[26]

***Hypovolemic Shock.*** Hypovolemic shock is defined as a decrease in intravascular volume that results in the fluid volume ineffectively filling the intravascular compartment.[36] Consequently, hypovolemic shock may evolve from many causes, such as internal and external hemorrhage, plasma volume loss in burns, third spacing of fluids, and decreased venous return.[27]

**Classifications of Hemorrhage.** As hemorrhage progresses, the cardiovascular system produces characteristic clinical manifestations that are classified according to approximate blood loss (Table 54-5).[15] The following hemorrhagic classifications are described in the conceptual framework of the Committee on Trauma of the American College of Surgeons' Advanced Trauma Life Support Course.[10]

Class I hemorrhage, or the early phase, is defined as a loss of as much as 750 mL of blood, or approximately 1% to 15% of the body's total blood volume. Minimal physiologic changes occur in heart rate, blood pressure, capillary refill, respiratory rate, and urinary output. However, the patient may have mild anxiety in response to the sympathetic nervous system.

Class II hemorrhage, or the moderate phase, is described as a loss of 750 to 1500 mL of blood, or approximately 15% to 30% of blood volume. In this phase, multiple incremental physiologic changes occur. The patient may have increased anxiety and restlessness as a result of cerebral stimulation by the sympathetic nervous system and subsequent catecholamine release. The heart rate may be higher than 100 bpm. Although minimal changes in blood pressure occur, peripheral vasoconstriction does develop, and a rise in diastolic blood pressure results, decreasing pulse pressure. Capillary refill is delayed slightly, and the skin is cool and pale. Finally, urinary output may be slightly depressed.

Class III hemorrhage, or the progressive phase, is described as a loss of 1500 to 2000 mL of blood, or a 30% to 40% loss of blood volume. These patients have signs of cerebral hypoperfusion, hypoxia, and acidosis that create a progressive reduction in the level of consciousness. The patient may be confused, agitated, and anxious, and the heart rate may be

| Table 54-5 | Identification of Hemorrhagic Shock | | | |
|---|---|---|---|---|
| | **Class I** | **Class II** | **Class III** | **Class IV** |
| % Blood loss | Up to 15%; 750 mL | 15%-30%; 750-1500 mL | 30%-40%; 1500-2000 mL | > 40%; > 2000 mL |
| Pulse rate | > 90 bpm | 100 bpm | 120 bpm | > 140 bpm |
| Capillary refill | Normal | Positive | Positive | Positive |
| Pulse pressure | Normal or increased | Decreased | Decreased | Decreased |
| Blood pressure | Normal; 90-100 SBP | Normal; < | Decreased; << | Decreased; <<< |
| Respirations | 14-20/min | 20-30/min | 30-40/min | > 35/min |
| Urine output | >30 mL/h | 20-30 mL/h | 5-15 mL/h | Negligible |
| Mental status | Slightly restless or anxious | Mildly restless and anxious | Anxious and confused | Confused, lethargic to unresponsive |
| **TREATMENTS** | | | | |
| Fluid replacement | Possibly | Always | Always | Always |
| Blood replacement | No | Possibly | Almost always | Always |

American College of Surgeons, Committee on Trauma: *Advanced trauma life support for doctors*, Chicago, 2004, ACS.
*SBP*, Systolic blood pressure.

higher than 120 bpm. The patient may have systolic and diastolic hypotension. Capillary refill time may be delayed more than 2 seconds. Deep rapid respirations result from the ensuing metabolic acidosis. As renal perfusion decreases, urinary output may be 5 to 15 mL/h.

Class IV hemorrhage is described as a blood loss of more than 2000 mL of blood, or approximately 40% of the body's blood volume. This significant blood loss profoundly impacts the trauma patient. The patient's level of consciousness may be lethargic, stuporous, or unresponsive. The heart rate may be 140 bpm or higher, and the peripheral pulses may be weak and difficult to palpate. The capillary refill time may be more than 10 seconds. The patient may have severe hypotension, and blood pressure may be difficult to obtain. The skin may be cold, clammy, diaphoretic, and even cyanotic. The respiratory rate is shallow, irregular, and higher than 35 breaths/min. Finally, no renal end-organ perfusion occurs, which results in anuria.[15]

According to the American College of Surgeons' Advanced Trauma Life Support Course, the treatment of patients with blood loss hemorrhage is infusion of crystalloids and possibly blood. A rough guideline for the total volume of replacement fluid is 3 mL of crystalloid for each 1 mL of blood loss.[10] This guideline is referred to as the 3:1 rule.[10] When the blood loss results in a class III hemorrhage, blood should be considered; the patient with a class IV hemorrhage needs blood administration and without aggressive measures dies within minutes. The goal is assessment of the patient's response to fluid resuscitation and evidence of adequate end-organ perfusion and oxygenation (e.g., urinary output, level of consciousness, and tissue perfusion). The same signs and symptoms that alert the presence of shock must be reassessed to determine the patient's response.[11] The first hour after injury is termed the "Golden Hour," in which treatment of shock successfully is associated with lower mortality.[26,27]

**Treatment.** The primary goal of treatment of patients with hypovolemic shock is fluid replacement. By filling the vascular "tank," the heart is able to generate adequate cardiac output and produce enough hydrostatic pressure to allow perfusion of the tissues.

***Cardiogenic Shock.*** Cardiogenic shock induced by inadequate cardiac output usually occurs in the trauma patient as a result of blunt injury to the heart muscle (e.g., contusions and ruptured heart or injury to heart valves or septa) or occasionally MI.[7] MIs, however, may either precipitate or precede the traumatic event. Consequently, the patient with a history of heart disease or age-related cardiac reserve limitations or who needs myocardial depressants, such as anesthesia, has a high propensity for cardiogenic shock.[26] Finally, this trauma patient population is also at greater risk for development of cardiac failure because of the rapid fluid resuscitation.

Cardiogenic shock is circulatory failure caused by a consequence of impairment of cardiac contractility, not by a loss of intravascular fluid volume. This impaired pumping ability of the heart may result from destruction of contractility of the ventricles, as in MI. Another cause of pump failure occurs from the disruption of normal conduction sequence, as in heart blocks or dysrhythmias. Myocardial depression that results from the release of vasoactive substances like myocardial depressant factor during septic shock causes dysfunction and decreased myocardial contractility.

Another method of classification of causes of cardiogenic shock is identification of the shock as either coronary or noncoronary. Rice[28] described coronary cardiogenic shock as an obstructive coronary artery disease process that interrupts blood flow and oxygen delivery to heart muscle cells, resulting in ischemia and death. The infarcted area of heart muscle is necrotic and dead and thus provides no function. Because the area of infarction and the surrounding area of ischemic heart muscle do not contract normally, the heart is unable to maintain forward blood flow or cardiac output.

Patients with acute MIs are at greatest risk of development of cardiogenic shock, especially when a significant portion (myocardial injury, >40%) of the left ventricle is involved. This loss of contractility reveals a low cardiac output, elevated left-ventricular filling pressure, peripheral vasoconstriction, and arterial hypotension. Another problem involves the volume of blood that accumulates in the left ventricle after systolic ejection and increases the left-ventricular filling pressure. This back-pressure mechanism causes the following sequence of events: (1) an increased left-atrial pressure; (2) an increased pulmonary venous pressure; and (3) an increased pulmonary capillary pressure that results in pulmonary interstitial edema and intraalveolar edema.[26] A small percentage of MIs, however, do involve the damaged right ventricle, which does not propel sufficient blood forward through the lungs into the left heart.[26] Again, cardiac output decreases, and systemic circulation is insufficient to maintain the body's needs.

As discussed previously, noncoronary cardiogenic shock may develop in the absence of coronary artery disease and heart muscle damage, such as with cardiomyopathies, valvular heart abnormalities, cardiac tamponade, and dysrhythmias.[26]

Cardiogenic shock is defined as shock from acute myocardial dysfunction, including the following clinical and diagnostic criteria: systolic blood pressure less than 80 mm Hg, or less than 30 mm Hg of baseline in the patient with hypertension; cardiac index less than 2.1 L/min/m$^2$; urinary output less than 20 mL/h; diminished cerebral perfusion evidenced by confusion or obtundation; and cold, clammy, cyanotic skin characteristic of a low cardiac output state.[14] However, classic signs and symptoms of cardiogenic shock, such as pulmonary congestion, edema, neck vein distention, and hepatic congestion, may not be seen in the trauma patient with coexisting acute hypovolemia.

Other clinical indicators may be obtained through hemodynamic monitoring. Cardiac, stroke, and left-ventricular stroke work indexes are decreased because of pump failure. Pulmonary artery and pulmonary capillary wedge pressures are increased, which indicates an increased left-ventricular end-diastolic pressure. Systemic vascular resistance is increased and reflects vasoconstriction. Systemic venous oxygen saturation is decreased because of decreased cardiac output and increased oxygen extraction from the capillary bed. Arterial blood gas determinations reveal respiratory and metabolic acidosis that is associated with hypoxemia. Consequently, cardiogenic shock is the most lethal and results in mortality rates that range from 80% to 100%.

**Treatment.** The importance of early recognition and treatment of cardiogenic shock cannot be overemphasized. Prompt improvement of myocardial oxygen supply and tissue perfusion, with a decrease in myocardial oxygen demand, is vital not only to minimization of heart damage but also to the trauma patient's chance of survival. The goals of treatment for cardiogenic shock are to establish an airway, maintain ventilation and oxygenation, provide proper positioning, relieve pain, correct acidosis, monitor urinary output, and deliver pharmacologic support to improve or correct cardiac rhythm. Furthermore, increasing cardiac output may be achieved with judiciously increasing intravascular volume to improve preload. The heart rate and myocardial contractility may be increased with the inotropic and vasoactive drugs such as epinephrine, dopamine, and dobutamine. Another goal of therapy is to decrease afterload, which may be accomplished by lowering peripheral vascular resistance. Other important pharmacologic agents that may be used in cardiogenic shock are vasopressors, vasodilators, adrenergic blocking agents, corticosteroids, digitalis, and thrombolytic agents.

When pharmacologic support fails to improve the oxygen supply-and-demand balance, alternative methods such as the intraaortic balloon pump and the right-ventricular and left-ventricular assist devices help increase myocardial oxygen supply, decrease myocardial $VO_2$, relieve pulmonary congestion, and improve organ perfusion.[26-28]

**Distributive Shock.** Distributive, or vasogenic, shock is an abnormal placement or a maldistribution of the vascular volume. Indeed, the heart's ability to pump blood, and the body's blood volume, is normal. Therefore, this category of shock describes a unique pathologic condition that exists within the vascular circulatory network and causes an alteration in blood vessels. The three types of distributive shock are neurogenic, anaphylactic, and septic.

**Neurogenic Shock.** Neurogenic shock reflects the domination of the parasympathetic nervous system and results in venous pooling and bradycardia. Neurogenic shock can occur from acute spinal cord injury or in patients who are paraplegic or quadriplegic and have a full bladder. Decreasing bladder pressure with catheterization helps resolve symptoms in the patient with non-acute spinal cord injury. Likewise, neurogenic shock is described as a tremendous increase in the vascular capacity such that even the normal amount of blood becomes incapable of adequately filling the circulatory system.[27,28] When the body has an increase in vascular capacity, the mean systemic pressure decreases, which causes a decreased venous return to the heart. Because the sympathetic nervous system causes vasoconstriction to maintain vascular tone, the loss of sympathetic enervation results in domination of the parasympathetic nerves, causing vascular dilation or "venous pooling." This massive vasodilation of veins occurs as a result of the loss of sympathetic vasomotor tone. Neurogenic shock, however, often is transitory and does not commonly occur.

Although neurogenic shock may be caused by deep general or spinal anesthesia, loss of sympathetic vasomotor tone in the trauma patient may occur directly from a brain concussion or contusion of the basal regions of the brain or from spinal cord injury above the level of T6.

Because massive unopposed vasodilation induces arterioles to dilate, decreasing peripheral vascular resistance, venules and veins also dilate and thus cause blood to pool in the venous vasculature and decrease venous return to the right heart.[26] Consequently, the following series of events occurs: (1) decreased ventricular filling pressure; (2) decreased stroke volume; (3) decreased cardiac output; (4) decreased blood pressure; (5) decreased peripheral vascular resistance; and (6) decreased tissue perfusion.

The clinical presentation in neurogenic shock is quite different from that in hypovolemic shock, even though the blood pressure is low. The patient is frequently bradycardic, and the skin is warm, dry, and even flushed. Hemodynamic monitoring reveals a decrease in cardiac output, as a result of a decrease in resistance in arteriolar vasculature, and also a decrease in venous tone.

**Treatment.** The treatment of neurogenic shock may require extensive volume expansion and the use of vasopressors, such as ephedrine. In the case of spinal anesthesia, the perianesthesia nurse should place the patient in a supine position and, if possible, decrease the head of the bed elevation and elevate the legs. Finally, the goal of treatment in neurogenic shock is to balance volume expansion with the titration of vasopressor administration.[26-30]

**Anaphylactic Shock.** Anaphylactic shock results from a severe antigen-antibody reaction. Although this type of shock is not commonly seen in the trauma patient, the condition may occur as an iatrogenic complication during resuscitation.[26-30] Other causes of anaphylactic shock are reactions to antibiotics, contrast media, and blood transfusions.

The pathophysiologic response of anaphylaxis relates to the systemic inflammatory response syndrome (SIRS) process and the activation of the complement and arachidonic cascades. The sequence of events involved in the development of anaphylactic shock are divided into three phases, as follows[26-31]:

1. The sensitization phase, in which immunoglobulin E antibody is produced in response to an antigen and binds to mast cells and basophils.
2. The activation phase, in which reexposure to the specific antigen triggers mast cells to release their vasoactive contents.
3. The effector phase, in which the complex response of anaphylaxis occurs as a result of the histamine and vasoactive mediators released by the mast cells and basophils.

These vasoactive mediators act on blood vessels and cause massive vasodilation and increased capillary permeability, which allows fluid to leak from the intravascular space to the interstitial space.[28]

Clinical symptoms of anaphylactic shock include conjunctivitis, angioedema, hypotension, laryngeal edema, urticaria, bronchoconstriction, dysrhythmias, and cardiac arrest. One or all of these symptoms may occur; therefore immediate and effective life-saving treatment must be initiated.

**Treatment.** The initial treatment of the patient in anaphylactic shock is identification and removal of the specific antigen that has caused the allergic reaction. Furthermore, if the patient is receiving an infusion of blood or blood products, the perianesthesia nurse should immediately discontinue the transfusion and initiate an intravenous infusion with normal saline solution. Administration of oxygen via facemask should be started. The initial pharmacologic agent of choice is epinephrine, a bronchodilator that helps restore vascular tone and increase arterial blood pressure.

Aminophylline may be administered to reduce bronchial constriction and wheezing and to minimize respiratory distress.[28] Diphenhydramine, an antihistamine, is another drug of choice. Corticosteroids may be used to decrease the inflammatory response. Finally, gastric acid blockers such as the $H_2$ blockers (pepcid, ranitidine) are given.

**Septic Shock.** Septic shock, the most common type of distributive shock, results from an acute systemic response, SIRS, to invading bloodborne microorganisms. The sepsis may be caused by gram-positive bacteria; however, the most common cause is gram-negative bacteria. Other pathogens that may cause septic shock are viruses, fungi, parasites, or *rickettsiae*. The trauma patient is predisposed to the following determinants that affect the outcome of septic shock: infection as a result of contaminated wounds, poor nutritional status, preexisting disease state, and altered integrity of the body's defense mechanisms.[28-30] Furthermore, sepsis-associated tissue damage is a major complication and remains the principal cause of death in the trauma patient who survives the first 3 days after injury.[7]

Septic shock is defined as a clinical syndrome that, on a continuum, begins with sepsis and ends with multisystem organ dysfunction or failure. Septic shock is primarily a complex cellular disease that results in a loss of autoregulation and in tissue dysfunction that occurs early and persists despite increased cardiac output. Interactions between bacterial toxins and the body's cellular, humoral, and immunologic systems are considered to activate the kinins and complement, arachidonic, and coagulation cascades, which generate other endogenous mediators that only intensify regional malperfusion.[28]

The profound hemodynamic instability of septic shock is revealed in the body's biphasic response. The first phase, or the hyperdynamic response, is characterized by a high cardiac output and a low systemic vascular resistance; the second phase, the hypodynamic response, reflects the classic shock picture with a low cardiac output and an extremely high systemic vascular resistance.[26-31] These phases are also referred to as early shock, or a warm hyperdynamic phase, and late shock, or a cold hypodynamic phase. During early shock, the patient's skin is pink, warm, and dry because of the increased cardiac output and peripheral vasodilation. With progressing shock, fluid leaks from the vascular compartment, and the patient has relative hypovolemia develop, with decreasing cardiac output and increasing peripheral vasoconstriction.[24] The clinical manifestations of late shock are cold clammy skin, decreased cardiac output, severe hypotension, and extreme vasoconstriction.[28]

In septic shock, the degree of myocardial depression is directly related to the severity of sepsis. Decreased force of contractions may be the result of the release of vasoactive chemical mediators, such as myocardial depressant factor, endotoxins, tumor necrosis factor, complement, leukotrienes, and endorphins.[26-31] Furthermore, decreased ventricular preload from increased capillary permeability augments the myocardial depression.

Rice[28,29] describes alterations in peripheral circulation as massive vasodilation that occur as a result of mediator activation of the bradykinins, histamines, endorphins, complement split products, platelet-activating factor, and prostaglandins.[26-31] Another aspect of altered circulation is observed in the maldistribution of blood volume that occurs when some tissues receive more blood flow than is needed and other tissues are deprived of needed oxygen and nutrients. Finally, increased capillary permeability causes reduced circulating blood volume, increased blood viscosity, hypoalbuminemia, and interstitial edema.[28]

One of the first target organs to be affected in septic shock is the lung.[26,31] Endotoxin stimulates the production of complement split products, producing bronchoconstriction, and the release of other vasoactive mediators that cause neutrophil and platelet aggregation to the lungs increases capillary permeability. Consequently, fluid collects in the interstitium and increases diffusion distance, decreases compliance, and thereby causes hypoxemia. Pulmonary vasoconstriction may be caused by thromboxane $A_2$, which augments capillary permeability and leads to acute respiratory distress syndrome or acute lung injury (ALI).

Septic shock also causes a profound alteration in metabolism. This metabolic dysfunction is attributed to the following: (1) increasing oxygen debt and rising blood lactate levels;

(2) sustained proteolysis; (3) altered gluconeogenesis with concurrent insulin resistance; and (4) liberation of free fatty acids.[26]

**Treatment.** The treatment of septic shock consists of identification and elimination of the focus of infection. With culturing of the blood, urine, sputum, wound drainage, and invasive lines, the organism can be identified, and the proper definitive antimicrobial therapy can be initiated. Hemodynamic monitoring ensures an accurate means to assess the patient's circulatory status and the patient's response to therapeutic interventions. Initially, the perianesthesia nurse may elect to use supplemental oxygen and encourage the patient to breathe deeply. However, as the shock state progresses, the patient's respiratory status becomes compromised. Aggressive ventilator support must be established to maintain adequate oxygenation and tissue perfusion. Proper selection of parenteral fluid administration is important not only in correcting the cause of shock but also in supporting tissue perfusion.[28-32]

Pharmacologic support, including the use of positive inotropes (primarily dopamine, dobutrex, norepinephrine) and vasodilators (primarily nipride and nitroglycerin), may be indicated to augment contractility, preload, and afterload. New evidence supports glycemic control to assist in control of the stress response.[32] Finally, promising research suggests that the use of arginine vasopressin in refractory septic shock, despite adequate fluid volume resuscitation and high-dose vasopressor therapy, helps restore mean arterial pressure and is catecholamine sparing in septic shock.[32]

***Obstructive Shock.*** Obstructive shock is caused by an obstructive source such as acute pulmonary embolism, dissecting aortic aneurysm, vena cava obstruction, cardiac tamponade, or tension pneumothorax. The result of all these pathologic mechanisms is decreased cardiac output from compression to the atria, which prevents the atrium from filling and thus leads to decreased stroke volume. Cardiac tamponade may compress the atria during diastole so that the atria cannot fill completely, and thus a decrease in stroke volume results. Displacement of the inferior vena cava can obstruct return of venous blood to the heart, building up pressure as in a tension pneumothorax. Clinical manifestations are in alignment with causative mechanisms.

**Treatment.** Interventions should be aimed toward correction of the cause. Tension pneumothorax may need a needle decompression and chest tube. Cardiac tamponade may need pericardiocentesis and surgical intervention. Without prompt and appropriate treatment, obstructive shock is fatal.

## FAMILY VISITATION IN THE POSTANESTHESIA CARE UNIT

The American Hospital Association is promoting patient and family–centered care and reuniting families with their loved ones in the hospital setting. A growing body of evidence supports visitation in the PACU.[33] The American Society of PeriAnesthesia Nurses has promulgated a Position Statement on Family Visitation in the PACU (Box 54-1).[33]

A collaborative inclusive approach to keeping families informed by the PACU nurse, such as notification by phone when the patient is admitted and interaction at regular timed intervals throughout the trauma patient's stay in the postanesthesia unit, promotes family bonding,

---

**Box 54-1  ASPAN's Position Statement on Visitation in Phase I Level of Care**

The American Society of PeriAnesthesia Nurses (ASPAN) has the responsibility for defining the practice of perianesthesia nursing. An integral part of this responsibility is to promote comfort and satisfaction among patients and families. The specialty of perianesthesia nursing encompasses the care of the patient and family/significant other along the perianesthesia continuum of care.

ASPAN sets forth this position statement to support the needs of both patients and families as it relates to family visitation in the Phase I level of care.

**BACKGROUND**

Historically, PACUs have been closed units. A patient's family waited anxiously while the patient recovered in the PACU. In recent years, there have been rapid advances in anesthesia management with shorter acting anesthetic agents and increased use of regional anesthetic techniques. There is a growing body of nursing research in support of family visitation and presence at the bedside. ASPAN supports the reevaluation of the needs of both patients and families while striving to maintain quality services across the continuum of care. In response to the concerns of many perianesthesia nurses from around the country, the Standards and

*Continued*

---

**Box 54-1   ASPAN's Position Statement on Visitation in Phase I Level of Care—cont'd**

Guidelines Committee conducted a review of literature and gathered information from various institutions to identify issues related to visitation in Phase I level of care.

A review of current nursing practice revealed a wide range of family visitation practices across the country ranging from no visitation, visitation for intensive care unit (ICU)/overnight patients, and visitation for pediatric patients only, to an open family visitation policy. Perianesthesia nurses also vary in their concerns regarding family visitation as it relates to:

1. Issues of patient confidentially and privacy.
2. Pain and comfort management.
3. Procedures done in Phase I level of care.
4. Potential for emergency situations.
5. Unclear family expectations regarding visitation guidelines.

A growing body of research supports the need of both patients and families for increased visitation in the ICUs. In addition, research directly related to the PACU setting reveals that family visitation in Phase I level of care benefits both patients and families. The concept of family visitation has gained increased acceptance by nurses when a well-developed visitation program is established.

**POSITION**

It is, therefore, the position of ASPAN that visitation in the Phase I level of care is supported and that perianesthesia nurses develop guidelines within their own settings to incorporate this into their practice.

Guidelines should include the following:

1. Appropriate education for patients and families regarding family visitation to maintain a safe and beneficial experience.
2. The confidentiality and privacy of all patients shall be maintained.
3. The visit will take place at an appropriate time for the patient, visitor, and clinical staff.
4. Perianesthesia nurses should work together with hospital administration to establish a well-organized family visitation program supported by appropriate personnel to meet the needs of families in this unique setting.

**EXPECTED OUTCOMES**

Perianesthesia nurses need to familiarize themselves with this position statement, current literature and research in support of family visitation.

Perianesthesia nurses should work together with hospital administration to develop organized methods of increasing communication with families throughout the perianesthesia experience and providing appropriate support personnel to establish a visitation program in Phase 1 level of care that meets the needs of patients, families, and clinical staff.

ASPAN, as the voice of perianesthesia nursing practice, must externalize this information by sharing this position statement with all disciplines that interface with the practice of perianesthesia patients and families.

**APPROVAL OF STATEMENT**

This statement was recommended by a vote of the ASPAN Board of Directors on April 5, 2003, and approved by a vote of the ASPAN Representative Assembly on April 6, 2003, in Albuquerque, NM.

Permission to publish from The American Society of PeriAnesthesia Nurses: A *position statement on visitation in phase 1 level of care*, Cherry Hill, NJ, 2006, ASPAN.

coping skills, and decreases family anxiety and stress. Although this approach may prove challenging, the benefits to the patient and family are numerous.

## SUMMARY

Each year thousands of children and adults have trauma injuries. These injuries occur within a short time but if not assessed and treated swiftly, may have profound long-term effects that affect functional outcomes and quality of life. The postanesthesia nurse must have astute nursing assessments that use critical thinking skills. Furthermore, this specialty nurse must also be cognizant of the mechanism of injury and the complex pathophysiologic responses from the trauma injuries. The focus of nursing care is on vigilant continuous assessments to ensure adequate oxygenation/ventilation and transport/perfusion of the tissues. The postanesthesia nurse must anticipate and identify the patient at risk of development of shock. Furthermore, prevention and effective management of shock must be the primary goal in care for the trauma patient. In addition, effective management of pain in the trauma patient is foremost. Consequently, the challenge of caring for the critically ill trauma patient demands that the postanesthesia nurse be familiar with current research and evidence-based practice guidelines that provides a framework for understanding and managing these trauma patients in the postanesthesia setting.

# REFERENCES

1. Spencer BL, Favand LR: Nursing care on the battlefield, *Am Nurse Today* 1(2):24-26, 2006.
2. Trunkey DD: History and development of trauma care in the United States, *Clin Orthropedic Relat Res* 347:36-46, 2000.
3. Department of Health and Human Services, Centers for Disease Control and Prevention: Surveillance summaries, *Morbidity Mortality Wkly Rep* 53(7):1-53, 2004.
4. Beachley M: Evolution of trauma cycle. In McQuillan KA, and Von Rueden KT, and Hartsock RL, et al, editor: *Trauma nursing: from resuscitation through rehabilitation*, ed 3, Philadelphia, 2002, Saunders.
5. Weigelt JA, Klein JD: Mechanism of injury. In McQuillan KA, and Von Rueden KT, and Hartsock RL, et al, editor: *Trauma nursing: from resuscitation through rehabilitation*, ed 3, Philadelphia, 2002, Saunders.
6. Childs SA: Musculoskeletal trauma: implications for the critical care nursing practice, *Crit Care Clin North Am* 6(3):483-490, 1994.
7. Emergency Nurses Association: *Trauma nursing core course*, ed 5, Des Plaines, Ill, 2004, Emergency Nurses Association.
8. Zuspan SJ: Mechanism of injury. In Maloney-Harmon PA, and Czerwinski SJ, editor: *Nursing care of the pediatric trauma patient*, St Louis, 2003, Science.
9. Childs SA: Nailgun injury, *Orthop Nurs* 10:60-66, 1991.
10. American College of Surgeons Committee on Trauma: *Advanced trauma life support for doctors*, Chicago, 2004, ACS.
11. Brenneman FD, Boulanger BR, McLellan BA: Measuring injury severity: time for a change? *J Trauma* 44(4):580-582, 1988.
12. Champion HR, Copes WS, Sacco WJ, et al: Improved predictions from severity characterization of trauma (AS-COT) over trauma and injury severity score (TRISS): results of an independent evaluation, *J Trauma* 40(1):42-49, 1996.
13. Hunt JP, Baker CC, Fakhry SM, et al: Accuracy of administrative data in trauma, *Surgery* 126(2):191-197, 1999.
14. Miller RD, editor: *Anesthesia*, ed 5, Philadelphia, 2004, Churchill Livingstone.
15. Flavell CM: Combating hemorrhagic shock, *RN*:vol. 26-30, 1994.
16. Kelley DM: Hypovolemic shock, *Crit Care Nurs Q* 28(1):1-19, 2005.
17. Revell M, Greaves I, Porter K: Endpoints to fluid resuscitation in hemorrhagic shock, *J Trauma Injury Infect Crit Care* 54(5):S63-S67, 2003.
18. Shackford SR, Bourguignon PR, Wald SL, et al: Hypertonic saline resuscitation of patients with head injury: a prospective randomized clinical trial, *J Trauma Injury Infect Crit Care* 50:44-58, 1998.
19. Mamaril M: Safety alert: dangerous communication gaps, *Breathline* 26(6):9, 2006.
20. Cohen SS: *Trauma nursing secrets*, Philadelphia, 2003, Hanley & Belfus, Inc.
21. Majchrzak C: Abdominal compartment syndrome: a case review, *JoPAN* 17(6):413-419, 2002.
22. Pasero C, McCaffery: Pain in the critically ill, *Am J Nurs* 102(1 part 1):59-60, 2002.
23. Bower TC, Vanderheyden BA: Analgesia, sedation, and neuromuscular blockade in the trauma patient. In McQuillan KA, and Von Rueden KT, and Hartsock RL, et al, editor: *Trauma nursing: from resuscitation through rehabilitation*, ed 3, Philadelphia, 2002, Saunders.
24. Scott M, Palmer S: *Trauma and posttraumatic stress disorder*, London, 1999, Cassell Academic.
25. Centers for Disease Control and Prevention: *Guidelines for the prevention of surgical wound infections*, Atlanta, 1982, U.S. Department of Health and Human Services.
26. Rivers EP, McIntyre L, Morro DC, et al: Early and innovative interventions for severe sepsis and septic shock: taking advantage of a window of opportunity, *CMAJ* 173(9):1-12, 2005.
27. Kearney ML: Imbalance of oxygen supply and demand. In Secour VH, editor: *Multisystem organ dysfunction & failure*, ed 2, St Louis, 1994, Mosby.
28. Ozawa K: Energy metabolism. In Cowley RA, and Trump BF, editor: *Pathophysiology of shock,*

*anoxia and ischemia*, Baltimore, 1982, Williams & Wilkins.

29. Rice V: Shock, a clinical syndrome: an update: I: an overview of shock, *Crit Care Nurse* 11:20-27, 1991.
30. Rice V: Shock, a clinical syndrome: an update: IV: nursing care of the shock patient, *Crit Care Nurse* 11:40-51, 1991.
31. Littleton MT: Pathophysiology and assessment of sepsis and septic shock, *Crit Care Nurs Q* 11:30-47, 1988.
32. Lee CS: Role of exogenous arginine vasopressin in the management of catecholamine-refractory septic shock, *Crit Care Nurse* 26(6):17-23, 2006.
33. American Society of PeriAnesthesia Nurses: *2006-2008 Standards of Perianesthesia Nursing*, Cherry Hill, NJ, 2006, ASPAN.

## BIBLIOGRAPHY

Barker SJ: Trauma and malignant hyperthermia, *AudioDigest Anesthesia* 43(1), 2001.
Benjamini E, Leskowitz S: *Immunology: a short course*, ed 2, New York, 1991, Wiley-Liss.
Chulay M, Guzzetta C, Dossey B: *AACN handbook of critical care nursing*, Stamford, Conn, 1996, Appleton & Lange.
Cowley RA, Trump BF: *Pathophysiology of shock*, anoxia and ischemia, Baltimore, 1982, Williams & Wilkins.

Department of Health and Human Services, Centers for Disease Control and Prevention: Surveillance summaries, *Morbidity Mortality Wkly Rep* 53(7):1-53, 2004.
McQuillan KA, Von Rueden KT, Hartsock RL, et al: *Trauma nursing: from resuscitation through rehabilitation*, Philadelphia, 2002, Saunders.
Miller RD, editor: *Anesthesia*, ed 5, Philadelphia, 2004, Churchill Livingstone.
Morton PG, Fontaine DK, Hudak CM, et al: *Critical care nursing: a holistic approach*, ed 8, Philadelphia, 2002, Lippincott Williams and Wilkins.
Peruzzi WT, Shapiro BA: Perioperative mechanical ventilation for trauma patients, *Semin Anesth* 13(3):226-246, 1994.
Revell M, Greaves I, Porter K: Endpoints to fluid resuscitation in hemorrhagic shock, *J Trauma Injury Infect Crit Care* 54(5):S63-S67, 2003.
Secour VH: *Multisystem organ dysfunction & failure*, ed 2, St Louis, 1994, Mosby.
Swearingen PL, Keen JH: *Manual of critical care nursing*, ed 4, St Louis, 2001, Mosby.
Urden KD, Stacy KM: *Priorities in critical care nursing*, ed 3, St Louis, 2000, Mosby.

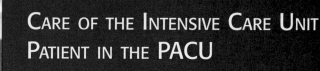

# 55

# CARE OF THE INTENSIVE CARE UNIT PATIENT IN THE PACU

*Myrna Eileen Mamaril, MS, RN, CPAN, CAPA*
*Mary Beth Flynn Makic, PhD, RN, CNS, CCNS, CCRN*

As the science of perianesthesia nursing has evolved and become increasingly more sophisticated, nursing educators, managers, and administrators have realized the importance of an economically sound evidence-based practice that continuously strives to provide safe quality care to the intensive care unit (ICU) patient in the postanesthesia care unit (PACU). However, recovery of the critically ill postoperative patient in the PACU often poses a myriad of challenges to the postanesthesia nurse and the PACU. Throughout the United States, divergent postanesthesia practices have existed in the provision of care for the surgical intensive care unit (SICU) patient. Operationally, ICU recovery must occur on a routine basis, regardless of prognosis or acuity in the appropriate care setting. Some PACU care of the postsurgical critical care patient may be sporadic or an exception to the norm. From a clinical and an administrative position, however, the PACU must provide the optimal standard of care to the SICU patient.[1] This chapter discusses the historic significance of critical care recovery, administrative issues in extended ICU care, innovative educational opportunities to ensure competent staff, and clinical strategies in caring for complex high-acuity critically ill patients. Because patient safety is essential in provision of care to low-volume high-risk patients, complex highly specialized ICU nursing care concentrates on neurosurgical, burn, and septic management during the postanesthesia period. Ultimately, postanesthesia care must be focused on provision of competent care with prevention of harm and keeping critically ill patients safe. Finally, when the SICU patient's condition becomes life-threatening, family presence during resuscitation is introduced as an end-of-life nursing intervention that promotes patient-family–centered care (PFCC).

## DEFINITIONS

**Extended Stay ICU Patients:** Critically ill surgical patients who have recovered from anesthesia but need to stay in the PACU an extended or prolonged period of time because of the severity of illness or the need to be watched for complications.

**Family Presence:** Families are provided the opportunity to be present in the PACU with their loved one during life-threatening situations or at the end-of life during cardiopulmonary resuscitation (CPR) or codes.

**Intensive Care Unit (ICU):** A hospital setting where critically ill patients are provided nursing care.

**Intensive Care Unit Boarders:** Critically ill surgical patients who have recovered from anesthesia in the PACU, have been designated ICU status, do not have an ICU bed, and are boarding in the PACU.

**Intensive Care Unit Overflow Patients:** Patients who have undergone anesthesia for surgical procedures, have recovered in the PACU, and are awaiting transfer to the ICU or SICU.

**Sepsis:** A systemic response to infection.

**Septic Shock:** Consists of a complex sepsis syndrome that is triggered by the inflammatory response that disrupts circulatory function and causes a decrease in tissue perfusion and inadequate oxygen and nutrients to the cells of the body. Septic shock is associated with hypotension, despite adequate fluid resuscitation that results in lactic acidosis; oliguria; acute alteration in level of consciousness; and other related symptoms.

**Surgical Intensive Care Unit (SICU):** A hospital setting for critically ill surgical patients who need specialized pulmonary, renal, cardiovascular, neurologic, or postoperative monitoring.

**Systemic Inflammatory Response Syndrome (SIRS):** A systemic response of the body that involves the activation of the inflammatory response and the mediators of inflammation, such as the mediated Immunoglobin E (IGE) mast/histamine response, complement system, clotting system, kinin system, fibrinolytic system, lymphokines, tumor necrosis factors, and other vasoactive inflammatory components that disrupt circulatory and organ function.

## HISTORIC SIGNIFICANCE OF CRITICAL CARE RECOVERY

During the late 1950s and early 1960s, intensive care units emerged in hospitals for close monitoring of the highest acuity of the critically ill patients. Before that time, the critically ill postsurgical patients were cared for in the units known as recovery rooms and also in inpatient wards. Critical care nursing was conceived to provide a setting in which the most acutely ill and injured patients received concentrated nursing care to enhance survival. Fifty years ago, ICUs were made up of a few specialized beds located at the end of or apart from an existing inpatient unit.[2]

Today, the design of ICUs is focused on individual rooms to promote an aesthetic therapeutic environment. The ICU provides patient privacy and is a unit focused on highly technical care that can also be family centered. In comparison, the interior design of the PACU has not changed much in 50 years. It is usually one large room in which individual patient units are separated by curtains.

## ADMINISTRATIVE ISSUES

### Financial Constraints

The 1990s brought increased financial constraints on hospitals and increased competiveness among hospitals. Governmental decisions to control cost rather than focus on quality patient care led to a dramatic shift in the types of patients that were admitted to hospitals. Only the sickest patients were eligible for admission, and the length of stay was compressed to the shortest possible time.[3] While hospital census dropped, ICU patient volumes were steadily increasing. Hospital mergers and closings occurred in many cities. During this same time, two significant changes developed: (1) patient acuity of critically ill patients admitted to hospitals was increased; and (2) the shortage of ICU nurses prompted hospital administrators to close ICU beds. ICU bed closures have had a serious impact on PACUs. PACUs were naturally chosen for critical care overflow because the environment of care included highly technical monitoring and many critical care–educated nursing staff. In addition, the retention of staff in the PACU was much higher with fewer vacancies. This choice seemed the ideal answer to a complex problem. Consequently, the PACUs were increasingly requested for recovery of SICU patients, and in many hospitals, the PACU was designated an ICU overflow unit until an ICU bed became available.

### Management Dilemmas

Nurse managers encounter numerous challenges between competing health care providers that relate to patient placement priority for ICU beds. These dilemmas are impacted by senior administration (chief operating officers, chief nursing officers, departmental medical officers of medicine and surgery, and emergency/trauma physicians). The dilemmas affect ancillary staff, families, patients, and the PACU staff nurses. The PACU manager is obligated to follow hospital policies and protocols. When senior administrators make decisions in the best interest of the hospital to keep the emergency departments and operating rooms open and to perform surgery for elective surgical cases regardless of high hospital census, the PACU becomes the relief valve for medical center admissions. Often, the hospitalized patients that occupy beds in the ICU are not ready for transfer to a lower level of care. This gridlock has a domino effect on the PACU beds. Emergency department patients who need critical care may be given priority status for ICU beds, as may "code" call patients from inpatient units. Some ICUs actually hold beds open for potential code call situations. As the inpatient and ICU surgical cases are completed, they too compete for the PACU available beds. Complications arise if the PACU is still holding ICU patients from the day before or from earlier in the morning. Eventually, the operating room (OR) schedule may grind to a halt because of the ensuing gridlocked beds. In some hospitals, the OR continues to perform surgery on critical care patients, with admission of more ICU overflow patients to an already stressed PACU. These SICU patients become known as "boarders," "extended stay," or "ICU overflow." Patients and families may voice intense dissatisfaction when the PACU is designated for ICU care.[1]

Recovery of the ICU patient who has an extended stay in the PACU may have serious physician repercussions. Anesthesiologists and surgeons become frustrated because they want to complete the elective surgical schedule. At times, their behaviors may strain relationships with the nurse manager. The lost surgical and anesthesia revenue may threaten the viability of the hospital if surgical cases continue to be delayed or cancelled. University hospitals also have graduate medical education and need to perform a required number of surgical or anesthesia cases per year to qualify for accreditation of the programs.

Other challenges that are encountered by medical staff may be the following issues that place the care of the ICU patient at risk. Medical intensivist management of the SICU patient may be delayed because of the physical location of the PACU or other commitments to patients in the ICU. Confusion may exist, regarding who to contact for medical or surgical problems. Another issue that frequently surfaces centers around the need to have medical consultations. PACU staff may believe that lack of timely medical care not only increases the stress of the nurse but ethically impacts the professional duty to provide safe timely quality care. Further delays in treatments may critically impact the patient's condition. Finally, the surgeon may become upset at hospital administration because the order was for the ICU patient to be admitted to the ICU for postoperative care and management.

The physical location of the PACU is always adjacent to the OR. However, more likely than not, the ICU is in a different area of the hospital. This situation may create delays in diagnostic care or treatment that otherwise is more expeditious if the patient is in the ICU. For example, respiratory therapy, pulmonary services, blood bank, and the critical care laboratories may be actually located in the ICU. Advanced practice nurses and physician assistants assigned to the ICU may not attend ICU patients in the PACU. The PACU may have to wait for the hospital's respiratory therapist or laboratory technician to come to the unit. If a computed tomographic (CT) scan or magnetic resonance imaging (MRI) scan is needed, the PACU nurse may not be able to transport the ICU patient in a timely manner because of assigned care of another postanesthesia patient. The ICU patient may need special medications or vasoactive intravenous drips that may not be immediately available to the nurse. Ancillary services play a vital role in the care and management of the ICU patient.

Intensive care unit patients emerging from anesthetic agents frequently request that their families visit in the PACU. Traditionally, PACUs have been considered large open units in which family visitation is severely limited because of other patients emerging from anesthesia. This type of policy may create intense conflict between the nurse and the family. Family expectations of a private room in which families may visit freely are not met. Furthermore, when the surgeon speaks about the critical nature of the surgery and the need to place the patient in the ICU, family anxiety increases. Families, however, frequently worry and may perceive the ICU as a sign of impending death, based on past experiences or those of others.[4] Understanding what critical care means to patients and families helps the nurse promote positive coping skills. Depending on the patient's physical condition, effective communication with the ICU patient may be challenging. Barriers to communication may relate to emergence from anesthesia; the patient's physical status; the existence of endotracheal tubes, which inhibit verbal communication; medications; or other conditions that alter cognitive function.[4,5] The critical care patient's anxiety may increase the stress response and further complicate the patient's recovery. Patients may consider that they have a "right" to see and visit with their family and may find significant emotional support for well being.

Managing and communicating with the ICU families in the PACU may be challenging. Depending on each patient's diagnosis and acuity, the SICU patient's family may be in crisis. If the patient's condition is critical, the family may have a high degree of stress, anxiety, blaming, or other disturbing behaviors. Families may be emotional and act out or exhibit disruptive outbursts. The staff nurse may believe that one's first duty is to provide care to the patient, not to the family. Time may go by quickly for the PACU nurse and not afford the family timely visits. Anxiety and worry mounts for the waiting family from little or no communication and from fear of the unknown. The PACU nurse needs to make a conscientious effort to effectively communicate with the family in a manner that promotes coping, personal growth, and adaptation to the ICU patient's critical condition (Box 55-1).[6]

## STAFFING ISSUES

The PACU nurses may express feelings of inadequacy related to critical care competencies. A PACU nurse may have no ICU nursing experience or outdated critical care experience. The critical care experience may have been generalized and not specific, or new technology may be foreign. Nurse-patient ratios may be exceeded for safe care. The PACU nurse may already be assigned one patient with simultaneous care for a newly admitted ICU patient with an unstable condition. Then, family members (frequently numerous) want to be present and are upset because visitation is limited or not allowed. PACU nurses may find themselves in the midst of ethical situations that involve conflict between the needs of the ICU patient's family members and the preferences of physicians and other health care providers. Consequently, this

## Box 55-1   PACU Nursing Actions for Families in Crisis

- Introduce the PACU Scope of Service.
- Assist the family in defining the SICU problem and condition.
- Aid in identifying sources of support for the family during hospitalization.
- Prepare the family for the PACU care environment, especially the effects of patients emerging from anesthesia, respect for other PACU patients, confidentiality, PACU equipment (i.e., cardiac monitors, ventilators, infusion pumps), and purpose of the equipment.
- Communicate with sincerity and compassion about the critical surgery or illness.
- Avoid false reassurance.
- Express confidence in the family's ability to deal with the situation.
- Try to understand the family's perspective about the patient's critical condition.
- Use a "one day at a time" approach and avoid encouraging the family to think of the "what ifs" of the patient's long-term outcome.
- Provide opportunities for the patient and family to make choices and feel useful.
- Guide the family in finding therapeutic ways to communicate with the patient.
- Ensure that the family receives information about significant changes in the patient's condition.
- Allow the family the opportunity to call the PACU and speak to the nurse anytime.
- Advocate adjusting visitation hours to accommodate the family's needs.
- Respect the patient's and family's spirituality.

Adapted from Norton C: The family's experience with critical illness. In Morton PG, Fontaine DK, Hudak CM, et al, editors: *Critical care nursing: a holistic approach*, ed 8, Philadelphia, 2005, Lippincott Williams & Wilkins.

PACU environment may be chaotic and not conducive for healing. Visitors may perceive the PACU as a suboptimal environment for a loved one. When PACU nursing staff perceive that safe patient care is becoming jeopardized or high risk, they should consult the nurse manager immediately.

As the nursing shortage in the United States became more severe, the ICU overflow patients in the PACU were becoming a standard of practice, rather than isolated incidents.[7] Reports from PACU nurses in different regions of the country communicated unsafe practices. Postanesthesia nurses turned to their

professional organization, the American Society of PeriAnesthesia Nurses (ASPAN), to voice their concerns about serious issues that affected the care they provided recovering ICU patients in the PACU. The ASPAN Standards and Guidelines Committee conducted a special review of the evidence to identify current nursing practice issues. The following trends in the care of ICU patients in the PACU were identified:

1. Staffing requirements identified for phase I PACUs may be exceeded during times when PACUs are used for ICU overflow patients.[1,5]
2. The phase I PACU nurse may be required to provide care to a surgical or nonsurgical ICU patient that the nurse has not been properly trained to care for or for whom the nurse has not had the required care competencies validated.[1,5]
3. Phase I PACUs may not be able to receive patients normally admitted from the operating room when staff is used to care for the ICU overflow patients.[1,5]
4. When the need to send ICU overflow patients to the phase I PACU does not occur regularly, both the PACU and the hospital management may not be properly prepared to deal with the admission and discharge of phase I PACU and ICU patients.[1,5]

The ASPAN invited the American Association of Critical Care Nurses (AACN) and the American Society of Anesthesiologists (ASA) to address the practice trend of caring for the ICU overflow patient in the PACU and to strategize to promote safe quality care regardless of where the SICU patient recovers from anesthesia. The collaborative Position Statement was promulgated by these three powerful specialty organizations (Box 55-2.).[1]

### Critical Care Educational Competencies

The postanesthesia nurse must have an in-depth knowledge of anesthesia agents, normal physiology, pathophysiology, and current surgical management to plan appropriate nursing interventions and care for the postanesthesia patient. Depending on the PACU nurse's critical care experience, competencies, skills, and available medical and nursing resources, the care and management may prove to be frustrating or threatening. However, one should remember that the PACU nurse is recognized for possessing critical care competencies and skills when caring for the vulnerable patient recovering from anesthesia and surgery. Likewise, the challenge of caring for the complex SICU patient may be a rewarding opportunity to use one's critical

**Box 55-2   Joint Statement on ICU Overflow**

**ISSUE**

A phase I postanesthesia care unit (PACU) is a critical care area that provides postanesthesia nursing care for patients immediately after operative and invasive procedures before discharge to the phase II ambulatory setting, the inpatient surgical unit, or the intensive care unit.

Perianesthesia nurses have identified concerns regarding the increasing use of the phase I PACU for the care of surgical and nonsurgical ICU patients when ICU beds are not available in the facility.

**PURPOSE**

As professional societies involved in the provision of care for operative and invasive procedures and critically ill patients, the American Society of PeriAnesthesia Nurses (ASPAN), the American Association of Critical-Care Nurses (AACN), and the American Society of Anesthesiologists (ASA) collaborated to develop criteria for the purposes of maintaining quality care in the PACU, ensuring quality care for the intensive care unit patient, and promoting the safe practice of perianesthesia nursing and critical care nursing.

ASPAN exists to promote quality and cost-effective care for patients, their families, and the community through public and professional education, research, and standards of practice. ASPAN has the responsibility for defining the practice of perianesthesia nursing. An integral part of this responsibility involves identifying the educational requirements and competencies essential to perianesthesia practice and recommending acceptable staffing requirements for the perianesthesia environment.

AACN was established to provide the highest quality resources to maximize nurse contributions to care for critically ill patients and their families. AACN provides and inspires leadership to develop standards and guidelines that establish work and care environments that are respectful, healing, and humane.

ASA was established to raise and maintain the standard of the medical practice of anesthesiology and improve the care of the patient during anesthesia and recovery and is involved in the provision of critical care medicine in the intensive care unit.

**BACKGROUND**

In response to concerns expressed by perianesthesia nurses around the country, the ASPAN Standards and Guidelines Committee conducted a review of current literature and perianesthesia nursing practice to identify issues related to the care of critically ill surgical and nonsurgical patients in phase I PACUs during times when all other ICU beds are full. The review identified the following trends:

1. Staffing requirements identified for phase I PACUs may be exceeded during times when PACUs are being used for ICU overflow patients.
2. The phase I PACU nurse may be required to provide care to a surgical or nonsurgical ICU patient that the nurse has not been properly trained to care for or for which the nurse has not had the required care competencies validated.
3. Phase I PACUs may be unable to receive patients normally admitted from the operating room when staff is being used to care for ICU overflow patients.
4. Because the need to send overflow patients to the phase I PACU does not occur regularly, both the PACU and the hospital management may not be properly prepared to deal with the admission and discharge of phase I PACU and ICU patients.

**STATEMENT**

Therefore, when admission of ICU overflow patients or prolonging the stay of the surgical ICU patient in the phase I PACU is necessary, ASPAN, AACN, and ASA recommend that the following criteria be met:

1. The primary responsibility for phase I PACU is to provide the optimal standard of care to the post-anesthesia patient and to effectively maintain the flow of the surgery schedule.
2. Appropriate staffing requirements should be met to maintain safe competent nursing care of the post-anesthesia patient and the ICU patient. Staffing criteria for the ICU patient should be consistent with ICU guidelines based on individual patient acuity and needs.
3. Phase I PACUs are by their nature critical care units, and as such, staff should meet the competencies required for the care of the critically ill patient. These competencies should include, but are not limited to, ventilator management, hemodynamic monitoring, and medication administration, as appropriate to the patient population.

*Continued*

SPECIAL CONSIDERATIONS

**Box 55-2   Joint Statement on ICU Overflow—cont'd**

4. Management should develop and implement a comprehensive resource utilization plan with ongoing assessment that supports the staffing needs for both the PACU and ICU patients when the need for overflow admission arises.
5. Management should have a multidisciplinary plan to address appropriate utilization of the ICU beds. Admission and discharge criteria should be used to evaluate the necessity for critical care and to determine the priority for admissions.

**EXPECTED ACTIONS**
ASPAN, AACN, and the ASA committees (Anesthesia Care Team, Critical Care Medicine, and Trauma Medicine) recognize the complexity of caring for patients in a dynamic health care environment where reduced availability of resources and expanding roles for the registered nurse have an impact on patient care. Thus, we encourage all members to actively pursue the education and development of competencies required for the care of the critically ill patient in the perianesthesia environment. We also encourage members to actively identify strategies for collaboration and problem solving to address complex staffing issues.

This information and position is to be shared with all individuals, organizations, and institutions involved in the care of the critically ill patient in the perianesthesia environment.

From ASPAN, AACN and ASA's Anesthesia Care Team Committee and Committee on Critical Care Medicine and Trauma Medicine: *A Joint Position Statement on ICU Overflow Patients,* September 1999.

thinking skills in making a difference in the outcome of the critically ill patient.

## Orientation and Basic Critical Care Competencies

The first steps in planning an orientation to the PACU is the interview process and subsequent hiring of the nurse who is motivated to learn many new skills. In addition, the nurse who seeks to be professionally challenged on a daily basis inspires and motivates the critical care preceptor. The PACU should never be viewed as a place to wind down or retire because nurses with that goal in mind are often immediately disappointed and dissatisfied with their new jobs. Many PACUs prefer to hire the nurse with critical care experience, although medical-surgical nurses are also hired, provided an adequate support system of nursing education exists during orientation and the length of orientation is such that the nurse without prior critical care experience has ample time to master the myriad of new skills essential to the new role.

Orientation to the PACU must focus on anesthesia and complications related to anesthetic agents, comorbidities, and surgery, because this subject area encompasses nearly all of the patient population in the PACU. But what about the critical care patient? All of the patients who arrive in the PACU, regardless of invasive lines and mechanical ventilation, must be viewed as having the potential to be a critically ill patient. Even a patient who has had a hernia repair or an appendectomy can become gravely ill. In addition

to this fact is the matter of the critically ill patient who arrives in the PACU before the final destination of the ICU. Thus, orientation and education must also focus on the following essentials:

- Cardiac monitoring, rhythm interpretation, electrocardiographic (ECG) interpretation
- Airway management
  - Bag, valve, mask management
  - Nasal and oral airways
  - Endotracheal tubes
  - Laryngeal mask airways
- Arterial blood gas (ABG) interpretation
- Mechanical ventilation
  - Modes
  - Appropriate tidal volumes
  - Concept of PEEP and pressure support
  - Adequate rate and methods of delivery
  - Assessment of adequate endotracheal tube placement
  - Adequate securing of endotracheal tubes per nursing policy
- Invasive monitoring equipment: both the care of and the assessment of the patient with:
  - Arterial lines
    - o Radial
    - o Brachial
    - o Femoral
  - Central lines
    - o Basic multiple lumen
    - o Advanced venous access devices (AVA)
  - Pulmonary artery catheters (PA lines)
    - o Assessment of correct placement
    - o Ability to perform cardiac outputs

- Interpretation of cardiac output, cardiac index, stroke volume, systemic vascular resistance, left ventricular stroke work index
- Titration of medications based on previous values
- Intracranial access (intracranial pressure [ICP])
  - Drainage
  - Monitoring
- Pharmacology
  - Anesthetic agents
  - Vasopressors
- Neurology
  - Neurologic assessments
  - ICP monitoring, cerebral perfusion pressures

Orientation should include the essentials of how to care for the patient who has all or some of the invasive monitoring equipment mentioned previously and how to assemble such equipment in preparation for insertion in the PACU. The PACU should have the necessary equipment readily available in the event that a patient's condition worsens and invasive procedures are to be performed in the PACU.

The main challenge in orienting the new hire to the critical care element of the PACU is access to these patients. A day in the operating room with an anesthesia provider who inserts a PA line and manages a critically ill patient, such as with a cardiac bypass case, can be helpful. An immersion in the ICU is another option, with the PACU registered nurse (RN) spending a week or so in the ICU shadowing an ICU nurse. A cardiothoracic ICU is ideal because this type of ICU admits patients frequently, similar to the PACU, and the orientee can learn the tasks of detangling lines, managing the newly vented patient, weaning the patient, initiating and titrating vasopressor medications, and other needed skills. The leadership team of the PACU should closely collaborate with the leadership team of the ICU to ensure that the PACU RN has an orientation either similar or identical to the orientation of the new hire in the ICU. If the ICU educator or clinical nurse specialist is providing education for the ICU staff, the PACU RNs should be encouraged to attend as well. Some ICUs use the online orientation program sponsored by the AACN. This program is called Essentials of Critical Care Orientation (ECCO). ECCO is a computer-based standardized orientation of critical care nursing. If the ICUs in the facility use this type of orientation program, the PACU hire might be helped by using it as well. If the ICU orientation consists of critical care courses, then the PACU orientee

should attend as well, after the essentials of perianesthesia nursing and PACU core competencies have been mastered.

But what about the experienced PACU nurse who is suddenly confronted with the increasing volume of critical care patients? Collaboration with the ICU leadership team is helpful, with the possible outcome of an opportunity to shadow an ICU nurse for one or several weeks to learn the basic care and management of the patient with both mechanical ventilation and invasive monitoring equipment that requires vasopressor support.

A competency-based orientation (CBO) checklist should be completed on both the new hire and the experienced PACU RN who receives any education in critical care as mentioned previously. The PACU leadership team must develop a standardized educational process with the requisite paper trail to safeguard the PACU RN, the hospital, and the PACU leadership team in the event of an untoward outcome.

In addition, if the facility sponsors an annual skills fair day, the PACU RN should complete or show similar competencies to the ICU RN, based on the patient population that the PACU cares for, even if that critical care population is rare. The care of a patient who is high risk and low volume is the most challenging for the RN.

The PACU RN should also be expected to complete the same annual competence assessment that is required of the ICU nurses. For example, if a dysrhythmia competency is developed for the ICU RN, the PACU RN should also be expected to complete it and it should be placed in the education folder.

### Advanced Critical Care Concepts

Understanding key advanced critical care concepts assists the PACU nurse in refining critical decision-making skills. The ICU patient who remains in the PACU for an extended period of time poses an enormous challenge in many aspects. Both the nursing and physician management of these patients can be difficult. The Standards of Care that are developed by the ICU and the facility and that are in place in the ICU should be readily available and implemented in the PACU. Included in these standards are:

- Frequency of line and tubing changes
- Frequency of endotracheal tube rotation
- Frequency of ICP/cerebral perfusion pressure (CPP) measurements
- Frequency of measurements of cardiac outputs/indexes, etc.
- Frequency of weighing the patient

SPECIAL CONSIDERATIONS

- Frequency of chest x-rays, ECGs, laboratory studies
- Use of a continuous cardiac output (CCO) type of PA catheter
- Use of warming devices for intravenous fluids or blood products
- Use of rapid infusers
- Frequency of, and ability to perform and manage, the calculation of oxygen consumption, oxygen demand, oxygen extraction ratios and other elements of oxyhemodynamic calculations (oxy-calcs)
- Various modes of mechanical ventilation, including pressure-controlled ventilation
- Use of and care of the patient with continuous infusions of muscle relaxants and twitch monitors
- Competency/knowledge of protocols in the prevention of ventilatory-acquired pneumonia (VAP)
- Competency/knowledge of protocols in the prevention of deep vein thrombosis (DVT)

### Creating a Specialized Critical Care Resource for the PACU

Many PACUs across the country only care for ICU patients sporadically. This situation occurs when the hospital census is high or when a surgical emergency presents. Specialized critical care educational resources strategically provide the PACU nurse with expert advisors when the critical time arises. This resourceful method may be accomplished in several ways. First, the PACU may recruit expertise from the unit. Second, the nurse manager may elect to request key leadership staff to orient and become competent and proficient in management of the care of specific patient populations.

Another innovative concept to achieving critical resources is cross training the PACU staff to the ICU and critical care nurses to the PACU. When the PACU admits a highly complex high-acuity SICU case and the primary nurse does not posses the knowledge or skill to provide care, an opportunity may exist to exchange nurses rather than patients to appropriately match the patient severity with the nurse's knowledge and competencies.

### CLINICAL STRATEGIES FOR THE COMPLEX ICU PATIENT

The PACU nurses are required to use critical decision-making skills in daily practice. Advanced life support competencies are mandated for PACU nurses who care for all vulnerable patients who are emerging from surgery and anesthesia. The foundation of PACU and critical care nursing is understanding anesthesia agents and human physiology that guides the postanesthesia nursing assessments and interventions. Foremost, the PACU nurses must ensure that adequate oxygenation/ventilation and transport/perfusion of the patient occur, regardless of unit: the ICU or the PACU. Impairment in oxygen delivery and utilization at the tissue level leads to global tissue hypoxia. Fundamental to recognition and treatment of global tissue hypoxia is knowledge of the principles of oxygen/ventilation and transport/perfusion and their etiologies and how they relate to postanesthesia care. The major differences lie in the complex pathophysiologic disease processes that occur in these critically ill patients. The following section of the chapter discusses the pathophysiology and clinical strategies in management of the care for three highly specialized high-acuity low-volume populations: the neurosurgical, burn, and septic ICU patients.

### COMPLEX SPECIALIZED CRITICAL CARE IN THE PACU

#### Postoperative Care of the Neurosurgical ICU Patient

The reasons for neurosurgical interventions are numerous. Some of the most common neurosurgical procedures that require intensive care monitoring after surgery include aneurysm clipping or coiling, tumor removal or debulking, lobectomy for seizure management, and cranial surgeries to manage increased intracranial pressure (ICP). The care of the patient who has had a neurosurgical procedure requires an understanding of the goals for the surgical procedure and continuous focused assessment for the presence of subtle neurologic changes in the patient after surgery. Specifically, the nurse should know: (1) the type of surgical procedure the patient underwent; (2) the length of the operative procedure and any known complications during the surgery; (3) the specific region of the brain in which the operation was performed; (4) the preoperative neurologic examination results to allow comparison with postoperative neurologic assessment results; and (5) the neurologic injury that is considered the primary insult and the negative effects of hypoxemia, hypotension, poor cerebral perfusion, hyperglycemia, hypocapnia, and cerebral edema that are responsible for secondary insults to the brain and further compromise to the patient's recovery.[8-13] Primary goals in the immediate phase of perioperative care of the patient focus on preserving cerebral blood flow through blood pressure management, optimizing tissue oxygenation, maintaining normothermia, and effectively treating cerebral edema.

***Brief Review of Intracranial Pressure.*** One of the greatest risks after surgery is increased ICP. Nurses who provide care to neurosurgical patients must be familiar with the pathophysiology of cerebral edema and interventions to attempt to minimize the negative effects of prolonged increased ICP. Cerebral insult of a variety of mechanisms causes chaos inside the cranial vault.[8] Edema and increased ICP are frequently a consequence of injury.

Intracranial pressure is the pressure normally exerted by cerebrospinal fluid (CSF) that circulates around the brain and spinal cord and within the cerebral ventricles.[11] Normal ICP is 0 to 10 mm Hg; however, 15 mm Hg is often considered the high end of normal range.[8,11,12] The cranial vault contains three primary elements: brain tissue (80%), CSF (10%), and blood (10%). The Monro-Kellie hypothesis treats the cranial vault as a closed compartment; thus, if one of these three components increases, reciprocal changes in the other two components must occur to maintain normal ICP.[8,11] For example, if brain tissue swells, CSF production may be decreased and or it is displaced into the basal subarachnoid cisterns and cerebral vasculature vasoconstricts to compensate for brain tissue edema.[11] Compliance refers to the ability of these compensatory mechanisms to attempt to maintain a steady relationship between volume and pressure within the cranial vault.[13] Displacement of CSF and vasoconstriction, however, is limited and when the limit is reached, ICP increases.

Intracranial pressure can be measured with an intraparenchymal catheter (ICP) bolt or a ventriculostomy. Both devises are surgically placed with sterile technique and should be transduced to a monitor to allow assessment of the ICP

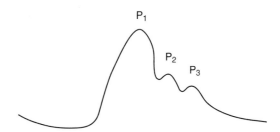

**Fig. 55-1**  Normal ICP wave form. *(From McQuillan KA, Von Rueden KT, Hartsock RL, et al: Trauma nursing: resuscitation through rehabilitation, 3 ed, Philadelphia, 2002, Saunders.)*

waveform. The intraparenchymal catheter displays a continuous ICP reading in addition to the ICP waveform. The ventriculostomy can be used to evacuate CSF and monitor ICP. The pulse wave arises primarily from arterial pulsations and to a lesser degree from the respiratory cycle.[11] Assessment of the ICP waveform provides valuable clinical information regarding cerebral compliance. The ICP waveform has three peaks known as $P_1$, $P_2$, and $P_3$ (Fig. 55-1). $P_1$ is the percussion wave and originates from pulsations of the arteries and chroid plexus; $P_2$ is the tidal wave and terminates in the dicrotic notch; and $P_3$ is the dicrotic wave, which immediately follows the dicrotic notch.[11] The $P_2$ wave is a reflection of intracerebral compliance; a rise in ICP is reflected by a progressive rise in $P_2$[11] and a concomitant rise in ICP numeric reading on the monitor (Fig. 55-2). Analysis of the ICP waveform along with the ICP value and neurologic assessment are used to determine interventions to reduce ICP.

Cerebral edema increases the pressure within the cranial vault, adversely increasing ICP. Cerebral edema may be vasogenic edema, cytotoxic edema, or interstitial edema. Vasogenic edema is an extracellular edema from increased capillary permeability and can develop around tumors or abscesses or with cerebral trauma.[11]

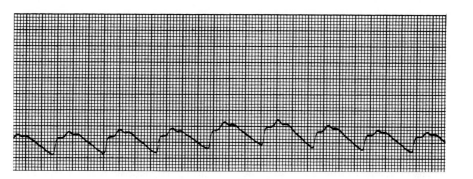

**Fig. 55-2**  Abnormal ICP wave form. $P_2$ is higher than $P_3$, which is indication of poor cerebral compliance. *(From McQuillan KA, Von Rueden KT, Hartsock RL, et al: Trauma nursing: resuscitation through rehabilitation, 3 ed, Philadelphia, 2002, Saunders.)*

Vasogenic edema may be treated with osmotic diuretics or, if the cause is tumors, corticosteroids are usually effective.[11] Cytotoxic edema occurs during states of poor cerebral perfusion, hypoxic or anoxic states that cause diffuse cerebral edema. Osmotic diuretics or hypertonic saline solution may be beneficial in treatment of acute states of cytotoxic edema.[14,15] Interstitial edema occurs with hydrocephalus, and the primary acute intervention is the removal of CSF though a ventriculostomy drainage device until the condition corrects itself or a surgical shunt is placed.[11]

Cerebral spinal fluid is a clear colorless fluid that fills the ventricles of brain and subarachnoid spaces of the brain and spinal cord. Most CSF is produced by the choroids plexus, which are located in the third and fourth ventricles of the brain. CSF is constantly produced at a rate or approximately 25 mL/h or 500 mL/d.[11] When the pressure within the brain exceeds 15 mm Hg, CSF production may slow or the brain displaces CSF to accommodate increases in brain tissue edema. Additional interventions may be the active removal of CSF through a ventriculostomy drain when the ICP exceeds a certain ICP parameter.

Cerebral blood flow (CBF) is the third component of intracranial pressure dynamics. The brain receives approximately 20% of the cardiac output and consumes 20% of the body's oxygen and 25% of the body's glucose.[8,11,14] When pressures within the cranial vault increase beyond normal ranges, the heart has more difficulty delivering nutrients to the brain. Factors that decrease cardiac output and function, increased blood viscosity, and hypotensive states significantly compromise effective cerebral blood flow. Cerebral vasculature is also influenced by changes in carbon dioxide levels in the blood. High levels of carbon dioxide ($PaCO_2$) cause cerebral vasculature dilation and increase blood flow, and decreased levels of $PaCO_2$ cause vasoconstriction of cerebral vasculature and decrease blood flow. However, reduction of $PaCO_2$ to less than 35 mm Hg reduces blood flow to the brain tissue and may exacerbate cerebral ischemia, further increasing ICP.[14] During states of elevated ICP, $PaCO_2$ may be artificially lowered through mechanical ventilation settings that cause hyperventilation to induce cerebral vasoconstriction. However, caution to avoid hyperventilation that lowers $PaCO_2$ less than 35 mm Hg is warranted to avoid worsening cerebral ischemia.

Autoregulation refers to the ability of the brain to maintain a constant CBF despite changes in the arterial perfusion pressure (systemic circulation). Autoregulation is a protective homeostatic mechanism of the brain that attempts to keep cerebral perfusion constant and generally continues to maintain CBF until the ICP exceeds 40 mm Hg.[11] Autoregulation provides a constant CBF flow by adjusting the diameter of blood vessels based on changes in the intracerebral pressure. It works synergistically with other protective mechanisms of the brain (e.g., reducing $PaCO_2$ and displacing CSF) to maintain CBF. Autoregulation, however, is limited as a compensatory mechanism. A critical point can be reached because of sustained increases in ICP, global or local diffuse injury, cerebral edema, ischemia, or inflammation.[11] If autoregulation is lost, reduced cerebrovascular tone occurs and the CBF becomes dependent on changes in systemic blood pressure. Thus, a primary goal in management of ICP is effective treatment of the cause of the increase in ICP so that autoregulation is maintained as a compensatory mechanism of CBF.

Cerebral perfusion pressure (CPP) is a parameter that is calculated from the mean arterial pressure (MAP) minus the ICP and is an indicator of general cerebral perfusion and CBF. Cerebral perfusion pressure becomes increasingly important when the patient loses autoregulatory homeostasis because of sustained increases in ICP. The minimal CPP necessary to maintain adequate perfusion is 60 to 70 mm Hg.[11,12,14,16] The optimal CPP remains an area of great controversy, however. Current guidelines suggest that a minimally acceptable CPP is 60 mm Hg and a more optimal CPP is 70 mm Hg, but efforts to achieve a CPP of more than 70 mm Hg should be avoided because higher CPP has been associated with more incidence of acute respiratory distress syndrome.[12] Because CPP is dependent on MAP, interventions to increase MAP may be necessary if ICP cannot be lowered to maintain effective cerebral perfusion during states of increased ICP. Vasoactive agents to support cardiac output and blood pressure are frequently administered to increase CPP to meet cerebral perfusion demands. Newer technology (LICOX) can be invasively introduced into the brain and cerebral vasculature to measure brain tissue oxygenation ($PtbO_2$).

Transient increases in ICP are dynamic temporary increases in ICP. Transient increases in ICP can be caused by coughing, pain, or excessive stimulation. Transient increases in ICP are associated with cerebral hypoxemic and ineffective cerebral perfusion states.[11] Signs and symptoms of transient increases in ICP of more than 15 mm Hg include headache, aphasia, changes in respiratory pattern (e.g., Cheyne-Stokes), changes in vital signs, decreases or changes in level of consciousness, motor dysfunction (e.g., hemiparesis), visual disturbances, and nausea and vomiting.[11,13,14] In addition sudden diuresis may indicate a disregulation of antidiuretic hormone related to ICP.

Consequences of increased ICP can be more devastating than the initial neurologic insult.[8] Nursing interventions need to focus on assessment of risk factors for increases in ICP and implementation and monitoring of the effects of interventions to reduce sustained increases in ICP.

***Postanesthesia Management of the Neurosurgical Patient.*** Postanesthesia management of the intensive care neurosurgical patient focuses on minimization of increases in ICP and continuous assessment of neurologic status. The goal of nursing care is to minimize secondary insults that are a consequence of ICP. A focused neurologic assessment to include level of arousal, orientation, motor skills, and a cranial nerve examination should be completed hourly for up to 12 hours or longer depending on the nature of the neurosurgical procedure. The nurse needs to assess for subtle changes in the neurologic assessment rather than looking for gross deviations from normal. Knowledge of the patient's neurologic assessment before surgery is important in establishing a baseline from which to base the immediate postoperative neurologic assessment. Another important variable in neurologic assessment is the nurse. Nurses should validate abnormal findings with each other because subtle changes may be hard to assess; and nurses should perform a neurologic assessment with each change of shift to ensure maximized consistency in the assessment of the neurosurgical patient. Basic assessments of cerebral dressings after surgery with observation for bleeding or presence of CSF fluid leakage are also part of the immediate perianesthesia nursing assessment. If the neurosurgical procedure was related to spinal pathology, the nursing assessment focuses on motor and sensory function of the patient. Management or prevention of edema and maintenance of body alignment remain the nursing priorities in the immediate postanesthesia period.

Monitoring of ICP, documentation and assessment of the ICP waveform at set intervals, and correlation of the neurologic assessment during elevations in ICP are important nursing assessment interventions. Immediate interventions to reduce ICP include elevating the head of the bed 30 degrees[8,17] and maintaining a neutral neck alignment. If noxious stimuli, environmental stimuli, or nursing activities are the cause of increase in ICP, limiting of noxious events such as venipuncture, suctioning, and nursing cares should be considered.

Maximization of oxygenation and ventilation is an important intervention in care for neurosurgical patients. Interventions to maximize oxygenation to achieve a $PaO_2$ greater than 60 mm Hg and normal $PaCO_2$ are important to ensure cerebral oxygen demands are met and cerebral vasoconstriction from hypocarbia is minimized.

Maintenance of an effective blood pressure and cardiac output to meet cerebral perfusion needs also is a primary nursing intervention. Medications to lower or raise blood pressure to optimize CPP are ordered for the neurosurgical patient. Immediately after surgery, the physician may want the blood pressure lower to minimize bleeding. If the neurologic examination becomes compromised when the blood pressure is lower, the nurse should notify the physician because this may be an indication of ineffective cerebral perfusion. Depending on the neurologic insult, the nurse either administers medications to lower the patient's blood pressure to prevent further intracerebral bleeding or administers medications to increase the patient's blood pressure to maximize cerebral perfusion and manage cerebral edema. Knowledge of the patient's pathology, neurosurgical procedure, and the neurologic examination results is a crucial assessment variable to help determine optimal blood pressure parameters.

Management of pain and sedation is an important nursing intervention during the perianesthesia care of the neurosurgical patient. Short-acting analgesics and sedation agents should be used to allow continued assessment of the patient's neurologic status. Maintaining normothermia or inducing mild hypothermia (core temperature, 33° C to 36° C) has been found to be neuroprotective in patients with cerebral injury.[12,18] For every decrease in temperature below normal, brain metabolism decreases by 7% to 10%.[13,18] Body temperature can be maintained or lowered with conventional air sources, ice, cooling blankets, or intravascular devices. Regardless of the method used to maintain normothermia or mild hypothermia, interventions should not induce shivering. Shivering can adversely increase metabolic demand and oxygen consumption needs beyond the benefits of lowering the patient's body temperature.[18]

The research on the negative effects of hyperglycemia in critical illness continues to mount. Hyperglycemia in critically ill patients has been described as a toxic metabolic milieu that slowly and insidiously results in increased morbidity and mortality.[9] Critical illness increases the secretion of counterregulatory hormones, such as glucagons, epinephrine, norepinephrine, and growth hormone, and results in an increase in hepatic glucose production, decrease in peripheral glucose uptake, and induction of a hyperglycemic state.[9] The hyperglycemia of critical illness is initially an adaptive response to stress; however, over time, it exacerbates the circulation of abnormal inflammatory mediators and worsens states of tissue ischemia.[19] Hyperglycemia has been found to worsen brain tissue acidosis with worsening of the ischemic state of brain tissue and extension of cerebral infarction size.[20] Thus, efforts to maintain normoglycemic states (serum glucose, 80 to 110 mg/dL) by administering intravenous insulin either intermittently or via continuous infusion is indicated in the management of the critically ill neurosurgical patient.

Care of the critically ill neurosurgical patient after surgical interventions requires that the nurse have a working knowledge of neuroanatomy, the surgical procedure, and monitoring of the patient for subtle changes in neurologic assessment and neurologic hemodynamics. Assessment of subtle changes in the neurologic assessment and correlation of changes to vital sign parameters and neurohemodynamics are essential in the treatment of critically ill neuroscience patients. Simple nursing interventions such as maintaining neutral head alignment, preventing shivering, and maintaining the head of the bed at more than 30 degrees, are effective first-line interventions in the treatment of patients with altered ICP. Other interventions focus on maximization of oxygenation, cardiac output, blood pressure, and prevention of infection. Technical knowledge related to ICP monitoring and ventriculostomy management is necessary to effectively monitor and treat changes in ICP. Finally, involving the family and ensuring they understand goals of care and interventions are important so that family-centered care is maximized throughout the patient's acute illness and recovery phase.

## Postoperative Care of the ICU Burn Trauma Patient

Deaths from fire and burns are the fifth most common cause of unintentional injury-related deaths in the United States.[21] According to the American Burn Association, approximately 1.1 million burn injuries require medical attention; 50,000 of these individuals need hospitalization, and 4500 individuals die of the burn injury.[22] An estimated 2670 individuals die in house fires and 14,050 patients are injured from fire-related injuries that cost $6.1 billion in direct property damage.[23,24] A small percentage of burn-injured patients, approximately 6%, do not survive; these patients have associated inhalation injury.[24,25] However, in the face of these sobering facts, the overall mortality and morbidity rates from burn injury have declined over the years because of advances in burn prevention strategies and medical interventions for this patient population. In the 1970s, a patient with a 50% total body surface area (TBSA) burn had an estimated 40% chance of survival; today, a patient with a 75% TBSA burn has a 50% chance of survival.[26] Elements that have been attributed to patient survival include more rapid response by emergency teams, efficiencies in transport to burn treatment facilities, advances in fluid resuscitation, improvements in wound coverage, better support of the hypermetabolic response to injury, advances in infection control practices, and improved treatment of inhalation injuries.[23,26,27]

Patients with burn injury have special needs throughout hospitalization. The American Burn Association (ABA)[22] has established guidelines to determine which burn-injured patients should be transferred to a specialized burn center to maximize treatment and decrease patient morbidity and mortality (Box 55-3).[22] Patients who meet the criteria outlined by the ABA should be transported to the nearest burn center to maximize patient survival and functional outcome.

### Brief Review of Burn Injury Pathophysiology.
Burn tissue injury is associated with the coagulation of cellular protein caused by exposure or

---

### Box 55-3   Criteria for Burn Center Transfer and Referral

- Second-degree burns greater than 10% TBSA
- Full-thickness burns greater than 5% TBSA
- Burns that involve the face, hands, feet, eyes, ears, or perineum
- Burns that could result in cosmetic or functional disability
- Circumferential burns of the chest or extremities
- Inhalation injury and associated trauma
- All chemical burns
- Electric burns
- Significant comorbid conditions (diabetes mellitus, chronic obstructive pulmonary disease, cardiac disease)

American Burn Association, www.ameriburn.org, accessed March 3, 2006.

contact with heat produced by thermal, electric, chemical, or radiation energy. The depth of coagulative tissue necrosis (depth of burn wound) depends on the intensity of the heat and length of time the tissues are exposed to the heat source. Thermal injury from flame, steam, scald, and contact with hot objects is the most frequent cause of burn injury. Inhalation injury is frequently associated with thermal injury when the victim is trapped in an enclosed space during the fire. Electric injury occurs when electric energy is converted into heat and causes tissue destruction as the current flows through the body. Electric current travels through the body along a path of least resistance, such as nerves, blood vessels, and muscles, sparing the skin except at the entry and exit points of the current.[28] Thus, most electric burn injuries result in deep internal tissue damage. Chemical injuries from either acidic or alkaline agents cause tissue destruction related to the type, strength, and duration of contact. Radiation burns are infrequent and usually are the result of medical radiation treatments or industrial accidents.

Regardless of what caused the burn injury, the tissue damage can be conceptualized as having three zones that represent the depth of tissue coagulation. Full-thickness burn is the deepest tissue injury in which full coagulation of the tissue proteins has occurred and causes irreversible tissue necrosis. Immediately surrounding the necrotic tissue area is the region or zone of stasis in which blood flow is impaired.[26,29] This region is considered a critical area because it may progress to tissue necrosis if tissue perfusion is inadequate during the burn fluid resuscitation period, which creates a larger burn wound injury. The outer zone of hyperemia has sustained minimal tissue injury and usually heals rapidly. Early goals of burn management focus on stopping the burning process and providing adequate fluid resuscitation to prevent the extension of burn injury from lack of perfusion.

When burn injury occurs, a myriad of local mediators are released by the body in response to the tissue insult. These mediators, such as histamine, serotonin, kinins, arachidonic acid metabolites, xanthine oxidase products, complement cytokines, and catecholamines cause arteriolar and venular dilation, increased microvascular permeability, and decreased perfusion.[26,29-31] Proteins leak from the intravascular space into the extravascular space and increase tissue oncotic pressure, creating edema.[32] Thromboxane $A_2$, a mediator that causes vasoconstriction, is also released by the body and may compromise perfusion to the burn injury area and cause

extension of the depth of burn tissue injury.[27,30] Concurrently, the coagulation system is activated, which causes platelet aggregation and activation of polymorphonuclear neutrophil (PMN) leukocytes and macrophages, which are essential to wound healing. The summation of the activation of the body's intense inflammatory response is vascular stasis and rapid formation of tissue edema.

In addition, the extensive loss of tissue and the exaggerated physiologic inflammatory and stress response associated with the burn injury, place the patient at risk for infection, hypothermia, hypercatabolism, and development of acute respiratory distress syndrome (ARDS), sepsis, systemic inflammatory response syndrome (SIRS), and multiple organ dysfunction syndrome (MODS).[33,34] The intensity of the metabolic changes experienced by burn patients is directly related to the extent of injury.[35] Metabolic demands increase by an estimated 30% in patients with an injury that covers 20% of the TBSA or more and by 100% in patients with burns that cover 50% of the TBSA or more.[35, 36] Primary goals in the management of a patient with burn injury focuses on: (1) providing adequate fluid resuscitation to restore circulating volume and minimize the conversion burn tissue injury to deeper full-thickness tissue injury; (2) optimizing tissue oxygenation and management of associated pulmonary insults; (3) preventing hypothermia; (4) preventing infection though topical antibiotics and excision and coverage of burn wounds; (5) maintaining nutritional support to maximize wound healing; and (6) effectively treating pain and emotional needs of the patient.

**Extent and Depth of Tissue Injury.** Burn injuries are described according to the extent and depth of tissue injury. Extent is the total amount of body surface area (TBSA) that has been injured, and depth is the severity of tissue necrosis. In the acute care setting, the percentage of TBSA is calculated with the Berkow[37] and Lund-Browder[38] formula. This assessment tool is used to estimate the amount of tissue injured by the thermal agent. The primary goal in estimating the TBSA of burn injury is to predict: morbidity/survival, physiologic response in relation to fluid shifts, fluid resuscitation requirement, and metabolic and immunologic responses. Burn wound depth describes tissue damage based on anatomic loss of the layers of the skin. Depth is estimated from the most external layers of the skin to the internal. Fig. 55-3 depicts the anatomic depth and nomenclature used to describe burn wound depth. Deep partial-thickness and full-thickness burn wounds require tissue grafting

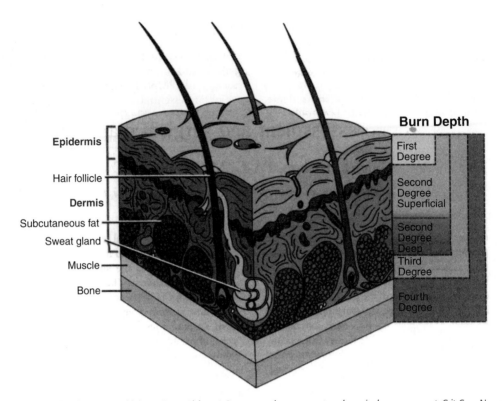

**Fig. 55-3** Depth of burn wound injury. *(From Bishop J: Burn wound assessment and surgical management,* Crit Care Nurse Clin North Am *16(1):145-177, 2004.)*

for effective healing, cosmesis, and prevention of infection with removal of devitalized tissue.

*Surgical and Postanesthesia Management of the Burn-injured Patient.* Current management involves the early excision of eschar (necrotic tissue) of deep partial-thickness and full-thickness burn wounds.[39] Typically, surgical débridement of eschar occurs within the first 48 hours after injury. The goal of surgery is to remove most of the devitalized tissue and cover wounds with either autografts or biologic or synthetic dressings that promote wound healing and closure. The operative plan involves removal of devitalized tissue and an evaluation of the wound bed before application of an autograft or synthetic dressing. If an autograft is used to cover the burn wound, it is important to realize the donor site for the autograft tissue is also a wound that requires observation after surgery. Physician orders and postoperative notes typically clearly identify the surgical procedure (e.g., excision, débridement, grafting technique) and type of wound coverage place on the burn wound.

Postanesthesia care of the burn wound (autograft or synthetic dressing) consists of limiting or immobilizing the area of the body where the wound is located. Frequently, the physician splints the wound or sutures the dressing in place

to minimize movement of the wound covering off of the fragile burn wound bed. In addition, observations for strikethrough or frank bleeding of the graft or donor site are required during the immediate postanesthesia period. Efforts to prevent friction and motion of the grafted area are necessary in the first 48 hours after surgery to prevent shearing of the graft from the wound bed. Simple interventions such as turning a patient or moving a patient off a stretcher onto a bed require utmost caution to preserve the graft adherence and successful coverage of the burn wound.

Other priorities focus on ensuring adequate fluid perfusion though effective management of intravenous fluids and vasoactive agents as needed. Efforts to maximize perfusion are necessary to enhance effective blood flow to the tissue bed. Evaluation of blood loss from the surgical procedure and insensible loss from the dressings need to be assessed, and blood products or fluids are adjusted to maintain mean arterial pressure greater than 70 mm Hg and urine output greater than 0.5 mL/kg/h. Continuous heart rate monitoring and trends are helpful in monitoring the cardiovascular response after surgery. The heart rate may be falsely elevated from a catecholamine response to the burn injury and surgery; however, changes in heart rate can be used to evaluate effectiveness of fluid replacement interventions.[39] Other invasive parameters such as pulmonary artery wedge pressure, central venous pressure, and mixed venous oxygen saturation may also provide helpful assessment data to evaluate effectiveness of tissue perfusion.[39,40] Acid-base balance can also provide valuable information on the effectiveness of fluid resuscitation after surgery and tissue perfusion. A base deficit is seen as metabolic acidosis and corrects to normal with adequate resuscitation. A base deficit of 6 mEq/L or more is an indicator of shock and has been associated with increased mortality.[34,41,42]

Patients with electric burn injury need additional attention and monitoring of heart rate and rhythm. As voltage passes through the patient's body, damage to the myocardial system is possible. These patients should be on continuous cardiac monitoring for up to 72 hours to assess for conduction disturbances and myocardial damage.[43]

Typically, if dysrhythmias occur, they are seen in the first few hours after injury. Myloglobinuria, however, is a serious complication that must be assessed and treated in electric burn–injured patients. Thus, fluid resuscitation to support the patient's perfusion and additional fluid to clear the kidneys of myloglobin are necessary during the postanesthesia period. Urine output of 75 to 100 mL/h or 1 to 2 mL/kg/h is usually necessary to treat myloglobinuria.[43]

Pulmonary assessment involves management of the ventilator to maximize oxygenation and ventilation. Third spacing and edema place the burn patient at risk for ARDS. Nursing interventions that monitor the ventilatory management of the patient, airway pressures, patient's tolerance of the ventilatory mode, and oxygenation parameters are important aspects of nursing care after surgery. The nurse should assess for early signs of ARDS by evaluating the patient's ventilatory airway pressures, changes in tidal volumes, and signs and symptoms of hypoxemia. The patient may need sedation or neuromuscular blocking agents to assist with ventilator efforts as the ARDS progresses. Pneumonia is a serious complication in a burn-injured patient. Nursing interventions to reduce ventilator-associated pneumonia are essential. Nursing interventions include assessment of the head of bed greater than 30 degrees, ideally 45 degrees; frequent oral care and toothbrushing with oropharyngeal suctioning; assessment of cuff pressure of the endotracheal tube; and assessment of enteral tube feeding tolerance.[44] Patients with inhalation injury are at greater risks of development of ARDS and pneumonia because of the direct injury to the lung parenchyma. Inhalation injury frequently requires more aggressive fluid resuscitation to support systemic perfusion; however, this may increase pulmonary third spacing. Serial bronchoscopy is frequently done to evaluate the severity of inhalation injury, and aggressive pulmonary suctioning is usually needed to assist with removal of debris and secretions.

Prevention of hypothermia and adverse effects of hypothermia such as electrolyte imbalances, tissue vasoconstriction, and coagulopathies are additional areas for nursing care focus. Application of convection air heating devices and thermal hats and warming of the patient's room can assist with preventing hypothermia. Care is needed, however, to prevent overshoot that causes hyperthermia. The burn patient cannot effectively regulate body temperature because of the tissue loss; thus, external temperature changes can greatly influence the patient's body temperature.

Maintenance of nutritional management through surgery and after surgery are also standards of care in the management of the burn patient. Typically, the patient has a postpyloric feeding tube in which low-dose continuous tube feeding is provided to the patient. Hypermetabolism associated with burn injury requires significant nutritional replacement strategies to meet metabolism demands and provide substrates for tissue healing.

The final nursing priority is effective management of pain. Burn patients have hypermetabolism in response to the injury and ongoing insults with surgical management for burn wound excision and wound coverage. Opioid infusions, usually morphine or fentanyl, are the mainstay for treatment of pain. The addition of continuous or intermittent (scheduled) anxiolytic agents is also beneficial with pain management.[45,46] Evidence-based pain assessment tools are needed to assess a patient's pain, and the patient may have a difficult time obtaining pain relief during the immediate postanesthesia period. Burn patients frequently have a tolerance to analgesic agents; thus, continuous infusions of analgesics and sedation agents titrated to desired pain and sedation responses for the patient provide optimal management after surgery. Efficacious postanesthesia management of the critically ill burn patient plays a vital role in the functional outcome and future rehabilitation.

## Postoperative Care of the Septic ICU Patient

Patients admitted and treated for sepsis in the emergency department, inpatient

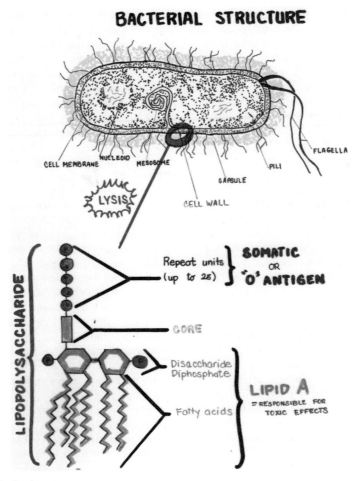

**Fig. 55-4**  Endotoxin drawing.

medical-surgical unit, or ICU are often transferred to the OR for surgery. The initial presentation is often nonspecific, and the severity may be deceiving. Critical illness may often be accompanied by localized or systemic infection. Patients may arrive with a relatively benign diagnosis, or clinically unapparent infection can progress within hours to a more devastating form of disease.[47] Sepsis is an acute systemic response to a bacteria invasion or to the toxins produced by bacteria (Fig. 55-4). It is associated with systemic inflammatory response syndrome (SIRS).[48,49] Sepsis is further defined as the presence of two or more SIRS criteria in the setting of documented or assumed infection.[48,49] Sepsis may precede the development of septic shock. According to Dellinger and colleagues,[48] abnormalities of temperature, heart rate, blood pressure, respiratory rate, and leukocyte count are clinical findings of SIRS (Box 55-4). The hallmark of severe sepsis is progressive organ perfusion and organ dysfunction. Septic shock results when the blood pressure falls and the

patient becomes hypotensive, despite adequate fluid resuscitation and vasopressor support. The transition from sepsis to septic shock occurs most often during the first 24 hours of hospitalization.[48] Although septic shock occurs from gram-positive or yeast infections, the most common cases are gram-negative endotoxins. This toxin-induced activation of the cellular, humoral, and immunologic defense systems initiates a cascade of the systemic inflammatory response evidenced by the generation of a variety of chemical mediators, including prostaglandins, endorphins, and kinins that modulate cellular and organ derangements associated with shock (Fig. 55-5).

***Pathophysiology of Septic Shock.*** Key to understanding septic shock is the profound hemodynamic instability. The nurse may witness two different dysfunctional patterns of the cardiovascular system as a consequence to sepsis. The first is characterized by high cardiac output (CO) and low systemic vascular resistance (SVR), and the second reveals a more

---

### Box 55-4 Sepsis Definitions

**Systemic inflammatory response syndrome (SIRS)** — includes 2 or more of:
- Temperature: $> 38°$ or $< 36°$ C
- Heart rate: $> 90$ beats/min unless the patient is taking medications to reduce the rate (a beta-blocker or calcium-channel blocker) or the heart is paced
- Respiratory rate: $> 20$ breaths/min (or $Paco_2 < 32$ torr) or mechanically ventilated
- Leukocyte count $> 12\,000/\mu L$ or $< 4000/\mu L$, or $> 10\%$ immature band forms

**Sepsis**
- Presence or presumed presence of an infection accompanied by evidence of SIRS

**Severe sepsis:** presence of sepsis, plus organ hypoperfusion or dysfunction
- Organ hypoperfusion; for example:
  - Increased blood lactate levels
  - Oliguria
  - Abnormal peripheral circulation, such as poor capillary refill, mottled skin
  - Acute alteration in mental status
- Dysfunction* of 1 or more organs, such as abnormalities of:
  - The hematologic system; e.g., thrombocytopenia, disseminated intravascular coagulation
  - The pulmonary system; e.g., acute respiratory distress syndrome
  - The renal system; e.g., acute renal failure
  - The gastrointestinal system with hepatic dysfunction; e.g., hyperbilirubinemia
  - The central nervous system; e.g., delirium

**Septic shock†**
- Presence of sepsis
- Refractory hypotension
  - A systolic blood pressure $< 90$ mm Hg
  - A mean arterial pressure $< 65$ mm Hg, or a 40 mm Hg drop in systolic blood pressure compared to baseline
  - Unresponsive to a fluid challenge of 20-40 mL/kg
- Vasopressor dependency after adequate volume resuscitation

From Rivers EP, McIntyre L, Morro DC, et al: Early and innovative interventions for severe sepsis and septic shock: taking advantage of window opportunity – Reprinted from, CMAJ 25-Oct-06; 173(9), Page(s) 1054-1065 by permission of the publisher. © Canadian Medical Association.
*Organs are considered to have failed when the organ dysfunction becomes most severe.
†Note that this is a standard definition. A patient may be in septic shock with a normal blood pressure if the baseline blood pressure is elevated (e.g., someone with a history of hypertension, diabetes, or vascular disease) or there is concomitant myocardial dysfunction.

classic shock with low CO and high SVR.[49] These two clinical findings reflect a hyperdynamic or hypodynamic shock state. The hyperdynamic response is termed early septic shock, and the hypodynamic response is the late septic shock that indicates a severe septic shock and is not reversible.

The term systemic inflammatory response syndrome (SIRS) was named to describe patients in whom the inflammatory response is fully and systemically activated.[50] Degrees of systemic activation of the inflammatory response result in damage to the tissues and organs. Vasodilation (that occurs and is a common finding in septic shock) is attributed to the inflammatory response of the vasoactive mediators (prostaglandins, kinins, histamines).[50] The blood-borne bacteria or endotoxins cause the activation of the complement cascade (C-reactive protein fragments), which is directly attributed to the humoral response of SIRS. These complement fragments cause the mast cells to degranulate liberating histamine, resulting in local vasodilation and capillary permeability. The activation of C-reactive protein fragments intensifies the mediators of inflammation and SIRS. During septic shock, activated neutrophils may synthesize leukotrienes and the oxygen free radicals that contribute to increased cell permeability and bronchoconstriction. Frequently, platelet abnormalities cause coagulopathies and ultimately cause profound thrombocytopenia.[50] Endotoxins have a direct effect by binding to the receptors on the platelets, stimulating degranulating and increasing platelet aggregation in the microvasculature. This devastating action creates thrombotic obstruction to flow in the pulmonary vasculature that results in adult respiratory distress syndrome (ARDS) and organ failure.

***Pulmonary Dysfunction.*** The lung is one of the chief target organs in septic shock. Transport and utilization of oxygen at the cellular and tissue levels are vital for survival (Fig. 55-6). ARDS is associated with an oxygen extraction defect that affects the utilization and delivery of oxygen to the tissues (Fig. 55-7). The subsequent formation of interstitial edema contributes to the inability to extract oxygen. In addition, the release of endoxin stimulates the inflammatory mediators. These mediators generate toxic oxygen metabolites, which damages the endothelium of the pulmonary vasculature and increases the permeability of the alveolar-capillary defect, resulting in ventilation/perfusion mismatch and impaired gas exchange.[50] Changes in lung compliance and impaired gas exchange are two pathophysiologic

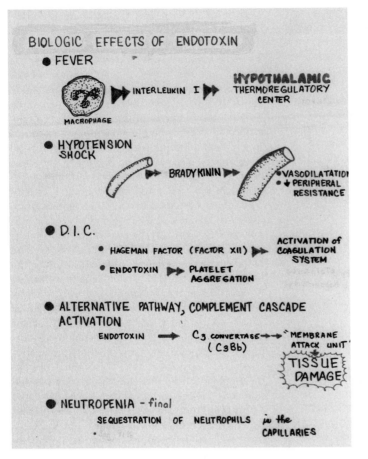

**Fig. 55-5** Mediators of inflammation.

abnormalities that may lead to the development of ARDS. Protracted oxygen debt may result in the development of multiple organ dysfunction syndrome (MODS) and eventual organ death.[50]

The goals in management of septic patients with ARDS are maximizing pulmonary gas exchange, optimizing oxygen delivery to the tissues, and preventing further organ injury.[50] The PACU nurse's role in ongoing vigilant assessments, interventions, and monitoring that help promote improved gas exchange and reduced oxygen demands provides a crucial key to better survival rates.

***Metabolic Dysfunction.*** The metabolic derangements that accompany septic shock are dependent on the severity and duration of the illness, which result in intensified transport and perfusion problems. Some of these abnormalities are manifested by: (1) mechanical obstruction of capillary beds by platelet aggregation; (2) vasoconstriction that causes shunting formation in the organs; (3) inflammatory mediator interaction, and (4) impaired cellular oxidative metabolism or oxygen debt to the tissues.[48-50] Increased lactic acidosis is persistent even though oxygen

consumption is consistently increased. Patients in septic shock need higher oxygen delivery because of the escalating metabolic demand. Sustained proteolysis is evidenced by high urinary nitrogen excretion.[51] Gluconeogenesis is increased; however, concurrent insulin resistance results in hyperglycemia in the hyperdynamic state of septic shock. In late septic shock, a profound hypoglycemia develops as glycogen stores are depleted and are insufficient to supply the body's demands.

**Steroid Therapy.** In the neurohumoral response to septic shock, many patients have an inadequate adrenal reserve. Although the physiologic mechanism is not fully understood, it is likely caused by the inflammatory cascade that leads to inadequate release of adrenocorticotropin. When compared with placebo, low-dose hydrocortisone that was administered to patients in septic shock decreased the requirements of vasopressors[52] and subsequently lowered mortality rate. Hydrocortisone has also shown a reduction in ARDS.

**Glycemic Control.** Tight glycemic control is directly related to decreased mortality in the postsurgical patient. This effect also included

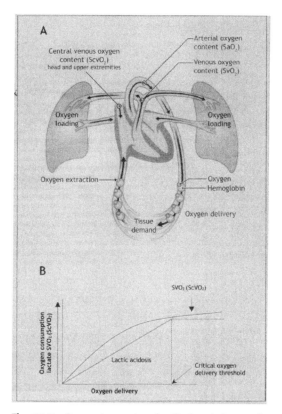

**Fig. 55-6** Oxygen transport and utilization during sepsis. *(From Rivers EP, McIntyre L, Morro DC, et al: Early innovative interventions for severe sepsis and septic shock: taking advantage of the window of opportunity,* Can Med Assoc J *173(9):1054-1065, 2005.)*

a significant reduction in organ failure. Thus, efforts to maintain normoglycemic states (serum glucose, 80 to 110 mg/dL) with administration of intravenous insulin either intermittently or via continuous infusion are indicated

in the management of the critically ill septic patient.

***Acute Renal Failure.*** Acute renal failure (ARF) is often associated with sepsis and septic shock. Postanesthesia nurses can have a major influence on the septic patient's morbidity and mortality related to ARF.[51] Generally, two pathophysiologic causes that occur are cellular ischemia related to hypoperfusion and the presence of SIRS. Mediators of inflammation, such as tumor necrosis factor (TNF), alpha interleukin-1 (IL-1), and interleukin-6, influence the hemodynamic consequences of sepsis and cause damage to the renal tubules.[53] The circulating bacterial endotoxins found in sepsis result in further renal deterioration.[53] Because the cause of prerenal acute renal failure is inadequate renal perfusion, often related to deficits in intravascular volume, prompt replacement of crystalloids and blood to correct this hypovolemic state is warranted. [53] In oliguric states, diuretics are frequently used. Furosemide, a loop diuretic, and mannitol, an osmotic diuretic, are used to prevent ARF. However, diuretics must be used with caution in patients with problems of hydration and electrolyte imbalance. Low-dose dopamine (1 to 3 μg/kg/min) may also be used as a renal diuretic. Management of acid-base, cardiovascular, and intake and output alterations is vital in preserving kidney function and preventing organ failure in the septic patient.[51,53]

***Postanesthesia Management of the Patient in Septic Shock.*** Advances within the last 5 years for the treatment of sepsis, severe sepsis, and septic shock have provided new therapeutic modalities.[52] Some studies have shown a significant mortality benefit within the first few hours of the presentation of severe sepsis ("Golden Hour" and "Silver Day") with hemodynamic optimization and resuscitation for

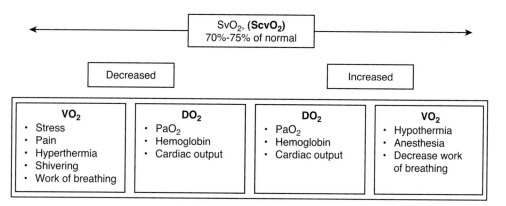

**Fig. 55-7** Clinical utilization and delivery of venous oxygen saturation ($SvO_2$ or $ScvO_2$) to tissues. *(From Rivers EP, McIntyre L, Morro DC, et al: Early and innovative interventions for severe sepsis and septic shock: taking advantage of the window of opportunity,* Can Med Assoc J *173(9):1054-1065, 2005.)*

SPECIAL CONSIDERATIONS

aggressive correction of septic shock and organ dysfunction.[47]

Postanesthesia care of the patient in septic shock must first focus on oxygenation and ventilation to ensure tissue perfusion. In sepsis, an impairment of oxygen extraction and utilization at the cellular level is seen. Further, the patient in septic shock may require higher than normal $PaO_2$. Consequently, nursing critical decision making should be aimed at optimizing ventilations. The patient may need frequent suctioning to remove secretions and careful monitoring of blood gases. Because ARDS frequently accompanies sepsis, the patient may need mechanical ventilation. New research shows that strategies to minimize oxygen demand through intubation, sedation, and analgesia with mechanical ventilation reduce the work of breathing and oxygen consumption by the respiratory muscles. In addition, experimental data revealed mechanical ventilation with large tidal volumes stretch the lung tissue and cause volume trauma that increases the inflammatory response that leads to acute lung injury.[52] Lower tidal volumes (6 mL/kg of estimated body weight versus 12 mL/kg of body weight) showed a 10% reduction in a 28-day mortality rate.[52] This reduction may be because lower tidal volumes limit lung tissue damage and may prevent biotrauma that further activates SIRS. Because sepsis is one of the most common causes of ARDS, institution of low tidal volume when lung injury or ARDS is suspected is prudent. The PACU nurse should frequently monitor the septic patient for decreased pulmonary compliance associated with airway hyperreactivity or pulmonary consolidation, which further impairs ventilation.[52]

Sepsis may be accompanied by myocardial suppression. Peripheral vasodilation, hypotension, and myocardial depression may significantly impede tissue perfusion. Therefore, end organ perfusion should be monitored with assessment of skin temperature, color, capillary refill, and peripheral pulses every hour. Because the mediators of inflammation activate the myocardial depressant factors and arterial vasodilation, pharmacologic support with a vasopressor-like dobutamine or dopamine is needed to increase myocardial contractility and systemic vascular resistance. Dobutamine may improve myocardial depression but may unmask underlying hypovolemia because it acts to increase contractility and reduce peripheral vascular resistance. Maintenance of oxygen transport to the tissues is essential. Tachycardia must be avoided to keep the heart rate at less than 100 bpm. Beta blocker therapy should be considered to minimize myocardial oxygen consumption and optimize

stroke volume. Finally, new research advocates use of vasopressin in the management of catecholamine refractory septic shock (Table 55-1).[52] Refractory septic shock is also termed late stage septic shock that is refractory to volume resuscitation and exogenous catecholamines.

**Sepsis Management Implications for the Postanesthesia Care Unit Nurse.** Management of the septic critically ill patient in the PACU can be challenging, even to the most experienced critical care nurse. The high mortality rate of septic shock emphasizes the importance of preventing and reversing the rapid progression of the disease.[54] Effective postanesthesia nursing care mandates knowledge of current sepsis research related to pathophysiology and clinical manifestations of SIRS. Understanding of the process of sepsis, severe sepsis, and septic shock sequelae is imperative. The PACU nurse must have a high degree of suspicion when the etiologies that predispose sepsis are seen in the recovering patient. Likewise, monitoring of the ICU patient vigilantly for signs and symptoms of decreased cardiac output and alterations in oxygenation and tissue perfusion provides key assessment information. Further, timely reporting is necessary of the subtle but significant critical changes in the patient's condition to the surgeon, anesthesiologist, or intensivist. New advancements in sepsis therapies should be used as evidence-based practice guidelines to care.

## FAMILY PRESENCE DURING RESUSCITATION

The impressive expertise of postanesthesia nurses is often taken for granted by both the nursing staff and medical colleagues.[55] The staff expect the patients under their care to do well. However, what does the staff do when the patient's condition becomes life threatening or even fatal? What happens in the PACU when things go wrong? Are these specialty nurses prepared for end-of-life nursing interventions? PACU nurses must become knowledgeable about the current evidence that emphasizes not only the needs of the patients but more importantly the needs of the surviving families.

The presence of a patient's family during resuscitation is emerging as an acceptable practice in the critical care setting. Critical care and emergency department (ED) nurses have been leaders in advocating family presence during resuscitation. In an article in 2001 entitled *Family Presence During Invasive and Resuscitation: Hearing the Voice of the Patient*, the authors reported an NBC Dateline Poll that showed 74% of 2464 respondents believed family members should be allowed to be in an

**Table 55-1  Evidence Review of Vasopressin Studies in Refractory Septic Shock**

| Reference | Year | Type of Study | Sample and treatment | Outcomes Beneficial | Outcomes Adverse |
|---|---|---|---|---|---|
| Landry et al | 1997 | Case control | 5 patients with septic shock AVP at 0.04 units/min | Increase in arterial blood pressure<br>Decrease or discontinuation of catecholamines<br>Increase in urine output | None |
| Landry et al | 1997 | Matched cohort | 19 patients with septic shock AVP at 0.04 units/min | Increase in arterial blood pressure<br>Decrease or discontinuation of catecholamines | Decrease in cardiac output |
| Malay et al | 1999 | Randomized controlled trial with isotonic sodium chloride solution | 10 patients with septic shock AVP at 0.04 untis/min | Increase in arterial blood pressure<br>Decrease or discontinuation of catecholamines | None |
| Tsuneyoshi et al | 2001 | Case control | 16 patients with septic shock AVP at 0.04 units/min | Increase in arterial blood pressure<br>Increase in urine output | None |
| Patel et al | 2002 | Double-blind randomized controlled trial with norepinephrine | 24 patients with septic shock AVP at 0.01-0.08 units/min | Increase in arterial blood pressure<br>Decrease or discontinuation of catecholamines<br>Increase in urine output | None |
| Dunser et al | 2003 | Randomized controlled trial with norepinehrine | 48 patients with vasodilatory shock AVP at 4 units/h | Increase in arterial blood pressure | Decrease in end-organ perfusion, hepatic |

*Continued*

**Table 55-1  Evidence Review of Vasopressin Studies in Refractory Septic Shock—cont'd**

| Reference | Year | Type of Study | Sample and treatment | Outcomes Beneficial | Outcomes Adverse |
|---|---|---|---|---|---|
| Van Haren et al | 2003 | Case control | 11 patients with septic shock<br>AVP at 0.04 units/min | Increase in arterial blood pressure | Decrease in end-organ perfusion, gastrointestinal, mucosal |
| Klinzing et al | 2003 | Case control | 12 patients with septic shock<br>AVP with dose adjusted until patient weaned off of norepinephrine | Increase in end-organ perfusion, hepatosplanchnic | Decrease in cardiac output<br>Decrease in end-organ perfusion, gastrointestinal, mucosal<br>Bradycardia |
| Morelli et al | 2004 | Case control | 15 patients with septic shock<br>1-mg bolus of AVP analog (terlipressin) | Increase in arterial blood pressure<br>Decrease or discontinuation of catecholamines<br>Increase in urine output<br>Increase in end-organ perfusion, gastrointestingal, mucosal | Decrease in cardiac output |
| Obritsch et al | 2004 | Retrospective | 102 patients with septic shock<br>AVP at 0.11–0.17 units/min | Increase in arterial blood pressure<br>Decrease or discontinuation of catecholamines | Bradycardia |
| Albanese et al | 2005 | Randomized controlled trial with norepinephrine | 20 patients with septic shock<br>Boluses of AVP analog (terlipressin) versus norepinephrine | Increase in arterial blood pressure<br>Increase in urine output | Decrease in cardiac output<br>Decrease in oxygen delivery |

From Lee CS: The role of exogenous arginine vasopressin in the management of catecholamine-refractory septic shock, *Crit Care Nurse* 26(6):17-29, 2006.
*AVP*, Arginine vasopressin.

ED during invasive procedures.[56] Today, evidence supports the multiple benefits of this practice to patients, families, and health care providers.[55-60] Patients feel family presence gives them the feeling of support, personhood, connectedness, and advocacy.[58,60] Research has repeatedly revealed that families have specific needs that include: (1) having honest, consistent, and thorough communication with health care providers; (2) being physically and emotionally close to their loved one; (3) feeling that the health care providers care about their loved one; and (4) visiting the patient frequently during a health-related crisis.[61] Both patients and families feel that they have a right to have families present during resuscitation.[62] Health care providers agree that family presence encourages professional behavior of staff at the bedside and facilitates end-of-life closure issues for families.[61-65] The Emergency Nurses Association (ENA) and the AACN have issued position statements in support of family presence during resuscitation.[66,67] PACU nurses need to expand their knowledge of family presence during resuscitation and adopt a holistic framework that provides the best possible outcomes for patients and families during the end of life.

The PACU nurse must remember the family when resuscitating an ICU patient in the PACU. The benefits far outweigh the risks in implementing family presence in the PACU. Research reveals that families perceive: (1) they have been supported; (2) everything was done for the patient; (3) patient-family connectedness was maintained; (4) the patient's personhood was respected; and (5) families coped better with death.[58-61]

## SUMMARY

The practice of providing postanesthesia care to the ICU patient in the PACU may be challenging and rewarding. Important administrative decisions to care for these critically ill patients must ensure safeguards to provide a comparable level of ICU care in the PACU. Key critical care education and clinical ICU competencies must be maintained. PACU nurses are recognized for their critical care skills and abilities in providing care to the ICU patient. This chapter has provided advanced clinical ICU nursing concepts in managing some of the highest risk high-acuity specialized complex cases (neurosurgery, burn, and septic shock). Finally, the introduction of family presence during resuscitation in the PACU advocates the family's right to be with the critically ill patient at the end of life.

## REFERENCES

1. American Society of Perianesthesia Nurses: *Standards of perianesthesia nursing practice*, Cherry Hill, NJ, 2006, American Society of Perianesthesia Nurses.
2. Fontaine DK: Impact of the critical care environment on the patient. In Morton PG, Fontaine DK, Hudak CM, et al, editors: *Critical care nursing: a holistic approach*, ed 8, Philadelphia, 2005, Lippincott Williams & Wilkins.
3. Ayres SA, Schlichtig R, Sterling MJ: *Care of the critically ill*, ed 3, Chicago, 1988, Yearbook Medical Publishers.
4. Bizek KS: The patient's experience with critical illness. In Morton PG, Fontaine DK, Hudak CM, et al, editors: *Critical care nursing: a holistic approach*, ed 8, Philadelphia, 2005, Lippincott Williams & Wilkins.
5. Happ MB: Communicating with mechanically ventilated patients: state of the science, *AACN Clin Iss* 12(2):247-258, 2001.
6. Norton C: The family's experience with critical illness. In Morton PG, Fontaine DK, Hudak CM, et al, editors: *Critical care nursing: a holistic approach*, ed 8, Philadelphia, 2005, Lippincott, Williams & Wilkins.
7. Johannes MS: A new dimension of the PACU: the dilemma of the ICU overflow patient, *J PeriAnesthesia Nurs* 9:297-300, 1994.
8. Bader MK: Gizmos and gadgets for the neuroscience intensive care unit, *J Neurosci Nurs* 38(4):248-260, 2006.
9. Paolina A, Garner K: Effects of hyperglycemia on neurologic outcome in stroke patients, *J Neurosci Nurs* 37(3):130-135, 2005.
10. Chesnut R: Management of brain and spine injuries, *Crit Care Clin* 20(1):25-55, 2004.
11. Hickey J: Intracranial hypertension: theory and management of increased intracranial pressure. In Hickey V, editor: *The clinical practice of neurological and neurosurgical nursing*, ed 5, Philadelphia, 2003, Lippincott Williams & Wilkins.
12. Blissitt P: Hemodynamic monitoring in the care of the critically ill neuroscience patient, *AACN Adv Crit Care* 17(3):327-340, 2006.
13. Bader MK, Littlejohns L: *AANN core curriculum for neuroscience nursing*, ed 4, St Louis, 2004, Mosby.
14. Censullo J, Sebastian S: Pentobarbital sodium coma for refractory intracranial hypertension, *J Neurosci Nurs* 35(5):252-262, 2003.
15. Johnson A, Criddle L: Pass the salt: indications for implications of using hypertonic saline, *Crit Care Nurse* 24(5):36-48, 2004.
16. Stevens W: Multimodal monitoring: head injury management using $SjvO_2$ and LICOX, *J Neurosci Nurs* 36(6):332-339, 2004.

17. Fan J: Effect of backrest position on intracranial pressure and cerebral perfusion pressure in individuals with brain injury: a systematic review, *J Neurosci Nurs* 36(5):278-288, 2004.

18. Lasater M: Intravascular temperature modulation in the neurosurgical critical care unit, *J Neurosci Nurs* 38(5):379-383, 2006.

19. Montori V, Bistrian B, McMahon M: Hyperglycemia in acutely ill patients, *JAMA* 288(17):2167-2169, 2002.

20. Alvarez-Sabin J, Molina C, Montaner J, et al: Effects of admission hyperglycemia on stroke outcome in reperfused tissue plasminogen activator-treated patients, *Stroke* 34:1235-1241, 2003.

21. Centers for Disease Control and Prevention: *Web-based Injury Statistics Query and Reporting System (WISQARS)*, available at www.ced.gov/ncipc/wisqars, accessed March 3, 2006.

22. American Burn Association: available at www.ameriburn.org, accessed March 3, 2006.

23. National Institutes of General Medical Sciences: Fact sheet: trauma, shock, burn and injury, available at www.nigms.nih.gov/factsheets/trauma_burn_facts, accessed March 3, 2006.

24. Ballesteros M, Jackson M, Martin M: Working toward elimination of residential fire deaths: the centers for disease control and prevention's smoke alarm installation and fire education program, *J Burn Care Rehabil* 26(5):434-439, 2005.

25. LaBorde P: Burn epidemiology: the patient, the nation, the statistics, and the data resources, *Crit Care Nurs Clin North Am* 16(1):13-25, 2004.

26. Wolf SE, Herndon DN: Burns and radiation injuries. In Mattox KL, Feliciano DV, Moore EE, editors: *Trauma*, ed 4, New York, 2000, McGraw-Hill.

27. Wolf SE, Herndon DN: Burns. In Townsend CM, Beauchamp RD, Evers BM, et al, editors: *Sabiston textbook of surgery: the biological basis of modern surgical practice*, ed 17, Edinburgh, 2004, Saunders.

28. Purdue GF, Hunt JL: Electrical injuries. In Herndon D, editor: *Total burn care*, ed 2, Edinburgh, 2002, Saunders.

29. Williams WG: Pathophysiology of the burn wound. In Herndon D, editor: *Total burn care*, ed 2, Edinburgh, 2000, Saunders.

30. Kramer GC, Lund T, Herndon DN: Pathophysiology of burn shock and burn edema. In Herndon D, editor: *Total burn care*, ed 2, Edinburgh, 2002, Saunders.

31. Marko P, Layon AJ, Caruso L, et al: Burn injuries, *Curr Opin Anaesthesiol* 16(2):183-191, 2003.

32. Demling RH: The burn edema process: current concepts, *J Burn Care Rehabil* 26(3):207-227, 2005.

33. Fitzwater J, Purdue GF, Hunt JL, et al: The risk factors and time course of sepsis and organ dysfunction after burn trauma, *J Trauma* 54(5):959-966, 2003.

34. Cumming J, Purdue GF, Hunt JL, et al: Objective estimates of the incidence and consequences of multiple organ dysfunction and sepsis after burn trauma, *J Trauma* 50(3):510-515, 2000.

35. Flynn MB: Nutritional support for the burn-injured patient, *Crit Care Nurs Clin North Am* 16(1):139-144, 2004.

36. Supple KG: Physiologic response to burn injury, *Crit Care Nurs Clin North Am* 16(1):119-126, 2004.

37. Berkow SG: A method for estimating the extensiveness of lesions (burns and scalds) based on surface area proportions, *Arch Surg* 8:138-142, 1924.

38. Lund CC, Browder NC: Estimation of areas of burns, *Surg Gynecol Obstet* 79:352-357, 1944.

39. Pereira C, Murphy K, Herndon D: Outcome measures in burn care: is mortality dead? *Burns* 20:761-771, 2004.

40. Rivers EP, Ander DS, Powell D: Central venous oxygen saturation monitoring in the critically ill patient, *Curr Opin in Crit Care* 7(3):204-211, 2001.

41. Ahrns KS: Trends in burn resuscitation: shifting the focus from fluids to adequate endpoint monitoring edema control, and adjuvant therapies, *Crit Care Clin North Am* 16(1):75-98, 2004.

42. Jeng JC, Jablonski K, Bridgeman A, et al: Serum lactate not base deficit, rapidly predicts survival after major burns, *Burns* 28:161-166, 2002.

43. Mann E, Makic MB: Burn injury. In Oman K, Koziol-McLain J, editors: *Emergency nursing secrets*, ed 2, St Louis, 2006, Mosby.

44. Metheny N, Clouse R, Chang Y, et al: Tracheobronchial aspiration of gastric contents in critically ill tube-fed patients: frequency outcomes, and risk factors, *Crit Care Med* 34(4):1007-1015, 2006.

45. Montgomery R: Pain management in burn injury, *Crit Care Nurs Clin North Am* 16(1):39-49, 2004.

46. Pasero C, McCafferery M: Pain in the critically ill, *Am J Nurs* 102(1 part 1):59-60, 2002.

47. Rivers EP, McIntyre L, Morro DC, et al: Early innovative interventions for severe sepsis and septic shock: taking advantage of the window of opportunity, *Can Med Assoc* 173(9):1054-1065, 2005.

48. Dellinger RP, Carlet JM, Masur H, et al: Surviving sepsis: campaign guidelines for the management of severe sepsis and septic shock, *Crit Care Med* 32:858-872, 2004.

49. Rivers E, Nyugen H, Havstad S, et al: Early goal-directed therapy in the treatment of severe sepsis and septic shock, *N Engl J Med* 345:1368-1377, 2001.

50. Flynn MB, McLeskey S: Shock, systemic inflammatory response syndrome, and multiple organ failure. In Morton PG, Fontaine DK, Hudak CM, et al, editors: *Critical care nursing: a holistic approach*, ed 8, Philadelphia, 2005, Lippincott Williams & Wilkins.

51. Agodoa L: Acute renal failure in the PACU, *J Perianesthesia Nurs* 17(6):377-383, 2002.

52. Lee CS: The role of exogenous arginine vasopressin in the management of catecholamine-refractory septic shock, *Crit Care Nurse* 26(6):17-29, 2006.

53. Price C: Acute renal failure: a sequelae of sepsis, *Crit Care Nurs Clin North Am* 6(2):359-373, 1994.

54. Kearney ML: Imbalance of oxygen supply and demand. In Secour VH, editor: *Multisystem organ dysfunction & failure*, ed 2, St Louis, 1994, Mosby.

55. Iacono M: Critical stress debriefing: application for perianesthesia nurses, *J PeriAnesthesia Nurs* 17(6):423-426, 2002.

56. Eichorn DJ, Meyer TA, Guzzetta CE: Family presence during invasive procedures and resuscitation: hearing the voice of the patient, *Am J Nurs* 101(5):48-53, 2001.

57. York NL: Implementing family presence protocol option, *Dimens Crit Care Nurs* 23(2):84-88, 2004.

58. Moreland P: Family presence during invasive procedures and resuscitation in the emergency department: a review of the literature, *J Emerg Nurs* 31(1):58-72, 2005.

59. Clark AP, Aldridge MD, Guzzetta CE, et al: Family presence during cardiopulmonary resuscitation, *Crit Care Nurs Clin North Am* 17(1):23-32, 2005.

60. Adridge MD, Clark AP: Making the right choice: family presence and the CNS, *Clin Nurse Specialist* 19(3):113-116, 2005.

61. Duran CR, Oman KS, Abel JJ, etal: Attitudes and beliefs about family presence: a survey of health care providers, families, and patients, *Am J Crit Care*. In Press, 2007.

62. Halm MA: Family presence during resuscitation: a critical review of the literature, *Am J Crit Care* 14(6):494-511, 2005.

63. Tucker T: Family presence during resuscitation, *Crit Care Nurs Clin North Am* 14:177-185, 2002.

64. Nibert AT: Teaching clinical ethics using case study family presence during cardiopulmonary resuscitation, *Crit Care Nurse* 25(1):38-44, 2005.

65. McGahey PR: Family presence during pediatric resuscitation: a focus on staff, *Crit Care Nurse* 22(6):29-34, 2002.

66. Emergency Nurses Association: *Position statement: family presence at the bedside during invasive procedures and cardiopulmonary resuscitation*, 2005, available at http://www.ena.ord, accessed January 8, 2006.

67. American Association of Critical Care Nurses: *Practice alert: family presence during CPR and invasive procedures*, 2005, available at http://www.aacn.org, accessed January 8, 2005.

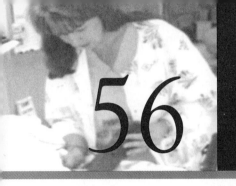

# 56

# BIOTERRORISM AND ITS IMPACT ON THE PACU

*Colleen Medley, BSN, RN, CPAN*

In the past 100 years, we have witnessed major developments in the protection of the health of humans. Many infectious disease threats have yielded to innovations in sanitation, water treatment plants, remarkable antibiotic discoveries, vaccines, and considerable understanding of the factors that affect our health. Smallpox has been eradicated from natural occurrence, and tuberculosis has been dramatically reduced. In this country, polio is quite rare. Deaths from childhood dysentery are few, and death in childbirth is uncommon. But some old problems remain, and new ones emerge. Until recent years, no one had heard of AIDS, Hantavirus, legionnaires' disease, or toxic shock syndrome. The latest threat is bioterrorism. The recent anthrax cases and the epidemic of fear that accompanied them created a substantial problem for many health professionals. Much time and effort have been spent in counseling and in reassuring our patients about this disease. The very infrastructure of the national public health system has been called into question.

## BIOLOGIC WARFARE

Biologic warfare has a long and ignoble history. In the 14th century, bodies of individuals who had died of plague were catapulted over the walls of cities in an effort to infect the defenders and thus attenuate the defenses. In the 18th century, blankets that had been used to wrap smallpox victims were subsequently distributed to Native Americans in an effort to reduce their numbers through the spread of disease.

In the 1940s, the United States established a biologic warfare program. In 1969, the offensive aspects of the program were disestablished as worldwide sentiment against biologic warfare increased. Behind the Iron Curtain, however, this was not so. In 1979, an incident involving the spread of anthrax from a production facility at Sverdlovsk revealed to the world the efforts by the Soviet Union to prepare offensive bioweapons. More recent defections from that political regime have led to further revelations about the extent of preparations for biologic warfare.

Numerous agents have been proposed over time. The intentional use of microorganisms, or toxins derived from living organisms, to produce death or disease in humans, animals, and plants have led to consideration of the agents in Box 56-1, which represent only a partial list.

Clearly, bioterrorist acts are, in many cases, quite unlike the usual "mass casualty" disasters that we have faced and with which we have considerable experience. In the case of an act like the destruction of the Murrah federal office building in Oklahoma in 1995 or an airplane crash like that in Lockerbie, Scotland, in 1988, all of the survivors are immediate and potential customers for the trauma service in hospital emergency rooms. But in the case of a bioterrorist release of an infectious disease agent or toxin, the effects may not be apparent for several days and may be widely distributed throughout the community. Victims of such an attack might turn up in widely dispersed emergency rooms and physician offices in ones, or twos, or threes and may not be immediately recognized as a mass casualty event. Each physician office must serve as an alert sentinel. In cases of bioterrorism, personnel from neither the fire department nor the police department are first responders. Practicing physicians and health professionals are the first responders.

In the event of a bioterrorist attack, such as the anthrax attacks on the East coast in October 2001, the impact on communities and hospitals largely depends on how effectively the local health department responds to the crisis. Expert local health officers at the head of strong health departments in Florida, New York, and Washington, DC, rapidly recognized the anthrax problem and used local, state, and federal resources to manage the problem effectively, thus limiting the adverse impact.

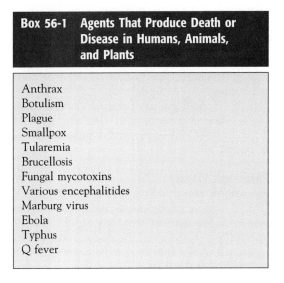

**Box 56-1** **Agents That Produce Death or Disease in Humans, Animals, and Plants**

Anthrax
Botulism
Plague
Smallpox
Tularemia
Brucellosis
Fungal mycotoxins
Various encephalitides
Marburg virus
Ebola
Typhus
Q fever

## Planning for Care

We must develop plans for early detection and streamlining responses to bioterrorism, avoiding duplication of effort and defining responsibilities and jurisdictional authority; develop a plan to administer mass vaccination and chemoprophylaxis, if they become necessary, with inclusion of both public and private resources; and develop, in conjunction with appropriate city, county, and state agencies and the Centers for Disease Control and Prevention, updated plans for quarantine, hospitalization, and evacuation procedures.

Planning for bioterrorism response should include the possibility that victims could number in the tens of thousands. Hospital capacity, generally numbering in the hundreds, would be quickly overrun; therefore, we must consider emergency use of stadiums, convention centers, school gymnasiums, hotels, nursing homes, and the like for care or quarantine.

*Reporting.* A major issue is reporting of cases, an important step in identification of a potential bioterrorist threat.

Disease reporting by physicians, emergency rooms, and laboratories is a key element in any bioterrorist threat detection system. Disease surveillance depends on accumulation of accurate timely reports of disease incidence; however, our system of disease reporting is widely held to be inefficient, incomplete, and irrelevant. When data are aggregated from several, or many, reporting sites, the true dimensions of a bioterrorist attack may be recognized. The timely collection of information, analysis, and pattern recognition can only be accomplished by a designated public health agency.

City and county governments must work through local health departments to ensure that efficient reporting mechanisms are in place and that a two-way flow of information exists to help provide incentives for collaboration by primary care providers. This reporting may include mechanisms for the health department to update area health professionals routinely with relevant information about immunization, local patterns of antibiotic resistance, seasonal changes in disease incidence monitored by the department, and information of immediate clinical relevance, such as rapid notification of a newly recognized outbreak of illness in the area. At best, these would be *active* reporting and surveillance systems, with providers communicating with local health authorities on a real-time basis.

Nonetheless, the effectiveness of any surveillance system depends on an available competent local health agency to collect and analyze data and (most importantly) to initiate appropriate and timely action to intervene.

*Response.* In the event of biowarfare introduction of a dramatic disease, the key is strong leadership by the health officer in a well-resourced local health department, strong personal reporting relationships with the local health professionals of the community, and cost-effective local surveillance systems.

Tremendous resources are being pumped into bioterrorist response systems. The Federal Bureau of Investigation (FBI), the Department of Defense, the Centers for Disease Control and Prevention, (CDC) the Federal Emergency Management Agency (FEMA), and states and municipalities are all receiving funds to develop their responses. Computerized communications systems, large quantities of antibiotic dosepacks, vaccines, decontamination systems, hazardous materials suits, and biosafety laboratories all can be made available on short notice. These vast resources are only called into play if an alert health professional detects an unusual situation and notifies the local health department. That local health department must have the epidemiologic and laboratory support to confirm or deny the possibility of a threat. Only then can this array of resources be called into play.

Strong local health departments and outfront local health officers generally are not in place over the country. This problem has been widely recognized. The need to upgrade our local health departments becomes obvious when bioterrorism is considered, but an upgrade would have salutary effects on all of the public health challenges that confront us, now and in the future.

## Anthrax

In the postanesthesia care unit (PACU), patients may appear with any of a wide variety of syndromes. Many, but not all of them, are related to the respiratory tract. For example, anthrax has three identifiable symptom clusters. *Bacillus anthracis*, a spore-forming bacterium, can lead to inhalational anthrax, which may appear much like a case of influenza, atypical pneumonia, or even pneumonic plague. In its classic form, it may appear in two phases. The first phase follows an incubation period of up to 6 days and is characterized by a nonspecific syndrome of fever, chills, weakness, muscle pain, headache, dyspnea, nonproductive cough (a diagnostic clue), and abdominal or chest pain. It then progresses to a second phase over 2 or 3 days, with progressive fever, diaphoresis, severe dyspnea, and possibly cyanosis. In 50% of cases, hemorrhagic meningitis occurs and leads to delirium, meningismus, obtundation, seizures, and coma. A further diagnostic clue is the finding of mediastinal widening, as revealed on chest radiographic or tomographic scan results. The patient may have stridor and subcutaneous edema of the upper thorax or neck. This syndrome may progress to obtundation and coma, with hypothermia, circulatory failure, and death within 2 to 3 days. Prompt treatment with antibiotics may result in survival.

For therapy of inhalational anthrax in an adult patient, the current recommendation is for ciprofloxacin 400 mg intravenously every 12 hours; if the bacterial strain is susceptible, therapy should continue with penicillin G, 8-12 million units intravenously every 4 to 6 hours, or doxycycline, 100 mg intravenously every 12 hours. High-dose intravenous penicillin conceivably gives improved penetration to the central nervous system in cases with meningitis.

Because of the deposition of spores into skin breaks or abrasions, the cutaneous form of anthrax is much less difficult to treat, although it may not be easily recognized. This form may be confused with various skin infections, insect bites, and nonspecific viral rashes. It is generally painless, although it may present with itching. With proper antibiotic therapy, death is uncommon.

Finally, the rarest form of anthrax, gastrointestinal anthrax, may occur when undercooked contaminated meat is consumed. The incubation period varies from 1 to 7 days. Gastrointestinal anthrax is characterized by acute inflammation of the gastrointestinal tract and may lead to ulcers in the upper tract (oropharynx) or in the terminal ileum or cecum. Presenting symptoms may include fever, sore throat, difficulty swallowing, nausea, vomiting, abdominal pain, bloody diarrhea, or total body sepsis. Mortality rates may be higher than 50%. The gastrointestinal disease can easily be confused with nonspecific gastroenteritis and other bacterial or viral syndromes.

Laboratory diagnosis of anthrax depends on a high index of suspicion so that the clinical microbiologist may be prepared for identification of *Bacillus anthracis*.

## Pneumonic Plague

Another disease that may be encountered in the PACU is pneumonic plague. One should suspect plague in the patient who has rapid onset of pneumonia, high fever, headache, and chills, combined with a history of exposure to possibly infected animals or fleas. The pneumonic form of the disease can spread by the dispersion of *Yersinia pestis* to the bloodstream from infected lymph nodes of the bubonic form of the disease or through inhalation of the bacilli (so-called primary plague pneumonia). Diagnosis is facilitated by the finding of bipolar or gram-negative coccobacilli on a smear from a lymph node, from aspirate from trachea or lung, or in the blood. The diagnosis may be confirmed with the more specific fluorescent-antibody test.

Pneumonic plague may be transmitted from person to person by droplets from the respiratory tract or spread on a face-to-face basis. Patients with pneumonic plague are highly infectious and should be placed on respiratory droplet isolation with eye protection. They should be kept in isolation until they have received 48 hours of antibiotic therapy and show improvement.

Rapid treatment cases of pneumonic plague is important. Recommended antibiotics include tetracycline, streptomycin, gentamicin, doxycycline, and chloramphenicol. Individuals who have had close contact with infected persons should be treated with appropriate antibiotics for 1 week.

## Botulism

The disease of botulism is caused not by the bacterium itself but by bacterial toxin produced by *Clostridium botulinum*, a spore-forming organism. The toxin is generally elaborated in anaerobic conditions and results in a syndrome characterized by the triad of descending flaccid paralysis with bulbar palsies, clear sensorium, and no fever. Initial symptoms may be the sudden onset of visual difficulties, which are the result of paralysis of cranial nerves. Paralysis may then progress downward and result in difficulty swallowing and dry mouth and manifestations of further paralysis of motor and autonomic nerves. The lack of fever and clear mentation are characteristic and frightening aspects of the disease. Most fatalities occur from respiratory failure, and those who survive may have respiratory symptoms for many years thereafter.

The diagnosis is confirmed with the demonstration of the botulinum toxin in the serum, gastric juices, or food. Because the standard test is a bioassay that requires several days to complete, clinical findings and a high index of suspicion are the best assets for diagnosis. Electromyogram may be useful in ruling out other paralytic conditions.

Most cases of botulism result from eating the preformed toxin in foods that have been canned or fermented at home or prepared unsafely. Uncommonly, toxins may be produced in wounds or in the gastrointestinal tract. Finally, the toxins theoretically may be distributed by a terrorist through aerosolization.

The management of cases of botulism consists largely of supportive care, augmented by immunization with botulism antitoxin (available from the Centers for Disease Control and Prevention). This antitoxin may reduce the severity of symptoms if administered sufficiently early in the course of the disease. Patients may need weeks or even months of respiratory care. Ventilatory support is the key to survival.

### Smallpox

Smallpox was eradicated worldwide in 1977, and the United States stopped routine vaccination in 1972. The reappearance of the disease would be highly indicative of a bioterrorist attack. Smallpox, caused by the variola virus, is highly infectious and spreads from person to person via respiratory nuclei, oral secretions, drainage from lesions, and direct contact with contaminated items like blankets. Five clinical syndromes of smallpox are seen. The classic clinical syndrome incubation period lasts approximately 7 to 20 days. The initial symptoms of high fevers, headache, backache, malaise, and vomiting closely resemble other acute viral illnesses, including influenza. During the first 2 to 3 days, the maculopapular rash is almost indistinguishable from chicken pox except for its centripetal evolution. The rash continues to evolve, and by day 8 or 9, the lesions start to crust and scabs begin to develop. The risk of transmission lasts until all the scabs have fallen off. Another clinical syndrome is the hemorrhagic form, which is characterized by diffuse hemorrhagic manifestations and a rapid progression to death. The flat type has a fatality rate of 95% and is characterized by a slow evolution of flat soft focal skin lesions and severe systemic toxicity. The nurse in the PACU is unlikely to encounter smallpox because this contagious systemic viral illness with its characteristic skin rash would likely be treated as an international emergency, with mandatory treatment at home in isolation conditions. Within the hospital setting, patients with smallpox would be under strict airborne isolation with a negative-pressure room with high-efficiency particle air filtration. No proven treatment exists for the disease. Supportive therapy includes hydration and electrolyte replacement for hypovolemia and shock. Patients with flat and hemorrhagic types may need mechanical ventilatory support as the incidence of pulmonary edema is higher. Contacts of cases should be vaccinated within 3 to 4 days because vaccination can decrease the severity of the disease. Cidofovir, an antiviral, has shown effectiveness in laboratory cultures when given in the first day or 2 and is a promising research development.

## SUMMARY

Other bacterial and viral agents may be encountered as a result of bioterrorist events, and the critical care unit should have a plan that is both responsive and flexible. In consideration of the large numbers of individuals who may need care, the establishment of temporary care units in various community locations may be necessary, with logistic support from a wide variety of sources. The use of mechanical ventilators may be augmented through manually assisted ventilation if large numbers of victims are identified. Perianesthesia nurses should develop plans that include other health professionals and perhaps even nonprofessionals who can be given immediate on-the-job training in operation of lifesaving techniques. Non–health care workers can supply logistic support, patient data recording, and appropriate security and crowd management.

The old adage applies in this case, as in so many others: "If we fail to plan, then we must plan to fail."

## BIBLIOGRAPHY

Arnon SS, Schechter R, Inglesby TV, et al: Botulinum toxin as a biological weapon: medical and public health management, *JAMA* 285(8):1059-1070, 2001.

Centers for Disease Control and Prevention: *Emergency preparedness*, available at http://www.bt.cdc.gov/, accessed March 11, 2007.

Chin J, editor: *Control of communicable diseases manual*, ed 17, Washington, DC, 2000, APHA.

Foster D: Smallpox as a biological weapon: implications for the critical care clinician, *Dimens Crit Care Nurs* 22(1):2-9, 2003.

Henderson DA, Inglesby TV, Bartlett JG, et al: Smallpox as a biological weapon: medical and public health management, *JAMA* 281(22):2127-2137, 1999.

Inglesby TV, Dennis DT, Henderson DA, et al: Plague as a biological weapon: medical and public health management, *JAMA* 283(17):2281-2290, 2000.

Inglesby TV, Henderson DA, Barlett JG, et al: Anthrax as a biological weapon: medical and public health management, *JAMA* 281(18):1735-1745, 1999.

Karwa M, Currie B, Kvetan V: Bioterrorism: preparing for the impossible or the improbable, *Crit Care Med* 33(Supp. 1):S75-95, 2005.

Schwartz MN: Recognition and management of anthrax: an update, *N Engl J Med* 345(22):1621-1626, 2001.

Shafazand S, Doyle R, Ruoss S, et al: Inhalational anthrax, *Chest* 116:1369-1376, 1999.

Steinhauer R: Bioterrorism, *RN* 65(3):48-55, 2002.

United States Department of Health and Human Services: available at www.hhs.gov, accessed March 11, 2007.

Varkey P, Poland GA, Cockerill FRIII, et al: Confronting bioterrorism: physicians on the front line, *Mayo Clinic Proc* 77(7):661-672, 2002.

# 57

## CARDIOPULMONARY RESUSCITATION IN THE PACU

*William Hartland, Jr., PhD, CRNA*

A nurse in the postanesthesia care unit (PACU) must be ever vigilant to the possibility of a patient who may need cardiopulmonary resuscitation (CPR). In January 2005, the International Consensus Conference on Cardiopulmonary Resuscitation and Emergency Cardiovascular Care Science with Treatment Recommendations was hosted by the American Heart Association (AHA) in Dallas. At this conference, Guidelines 2000 for Cardiopulmonary Resuscitation and Emergency Cardiovascular Care were updated and revised.[1]

This chapter looks at cardiopulmonary resuscitation based on the 2005 AHA guidelines for CPR and emergency cardiovascular care (ECC) as it applies to the PACU. Although this chapter highlights the responsibilities of the health care provider during a cardiopulmonary emergency, it is not designed to replace formal training in either basic life support (BLS) or advanced cardiopulmonary life support (ACLS).

## ETHICAL ISSUES RELATED TO CARDIOPULMONARY RESUSCITATION

Many patients are increasingly concerned about the inappropriate use of life-sustaining procedures that can have a dramatic effect on the length and quality of life. Consequently, increasing numbers of patients place limitations on medical treatments that may impact their lives in the future, which is accomplished with living wills, advanced directives, Do Not Attempt Resuscitation orders (DNAR), and the no-CPR Program. Living wills allow a person to express preferences concerning end-of-life medical care. Some states have adopted DNAR and no-CPR programs with focus on the use or extent of resuscitation efforts. Advanced directives are usually prepared by the physician attending critically/terminally ill patients who are unable to make decisions for themselves. These directives are based on the patient's living will, if one exists. The patient's right to limit medical interventions is firmly established in modern medical practice.[2,3] The operating room, however, is one

area in which restrictions on cardiopulmonary resuscitation have caused considerable ethical conflicts between patients and health care providers.

Approximately 75% of all cardiac arrests in the operating room are related to specific anesthesia or surgical causes, such as an accidental overdose of an anesthetic agent. Resuscitation has been found to be highly successful. In such instances, many health care providers view honoring DNARs as failure to treat a reversible process and thus similar to committing murder.[3,4] One could argue that the same ethical dilemma exists in the PACU because this unit is so closely aligned with surgery. All the ethical dilemmas concerning DNARs that may arise in the PACU and other topics related to advanced directives are beyond the scope of this chapter. The PACU nurse must be familiar with the institution's policies and guidelines concerning these issues.

## CARDIOPULMONARY RESUSCITATION

### Urgency of Cardiopulmonary Resuscitation

During cardiopulmonary arrest, time is a major factor that influences patient outcomes. The probability of survival decreases rapidly with each minute of cardiopulmonary compromise. The survival rate from cardiac arrest caused by ventricular tachycardia decreases approximately 7% to 10% for each minute the patient is deprived of defibrillation. At 12 minutes, this survival rate decreases to 2% to 5%. CPR plus defibrillation within 3 to 5 minutes of patient collapse can produce survival rates as high as 49% to 75%.[1] Therefore, the PACU nurse must respond quickly and efficiently during all cardiopulmonary emergencies.[5,6]

### Indications for Resuscitation

Numerous precipitating events are associated with cardiopulmonary arrest. These events include respiratory compromise, circulatory/cardiac compromise, metabolic imbalances, medication/anesthetic overdoses or toxicity, and anaphylaxis. All these events can occur in the PACU.

Respiratory compromise appears to be the primary cause of morbidity in the PACU. Respiratory compromise can result from residual anesthesia, upper airway obstruction, laryngeal edema, laryngospasm, bronchospasm, noncardiogenic pulmonary edema, and aspiration.

One of the most common causes of upper airway obstruction in the postanesthetic patient results from mechanical obstruction from the tongue. This situation occurs when the tongue falls back into a position that mechanically obstructs the pharynx and thus blocks the passage of air to and from the lungs. The underlying cause of this obstruction may be the result of residual anesthetics, narcotics, or muscle relaxants administered during surgery. The tongue may also be edematous from surgical manipulation, anatomic deformities, or allergic reaction. Clinical signs of this type of obstruction include snoring, flaring of the nostrils, use of accessory muscles for ventilation, retraction of the intercostal spaces and suprasternal notch, asynchronous movements of the chest and abdomen, tachycardia from hypoxia, and decreased oxygen saturation.[7] Arterial carbon dioxide pressure ($PaCO_2$) increases 6 mm Hg during the first minute of total obstruction, with an additional 3 to 4 mm Hg increase each passing minute.[8] If the obstruction is not corrected, the patient's condition continues to deteriorate and may lead to cardiopulmonary arrest. This occurrence is especially tragic when the obstruction could have been corrected by simply stimulating the patient to take deep breaths or by repositioning the airway via a chin lift or jaw thrust. More advanced measures may include the use of a nasal or oral airway; one should remember that the nasal airway is usually less stimulating and thus tolerated better in the patient emerging from general anesthesia. If the obstruction remains unrelieved, advanced airway management procedures with the esophageal-tracheal Combitube, laryngeal mask airway (LMA), or endotracheal tube (ETT) may be indicated. Obviously, prevention of cardiopulmonary arrest is more desirable than treatment. When a cardiopulmonary arrest does occur, emergency procedures must be administered rapidly and decisively before irreversible damage occurs.

### Emergency Equipment

The perianesthesia nurse, faced with a cardiopulmonary event, has an advantage over a layman or health care provider faced with a similar event outside the hospital. This advantage is rooted in the fact that the perianesthesia nurse has immediate access to numerous resources to aid in the diagnosis and treatment of an actual or pending adverse cardiopulmonary event. These resources include the immediate availability of various monitoring modalities, emergency medications, essential emergency equipment, and access to the patient's medical history, which can give valuable insight into possible underlying causes and pathology leading up to the adverse event. Another advantage is the availability of assistance and consultation from other health care providers.

The routine use of various monitoring modalities in the PACU is invaluable to nurses for the diagnosis of many developing patient complications that could precipitate a cardiopulmonary arrest. The use of pulse oximetry, for example, can be extremely helpful in the diagnosis of problems concerning patient oxygenation, as in the case of a progressing airway obstruction. The routine use of an ECC monitor allows the PACU nurse to identify life-threatening arrhythmias such as pulseless ventricular tachycardia (VT), ventricular fibrillation (VF), or asystole. Both of these monitoring methods provide the PACU nurse with a more definitive means of diagnosis and opportunity for early intervention.

All advanced cardiac life support equipment should be immediately available to the perianesthesia nurse. This equipment is usually found on a designated code cart or tray that is located in a designated area of the PACU. The cart should contain such emergency items as a defibrillator/monitor, emergency pharmacologic agents, equipment for circulatory and airway/respiratory management, and specialty trays for various emergency procedures. Usually the individual unit or health care institution establishes the general setup and contents of the cart. Each perianesthesia nurse must be familiar with not only the location of the cart but also with its contents and their proper use. The immediate availability of necessary emergency equipment and pharmacologic agents is essential for any possibility of patient survival.

### Steps in Cardiopulmonary Resuscitation

Usually some event occurs that leads the perianesthesia nurse to suspect a possible cardiopulmonary arrest. This event could be in the form of a witnessed or unwitnessed collapse of a patient. In the PACU, this event may involve the development of a life-threatening arrhythmia such as VT, VF, or asystole. At the first sign of potential trouble, the nurse should immediately assess the responsiveness of the patient.[9] No nurse wants to prematurely initiate a code and start CPR only to find out that the patient had fallen asleep and that one of the electrocardiographic (ECG) leads was loose or disconnected. If a lone PACU nurse finds an unresponsive adult patient, the nurse should immediately activate the unit's emergency response system, get a defibrillator (if available), and return to the victim to provide CPR and defibrillation if needed. When two or more rescuers are present, one should begin CPR while another activates the emergency response system and retrieves a defibrillator. Activation of the emergency response system brings help in the form of necessary emergency equipment and essential personnel to the patient's bedside. Assistance from other health care team members serves many purposes, including the ability to perform many essential tasks simultaneously, availability of various knowledge backgrounds and experience levels for consultation, and overall support. Nursing personnel should be thoroughly familiar with the unit's specific protocols for initiating a code and obtaining needed assistance.

Once unresponsiveness has been confirmed and the emergency system activated, the PACU nurse should immediately proceed with the AHA's Primary and Secondary ABCD Surveys. The primary survey is associated with the AHA's BLS, whereas the secondary survey involves ACLS procedures. Each of these surveys consists of four steps identified as the ABCDs of cardiopulmonary resuscitation. The ABCDs of the primary survey consist of Airway, Breathing, Circulation, and Defibrillation. The ABCDs of the secondary survey stand for Airway, Breathing, Circulation, and Differential Diagnosis.[2,10]

## Primary ABCD Survey

*A: Primary Airway.* The first step in the primary survey is Airway assessment. In this step, the patient's airway is manually opened and breathing is assessed. Most postoperative airway obstructions result from the mechanical obstruction of a patient's tongue and epiglottis obstructing the pharynx.[7] When a patient is unresponsive, possibly from residual anesthesia, decreased muscle tone may result in obstruction of the pharynx with the tongue and epiglottis. Because the tongue is attached to the lower jaw, the tongue can be lifted away from the back of the throat by moving the lower jaw forward, thus relieving the obstruction. To rule out the possibility of an airway obstruction, the nurse should mechanically open the patient's airway, which can be accomplished in a number of ways, depending on the patient's condition. Unless medically contraindicated, as in the case of a

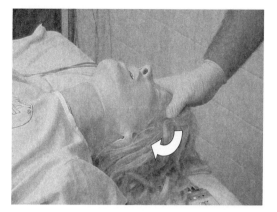

**Fig. 57-1** *Head tilt:* Patient's head is tilted backwards and neck is hyperextended. This maneuver is contraindicated in presence of possible cervical injury. *(Courtesy Department of Nurse Anesthesia, Virginia Commonwealth University, Richmond.)*

suspected neck injury, the PACU nurse can open the patient's airway by performing the head tilt–chin lift maneuver. The head tilt maneuver is accomplished by simply tilting the patient's head backward and hyperextending the neck (Fig. 57-1). As stated previously, this maneuver should not be performed if the patient is suspected of having a cervical injury. The chin lift involves placing two fingers under the bony portion of the lower jaw, near the chin, and pushing the patient's chin upward with moderate pressure (Fig. 57-2). The head tilt–chin lift maneuver is simply a combination of both these maneuvers (Fig. 57-3). If a cervical spine injury is suspected, the airway should be opened with the jaw thrust maneuver. To perform the jaw thrust, the rescuer is positioned at the head

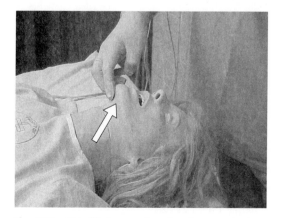

**Fig. 57-2** *Chin lift:* Rescuer places two fingers under bony portion of lower jaw, near chin, and pushes patient's chin upward with moderate pressure. *(Courtesy Department of Nurse Anesthesia, Virginia Commonwealth University, Richmond.)*

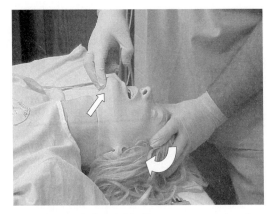

**Fig. 57-3**   Head tilt and chin lift maneuvers are often done collectively. *(Courtesy Department of Nurse Anesthesia, Virginia Commonwealth University, Richmond.)*

of the patient. The rescuer places one hand on each side of the patient's head and grasps the angles of the patient's lower jaw and lifts with both hands (Fig. 57-4). If the jaw thrust does not open the airway in a patient with a suspected cervical spine injury, the head tilt–chin lift maneuver may be used because adequate ventilation is a priority in CPR.[1] As with any procedure outlined in this chapter, the perianesthesia nurse should be familiar with the individual institution's policies.

Many times, in the case of an obstruction, these maneuvers are all that is necessary for spontaneous respirations to occur. As soon as the airway is opened, breathing should be assessed. This assessment can be accomplished by simply observing chest rise, listening for

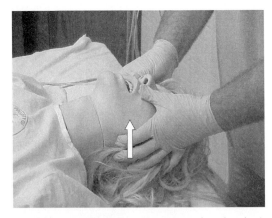

**Fig. 57-4**  *Jaw thrust:* Rescuer grasps angles of patient's lower jaw and lifts with both hands. Jaw thrust can be done with head tilt *(as pictured)* or alone without head tilt. Jaw thrust without head tilt is technique of choice for patient with suspected neck injury because it causes least movement of cervical spine. *(Courtesy Department of Nurse Anesthesia, Virginia Commonwealth University, Richmond.)*

ventilatory sounds, or feeling for air movement at the patient's nose and mouth.[1]

**B: Primary Breathing.** If no ventilations are detected, the perianesthesia nurse should progress to the second step of the survey: Breathing. In this step, the patient should be immediately given two breaths, each over 1 second. These two initial breaths can be performed with the use of a bag-mask device, such as an Ambu-Bag, which should be connected to a minimum supplemental oxygen source of 10 to 12 L/min as soon as possible.

If continuous ventilation is indicated, the following guidelines should be followed. For the adult patient, rescue breathing without chest compressions should be administered at 10 to 12 breaths/min. Rescue breaths with chest compressions should be administered at 8 to 10 breaths/min. A sufficient tidal volume should be delivered to produce visible chest rise. Rapid or forceful breaths should be avoided because they may cause increased thoracic pressure, decreased venous return, diminished cardiac output, and gastric inflation. Infants and children 1 to 8 years of age, with perfusing rhythms (pulses present) but not breathing, should be ventilated approximately 12 to 20 times/min (one breath every 3 to 5 seconds) at a large enough volume to raise the chest on inspiration.[1,2]

If for some reason a bag-valve-mask system is not available, the PACU nurse should have access to a mouth-to-patient barrier device so ventilation can be started until appropriate airway support devices can be secured. With use of these barrier devices, the rescuer must be sure to maintain a patent airway and an airtight seal to adequately ventilate the patient. When ventilating an infant, the rescuer must remember that an infant's neck is very pliable. If the infant's head is forcefully flexed, the rescuer may actually create an airway obstruction.

During the initial ventilation of the patient, a second rescuer should assess the adequacy of the ventilation by auscultation of the chest. If a second rescuer is not present, the primary rescuer should check to see whether the chest rises and falls and whether air escapes during expiration. If properly trained personnel are available and the patient cannot be ventilated with these methods, advanced airway techniques such as LMA, Combitube, or endotracheal intubation should be performed immediately.

**C: Primary Circulation.** After the initial two slow breaths have been given, the rescuer should move to the third step of the survey: Circulation. During this step, the patient's

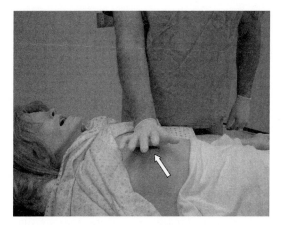

**Fig. 57-5** To begin external cardiac compressions, rescuer should place heel of one hand over lower half of patient's sternum, between nipples in center of chest. *(Courtesy Department of Nurse Anesthesia, Virginia Commonwealth University, Richmond.)*

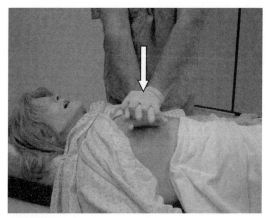

**Fig. 57-6** Rescuer's free hand should be placed on top of hand already positioned on patient's chest so hands are over-lapped and parallel. Rescuer should keep arms straight and shoulders directly over adult patient's sternum while pressing down on sternum a minimum of 1.5 to 2 inches. *(Courtesy Department of Nurse Anesthesia, Virginia Commonwealth University, Richmond.)*

circulatory status should be evaluated, which is accomplished with assessment of the patient's pulse. For an adult and child, this assessment is accomplished by feeling the carotid artery for no more than 10 seconds. With an infant, the brachial artery should be checked first. If no pulse is detected, chest compressions should be started immediately.[9]

External cardiac compression should be performed with the patient in a horizontal position on a firm surface and the lower extremities elevated to promote venous return. The rescuer should be positioned at the patient's side. To begin compressions, the rescuer should place the heel of one hand on the center (middle) of the chest between the patient's nipples (Fig. 57-5). The rescuer's free hand should be placed on top of the hand already positioned on the patient's chest. The rescuer should keep the arms straight with shoulders directly over the adult patient's sternum. The sternum should be depressed approximately 1.5 to 2 inches (Fig. 57-6). Rescuers should "push hard, push fast" at a rate of 100 compressions/min. Evidence appears to support the premise that this rapid compression rate effectively benefits the patient in terms of blood flow and blood pressure. The chest should be allowed to completely recoil after each compression. Interruptions to chest compression should be minimized to as few as possible.[1]

In children, the sternum is compressed with the heel of one hand only. In infants, the sternum is compressed with the tips of two fingers for one rescuer or the thumbs of the encircling hands of the rescuer when two rescuers are present (Figs. 57-7 and 57-8). In infants and

children, a rate of 100 compressions/min is also recommended.[9]

If external cardiac compression is done correctly, systolic blood pressure reaches 60 to 80 mm Hg and diastolic pressure is zero. Mean blood pressure in the carotid artery seldom exceeds 40 mm Hg. Cardiac output from chest compression is approximately one fourth to one third normal. As a result, compressions must be regular, smooth, and uninterrupted.[1]

External cardiac compression must be combined with ventilation of the lungs. Evidence suggests that adult cardiopulmonary

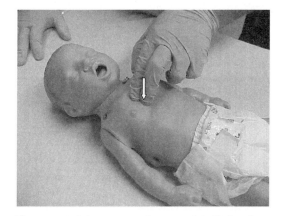

**Fig. 57-7** In infants, sternum is compressed with tips of two fingers when only one rescuer is present, which frees rescuer's other hand to open the airway for ventilations. *(Courtesy Department of Nurse Anesthesia, Virginia Commonwealth University, Richmond.)*

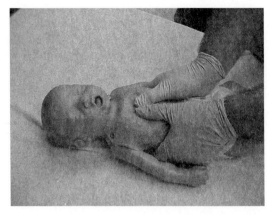

**Fig. 57-8**  If two rescuers are present, one rescuer can perform compressions with thumbs of encircling hands while other rescuer performs ventilations. *(Courtesy Department of Nurse Anesthesia, Virginia Commonwealth University, Richmond.)*

arrest patients are more likely to survive if a higher number of chest compressions are delivered even if the patient receives fewer ventilations. Because coronary perfusion pressure gradually rises with consecutive compressions, a ratio of 30 compressions to 2 ventilations is recommended for adults whether one or two rescuers are present. When the patient is a child or infant, one rescuer should use a 30:2 compression/ventilation ratio and two rescuers should use a 15:2 compression/ventilation ratio.

Once the patient's airway is secured and protected, as is the case with oral tracheal intubation, a continuous and uninterrupted compression rate of 100 compressions/min should be maintained. Ventilations, 6 to 8 breaths/min, should be simultaneously delivered without interruption of the compression rate. For assessment of the effectiveness of chest compressions, the nurse ventilating the

patient should periodically check the patient's pulse during compressions. The patient should be rapidly assessed for spontaneous breathing and circulation approximately every 5 cycles (2 minutes) of CPR. During this assessment, chest compressions should be interrupted for no longer than 10 seconds.[1]

If adequate spontaneous circulation returns without spontaneous breathing, compressions should be terminated, but ventilations should continue. The adult patient should be ventilated at a rate of 1 breath every 5 to 6 seconds. A child or infant should be ventilated at a rate of 1 breath every 3 to 5 seconds. If the patient is attempting to breathe but spontaneous ventilations are inadequate, the nurse can assist the patient with the bag-mask device.[9] This assistance is accomplished with ventilation when the patient attempts to inhale. Depending on the adequacy of the patient's own ventilations, the rescuer can assist with every ventilation, every other ventilation, or as needed. Once the patient's spontaneous ventilations are adequate, positive-pressure ventilation can be discontinued, but supplemental oxygen should be continued via a mask or nasal cannula. A summary that compares resuscitation interventions across age groups is presented in Table 57-1.

***D: Primary Defibrillation.*** Once ventilation and compressions have been initiated, the rescuer's attention should move toward Defibrillation, the most important determinant for survival in adult VF/VT. If the patient is not already being monitored, the patient should be connected to an ECG monitor or defibrillator with monitoring capabilities. Rhythm assessment is imperative for the detection of VF or VT. The PACU nurse must remember that for each minute of persistent VF, the patient's chance of survival decreases. Survival rates are highest when immediate CPR is provided and

| Table 57-1 | A Health Care Provider's Comparison of Ventilation and Chest Compressions for Infant, Child, and Adult Patients | | |
|---|---|---|---|
| | **Infant** | **Child** | **Adult** |
| Ventilations without compressions (approximate) | 12-20/min | 20/min | 10-12/min |
| Compressions (approximate) | 100/min | 100/min | 100/min |
| Compression depth (approximate) | 1/3 to 1/2 depth of chest | 1/3 to 1/2 depth of chest | 1.5 to 2 inches |
| Compression/ventilation ratio | 30:2 (1 rescuer) 15:2 (2 rescuers) | 30:2 (1 rescuer) 15:2 (2 rescuers) | 30:2 (1 or 2 rescuers) |

defibrillation is performed within 3 to 5 minutes. Once VF/VT have been identified, the defibrillation sequence should start immediately.[1]

Although automated external defibrillators (AEDs) are gaining popularity in hospital settings, conventional defibrillators are still used in many PACUs and other hospital specialty areas. Perianesthesia nurses must have a working knowledge of all defibrillators available in their respective units whether they are the older monophasic or newer biphasic models.

When the nurse uses the conventional (manual) defibrillator, basic protocol should be followed. On arrival to the patient's bedside, the defibrillator should be immediately turned on. CPR should be continued while the defibrillator is charging. In determination of energy settings for the unit's defibrillator, the nurse should follow the manufacturer's recommendations and the institution's protocol. A manual biphasic device should be charged according to the manufacturer's or institution's protocol (typically 120 to 200 J). If this protocol is unknown, the biphasic device should be charged to 200 J. A monophasic device should be charged to 360 J. AEDs are device specific in the charge they deliver.

With conventional defibrillators, the lead selection switch should be switched to "paddles." If monitor leads are used, lead I, II, or III should be selected. Paddles should have gel or paste made specifically for defibrillation applied to them before they are positioned on the patient's chest. This gel or paste maximizes current flow by reducing transthoracic impedence between the paddles and the patient's chest. If the defibrillator uses adhesive conductor pads instead of paddles, they should be positioned on the patient's chest at this time. One paddle or pad should be positioned just to the right of the patient's upper sternal border, below the clavicle. The second paddle or pad should be placed on the left side of the patient's chest slightly to the left of the nipple with the center of the electrode in the midaxillary line (Fig. 57-9). Often the defibrillator's manufacturer marks the paddles or pads to designate position on the patient. Once positioned, the monitor display should be visually checked for rhythm assessment. If VF or VT is present, the operator should announce to all team members that the defibrillator is being charged and everyone should stand clear. The charge button on the defibrillator or apex paddle should be pressed. As soon as the defibrillator is charged, the operator should firmly announce to all present that the patient is about to be shocked. To protect fellow rescuers,

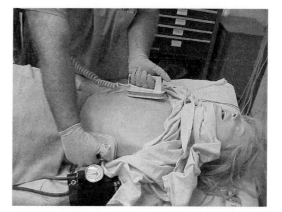

**Fig. 57-9** During defibrillation, operator should apply approximately 25 lbs of pressure on paddles while simultaneously pressing both paddle discharge buttons with rescuer's thumbs. *(Courtesy Department of Nurse Anesthesia, Virginia Commonwealth University, Richmond.)*

no one should be in direct or indirect contact with the patient during defibrillation, which means that no one is touching the patient or any item or apparatus in contact with the patient, including the stretcher or bed. If an individual is in direct or indirect contact with the patient during defibrillation, the electric shock may pass through the individual and the patient. To alleviate this danger, the AHA suggests the following chant be used. First, the defibrillator operator states loudly and clearly, "I am going to shock on three. One, I'm clear." At this time, the operator checks to be sure he or she is clear of any contact with the patient. Next, the operator states, "Two, you're clear," and makes a visual check to ensure that no one else is touching the patient or any item that is in contact with the patient. Finally, the operator states, "Three, everybody's clear." At this point, the operator checks everyone, including himself or herself, one last time before administering the shock to the patient. If pads are used instead of paddles, pressing the defibrillator discharge button discharges the defibrillator. With paddles, the operator should apply approximately 25 lbs of pressure on the paddles while simultaneously pressing both paddle discharge buttons.[10]

After the charge has been delivered to the patient, CPR should be immediately resumed and continued for 5 cycles, after which the patient's rhythm should be again evaluated.[1] As long as VF/VT persist, attempts to defibrillate must continue. The PACU nurse must remember that as long as the patient's myocardium has the energy to produce VF/VT, it should have the energy to produce a perfusing rhythm.[2]

As soon as the primary survey has been completed, the secondary survey must be addressed. The secondary survey builds on the primary survey, with more advanced assessments and treatments. In the presence of more than one rescuer, which is usually the case in the PACU, the secondary survey can often be started before the primary survey is complete.

## Secondary ABCD Survey

**A: Secondary Airway.** Determination should be made concerning the need for an advanced airway. Because the insertion of an advanced airway may necessitate the interruption of chest compressions for many seconds, the rescuer must weigh the need for compressions against the need for an advanced airway device. Deference of insertion of an advanced airway until the patient fails to respond to initial CPR and defibrillation or shows return of spontaneous circulation is acceptable. Recommended advanced airway devices include: LMAs, esophageal-tracheal Combitubes, and endotracheal tubes. All three of these advanced airways should only be used by a rescuer who is properly trained and experienced with the techniques. In many institutions, endotracheal intubations performed in the PACU are usually the responsibility of an anesthesiologist or certified registered nurse anesthetist (CRNA).

**B: Secondary Breathing.** Once the patient's airway is secured, proper placement of the advanced airway device should be confirmed. This confirmation is especially critical when endotracheal intubation is performed because of the high risk of tube misplacement, displacement, and obstruction. Confirmation of proper endotracheal tube placement should be assessed with auscultation of the lungs to determine whether breath sounds are present and bilaterally equal in both lungs. Auscultation over the epigastric region is an additional means of assessment of accidental esophageal intubation. In addition to auscultation, a confirmation device such as an exhaled $CO_2$ detector or an esophageal detector device should also be used. If a capnogram is available, the presence of end-tidal carbon dioxide should be confirmed along with oxygen saturation with an oxygen saturation monitor. Once proper tube placement has been confirmed, the tube should be secured in place to prevent dislodgement, which can be accomplished with tape or specially designed endotracheal tube holders.[1]

**C: Secondary Circulation.** If not already present, intravenous or intraosseous access should be secured and the patient should be connected to an ECG monitor. Cardiac rhythm analysis should be performed with appropriate pharmacologic interventions. Vital signs such as blood pressure, pulse rate, and temperature should also be monitored and assessed.[1]

In the case of VT/VF, we have seen from the primary survey that one shock is delivered. Immediately after this shock, CPR is continued for 5 cycles (approximately 2 minutes), at which time the patient's rhythm is evaluated. If the VT/VF persist, the patient should be shocked once again with CPR immediately following. When intravenous or intraosseous access is available, a vasopressor (epinephrine 1 mg, repeated every 3 to 5 minutes or 1 dose of vasopressin 40 units to replace the first or second dose of epinephrine) should be given during CPR before or after the shock.[1] Additional pharmacologic interventions that might be considered include the administration of such drugs as amiodarone, lidocaine, and magnesium.[1]

**D: Differential Diagnosis.** The differential diagnosis consists of determining the underlying cause of the arrest. The primary purpose of the differential diagnosis is identification of reversible causes that have a specific therapy. For the perianesthesia nurse, this diagnosis may involve looking at the patient's preoperative history and physical condition, preoperative and postoperative laboratory values, postoperative diagnosis, surgical procedure performed, and condition on arrival into the PACU. It should also involve the patient's intraoperative course, including unexpected surgical events such as excessive blood loss, fluid replacement, pharmacologic management, and any other intraoperative surgical/anesthetic events. Any of these factors may add some insight into the underlying question of why the patient had arrest. Potentially reversible causes of an arrest may include hypovolemia, hypoxia, acidosis, hypokalemia, hyperkalemia, hypoglycemia, hypothermia, drug overdoses, cardiac tamponade, tension pneumothorax, coronary/pulmonary thrombosis, and trauma. The perianesthesia nurse should remember that successful resuscitation outcomes usually depend on the discovery and treatment of these or other reversible underlying causes.[10]

## Asystole

Thus far, this discussion of the AHA's primary and secondary surveys has focused on pulseless ventricular tachycardia and ventricular fibrillation. The following examines another common arrhythmia: asystole. The perianesthesia nurse may commonly check a patient only to notice that the patient's rhythm on the ECG monitor is flat or straight-line. The nurse should remember that asystole is a specific diagnosis but that a flat line is not.[2] Many nonphysiologic reasons could explain why the monitor may be flat or straight-line. One of the most common causes is that one of the monitor leads becomes disconnected or unplugged. Monitor failure or an insufficient gain setting may also cause a straight-line wave. Although it lacks significant confirmation in human studies, a theory called "VF-has-a-vector" states that VF may present as a flat line in any lead recording at 90 degrees to the VF waves that are moving through the myocardium with a specific vector. This theory can be ruled out with selection of different leads on the ECG monitor.[10] A change in lead selection may also assist the nurse in identification of a disconnected lead.

A straight-line ECG rhythm may also indicate that the patient is in cardiopulmonary arrest. The PACU nurse should approach this situation in the same way as other potential cardiopulmonary emergencies with use of the AHA's primary and secondary ABCD surveys. The first step to be taken is to assess patient consciousness. If the patient is awake and talking, without any distress, true asystole is unlikely. With assessing consciousness, the nurse may find the patient was merely sleeping and inadvertently disconnected one of the monitor leads. If, however, the nurse confirms that the patient is unconscious and unresponsive, help should be called by activating the unit's emergency response system. The nurse should then immediately move into the primary ABCD survey. At the beginning of the primary survey, asystole has not been established as a definite diagnosis. The possibility exists that the patient is actually in VT or VF in addition to having a disconnected monitor lead. A disconnection should be discovered during the defibrillation stage of the survey. During this stage, the patient is connected to a monitor/defibrillator to assess the necessity of defibrillation. If during the primary survey the patient is confirmed to be in VT/VF instead of asystole, defibrillation should be performed immediately. If the patient is confirmed to be in true asystole, defibrillation is not recommended.[1]

At this time, no valid adult human research data support the use of defibrillation in the asystole patient. During asystole, shocks may be harmful from producing a "stunned heart" and profound parasympathetic discharge. As a result, the AHA considers the practice of empiric shocking of asystole to have no evidence of support and to be harmful to the patient.[10] The

perianesthesia nurse should consult the unit's or institution's policy concerning this practice.

Steps that should be followed with confirmed asystole include uninterrupted CPR with epinephrine 1 mg intravenous (IV)/intraosseous (IO) push every 3 to 5 minutes. Vasopressin 40 units IV/IO may be given as a replacement for the first and second dose of epinephrine. Atropine 1 mg IV/IO should be considered for asystole every 3 to 5 minutes, with a maximum of three doses. Drugs should be delivered immediately after rhythm assessments without interruption of CPR. After drug administration and approximately five cycles of CPR, the patient's rhythm should be reassessed. During this process, the rescuers must always remember to continuously search for and treat identified reversible causes of the arrest as outlined in the secondary survey's differential diagnosis.[1]

## PHARMACOLOGIC THERAPY

The following short summary is based on the AHA's recommendations concerning various drugs that are commonly used during cardiovascular resuscitation.[1,2] As the PACU nurse is aware, a thorough understanding of each drug, including its indications, contraindications, interactions, dosage, and adverse reactions, should be obtained before its use. The nurse also must have the same understanding for all additional drugs found in the unit's code cart.

### Epinephrine
The adrenergic effect of epinephrine increases myocardial and cerebral blood flow and may improve return of spontaneous circulation during CPR. The recommended dose of epinephrine hydrochloride is 1.0 mg (10 mL of a 10:000 solution) IV every 3 to 5 minutes during resuscitation. Epinephrine may also be administered via the endotracheal tube if IV/IO access has not been secured. Although the optimal dose for tracheal delivery is unknown, a dose 2 to 2.5 times the IV dose may be needed. Only a physician trained in this technique should perform intracardiac injection of this drug. With the increased risk of coronary artery laceration, cardiac tamponade, and pneumothorax, intracardiac injection of epinephrine should only be used during open cardiac massage or when other routes of administration are unavailable.[1]

### Vasopressin
Vasopressin is a naturally occurring antidiuretic hormone. In high doses, higher than those needed for antidiuretic effects, vasopressin acts

as a nonadrenergic peripheral smooth muscle vasoconstrictor. Vasopressin has been found useful as an alternative to epinephrine for the treatment of adult shock-refractory VF and encouragement of the return of spontaneous circulation in the event of asystole or pulseless electric activity. For patients in pulseless arrest, the recommended one time adult dose of vasopressin is 40 units IV/IO, which can be given to replace the first or second dose of epinephrine.[1]

### Lidocaine

Lidocaine is useful as an antiarrhythmic agent for the treatment of ventricular ectomy, VT, and VF. During a cardiac arrest, it is administered as a bolus of 1.0 to 1.5 mg/kg IV/IO, not to exceed 3 mg/kg. The administration of a prophylactic continuous infusion after circulation has been restored is controversial. If it is used, the infusion can be administered up to a maximum rate of 4 mg/min. Side effects include slurred speech, muscle twitching, altered consciousness, respiratory compromise, seizures, and tachycardia.[1]

### Magnesium

Magnesium is only used during a cardiac arrest when the arrhythmias are suspected to be caused from magnesium deficiency or in the presence of torsades de pointes. The usual dose in these states is 1 to 2 g diluted in D5W over 5 to 60 minutes. Rapid infusion of magnesium can cause clinically significant hypotension and possible asystole.[1]

### Procainamide

Procainamide hydrochloride is used to suppress both atrial and ventricular arrhythmias by slowing conduction in myocardial tissue. It should be considered as one of several drugs that may be used for stable monomorphic VT, atrial fibrillation/flutter, and atrioventricular reentrant narrow-complex tachycardias. The infusion dosage of procainamide is 20 mg/min for non-VT arrest. Administration of procainamide should be stopped when the dysrhythmia is suppressed, when the QRS complex is widened by 50%, when hypotension occurs, or when the maximum total dose of the procainamide reaches 17 mg/kg. Bolus administration of the drug can result in toxic concentrations and significant hypotension. Procainamide should be used with caution in patients with preexisting QT prolongation.[1]

### Atropine Sulfate

Atropine sulfate as an anticholinergic agent is useful in the treatment of symptomatic sinus bradycardia. It may also be useful with AV block at the nodal level and ventricular asystole. Atropine sulfate should not be used when Mobiz type II block is suspected. It should always be used with caution in a patient with an acute myocardial infarction because acceleration of heart rate may increase ischemia. The recommended dose of atropine sulfate in the presence of bradycardia is 0.5 to 1.0 mg IV/IO every 3 to 5 minutes up to a total dose of 0.04 mg/kg. For asystole and slow pulseless electric activity, a dose of 1.0 mg is administered IV/IO. This dose may be repeated in 3 to 5 minutes if asystole persists, up to a maximum dose of 0.03 to 0.04 mg/kg.[1]

### Sodium Bicarbonate

Hyperventilation corrects respiratory acidosis by removing carbon dioxide. Acidemia during cardiac arrest and resuscitation primarily results from low blood flow. For maintenance of acid base balance, adequate alveolar ventilation and tissue perfusion must be maintained during cardiac arrest. Clinical/laboratory data have not conclusively shown that acidosis interferes with defibrillation, restoration of spontaneous circulation, or short-term survival. Few data indicate that the use of buffers improves outcome. The data do, however, indicate that bicarbonate can compromise coronary perfusion pressure and induce hypernatremia. In addition, it can exacerbate central venous acidosis and cause adverse effects from extracellular alkalosis.[1]

Sodium bicarbonate can be beneficial in patients with hyperkalemia, tricyclic/phenobarbitone overdose, or preexisting metabolic acidosis. Bicarbonate may also have some benefit during long resuscitative efforts or when confirmed interventions such as defibrillation, cardiac compressions, and intubation have been ineffective. If used, bicarbonate should be administered with an initial dose of 1 mEq/kg. Administration of bicarbonate should be guided with blood gas analysis or laboratory measurement.[1]

## SUMMARY

Whenever a possible cardiopulmonary emergency exists, the perianesthesia nurse should immediately institute the AHA's primary and secondary ABCDs of cardiopulmonary resuscitation. First, consciousness must be assessed. If the patient is unconscious, help must be called and the primary survey of **A**irway, **B**reathing, **C**irculation, and **D**efibrillation efficiently followed. Immediately after the primary survey, the secondary survey of advanced **A**irway, **B**reathing, **C**irculation, and **D**ifferential Diagnosis should be performed.

A cardiopulmonary emergency is not an event that any health care provider looks forward to facing. It is, however, an event that is more common in highly specialized acute nursing units such as the PACU. As such, every nurse working in the PACU must always be prepared for such life-threatening emergencies.

## REFERENCES

1. AHA: 2005 American Heart Association guidelines for cardiopulmonary resuscitation and emergency cardiovascular care, part 4: adult basic life support, *Circulation* 112(Suppl IV):19-IV-24, 2005.
2. Cummins RO, editor: *ACLS provider manual*, Dallas, 2001, American Heart Association.
3. Barash P, Cullen B, Stoelting R: *Clinical anesthesia*, ed 3, Philadelphia, 1997, JB Lippincott.
4. Walker R: DNR in the OR: resuscitation as an operating room risk, *JAMA* 266:2407, 1991.
5. Cummins R, Ornato J, Thies W, et al: Improving survival from sudden cardiac arrest: the 'chain of survival' concept, *Circulation* 83:1833-1847, 1991.
6. Cummins R: From concept to standard-of-care? Review of the clinical experience with automated external defibrillators, *Ann Emerg Med* 4:721-727, 1993.
7. Odom J: Airway emergencies in the post anesthesia care unit, *Post Anesth Care Nurs* 28:483-491, 1993.
8. Nagelhout J, , Zaglaniczny K, , editors: *Nurse anesthesia*, ed 2, Philadelphia, 2000, Saunders.
9. Aufderheide TP, Stapleton ED, editors: *Instructor's manual: basic life support*, Dallas, 2000, American Heart Association,
10. The American Heart Association in collaboration with the International Liaison Committee on Resuscitation: Guidelines 2000 for cardiopulmonary resuscitation and emergency cardiovascular care, international consensus on science, *Circulation* 102(Suppl I):8, 2000.

## BIBLIOGRAPHY

Graham-Garcia J, Heath J, Andrews J: Defibrillation and biphasic shocks: implications for perianesthesia nursing, *J PeriAnesthesia Nurs* 20(1):23-33, 2005.

# INDEX

*Note: Entries followed by "b" denote boxes; "f" figures; "t" tables.*

## Numbers

1-Deamino-8-D-arginine vasopressin. See DDVAP (desmopressin).
3', 5'-adenosine monophosphate, 162–163, 229–230
5-HT₃ receptor antagonists, 268t, 270t, 308

## A

A/C (assisted/control) ventilation, 397t
AACCN (American Association of Critical Care Nurses), 13b, 16t
AACN (American Association of Colleges of Nursing), 13b, 784–786, 785b–786b
AANA (American Association of Nurse Anesthetists), 13b, 105–106
AAROD (anesthesia-assisted rapid opiate detoxification), 316–317
AARP (American Association of Retired Persons) demographics, 717
ABA (American Burn Association), 792–795
Abbreviated Injury Scale. See AIS (Abbreviated Injury Scale).
ABCD surveys, 767, 813–818
  primary, 813–818, 813f–816f, 816t
  secondary, 818–819
  shock trauma and, 767
Abdominal cavity related organ surgery, 599–601. See also GI (gastrointestinal), abdominal, and anorectal surgical patients.
  biliary tract, 600–601, 601f
  liver, 599–600, 599f
  spleen, 600
Abdominal compartment syndrome. See ACS (abdominal compartment syndrome).
Abdominal distention, 606
Abdominal gynecologic surgery, 624–625
Abdominal myomectomy, 617–618
Abdominal surgery, 592–595, 592f, 617–618. See also GI (gastrointestinal), abdominal, and anorectal surgical patients.
Abdominoperineal resection, 598
Abdominoplasty, 636
Abducens cranial nerve (VI), 129t
Abduction pillows, 551
ABI (ankle-brachial index), 539, 543, 543b
Abnormal pulmonary function, 201
ABO/Rh typing, 225
Above all, do no harm (Primum non nocere), 103–104
ABPANC (American Board of Perianesthesia Nursing Certification), 13b
Abscess infections, 60t
Absorption, 271, 276, 665–667
Abstinence syndrome, 742

ACC (American College of Cardiology), 718–719
Access-related factors, 3, 76
Accolate (zafirlukast), 271t
ACE (angiotensin-converting enzyme) inhibitors, 264t–265t, 270t
Acetaminophen, 443–445
Acetazolamide (Diamox), 213, 483t
Acetonuria, 206
Acetylcholine. See ACh (acetylcholine).
Acetylcholine receptors. See ACh (acetylcholine) receptors.
Acetylcholinesterases, 319–320, 319f
Acetylcysteine (Mucomyst), 271t
ACh (acetylcholine), 222–223, 471t, 483t
ACh (acetylcholine) receptors, 680, 684–685
Achalasia, 236–237
Achlorhydria, 236
Acid-base
  balance, 210–211
  buffers, 269
  relationships, 191–193, 192b–193b
Acidemia, 170
Acidosis, 193–194, 193b, 211, 410, 681
Acidosis, respiratory, 681
Acinetobacter baumannii, 58
ACLS (advanced cardiac life support), 16–17, 19, 19b, 408, 476
Acoustic cranial nerve (VIII), 129t
Acquired immunity, 250–254
  active, 250–251
  passive, 250–251
Acquired immunodeficiency syndrome. See AIDS (acquired immunodeficiency syndrome)
Acromegaly, 230
ACS (abdominal compartment syndrome), 769–770, 769t
ACS (American College of Surgeons), 105–106, 764–765, 772–773
ACS (anticholinergic syndrome), 412–413
ACTH (adrenocorticotropin), 230–233
Action mechanisms
  of epidural anesthetics, 349
  of nonopioid IV anesthetics, 293–294
    GABA interactions, 293–294
    muscarinic receptor interactions, 293–294
    postsynaptic neuron interactions, 293
  of opioids, 307
  of spinal anesthetics, 347, 347f
Action potentials, 318, 338–339
Actiq, 449
Activated coagulation times. See ACTs (activated coagulation times).
Activated partial thromboplastin times. See APTTs (activated partial thromboplastin times).
Active immunity
  acquired, 250–251
  passive, 250–251
Active learning, 390, 392–393
Active warming measures, 748
ACTs (activated coagulation times), 533

Actual costs, 76
Acute conditions and disorders
  distress, 387
  hepatic failure, 242
  lung injury. See ALI (acute lung injury).
  MH, 756–757, 757b. See also MH (malignant hyperthermia).
  MI, 403, 409, 409f. See also MI (myocardial infarction).
  pancreatitis, 243–244
  renal failure. See ARF (acute renal failure).
  respiratory distress syndrome. See ARDS (acute respiratory distress syndrome).
  tubular necrosis, 214
AD (Alzheimer's disease), 722–723
Adalat (nifedipine), 162–163, 268t
Addisonian crisis, 234
Addison's disease, 234
Additive effects, 260
Adenocarcinoma, 626
Adenohypophysis hormones, 230–231
Adenoidectomy. See T&A (tonsillectomy and adenoidectomy).
Adenosine
  Adenocard, 264t
  monophosphate. See AMP (adenosine monophosphate), cyclic.
  triphosphate. See ATP (adenosine triphosphate).
Adenotonsillar hypertrophy, 714
Adenovirus infection, 60t
ADH (antidiuretic hormone), 209, 209f, 219, 231, 270t
ADH (antidiuretic hormone)/vasopressin, 231
Adjustable-positive relief valves. See APR (adjustable-positive relief) valves.
Administration for Children and Families, 73, 73f
Administration on Aging, 73, 73f
Administration routes and techniques. See also Pharmacology principles.
  aerosolized, 263
  for epidural anesthetics, 349
  for inhalation anesthesia, 286–287, 286f–287f
    anesthesia machines, 286–287, 286f–287f
    APR valves, 281
    Bain anesthesia circuits, 286–287, 287f
    circle systems, 286–287
    scavenger systems, 281
    solubility coefficients and, 281
    vaporizers, 281
  intramuscular, 262
  IV, 262–263, 313–316, 315t–316t
  for opioid IV (intravenous) anesthetics, 262–263, 313–316, 315t–316t
    epidural routes, 313–314
    intrathecal routes, 313–314
    MEAC and, 314–315
    PCA, 314–315, 315t

823

Brethine (terbutaline), 270t–271t
Bretylium (Bretylol), 264t, 272t
Brevibloc (esmolol), 166t, 168, 265t
Brevital Sodium (methohexital), 267t, 294–295
Brice questionnaire, 411, 411b
Bright's disease, 206
British Anaesthetic and Recovery Nurses Association. *See* BARNA (British Anaesthetic and Recovery Nurses Association).
Broca's area, 124–125, 124f
Bronchi and lungs, 175–176, 175t, 176f
Bronchiectasis, 170
Bronchiolitis, 60t
Bronchodilators, 264t, 267t, 279t, 681
Bronchoscopes, 488–490
Bronchoscopes, fiberoptic, 489f, 703
Bronchospasms, 170, 405, 489–490, 680–681, 812–813
Bronkosol (isoetharine), 270t
Brucellosis, 807b
BSA (body surface area), 148
BSIs (bloodstream infections), 66–67
BTs (bleeding times), 156
Bubonic plague, 62t
Budesonide (Rhinocort), 271t
Buffers, neutralizing, 270t
Bumetanide (Bumex), 212, 264t
Bumex (bumetanide), 212, 264t
Bundle of His-Purkinje, 154
Bupivacaine (Marcaine, Sensorcaine), 264t, 340t, 342, 445–446, 451t, 756b
Buprenorphine (Buprenex), 445, 446t
*Burkholderia cepacia*, 63t
Burn trauma patients, 248–249, 792–795, 792b, 794f
Burnout and stress issues, 26–29, 27b–28b
Burns, 644–651. *See also* Thermally-injured patients.
    classification of, 645–647
        full-thickness, 645
        partial-thickness, 645
        partial thickness, deep dermal, 645
        partial-thickness, superficial, 645
        superficial, 645
    definitions for, 644
    extent estimation methods, 645–647, 646f
        Lund and Browder chart, 645–646, 646f
        percentages, 645–646, 646f
        rule of nines, 646, 646f
    fundamentals of, 644, 650
    injury types, 645–647
        chemical injuries, 645–647
        cold injuries and, 645–646
        electric injuries, 645–646
    integumentary system and, 644–645
    PACU-specific contexts for, 650
    pathophysiology of, 647–648
    research resources for, 650–651
    wound management for, 648–650
Bursa dependent cells, 250
Butisol, 739t
Butorphanol (Stadol), 264t, 311–312, 312t, 446t, 742
Butyl nitrite, inhaled, 744–745
Butyrophenones, 299–301, 300b
    droperidol (Inapsine), 299–301
    haloperidol (Haldol), 299, 300b
Bypass procedures
    axillofemoral, 541–542, 542f
    cardiac, 508–523
        CABG, 513–514, 514f, 517t
        effects of, 510t
        female patient guidelines, 515b

Bypass procedures–cont'd
        MICB, 508f
    femoral-femoral, 541–542, 542f
    gastric, 589–590, 590f, 597. *See* RGB (resectional gastric bypass) surgery.
    Roux-en-Y gastric, 589
    vascular, 538

**C**
C-Bloc systems, 444–453, 452b
C-section (Cesarean section), 617, 619–620
    classic, 617
    low segment, 617
CABG (coronary artery bypass grafting), 513–514, 514f, 517t
CAD (coronary artery disease), 408–409, 513–514
Caffeine, 162, 701
Calan (verapamil), 162–163, 168, 270t, 272t
Calcineurin inhibitors, 609b
Calcitonin, 232
Calcium
    channel blockers, 162–163, 265t, 268t, 270t
    chloride, 757b
    definitions of, 222
    imbalances, 387t
Calices, 206–208, 207f
Call for help component, 46b, 48–49. *See also* ERR WATCH principles.
Calwell-Luc operation, 459
Candidiasis, 63t
Cannabinoids, 741t, 744
Cannulation sites, 506–509, 506f–507f
CAPA (Certified Ambulatory Perianesthesia) nurses, 13b–14b, 14–17, 16t
Capacities, lungs, 176–178, 177f–178f, 177t
Capnography, 360, 366–369, 367f–369f, 818
Capoten (captopril), 264t
Captopril (Capoten), 264t
Carbocaine (mepivacaine), 267t, 340t, 342, 451t
Carbon dioxide
    ETCO$_2$, 360, 366–369, 713–714
    lasers, 668t–669t
    responses, 197–198, 197f
Carbonic anhydrase inhibitors, 213
Carboxyhemoglobin, 682
Carcinomas, breast, 626–628
    adenocarcinoma, 626
    DCIS, 626, 628
    IDC, 626–627
    ILC, 627
    LCIS, 627
    medullary, 627–628
    tubular, 628
Cardiac arrest, 148
Cardiac catheterization, 503–504
Cardiac cycle, 149–150, 150f
Cardiac index. *See* CI (cardiac index).
Cardiac massage, open, 819
Cardiac output. *See* CO (cardiac output).
Cardiac surgical intensive care units. *See* CSICUs (cardiac surgical intensive care units).
Cardiac surgical patients, 496–537
    AS and, 500, 502f, 503–504
    AI and, 499–500, 500f
    annuloplasty and, 498–499, 498f–499f
    aortic aneurysm and, 499
    aortic dissection and, 499
    ASDs and, 500–504, 501f, 503f
    balloon procedures, 503, 520–521

Cardiac surgical patients–cont'd
    IABPs, 520–521
    valvotomy, 503
    valvuloplasty, 503
    bicuspid aortic valves and, 503–504
    bypass procedures, 508–523
        CABG, 513–514, 514f, 517t, 523
        effects of, 510t
        female patient guidelines, 515b
        MICB, 508f
    CAD and, 513–514, 531–532
    cannulation sites and, 506–509, 506f–507f
    cardiac catheterization and, 503–504
    cardioplegia and, 504
    coarctation and, 505
    commissurotomy, 505, 518
    complications, 531–535
        AF, 506–507, 532
        cardiac tamponade, 532
        cardiovascular system, 531–533
        CHF, 531–532
        dysrhythmias, 532
        hemorrhage, 533
        inadequate volume status, 533–534
        infection, 533
        MI, 531–533
        myocardial contractility, 531–532
        noncardiac, 533–535
        peripheral vasoconstriction, 532
        sternal wound dehiscence, 533
    congenital heart disease and, 505–507
    coronary angiography and, 503–504
    CSICUs and, 496–497
    De Vega technique and, 498–499
    definitions of, 498–523, 503–504
    dysrhythmia surgery and, 506–507
    extra corporeal circuit and, 506f
    fundamentals for, 496–498, 497t, 535
    grafts and, 498–505
        allografts, 498, 498f
        aortocoronary bypass, 500–501, 501f
        Dacron, 499
        endovascular stent, 499
        homografts, 498, 498f
        prosthetic, 499, 505
    heart valves, biologic vs. mechanical, 518–520, 519f–520f
    hypothermia and, 507–509
    ICDs and, 509
    IHSS and, 500
    IMAs and, 513–514, 514f, 515b
    intraoperative considerations for, 523
    ligamentum arteriosum and, 505
    LOS considerations for, 496–497
    LVADs and, 520–521
    LVH and, 500
    magnetic resonance arteriography and, 504
    MICS and, 509
    MIS and, 509, 516f
    MR and, 509–513, 511f, 513f
    MS and, 512–513, 512f
    myocardial protection techniques and, 513–514
    myocardial revascularization and, 500, 513–514
    New York Heart Association functional classification system, 518
    off-pump procedures and, 509, 509b, 514–515, 516f, 517t
    ostium primum lesions and, 503
    ostium secundum defects and, 501–503
    patient education considerations, 497t, 517t
    PDA and, 505, 514–515
    pericardiectomy and, 514–515